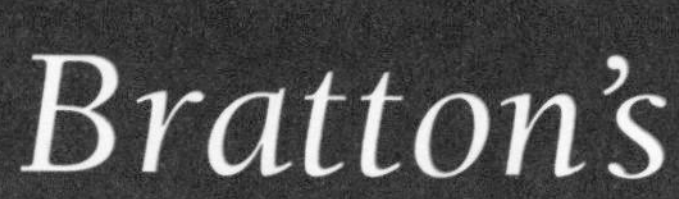

Family Medicine Board Review

THIRD EDITION

Bratton's

Family Medicine Board Review

THIRD EDITION

Robert L. Bratton, M.D.
Chair and Associate Professor
Department of Family Medicine
Mayo Clinic Arizona
Scottsdale/Phoenix

Wolters Kluwer | Lippincott Williams & Wilkins
Health
Philadelphia • Baltimore • New York • London
Buenos Aires • Hong Kong • Sydney • Tokyo

Acquisitions Editor: Sonya Seigafuse
Developmental Editor: Jenny Koleth
Managing Editor: Nancy Winter
Project Manager: Jennifer Harper
Manufacturing Coordinator: Kathleen Brown
Marketing Manager: Kimberly Schonberger
Art Director: Risa Clow
Production Services: GGS Book Services
Printer: RR Donnelley

530 Walnut Street
Philadelphia, PA 19106 USA
LWW.com

Printed in China

Library of Congress Cataloging-in-Publication Data

Bratton, Robert L.
Bratton's family medicine board review/Robert L. Bratton.—3rd ed.
p. ; cm.
Rev. ed. of: Family practice board review/Robert L. Bratton. 2nd ed. c2002.
Includes bibliographical references and index.
ISBN–13: 978-0-7817-7287-7
ISBN–10: 0-7817-7287-7
1. Family medicine—Examinations, questions, etc. I. Bratton, Robert L. Family practice board review. II. Title. III. Title: Family medicine board review.
[DNLM: 1. Family Practice—Examination Questions. WB 18.2 B824b 2007]
RC58.B73 2007
610.76—dc22

2007003322

To purchase additional copies of this book, call our customer service department at (800) 638-3030 or fax orders to (301) 223-2320. International customers should call (301) 223-2300.

Visit Lippincott Williams & Wilkins on the Internet at LWW.com. Lippincott Williams & Wilkins customer service representatives are available from 8:30 am to 6pm, EST.

10 9 8 7

RRS0908

This book is dedicated to my beautiful children, Davis Elizabeth and Robert Lisle, Jr., and to my wonderful wife, Linda. I appreciate your loving support while I prepared this study guide.

Contents

Preface

Bratton's Family Medicine Board Review, Third Edition, is a directed review of important topics that typically appear on American Board of Family Medicine (ABFM) in-training examinations, board certification examinations, and recertification examinations. This material is not intended for a comprehensive review but, instead, should direct the examinee to areas of weakness that may need further review.

Family medicine is a broad field, and to provide a complete, comprehensive review of all topics that may be covered is extremely time consuming if not impossible. Several other courses attempt to provide this type of review; however, this book is more abbreviated and focuses on topics that are commonly found on board examinations.

Adequate preparation for any test is the key to success and rewarding results. Given this, we all know the importance of practice tests and the benefits of testing our knowledge base before the actual examination. This review book is structured for the examinee with limited time and resources for review and should be used only by those individuals with an established foundation of knowledge within the field of family medicine. Its primary purpose is to identify areas of weakness that can be improved on.

Each edition attempts to update the existing information and revise any changes that have occurred in the medical field. The ABFM restructures the examination on a yearly basis, so it is important to visit its Website, *www.theabfm.org,* to get updates on the structure of each examination. I hope that you will find this book enlightening and, most of all, beneficial in your studies for the ABFM examinations. If you have any suggestions to help improve this material, please contact me with your suggestions at rbrat@lexclin.com. Our goal is to help you pass your examination. Good luck!

Acknowledgments

Special thanks to Ms. Sonya Seigafuse and Ms. Nancy Winter (and many others) of Lippincott Williams & Wilkins, and Ms. Jenny Koleth for all their hard work and guidance preparing this study guide.

Registration for Examinations

Residency In-Training Examinations

Registration for the in-training examination for residents in training is unnecessary, because it is handled by your Department of Family Medicine. Your residency director has all the details. The test is administered annually to each resident during the 3 years of residency training. All residents receive the same test; however, grading is based on your level of training. There are no pass or fail scores. The examination is given in the first 2 weeks of November, and your residency program usually makes the necessary arrangements to relieve you of your responsibilities for the half-day during which you are tested. The purpose of this is to assess objectively your education and your knowledge base as you progress through your residency training. Your scores are reported to you (within 3 months) with computerized results that compare your results with those of your respective peers in training. Your scores are also reported to your residency director, so that he or she may track your educational development.

Board Certification and Recertification Examinations

All candidates for board certification must complete the residency training guidelines set forth by the American Board of Family Medicine (ABFM). Registration for board certification and recertification is done by contacting

American Board of Family Medicine
2228 Young Drive
Lexington, Kentucky 40505-4294
Telephone: 859-269-5626 or 888-995-5700
Website: http://www.theabfm.org

Your residency program is able to assist you in your process of initial certification; however, the arrangements for recertification are the responsibility of each physician. The ABFM sends you information about the dates and sites of testing. The examination is held annually in testing centers throughout the country on various dates in July and August. As stated in the ABFM Booklet of Information, September 1996, "The American Board of Family Medicine Certification and Recertification Examinations are tests of cognitive knowledge and problem-solving abilities relevant to Family Medicine. Appropriate subject areas of the following disciplines are included: Internal Medicine, Surgery, Obstetrics, Community Medicine, Pediatrics, Psychiatry and Behavioral Sciences, Geriatrics and Gynecology. Elements of the examinations include but are not limited to, diagnosis, management, and prevention of illness."

Recertification involves submission of the formal application obtained from the ABFM, documentation of required continuing medical education hours, assessment of licensure status, newly required self-assessment modules (SAMs) for Maintenance of Certification (MOC), and successful completion of the recertification examination. More information is available by contacting the ABFM office or accessing the Website.

Test-Taking Tips

Introduction

Just when we thought all of the standardized tests that we dreaded in high school, college, and medical school were behind us, the American Board of Family Medicine (ABFM) requires an in-training examination (in some cases referred to as the *in-service examination*) yearly during our residency training. In addition to those tests, the ABFM requires a board examination at the end of our residency training that we must pass to receive board certification. Finally, the ABFM now requires diplomates to pass a recertification examination every 10 years after residency training, not to mention new guidelines for Maintenance of Certification, including self-assessment modules (SAMs). It's obvious that we're never going to get away from this anxiety-provoking and stressful testing of our knowledge and skills, so it is best to learn some tips to help improve our test scores.

Obviously, all of us are fairly good at test taking, or we never would have made the long journey through college and medical school. But it is always helpful to review some of the basics. The following are some general guidelines for taking the in-training, board, and recertification examinations.

Prepare for the Examination

Although most who sit for the ABFM examinations pass, they should not be taken for granted. A poor score could result in not becoming board certified or losing board certification status (thus prohibiting hospital privileges in many areas). In addition, for residents who perform poorly on their in-training examination, their efforts may give rise to a closer eye and perhaps different attitude toward their overall performance as they progress through their residency training.

I suggest a structured study program that you begin at least 6–8 weeks before the examination. Some individuals may need longer; however, if the review process takes too long, you may forget some of the material before the test. Each night during the week (reserving the weekends for family, friends, and rest), I suggest reviewing for 2–3 hours with scheduled breaks. During the week before the test, I suggest a brief "cramming period" that covers the topics you have reviewed over the previous 6 weeks, to refresh and fine tune your memory bank just before the test.

This study guide is meant to guide the reader to areas of weakness. If there is a topic that you do not feel comfortable with, I suggest further studying with other, more comprehensive texts. This study guide is meant to highlight topics previously covered by ABFM tests, and is not an exhaustive review of all information.

Registration Materials

Once you have inquired about the certification/recertification examination, you will receive registration information that asks for your preferred testing site. Before the test, you will receive additional material that includes your assigned testing site and a registration number. Make sure you bring the information including your registration number and photo identification along with an additional form of identification to the test site on the day of the test. Failure to do this may prevent you from taking the test, or it may delay you in the on-site registration process. This is not required for in-training residency examinations.

Review the Structure of the Test

Although your knowledge of the topics covered is the most important aspect of the test, it is also important to be familiar with the structure of the test, including the types of questions and sections as well as the time allotted for each section.

New Differences between the In-Training Examination and the Certification/Recertification Examination

Recently, the ABFM has converted the certification/recertification examination to a computer-based exam. Examinees are currently tested at Pearson/VUE test centers across the country on various days in July and August, and again in December. The structure of the exam is all multiple-choice questions (the true–false Clinical Set questions have been removed). In contrast, the In-Training Examination remains a written exam that is taken at a site designated by your residency program. The format consists of multiple-choice type questions and true–false questions associated with clinical set questions. Stay tuned . . . many new changes may occur to both the certification/recertification and In-Training Examination over the next few years. The American Board of Family Medicine website can be accessed at www.theabfm.org and is an excellent resource for further information and more practice test questions.

Structure of the In-Training Examination for Residents

There is now one booklet for the in-training examination, and the entire examination lasts approximately 4 hours. The test begins around 8:30 AM, after instructions are given by designated proctors. The entire test is now single-best-answer multiple-choice questions; each question has four or five options for each question. Time allowed for this section is usually 2.5–3 hours, and the time is usually displayed so that you can check your progress. There is no penalty for guessing, so if you reach the end of the test and are short of time, make sure you have answered all the questions.

Clinical set questions have recently been eliminated, but the study questions and answers that are covered in this book will help you to study various topics in a different format.

Structure of the Certification/Recertification Examination for Physicians

The certification and recertification examinations have recently been modified and are all computer-based. All questions are multiple choice and the clinical set problems commonly seen on the in-training examination have been removed. The certification/recertification examination lasts a full day. The question count may be variable, but there are about 120 (general) questions that include all aspects of Family Medicine, followed by 40 questions associated with each module you select, for a total of 200 questions during the morning session. In the afternoon, there are approximately 150 questions that are general family-medicine-type questions. Some questions are not counted in your grade, and are simply experimental questions that the ABFM is testing. You are not told which questions these are.

Most test sites start the examination at 8:30 AM and finish at 5:00 PM, with a 90-minute lunch period. During the morning session of the examination, all candidates (both certification and recertification) are tested over the same material. During the second part of the morning session, the recertification examinee must select two modular examinations from the following areas—Ambulatory Family Medicine, Child and Adolescent Care, Women's Health, Maternity Care, Emergent/Urgent Care, Hospital Medicine, and Sports Medicine—from which their questions are derived. The choice of modular examinations is made during the application process.

Although the clinical set type questions have been eliminated, they should continue to be useful in your preparation for the examination.

Pictorial Atlas

The Pictorial Atlas portion of this book is a section included in the resident's in-training examination. The section is composed of multiple-choice questions that make reference to a photograph, radiograph, audiogram, blood smear, or electrocardiogram tracing. Examinees are asked to select the single best answer for each question, which usually involves making a diagnosis based on observation of common findings.

Familiarize Yourself with the Test Site for the In-Training Examination

Each residency program provides the in-training examination at its institution. To adequately prepare, it is a good idea to find out where the test is going to take place and locate the room and nearby restrooms before the day of the test. It may also be important to listen for any distractions, such as nearby construction or loud traffic, which may be distracting during the test. In these situations, earplugs may be helpful. Weather is also a consideration. I remember distinctly in Rochester, Minnesota, where I did my residency (many years ago), that we had a bad snowstorm the night before our in-training examination and many residents were late arriving at the test site; one of our residents who lived in a rural area did not make it at all. So, if the weather threatens, it may be wise to make arrangements for an alternative place to stay the night before the test. Other suggestions include arranging call schedules so that you are not on call the night before the test. On many rotations, there are residents in other fields who are not taking the test and could take calls the night before the test. Think ahead and discuss this with your chief resident or supervising staff well in advance of the rotation. In most cases, your residency director will arrange this for you.

Board and Recertification Examinations

The certification and recertification examinations are usually given on various days in July and August. These tests are given at specific locations (currently at Pearson /VUE testing centers) across the United States and may require a significant amount of traveling to reach the location. You can select your site of testing from a list of locations that is accessed through the ABFM website at the time of registration. Remember that it is very important to register early to ensure that you get your first choice of location. On arrival, you are photographed and fingerprinted for access to and from the testing site. You must have two forms of identification (one with photo) when you check in.

Because of the travel that may be involved, it is extremely important to arrive in plenty of time at your destination and locate the testing site. Also, if possible, arrange your call schedule with your partners to allow plenty of sleep the week before the test.

Prepare for Comfort

The in-training, board, and recertification examinations require you to sit for extended periods, often at a hard and uncomfortable desk. Prepare yourself. You may want to consider a lightweight jacket or sweater in case it gets cold, and loose-fitting clothing with comfortable shoes. Also, don't forget your glasses. You are *not* allowed to take in any additional snacks or material, or even your watch into the testing room for the certification/recertification examination. These are to be left in a secure locker provided by the testing site. The testing site does offer hard candy or mints and you are given a small white erasable board with a magic marker for making notes or doing calculations. Make sure you use the bathroom before entering the testing room; having to leave requires you to raise your hand and the proctor must log you out from your computer and allow you to leave the room and then fingerprint you when you return; needless to say, it can be an ordeal. While in the examination room, you are seated facing the outer wall at a small, isolated cubicle with fellow test-takers at your left and right. A proctor is seated behind a glass enclosure and observes all who are taking the test. Additionally, you are monitored by video cameras during the examination. Approximately 20 people took the examination when I did.

Diet and Exercise

As we all know, food and exercise are important. I firmly believe that a regular exercise program during the weeks of preparation can help you to retain the information you have studied and put you in a better frame of mind for the test. I also think a well-rounded diet can help fuel the brain with high-octane energy that helps those brain cells retain information. Think of the test as a marathon, and avoid high-fat meals. Choose healthy foods, especially the night before the test. Also, avoid alcohol and its deleterious effect on sleep during your preparation.

On the morning of the test, I suggest a light meal. I also suggest that you take your lunch for the board and recertification examinations; this is not necessary for the in-training examination, because you are usually through with the test at around 1:00 PM. Pack your own lunch and find a quiet place to enjoy your meal and relax.

Sleep

Adequate sleep is imperative as you prepare for any test, and this test is no exception. The mind works better when it is rested. Unfortunately, adequate sleep is not always possible for residents in training and physicians in practice. If at all possible, try to arrange your schedule so that it allows for maximal sleep during your preparation, and, as mentioned previously, make sure you are not on call the night before the test. Try to maintain a regular schedule with bedtime and awakening at the same time during the weeks before your test.

Miscellaneous Items Not to Forget

Bring along aspirin, ibuprofen, or acetaminophen if a headache should occur during the test. Cough drops and allergy medication (non-sedating) should be remembered. Remember that calculators or watches are not allowed, and beeping electronic devices or cellular phones should be left at home. Earplugs may help mute unwanted noises that distract you. I'll always remember that while I was taking an in-training examination, a test-taker sitting in front of me had the sniffles for the entire day. At one point, I could no longer focus on the questions but instead was anticipating this person's next mucus-filled nasal inhalation. It just about rattled me to the point where I walked out, and so I've never taken a test without bringing earplugs since.

Selecting a Seat

For the in-training examination, it is important to choose the seat where you will spend the next several hours, if allowed. Try to select a seat close to the center, so those who finish testing early will not have to climb over you to get out of the room, and with adequate lighting overhead. Some rooms are very dark with poor lighting. Also, try to locate yourself away from doors where passing traffic may be disruptive. You are *not* allowed to select a seat for the certification or recertification examination; instead, you are assigned a seat when you check in.

Relax

Anxiety is a natural response when faced with a test situation. The important thing is to not let anxiety affect your performance deleteriously. If your anxiety has adversely affected your performance in the past, you may want to consider a β-blocker to help reduce your anxiety. I would strongly suggest that you undergo a trial several times before you use them during the test to make sure you do not react adversely to them. But, in most cases, simple relaxation techniques, such as exercising, deep breathing, meditation, or biofeedback, can be used. Remember that a little anxiety is usually good for you and helps to improve your performance.

Tips for the Actual Test

Listen to and Read the Instructions

Listen carefully to the instructions and ask questions if you do not understand something. In addition, take a minute to read the instructions and sample question before starting. Also, for the in-training exam, make sure you adequately color in your responses with a #2 pencil on the answer sheet, and make sure there are no stray marks on the answer sheet when you have completed the test. Another precaution is to make sure that at the end of the booklet there is a statement that the section has ended. A fellow resident of mine finished his test early and left only to discover there was a misprint, and he was missing two pages of the test. For the certification and recertification examination, it is important to read all the instructions. This is done at the beginning of each section, and there is no formal explanation by the proctor.

Answer the Easiest Questions First

Start at the first question of the section and answer all the questions you can with reasonable certainty. If there is a difficult question you are unsure of, skip it, and return to it when you have finished the section. Don't spend an excessive amount of time on one question and risk not being able to answer easy questions at the end of the test because you ran out of time. Circle or mark the questions you skip, and be very careful on the answer sheet that you skip the number you have omitted. It is an empty feeling when you get to the end of the answer sheet and realize you have answered in the wrong row for the last 50 questions. To help prevent this, I usually check the numbers of the questions in the test book to the number on the answer sheet each time I turn a page of the test booklet. The computerized certification/recertification examination does allow you to flag questions that you are unsure of the answer to so you can return to them.

Check Your Pace

Throughout the test, you will receive reminders of the time. On the computerized test, you see the time in a small box at the bottom of the screen. Pay attention to these reminders, and adjust your pace as necessary. Having your own watch is helpful (although not allowed during the certification/recertification examination). In some situations, there may not be a clock available, but only announcements of how much time is left.

Guess If You Do Not Know the Answer

You are penalized only for an incorrect or unanswered question; therefore, all questions should be answered even if they require a guess. Remember that any answer is better than no answer. If you are unsure of an answer, try to narrow the options down to two or three selections and choose from them. Also, it is important to remember that if the question uses absolute terminology, such as *always, never, all,* or *none,* it usually is a false response. Very little in the world of medicine is absolute.

Review Your Answers

If time allows during the multiple-choice question section, review your work. There is an old saying that goes, "You should always stick with your first impression." For a multiple-choice test, this is not always the case. If after further consideration you feel you must change the answer, go ahead.

Try to Anticipate the Answers

Before looking at the choices available for the answers, try to answer the question. Then see if your answer matches one of the selections given. This allows more certain responses for questions and helps save time.

Do Not Read Extra Meaning into the Questions

The ABFM is not interested in structuring questions to try to outsmart the test taker. Questions are designed to be fair and not have hidden agendas. Take questions literally and do not imply hidden meanings.

Above all, the most important thing to remember is to remain confident that you can perform well on the test. The mind can work miracles, and a positive attitude with confidence can be achieved with adequate preparation. Remember that a test gives you the opportunity to show what you know. Do not think of it as a test of what you do not know. Study and prepare yourself, and these tests will be nothing more than time away from your practice. Once the test has been completed, take some time to reward yourself (and your family) for the hard work you've done in preparation. After all, you deserve it!

Bratton's

Family Medicine Board Review

THIRD EDITION

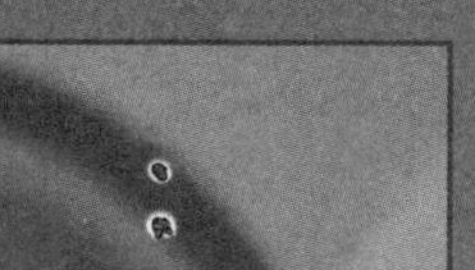

Chapter 1

Internal Medicine

Questions

Each of the following questions or incomplete statements is followed by four or five suggested answers or completions. Select the ONE BEST ANSWER in each case.

1. Which of the following is considered first-line therapy for primary dysmenorrhea?

A) Nonsteroidal anti-inflammatories (NSAIDs)
B) Selective serotonin receptor inhibitors (SSRIs)
C) Antiestrogens
D) Acupuncture
E) Tricyclic antidepressants

Answer and Discussion

The answer is A. Primary dysmenorrhea is associated with cramping pain in the lower abdomen occurring just before and/or during menstruation, in the absence of other conditions such as endometriosis. The initial presentation of primary dysmenorrhea typically occurs in adolescence. The condition is associated with increased production of endometrial prostaglandin, resulting in increased uterine tone and stronger, more frequent uterine contractions. A diagnostic evaluation is unnecessary in women with typical symptoms and in the absence of risk factors for secondary causes. NSAIDs are the most effective treatment, with the addition of oral contraceptive pills when necessary. About 10% of affected women do not respond to these measures. In these cases it is important to consider secondary causes of dysmenorrhea in women affected. Acupuncture is also used as an alternative treatment.

Rakel RE, Bope ET. *Conn's Current Therapy 2005*. Philadelphia: Elsevier/Saunders; 2005:1213–1214.

> Nonsteroidal anti-inflammatory medications are the most effective treatment for primary dysmenorrhea.

2. You are called to see an infant in the newborn nursery. The child was delivered 60 hours prior to your visit. The child appears jaundiced but otherwise healthy. A total serum bilirubin level is measured at 18 mg/dL. Appropriate treatment includes

A) observation
B) stop breast feeding and switch to formula feedings
C) begin phototherapy
D) perform a septic workup
E) start IV hydration

Answer and Discussion

The answer is C. Hyperbilirubinemia is very common in term newborns. Current recommendations include the following: phototherapy should be instituted when the total serum bilirubin level is >=15 mg/dL (257 μmol/L) in infants 25 to 48 hours old, 18 mg/dL (308 μmol /L) in infants 49 to 72 hours old, and 20 mg/dL (342 μmol/L) in infants older than 72 hours. It is unlikely that term newborns with hyperbilirubinemia have serious underlying pathology. Physiologic jaundice peaks on the third or fourth day and declines over the first week following birth. Infants who are breast fed are more likely to develop physiologic jaundice because of relative caloric deprivation in the first few days of life. If jaundice occurs in breast-fed infants, feedings should be increased to more than ten times/day. In some cases formula supplementation may be necessary. Pathologic jaundice occurs if it presents within the first 24 hours after birth, the total serum bilirubin level rises by >5 mg/dL (86 μmol/L) per day or is >17 mg/dL (290 μmol/L), or an infant has signs and symptoms suggestive of serious illness. The management consists of excluding pathologic causes of hyperbilirubinemia and initiating treatment to prevent harmful neurotoxicity.

Porter ML, Dennis BL. Hyperbilirubinemia in term newborn. *Am Fam Physician*. 2002;65:599–606, 613–614.

3. Which of the following p values reflects the best chance that the findings are not the result of chance?

A) p value <0.005
B) p value <0.001
C) p value <0.05
D) p value <0.01
E) p value = 1

Answer and Discussion

The answer is B. The p value is defined as the measured probability of a finding occurring (i.e., rejecting the null hypothesis) by chance alone given that the null hypothesis is actually true. By convention, a p value <0.05 is often considered significant. ["There is less than a 5% probability that the finding (null hypothesis rejected) was due to chance alone."]

Rind DM. Proof, *p*-values, and hypothesis testing. Up to Date version 14.1. Accessed 6/6/06. Available at http://uptodateonline.com.

4. Which of the following statements is true regarding influenza?
A) Treatment with antivirals should be initiated within 48 hours of the onset of symptoms.
B) Anitiviral agents reduce the duration of fever by 1 week.
C) Amantadine is effective for both influenza types A and B.
D) Prophylactic therapy is the single most important measure to prevent influenza outbreaks.
E) Amantadine is the only agent approved for prophylaxis.

Answer and Discussion

The answer is A. Influenza causes significant morbidity and mortality and is responsible for considerable medical expenditures especially in the elderly. Vaccination is the single most important public health measure to prevent this illness. Amantadine (Symmetrel) and rimantadine (Flumadine) are older antiviral agents (called M2 inhibitors) that have been important medications in the prevention and treatment of influenza A outbreaks. They are not effective for influenza B. Zanamivir (Relenza) and oseltamivir (Tamiflu) are newer agents (neuraminidase inhibitors) indicated for the treatment of both influenza A and B. Oseltamivir (Tamiflu) is the only neuraminidase inhibitor currently approved for prophylaxis. For antiviral agents to be effective, they must be initiated within 48 hours of the onset of influenza symptoms. Antiviral agents reduce the duration of fever and illness by 1 day and also reduce the severity of some symptoms. Use of amantadine or rimantadine is appropriate if influenza virus A is determined to be the predominant agent in a particular year or location. For optimal use of antiviral agents, patients with influenza symptoms must present early, and family physicians must accurately and rapidly diagnose the illness. Rimantadine is metabolized in the liver and therefore should be used with caution in patients with liver disease.

Montalto NJ, Gum KD, Ashley JV. Updated treatment for influenza A and B. *Am Fam Physician*. 2000;62:2467–2476.

5. Primary insomnia is usually associated with
A) sleep apnea
B) restless legs syndrome
C) periodic limb movements
D) circadian rhythm sleep disorders
E) none of the above

Answer and Discussion

The answer is E. *Insomnia* is defined as inadequate or poor-quality sleep characterized by one or more of the following: difficulty falling asleep, difficulty maintaining sleep, waking up too early in the morning, or sleep that is not refreshing. Insomnia also involves daytime consequences such as fatigue, difficulty concentrating, and irritability. Periods of insomnia lasting between 1 night and a few weeks are defined as acute insomnia. Chronic insomnia refers to sleep difficulty occurring at least 3 nights per week for 1 month or more. Insomnia may be associated with specific sleep disorders, including restless legs syndrome, periodic limb movement disorder, sleep apnea, and circadian rhythm sleep disorders. Restless legs syndrome is characterized by unpleasant sensations in the legs or feet that are temporarily relieved by movement. Symptoms are worse in the evening, especially when a person is lying down and remaining still. The sensations cause difficulty falling asleep and are often accompanied by periodic limb movements. Periodic limb movement disorder is characterized by bilateral repeated and rhythmic, small-amplitude jerking or twitching movements in the lower extremities and, less frequently, in the arms. These movements occur every 20 to 90 seconds and can lead to awakenings, which are usually not noticed by the patient. Often the patient reports that sleep is not refreshing. In many cases, the bed partner is more likely to report the movement problem. Obstructive sleep apnea is most commonly associated with snoring, daytime sleepiness and obesity but occasionally presents with insomnia. Circadian rhythm sleep disorders including sleep-work insomnia are characterized by an inability to sleep because of a disturbance between the circadian sleep rhythm and the desired or required sleep schedule. Primary insomnia occurs in the absence of the previously mentioned conditions. When the insomnia persists beyond 1 or 2 nights or becomes predictable, treatment should be considered. Pharmacologic treatment is usually effective, especially short-acting hypnotics. Sleep hygiene measures may also be useful. Chronic insomnia may be more difficult to treat. Because chronic insomnia is often multifactorial in etiology, a patient may need multiple treatment modalities, including medication (antidepressants, antihistamines, melatonin) and behavioral therapy. If an underlying medical or psychiatric condition is identified, this condition should be treated first.

National Heart, Lung, and Blood Institute Working Group on Insomnia. Insomnia: assessment and management in primary care. *Am Fam Physician*. 1999; 59(11):3029–3039.

6. A 65-year-old man presents to your office and reports urinary incontinence. Examination reveals an enlarged prostate. You suspect overflow incontinence. Which of the following measurements of post-void residual (PVR) volumes would represent the threshold for a normal amount?
A) 50 ml
B) 100 ml
C) 200 ml
D) 500 ml
E) 1000 ml

Answer and Discussion

The answer is A. Urge incontinence results from bladder contractions that exceed the ability of the brain to prevent them. Causes include inflammation or irritation within the bladder resulting from calculi, malignancy, infection, or atrophic vaginitis–urethritis. Other central causes include stroke, Parkinson's disease or dementia, drugs such as hypnotics or narcotics, or metabolic disorders such as hypoxemia and encephalopathy. Additionally, urge incontinence can occur when ambulation is impaired, making it difficult for patients to get to the bathroom in time. This condition is referred to as *"functional" incontinence.*

Stress incontinence is caused by a malfunction of the urethral sphincter that causes urine to leak from the bladder when intra-abdominal pressure increases, such as during coughing or sneezing. Causes for stress incontinence include pelvic prolapse, urethral hypermobility, or displacement of the urethra and bladder neck from their normal anatomic alignment. Stress incontinence can also occur as a result of intrinsic sphincter deficiency, in which the sphincter is weak because of a congenital condition or denervation resulting from alpha-adrenergic blocking drugs, surgical trauma, or radiation damage. Overflow bladder incontinence occurs as a result of urine retention with bladder distention. Urine collects in the bladder until maximum bladder capacity is reached. It then leaks as a result of "overflow," usually manifesting as dribbling. Increased intra-abdominal pressure may also cause loss of urine, so that overflow incontinence sometimes mimics stress incontinence.

Overflow incontinence can be caused by medications that relax the bladder detrusor muscle (e.g., anticholinergic agents, calcium-channel blockers). It can also be caused by denervation of the detrusor resulting from a neurologic abnormality that affects bladder innervation (e.g., diabetic neuropathy) or because of damage to bladder innervation (e.g., tumors, radiation, surgery). Additionally, overflow incontinence can be caused by obstructed urinary outflow resulting from prostate enlargement, fecal impaction, urethral stricture, or urethral constriction related to alpha-adrenergic agonist medications.

The workup should include a urinalysis, which can identify acute urinary tract infection and diabetes-induced glycosuria, both of which can cause or aggravate urge incontinence. These conditions are reversible with treatment. If appropriate, a urine culture should also be obtained. The basic evaluation of urinary incontinence should also include measurement of PVR urine volume to detect urinary retention (i.e., overflow bladder). PVR volume measurement can detect retention caused by potentially reversible factors (e.g., anticholinergic or other drugs, fecal impaction). Urinary retention not obviously resulting from a transient cause generally requires further evaluation, including cystometry, to determine why the bladder does not empty properly. The PVR urine volume can be measured by one of two methods. The first and most common method is "in and out" urethral catheterization after the patient has urinated to empty the bladder. The quantity of urine obtained is measured. PVR volume can also be measured with pelvic ultrasonography. Ultrasonography is a useful alternative to catheterization, especially for measuring the PVR volume in men with suspected prostate obstruction, because catheterizing these patients may cause urinary infection or obstruction. Normally, <50 mL of residual urine is present after voiding. Volumes of >200 mL are abnormal. Intermediate volumes (50 to 200 mL) are considered equivocal, and the test should be repeated. Other tests include office cystometry and office stress testing. Office cystometry consists of aliquots of sterile saline that are infused into the bladder via a catheter with an open syringe attached to the catheter. Contractions are detected by monitoring the fluid level that appears in the syringe after several aliquots of water have been instilled. A rise and fall in the fluid level indicates pressure changes (i.e., contractions) within the bladder. Severe feelings of urgency or bladder contractions at <300 mL of bladder volume constitute a presumptive diagnosis of urge incontinence. For the diagnosis of urge incontinence, simple cystometry can be used. In this test the patient lies supine on the examination table with a full bladder and coughs forcefully. The physician places a gauze pad in front of the perineum. If urine leaks onto the gauze pad during coughing, a presumptive diagnosis of stress incontinence is made. The physician then places his or her fingers on either side of the patient's urethra and elevates the structure. The patient is then asked to cough. In patients with stress incontinence, urethral elevation prevents further urine leakage. If no incontinence is noted in the supine position, the maneuvers should be repeated with the patient standing. If no incontinence occurs in either position, the patient probably does not have stress incontinence.

Weiss BD. Diagnostic evaluation of urinary incontinence in geriatric patients. *Am Fam Physician*. 1998;57:2675–2688.

7. Which of the following is considered a risk factor for retinal detachment?
A) Glaucoma
B) Diabetic retinopathy
C) Hyphema
D) Myopia

Answer and Discussion

The answer is D. Retinal detachment is a preventable cause of vision loss. It is relatively common after the age of 60. There are three types of retinal detachments: exudative, tractional, and rhegmatogenous. The most common type is rhegmatogenous, which results from retinal breaks caused by vitreoretinal traction. Exudative (or serous) retinal detachment results from the accumulation of serous and/or hemorrhagic fluid in the subretinal space because of hydrostatic factors (e.g., severe acute hypertension), or inflammation (e.g., sarcoid uveitis), or neoplastic effusions. Exudative retinal detachment generally resolves with adequate treatment of the underlying disease, and restoration of normal vision is often excellent. Tractional retinal detachment occurs via centripetal mechanical forces on the retina, usually mediated by fibrotic tissue resulting from previous hemorrhage, injury, surgery, infection, or inflammation. Risk factors for retinal detachment include advancing age, previous cataract surgery, myopia, and trauma. Other eye conditions including hyphema, glaucoma, and diabetic retinopathy are not considered risk factors for retinal detachment. Patients typically present with symptoms such as light flashes, floaters, peripheral visual field loss, and blurred vision. Retinal tears may occur without symptoms, but often photopsia (light flashes) is noted. Photopsia results from vitreoretinal traction. When the retina tears, blood and retinal pigment epithelium cells may enter the vitreous cavity and are perceived as "floaters." Immediate intervention can prevent retinal detachment. Patients with the acute onset of flashes or floaters should be referred to an ophthalmologist.

Gariano RF, Chang-hee K. Evaluation and management of suspected retinal detachment. *Am Fam Physician*. 2004;69: 1691–1698.

8. Which of the following medications is considered the treatment of choice for *Bordetella pertussis* infection?
A) Penicillin
B) Ciprofloxacin
C) Azithromycin
D) Tetracycline
E) Cefuroxime

Answer and Discussion

The answer is C. Recent epidemiologic studies have shown that the incidence and prevalence of *Bordetella pertussis* infection in adults are much greater than previously reported. In studies of adults with chronic cough, 20% to 25% were found to have serologic evidence of recent *B. pertussis* infection. However, pertussis is rarely considered in adults because the signs and symptoms are nonspecific. Apart from a prolonged cough, there are no specific symptoms suggestive of pertussis in older individuals who have been immunized. With this in mind, pertussis should be considered in the differential diagnosis of persistent cough in previously immunized children and adults. Administration of erythromycin or other macrolide (azithromycin or clarithromycin) may be a consideration in patients presenting with persistent cough. Prophylaxis of exposed persons before culture or serologic results are available would be another consideration. Early treatment with a macrolide should limit the spread of infection to persons whose immunity has waned or in unimmunized children. The acellular vaccine may allow booster immunization, which can be a method of preventing *B. pertussis* infection after immunity from the pertussis vaccination has waned.

Yaari E, Yafe-Zimerman Y, Schwartz SB, et al. Clinical manifestations of *Bordetella pertussis* infection in immunized children and young adults. *Chest*. 1999;115:1254–1258.

9. Which of the following is associated with reducing the risk of falls in elderly patients?
A) Vitamin C
B) Vitamin D
C) Folate
D) Vitamin B_{12}
E) Calcium

Answer and Discussion

The answer is B. Falls are a major cause of injury-related visits to emergency departments in the United States, and the primary cause of accidental deaths in persons older than 65 years. The mortality rate for falls increases dramatically with age in both sexes and in all racial and ethnic groups. Falls can be an indication of poor health and declining function, and they are often associated with significant morbidity. More than 90% of hip fractures occur as a result of falls, with most of these fractures occurring in persons older than 70 years of age. Risk factors for falls in the elderly include increasing age, arthritis, medication use (more than four medications, including tricyclic antidepressants, neuroleptics, benzodiazepines, and type IA antiarrythmics), cognitive impairment (dementia and depression), and sensory deficits. Outpatient evaluation of a patient who has fallen includes a focused history with an emphasis on medications, a directed physical examination, and tests of postural control and overall physical function. Treatment is directed at the underlying cause of the fall, with the goal to return the patient to baseline function. Vitamin D deficiency has been associated with an increased risk of falls, and empiric supplementation can reduce the risk.

Fuller GF. Falls in the elderly. *Am Fam Physician*. 2000; 61:2159–2168, 2173–2174.

10. An 18-year-old high school student presents with her mother to your office. Mom reports her daughter is binge eating and purging in order to lose weight. You suspect bulimia. Of the medications listed, which would be best indicated in treatment of the condition?
A) Sertraline (Zoloft)
B) Paroxetine (Paxil)
C) Fluoxitene (Prozac)
D) Venlafaxine (Effexor)
E) Buproprion (Wellbutrin)

Answer and Discussion

The answer is C. Persons affected by anorexia nervosa eventually become visibly recognizable because of their severely underweight status. In contrast, those affected by bulimia are typically of normal weight and are not as easily detected. This disorder is characterized by binge eating and purging. Bulimia is most common in late adolescent females. Associations with other psychiatric disorders is common, and patients with personality disorders (e.g., borderline, narcissistic, and antisocial disorders) have a worse prognosis. Most bulimics purge by vomiting, although abuse of laxatives or diuretics can also occur. The number of times a bulimic patient purges can vary widely, from as seldom as once or twice weekly to as often as ten times per day. Repeatedly induced vomiting can lead to the loss of dental enamel, increased dental caries, swollen salivary glands, Mallory–Weiss esophageal tears, and gastroesophageal reflux. Laxative abusers can develop constipation on withdrawal of laxatives. The typical electrolyte abnormalities associated with bulimia are hypokalemia and metabolic acidosis. Although severe hypokalemia in an otherwise healthy young female suggests bulimia, most patients who purge do not develop electrolyte abnormalities. As a result, screening for hypokalemia or other electrolyte disturbances is not a sensitive means for detecting bulimia. Treatment of the complications associated with bulimia is usually possible, but the underlying disorder can be challenging to treat successfully. Fluoridated mouthwash and toothpaste can help prevent dental caries, and the use of sour candies may decrease salivary gland swelling. Antacid medications help reduce gastroesophageal reflux symptoms, and nonstimulant laxatives may be used to decrease constipation in those with stimulant laxative abuse. Oral replacement of potassium is typically accomplished with 40 to 80 mEq per day of supplementary potassium, until a normal serum potassium level is achieved. Patients with severe hypokalemia and metabolic alkalosis need volume repletion with intravenous normal saline to allow normalization of potassium levels. Cognitive–behavioral therapy has demonstrated efficacy in the treatment of bulimia, but relapse is common. Disturbances in serotonergic systems have been suggested as contributing to bulimia. The selective serotonin reuptake inhibitor fluoxetine is the only medication that has been approved by the U.S. Food and Drug Administration for treatment of bulimia. Higher dosages of fluoxetine (more than required to treat depression), up to 60 mg daily, may be necessary for effective control. Even with a combination of psychotherapy and pharmacologic treatment, remission rates are high.

Mehler PS. Bulimia nervosa. *N Engl J Med*. 2003;349:875–881.

> The selective serotonin reuptake inhibitor fluoxetine is the only medication that has been approved by the U.S. Food and Drug Administration for treatment of bulimia.

11. The Health Insurance Portability and Accountability Act (HIPAA) standards ensure that
A) patients have control and access to their medical records
B) insurance companies have unlimited access to health information
C) physicians can protect themselves from liability
D) attorneys have unrestricted access to health-care records

Answer and Discussion

The answer is A. HIPAA is three sets of standards (1. Transactions and Code Sets; 2. Privacy; and 3. Security) developed by the Department of Health and Human Services in 1996. The goals of the standards are to simplify the administration of health insurance claims and lower costs; give patients more control and access to their medical information; and protect individually identifiable medical information from real or potential threats of disclosure or loss. Privacy and security are closely related. *Privacy* is the patient's right over the use and disclosure of his or her own personal health information. Privacy includes the right to determine when, how, and to what extent personal information is shared with others. The HIPAA privacy rules grant new rights to patients to gain access to and control the use and disclosure of their personal health information. *Security* is the specific measures a health-care provider must take to protect personal health information from unauthorized breaches of privacy, as in situations where information is stolen or sent to the wrong person in error. Security also includes measures taken to ensure against the loss of personal health information, as in situations where a patient's records are lost or destroyed by accident. The HIPAA privacy rules require general security measures be put in place, and the proposed security rules follow a detailed and comprehensive set of activities to guard against unauthorized disclosure of personal health information stored or transmitted electronically or on paper.

Kibbe DC. A problem-oriented approach to the HIPAA security standards family practice management. *Fam Pract Manag.* July/August. 2001;8(7):37–43.

12. Which statement regarding visual screening in children is correct?

A) Visual screening is not indicated until age 5.
B) Visual acuity can be assessed by the Random Dot E test.
C) Stereopsis can be measured by the Tumbling E test.
D) Strabismus can be assessed with the cover test during the first year of life.
E) Visual screening can be reliably assessed at age 2.

Answer and Discussion

The answer is D. The U.S. Preventive Services Task Force (USPSTF) recommends screening to detect amblyopia, strabismus, and defects in visual acuity in children younger than age 5 years. The USPSTF found no evidence of harm associated with screening, and concluded that the benefits of screening are likely to outweigh any potential harms. The most common causes of visual impairment in children are (1) amblyopia and its risk factors and (2) refractive error not associated with amblyopia. *Amblyopia* refers to reduced visual acuity without a detectable organic lesion of the eye and is associated with risk factors that interfere with normal binocular vision, such as strabismus (ocular misalignment), anisometropia (a large difference in refractive power between the two eyes), cataract (lens opacity), and ptosis (eyelid drooping). Refractive error not associated with amblyopia principally includes myopia (nearsightedness) and hyperopia (farsightedness). Various tests are used to identify visual defects in children, and the choice of tests is determined by the child's age. During the first year of life, strabismus can be assessed by the cover test and the Hirschberg light reflex test. Screening children younger than age 3 years for visual acuity is more challenging than screening older children, and typically requires testing by specially trained personnel. Traditional vision testing requires a cooperative, conversive child and cannot be performed reliably until ages 3 to 4 years. In children older than age 3 years, stereopsis (the ability of both eyes to function together) can be assessed with the Random Dot E test or Titmus Fly Stereotest; visual acuity can be assessed by tests such as the HOTV chart, Lea symbols, or the tumbling E.

U.S. Preventive Services Task Force. Screening for visual impairment in children younger than five years: recommendation statement. *Ann Fam Med.* 2004;2:263–266.

13. Which of the following tumor markers is correct for the condition?

A) CA (cancer antigen) 27.29 for metastatic cervical cancer
B) CA (cancer antigen) 125 for hepatic carcinoma
C) AFP (alpha-fetoprotein) for ovarian carcinoma
D) CA (cancer antigen) 19-9 for pancreatic cancer
E) β-hCG (beta unit of human chorionic gonadotropin) for ovarian cancer

Answer and Discussion

The answer is D. Recognized tumor markers are most appropriate for monitoring response to therapy and detecting early recurrence. Cancer antigen (CA) 27.29 is most often used to follow response to therapy in patients with metastatic breast cancer. CA 27.29 is highly associated with breast cancer, although levels are elevated in several other malignancies (colon, gastric, hepatic, lung, pancreatic, ovarian, and prostate cancers). CA 27.29 also can be found in patients with benign disorders of the breast, liver, and kidney, and in patients with ovarian cysts. CA 27.29 levels higher than 100 units per mL are rare in benign conditions.

Carcinoembryonic antigen (CEA) is used to detect relapse of colorectal cancer. CEA elevations also occur with other malignancies. Nonmalignant conditions associated with elevated CEA levels include cigarette smoking, peptic ulcer disease, inflammatory bowel disease, pancreatitis, hypothyroidism, biliary obstruction, and cirrhosis. Levels exceeding 10 ng/mL are rarely due to benign disease. Fewer than 25% of patients with disease confined to the colon have an elevated CEA level. Therefore, CEA is not useful in screening for colorectal cancer or in the diagnostic evaluation of an undiagnosed illness. A CEA level should be utilized only after malignancy has been diagnosed.

CA 19-9 may be helpful in diagnosing pancreatic abnormalities. Levels >1,000 units/mL are correlated with pancreatic cancer. Benign conditions such as cirrhosis, cholestasis, cholangitis, and pancreatitis can also result in CA 19-9 elevations, although values are usually <1,000 units/mL.

CA 125 is useful for evaluating pelvic masses in postmenopausal women, monitoring response to therapy in women with ovarian cancer, and detecting recurrence of ovarian carcinoma. Postmenopausal women with asymptomatic palpable pelvic masses and CA 125 levels >65 units/mL likely have ovarian cancer. Because premenopausal women have more benign causes of elevated CA 125 levels, testing for the marker is less useful in this population.

Alpha-fetoprotein (AFP) is a marker for hepatocellular carcinoma. It is used to screen highly selected populations and to assess hepatic masses in patients at particular risk for developing hepatic malignancy.

Testing for the β-subunit of human chorionic gonadotropin (β-hCG) is an integral part of the diagnosis and management of gestational trophoblastic disease. Combined AFP and β-hCG testing is an essential adjunct in the evaluation and treatment of nonseminomatous germ cell tumors, and in monitoring the response to therapy. AFP and β-hCG are useful in evaluating potential origins of poorly differentiated metastatic cancer.

PSA is used to screen for prostate cancer and detects recurrence of the malignancy.

Perkins GL, Slater ED, Sanders GK, et al. Serum tumor markers. *Am Fam Physician*. 2003;68:1075–1082.

14. A 27-year-old female presents for her annual examination. Her BMI is 31 and she has hirsutism and reports difficulty with conception. Her periods are irregular. Based on her likely diagnosis, which of the following malignancies is she most at increased risk for?
A) Ovarian carcinoma
B) Colon cancer
C) Pancreatic cancer
D) Endometrial carcinoma
E) Breast cancer

Answer and Discussion

The answer is D. Polycystic ovary syndrome (PCOS) is the most common endocrine abnormality in women of reproductive age. The syndrome is associated with chronic anovulation, abnormal menstrual bleeding, and infertility. Macrovascular diseases such as type 2 diabetes mellitus, hypertension, and atherosclerotic heart disease are more likely in women with PCOS. In addition, chronic anovulation predisposes women to endometrial hyperplasia and carcinoma. Symptoms that prompt females to seek attention include irregular menses, hirsutism, or infertility. The earliest manifestations of PCOS are noted around the time of puberty. Adolescent girls affected with PCOS often have early puberty and show hyperandrogenism and insulin resistance. In the early reproductive period, chronic anovulation results in difficulty with fertility. If pregnancy is achieved, it frequently terminates in spontaneous, first-trimester loss or is associated with gestational diabetes. More than 50% of those affected are obese. Abnormal androgen production declines as menopause approaches (as it does in women without PCOS), and menstrual patterns may normalize. However perimenopausal and postmenopausal women with a history of PCOS have increased rates of type 2 diabetes, hypertension, and coronary artery disease compared with control patients. PCOS appears to follow a familial distribution. LH and FSH levels are often elevated in PCOS, with the LH:FSH ratio greater than 3:1. Individualized therapy should incorporate steroid hormones, antiandrogens, and insulin-sensitizing agents (metformin). Weight loss by way of reduced carbohydrate intake and exercise is the most important intervention; this step alone can restore menstrual regularity and fertility, and provide long-term prevention against diabetes and heart disease.

Richardson MR. Current perspectives in polycystic ovary syndrome. *Am Fam Physician*. 2003;68:697–704.

15. Most cases of infant botulism are related to the ingestion of
A) honey
B) peanut butter
C) whole milk
D) mayonnaise
E) eggs

Answer and Discussion

The answer is A. Although rare, the majority of cases of infant botulism are diagnosed in the United States. An infant acquires botulism by ingesting *Clostridium botulinum* spores, which are found in soil or honey products. The spores develop into bacteria that colonize the bowel and produce toxin. As the toxin is absorbed, it irreversibly binds to acetylcholine receptors on motor nerve terminals at neuromuscular junctions, leading to progressive weakness, hypotonia, and hyporeflexia, with associated bulbar and spinal nerve abnormalities. Symptoms of infant botulism include constipation, lethargy, a weak cry, poor feeding, and dehydration. A high level of suspicion is important for the diagnosis and prompt treatment of infant botulism, because this disease can quickly progress to respiratory failure and possibly death. Diagnosis is confirmed by isolating the organism or toxin in the stool and finding the classic triad of electromyogram patterns, including the following:

1. Compound muscle action potentials of decreased amplitude in at least two muscle groups
2. Tetanic and post-tetanic facilitation defined by an amplitude >120% of baseline
3. Prolonged post-tetanic facilitation >120 seconds and absence of post-tetanic exhaustion

Treatment consists of nutritional and respiratory support until new motor endplates are regenerated, which results in spontaneous recovery. Neurologic sequelae are seldom seen.

Cox N, Hinkle R. Infant botulism. *Am Fam Physician*. 2002; 65:1388–1392.

16. Of the following conditions, which is related to the development of osteoporosis in men?
A) Prolactinoma
B) Hypogonadism
C) Prostate cancer
D) Renal stones
E) Inguinal hernia

Answer and Discussion

The answer is B. Men, like women, are at risk of developing osteoporosis that may lead to increased risk of fractures. According to bone density studies in men with low levels of testosterone, hypogonadism is an independent risk factor for osteoporosis. When testosterone is replaced, bone density has been shown to increase. Bone density is a popular and easy way to measure the degree of osteoporosis, but it does not provide complete information about fracture risk. Alterations of bone architecture represent increased risk of fracture, even in men with minimal evidence of osteoporosis. Alternative ways to examine bone microarchitecture include quantitative computed tomography and high-resolution magnetic resonance microimaging (μMRI). The latter test has been called "the *virtual bone biopsy*," and better demonstrates the integrity of the trabecular network. The only approved treatments for male osteoporosis are alendronate (Fosamax) and recombinant parathyroid hormone. Testosterone is often prescribed, but should not be used in men with a history of prostate cancer for obvious reasons.

Benito M, Gomberg B, Wehrli FW. Deterioration of trabecular architecture in hypogonadal men. *J Clin Endocrinol Metab*. 2003;88:1497–1502.

17. In patients treated with disulfiram (Antabuse) for alcohol abuse, which test is necessary for monitoring during treatment?
A) Alkaline phosphatase
B) Amylase
C) Creatinine
D) Alanine aminotransferase (ALT)
E) Ammonia level

Answer and Discussion

The answer is D. In the United States, disulfiram (Antabuse), acamprosate (Campral), and naltrexone (Revia) are approved for the treatment of alcohol dependence. Although disulfiram is reported to be effective as an aversive drug, placebo-controlled clinical trials have been inconclusive. Disulfiram inhibits the metabolism of anticoagulant drugs, phenytoin, and isoniazid. This drug should be used cautiously in patients with liver disease and is contraindicated during pregnancy and in patients with ischemic heart disease. Disulfiram can cause hepatitis, and therefore monitoring of liver function studies is essential. Acamprosate is a newer agent that works by its affect on the GABA system. Side effects include diarrhea, insomnia, anxiety, depression, pruritus, and dizziness. The third drug approved for use in the treatment of alcohol dependence is the opioid antagonist naltrexone. Naltrexone is believed to reduce consumption of alcohol and increase abstinence by reducing the craving for alcohol. The rate of relapse is highest within the first 90 days of abstinence, and it is during this time that naltrexone may be beneficial. Daily dosages may range from 25 to 100 mg. Side effects include nausea, headache, anxiety, and sedation. Naltrexone can be hepatotoxic at higher dosages and should be used with caution in patients with chronic liver disease. Selective serotonin reuptake inhibitors (SSRIs), including fluoxetine and sertraline, have been found to decrease alcohol intake in heavy drinkers without a history of depression. However, in some trials SSRIs were found to be no more effective than a placebo. Any drug therapy should be combined with psychotherapy or group therapy to help address the social and psychologic aspects of alcohol dependence.

Swift RM. Drug therapy for alcohol dependence. *N Engl J Med.* 1999;340:1482–1490.

Disulfiram can cause hepatitis and therefore monitoring of liver function studies is essential.

18. The test of choice for the diagnosis of ureteral obstruction secondary to renal lithiasis is

A) noncontrast helical computed tomography
B) ultrasound
C) intravenous pyelogram
D) magnetic resonance imaging
E) plain radiographs

Answer and Discussion

The answer is A. The most common cause of the sudden onset of flank pain in adults is acute urolithiasis. Identification of a stone in the ureter with resultant partial or complete ureteral obstruction confirms the suspected diagnosis. In the past, intravenous pyelography (IVP) has been the classic diagnostic test of choice. Noncontrast helical computed tomography (CT), which was introduced in 1994, has the advantages of avoiding contrast exposure, identifying radiolucent calculi, evaluating nearby structures, and requiring a shorter time for examination. Intravenous urograms provide only gross images of the kidneys and miss other local pathology. When noncontrast helical CT is readily available, the amount of time required to evaluate patients is reduced, and potential contrast complications that may occur with conventional radiologic imaging are avoided. As a result, helical CT is a better test for assessing acute urolithiasis. Abdominal ultrasound has a high specificity in evaluating stones but its sensitivity is lower than helical CT. Plain films are used to follow patients with known radiopaque (i.e., calcium) stones.

Worster A, Preyra I, Weaver B. The accuracy of noncontrast helical computed tomography versus intravenous pyelography in the diagnosis of suspected acute urolithiasis: a meta-analysis. *Ann Emerg Med.* 2002;40:280–286.

19. Which of the following infections is least likely in a patient with chronic obstructive pulmonary disease (COPD)?

A) *Streptococcus pneumoniae*
B) *Haemophilus influenzae*
C) *Moraxella catarrhalis*
D) *Mycoplasma pneumoniae*

Answer and Discussion

The answer is D. The American Thoracic Society (ATS) defines COPD as a disease process involving progressive chronic airflow obstruction because of chronic bronchitis, emphysema, or both. Chronic bronchitis is defined clinically as excessive cough and sputum production on most days for at least 3 months during at least 2 consecutive years. Emphysema is characterized by chronic dyspnea resulting from the destruction of lung tissue and the enlargement of air spaces. Asthma, which features airflow obstruction, airway inflammation, and increased airway responsiveness to various stimuli, may be distinguished from COPD by reversibility of pulmonary function deficits. Acute exacerbations of COPD are treated with oxygen (in hypoxemic patients), inhaled β_2 agonists, inhaled anticholinergics, antibiotics, and systemic corticosteroids. Theophylline may be considered in patients who do not respond to other bronchodilators.

Antibiotic therapy is directed at the most common pathogens, including *Streptococcus pneumoniae*, *Haemophilus influenzae,* and *Moraxella catarrhalis.* Mild to moderate exacerbations of COPD are usually treated with broad-spectrum antibiotics such as doxycycline, trimethoprim–sulfamethoxazole, and amoxicillin–clavulanate potassium. Treatment with extended-spectrum penicillins, fluoroquinolones, third-generation cephalosporins, or aminoglycosides may be considered in patients with severe exacerbations. The management of chronic stable COPD includes smoking cessation and oxygen therapy. Inhaled β_2 agonists, inhaled anticholinergics, and systemic corticosteroids are also used in patients with chronic stable disease. Inhaled corticosteroids decrease airway reactivity and can reduce the use of health-care services for management of respiratory symptoms. Avoiding acute exacerbations helps to reduce long-term complications. Long-term oxygen therapy, regular monitoring of pulmonary function, and referral for pulmonary rehabilitation are often utilized and can improve the quality of life and reduce hospitalizations. Influenza and pneumococcal vaccines should be administered. Selected patients who do not respond to standard therapies may benefit from lung reduction surgery.

Hunter MH, King DE. COPD: management of acute exacerbations and chronic stable disease. *Am Fam Physician.* 2001;64:603–612, 621–622.

20. A 2-year-old child is brought into your office. Mom reports the boy fell off his bed and has been limping for the last 3 days. He did hit his head, but had no loss of consciousness and has been acting normally since his fall. You note retinal hemorrhages and several areas of bruising on the head, legs, thighs, and arms in varying stages of healing. The most likely cause is

A) autism
B) abuse
C) hemophilia

D) leukemia
E) poor coordination

Answer and Discussion

The answer is B. Determining whether head injuries in children are accidental or a result of physical abuse is very important. Children with head injuries related to abuse tend to be younger than those with accidental injuries. Boys are more frequently affected. Subdural hematoma, subarachnoid hemorrhage, and retinal hemorrhage are more common in abused children. Child abuse should be strongly suspected when such injuries are present in a child without a history of a fall or with a history of a fall from a relatively low height. Multiple injuries in various stages of healing should also alert the clinician to the possibility of abuse. A skeletal survey for children younger than 3 years should be performed when inflicted head injuries are suspected.

Reece RM, Sege R. Childhood head injuries: accidental or inflicted? *Arch Pediatr Adolesc Med.* 2000;154:11–15.

21. A 65-year-old with a history of chronic atrial fibrillation is being monitored while on warfarin therapy. The nurse calls to inform you the patient's International Normalized Ratio (INR) is measured at 7. He has no active signs of bleeding, but is at increased risk of bleeding. Appropriate management at this time includes

A) stop warfarin, observe, and repeat INR in 3 days
B) stop warfarin and observe; repeat INR in 24 hours
C) stop warfarin, give vitamin K, and repeat INR in 24 hours
D) stop warfarin, give vitamin K and fresh frozen plasma with daily INRs

Answer and Discussion

The answer is C. Warfarin inhibits the formation of clotting factors II, VII, IX, and X. The drug is highly protein-bound to albumin. Because of this inverse relationship between the levels of albumin and free warfarin, acutely ill with poor nutritional states and postoperative patients may need lower dosages of warfarin. The INR is the patient's prothrombin time divided by the mean of the normal prothrombin time, with this ratio raised to the international sensitivity index. After starting warfarin therapy, a steady-state response is not typically achieved for approximately 2 weeks. A dosage of 4 to 5 mg/day is typical, although the required dosage may be variable (as low as 0.5 mg or as high as 50 mg/day). Elderly patients should start at a lower dosage. Checking the INR approximately 24 hours after the first dose can help determine the second dose. If there has been little or no rise in the INR (which is to be expected), a 5-mg dose on the second day should be safe. If an INR is not available on the day after the first dose, it can be obtained on days 2, 3, or 4. If the initial INR (on days 1 through 4) is high, the patient is likely sensitive to warfarin's effects; therefore, a lower dose should be given. Patients who are restarting warfarin therapy after a time off the drug can safely begin with their previous maintenance dose. Guidelines recommend that the INR be checked at least four times during the first week of therapy. This frequency could then be gradually decreased, based on the stability of the INR. Because the risk of bleeding is greatest in the first 6 to 12 weeks of treatment, checking the INR weekly is appropriate. The maximum time between tests should be no more than 4 to 6 weeks. If a patient's INR has been stable and then fluctuates by more than 0.2 below or 0.4 above the goal INR, the patient should be evaluated for the cause of the change. Associated causes include laboratory error, noncompliance, drug interactions with warfarin, dietary interactions, or a change in the patient's health. If no reversible cause is found, a change in dosage may be made, with a repeat INR within 2 weeks. Close follow-up with repeated testing is needed, because the patients who have the most variation in results are most likely to develop bleeding or thromboembolism. In asymptomatic patients whose INR is elevated, temporary discontinuation of the drug is often used, but administration of vitamin K shortens the time to return to the target INR. There is indirect evidence that use of vitamin K is associated with a lower incidence of hemorrhage. Oral vitamin K is effective and may have fewer risks than the parenterally administered form. When a patient's INR is between 5 and 9, the recommendations include temporary discontinuation of warfarin therapy. If the patient is at risk for hemorrhage (e.g., is taking NSAIDs), low-dose oral vitamin K (1.0 to 2.5 mg) also should be given. However, the lowest dose available in tablet form is 5 mg, and often only 1 or 2 mg is needed. The parenteral form can be given orally and mixed in a flavored drink if needed. If the patient cannot be treated orally, 0.5 to 1 mg of intravenous vitamin K should be administered. For INRs of 9 or higher, vitamin K also should be given at a higher dose (2.5 mg intravenously or 5 mg orally). A repeat INR should be obtained within 24 hours. Additional vitamin K may be needed, depending on the result of the repeat INR. If the INR is elevated and the patient is bleeding, fresh-frozen plasma or a concentrate of clotting factors should be administered. A repeat INR should be obtained shortly after the fresh-frozen plasma is given. Additional fresh-frozen plasma may be needed because of its short duration of action. A large dose of vitamin K (10 mg) should also be given. Additional vitamin K may be necessary because the half-life of warfarin is longer than the half-life of vitamin K. Daily INR measurements should be instituted.

Gage BF, Fihn SD, White RH. Management and dosing of warfarin therapy. *Am J Med.* 2000;109:481–488.

22. A 55-year-old man is returning to discuss blood tests from his recent general examination. His PSA increased from 2.6 to 3.4. He does report a mild decrease in his urinary flow and gets up two times a night. Examination confirms a mildly enlarged prostate without nodules. Appropriate management at this time includes

A) further evaluation to exclude malignancy
B) observation and reassurance
C) use of alpha blockers to improve urinary flow
D) use of a 5-alpha reductase inhibitor

Answer and Discussion

The answer is A. Prostate cancer screening should be performed at the age of 50 years in those who wish to undergo evaluation and at normal risk for development of disease. Annual examinations can then be considered. In patients with PSA values between 4 and 10 ng/mL, the PSA velocity and percentage of free PSA can be used in making clinical decisions. A velocity of 0.75 ng/mL per year is predictive of cancer. When <10% of PSA is unbound, the positive predictive value for prostate cancer is 55%, compared with 8% when >25% of PSA is unbound. Prostate cancer screening probably should not be done once patients are over the age of 70 or if they develop a significant underlying medical illness or other incurable malignancy that decreases their life expectancy to <10 years. The issue of screening for prostate cancer remains very controversial and should be individualized to each patient.

Perkins GL. Serum tumor markers. *Am Fam Physician.* 2003; 68:1075–1082.

23. Type II renal tubular acidosis is associated with
A) the proximal tubules have decreased ability to absorb bicarbonate
B) urine pH that is normal when plasma bicarbonate levels are normal
C) chronic metabolic alkalosis
D) plasma bicarbonate levels that are easily restored with supplementation
E) hyperkalemia

Answer and Discussion

The answer is A. Type I (distal) renal tubular acidosis (RTA) is a disorder that affects adults and is considered a familial disorder in children. Sporadic cases may be primary (especially in women) or secondary (e.g., to an autoimmune disease such as Sjögren's syndrome; medications including amphotericin B or lithium therapy; kidney transplantation; nephrocalcinosis; renal medullary sponge kidney; chronic renal obstruction). Familial cases may be autosomal dominant and are often associated with hypercalciuria. In type I RTA, the urine pH is never <5.5.

Type II (proximal) RTA is associated with several inherited diseases (e.g., Fanconi's syndrome, fructose intolerance, Wilson's disease, Lowe's syndrome), multiple myeloma, vitamin D deficiency, and chronic hypocalcemia with secondary hyperparathyroidism. It may occur after renal transplant, exposure to heavy metals, and after treatment with certain medications, including acetazolamide, sulfonamides, tetracycline, and streptozocin.

In type II RTA, the ability of the proximal tubules to reabsorb HCO_3^- is decreased, so that urine pH is >7 at normal levels of plasma HCO_3^-, but may be <5.5 at low levels of plasma HCO_3^- Type III RTA is a combination of types I and II and is seldom seen.

Type IV RTA is a condition associated with mild renal insufficiency in adults with diabetes mellitus, HIV nephropathy, or interstitial renal damage [systemic lupus erythematosus (SLE), obstructive uropathy, sickle cell disease]. It also may be produced by drugs that interfere with the renin–aldosterone system (e.g., NSAIDs, ACE inhibitors, potassium-sparing diuretics, trimethoprim). Aldosterone deficiency or unresponsiveness of the distal tubule to aldosterone results in type IV RTA. This reduces potassium excretion, causing hyperkalemia, which reduces ammonia production and acid excretion by the kidney. Urine pH is usually normal.

Types I and II RTA are associated with chronic metabolic acidosis, mild volume loss, and hypokalemia. Hypokalemia may lead to muscle weakness, hyporeflexia, and paralysis. Type I RTA has decreased citrate excretion in the urine, increased mobilization of bone calcium, and hypercalciuria, which results in osteopenia, bone pain, and kidney stones or nephrocalcinosis. Renal parenchymal damage and chronic renal failure may develop. Type IV RTA is usually asymptomatic with only mild acidosis, but cardiac arrhythmias or paralysis may develop if hyperkalemia is extreme. Sodium bicarbonate relieves symptoms and prevents or stabilizes renal failure and bone disease. In adults with type I RTA, sodium bicarbonate eliminates acidosis and reduces the occurrence of kidney stones. In type II RTA, the plasma HCO_3^- cannot be restored to the normal range. HCO_3^- replacement should exceed the acid load of the diet. Additional HCO_3^- replacement increases potassium bicarbonate losses in the urine. Bicitra or Polycitra-K can be substituted for sodium bicarbonate and may be better tolerated. Potassium supplements may be required in patients who become hypokalemic when given sodium bicarbonate, but are not recommended in patients with normal or high serum potassium levels. In type IV RTA, the hyperkalemia is treated with fluid administration and potassium-depleting diuretics. A few patients may need mineralocorticoid replacement therapy.

Beers MH, Porter RS, eds. *The Merck manual of diagnosis and therapy,* Merck Research Laboratories, 18th ed. Whitehouse Station, NJ: Merck & Co.; 2006:2026–2028.

24. Which of the following is considered a first line medication in the treatment of hypertension?
A) Chlorthalidone
B) Lisinopril
C) Clonidine
D) Losartan
E) Amlodipine

Answer and Discussion

The answer is A. The Antihypertensive and Lipid-Lowering Treatment to Prevent Heart Attack Trial (ALLHAT) was a randomized, double-blind, multicenter clinical trial comparing the efficacies of various antihypertensive treatments in decreasing rates of coronary heart disease (CHD). The antihypertensives used in the trial included amlodipine, a calcium-channel blocker; lisinopril, an angiotensin-converting enzyme (ACE) inhibitor; doxazosin, an alpha-blocker; and chlorthalidone, a thiazide diuretic. The study showed similar mortality rates and no improvement in CHD risk in all treatment groups. Chlorthalidone (a diuretic) was found to be superior in preventing one or more major forms of cardiovascular disease, including stroke and heart failure. These findings resulted in the recommendation that diuretics be the first line drug of choice and a part of any multidrug antihypertensive regimen. Although the rates of primary outcomes, including fatal CHD and nonfatal myocardial infarction, were the same in the chlorthalidone, amlodipine, and lisinopril groups, the study's secondary endpoints such as heart failure showed the superiority of diuretics, specifically chlorthalidone. The diuretic users had a small increase in serum glucose levels, but this increase did not affect adverse outcomes. Thiazide-associated diabetes also has been shown to be reversible with good potassium balance, weight control, and increased physical activity. Thiazide-based treatments for hypertension are less expensive, and the additional laboratory monitoring for hypokalemia or hypoglycemia is probably no more than that required during ACE-inhibitor administration. Although ALLHAT has legitimate limitations, its conclusions appear valid. The newer antihypertensive agents tested are not superior to diuretics in the prevention of cardiovascular disease. These newer drugs are more expensive and appear to be less effective in preventing heart failure. Diuretics appear to be the preferred first-step drug and an important part of any multidrug regimen for the treatment of hypertension.

Davis BR, Furberg CD, Wright JT Jr. ALLHAT: setting the record straight. *Ann Intern Med.* 2004;141:39–46.

Based on the ALLHAT trial, diuretics should be the first-line drug of choice when treating hypertension and a part of any multidrug antihypertensive regimen.

25. Which of the following drugs offers protection from osteoporosis?
A) Hydrochlorothiazide
B) Metoprolol

C) Enalapril
D) Verapamil
E) Losartan

Answer and Discussion

The answer is A. In healthy elderly adults, low-dose hydrochlorothiazide preserves bone mineral density at the hip and spine. Although the effects appear modest at 3 years, if accumulated over 10 to 20 years, the use of diuretics provides one-third reduction in risk for hip fracture. Of the following list, none of the others provides this protection.

LaCroix AZ, Ott SM, Ichikawa L, et al. Low-dose hydrochlorothiazide and preservation of bone mineral density in older adults, a randomized, double-blind, placebo-controlled trial. *Ann Int Med.* 2000; 133(7):516–526.

26. Obsessive–compulsive disorder (OCD) is characterized by recurrent obsessions and compulsive behaviors such as repeated hand washing and checking routines. Which of the following statements regarding the disorder is true?
A) Patients affected rarely know they are affected.
B) Serotonin reuptake inhibitors are often first-line therapy.
C) Cognitive–behavioral therapy is rarely helpful in treatment.
D) Structural changes are not found in the brain.
E) Successful treatment leads to symptom resolution.

Answer and Discussion

The answer is B. OCD typically appears during the young adult years and has a chronic variable course. Although treatment can lessen the severity of the disorder, patients typically have some residual symptoms. It often is many years before affected patients are properly diagnosed and treated. OCD appears to have a genetic basis. Although some neurologic findings have been associated with OCD, such as increased gray matter and decreased white matter on brain imaging, the diagnosis remains a clinical one. Patients with OCD are plagued by recurrent obsessions and often perform compulsive washing and checking rituals in an attempt to deal with the anxiety provoked by their obsessions. Those affected by OCD usually are aware that their behavior is irrational and may spend a lot of effort to hide their symptoms from others. Cognitive–behavioral therapy usually is utilized in the treatment of OCD. In most patients, combining medication with behavioral therapy produces the best results. Selective serotonin reuptake inhibitors (SSRIs) generally are utilized first, with other psychotropic agents added if initial therapy fails. The optimal SSRI dosage for OCD tends to be higher than the dosage used to treat depression, and an adequate trial of medication may take up to 12 weeks.

Jenike MA. Obsessive–compulsive disorder. *N Engl J Med.* 2004;350:259–265.

27. An ankle–brachial index of _____ is considered normal.
A) 0.95
B) 0.75
C) 0.50
D) 0.25
E) 0.15

Answer and Discussion

The answer is A. Symptoms of claudication include a pain, ache, cramp, or tired feeling that occurs on walking. They are most common in the calf but may occur in the foot, thigh, hip, or buttocks. The condition is worsened by walking rapidly or uphill and usually relieved in 1 to 5 minutes by rest (sitting is not necessary); the patient can walk the same distance again before pain recurs. Disease progression is indicated by a reduction in the distance that the patient can walk without symptoms. Eventually, ischemic pain may occur at rest, beginning in the most distal parts of a limb as a severe, unrelenting pain aggravated by elevation and often interfering with sleep. If intermittent claudication is the only symptom, the extremity may appear normal, but the pulses are reduced or absent. The level of arterial occlusion and the location of intermittent claudication closely correlate (e.g., aortoiliac disease frequently causes claudication in the buttocks, hips, and calves, and the femoral pulses are reduced or absent). In males, impotence is common and depends on the location and extent of occlusion. In femoropopliteal disease, claudication is typically in the calf, and all pulses below the femoral are absent. In patients with small vessel disease (e.g., thromboangiitis obliterans, diabetes mellitus), femoropopliteal pulses may be present, but foot pulses are absent. Pallor of the involved foot after 1 to 2 minutes of elevation, followed by redness on dependency, helps confirm arterial insufficiency. Normal venous filling time with dependency after elevation is 15 seconds. If symptoms of claudication occur with good distal pulses, spinal stenosis should be considered. A severely ischemic foot is painful, cold, and often numb. In chronic cases, the skin may be dry and scaly, with poor nail and hair growth. As ischemia worsens, ulceration may appear (typically on the toes or heel, occasionally on the leg), especially after local trauma. Edema is usually not present unless the patient has kept the leg in a dependent position for pain relief. More extensive blockage may compromise tissue viability, leading to necrosis or gangrene. Ischemia with redness, pain, and swelling of the foot on dependency may mimic cellulitis or venous insufficiency. Although arterial occlusion in the extremities can usually be diagnosed clinically, noninvasive tests confirm the diagnosis and are useful in follow-up. Invasive tests can document the location and extent of disease if angioplasty, local fibrinolytic therapy, or surgical bypass is contemplated. Doppler ultrasonography is most widely used. Arterial stenosis and occlusion can be detected using a velocity detector (Doppler probe). A colored signal shows the direction of flow (color Doppler). The simplest method for estimating blood flow to the lower extremities is to compare systolic BP at the level of the ankle with brachial systolic pressure (ankle–brachial indices). During this procedure, a blood pressure cuff is applied to the ankle, inflated above brachial systolic pressure, and deflated slowly. Ankle systolic blood pressure can be obtained accurately with a Doppler probe placed over the dorsalis pedis or posterior tibial arteries. This blood pressure at rest normally is >= 90% of the brachial systolic pressure; with mild arterial insufficiency, it is 70% to 90%; with moderate insufficiency, 50% to 70%; and with severe insufficiency, <50%.

Beers MH, Porter RS, eds. *The Merck manual of diagnosis and therapy,* Merck Research Laboratories, 18th ed. Whitehouse Station, NJ: Merck & Co.; 2006:749–750.

28. A secondary cause of restless legs syndrome (RLS) is
A) vitamin B_{12} deficiency
B) heavy metal intoxication
C) alcohol abuse
D) iron deficiency
E) bismuth overdose

Answer and Discussion

The answer is D. RLS is a neurologic movement disorder that is often associated with a sleep disturbance. Patients with RLS have an irresistible urge to move their legs, which is usually secondary to uncomfortable sensations that are worse during periods of inactivity and often interfere with sleep. It is estimated that between 2% and 15% of the population may experience symptoms of RLS. Primary RLS may have a genetic origin. Secondary causes of RLS include iron deficiency, neurologic lesions, pregnancy, and uremia. RLS also may occur secondarily to the use of certain medications. The diagnosis of RLS is based primarily on the patient's history. Pharmacologic treatment of RLS includes dopaminergic agents, opioids, benzodiazepines, and anticonvulsants.

National Heart, Lung, and Blood Institute Working Group on Restless Legs Syndrome. Restless legs syndrome: detection and management in primary care. *Am Fam Physician.* 2000; 62:108–114.

29. In appropriate patients, thrombolytic therapy can be given up to ______ after onset of stroke symptoms.

A) 1 hour
B) 2 hours
C) 3 hours
D) 24 hours
E) 36 hours

Answer and Discussion

The answer is C. Transient ischemic attack (TIA) is considered a significant warning sign of impending stroke. It is crucial to recognize these events to prevent permanent disability or death in affected individuals. The 90-day risk of stroke after a TIA has been estimated to be approximately 10%, with one half of strokes occurring within the first 2 days of the attack. The 90-day stroke risk is even higher when a TIA results from internal carotid artery disease. Most patients reporting symptoms of TIA should be referred to an emergency department for further evaluation. Patients who arrive at the emergency department within 180 minutes of symptom onset should undergo evaluation to determine if they are candidates for thrombolytic therapy. Initial testing should include complete blood count with platelet count, prothrombin time, International Normalized Ratio, partial thromboplastin time, and electrolyte and glucose levels. Computed tomographic scanning of the head should be performed immediately to ensure that there is no evidence of brain hemorrhage or mass. Risk factors for stroke should be evaluated in patients who have had a TIA. Blood pressure, lipid levels, and diabetes mellitus should be controlled. If indicated, smoking cessation and weight loss are also important. Angiotensin-converting enzyme inhibitor therapy may help prevent stroke. Aspirin is the treatment of choice for stroke prevention in patients who do not require anticoagulation. Clopidogrel (Plavix) is an alternative therapy in patients who do not tolerate aspirin. Atrial fibrillation, a known cardioembolic source (confirmed thrombus), or a highly suspected cardioembolic source (e.g., recent large myocardial infarction, dilated cardiomyopathy, mechanical valve, rheumatic mitral valve stenosis) are indications for anticoagulation with warfarin therapy.

Solenski NJ. Transient ischemic attacks: Part I. Diagnosis and evaluation. *Am Fam Physician.* 2004;69:1665–1674, 1679–1680.

Solenski NJ. Transient ischemic attacks: Part II. Treatment. *Am Fam Physician.* 2004;69:1681–1688.

30. Of the following, which is *least* likely to be seen in strep throat?

A) Fever
B) Malaise
C) Tonsilar exudates
D) Palatine petechiae
E) Rhinorrhea

Answer and Discussion

The answer is E. Sore throat is one of the most common reasons for visits to family physicians. Although most patients with sore throat have an infectious cause (pharyngitis), <20% have a clear indication for antibiotic therapy (i.e., group A β—hemolytic streptococcal infection). Viral pharyngitis is the most common cause of sore throat. Infectious mononucleosis is most common in patients 15 to 30 years of age. Patients typically present with fever, sore throat, and malaise. On examination, there is pharyngeal redness with exudates. Posterior cervical lymphadenopathy is common in patients with infectious mononucleosis, and its absence makes the diagnosis much less likely. Hepatosplenomegaly also may be present. If these patients are treated with amoxicillin or ampicillin, 90% develop a classic maculopapular rash. Patients with bacterial pharyngitis generally do not have rhinorrhea, cough, or conjunctivitis. Children younger than 15 are more likely to have strep throat. Symptoms of strep throat may include pharyngeal erythema and swelling, tonsillar exudate, edematous uvula, palatine petechiae, and anterior cervical lymphadenopathy. Untreated, strep pharyngitis lasts 7 to 10 days. Patients with untreated streptococcal pharyngitis are infectious during the acute phase of the illness and for 1 additional week. Antibiotic therapy shortens the infectious period to 24 hours, reduces the duration of symptoms by about 1 day, and prevents most complications. The incidence of complications with strep infection, such as rheumatic fever and peritonsillar abscess, is low. Peritonsillar abscess occurs in <1% of patients treated with antibiotics. Patients with peritonsillar abscess typically have a toxic appearance and may present with a muffled voice, fluctuant peritonsillar mass, and asymmetric deviation of the uvula.

Vincent MT, Celestin N, Hussain AN. Pharyngitis. *Am Fam Physician.* 2004;69:1465–1470.

31. Angioneurotic edema is associated with the use of

A) ACE inhibitors
B) beta blockers
C) loop diuretics
D) alpha-receptor blockers
E) calcium-channel blockers

Answer and Discussion

The answer is A. Angioneurotic edema, which occurs in 0.1% to 0.2% of patients, usually develops within the first week of therapy but can occur at any time. This life-threatening adverse effect also occurs with angiotensin II–receptor blockers, but to a lesser extent. Any patient with a history of angioneurotic edema, whether related to an ACE inhibitor, angiotensin-receptor blockers, or another cause, should not be given an ACE inhibitor. Other contraindications include pregnancy, renal artery stenosis, and previous allergy to ACE inhibitors.

Bicket DP. Using ACE inhibitors appropriately. *Am Fam Physician.* 2002;66:461–468, 473.

32. Genital warts

A) rarely resolve spontaneously
B) are treated based on cost, convenience, and adverse affects
C) do not remain in tissue after treatment
D) are treated with an alternative method if a single treatment fails to eradicate the wart

Answer and Discussion

The answer is B. Untreated visible genital warts may resolve spontaneously, remain the same, or increase in size. The primary treatment goal is removal of symptomatic warts. Some evidence suggests that treatment also may reduce the persistence of human papillomavirus (HPV) DNA in genital tissue, and therefore may reduce the incidence of cervical cancer. The choice of therapy is based on the number, size, site, and morphology of lesions, as well as patient preference, treatment cost, convenience, adverse effects, and physician experience. Assuming that the diagnosis is certain, switching to a new treatment modality is appropriate if there is no response after three treatment cycles. Routine follow-up at 2 to 3 months is advised to monitor response to therapy and evaluate for recurrence. Treatment methods can be chemical or ablative.

Kodnar CM, Nasraty S. Management of genital warts. *Am Fam Physician.* 2004;70:2335–2342, 2345–2346.

33. When is a comprehensive evaluation necessary when a patient is affected by a deep venous thrombosis (DVT)?

A) 45-year-old male with an idiopathic DVT
B) 65-year-old with a recent transatlantic flight and DVT of left thigh
C) 55-year-old who develops a calf DVT after a 4-hour car ride
D) 75-year-old with a history of non-small-cell cancer of lung with left leg DVT
E) 72-year-old with a right thigh DVT and no history of travel

Answer and Discussion

The answer is A. Treatment goals for DVT include stopping clot propagation and preventing the recurrence of thrombus, the occurrence of pulmonary embolism, and the development of pulmonary hypertension, which can be a complication of multiple recurrent pulmonary emboli. About 30% of patients with DVT or pulmonary embolism have a thrombophilia. A comprehensive evaluation is suggested in patients younger than 50 years with an idiopathic episode of DVT, patients with recurrent thrombosis, and patients with a family history of thromboembolism. Intravenous administration of unfractionated heparin followed by oral administration of warfarin remains the mainstay of treatment for deep venous thrombosis. Subcutaneous low-molecular-weight (LMW) heparin is at least as effective as unfractionated heparin given in a continuous intravenous route. LMW heparin is the agent of choice for treating DVT in pregnant women and patients with cancer. Based on validated protocols, warfarin can be started at a dosage of 5 or 10 mg/day. The intensity and duration of warfarin therapy depends on the individual patient, but treatment of at least 3 months usually is required. Some patients with thrombophilias require lifetime anticoagulation. Treatment for pulmonary embolism is similar to that for DVT. Because of the risk of respiratory failure and hemodynamic instability, in-hospital management is advised. Unfractionated heparin commonly is used, although LMW heparin is safe and effective. Thrombolysis is used in patients with massive pulmonary embolism. Subcutaneous heparin, LMW heparin, and warfarin have been approved for use in surgical prophylaxis. Elastic compression stockings are useful in patients at lowest risk for thromboembolism. Intermittent pneumatic leg compression is a useful adjunct to anticoagulation and an alternative when anticoagulation is contraindicated.

Razmi DW, Leeper KV. DVT and pulmonary embolism: Part II. Treatment and prevention. *Am Fam Physician.* 2004;69: 2841–2848.

34. Which of the following statements is correct concerning hepatitis C virus (HCV)?

A) There is no risk to infants if the mother is affected.
B) There is no risk associated with sexual intercourse with an individual with hepatitis C.
C) Cesarean section should be performed on mothers who test positive for hepatitis C to prevent transmission to the newborn.
D) Hepatitis C can be spread by contaminated water supplies.
E) Hepatitis C does not appear to be transmitted in breast milk.

Answer and Discussion

The answer is E. In an effort to reduce the risk of transmission to others, HCV positive patients should be advised not to donate blood, organs, tissue, or semen; not to share toothbrushes, dental appliances, razors, or other personal care articles that might have blood on them; and to cover cuts and sores on the skin to keep from spreading infectious blood or secretions. HCV positive patients with one long-term, steady sex partner do not need to change their sexual practices. They should, however, discuss the risk (which is low but not absent) with their partner. If they want to lower the small chance of spreading HCV to their partner, they may decide to use barrier precautions such as latex condoms. HCV positive women do not need to avoid pregnancy or breast feeding. Potential, expectant, and new parents should be advised that about 5 of every 100 infants born to HCV infected women become infected. This infection occurs at the time of birth, and no treatment has been shown to prevent the transmission. There is no evidence that the method of delivery is related to transmission; therefore, the need for cesarean section versus vaginal delivery should not be determined on the basis of HCV infection status. Limited data on breast feeding indicate that it does not transmit HCV, although it may be prudent for HCV-positive mothers to abstain from breast feeding if their nipples are cracked or bleeding. Infants born to HCV positive women should be tested for HCV infection and, if positive, evaluated for the presence or development of chronic liver disease. HCV is not spread by sneezing, hugging, coughing, food or water, sharing eating utensils or drinking glasses, or casual contact. Persons should not be excluded from work, school, play, child care, or other settings on the basis of HCV infection status. HCV positive persons should be evaluated to assess for biochemical evidence of chronic liver disease. These patients should be assessed for severity of disease and possible treatment according to current practice guidelines in consultation with, or by referral to, a specialist knowledgeable in this field.

Moyer LA, Mast EE, Alter MJ. Hepatitis C: Part II. Prevention, counseling and medical evaluation. *Am Fam Physician.* 1999;59:349.

HCV-positive women do not need to avoid pregnancy or breast-feeding.

35. Which of the following classes of drugs can be used safely with nonsteroidal anti-inflammatory drugs (NSAIDs) without needing to closely monitor the patient's renal function, potassium levels, and/or blood pressure?
A) Angiotensin-converting enzyme (ACE) inhibitors
B) Calcium-channel blockers
C) Diuretics
D) β-Blockers

Answer and Discussion

The answer is B. Combined use of NSAIDs and hypertensive medication (i.e., diuretics, β-blockers α-blockers, and ACE inhibitors) may decrease the effectiveness of antihypertensive medication and cause serious complications. Thus, when using the two in combination, renal function, potassium levels, and blood pressure should be monitored. Calcium-channel blockers and central α agonists can usually be used without these concerns.

Oparil S, Calhoun DA. Managing the patient with hard-to-control hypertension. *Am Fam Physician.* 1998;57:1018.

36. Which of the following statements about sunscreens and sun exposure is true?
A) The most dangerous rays are the ultraviolet A (UVA) type.
B) Sunscreens with a skin protection factor of 10 are adequate protection.
C) Patients allergic to thiazide diuretics may react adversely to *para*-aminobenzoic acid (PABA).
D) Steroids should be avoided in patients with sunburns because of their immunosuppressant properties.
E) Repeated use of sunscreens can increase the risk of sun poisoning.

Answer and Discussion

The answer is C. Sun-produced UV light is divided into two types of rays: UVA (2,800 to 3,200 nm) and UVB (280 to 320 nm). The dangerous rays are in the UVB range. Sunscreens of at least skin protection factor 15 (and preferably SPF-30) should be used when persons are exposed to the sun. *para*-aminobenzoic acid, which is used in many sunscreens, is very effective at preventing sunburns. Unfortunately, patients with sensitivities to thiazides, benzocaine, or sulfonamides may react adversely to *para*-aminobenzoic acid. In most cases, sunburn is prevented with simple precautions. Sunburn (usually a first-degree burn) appears within the first 24 hours and can be very painful. Sunburn is treated with cold-water compresses. In severe cases, sunburns can be treated with steroids.

Medical Letter Consultants. Sunscreens: are they safe and effective? *Med Lett Drugs Ther.* 1999;41(1052):43–44.

37. Which of the following tests can be used in the diagnosis of celiac sprue?
A) Shilling's test
B) String test
C) Xylose absorption test
D) Withdrawal of lactose from the diet to monitor for improvement of symptoms
E) Scotch tape test

Answer and Discussion

The answer is C. Celiac sprue is an inherited disorder that is characterized by an intolerance to gluten, a cereal-type protein found in wheat, rye, oats, and barley. Symptoms in infancy include colic, failure to thrive, and, in severe cases, iron deficiency anemia with the development of edema. In adults, symptoms include abdominal bloating and discomfort, with diarrhea, anemia, weight loss, arthralgias, and edema. Laboratory findings usually include iron deficiency anemia (in children), folate deficiency anemia (in adults), low protein levels, and electrolyte abnormalities. Antigliadin IgA and IgG antibodies are elevated in >90% of patients; however, they are nonspecific. IgA endomysial antibodies are more specific for celiac sprue and are the best screening test for celiac disease. Tissue transglutinase autoantibody by ELISA is a newer serologic test for celiac sprue. Steatorrhea is usually present, and coagulation studies may be abnormal. Diagnosis is accomplished through the following:

1. Biopsy of the jejunum, which shows a flat mucosa with a loss of intestinal villi
2. A D-xylose absorption test, which shows an abnormal result indicating malabsorption
3. Withdrawal of gluten from the diet, which results in a significant improvement in symptoms
4. Fecal fat estimation for 72 hours is elevated (>7 g/day)

Treatment involves dietary counseling to avoid gluten-containing foods and supplementary vitamins. In severe cases, corticosteroids are used to induce a refractory stage.

Ferri F. *Ferri's Clinical Advisor, Instant Diagnosis and Treatment.* Philadelphia: Elsevier/Mosby; 2006:529.

38. Pregnant women should avoid contact with cat litter because of the risk for developing
A) *Cryptococcus*
B) *Cytomegalovirus*
C) *Toxoplasmosis*
D) *Coccidioidomycosis*
E) *Erythema infectiosum*

Answer and Discussion

The answer is C. *Toxoplasmosis* is a granulomatous disease caused by the protozoan *Toxoplasmosis gondii,* which affects the CNS. The disease is extremely common, and affected patients are usually asymptomatic. Symptoms, when present, mimic mononucleosis and include malaise, fever, myalgias, rashes, and cervical and axillary lymphadenopathy. Laboratory and physical findings include mild anemia, leukopenia, lymphocytosis, elevated liver function tests, and hypotension. A more severe form may occur in patients with AIDS or other patients who are immunocompromised; complications include hepatitis, pneumonitis, meningoencephalitis, and myocarditis. Chronic toxoplasmosis can lead to retinochoroiditis, persistent diarrhea, muscular weakness, and headache. Congenital toxoplasmosis can lead to spontaneous abortion or stillbirths. A multitude of congenital defects may occur, including blindness and severe mental retardation. Diagnosis is usually made by serologic tests with fluorescent antibody techniques. CT examination of the brain may show enhancing lesions, and biopsies can be taken to look for the organisms microscopically. Treatment is reserved for more severe cases and consists of the combined use of pyrimethamine, sulfadiazine, and folinic acid (leucovorin). Immunocompromised patients require maintenance treatment for life. Because the protozoan is found in cat feces, pregnant women should avoid handling cat litter.

Goldman L, Ausiello D, eds. *Cecil textbook of medicine,* 22nd ed. Philadelphia: WB Saunders; 2004:2088–2092.

39. Pain associated with the distal second metatarsal head is most likely a result of
A) Morton's neuroma
B) Jones fracture
C) March fracture
D) metatarsalgia
E) gout

Answer and Discussion

The answer is D. Metatarsalgia is characterized by pain and sometimes swelling associated with the second (and, less commonly, the third) metatarsal head. The pain is secondary to a synovitis that affects the joint. Patients with hammertoes are at an increased risk because of stress placed at the head of the metatarsals. In most cases, radiographs are normal; however, more severe cases may show subluxation or dislocation of the metacarpal joint. NSAIDs, hot soaks, and metatarsal pads may help; however, if subluxation or dislocation is present, surgery may be necessary.

Ferri F. *Ferri's Clinical Advisor, Instant Diagnosis and Treatment.* Philadelphia: Elsevier/Mosby; 2006:529.

40. Desensitization immunotherapy may be used in the treatment of
A) chronic urticaria
B) hymenoptera allergies
C) atopic dermatitis
D) milk allergy
E) none of the above

Answer and Discussion

The answer is B. Desensitization immunotherapy is used in the treatment of severe allergic rhinitis and bee-sting (hymenoptera) allergies. The patient is given gradually increasing concentrations of the allergen over an increasing period. Typically, there is a decrease in the mast cell response with a decrease in histamine production when the patient is exposed to the allergen. In addition, IgE levels decrease. In most cases, the injections are continued year-round and may be spaced out as the desired response occurs. Injections should always be given in the presence of a physician, and appropriate equipment must be available to treat potential anaphylaxis. Patients must be observed for at least 30 minutes after administration of the injections. Desensitization immunotherapy is not appropriate for the treatment of chronic urticaria, milk allergies, or atopic dermatitis.

Beers MH, Porter RS, eds. *The Merck manual of diagnosis and therapy,* Merck Research Laboratories, 18th ed. Whitehouse Station, NJ: Merck & Co.; 2006:1356–1357.

41. A 16-year-old boy is brought to the emergency room after suffering a seizure. He is tachycardic and hypertensive, and has a temperature of 38.6°C. Physical examination shows that the patient is in a postictal state and has a nasal septum perforation. Electrocardiogram (ECG) findings suggest acute myocardial infarction. Friends of the patient report recent cocaine use. Which of the following drugs is indicated?
A) Flumazenil
B) Phentolamine
C) Dexfenfluramine
D) Propranolol
E) Phenytoin

Answer and Discussion

The answer is B. Cocaine is a strong narcotic stimulant that is often abused. Its mechanism of action involves the increased release of norepinephrine and the blockage of its reuptake. Effects of cocaine begin within 3 to 5 minutes (within 8 to 10 seconds with smoking "crack" cocaine), and peak effects occur at 10 to 20 minutes. The effects rarely last more than 1 hour. Cocaine toxicity is characterized by seizures; hyperpyrexia; tachycardia; mental status changes, including paranoid behavior; hypertension; cerebrovascular accidents; myocardial infarctions; and rhabdomyolysis. Nasal septum perforation may also occur. In most cases, treatment involves the use of diazepam for neurologic symptoms and phentolamine for severe tachyarrhythmias and observation. Nitroprusside can be used for hypertensive crisis. The use of β-blockers is not recommended; other complications, such as cerebrovascular accidents, rhabdomyolysis, and myocardial infarctions, should be managed in a conventional manner. Fortunately, cocaine has a short half-life and symptoms are usually self-limited. Individuals who use cocaine may become rapidly addicted.

Rakel RE, Bope ET. *Conn's Current Therapy 2005.* Philadelphia: Elsevier/Saunders; 2005:1352–1353.

42. Goodpasture's syndrome is associated with
A) osteoporosis and renal lithiasis
B) pathologic fractures and thyroiditis
C) hepatitis and recurrent cystitis
D) pulmonary hemorrhage and glomerulonephritis
E) pica and angioedema

Answer and Discussion

The answer is D. Goodpasture's syndrome is a condition manifested by pulmonary hemorrhages and progressive glomerulonephritis. Circulating basement membrane antibodies are responsible for the renal and pulmonary abnormalities. Patients with Goodpasture's syndrome are typically young males (5 to 40 years; male:female ratio of 6:1); however, there is a bimodal peak at approximately 60 years of age. Men and women are equally affected at older ages. Symptoms include severe hemoptysis, shortness of breath, and renal failure. Laboratory findings include iron deficiency anemia, hematuria, proteinuria, cellular and granular casts in the urine, and circulating antiglomerular antibodies. Chest radiographs show progressive, bilateral, fluffy infiltrates that may migrate and are asymmetrical. Renal biopsy may be necessary to make the diagnosis. Treatment involves high-dose steroids, immunosuppression, and plasmapheresis, which may help preserve renal function. If significant injury to the kidneys occurs, then dialysis or transplant may be necessary. Untreated, Goodpasture's syndrome can be fatal.

Kasper DL, Braunwald E, Fauci AS, et al., eds. *Harrison's principles of internal medicine,* 16th ed. New York: McGraw-Hill; 2005:1560, 1676–1683.

> Goodpasture's syndrome is a condition manifested by pulmonary hemorrhages and progressive glomerulonephritis. Circulating basement membrane antibodies are responsible for the renal and pulmonary abnormalities.

43. Black cohosh has been advocated to treat
A) muscle and joint pain
B) the common cold

C) depression
D) menopausal symptoms
E) osteoporosis

Answer and Discussion

The answer is D. The herb black cohosh, or *Actaea racemosa* (formerly named *Cimicifuga racemosa*), is native to North America. The roots and rhizomes of this herb are widely used in the treatment of menopausal symptoms and menstrual dysfunction. Although the clinical trials on black cohosh are of insufficient quality to support definitive statements, this herbal medicine may be effective in the short-term treatment of menopausal symptoms. The mechanism of action is unclear, and early reports of an estrogenic effect have not been proved in recent studies. Although black cohosh may be useful in treating some menopausal symptoms, there is currently no evidence regarding any protective effect of black cohosh against the development of osteoporosis. Adverse effects are extremely uncommon, and there are no known significant adverse drug interactions.

Kligler B. Black cohosh. *Am Fam Physician*. 2003;68:114–116.

44. Smoking "crack cocaine"
A) has become a major health problem in urban middle-class populations
B) leads to physical dependence
C) is more common than snorting cocaine
D) can lead to tolerance
E) produces a stereotypical withdrawal syndrome

Answer and Discussion

The answer is D. Although the majority of cocaine in the United States is snorted intranasally, smoking crack cocaine has been widely publicized. The imported hydrochloride salt is converted to a more volatile form, usually by adding sodium bicarbonate, water, and heat. The converted material is combusted, and the resultant smoke inhaled. The onset of effect is faster, and intensity of the "high" is increased. Tolerance occurs, but physical dependence has not been confirmed; no stereotypical withdrawal syndrome occurs when the drug is discontinued. However, the tendency to continue taking the drug is strong. Use of crack by the urban poor and the criminal market for crack have become one of the most feared problems of drug abuse. Despite frequent predictions, crack use has not expanded to the suburbs or the urban middle class. Its continued use still occurs primarily in poor Americans.

Beers MH, Porter RS, eds. *The Merck manual of diagnosis and therapy,* Merck Research Laboratories, 18th ed. Whitehouse Station, NJ: Merck & Co.; 2006:1693–1694.

45. A recognized complication of sleep apnea is
A) hyperlipidemia
B) diabetes mellitus
C) restless legs syndrome
D) migraines
E) congestive heart failure

Answer and Discussion

The answer is E. Obstructive sleep apnea occurs most often in moderately or severely obese persons. Men are affected more often than women (4% of men and 2% of women in middle age). Upper airway narrowing leads to obstruction during sleep. In severely obese persons, a combination of hypoxemia and hypercapnia may induce central apnea as well. By definition, apneic periods last at least 10 seconds (some for 2 minutes). Repeated nocturnal obstruction may cause recurring cycles of sleep, obstructive choking, and arousal with gasping for air. Daytime drowsiness usually results from the repeated cycles. Similar but less-pronounced cycles occur in non-obese persons, possibly secondary to developmental or congenital abnormalities of the upper airway. Complications of sleep apnea include cardiac abnormalities (e.g., sinus arrhythmias, extreme bradycardia, atrial flutter, ventricular tachycardia, heart failure), hypertension, excessive daytime sleepiness, morning headache, and slowed mentation. The mortality rate from stroke and MIs is significantly higher in persons with obstructive sleep apnea than in the general population.

Rakel RE, Bope ET. *Conn's Current Therapy 2005*. Philadelphia: Elsevier/Saunders; 2005:262–265.

46. Which of the following medications is effective for restless legs syndrome?
A) Levodopa/carbidopa
B) Diltiazem
C) Phenytoin
D) Haloperidol
E) Vitamin B_6

Answer and Discussion

The answer is A. Restless legs syndrome (RLS) is a relatively common problem seen by family physicians. The condition is characterized by repeated movements and paresthesias of the lower extremities (occasionally the arms). Patients may describe a tingling irritation or a drawing or crawling sensation that prevents the onset of sleep or they may disturb sleep. The symptoms are often relieved by movement. Laboratory and neurologic tests are normal. Associated conditions include iron deficiency, diabetes, uremia, pregnancy, rheumatoid arthritis, vitamin B_{12} deficiency, and polyneuropathy. Treatment includes the use of ropinirole (Requip), pramipexole (Mirapex), pergolide (Permax), levodopa/carbidopa (Sinemet), gabapentin (Neurontin), carbamazepine (Carbatrol), and other antiepileptics, opiates, and benzodiazepines.

Ferri F. *Ferri's Clinical Advisor, Instant Diagnosis and Treatment*. Philadelphia: Elsevier/Mosby; 2006:731–732.

47. Which of the following forms of hepatitis does NOT have a chronic state?
A) Hepatitis A
B) Hepatitis B
C) Hepatitis C
D) Hepatitis D

Answer and Discussion

The answer is A. Hepatitis is an inflammation of the liver that is characterized by nausea, anorexia, fever, right-upper abdominal discomfort, jaundice, and marked elevation of liver function tests. The condition is usually classified into the following types:

- *Hepatitis A.* Also known as infectious hepatitis, the causative agent is an RNA virus. The disease is common and often presents subclinically. It is estimated that as much as 75% of the U.S. population has positive antibodies to hepatitis A. The onset of clinical symptoms is usually acute, and children and young adults are usually affected. The transmission is via a fecal–oral route and has been linked to the consumption of contaminated shellfish (e.g., raw oysters). The course of the disease is usually mild, and the prognosis is usually excellent. There is neither an associated chronic state nor a carrier state. The diagnosis is made by the detection of elevated levels of IgM antibodies, which indicate active disease, and IgG antibodies, which indicate previous disease. Most cases require no special treatment other than supportive care, and symptoms usually resolve after several weeks. The disease can be prevented by administering Ig to those who are in close contact with those affected. Immunization, especially for travelers, is recommended to specifically prevent hepatitis A.

- *Hepatitis B.* This DNA viral disease is more severe than hepatitis A and causes more complications. It affects as much as 10% of the U.S. population. The infective Dane particle consists of a viral core and outer surface coat. The disease often develops insidiously and can affect persons of all ages. It is transmitted parenterally (through infected blood transfusions or infected needles used by intravenous drug abusers) and through sexual contact (especially in sexually active young adults and homosexuals). The symptoms are often severe and can be devastating to elderly patients or those who are debilitated. Approximately 10% of cases become chronic; up to 30% of affected patients become carriers of the virus after they are infected. The detection of the hepatitis B surface antigen (formerly known as the Australian antigen) supports the diagnosis of acute illness, and values become positive between 1 and 7 weeks before the symptoms become evident. The hepatitis B antibody appears weeks to months after the development of the clinical symptoms. The presence of a hepatitis B surface antibody indicates previous disease and represents immunity. Those who have received hepatitis B vaccination also have positive titers if they are immune. An anticore antibody (IgM) usually develops at the onset of the illness, and the IgG anticore antibody (which develops shortly after IgM appears) can be used as a marker for the disease during the "window period," which occurs when the hepatitis B surface antigen disappears and before the hepatitis B surface antibodies appear. The hepatitis B e antigen is found in those who are hepatitis B surface antigen–positive; its presence is associated with greater infectivity and a greater chance of progression to the chronic state. The delta agent (hepatitis D) is a separate virus that may coexist with hepatitis B; it is usually associated with a more severe case of hepatitis B and in cases of chronic hepatitis B in which there is reactivation of the virus. Prophylaxis of hepatitis B can be achieved with hepatitis B vaccine given at 1 month and 6 months after the initial injection, for a total of three injections. Persons exposed to hepatitis B (e.g., by needle stick) should also receive hepatitis B Ig at the time of exposure.
- *Hepatitis C.* This disease (also known as *non-A, non-B hepatitis*, or *post-transfusion hepatitis*) accounts for as many as 40% of the cases of hepatitis in the United States. It is the main indication for liver transplant in the United States when cirrhosis is present. The disease is transmitted by infected blood, and is commonly seen in intravenous drug abusers and those who had blood transfusions infected with the virus. The disease is usually insidious in its presentation, and the severity is variable. As many as 50% of these patients may develop chronic disease, which may eventually lead to cirrhosis. The diagnosis is made by serologic means, and pegylated α-interferon and ribavirin have been used for treatment.
- *Hepatitis E.* The transmission is similar to the hepatitis A virus. The disease is found in India and Southeast Asia, Africa, and Mexico. Cases in the United States are usually related to travel to these endemic areas. Hepatitis E virus is associated with a high fatality in pregnant women.
- Chemical hepatitis. This condition has been associated with the use of excessive alcohol, high-dose acetaminophen, halothane, carbon tetrachloride, INH, and birth control pills.

Ferri F. *Ferri's Clinical Advisor, Instant Diagnosis and Treatment.* Philadelphia: Elsevier/Mosby; 2006:372–379.

48. Which of the following factors is included in the criteria for administering streptokinase with myocardial infarction?

A) Cardiogenic chest pain lasting at least 6 hours
B) ECG changes of at least 1 to 2 mm of ST elevation in two adjacent precordial leads
C) Streptokinase should not be administered 6 hours after the onset of chest pain
D) Q waves noted in the lateral precordial leads

Answer and Discussion

The answer is B. Streptokinase is a thrombolytic agent administered during myocardial infarction. In the Second International Study of Infarct Survival, there was a 23% reduction in vascular death for those given streptokinase compared with those given a placebo. Allergic reactions consisting of skin rashes and fever may be seen in 1% to 2%. Hypotension occurs in 10% of patients. Because of the development of antibodies, patients previously treated with streptokinase should be given recombinant tissue-plasminogen activator (alteplase) or reteplase plasminogen activator. The criteria for consideration of thrombolytics include chest pain (consistent with cardiogenic pain) for at least 30 minutes' duration and ECG changes that show at least 1 to 2 mm of ST elevation in two adjacent precordial leads. Medication should be given within 12 hours for maximal benefit. Although extremely variable depending on the source, the following is a list of absolute contraindications to thrombolytics:

- History of intracranial hemorrhage
- Uncontrolled hypertension defined as systolic blood pressure (SBP) >180 mm Hg or diastolic blood pressure (DBP) >100 mm Hg
- Recent surgery (1 month or less)
- Recent vascular puncture in a noncompressible region (<2 weeks)
- Unclear mental status
- Active gastrointestinal (GI) bleeding
- Aortic dissection
- Acute pericarditis
- Prolonged (>10 minutes) cardiopulmonary resuscitation

Relative contraindications include:

- Prior stroke (nonhemorrhagic)
- Major surgery (3 months or less)
- Pregnancy
- Bleeding diasthesis
- Active peptic ulcer disease

Minor hemorrhage, menstruation, and diabetic retinopathy are not contraindications to fibrinolytic therapy. Of the list of thrombolytic medications, streptokinase is the least expensive but has the highest incidence of side effects, including allergic reactions and hypotension.

Rakel RE, Bope ET. *Conn's Current Therapy 2005*. Philadelphia: Elsevier/Saunders; 2005:404.

49. A 48-year-old alcoholic stops drinking 2 days before presenting to his physician. He is diaphoretic, nauseated, tachycardic, anxious, and hypertensive. The most appropriate management is to

A) prescribe diazepam and refer the patient to a drug treatment program
B) hospitalize the patient, administer diazepam, and closely observe his condition
C) administer disulfiram and diazepam and follow up with the patient in 1 week
D) reassure the patient, compliment his decision to stop drinking, and explain the symptoms that are to be expected
E) refer the patient to psychiatry

Answer and Discussion

The answer is B. Symptoms of alcohol withdrawal usually occur 6 to 48 hours after the last alcoholic drink. These symptoms include sweating, anxiety, tremor, weakness, gastrointestinal (GI) discomfort, hypertension, tachycardia, fever, and hyperreflexia. Other symptoms include hallucinations and, in severe cases, delirium tremens that are characterized by disorientation with hallucinations, drenching sweats, severe tremors, and electrolyte disturbances that can lead to seizures. Treatment involves hospitalization and close observation. Antianxiety medications, including chlordiazepoxide, lorazepam, diazepam, midazolam, and oxazepam, are used for treatment and are slowly tapered to prevent withdrawal-related symptoms. Oral multivitamin supplementation with thiamine, folate, and pyridoxine is also recommended. Disulfiram is not used for alcohol withdrawal but can be used in the treatment of alcoholism to help discourage further drinking.

Ferri F. *Ferri's Clinical Advisor, Instant Diagnosis and Treatment*. Philadelphia: Elsevier/Mosby; 2006:36–38.

50. Which of the following statements about Burner's syndrome is true?

A) The mechanism of injury involves acute hyperextension of the shoulder while the neck and head are forced in the same direction.
B) Symptoms include temporary weakness, pain, paresthesias, and decreased sensation of the distal extremity.
C) The injury involves traction forces on the spinal cord's dorsal columns.
D) Most cases cause permanent neurologic deficits.
E) The condition is associated with overuse injury of the knees.

Answer and Discussion

The answer is B. Burner's syndrome is seen mostly in football players and results from a tackling or blocking injury. The injury occurs when the contact shoulder is depressed and the head and neck are forced in the opposite direction of contact. The traction-type forces placed on the brachial plexus lead to variable symptoms of weakness, pain, paresthesias, limited motion, and decreased sensation of the affected extremity. Diminished reflexes may also be seen. The condition should be treated with caution, and cervical disc or bony injury should be ruled out. In most cases, the symptoms last only a few minutes; however, the athlete should not return to play until a complete evaluation can be performed and the symptoms resolve.

Kuhlman GS, McKeag DB. The "Burner": A common nerve injury in contact sports. *Am Fam Physician*. 1999;60: 2035–2042.

> Burner's syndrome occurs when the contact shoulder is depressed and the head and neck are forced in the opposite direction of contact. The traction-type forces placed on the brachial plexus lead to variable symptoms of weakness, pain, paresthesias, limited motion, and decreased sensation of the affected extremity.

51. Which of the following indicates a therapeutic effect for β-blockers

A) Pupillary constriction
B) Drug level within the acceptable range
C) Heart rate between 60 and 70 bpm
D) Generalized fatigue
E) Peripheral cyanosis

Answer and Discussion

The answer is C. β-Blockers (e.g., propranolol, metoprolol, labetalol, nadolol) are used in the treatment of hypertension. They are considered a negative inotrope and chronotrope. In most cases, they are best suited for young patients who have a hyperdynamic cardiac status. β-Blockers should be used cautiously in patients with the following:

- Asthma and COPD, because nonselective β-blockers can induce bronchoconstriction
- Diabetes, because β-blockers can blunt the response of hypoglycemia
- History of CHF, because β-blockers can decrease cardiac output (however, recent evidence supports cardioselective β-blocker use in CHF with systolic dysfunction)
- Bradycardia or heart block

Other side effects include fatigue, impotence, impaired glucose tolerance, and rebound tachycardia and hypertension (if the drug is abruptly discontinued). β-Blockers are also used for migraine prophylaxis and to treat performance anxiety and tachycardia. Newer evidence supports that β-blockers are not deleterious for patients with depression as once thought. Finally, β-blockers are also used after myocardial infarction to improve survival; they reduce myocardial oxygen demand by decreasing heart rate and contractility. Additionally, they should be given prior to surgery in those at risk for cardiac events. A therapeutic dose is determined by a recorded heart rate of 60 to 70 bpm.

Beers MH, Porter RS, eds. *The Merck manual of diagnosis and therapy*, Merck Research Laboratories, 18th ed. Whitehouse Station, NJ: Merck & Co.; 2006:387.

52. A 54-year-old woman presents to your office with complaints of frequent sweating episodes, palpitations, nervousness, and sensitivity to heat with increased appetite and weight loss. The most likely diagnosis is
A) hypothyroidism
B) menopause
C) Addison's disease
D) hyperthyroidism
E) Cushing's disease

Answer and Discussion

The answer is D. The manifestations of hyperthyroidism are numerous and include the following: goiter; widened pulse pressure; tachycardia; warm, moist skin; tremor; atrial fibrillation; nervousness; frequent diaphoresis; sensitivity to heat; palpitations; exophthalmos; pretibial myxedema; increased appetite with weight loss; diarrhea; and insomnia. The hallmark findings of Graves' disease include the triad of goiter, exophthalmos, and pretibial myxedema. Anemia, present with hypothyroidism, is not seen with hyperthyroidism.

Ferri F. *Ferri's Clinical Advisor, Instant Diagnosis and Treatment.* Philadelphia: Elsevier/Mosby; 2006:432.

53. Which of the following statements about altitude sickness is true?
A) Most people are affected at altitudes between 5,000 and 7,500 ft.
B) Dehydration is rarely an associated condition.
C) The most common symptom is headache.
D) Hydrochlorothiazide is used for prophylaxis.
E) A high carbohydrate diet can help prevent symptoms.

Answer and Discussion

The answer is C. As altitude increases, the partial pressure of oxygen decreases. Approximately 20% of people experience symptoms ascending to more than 8,000 ft in less than 1 day, and 80% show some symptoms at altitudes higher than 12,700 ft. Symptoms include headache (most common), impaired concentration, nausea, vomiting, fatigue, dyspnea and hyperventilation, palpitations, and insomnia. Any type of physical exertion usually aggravates the symptoms, and excessive hyperventilation leads to dehydration. In severe cases, pulmonary and cerebral edema can occur. Treatment involves hydration and usually only symptomatic measures, along with the avoidance of alcohol and a high carbohydrate diet. Prophylaxis with acetazolamide (a carbonic anhydrase inhibitor) helps prevent respiratory alkalosis, which contributes to the symptoms.

Kasper DL, Braunwald E, Fauci AS, et al., eds. *Harrison's principles of internal medicine,* 16th ed. New York: McGraw-Hill; 2005:205, 1617.

54. Anemia that is seen in patients with chronic renal disease is usually caused by insufficient
A) iron stores
B) vitamin B_{12}
C) renin levels
D) erythropoietin levels
E) folate stores

Answer and Discussion

The answer is D. Serum recombinant erythropoietin is used to treat refractory anemia in patients with chronic renal disease. The synthetic drug replaces erythropoietin that is normally produced by the kidneys. Although extremely expensive, the drug may be indicated if the patient has significant anemia that is not caused by other factors. The major side effect is hypertension, which must be monitored at regular intervals. Other side effects include polycythemia, with the possible development of thromboembolism, stroke, and myocardial infarction. The drug does not appear to accelerate the preexisting renal disease. Close monitoring of serum Hb is necessary with the use of erythropoietin. Iron supplementation must be given to achieve an adequate erythropoietin response.

Beers MH, Porter RS, eds. *The Merck manual of diagnosis and therapy,* Merck Research Laboratories, 18th ed. Whitehouse Station, NJ: Merck & Co.; 2006:1031.

55. Which of the following statements is true of Lyme disease?
A) The disease is transmitted by the bite of a common wood tick.
B) The second stage may be characterized by fever, malaise, a stiff neck, back pain, and erythema chronicum migrans.
C) The first stage may involve carditis with atrioventricular (AV) block or pericarditis, peripheral neuropathies, and meningitis.
D) Treatment may be accomplished with tetracycline or doxycycline.
E) It is predominant in the South Central and Western regions of the United States.

Answer and Discussion

The answer is D. Caused by the spirochete *Borrelia burgdorferi,* Lyme disease is transmitted by the bite of the deer tick (*Ixodes dammini*). Although reported in most states, it appears to be predominant in the Great Lakes area and the western and northeastern United States. The symptoms occur in three stages:

1. *First stage.* This stage usually begins with malaise, fever, headache, stiff neck, and back pain. Generalized lymphadenopathy with splenomegaly occurs, and a large annular erythematous lesion forms at the bite site and shows central clearing (erythema chronicum migrans). Multiple lesions may occur and affect other areas of the body. The lesions are warm but not often painful. As many as 25% may not exhibit skin manifestations. These symptoms usually appear within a few days to up to 1 month after the tick bite.
2. *Second stage.* This is the disseminated stage. Complications include carditis with AV block, palpitations, dyspnea, chest pain, and syncope. Pericarditis may also occur. Neurologic manifestations, including peripheral neuropathies and meningitis, are sometimes present. Large-joint arthritis is also common.
3. *Chronic phase.* After the second stage, a chronic phase may result. This phase is predominantly characterized with intermittent attacks of oligoarthritis lasting weeks to months. Other symptoms include subtle neurologic abnormalities (e.g., memory problems, mood or sleep disorders). Diagnosis is usually made by the clinical presentation; however, an enzyme-linked immunosorbent assay followed by Western blot for positive results can help in the diagnosis but is somewhat unreliable.

Treatments for early disease include tetracycline, cefuroxime axetil, doxycycline, and amoxicillin. Azithromycin is less effective than other medications. Ceftriaxone is recommended for late disease. A single dose of doxycycline has been shown to reduce the likelihood of Lyme disease after a deer tick bite. A moderately effective recombinant vaccine for the prevention of Lyme disease has been removed from the market.

Kasper DL, Braunwald E, Fauci AS, et al., eds. *Harrison's principles of internal medicine,* 16th ed. New York: McGraw-Hill; 2005:995.

Beers MH, Porter RS, eds. *The Merck manual of diagnosis and therapy,* Merck Research Laboratories, 18th ed. Whitehouse Station, NJ: Merck & Co.; 2006:1480.

56. Which of the following conditions would disqualify a patient from passing a Department of Transportation (DOT) examination?
A) Diabetic taking insulin
B) Blood pressure reading of 160/90 mm Hg
C) Vision 20/40 in both eyes
D) Use of a hearing aid
E) Field of vision measured at 70 degrees in each eye

Answer and Discussion

The answer is A. Many physicians perform DOT physical examinations. The following are disqualifying conditions: A diabetic patient taking insulin cannot be certified for interstate driving. However, a driver who has diabetes controlled by oral medications and diet may be qualified if the disease is well controlled and the driver is under medical supervision. If diabetes is untreated or uncontrolled, certification should not be given.

From a cardiac standpoint, any condition known to be accompanied by sudden and unexpected syncope, collapse, or congestive heart failure is disqualifying. Conditions such as myocardial infarction, angina, and cardiac dysrhythmias should, in most cases, be evaluated by a cardiologist before certification is issued. Holter monitors and exercise stress tests may be needed when a driver has multiple risk factors. Tachycardia or bradycardia should be investigated to rule out underlying cardiac disease. Asymptomatic dysrhythmia with no underlying disease process should not be disqualifying.

From a pulmonary perspective, if a driver has clear symptoms of significant pulmonary disease, basic spirometry and lung volume tests are recommended. If the forced expiratory volume in 1 second (FEV_1) is <65% of predicted value, the forced vital capacity (FVC) is less <60% of predicted, or the ratio of FEV_1 to FVC is <65%, pulse oximetry should be performed. If pulse oximetry on room air is <92%, an arterial blood gas measurement is recommended. If the partial pressure of arterial oxygen is <65 mm Hg or the partial pressure of arterial carbon dioxide is >45 mm Hg, disqualification is recommended.

With regards to blood pressure: If the blood pressure is 160/90 mm Hg or lower, a full 2-year certification is appropriate. If the blood pressure is >160/90 mm Hg (either systolic or diastolic) but <181/105 mm Hg, temporary certification may be granted for 3 months to allow time for the driver to be evaluated and treated. If the initial pressure is 181/105 mm Hg or higher, the driver should not be certified. Once the driver's blood pressure is under control, certification can be issued for no more than 1 year at a time. Several readings should be taken over several days to rule out "white coat" hypertension. Significant target organ damage and additional risk factors increase the risk of sudden collapse and should be disqualifying.

Vision must be at least 20/40 in each eye with or without correction. Certification can be given once vision has been corrected, but not until. The driver should be advised to have his or her eyes evaluated, obtain corrective lenses, and then return for certification. Field of vision must be at least 70 degrees in each eye. Color vision must allow recognition of standard traffic signals (i.e., red, green, and amber).

The driver should pass a whispered voice test at 5 feet in at least one ear. A hearing aid may be worn for the test. If the test result is questionable, an audiogram is recommended. The better ear must not have an average hearing loss of more than 40 dB at 500, 1,000, and 2,000 Hz (to obtain an average, add the three decibel losses together and divide by 3).

Pommerenke F, Hegmann K, Hartenbaum NP. DOT examinations: practical aspects and regulatory review. *Am Fam Physician.* 1998;58(2):415–426.

57. A 45-year-old female presents to your office with petechiae noted on the lower extremities. A platelet count is obtained and noted to be 10,000. Which of the following conditions would not be associated with her thrombocytopenia?
A) Epistaxis
B) Hemarthrosis
C) Vaginal bleeding
D) Mucosal bleeding in the mouth
E) Ecchymosis at the site of minor trauma

Answer and Discussion

The answer is B. Thrombocytopenia is caused by decreased platelet production, splenic sequestration of platelets, increased platelet destruction or use, or dilution of platelets. Severe thrombocytopenia results in a characteristic pattern of bleeding: multiple petechiae in the skin, often most evident on the lower legs; scattered small ecchymoses at sites of minor trauma; mucosal bleeding [epistaxis, bleeding in the GI and genitourinary (GU) tracts, vaginal bleeding]; and excessive bleeding following surgical procedures. Heavy GI bleeding and bleeding into the central nervous system (CNS) may be life threatening. Thrombocytopenia does not cause massive bleeding into tissues (e.g., deep visceral hematomas, hemarthroses), which is characteristic of bleeding secondary to coagulation disorders such as hemophilia. Medications associated with thrombocytopenia include: heparin (up to 5%, even with very low doses), quinidine, quinine, sulfa preparations, oral antidiabetic drugs, gold salts, and rifampin.

Beers MH, Porter RS, eds. *The Merck manual of diagnosis and therapy,* Merck Research Laboratories, 18th ed. Whitehouse Station, NJ: Merck & Co.; 2006:1064–1072.

58. Iron deficiency anemia is associated with
A) hyperchromic, macrocytic features
B) elevated serum iron levels
C) increased total iron-binding capacity (TIBC)
D) increased ferritin levels
E) normal bone marrow biopsy results

Answer and Discussion

The answer is C. Iron deficiency anemia produces a hypochromic, microcytic anemia. Causes include excessive menstruation, GI blood loss, inadequate iron consumption, malabsorption, pregnancy, or excessive growth in the absence of adequate iron consumption during infancy. Symptoms may include generalized weakness and fatigue, facial pallor, glossitis, cheilosis, and angular stomatitis. In chronic, severe cases patients may have pica (e.g., craving for dirt, paint), pagophagia (craving for ice), or dysphagia associated with a postcricoid esophageal web. Physical examination may show skin pallor, dry brittle nails, and tachycardia with perhaps a flow murmur. Laboratory tests show a depressed Hb with microcytic, hypochromic features; low serum iron concentration; low ferritin; and increased transferrin (TIBC). Bone marrow aspiration shows diminished iron stores with small, pale red blood cells. Only when the hematocrit falls below 31% to 32% do the red blood cell (RBC) indices become microcytic. Treatment is the administration of iron replacement for 6 to 12 months until iron stores are replenished. The addition of ascorbic acid enhances iron absorption without increasing gastric distress.

Goldman L, Ausiello D, eds. *Cecil textbook of medicine,* 22nd ed. Philadelphia: WB Saunders; 2004:1003–1006.

59. Which of the following is not indicated in the emergent treatment of thyroid storm?

A) Propylthiouracil
B) Supersaturated potassium iodine
C) Propranolol
D) Aspirin
E) Acetaminophen

Answer and Discussion

The answer is D. Thyroid storm is a life-threatening condition seen in patients with hyperthyroidism. The condition is usually precipitated by stress, illness, or manipulation of the thyroid during surgery. Signs and symptoms include diaphoresis, tachycardia, palpitations, weight loss, diarrhea, fever, mental status changes, weakness, and shock. Treatment should be provided immediately and includes propylthiouracil, supersaturated potassium iodine, and propranolol. Other measures involve fluid replacement and control of fever with acetaminophen and cooling blankets. Avoid aspirin, because it may increase T3 and T4 by reducing protein binding. Steroids may also be given to help prevent the conversion of T3 and T4 peripherally. The definitive therapy after control of the thyroid storm involves ablation of the thyroid gland with iodine-131 or surgery. After treatment, many patients become hypothyroid and may require replacement therapy.

Goldman L, Ausiello D, eds. *Cecil textbook of medicine,* 22nd ed. Philadelphia: WB Saunders; 2004:1401.

60. Which of the following ECG findings is associated with sudden cardiac death?

A) Prolonged QT interval
B) First-degree AV block
C) Sinus arrhythmia
D) Right bundle branch block
E) Premature ventricular contractions

Answer and Discussion

The answer is A. A prolonged QT interval is a common entity associated with sudden arrhythmia death syndrome. Arrhythmias may be induced in normal hearts by medications; electrolyte abnormalities (e.g., hypokalemia, hypomagnesemia); myocarditis; and endocrine, central nervous system, or nutritional disorders. These arrhythmias are associated with prolongation of the QT interval. A group of inherited gene mutations has been identified associated with cardiac ion channels that cause long QT syndrome and carry an increased risk for sudden death. Some of the highest rates of inherited long QT syndrome occur in Southeast Asian and Pacific Rim countries. The average age of persons who die of long QT syndrome is 32 years; men are more commonly affected. In addition to a prolonged QT interval, which occurs in some but not all persons with long QT syndrome, another characteristic electrocardiographic abnormality is the so-called Brugada sign (an upward deflection of the terminal portion of the QRS complex). Most cardiac events are precipitated by vigorous exercise or emotional stress, but they also can occur during sleep. Torsades de pointes and ventricular fibrillation are the usual fatal arrhythmias. Long QT syndrome should be suspected in patients with recurrent syncope during exertion and those with family histories of sudden, unexpected death. Not all persons with long QT syndrome have warning symptoms or identifiable electrocardiographic abnormalities, and they may present with sudden death. β-Blockers, potassium supplements, and implantable defibrillators have been used for treatment of long QT syndrome. Identifying the specific gene mutation in a given patient with long QT syndrome can help guide prophylactic therapy.

Meyer JS, Mehdirad A, Salem BI, et al. Sudden arrhythmia death syndrome: importance of the long QT syndrome. *Am Fam Physician.* 2003;68:483–488.

> Long QT syndrome should be suspected in patients with recurrent syncope during exertion and those with family histories of sudden, unexpected death.

61. A *felon* is defined as a

A) infection of the distal pulp space of a phalanx
B) herpetic infection associated with a phalanx
C) fracture involving the proximal fifth metatarsal
D) superficial infection of the nail bed
E) hypertrophic changes noted in gout

Answer and Discussion

The answer is A. A felon is an infection of the pulp space of a phalanx. A felon usually is caused by inoculation of bacteria into the fingertip through a penetrating trauma. The most commonly affected digits are the thumb and index finger. Predisposing causes include splinters, bits of glass, abrasions, and minor trauma. A felon also may arise when an untreated paronychia spreads into the pad of the fingertip. The most common site is the distal pulp, which may be involved centrally, laterally, and apically. The septa between pulp spaces ordinarily limit the spread of infection, resulting in an abscess, which creates pressure and necrosis of adjacent tissues. The underlying bone, joint, or flexor tendons may become infected, and intense throbbing pain and a swollen pulp are present. If diagnosed in the early stages of cellulitis, a felon may be treated with elevation, oral antibiotics, and warm water or saline soaks. Radiographs should be obtained to evaluate for osteomyelitis or a foreign body. Tetanus prophylaxis should be administered when necessary. If fluctuance is present, incision and drainage are appropriate along with administration of appropriate antibiotics (usually a cephalosporin or anti-staphylococcal penicillin).

Clark DC. Common acute hand infections. *Am Fam Physician.* 2003;68:2167–2176.

62. Which of the following statements about hyperglycemic hyperosmolar nonketotic coma is true?
A) It is usually associated with type I adult-onset diabetes mellitus.
B) It is associated with fluid overload.
C) Associated laboratory findings include elevated serum lactate.
D) Treatment involves intravenous administration of glucose.
E) Treatment involves fluid administration.

Answer and Discussion

The answer is E. Hyperosmolar nonketotic coma secondary to hyperglycemia usually occurs in patients with type II adult-onset diabetes mellitus. The condition occurs when serum glucose is elevated, leading to osmotic diuresis and the development of dehydration without ketosis. In most cases, the condition affects elderly, mildly obese patients who fail to keep adequate fluid intake to make up for the osmotic diuresis. Complications include mental status changes with the development of coma, acute renal failure, thrombosis, shock, and lactic acidosis. Diagnosis depends on the detection of plasma glucose >600 mg/dL, serum lactate >5 mmol, and a serum osmolality >320 mOsmol/kg. Sodium and potassium levels are usually normal; however, BUN and creatinine are markedly elevated. Treatment consists of fluid replacement (usually approximately 10 L) with potassium supplementation and the cautious administration of insulin. Triggering conditions such as infection, myocardial infarction, or stroke should be ruled out. Unfortunately, the mortality rate for hyperglycemic hyperosmolar nonketotic coma approaches 50% if not treated immediately.

Goldman L, Ausiello D, eds. *Cecil textbook of medicine,* 22nd ed. Philadelphia: WB Saunders; 2004:1442.

63. Which of the following statements about giardiasis is true?
A) Transmission occurs through fecal–oral contamination.
B) Chlorination of drinking water kills the cyst.
C) Diagnosis can be achieved by peripheral blood smears.
D) The cyst form is responsible for symptoms.
E) Asymptomatic carriers do not require treatment.

Answer and Discussion

The answer is A. *Giardia lamblia* is the causative agent in parasitic giardiasis. Most cases are asymptomatic. However, these patients pass infective cysts and must be treated. Symptoms occur 1 to 3 weeks after infection and include foul-smelling watery diarrhea, flatulence, abdominal cramps and distention, and anorexia. Outbreaks in day schools, nursing homes, and institutions for the mentally retarded are common. Transmission is through a fecal–oral route. The infective form is the cyst, and trophozoites are responsible for the symptoms. Cysts are transmitted in contaminated food or water. *Giardia* cysts are resistant to chlorination; therefore, filtration is used to clear cysts from drinking water supplies. *Giardia* is sensitive to heat, thus bringing water to a boil is effective before consumption. Diagnosis is accomplished by detecting cysts or the parasite in the stool (usually three samples) or in duodenal contents (by using endoscopy, the swallowed-string test, or Enterotest). Treatment includes metronidazole and furazolidone. The medication is available in suspension, making it useful for children. Close contacts should also be tested, especially when recurrent infections are found. Although *Giardia* is most commonly associated with beavers, there is evidence of sporadic transmission between infected dogs and people.

Goldman L, Ausiello D, eds. *Cecil textbook of medicine,* 22nd ed. Philadelphia: WB Saunders; 2004:2095–2096.

64. A 32-year-old sportsman who recently attended a wild-game feed banquet consumed summer sausage made from bear meat. He complains of abdominal discomfort, diarrhea, and muscle tenderness. The most likely diagnosis is
A) trichinosis
B) salmonellosis
C) giardiasis
D) ascariasis
E) shigellosis

Answer and Discussion

The answer is A. Trichinosis is a parasitic infection caused by the roundworm *Trichinella spiralis*. The condition results from eating inadequately prepared or raw pork, bear, or walrus meat that contains the encysted larva. Many cases are linked to the consumption of contaminated summer sausage. Many patients are asymptomatic; however, some may exhibit diarrhea, abdominal discomfort, and a low-grade fever. Ocular symptoms may also occur with edema of the eyelids, photophobia, and retinal or subconjunctival hemorrhages. Muscle soreness and urticaria may also be associated with the parasitic infection. Laboratory studies show an increasing eosinophilia with a leukocytosis. Diagnosis can be made by muscle biopsy showing the larva or cysts, serologic tests, or enzyme-linked immunosorbent assay (ELISA) tests. Treatment is accomplished with thiabendazole with variable response. For severe cases, corticosteroids may be indicated. Complications include myocarditis, meningitis, and pneumonitis. The prognosis is usually good. Most cases can be avoided by thoroughly cooking pork before consumption.

Goldman L, Ausiello D, eds. *Cecil textbook of medicine,* 22nd ed. Philadelphia: WB Saunders; 2004:2116.

65. A 24-year-old long-distance runner has been training for a track meet. He reports localized pain, especially at night, and mild swelling over his proximal left tibia that has not responded to anti-inflammatory agents or ice therapy. Radiographs of the area are normal. The most likely diagnosis is
A) stress fracture
B) shin splints
C) osteoid osteoma
D) gastrocnemius tear
E) iliotibial band (ITB) syndrome

Answer and Discussion

The answer is A. Stress fractures usually involve the tibia (commonly in the proximal two-thirds of the bone) and fibula (usually 5 to 7 cm above the lateral malleolus) after prolonged and repeated use. Stress fractures account for up to 10% of all sports injuries. Long-distance runners or athletes who are inadequately conditioned are frequently affected. Symptoms include pain over the lower leg in the affected area; the pain usually improves with rest but recurs with repeated activity. Localized erythema and swelling may occur over the fracture site. Night pain is a common feature, which should alert the clinician to the possibility of a stress fracture. Radiographs are normal in many cases; however, technetium bone scans can be used to demonstrate the fracture. Bone scans are the most cost-effective means to diagnose stress fractures. The MRI is also very sensitive but is more expensive. Treatment of stress fractures includes rest from exercise or competition for 6 to 8 weeks. Those who experience pain with ambulation or cannot adhere to limited activity for 6 to 8 weeks should be in a walking cast for 4 to 6 weeks. When patients resume their activity, they should begin slowly and gradually work back to their normal routines. If pain should recur, nonunion of the fracture should be suspected and the athlete should be referred to an orthopedist. The athlete may return to competition after 14 days without pain and no pain with gradual return to activity.

Johnson R. *Sports Medicine in Primary Care*. Philadelphia: WB Saunders Company; 2000:174–181.

66. Which of the following statements about familial periodic paralysis is true?
A) It is an autosomal-recessive transmitted disorder.
B) It involves disturbances of potassium regulation.
C) It is associated with permanent muscle weakness.
D) It is aggravated by administration of acetazolamide.
E) It most commonly affects the elderly.

Answer and Discussion

The answer is B. Familial periodic paralysis is an autosomal-dominant transmitted disorder that is characterized by episodes of paralysis, loss of deep tendon reflexes, and failure of the muscles to respond to electrical stimulation. Onset is usually early in life; episodic weakness beginning after age 25 years is almost never due to periodic paralysis. There is no alteration in mental status—patients remain alert during attacks. Muscle strength is normal between attacks. There are two basic types:

1. *Hypokalemic*. Attacks usually begin in adolescence. Symptoms occur the day after vigorous exercise. The symptoms are usually mild and may affect particular muscle groups (proximal muscles) or involve all extremities at once. Oropharyngeal and respiratory muscles are unaffected. The weakness usually lasts 24 to 48 hours. Meals high in carbohydrates and sodium may precipitate the attacks.
2. *Hyperkalemic*. Attacks usually occur earlier in childhood. They are shorter in duration, more frequent, and less severe. Attacks are usually associated with myotonia. Most patients are actually normokalemic during the attacks; however, the administration of potassium can precipitate the attack—thus the name.

Diagnosis is made by the history, and serum potassium levels should be drawn during the attacks to determine the specific type of paralysis. Provocative testing with glucose and insulin can be used (in hypokalemic forms) with caution in those who have infrequent attacks. The treatment of choice for both types is acetazolamide. Potassium chloride may help abort hypokalemic attacks; calcium gluconate and furosemide may help abort hyperkalemic attacks.

Beers MH, Porter RS, eds. *The Merck manual of diagnosis and therapy*, Merck Research Laboratories, 18th ed. Whitehouse Station, NJ: Merck & Co.; 2006:1245, 1248.

67. Crohn's disease is associated with which of the following?
A) Inflammation limited to the superficial layer of the bowel wall
B) The affinity to involve the rectosigmoid junction
C) Decreased risk of colon cancer
D) Continuous mucosal areas of ulceration that affect the anus
E) Fistula formation

Answer and Discussion

The answer is E. Crohn's disease is characterized by a transmural inflammation of the GI tract. It may affect any part of the GI tract but is usually associated with the terminal ileum, the colon, or both. On colonoscopy, areas of ulceration and submucosal thickening give the bowel a cobblestone appearance, with some skipped areas of normal bowel. In addition to the transmural inflammation, there are granulomas, abscesses, fissures, and fistula formation. Symptoms include fever, weight loss, abdominal pain (usually the right-lower quadrant), diarrhea (rarely with associated blood), and growth retardation in children. In children, Crohn's disease is more common than ulcerative colitis. Complications include intestinal obstruction; toxic megacolon, which is usually more common in ulcerative colitis; malabsorption, particularly associated with fat-soluble vitamins and especially vitamin B_{12}; intestinal perforation; fistula formation; and development of gall and kidney stones. There is also an increased risk—five times the average—for bowel cancer. Other areas may be affected, including the following:

- Joints: arthritis, ankylosing spondylitis
- Skin: erythema nodosum, aphthous ulcers, pyoderma gangrenosum
- Eyes: episcleritis, iritis, uveitis
- Liver: fatty liver, pericholangitis

The diagnosis is usually made with colonoscopy or flexible sigmoidoscopy with biopsy or with x-ray contrast studies (usually avoided in acute stages because of the risk of developing toxic megacolon with barium). Treatment involves the use of oral corticosteroids or steroid enemas, ciprofloxacin, metronidazole, antidiarrheal agents, and sulfasalazine (Azulfidine), olsalazine (Dipentum), or mesalamine (Asacol, Pentasa, Rowasa), all three of which contain 5-aminosalicylic acid. Infliximab (Remicade) is a new drug that has been approved for the treatment of Crohn's disease. The drug is a potent antibody to tumor necrosis factor that is elevated in patients with Crohn's disease and can help close fistulas in up to 60% of patients. In severe cases, total parenteral nutrition may be necessary with surgery to remove the ulcerated bowel.

Knutson D, Greenberg G, Cronau H. Management of Crohn's disease. *Am Fam Physician*. 2003;68:707–714, 717–718.

Goldman L, Ausiello D, eds. *Cecil textbook of medicine,* 22nd ed. Philadelphia: WB Saunders; 2004:861–867.

68. A 68-year-old patient is seen for a general examination. Current recommendations for immunizations include
A) tetanus booster every 5 years
B) influenza vaccination yearly
C) pneumococcal vaccination yearly
D) hepatitis booster every 5 years
E) meningococcal vaccination

Answer and Discussion

The answer is B. Adult immunizations should include tetanus immunization every 10 years and influenza vaccination yearly beginning at age 50. Pneumococcal immunization should be given at age 65 years. Those at high risk receiving pneumococcal vaccination before age 65 years and after 5 years may require boosters. Vaccination can be started earlier in patients at high risk for disease (e.g., patients who are immunocompromised, those with chronic lung disease or diabetes). Patients who do not have functional spleens should receive pneumococcal, meningococcal, and influenza immunization.

Centers for Disease Control and Prevention website. Summary of adolescent/adult immunization recommendations. Available at: http://www.cdc.gov/nip/recs/adult-schedule.pdf. Accessed 6/5/06.

69. A 10-year-old female is brought in by her mother. The child was bitten on the finger by the neighbor's cat 1 hour ago. There are small puncture bites with minimal inflammation at the site. She is allergic to penicillin. Appropriate management at this time includes

A) observation only
B) topical antibiotic ointment
C) oral doxycycline (Vibramycin)
D) IV ceftriaxone (Rocephin)
E) oral amoxicillin–clavulanate (Augmentin)

Answer and Discussion

The answer is C. The oral flora of humans and animals contains a mixture of potential pathogens: *Eikenella corrodens* is frequently isolated from human bites, and *Pasteurella multocida* from many animal bites, particularly those of cats. Amoxicillin–clavulanate potassium (Augmentin) is the antibiotic of choice for both dog and cat bites when infection is present. For patients who are allergic to penicillin, doxycycline (Vibramycin) is an acceptable alternative, except for children younger than 8 years and pregnant women. Erythromycin can also be used, but the risk of treatment failure is greater because of antimicrobial resistance. Other acceptable combinations include clindamycin (Cleocin) and a fluoroquinolone in adults or clindamycin and trimethoprim–sulfamethoxazole (Bactrim, Septra) in children. When compliance is a concern, daily intramuscular injections of ceftriaxone (Rocephin) are appropriate. All bite injuries are potentially dangerous and can cause significant infection. They should be debrided surgically, with the wounds left open. Currently there is insufficient evidence to support antibiotic prophylaxis in dog and cat bites, and minimal evidence supports its use for human bites. However, there is evidence that antibiotics reduce the risk of infection in hand bites.

Turner TW. Do mammalian bites require antibiotic prophylaxis? *Ann Emerg Med.* 2004;44:274–246.

Beers MH, Porter RS, eds. *The Merck manual of diagnosis and therapy,* Merck Research Laboratories, 18th ed. Whitehouse Station, NJ: Merck & Co.; 2006:2638–2639.

70. The treatment of choice for leishmaniasis is

A) mebendazole
B) quinine
C) doxycycline
D) ciprofloxacin
E) antimonial compound

Answer and Discussion

The answer is E. The condition *leishmaniasis* refers to various clinical syndromes caused by a protozoa species. Leishmaniasis is endemic in many of the tropics, the subtropics, and southern Europe. It is typically a vector-borne disease, with rodents and canids as common reservoir hosts and humans as incidental hosts. In humans, visceral, cutaneous, and mucosal leishmaniasis results from infection of macrophages throughout the reticuloendothelial system, in the skin, and in the nasal and oropharyngeal mucosa. *Leishmania* parasites are transmitted by the bite of female sandflies. The transmission of *Leishmania* species typically is localized because of the limited area that sandflies inhabit. Typically these insects remain within a few hundred yards of their breeding ground. They are found in dark, moist places in areas ranging from deserts to rain forests. Many reside in debris or rubble near structures. The primary lesion at the site of an infected sandfly bite is small and usually not noticed. Parasites travel from the skin through the bloodstream to the lymph nodes, spleen, liver, and bone marrow. Clinical signs develop gradually after 2 weeks up to 1 year later. The typical syndrome consists of fevers, hepatosplenomegaly, pancytopenia, and polyclonal hypergammaglobulinemia with reversed albumin/globulin ratio. In up to 10% of patients, twice-daily temperature spikes occur. Death can occur within 1 to 2 years in a majority of untreated symptomatic patients. A subclinical form with vague minor symptoms resolves spontaneously in a majority of patients and can progress to full-blown visceral leishmaniasis in one-third of cases. Those infected are resistant to further attacks unless they are immunocompromised. One to 2 years after apparent cure, some patients develop nodular cutaneous lesions full of parasites, which can last for years and is often treated as folliculitis. Treatment consists of a regimen of antimonial compounds. Toxicity including myalgia, arthralgia, fatigue, elevated liver function tests, pancreatitis, and electrocardiographic abnormalities are more common as the length of treatment progresses but usually does not limit treatment and is reversible. Alternatives include amphotericin B and pentamidine. Many other agents have been recommended as alternatives or adjuncts to antimonial compounds often on the basis of suboptimal data.

Kasper DL, Braunwald E, Fauci AS, et al., eds. *Harrison's principles of internal medicine,* 16th ed. New York: McGraw-Hill; 2005:1233, 1236–1237.

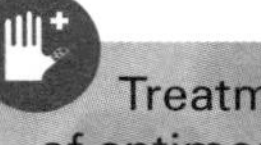

Treatment of leishmaniasis consists of a regimen of antimonial compounds.

71. Which of the following statements is true regarding glaucoma?

A) Intraocular pressure is diagnostic for glaucoma.
B) Glaucoma suspects have normal intraocular pressure.
C) Measurement of intraocular pressures by primary care physicians to screen for glaucoma is not recommended.
D) Prostaglandin eye drops are contraindicated in the treatment of glaucoma.
E) Laser treatment is the treatment of choice once glaucoma is identified.

Answer and Discussion

The answer is C. Glaucoma is the second most common cause of legal blindness in the United States. Open-angle glaucoma is a condition that involves progressive optic neuropathy characterized by enlarging optic disc cupping and visual field loss. Most patients are asymptomatic. Patients at increased risk for open-angle glaucoma include African Americans over 40 years of age, Whites older than 65 years, a personal history of diabetes or severe myopia, and persons with a family history of glaucoma. Elevated intraocular pressure is a risk factor for open-angle glaucoma, but it is not diagnostic. Some patients with glaucoma have normal intraocular pressure (i.e., normal-pressure glaucoma), and many patients with elevated intraocular pressure do not have glaucoma (i.e., glaucoma suspects). Screening patients for glaucoma by the primary physician is not recommended. Formal visual field testing (perimetry) by vision care is the mainstay of glaucoma diagnosis and management. Nonspecific β-blocker or prostaglandin analog eye drops generally are the first-line treatment to reduce intraocular pressure. Laser treatment and surgery usually are reserved for patients in whom medical treatment has failed. Without treatment, open-angle glaucoma can result in irreversible vision loss.

Distelhorst JS, Hughes GM. Open-angle glaucoma. *Am Fam Physician.* 2003;67:1937–1944, 1950.

72. Which of the following statements about acetaminophen overdose is correct?
A) Symptoms include extremity pain with physical findings of peripheral neuropathy.
B) Toxic effects rarely occur with ingestion of greater than 140 to 150 mg/kg of acetaminophen.
C) Elevations in liver tests peak 3 to 4 hours after ingestion.
D) Blood levels obtained 4 hours after ingestion determine treatment.
E) Treatment involves the use of deferoxamine.

Answer and Discussion

The answer is D. Acetaminophen overdose is not uncommon. Most cases involve children younger than 6 years. Toxic effects occur when the doses exceed 140 to 150 mg/kg or a total dose of 7.5 g. The drug primarily affects the liver 24 to 72 hours after ingestion by depleting glutathione stores and causing hepatocellular necrosis. Symptoms include nausea, vomiting, and right-upper quadrant abdominal pain. Acetaminophen levels should be checked 4 hours after ingestion and plotted on the Rumack–Matthew nomogram. Peak aspartate aminotransferase, alanine aminotransferase (ALT), bilirubin, and prothrombin time (PT) values are seen 3 to 4 days after ingestion. Treatment, including emesis induced by syrup of ipecac, gastric lavage, and administration of activated charcoal, should be initiated as soon as possible. A 4-hour acetaminophen level greater than 150 μg/mL requires administration of the antidote acetylcysteine (Mucomyst). For maximal therapeutic effect, *N*-acetylcysteine should be administered within 8 hours of acetaminophen ingestion.

Linden CH, Rumack BH. Acetaminophen overdose. *Emerg Med Clin North Am.* 1984;2:103–115.

Goldman L, Ausiello D, eds. *Cecil textbook of medicine,* 22nd ed. Philadelphia: Saunders; 2004:908–909.

73. Which of the following statements about chronic fatigue syndrome is true?
A) Antibiotics may be beneficial.
B) Antidepressants may be beneficial.
C) The disease is most likely linked to the Epstein–Barr virus (EBV).
D) Symptoms rarely improve.
E) Bed rest is usually beneficial.

Answer and Discussion

The answer is B. Chronic fatigue syndrome is a poorly understood constellation of symptoms that includes generalized fatigue, sore throat, tender lymphadenopathy, headaches, and generalized myalgias. The disease does not appear to be associated with chronic infections of EBV or Lyme disease. It does appear to be associated with underlying psychiatric disorders, such as somatization disorder, depression, and anxiety. Chronic fatigue syndrome has no pathognomonic features and remains a constellation of symptoms and a diagnosis of exclusion. Patients with this constellation of symptoms should receive supportive therapy and be encouraged to gradually increase their exercise program within their limits and participate in their usual activities. Alternative medicines and vitamins are popular with many chronic fatigue syndrome patients but generally are not very helpful. The use of antibiotics or antiviral agents is contraindicated. In some cases, patients may respond to antidepressant medications. Given enough time, most patients improve.

Ferri F. *Ferri's Clinical Advisor, Instant Diagnosis and Treatment.* Philadelphia: Elsevier/Mosby; 2006:57.

74. Chronic gingivitis as a result of chronic plaque buildup can initially lead to
A) periodontitis
B) dental caries
C) glossitis
D) oropharyngeal cancer
E) oropharyngeal candidiasis

Answer and Discussion

The answer is A. Periodontitis is the most common cause of tooth loss. It occurs when chronic gingivitis (a result of bacterial plaque buildup) leads to loss of supporting bone around the tooth root. Symptoms include deepening of the gingival pockets between the teeth with the accumulation of calculus deposits. The gums soon lose their attachment to the tooth, and bone loss occurs. Bacteria accumulate in the gingival pockets and can lead to progression of the disease. Later in the course of the disease, the gums recede and eventually tooth loss occurs. Treatment involves dental referral and, in severe cases, surgery. Regular dental visits twice yearly and proper brushing and flossing techniques help prevent plaque buildup.

Douglass AB, Douglass JM. Common dental emergencies. *Am Fam Physician.* 2003;67:511–516.

75. Which of the following medications is contraindicated in pregnancy?
A) Lisinopril
B) Penicillin
C) Acetominophen
D) Alpha methyldopa

Answer and Discussion

The answer is A. Women of childbearing age should be warned to notify their physicians as soon as possible if they become pregnant during ACE-inhibitor therapy. ACE inhibitors are not considered teratogenic if they are discontinued during the first trimester (class C), but they are considered teratogenic in the second and third trimesters (class D).

Bicket DB. Using ACE inhibitors appropriately. *Am Fam Physician.* 2002;66:461–468, 473.

76. A 48-year-old woman presents to your office complaining of blurred vision and pain associated with the right eye. The patient also reports seeing halos around light sources as well as nausea, abdominal pain, and vomiting. Physical examination shows

her right eye is red and the pupil is dilated. The most likely diagnosis is
A) angle-closure glaucoma
B) Graves' disease
C) digoxin toxicity
D) hyphema
E) atropine poisoning

Answer and Discussion

The answer is A. Glaucoma is classified into two types: open-angle and angle-closure.

- *Open-angle type* (90% of cases) results when the rate of aqueous fluid outflow is decreased and the ocular pressure is consistently increased, giving rise to optic atrophy with loss of vision. The disease usually is bilateral, affects African Americans more commonly than Whites, and appears to have genetic predisposition. Examination may show optic disc cupping and an increase in intraocular pressure (normal: 10 to 21 mm Hg). The diagnosis should not be based on one reading. Treatment involves the use of intraocular β-blockers, such as timolol and pilocarpine. Surgical therapy may be necessary for patients whose conditions do not respond appropriately to medical treatment.
- *Angle-closure glaucoma* is less common, often more acute in onset, and is associated with a narrow anterior chamber and pupillary dilation that obstructs the normal flow of aqueous fluid. The condition constitutes an ophthalmologic emergency and is associated with stress, dark rooms, and pupillary dilation by medication used to perform eye examinations. Most patients experience pain and blurred vision with halos around lights. They may also present with abdominal pain and vomiting. Physical examination shows an eye that is red with the pupil dilated and unresponsive to light. Untreated, the condition can lead to blindness in 2 to 5 days. Treatment involves medication (miotics and carbonic anhydrase inhibitors) and laser peripheral iridectomy.

Patients older than 65 years should be screened for glaucoma every 1 to 2 years, or every year if there is a strong family history for glaucoma. African-American individuals should be screened at an earlier age (40 years). The report of the United States Preventative Services Task Force does not recommend the routine performance of tonometry by primary care physicians. Instead, primary care physicians are encouraged to refer to an eye specialist for screening.

Goldman L, Ausiello D, eds. *Cecil textbook of medicine,* 22nd ed. Philadelphia: WB Saunders; 2004:2414.

77. The ligament most commonly injured with an ankle sprain is the
A) anterior talofibular ligament
B) fibulocalcaneal ligament
C) posterior talofibular ligament
D) deltoid ligament

Answer and Discussion

The answer is A. Ankle sprains are graded according to the following criteria:

- *Grade 1:* Mild sprain with no evidence of ligamentous tear; associated with mild pain and swelling
- *Grade 2:* Moderate sprain with evidence of partial tear of ligaments; associated with moderate swelling, ecchymosis, and difficulty ambulating
- *Grade 3:* Severe sprain with evidence of a complete tear of the ligament; associated with significant swelling, ecchymosis, ankle instability, and the inability to walk

The ligaments involved include the anterior talofibular (which is the most commonly affected), the fibulocalcaneal, and the posterior talofibular ligament. A positive drawer sign (movement of the talus forward) indicates rupture of the anterior talofibular ligament. Treatment for grades 1 and 2 sprains involves rest, ice, compression, elevation (RICE), use of air casts and splints, and NSAIDs followed by early mobilization and physical therapy, which emphasizes strengthening and proprioceptive training. Grade 3 sprains require surgical referral. High-ankle sprains involve injury to the syndesmosis, the thick ligament between the distal tibia and fibula. Recovery time is increased with these injuries.

Snider RK, ed. *Essentials of musculoskeletal care.* Rosemont, IL: American Academy of Orthopedic Surgeons; 1997:390–393.

78. Of the following, the medication of choice for refractive hiccups is
A) chlorpromazine
B) acetazolamide
C) gabapentin
D) chloral hydrate
E) clonidine

Answer and Discussion

The answer is A. Hiccups are sudden, repeated, involuntary contractions of the diaphragm followed by abrupt closure of the glottis. They result from stimulation of the efferent and afferent nerves that innervate the diaphragm. Causes include excitement, alcohol consumption, and gastric distention caused by overeating. Low CO_2 levels tend to accentuate hiccups, and high levels tend to prevent them. Advocated symptomatic treatment includes breathing into a paper bag, rapidly drinking a glass of water, swallowing dry bread, holding one's breath, or consuming crushed ice. In addition, gastric decompression may provide relief. For refractive hiccups, chlorpromazine may be given orally or intravenously. Other medications include phenobarbital, scopolamine, chlorpromazine, metoclopramide, and narcotics. In severe cases, surgery to disrupt the phrenic nerve or to inject the phrenic nerve with a procaine solution may be performed.

Beers MH, Porter RS, eds. *The Merck manual of diagnosis and therapy,* Merck Research Laboratories, 18th ed. Whitehouse Station, NJ: Merck & Co.; 2006:70.

79. Which of the following organisms is responsible for the development of pseudomembranous colitis?
A) *Escherichia coli*
B) *Clostridium difficile*
C) *Pseudomonas aeruginosa*
D) Methicillin-resistant *Staphylococcus aureus*
E) *Enterococcus faecalis*

Answer and Discussion

The answer is B. Pseudomembranous colitis is characterized by profuse, watery diarrhea; abdominal cramps; low-grade fevers; and, occasionally, hematochezia. The etiologic agent is *C. difficile,* which produces a toxin that causes the lesions affecting the colon. The condition is thought to be associated with antibiotic use in the preceding 2 to 3 weeks (in some cases up to 6 weeks);

however, antibiotic use is not necessary for the condition to occur. The diagnosis may be achieved by a laboratory stool test, which isolates the *C. difficile* toxin. Sigmoidoscopy or colonoscopy usually shows characteristic yellowish-white plaques. Treatment includes the use of metronidazole or vancomycin (which is more expensive). Complications include dehydration, electrolyte imbalances, intestinal perforation, toxic megacolon, and, in severe cases, death. Relapse may occur in up to one-third of patients after treatment.

Goldman L, Ausiello D, eds. *Cecil textbook of medicine,* 22nd ed. Philadelphia: WB Saunders; 2004:1836–1838.

80. Dermatomyositis is associated with which of the following?
A) Generalized morbilliform rash
B) Underlying malignancy
C) Elevated lipids
D) Distal muscle weakness
E) Inflammatory bowel disease

Answer and Discussion

The answer is B. Dermatomyositis is a systemic connective tissue disease that involves inflammation and degeneration of the muscles. Females are affected more than males at a 2:1 ratio. Although the disease may occur at any age, it occurs most commonly in adults 40 to 60 years of age and in children 5 to 15 years of age. The cause is unknown. In adult cases (15% of men older than 50 and a smaller proportion affecting women), there is an underlying malignant tumor, which may give rise to an autoimmune reaction and lead to an attack of tumor antigens with similar muscle antigens. Symptoms include symmetric proximal muscle weakness, muscular pain, violaceous, flat-topped papules over the dorsal interphalangeal joints (Gottron's papules), purple-red discoloration of the upper eyelids (heliotropic rash), polyarthralgia, dysphagia, Raynaud's phenomenon, fever, and weight loss. Interstitial pneumonitis with dyspnea and cough may occur and precedes the development of myositis. Cardiac involvement may be detected when ECG tracings show arrhythmias or conduction disturbances. Laboratory findings include increased erythrocyte sedimentation rate (ESR), positive antinuclear antibodies and/or lupus erythematosus (LE) preparation test, and elevated creatinine kinase (most sensitive and useful marker) and aldolase. Diagnosis is confirmed by electromyography and muscle biopsy. Initial treatment consists of steroids. Patients who fail to respond can be given immunosuppressive agents such as methotrexate, cyclophosphamide, and chlorambucil. After the diagnosis of dermatomyositis is made, an effort should be made to uncover an occult malignancy. Dermatomyositis associated with malignancy often remits once the tumor is removed.

Kasper DL, Braunwald E, Fauci AS, et al., eds. *Harrison's principles of internal medicine,* 16th ed. New York: McGraw-Hill; 2005:2540.

After the diagnosis of dermatomyositis is made, an effort should be made to uncover an occult malignancy.

81. Of the following medications, which is most effective in relieving premenstrual dysphoric disorder?
A) Spironolactone
B) Bromocriptine
C) Amitryptyline
D) Fluoxetine
E) Oral contraceptives

Answer and Discussion

The answer is D. Treatment of premenstrual syndrome involves multiple treatment options. Fluid retention may be treated by reducing sodium intake and using a thiazide diuretic starting just before symptoms are expected. Counseling may help the woman and her partner cope with PMS, and the woman's activities can be modified to reduce stress. Hormonal manipulation is effective in some cases. Medications include oral contraceptives; progesterone by vaginal suppository or by injection for 10 to 12 days premenstrually; a long-acting progestin; or a gonadotropin-releasing hormone agonist with low-dose estrogen-progestin "add-back" therapy to eliminate cyclic changes. Benzodiazepines may be used for anxiety, irritability, nervousness, and lack of control, especially if patients cannot alter their stressful environments. Spironolactone, bromocriptine, and monoamine oxidase inhibitors are not beneficial. Selective serotonin reuptake inhibitors (e.g., fluoxetine or sertraline 50 mg) are the most effective drugs in the management of premenstrual dysphoric disorder.

Beers MH, Porter RS, eds. *The Merck manual of diagnosis and therapy,* Merck Research Laboratories, 18th ed. Whitehouse Station, NJ: Merck & Co.; 2006:2080.

82. A 65-year-old woman presents with glossitis, weight loss, paresthesias, and diarrhea. Laboratory tests show a macrocytic anemia. The most likely cause is
A) iron deficiency anemia
B) thalassemia
C) pernicious anemia
D) multiple myeloma
E) colon cancer

Answer and Discussion

The answer is C. Vitamin B_{12} (cobalamin) deficiency is associated with several different conditions, including pernicious anemia (lack of intrinsic factor required for vitamin B_{12} absorption), celiac sprue, Crohn's disease, and previous gastrectomy. Causes for vitamin B_{12} deficiency include inadequate diet, inadequate absorption, inadequate use, increased requirement, and increased excretion. Symptoms include glossitis, anorexia, weight loss, paresthesias, ataxia, dementia, neuropsychiatric changes, and diarrhea. Signs include a macrocytic anemia, tachycardia, abnormal reflexes, positive Romberg sign, and abnormal positional and vibratory sensation. Laboratory findings show low vitamin B_{12} levels and reticulocyte counts. Mild thrombocytopenia, leukopenia, elevated lactate dehydrogenase, and indirect bilirubin levels due to ineffective erythropoiesis are seen. The Shilling test is used for additional information in the diagnosis. Treatment consists of removing the underlying cause of vitamin B_{12} deficiency. Vitamin replacement therapy can be used. Iron deficiency, which coexists in up to one-third of patients, should be ruled out. The recommended daily allowance is 2 μg. Vitamin B_{12} is usually used slowly and, unless there is absence of the vitamin for months, there are sufficient stores to prevent deficiency. A strict vegetarian diet avoids the consumption of meat, dairy products, seafood, and poultry (including eggs). Unfortunately, vegetarians often lack adequate vitamin B_{12}; physicians should look for deficiencies in this population. Meat substitutes, enriched yeast, and soybean milk are alternative sources for vitamin B_{12}.

Kasper DL, Braunwald E, Fauci AS, et al., eds. *Harrison's principles of internal medicine,* 16th ed. New York: McGraw-Hill; 2005:2404.

Ferri F. *Ferri's Clinical Advisor, Instant Diagnosis and Treatment.* Philadelphia: Elsevier/Mosby, 2006:57.

83. Which of the following is NOT considered a risk factor for myocardial infarction?
A) Alcoholism
B) Homocystinemia
C) Type A personality
D) Male sex
E) Obesity

Answer and Discussion

The answer is A. Risk factors for myocardial infarction include

- Hypertension
- Hyperlipidemia—particularly high total cholesterol, high LDL cholesterol, and low HDL cholesterol
- Cigarette smoking
- Diabetes mellitus
- Obesity (increased weight for height)
- Male gender
- Family history of coronary artery disease (CAD)
- Sedentary lifestyle
- Type A personality
- Increased age
- Postmenopausal
- Homocystinemia

Kasper DL, Braunwald E, Fauci AS, et al., eds. *Harrison's principles of internal medicine,* 16th ed. New York: McGraw-Hill; 2005:1430–1433.

84. A 55-year-old business executive presents to your office complaining of a 4-week history of daily headaches. He describes the headache as being pronounced in the morning on awakening, associated with nausea and vomiting. The most likely diagnosis is
A) classic migraine headache
B) cluster headache
C) brain tumor
D) sinus headache
E) muscle tension headache

Answer and Discussion

The answer is C. There are several types of headache associated with specific clinical histories. The following are some common types and their distinguishing features:

- *Migraine headaches.* These usually affect young women (but can affect men) and are pulsating and unilateral in location. They occur infrequently, are throbbing, and are associated with photophobia (in some cases an aura preceding the headache), nausea, and vomiting; sleep usually provides relief. They typically last 4 to 72 hours.
- *Headaches associated with tumors.* Pain occurs daily, becomes more frequent and severe as time passes, and may be associated with focal neurologic deficits or visual disturbances. Patients may report pain more in the morning on awakening, nausea, vomiting, or the pain may be worse with bending over.
- *Headaches associated with sinus headaches.* These are usually associated with facial pain or pressure in the sinus area, fever, and purulent sinus drainage.
- *Muscle-tension headaches.* These are associated with a bandlike tightness that encircles the scalp area, usually occurring on a daily basis and usually worse at the end of a workday.
- *Cluster headaches.* More common in middle-age men, these headaches are usually described as a unilateral, sharp (i.e., "feels like an ice pick"), agonizing pain located in the orbital area, in many cases occurring 2 to 3 hours after the patient falls asleep; they are associated with tearing, nasal congestion, rhinorrhea, and autonomic symptoms on the same side as the headaches. Frequency of attacks ranges from one to eight daily.

Ferri F. *Ferri's Clinical Advisor, Instant Diagnosis and Treatment.* Philadelphia: Elsevier/Mosby; 2006:358–361.

85. Which of the following statements about sickle cell anemia is true?
A) The disease is a sex-linked, recessive, inherited disorder.
B) The condition is related to a defective β chain with sickling under conditions of low CO_2.
C) Hydroxyurea is contraindicated for patients with sickle cell anemia.
D) Patients with sickle cell should receive pneumococcal vaccination.
E) Individuals with sickle cell should avoid influenza vaccination.

Answer and Discussion

The answer is D. Sickle cell anemia is an autosomal-dominant inherited hemolytic anemia that predominantly affects African Americans (approximately 8% of the African-American population). Because of a defective β chain (valine is substituted for a glutamic acid in the sixth position of the β chain), blood cells tend to sickle under conditions of low PO_2. The condition is manifested in a milder heterozygote form (referred to as sickle cell trait) and in the more severe homozygote form. Signs and symptoms include anemia, jaundice, arthralgias, fever, painful aplastic crises that are characterized by severe abdominal and joint pain, poor-healing ulcers associated with the pretibial area, nausea, vomiting, hemiplegia, and cranial nerve palsies. Other manifestations include pulmonary and renal dysfunction, cardiomegaly, hepatosplenomegaly, cholelithiasis, and aseptic necrosis of the femoral heads. Heterozygous individuals are usually unaffected by these complications. Laboratory findings include normocytic, normochromic anemia with a peripheral smear showing sickled red cells with Howell–Jolly bodies and target cells; leukocytosis with a left shift; thrombocytosis; elevated bilirubin levels; and elevated urinary and fecal urobilinogen. ESRs are usually normal. Diagnosis is usually made by Hb electrophoresis demonstrating HbS chains. Heterozygous individuals usually show HbA and HbS chains. Treatment is symptomatic and may include transfusions in severe cases, hydration, pain control, and possible corticosteroids. More recently, hydroxyurea has been used in the treatment of sickle cell anemia. Most crises are precipitated by infections, and treatment should provide coverage for these infections. Because of splenic dysfunction, those affected are at an increased risk for bacterial infections, particularly pneumococcal and Salmonella infections; therefore, they should receive the pneumococcal (Pneumovax) vaccine. Genetic counseling should also be instituted for those affected. Life spans may be shortened for those affected but have been increasing.

Steinberg MH, Barton F, Castro O. Effect of hydroxyurea on mortality and morbidity in adult sickle cell anemia. Risks and benefits up to 9 years of treatment. *JAMA*. 2003; 289:1645–1651.

Ferri F. *Ferri's Clinical Advisor, Instant Diagnosis and Treatment*. Philadelphia: Elsevier/Mosby; 2006:779–780.

86. Which of the following statements about hereditary angioedema is true?
A) It is related to excessive amyloid deposition.
B) It is caused by a deficiency of the C1 esterase inhibitor.
C) Attacks are triggered by antihistamines.
D) Treatment involves dehydroepiandrosterone (DHEA) administration.

Answer and Discussion

The answer is B. Hereditary angioedema is an autosomal-dominant transmitted genetic disorder that is related to a deficiency of C1 esterase inhibitor or, less commonly, to inactive C1 esterase inhibitor that is involved in the first step of complement activation. Symptoms include pruritus; urticarial rashes; abdominal pain; and, in severe cases, bronchoconstriction, which can be life threatening. Attacks are usually triggered by stress, trauma, or illnesses. Diagnosis is made by detection of low C4 levels or deficiency of the C1 esterase inhibitor by immunoassay. Treatment involves the use of antihistamines, glucocorticoids, and epinephrine (in severe cases). Fresh frozen plasma given before procedures can be used for short-term prophylaxis. Other medications used to prevent attacks include the androgens: methyltestosterone, danazol, and stanozolol. In addition, the C1 esterase inhibitor concentrate may be given directly in life-threatening cases.

Ferri F. *Ferri's Clinical Advisor, Instant Diagnosis and Treatment*. Philadelphia: Elsevier/Mosby; 2006:65–66.

87. Which of the following statements best describes astereognosis?
A) Loss of the ability to carry out movements in the absence of paralysis or sensory deficits.
B) Inability to recognize smells.
C) Loss of the ability to express oneself by speech.
D) Loss of the ability to recognize objects by touch.
E) Loss of ocular coordination.

Answer and Discussion

The answer is D. *Astereognosis* is the loss of the ability to recognize objects by the sense of touch. The loss of the ability to carry out movements in the absence of paralysis or sensory deficits is called *apraxia*. Inability to recognize sensory stimuli is called *agnosia*; subgroups include auditory, visual, olfactory, gustatory, and tactile agnosias. The loss of the ability to express oneself by speech or written language is called *aphasia*.

Wiebers DO, Dale AJD, Kokmen E, et al., eds. *Mayo Clinic examinations in neurology*. New York: Mosby; 1998:44, 52, 54, 80–81.

88. Which of the following lung cancers is most commonly associated with the syndrome of inappropriate secretion of antidiuretic hormone (SIADH)?
A) Squamous cell carcinoma
B) Small-cell (oat-cell) carcinoma
C) Large-cell carcinoma
D) Adenocarcinoma
E) Mesothelioma

Answer and Discussion

The answer is B. Lung cancer is often associated with a paraneoplastic syndrome, which occurs as a result of cancer and is extrapulmonary. The following are some common neoplastic syndromes:

- *Squamous cell:* hypercalcemia
- *Small cell:* Cushing's syndrome, SIADH with hyponatremia, myasthenic syndrome, Eaton–Lambert syndrome, peripheral neuropathy, subacute cerebellar degeneration
- *Large cell:* gynecomastia
- *Adenocarcinoma:* clubbing, thrombophlebitis, marantic endocarditis, periostitis, or hypertrophic osteoarthropathy

In addition, all of the previously mentioned lung cancers may be associated with dermatomyositis, disseminated intravascular coagulation, eosinophilia, thrombocytosis, and acanthosis nigricans.

Beers MH, Porter RS, eds. *The Merck manual of diagnosis and therapy*, Merck Research Laboratories, 18th ed. Whitehouse Station, NJ: Merck & Co.; 2006:1150–1153.

89. The best medication to use in the emergent treatment of supraventricular tachycardia is
A) digoxin
B) verapamil
C) adenosine
D) diltiazem
E) isoproterenol

Answer and Discussion

The answer is C. Treatments for stable patients with supraventricular tachycardia (also referred to as regular *narrow QRS tachycardias*) include vagal maneuvers such as Valsalva maneuvers; coughing; activation of gag reflex; carotid sinus massage; and placing an ice bag to the face or swallowing ice-cold water, which can be extremely effective. Unilateral carotid sinus massage, one of the more common methods used, should be given at the angle of the jaw on one side for 3 to 5 seconds. Patients with a history of carotid artery disease are at increased risk for the dislodgment of plaque, which may lead to stroke. Adenosine (Adenocard) and verapamil (Isoptin) administered intravenously are also effective if the previously mentioned measures fail to succeed. Adenosine is preferred because of its rapid onset of action and short half-life. For unstable patients, low-energy electrical cardioversion is the treatment of choice. Most patients troubled by this arrhythmia are candidates for radiofrequency ablation.

Beers MH, Porter RS, eds. *The Merck manual of diagnosis and therapy*, Merck Research Laboratories, 18th ed. Whitehouse Station, NJ: Merck & Co.; 2006:700–702.

> Adenosine is the preferred treatment of supraventricular tachycardia (SVT) because of its rapid onset of action and short half-life.

90. Which of the following effects distinguishes aspirin from acetaminophen?
A) Analgesic properties
B) Antipyretic properties
C) Anti-inflammatory properties
D) Amnestic properties
E) Antipruritic properties

Answer and Discussion

The answer is C. Aspirin (acetylsalicylic acid) is the drug of choice for mild-to-moderate pain. It has antipyretic and anti-inflammatory properties (unlike acetaminophen, which has no anti-inflammatory properties). The major side effect is gastric irritation, which can be reduced by using an enteric-coated aspirin and taking the medication with meals. Tinnitus has also been associated with chronic aspirin use. Aspirin's mode of action is accomplished by the inhibition of prostaglandin synthesis by permanently acetylating cyclooxygenase. Because platelet function is irreversibly inhibited, bleeding times are prolonged as much as 1 to 2 weeks. Aspirin can evoke an anaphylactic response in some individuals, especially in those with a history of asthma and nasal polyps, and, thus, should be avoided. Aspirin use should also be avoided in children and teenagers with viral febrile illnesses (e.g., chickenpox, infectious mononucleosis, viral influenza) because of the risk of Reye's syndrome. Some studies have suggested aspirin use may help prevent adenomatous colon polyp development or regression. Also, prophylactic aspirin use has been advocated to help prevent myocardial infarction and stroke.

Rakel RE, Bope ET. *Conn's Current Therapy 2005*. Philadelphia: Elsevier/Saunders; 2005:30–31, 402, 406.

91. A 56-year-old man presents to your office with complaints of "chronic" diarrhea. He states that he has had loose stools for the last 2 days. He denies blood in the stool, fever, and has no weight loss and no recent travel. Appropriate management at this time includes
A) observation
B) check stool cultures
C) colonoscopy
D) stool fat studies

Answer and Discussion

The answer is A. Chronic diarrhea is a common and sometimes difficult problem encountered by physicians and patients. The condition is defined as diarrhea that continues for >4 weeks. The problem occurs in 1% to 5% of the population. Patients often present late in their course, after other symptoms such as weight loss, rectal bleeding, and abdominal pain have developed. Diarrhea results from incomplete absorption of water from the bowel lumen because of a reduced rate of water absorption or osmotically induced luminal retention of water. Even mild changes in absorption can cause loose stools. The three available management strategies are test and treat; categorize, test, and treat; and empiric therapy. The "test and treat" plan is useful when the history and physical examination yield a high probability of a specific diagnosis. When the evaluation is less clear, it is impractical to test for every possible etiology. A "categorize, test, and treat" plan is useful because the presentation often is nonspecific. Diarrhea can be categorized as watery, fatty, or inflammatory based on gross stool or microscopic examination. Once the diarrhea is categorized, further testing becomes more specific. An "empiric therapy" plan avoids determining a diagnosis and simply treats the symptoms. This is a reasonable approach, assuming serious causes for the diarrhea have been excluded. Patients must be monitored closely when this plan is followed.

Schiller LR. Chronic diarrhea. *Gastroenterology.* 2004;127: 287–293.

92. A 20-year-old otherwise healthy woman presents with cloudy urine, burning on urination, and urinary frequency. The patient has no allergies. Physical examination shows the patient is afebrile. She has mild suprapubic pain with palpation but no costovertebral angle tenderness. Urinalysis is positive for nitrites and leukocyte esterase. Which of the following is the most appropriate treatment?
A) Hospitalize the patient and administer intravenous antibiotics.
B) Administer macrolide-containing antibiotics on an outpatient basis.
C) Administer sulfa-containing antibiotics plus phenazopyridine (Pyridium) on an outpatient basis.
D) Advise the patient to increase fluid intake, especially with cranberry juice.
E) Arrange for an intravenous pyelogram.

Answer and Discussion

The answer is C. Urinary tract infections are more common in sexually active women. Symptoms include dysuria, urinary frequency, enuresis, incontinence, suprapubic tenderness, flank pain, or costovertebral angle tenderness (which usually indicates pyelonephritis). Gram-negative bacteria that originate from the intestinal tract (i.e., *Escherichia coli, Staphylococcus saprophyticus, Klebsiella, Enterobacter, Proteus, Pseudomonas*) are usually the causative organisms. Diagnosis is accomplished by microscopic or dipstick evaluation of a clean-catch midstream urine sample. Urine culture confirms the diagnosis. Treatment is oral (and in most cases sulfa-containing) antibiotics. With no complicating clinical factors, reasonable empiric treatment for presumed cystitis before organism identification is a 3-day regimen of any of the following: oral TMP-SMX, TMP, norfloxacin, ciprofloxacin, ofloxacin, lomefloxacin, or enoxacin. With complicating factors of diabetes, symptoms for more than 7 days, recent urinary tract infection, use of diaphragm, and postmenopausal women, a 7-day regimen can be considered using the same antibiotics. Phenazopyridine hydrochloride (Pyridium) may be necessary for 1 to 3 days if significant dysuria is present. Affected patients should also be encouraged to increase their fluid intake.

Mehnert-Kay SA. Diagnosis and management of uncomplicated urinary tract infections. *Am Fam Physician.* 2005;72: 451–456, 458.

93. Treatment of severely infected diabetic foot ulcers should involve
A) topical antibiotics
B) débridement only
C) débridement with systemic antibiotics
D) débridement with topical antibiotics
E) none of the above

Answer and Discussion

The answer is C. Diabetic foot ulcers usually result from large vessel disease, microvascular disease, neuropathies, or a combination of all three. Ulcers associated with large vessel disease tend to affect the distal tips of the toes, whereas those secondary to neuropathy typically occur on the weight-bearing surfaces. Smoking and heavy alcohol abuse can increase the risk of diabetic ulcers. Prevention is the key to treatment. All diabetic patients should be instructed about foot care, and their feet should be examined regularly. Organisms that typically infect diabetic ulcers include *Staphylococcus*, *Streptococcus*, anaerobes, and gram-negative organisms. Severe infections may involve methicillin-resistant *Staphylococcus aureus* and *Pseudomonas* infections. Cultures should be taken from the débrided ulcer base or from purulent drainage. Oral antibiotics may be adequate for mild infections. However, if the infection is severe, débridement and systemic antibiotics are usually necessary. Topical antibiotics provide little help in the treatment of such infections.

Kasper DL, Braunwald E, Fauci AS, et al., eds. *Harrison's principles of internal medicine,* 16th ed. New York: McGraw-Hill; 2005:2169.

94. A 13-year-old boy with asthma complains of shortness of breath and wheezing during physical education class. Otherwise the child has no symptoms. The most appropriate treatment is

A) oral steroid therapy
B) inhaled steroids before exercise
C) inhaled β agonist before exercise
D) long-acting β agonist
E) anxiolytic medication

Answer and Discussion

The answer is C. Exercise-induced asthma occurs mainly in patients already diagnosed with asthma. Wheezing usually begins shortly after the initiation of exercise and can be debilitating and limit participation. Use of β2-agonist inhalers before exercise is one of the most beneficial preventive measures for wheezing. Other preventive measures include a slow warm-up and the avoidance of very warm and very cold conditions. Many professional and Olympic athletes are affected with exercise-induced asthma but are able to compete with little or no problem.

Kasper DL, Braunwald E, Fauci AS, et al., eds. *Harrison's principles of internal medicine,* 16th ed. New York: McGraw-Hill; 2005:1511.

95. A 30-year-old man with human immunodeficiency virus (HIV) infection and a CD4 count of 150/mm^3 should

A) start antiviral medication
B) have additional follow-up tests in 1 month
C) have additional follow-up tests in 3 months
D) have additional follow-up tests in 6 months
E) have tests repeated in 1 year

Answer and Discussion

The answer is A. The CD4 count is a marker for T-helper cells and is used in the treatment of HIV. Once the patient has been diagnosed with HIV, the CD4 count should be measured and followed. Typically, there is a diurnal variation in the CD4 count; therefore, it should be measured at the same time with each determination. Plasma viral load (PVL) is also used to determine treatment in HIV. The major guidelines vary slightly in the PVL and CD4$^+$ cell cutoff values that are used for recommendations on starting, considering, or deferring antiretroviral drug therapy (ART). ART is *recommended* for all patients with a history of AIDS-defining illness or severe symptoms of HIV infection regardless of CD4 cell count. ART is also *recommended* for asymptomatic patients with a CD4 count <200 cells/μL. Therapy *should be offered* to asymptomatic patients with CD4 cell counts of 201 to 350 cells/μL. The urgency of treatment recommendations may be based on various factors, including

- Rate of CD4 cell decline
- Plasma HIV RNA >100,000 copies/mL
- Patient interest
- Risk of toxicity

Therapy should probably be *deferred* for asymptomatic patients with CD4 cell counts of >350 cells/μL and plasma HIV RNA <100,000 copies/mL.

The question of when to initiate ART in asymptomatic patients remains an area of research and debate. It is clear that ART should be initiated before the CD4 count declines to <200 cells/μL, if at all possible. However, it is not yet known at what CD4 threshold >200 cells/μL, therapy should be started, as the long-term risks of ARVs may be substantial in some patients. With the increasing availability of ARV regimens that are more tolerable, are composed of fewer pills, and have easier dosing schedules, some clinicians are choosing to initiate therapy earlier in the course of HIV infection. CD4$^+$ cell counts and HIV RNA levels are important tools for evaluating treatment response. A minimum of two CD4$^+$ cell counts and PVL measurements should be obtained on separate visits before treatment is changed. Ideally, the HIV RNA level should decline rapidly after antiretroviral drug therapy is initiated. Guidelines on the expected PVL reductions vary. A typical goal is a 1- to 2-log reduction within 4 to 8 weeks (e.g., from 50,000 copies/mL to 500 copies/mL). Failure to achieve the target level of <50 copies/mL after 16 to 24 weeks of treatment should prompt consideration of drug resistance, inadequate drug absorption, or poor compliance. Maximal viral suppression often takes longer in patients with higher baseline HIV RNA levels (e.g., >100,000 copies/mL). HIV RNA levels should be obtained periodically during antiretroviral drug therapy, although precise data are not available on the optimal frequency of such monitoring.

Data from HIV/AIDS Treatment Information Service website. Guidelines for the use of antiretroviral agents in HIV-infected adults and adolescents. Available at: http://www.hivatis.org. Accessed 6/5/06.

96. Which of the following factors is associated with dysplastic nevi syndrome?

A) No genetically related transmission.
B) Scattered moles with benign appearance.
C) Increased risk for malignant transformation.
D) The number of lesions noted at birth remains the same over time.
E) Excessive vitamin A ingestion.

Answer and Discussion

The answer is C. Dysplastic nevi syndrome is a condition that is inherited as an autosomal-dominant disease. Usually more than two family members are affected; however, sporadic cases do occur. Patients are affected with numerous (in some cases >100) irregular, large moles. These moles are abnormal in appearance and show variegation of color. The moles more commonly occur on covered areas such as the breast, buttocks, and scalp. Unlike common moles, dysplastic nevi continue to appear as the patient ages. These patients are at increased risk for the development of melanoma. Patients should be counseled to avoid sun exposure, and any suspicious lesion or change in nevi should warrant a biopsy. Photographs of the patients can help determine if there are any changes in nevi.

Kasper DL, Braunwald E, Fauci AS, et al., eds. *Harrison's principles of internal medicine,* 16th ed. New York: McGraw-Hill; 2005:498–500.

97. The proportion of patients with a disease in whom a test result is positive is referred to as
A) the *p* value
B) sensitivity
C) specificity
D) reliability
E) variability

Answer and Discussion

The answer is B. *Sensitivity* is defined as the proportion of people who are affected by a given disease and who also test positive for that disease. For example, the proportion of patients who actually have coronary artery disease (CAD) and also test positive with a treadmill exercise test would be defined as the sensitivity. Typically, the sensitivity for treadmill exercise testing is 72% to 96%.

Mark DB. Chapter 2: Decision-making in clinical medicine. Available at Harrison's Online website (http://www.harrisons-online.com). Accessed 6/5/06.

Sensitivity is defined as the proportion of people who are affected by a given disease and who also test positive for that disease.

98. An intensely pruritic, vesicular rash that is localized to the upper extremity is most likely
A) herpes zoster
B) poison ivy
C) *Staphylococcus* infection
D) atopic dermatitis
E) varicella

Answer and Discussion

The answer is B. Exposure to poison ivy, poison oak, or poison sumac can cause an intensely pruritic vesicular rash. The patient often recalls an exposure to the plants within 24 to 48 hours, and the extremities are often affected. The condition is a result of a delayed hypersensitivity reaction that may take several days to appear. Management should include thorough washing with soap and water, preferably within 10 minutes of exposure, as this may prevent dermatitis. All contaminated clothes should be removed as soon as possible and cleaned. Frequent baths using colloidal oatmeal also relieve symptoms. Treatment of mild to moderate rash includes application of cool compresses or diluted aluminum acetate solution such as Burow's solution or calamine lotion. Use of topical antihistamines and anesthetics should be avoided because of the possibility of increased sensitization. Early application of topical steroids is useful to limit erythema and pruritus. However, occlusive dressings should be avoided on moist lesions. Refractory dermatitis can be treated with oral corticosteroids such as prednisone, with an initial dosage of 1 mg/kg/day, slowly tapering the dosage over 2 to 3 weeks. Shorter courses of steroids may be followed by severe rebound exacerbations shortly after drug therapy is discontinued. Oral antihistamines may help reduce pruritus and provide sedation, when needed.

Lee NP, Arriola ER. Poison ivy, oak, and sumac dermatitis. *West J Med.* 1999;171:354–355.

99. The presence of polymorphonuclear cells in stool samples most likely supports the diagnosis of a
A) bacterial infection
B) viral infection
C) parasitic infection
D) fungal infection

Answer and Discussion

The answer is A. *Acute diarrhea* is defined as stools occurring with increased frequency or decreased consistency. There are many different organisms. Bacterial agents include *E. coli, Salmonella, Shigella, Campylobacter, Clostridium, Yersinia,* and *Vibrio cholera.* Viral agents include rotavirus, enterovirus, and Norwalk agent. Parasitic infections include *Giardia lamblia, Entamoeba histolytica, Cryptosporidium,* and *Strongyloides.* Fungal agents include *Candida, Histoplasma,* and *Actinomyces.* Diagnosis is accomplished with stool culture and sensitivity studies; however, the presence of polymorphonuclear cells supports a bacterial cause. In most cases of acute diarrhea, the use of antibiotics is unnecessary; however, the empiric use of antibiotics, including TMP-SMX, ciprofloxacin, or erythromycin, may be appropriate (although controversial) in severe cases in which stool cultures are pending, especially for those at risk for transmitting the offending organism to others.

Beers MH, Porter RS, eds. *The Merck manual of diagnosis and therapy,* Merck Research Laboratories, 18th ed. Whitehouse Station, NJ: Merck & Co.; 2006:77–80.

100. Café-au-lait spots are associated with which of the following disorders?
A) Peutz–Jeghers syndrome
B) Neurofibromatosis
C) Dysplastic nevus syndrome
D) Addison's disease

Answer and Discussion

The answer is B. The following are skin abnormalities noted in patients affected with the following disease processes:

Neurofibromatosis (von Recklinghausen's disease)	Café-au-lait spots
Peutz–Jeghers syndrome	Hyperpigmentation around the oral cavity, hamartomas of the intestine
Dysplastic nevus syndrome	Multiple pigmented nevi
Hypoadrenocorticism (Addison's disease)	Hyperpigmentation of the gin giva, areola of the nipples, labia, and linea alba of the abdomen

Fitzpatrick TB, Johnson RA, Polano MK, et al., eds. *Color atlas and synopsis of clinical dermatology, common and serious diseases*, 2nd ed. New York: McGraw-Hill; 1994:448–492.

101. Which of the following tests is most helpful in distinguishing fever of unknown origin (FUO) from factitious fever?
A) Urinalysis
B) Chest x-ray
C) Rheumatoid factor
D) Blood cultures
E) Sedimentation rate

Answer and Discussion

The answer is E. FUO is defined as a fever higher than 101°F (38.3°C) on at least three occasions, accompanied by an illness that lasts longer than 3 weeks, and the diagnosis is uncertain after 3 days of hospitalization, although most workups are now done in the outpatient setting. Causes include infection, neoplasm, drugs, collagen vascular disease, vasculitis, and factious fever. Laboratory tests include CBC, urinalysis with culture, blood cultures, chest radiography, HIV testing, serum protein electrophoresis, sedimentation rate, serology tests, ANA, rheumatoid factor, and thyroid tests. The ESR may be helpful in distinguishing real disease from a factious fever. A good history and physical examination are imperative in the evaluation of a patient with FUO and helps direct further testing. Observing the temperature pattern can be helpful. Disease states such as malaria, babesiosis, Hodgkin's disease, and cyclic neutropenia have patterns, whereas factitious fever often has no pattern.

Ferri F. *Ferri's Clinical Advisor, Instant Diagnosis and Treatment.* Philadelphia: Elsevier/Mosby; 2006:318.

102. Which of the following test results supports the diagnosis of Graves' disease?
A) Decreased thyroid-stimulating hormone (TSH)
B) Increased TSH
C) Decreased thyroxine (T4) levels
D) Decreased triiodothyronine (T3) levels
E) None of the above

Answer and Discussion

The answer is A. Graves' disease is the most common form of hyperthyroidism seen predominantly in women between 20 and 40 years of age. The condition, also known as *toxic diffuse goiter,* is characterized by a triad of symptoms, including goiter, exophthalmos, and pretibial edema. Patients affected may report palpitations, tachycardia, heat intolerance with excessive sweating, weight loss, emotional lability, weakness and fatigue, diarrhea, or menstrual irregularities. Laboratory findings include a decreased sensitive TSH (sTSH) and positive thyroid-stimulating antibodies (which are thought to bind to the TSH receptors and stimulate the gland to hyperfunction). T4 levels are usually elevated, but in rare cases may be normal with increased T3 levels. Treatment involves the use of propylthiouracil or methimazole, inorganic iodine, propranolol (especially in thyroid storm), radioactive iodine (but not in pregnant patients), and surgery.

Beers MH, Porter RS, eds. *The Merck manual of diagnosis and therapy,* Merck Research Laboratories, 18th ed. Whitehouse Station, NJ: Merck & Co.; 2006:1195–1200.

103. A 45-year-old man is seen in your clinic. The patient has known cirrhosis, diabetes, and complains of multiple joint pain. Examination shows a bronze discoloration of the skin and testicular atrophy. Laboratory values show a serum iron of 500 μg/dL, serum ferritin of 2,000 ng/mL, and a transferrin saturation of 80%. The most likely diagnosis is
A) alcoholism
B) hemochromatosis
C) Wilson's disease
D) Gilbert's disease
E) Hepatitis C

Answer and Discussion

The answer is B. Hemochromatosis is a result of excessive iron deposition in the body (hemosiderosis) that leads to damage of bodily tissues. Primary hereditary hemochromatosis is an autosomal-recessive trait that is associated with defects on chromosome 6. It is the most common form of hemochromatosis, affecting approximately 5 in 1,000 persons. Complications include

- Cirrhosis
- Diabetes mellitus
- Multiple joint pain
- Abdominal pain
- Chondrocalcinosis
- Bronze discoloration of the skin
- Cardiomyopathy that may result in cardiac enlargement, CHF, and cardiac arrhythmias
- Hepatomas
- Pituitary dysfunction leading to testicular atrophy and decreased sexual drive

The onset is usually in the fourth and fifth decades of life. The condition is rare before middle age. Diagnosis in women usually occurs after menopause, because menstrual blood loss helps provide protection from iron overload. Laboratory findings show serum iron >300 mg/dL, serum ferritin >1,000 ng/mL, and transferrin saturation >50%. Liver biopsy confirms the diagnosis when hepatic siderosis and cirrhosis is suspected. Treatment involves phlebotomy (500 mL/week = 200 to 250 mg iron) to remove excess iron from the body and the chelating agent deferoxamine in severe cases, which promotes urinary excretion of iron. Family members of those affected should be screened for hemochromatosis with HLA typing and iron studies.

Brandhagen DJ, Fairbanks VF, Baldus W. Recognition and management of hereditary hemochromatosis. *Am Fam Physician.* 2002;65:853–860, 865–866.

104. Acromegaly is associated with which of the following factors?
A) Excessive cortisol secretion
B) Lack of adequate parathyroid hormone
C) Excessive growth hormone
D) Thyroid dysfunction
E) Excessive gastrin secretion

Answer and Discussion

The answer is C. The condition of acromegaly is associated with an excessive amount of growth hormone, which in most cases is caused by a pituitary tumor. If there is excessive growth hormone secretion before closure of the epiphyses during childhood, then the condition of excessive skeletal growth is referred to as gigantism. When excessive growth hormone occurs in adulthood, it is usually between the third and fifth decades and is referred to as *acromegaly.* Associated conditions include coarsening of facial features with increased hand, foot, jaw, and cranial size; macroglossia; wide spacing of the teeth; deep voice; excessive coarse hair growth; thickening of the skin; excessive sweating as a result of increased number of sweat glands; and neurologic symptoms, including headaches, peripheral neuropathies, muscle weakness, and arthralgias. Insulin resistance is common; diabetes occurs in 25% of patients. CAD, cardiomyopathy with arrhythmias, left ventricular dysfunction, and hypertension occur in 30% of patients. Sleep apnea occurs in 60%. Acromegaly is also associated with an increased risk of colon polyps and colonic malignancy. The diagnosis is made by detecting elevated levels of growth hormone after the administration of a 100-g glucose load. Because of the pulsatility of growth hormone secretion, a single random growth hormone level is not useful. Further diagnostic tests include MRI and CT scanning. Treatment is usually surgery; however, radiation is considered in some patients to treat pituitary tumors. Bromocriptine and a long-acting somatostatin analog (e.g., octreotide acetate) may also be used as adjuncts to surgery to help shrink the tumor.

Kasper DL, Braunwald E, Fauci AS, et al., eds. *Harrison's principles of internal medicine,* 16th ed. New York: McGraw-Hill; 2005:2090.

105. Which of the following signs is associated with Achilles tendonitis?
A) Hyperpronation
B) Gynecoid pelvis
C) Increased Q angle
D) Lateral collateral ligament instability

Answer and Discussion

The answer is A. Achilles tendonitis occurs with repeated stress to the Achilles tendon. Precipitating factors include brisk walking, running, jumping, or hiking. Although known as *Achilles tendonitis,* it is usually the tissue surrounding the tendon that is responsible for the inflammation and pain. Persons who exercise or compete in low-heel shoes and those who hyperpronate their feet are at increased risk for Achilles tendonitis. Patients report pain in the heel and leg discomfort when the Achilles tendon is used. Physical findings include pain with palpation over the Achilles tendon approximately 3 cm above the insertion site on the calcaneus. Treatment goals are to decrease the inflammation associated with the inflamed structures and to reduce the stress on the Achilles tendon. Treatment includes NSAIDs, 1/2-in. heel lifts, and strengthening and stretching exercises of the gastrocnemius and soleus muscles. For patients with hyperpronation, a soft navicular pad and 1/8-in. medial wedge may help prevent excessive pronation.

Mazzone MF, McCue T. Common conditions of the Achilles tendon. *Am Fam Physician.* 2002;65:1805–1810.

106. Which of the following statements about systolic hypertension is true?
A) It represents relatively little risk to the patient.
B) It is defined as a systolic pressure >140 mm Hg with a diastolic pressure >100 mm Hg.
C) It does not increase the risk of stroke.
D) It is often caused by mitral regurgitation.
E) It is more dangerous to elderly patients than an elevated diastolic pressure.

Answer and Discussion

The answer is E. Systolic hypertension is a condition that usually affects the elderly. The condition is defined as a systolic blood pressure >140 mm Hg and diastolic pressure <90 mm Hg. The cause is the loss of elasticity of the arteries that occurs with aging. Other causes include thyrotoxicosis, arteriovenous fistulas, or aortic regurgitation. Untreated systolic hypertension can lead to an increased risk for stroke and cardiovascular disease. Data from the Framingham study and the Multiple Risk Factor Intervention Trial indicated the importance of isolated systolic hypertension in the development of coronary heart disease (CHD). These trials concluded that elevated systolic blood pressure in the elderly was probably of more significance than elevated diastolic blood pressure. In other words, a systolic blood pressure of 160 mm Hg with a diastolic blood pressure of 85 mm Hg posed a greater risk for cardiovascular disease than a systolic blood pressure of 135 to 140 mm Hg and a diastolic blood pressure of 95 mm Hg. Isolated systolic hypertension, defined as a blood pressure of >140 mm Hg systolic and <90 mm Hg diastolic, occurs in more than 30% of women older than 65 years and in more than 20% of men of the same age. Treatment involves lifestyle changes (e.g., exercise, sodium restriction, weight loss) and the use of hypertensive medications. In most instances, low-dose diuretic therapy should be used as initial antihypertensive therapy in the elderly. A long-acting dihydropyridine calcium channel blocker may be used as alternative therapy in elderly patients with isolated systolic hypertension. Diabetics benefit from ACE inhibitors. In some cases, systolic hypertension may be more difficult to control than essential hypertension.

Kasper DL, Braunwald E, Fauci AS, et al., eds. *Harrison's principles of internal medicine,* 16th ed. New York: McGraw-Hill; 2005:1468.

107. Which of the following statements is true regarding pneumococcal (Pneumovax) vaccination?
A) Healthy individuals older than 50 years should receive the vaccine.
B) Medicare does not cover the cost of pneumococcal (Pneumovax) vaccination.
C) Adults with previous splenectomy should not receive pneumococcal (Pneumovax) vaccination.
D) Children younger than 2 years with sickle cell anemia should receive pneumococcal (Pneumovax) vaccination.
E) Boosters are recommended for individuals older than 65 years if they received their first dose more than 5 years prior to their last injection.

Answer and Discussion

The answer is E. The pneumococcal (Pneumovax) vaccine is made from the polysaccharides of 23 different strains of bacterial pneumonia. The vaccine is recommended for patients older than 65 years, individuals with underlying pulmonary disease or chronic debilitating diseases (e.g., diabetes, liver and renal disease, cardiac disease, lymphoma, transplant patients, HIV patients), and those without a spleen. The vaccine is given intramuscularly or subcutaneously and is not recommended during an acute illness. Antigenic response occurs 2 to 3 weeks after vaccination. Adverse reactions include local irritation or soreness, erythema, induration, low-grade fever, rash, myalgia, and arthralgia; in severe reactions (less than 1%), anaphylaxis or nerve disorders may occur. Children younger than 2 years should not receive the vaccine. Since 1981, Medicare has covered the cost of pneumococcal vaccine (Pneumovax). One-time boosters are recommended for individuals older than 65 years if they received their first dose more than 5 years prior. Other individuals at high risk who received pneumococcal vaccination more than 5 to 10 years prior may require boosters. The vaccine has been determined to be cost-effective for all ages.

Centers for Disease Control and Prevention website. Summary of adolescent/adult immunization recommendations. Available at: http://www.cdc.gov/nip/recs/adult-schedule.pdf. Accessed 6/5/06.

108. Cigarette smoking is associated with increased risk of all of the following EXCEPT:
A) bladder cancer
B) osteoporosis
C) peptic ulcer disease
D) Alzheimer's disease
E) cervical cancer

Answer and Discussion

The answer is D. Cigarette smoking is a severe health-related problem throughout the world. Smokers typically live 5 to 8 years less than nonsmokers. They have an increased risk of cancer of the lung, mouth, throat, esophagus, pancreas, kidney, bladder, and cervix. In addition, they are at increased risk for the development of peptic ulcer disease and osteoporosis. Furthermore, they have an increased risk of heart diseases and chronic lung disease. Mothers who smoke during their pregnancy typically have smaller babies. All patients who smoke should be encouraged to stop. The physician should always ask about smoking; if the patient does smoke, there should be an attempt by the physician to motivate the patient to stop. Setting a stop date may be helpful, and follow-up is necessary to provide support and reinforce the patient's commitment to stop. Nicotine-containing patches and gum can also be used to wean people from their nicotine dependence. Bupropion (Zyban) also has been used to help relieve nicotine withdrawal. Bupropion hydrochloride, also marketed as an antidepressant, has been reintroduced in a sustained-release formulation to be used as a smoking cessation aid. Bupropion potentiates the effects of norepinephrine and dopamine. Dopamine has been associated with the rewarding effects of addictive substances. It is postulated that inhibition of norepinephrine reuptake might lead to a decrease in withdrawal symptoms. Bupropion does not have a sedating effect, although agitation and insomnia have been commonly reported in patients taking the drug for depression. It is not frequently associated with sexual dysfunction, weight gain, or anticholinergic effects. Tremor, rash, and a few anaphylactoid reactions have been reported. Panic symptoms and psychotic reactions have been reported in patients taking bupropion and fluoxetine concurrently. Bupropion is contraindicated in patients taking monoamine oxidase inhibitors or ritonavir. Carbamazepine increases the metabolism and decreases the antidepressant effect of bupropion. The recommended dosage in patients attempting smoking cessation is 150 mg once daily for 3 days and then twice daily for 7 to 12 weeks or longer. This regimen may be accompanied by nicotine replacement therapy. Patients are advised to stop smoking during the second week of treatment. The manufacturer offers a counseling and support service.

Medical Letter Consultants. Bupropion (Zyban) for smoking cessation. *Med Lett Drugs Ther.* 1997;39(1007);77–78.

> Bupropion hydrochloride, also marketed as an antidepressant, has been reintroduced in a sustained-release formulation to be used as a smoking cessation aid.

109. A 45-year-old female presents with persistent nasal symptoms for the last 6 weeks. She has been treated with an extended course of antibiotics but despite therapy her symptoms remain. She is afebrile and otherwise looks well. Appropriate management at this time includes
A) additional 2-week course of antibiotic therapy
B) plain films of the sinuses
C) CT scan of the sinuses
D) MRI of the sinuses
E) laboratory evaluation including a CBC and blood cultures

Answer and Discussion

The answer is C. Rhinosinusitis is typically divided among four subtypes: acute, recurrent acute, subacute, and chronic, based on patient history and a limited physical examination. In most cases, therapy is administered based on this classification. Antibiotic therapy along with hydration and decongestants is indicated for 7 to 14 days in patients with acute, recurrent acute, or subacute bacterial rhinosinusitis. For patients with chronic disease, the same treatment regimen is indicated for an additional 4 weeks or more, and a nasal steroid may also be prescribed if inhalant allergies are suspected as an etiologic agent. Nasal endoscopy and computed tomography of the sinuses are reserved for circumstances that include a failure to respond to therapy as expected, spread of infection outside the sinuses, a question of diagnosis, and when surgery is being considered. Laboratory tests are rarely needed and are reserved for patients with suspected allergies, cystic fibrosis, immune deficiencies, mucociliary disorders, and similar disease states. Findings on endoscopically guided culture obtained from the middle meatus correlate 80% to 85% of the time with results from the more painful antral puncture technique, and is performed in patients who fail to respond to the initial antibiotic selection. Surgery is indicated for extranasal spread of infection, evidence of mucocele or pyocele, fungal sinusitis, or obstructive nasal polyposis, and is often performed in patients with recurrent or persistent infection not resolved by drug therapy.

Osguthorpe JD. Adult rhinosinusitis: diagnosis and management. *Am Fam Physician.* 2001;63:69–76.

110. A 56-year-old smoker with recently diagnosed small-cell carcinoma of the lung presents with increasing muscle contraction with repeated nerve stimulation. The most likely diagnosis is
A) Eaton–Lambert syndrome
B) myasthenia gravis
C) tetanus
D) polymyalgia rheumatica
E) Parkinson's disease

Answer and Discussion

The answer is A. Eaton–Lambert syndrome is a neurologic disorder that results from inadequate release of acetylcholine from the presynaptic nerve endings. Often associated with a paraneoplastic syndrome (e.g., small-cell or oat-cell carcinoma of the lung), the condition causes weakness and sometimes pain associated with the proximal muscles, paresthesia, impotence, and ptosis. Reflexes are usually reduced or absent. Diagnosis is made by showing increasing muscle contraction with repeated nerve stimulation, unlike myasthenia gravis, in which decreased muscle contraction with repeated nerve stimulation is seen. Special care must be taken to rule out underlying malignancy. The treatment is to identify and treat any underlying malignancy. Guanidine has also been shown to help acetylcholine release from the presynaptic membrane; however, side effects (bone marrow suppression) may limit its use. Other treatment includes the use of immunosuppressant medication (e.g., steroids, azathioprine) and plasmapheresis. Anticholinesterase medications (e.g., pyridostigmine, neostigmine) are variably effective.

Beers MH, Porter RS, eds. *The Merck manual of diagnosis and therapy,* Merck Research Laboratories, 18th ed. Whitehouse Station, NJ: Merck & Co.; 2006:1184.

111. Which is *not* generally a characteristic of a suspicious skin lesion?
A) Asymmetric border
B) Bleeding
C) Color change
D) Variegation of color
E) Diameter less than 5 mm

Answer and Discussion

The answer is E. Skin lesions that represent concern usually possess certain characteristics, including

A = Asymmetric and irregular borders
B = Bleeding or ulceration; persistent itching or tenderness
C = Color change or variegation of color
D = Diameter >6 mm

If any of these criteria are met, the lesion should be biopsied and sent for pathologic examination. Large, raised, and pigmented congenital lesions should also be biopsied. Patients who have a history of dysplastic nevi syndrome are at increased risk for the development of melanoma, particularly if a family member has been affected.

Jerant AF, Johnson JT, Sheridan CD, et al. Early detection and treatment of skin cancer. *Am Fam Physician.* 2000;62: 357–368, 375–376, 381–382.

112. Which of the following conditions is a contraindication to influenza vaccination?
A) Allergy to eggs
B) Allergy to red dye
C) Allergy to penicillin
D) Allergy to milk
E) Allergy to dust mites

Answer and Discussion

The answer is A. Influenza immunizations are administered yearly to help prevent outbreaks of different strains of viral influenza. The inactivated vaccine is derived from purified egg protein, which harbors the viral protein. The vaccine is developed based on the preceding year's outbreak of virus, those viruses seen in other parts of the world, and the antibody response of persons previously vaccinated. Persons who are allergic to eggs or neomycin (a component of the vaccine) should not receive the vaccine. In those individuals, amantadine may be considered. Protective vaccine should be administered to immunocompromised individuals; individuals with underlying medical conditions such as asthma, COPD, and diabetes; and individuals older than 50 years. (Other recommendations follow.) Otherwise healthy patients may also elect to receive vaccination. Side effects, including fever, fatigue, cough, and headache, are no more common in those who received a placebo in double-blinded studies; however, arm soreness was reported more frequently in vaccine recipients.

Recommendations for the administration of influenza vaccine include the following categories and specific indications:

Age

- Persons 6 months or older with an underlying medical condition (e.g., cardiac, pulmonary) who are at increased risk for complications of influenza or who required regular medical follow-up or hospitalization during the preceding year (see Medical conditions as follows)
- Healthy children ages 6–23 months and close contacts of healthy children ages 6–23 months
- Persons 50 years or older
- Any person 6 months or older to reduce the chance of influenza infection

Occupations

- Physicians, nurses, and other personnel in hospital and outpatient care settings, including emergency response workers
- Employees of health-care facilities (e.g., nursing homes, chronic care facilities) who have contact with residents
- Persons who provide home care to people in high-risk groups

Medical conditions

- Alcoholism and alcoholic cirrhosis
- Long-term aspirin therapy in children and teenagers (6 months to 18 years of age) who may be at risk for Reye's syndrome after influenza virus infection
- Chronic cardiovascular disorders in adults and children
- Hemoglobinopathies
- Immunocompromised conditions (e.g., congenital immunodeficiency, malignancy, HIV infection, organ transplantation, immunosuppressive therapy)
- Chronic metabolic diseases (e.g., diabetes)
- Chronic pulmonary diseases, including asthma and COPD
- Chronic renal dysfunction
- Pregnancy beyond 14 weeks of gestation during the influenza season
- Pregnancy in women with medical conditions that increase their risk for complications from influenza, regardless of trimester
- Persons who can transmit influenza to high-risk individuals
- Household members (including children) in close contact with persons who are at high risk for influenza
- Residents of nursing homes and other chronic care facilities, regardless of age, who have chronic medical conditions

Vaccination ideally should occur approximately 2 weeks before chemotherapy or immunosuppressive therapy is started. If a patient is vaccinated during or within 2 weeks before the initiation of immunosuppressive therapy, influenza vaccine should be given again approximately 3 months after treatment ends.

Data from Advisory Committee on Immunization Practices. Prevention and control of influenza: recommendations of the Advisory Committee on Immunization Practices (ACIP). CDC website at www.cdc.gov, accessed 6/5/06.

Montalto NJ, Gum KB, Ashley JV. Updated treatment for influenza A and B. *Am Fam Physician.* 2000;62:2467–2476.

113. A 41-year-old business executive presents to your office and complains of palpitations and shortness of breath. After further questioning, he admits to heavy alcohol consumption the previous evening. On examination, he is found to have an irregular heartbeat of 130 bpm. The most likely diagnosis is
A) ventricular tachycardia
B) ventricular fibrillation
C) premature ventricular contractions (PVCs)
D) atrial fibrillation
E) Wolff-Parkinson-White syndrome

Answer and Discussion

The answer is D. Atrial fibrillation is the most common cardiac arrhythmia. It is characterized on ECG by the absence of P waves and an irregular ventricular rhythm. The atrial rate can range from 400 to 600 bpm, whereas the ventricular rate usually ranges from 80 to 180 bpm in the untreated state. Causes include thyrotoxicosis, rheumatic or ischemic heart disease, hypertension, pericarditis, chest trauma, or excessive alcohol intake. The major risk associated with atrial fibrillation is stroke secondary to embolic complications. Rapid ventricular response of atrial fibrillation requires treatment with rate-controlling calcium-channel blockers, β-blockers, or digoxin to achieve rate control. Elective medical cardioversion may be considered for stable patients. Patients in whom medical conversion fails or whose conditions are unstable may need electrical cardioversion. Patients with long-standing atrial fibrillation (longer than 6 months) have less chance for success than those who have new or relatively new onset. Anticoagulation therapy with warfarin can decrease the risk of stroke and is recommended before any attempt at cardioversion if there is risk for thrombus formation. Patients with chronic atrial fibrillation who are at low risk for bleeding may be treated with warfarin; others may be treated with aspirin therapy. Antiarrhythmics may be needed to treat resistant cases. The risk of embolism during cardioversion in unanticogulated patients is 1% to 7%; however, this risk can be minimized with anticoagulation for 4 weeks before and after cardioversion. Recent studies demonstrate no reductions in either mortality or stroke rates between those patients managed with simple rate control and anticoagulation, compared with those receiving cardioversion with rhythm maintenance using antiarrhythmic medication.

Rakel RE, Bope ET. *Conn's Current Therapy 2005*. Philadelphia: Elsevier/Saunders; 2005:340–344.

114. The most common cause of superior vena cava syndrome is
A) carcinoma of the lung
B) aortic aneurysm
C) tuberculosis
D) metastatic carcinoma from a distant site
E) constrictive pericarditis

Answer and Discussion

The answer is A. Superior vena cava syndrome results from compression of the superior vena cava by a neoplastic process (90% of cases) and less commonly by inflammatory states. Other causes include benign tumors, aortic aneurysm, thyroid enlargement, thrombosis of a central venous line, and fibrosing mediastinitis. Lung cancer, particularly small-cell and squamous-cell type, is the most common associated malignancy. The condition causes the obstruction of venous drainage to the heart and leads to dilation of collateral veins of the upper chest and neck. Signs include plethora and swelling of the face, neck, and upper torso. Edema of the conjunctiva, shortness of breath in a supine position, and CNS disturbances, including headache, dizziness, stupor, and syncope, may be seen. Acute development of symptoms indicates a poor prognosis. The diagnosis of superior vena cava syndrome is essentially a clinical one. Chest x-rays may show widening of the mediastinum, particularly on the right, but the best confirmatory test is CT. The MRI has no advantages over CT. The one potentially life-threatening complication of a superior mediastinal mass is tracheal obstruction. Treatment includes steroids, chemotherapy, and radiation to the tumor. Although the most common cause of this syndrome is metastasized carcinoma of the lung, other less common infectious causes include tuberculosis, histoplasmosis, and constrictive pericarditis.

Kasper DL, Braunwald E, Fauci AS, et al., eds. *Harrison's principles of internal medicine,* 16th ed. New York: McGraw-Hill; 2005:575–576.

115. A construction worker presents with pain over the lateral elbow. He reports that he has been using a hammer more often, and this seems to aggravate his discomfort. The most likely diagnosis is
A) carpal tunnel syndrome
B) rotator cuff dysfunction
C) lateral epicondylitis
D) ulnar nerve entrapment
E) biceps tendonitis

Answer and Discussion

The answer is C. Tennis elbow is usually caused by overuse, repeated trauma, strain, or exercise that involves the upper extremity and a gripping motion. Although associated with playing tennis, it may affect baseball players, golfers, and racquetball enthusiasts, as well as carpenters, assembly-line workers, and electricians, all of whom repeatedly extend the wrist and rotate the forearm. The cause of pain originates at the extensor origin of the extensor carpi radialis brevis in the area of the lateral epicondyle. Symptoms include pain in the area of the lateral epicondyle but may also include the extensor surface of the forearm. In more severe cases, swelling and erythema may be noted. Pain is exacerbated by passively flexing the fingers and wrist with the elbow fully extended. Radiographs are usually negative; however, calcification may be noted in chronic cases. The condition should be distinguished from radial nerve entrapment syndrome (pain with middle finger extension and forearm supination with the elbow fully extended) and posterior interosseous nerve syndrome (pain located more distally over the forearm supinator muscle). Treatment includes NSAIDs, rest of the affected arm, ice therapy, and a volar wrist splint that immobilizes the wrist and prevents flexion and extension. If this treatment does not provide relief, a steroid injection of 1 mL of 1% lidocaine and 0.5 mL of corticosteroid should be attempted. Once the inflammation has been controlled, a constricting band can be used over the proximal forearm to help prevent recurrence. In addition, rehabilitation exercises should be instituted. In severe cases, orthopedic referral may be necessary for possible surgical treatment.

Chumbley EM, O'Connor FG, Nirschl RP. Evaluation of overuse elbow injuries. *Am Fam Physician;* 2000;61:691–700.

116. Which of the following is a characteristic of Marfan's syndrome?
A) Autosomal-recessive transmission
B) Decreased mobility of joints

C) Arm span less than height
D) Aortic dilatation with possible rupture
E) Café-au-lait spots

Answer and Discussion

The answer is D. Marfan's syndrome is an autosomal-dominant transmitted disorder that affects the connective tissue and results in abnormalities associated with the eyes, bones, and cardiovascular system. Up to 25% of all cases may develop from spontaneous mutations. Symptoms include tall stature with arm span exceeding height, arachnodactyly, dislocation of the ocular lens, high-arched palate, pectus excavatum, and hyperextensibility of joints. Complications of the condition include myopia; spontaneous detachment of the lens; and cardiac defects, including aortic regurgitation, mitral valve prolapse (MVP), mitral regurgitation, and aortic dilatation with aortic dissection and rupture (the most common cause of cardiovascular death). Patients affected are at increased risk of endocarditis. Treatment is directed toward the cardiovascular findings. An echocardiogram can help determine cardiac involvement. In some cases, β-blockers may help protect the aorta. Surgery is reserved for those with aortic dilatation or aortic valve dysfunction. New DNA diagnostic tests for mutations in fibrillin-1 and fibrillin-2 can help determine which patients affected with Marfan's are at increased risk for aortic aneurysm. Scoliosis may require bracing or surgery for severe cases.

Kasper DL, Braunwald E, Fauci AS, et al., eds. *Harrison's principles of internal medicine,* 16th ed. New York: McGraw-Hill; 2005:2329.

117. Third-generation cephalosporins differ from first-generation cephalosporins in their increased effectiveness against
A) gram-positive organisms
B) gram-negative organisms
C) anaerobic organisms
D) parasites
E) fungi

Answer and Discussion

The answer is B. Cephalosporins are antibiotics that have a similar chemical structure as the penicillins. They are bacteriocidal and cover gram-positive organisms; second-generation and third-generation cephalosporins also cover gram-negative organisms. As a group, the cephalosporins' mechanism of action is the inhibition of cell wall synthesis. Inflammation increases their absorption, and they are active against a wide spectrum of organisms with relatively few side effects. Some of the cephalosporins, especially third-generation ones, are concentrated enough in the CSF to treat meningitis. Because of their similarity to penicillin, there is a 2% to 3% cross-reactivity in those allergic to penicillin. Unfortunately, there are no predictable skin tests that can test for allergic reactions. Therefore, use of cephalosporins in patients with penicillin allergies should be monitored closely. If the patient has had a severe, immediate reaction to any of the cillin-type medications, it is necessary to use extreme caution prescribing cephalosporins; alternative antibiotics should be strongly considered.

Beers MH, Porter RS, eds. *The Merck manual of diagnosis and therapy,* Merck Research Laboratories, 18th ed. Whitehouse Station, NJ: Merck & Co.; 2006:1427–1428.

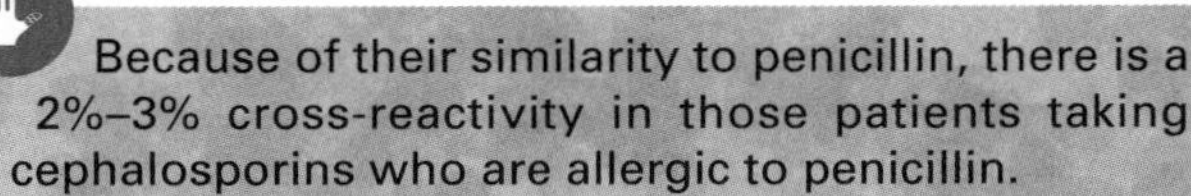

Because of their similarity to penicillin, there is a 2%–3% cross-reactivity in those patients taking cephalosporins who are allergic to penicillin.

118. During which of the following stages of sleep does most dreaming occur?
A) Stage 1 non–rapid eye movement (REM) sleep
B) Stage 2 non-REM sleep
C) Stage 3 non-REM sleep
D) Stage 4 non-REM sleep
E) REM sleep

Answer and Discussion

The answer is E. There are two distinct states of sleep: REM sleep and non-REM sleep, which make up 75% to 80% of sleep. Based on electroencephalographic (EEG) patterns, non-REM sleep can be classified into stages 1, 2, 3, and 4. Necessary for survival, sleep is a cyclical phenomenon. There are four to five REM periods nightly that always follow non-REM sleep and end each cycle. REM sleep, which accounts for 25% (or 1.5 to 2 hours) of the night's sleep, is the period of sleep in which most dreaming occurs. The first period of REM sleep occurs approximately 1.5 to 2 hours after sleep has occurred and lasts approximately 10 minutes. A night's sleep cycles through the different stages and reenters REM stage three or four times for longer periods (15 to 45 minutes), usually in the last several hours of sleep. Non-REM sleep is characterized by slow waves on EEG, with stage 4 being the deepest stage of sleep. REM sleep is characterized by low-voltage, fast activity on EEG. Most night terrors, sleep walking, and sleep talking occur during stage 4 sleep. In REM, sleep muscle tone is decreased, but depth of respiration is increased. As patients become older, the length of REM sleep remains the same; however, there are significant decreases in stages 3 and 4 sleep and an increase in wakeful periods during the night. In addition, it takes elderly patients a longer period to fall asleep. Wakefulness is characterized by alpha wave activity on EEG.

Kasper DL, Braunwald E, Fauci AS, et al., eds. *Harrison's principles of internal medicine,* 16th ed. New York: McGraw-Hill; 2005:153–154.

119. Treatment for uncomplicated infectious mononucleosis should be
A) intravenous antiviral medication
B) oral antiviral therapy (acyclovir or ganciclovir)
C) oral steroids
D) empiric antibiotic treatment
E) symptomatic treatment only

Answer and Discussion

The answer is E. Infectious mononucleosis is caused by the double-stranded EBV, a member of the Herpesviridae family. The incidence is highest in young adults 15 to 35 years of age. Asymptomatic infections are common, and most adults are seropositive to the EBV. Symptoms include fever, headache, generalized fatigue, and malaise. Signs include lymphadenopathy (especially the posterior cervical chain), splenomegaly, hepatomegaly, jaundice, periorbital edema, exudative pharyngitis, palatine petechiae, and rash. Laboratory findings show a lymphocytosis with 20% or more atypical lymphocytes (Downey lymphocytes), a positive heterophile agglutination (Monospot) test after the second week of illness, and a heterophile titer greater than 1:56. Liver function tests are usually elevated. Other laboratory findings may include granulocytopenia, thrombocytopenia, and hemolytic anemia in complicated cases. No specific treatment is recommended for mild cases, and symptoms usually improve in 2 to 4 weeks. In severe cases in which the pharyngitis threatens to obstruct the patient's airway, a 5-day course of steroids may be beneficial. Specific antiviral therapies (acyclovir or ganciclovir) do not appear to be clinically beneficial. Treatment with amoxicillin or ampicillin may lead to a severe maculopapular rash and should be avoided. If the patient has evidence of splenomegaly, contact sports should be avoided until the splenomegaly has resolved. Mononucleosis-type infections may occur more than once but are generally caused by sequential infections with different pathogens rather than by reactivated EBV infections. EBV infections can become reactivated when patients are immunosuppressed (during corticosteroid or cyclosporine therapy) or develop immune deficiencies (e.g., HIV).

Ebell MH. Epstein Barr virus infectious mononucleosis. *Am Fam Physician.* 2004;70:1279–87, 1289–1290.

120. A 65-year-old man presents with increasing shortness of breath over the previous 5 years. Further history reveals that the patient worked for many years in a factory that produced fluorescent lights. On examination, the patient has granulomas affecting the skin and conjunctiva. A chest radiograph shows evidence of parenchymal infiltrates and intra-alveolar edema with mediastinal lymphadenopathy. The most likely diagnosis is

A) coccidioidomycosis
B) berylliosis
C) tuberculosis
D) sarcoidosis
E) asbestosis

Answer and Discussion

The answer is B. Chronic inhalation of beryllium compounds and their products can result in a disease characterized by granulomas that affect primarily the lungs but also the skin and conjunctivae. Beryllium is found in electronics and chemical plants, aerospace factories, beryllium-mining sites, and industries in which fluorescent lights are manufactured. Changes that occur in the lungs include diffuse parenchymal inflammatory infiltrates with the development of intra-alveolar edema. The hallmark finding is a granulomatous reaction involving the hilar lymph nodes and pulmonary parenchyma, which is indistinguishable from sarcoidosis. Symptoms of the disease include dyspnea with shortness of breath, cough, and weight loss. Chest radiographs usually show diffuse alveolar consolidation with hilar lymphadenopathy. The prognosis of the disease is variable and ranges from mild pulmonary symptoms to extreme respiratory compromise and even death. Chronic exposure tends to cause a progressive decrease in pulmonary function with the development of right heart failure and cor pulmonale. Treatment is usually supportive. Steroids have been used with little benefit in chronic cases but may be used for acute berylliosis. Those exposed to beryllium dust should be counseled to protect themselves with masks and should take measures to avoid exposure. A pulmonary function test may be helpful in determining the extent of damage and the progression of disease.

Beers MH, Porter RS, eds. *The Merck manual of diagnosis and therapy,* Merck Research Laboratories, 18th ed. Whitehouse Station, NJ: Merck & Co.; 2006:472–473.

121. Which of the following drugs is associated with drug-induced lupus erythematosus (LE)?

A) Hydralazine
B) Azithromycin
C) Metoprolol
D) Digoxin
E) Penicillin

Answer and Discussion

The answer is A. Drug-induced LE is associated with the use of procainamide (most common), hydralazine, INH, penicillamine, sulfonamides, quinidine, thiouracil, methyldopa, and cephalosporins. All patients with drug-induced LE have positive reactions to ANA testing; however, they usually do not have positive reactions to antibodies to double-stranded DNA. Other laboratory findings supporting drug-induced lupus include anemia, leukopenia, thrombocytopenia, positive rheumatoid factor, positive cryoglobulins, positive lupus anticoagulants, false-positive Venereal Disease Research Laboratory (VDRL) test results, and positive results on a direct Coombs' test. Signs and symptoms include polyarthralgias, fever, butterfly rash affecting the facial area, alopecia, photosensitivity, pleurisy, proteinuria, and glomerulonephritis. In most cases, the symptoms disappear when the medication is discontinued. Steroids may be necessary for severe cases.

Kasper DL, Braunwald E, Fauci AS, et al., eds. *Harrison's principles of internal medicine,* 16th ed. New York: McGraw-Hill; 2005:1960.

122. Which of the following medications is used for the treatment of pseudomembranous colitis?

A) Metronidazole
B) Amphotericin B
C) Ketoconazole
D) Acyclovir
E) Intravenous vancomycin

Answer and Discussion

The answer is A. Overgrowth of *Clostridium difficile* in the intestine gives rise to a condition known as *pseudomembranous colitis.* The condition results from the use of antibiotics (especially clindamycin, ampicillin, and cephalosporins) usually 2 days to 6 weeks after administration. In some cases, it may occur without recent antibiotic use. Symptoms include watery diarrhea, abdominal cramps, tenesmus, low-grade fever, and, in some cases, hematochezia. Physical findings may include a tender, distended abdomen with hyperactive bowel sounds. *C. difficile* may be present in as much as 3% to 8% of healthy asymptomatic carriers. Diagnosis is made by the detection of *C. difficile* toxin in the stool and sigmoidoscopy or colonoscopy findings consisting of yellowish-white plaques of exudate with alternating areas of normal bowel mucosa. If the exudate is removed, bleeding often occurs from the affected mucosa. Not all affected patients have the identifiable lesions. Treatment involves the use of metronidazole. For infections unresponsive to metronidazole, oral vancomycin can be used. Mild cases can be treated with cholestyramine resin. *Saccharomyces boullardii* yeast may also be helpful in treatment. Complications include dehydration with electrolyte imbalances, intestinal perforation, toxic megacolon, and, in severe cases, death. Relapses may occur in up to 20% of cases.

Beers MH, Porter RS, eds. *The Merck manual of diagnosis and therapy,* Merck Research Laboratories, 18th ed. Whitehouse Station, NJ: Merck & Co.; 2006:1500.

123. Which of the following is a distinguishing feature between drug-induced and idiopathic systemic lupus erythematosis (SLE)?
A) In drug-induced lupus, there is an absence of antibodies to double-stranded DNA.
B) In drug-induced lupus, there are increased levels of complement.
C) In idiopathic SLE, a butterfly facial rash is seen.
D) Renal and central nervous system (CNS) involvement are common with drug-induced SLE.
E) There are no differences seen between the two conditions.

Answer and Discussion

The answer is A. Several drugs are known to cause a lupus-like syndrome; two of the most common are procainamide and hydralazine. Approximately 50% of patients receiving procainamide are ANA positive, and approximately 50% of those develop lupus-like symptoms. Most patients with drug-induced SLE do not have antibodies to double-stranded DNA, and they rarely have depressed levels of complement, which can distinguish drug-induced SLE from idiopathic SLE. Other laboratory abnormalities seen with drug-induced SLE include anemia, thrombocytopenia, and leukopenia. Additional findings include a positive rheumatoid factor, false-positive VDRL result, and positive direct Coombs' test. In most cases, the symptoms resolve once the medication is discontinued; however, steroid administration may be needed in severe cases. Most symptoms are completely resolved in 6 months, but ANA test results may remain positive for years. Most affected patients complain of arthralgias, myalgias, fever, and pleuritic chest pain. Renal and CNS involvement are rare with drug-induced SLE. Other medications associated with drug-induced lupus include chlorpromazine, methyldopa, and INH.

Klippel JH, ed. *Primer on the rheumatic diseases,* 11th ed. Atlanta: Arthritis Foundation; 1997:255–256.

124. The drug of choice to treat methicillin-resistant *S. aureus* is
A) penicillin
B) dicloxacillin
C) cefuroxime
D) vancomycin
E) metronidazole

Answer and Discussion

The answer is D. Methicillin-resistant *S. aureus* infection is becoming more common in hospitals and nursing homes. Increasingly, *S. aureus* infections are resistant to methicillin treatment. Burn victims, intravenous drug abusers with endocarditis, and elderly immunocompromised patients in institutionalized nursing homes are the most frequently affected groups. The most common reservoir is the nasal mucosa and oropharynx. Isolates are usually resistant to all the -cillin-type antibiotics and the cephalosporins. Intravenous vancomycin is the drug of choice for severe infections until results of susceptibility testing are known. Other medications used include trimethoprim–sulfamethoxazole (TMP-SMX), linezolid, doxycycline, and clindamycin. Duration of therapy is based on the patient's response but is usually 2 to 4 weeks. Colonization occurs in approximately 50% of treated patients. Asymptomatic colonization with methicillin-resistant *S. aureus* does not require systemic treatment; however, patients affected should be isolated.

Mouton CP, Bazalda OV, Pierce B, et al. Common infections in older adults. *Am Fam Physician.* 2001;63:257–268.

Kasper DL, Braunwald E, Fauci AS, et al., eds. *Harrison's principles of internal medicine,* 16th ed. New York: McGraw-Hill; 2005:1539.

125. Ramsay Hunt syndrome is associated with
A) herpes zoster infection affecting the geniculate ganglion of the facial nerve
B) spinothalamic disruption leading to loss of motor function in the lower extremities
C) spontaneous progressive demyelination of motor neurons
D) autoimmune destruction of norepinephrine receptors in the thalamus

Answer and Discussion

The answer is A. Ramsay Hunt syndrome is a disorder caused by the herpes zoster virus that affects the geniculate ganglion of the facial nerve. The syndrome can give rise to ipsilateral facial nerve palsy and can be distinguished from Bell's palsy by the development of vesicular herpetic lesions that affect the pharynx, external auditory canal, and, occasionally, the eighth cranial nerve. Patients report painful lesions and lose their sense of taste associated with the anterior two-thirds of the tongue.

Kasper DL, Braunwald E, Fauci AS, et al., eds. *Harrison's principles of internal medicine,* 16th ed. New York: McGraw-Hill; 2005:195, 1043, 2436.

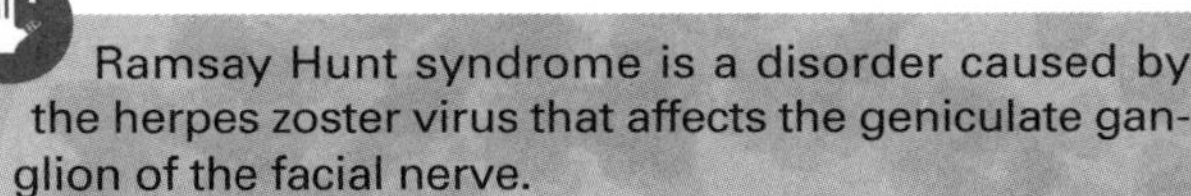

Ramsay Hunt syndrome is a disorder caused by the herpes zoster virus that affects the geniculate ganglion of the facial nerve.

126. A 10-year-old jumped off the high dive at a local swimming pool and presents to your office complaining of severe right-sided ear pain after landing on that side when he hit the water. You have seen him for this problem for the last 12 weeks, but a small perforation remains in the tympanic membrane. There is no sign of infection. Appropriate treatment at this point consists of
A) continued observation
B) an audiogram to document hearing
C) steroid otic drops
D) antibiotic ear drops and no water exposure
E) referral to an ear-nose-throat specialist

Answer and Discussion

The answer is E. Rupture of the tympanic membrane can be caused by placing objects (e.g., cotton swabs, twigs, pencils) in the ear canal, excessive positive pressure applied to the ear (e.g., explosions, loud noises), swimming, diving, or excessive negative pressure (e.g., kiss over the ear); it can be iatrogenically produced by a ventilating tube. Symptoms of traumatic rupture include a sudden severe pain followed by, in some cases, bleeding from the ear. Hearing loss and tinnitus are also usually present. Vertigo suggests damage to the inner ear. Treatment involves gentle removal of debris and blood from the otic canal and earplugs to provide protection when bathing or shampooing. Antibiotic eardrops are indicated only if there has been contamination by water or debris. Oral antibiotics can be used prophylactically to prevent infection but are generally unnecessary. Pain medication may be necessary for the first few days. Persistent perforation for more than 10 to 12 weeks is an indication for otolaryngology referral. An audiogram should be performed after treatment to document the return of hearing.

Beers MH, Porter RS, eds. *The Merck manual of diagnosis and therapy,* Merck Research Laboratories, 18th ed. Whitehouse Station, NJ: Merck & Co.; 2006:802.

127. A 50-year-old woman presents to your office complaining of nausea, diarrhea, muscle pains, urticaria, and generalized fatigue. Laboratory results show an eosinophilia. Further history reveals she has been eating summer sausage. The most likely diagnosis is
A) *Salmonella* infection
B) *Giardia* infection
C) trichinosis
D) pinworm infection
E) tularemia

Answer and Discussion

The answer is C. Trichinosis is a parasitic infection caused by the roundworm *T. spiralis*. The parasite's larvae are sometimes found in pork and occasionally in beef. The condition results from ingestion of inadequately cooked pork, wild boar, or bear products. The infection occurs worldwide but is relatively rare in the United States. Outbreaks have been linked to the consumption of inadequately prepared summer sausage. The life span of the parasite includes a larval phase that is found in inadequately cooked food. The larvae mature once in the host and mate. The females then burrow into the intestines and begin producing thousands of larvae daily. The larvae are carried to the lymphatics and by the bloodstream to multiple organs and tissues. Only the larvae that reach skeletal muscle survive. In the muscle they grow, coil up, and become encysted. Eventually they may calcify. Symptoms may be absent or mild and include nausea, diarrhea, abdominal discomfort, fever, eye pain, periorbital edema, muscle soreness and pain, urticaria, subungual hemorrhages, weakness, and generalized fatigue. Eye pain and photophobia usually precede myalgias. Laboratory results show eosinophilia, and a muscle biopsy may show the larvae or cysts. Creatine phosphokinase and lactate dehydrogenase are elevated in 50% of patients and correlate with abnormal EMGs. An enzyme-linked immunosorbent assay (ELISA) and bentonite flocculation test are highly sensitive and specific for the detection of trichinosis after 2 to 3 weeks. The parasite is rarely found in stool, blood, or CSF. Treatment involves symptomatic measures to control muscle discomfort. In most cases the infection is self-limited, often requiring only symptomatic and supportive treatment. Corticosteroids may be used in severe cases with myocardial involvement. Thiabendazole or mebendazole eliminate the adult worms from the GI tract but they have no effect on encysted larvae. In most cases, the prognosis is good. Those with myocardial involvement are at greater risk for complications.

Beers MH, Porter RS, eds. *The Merck manual of diagnosis and therapy,* Merck Research Laboratories, 18th ed. Whitehouse Station, NJ: Merck & Co.; 2006:1554–1555.

128. A 62-year-old woman presents to your office complaining of unilateral headache, temporal area tenderness, and visual disturbances. Laboratory tests show mild anemia and a sedimentation rate of 110 mm/hour. The most appropriate management includes
A) CT scan of the head
B) initiation of high-dose steroids
C) referral to an ophthalmologist
D) MRI of the head
E) initiation of NSAIDs

Answer and Discussion

The answer is B. Polymyalgia rheumatica is a generalized inflammatory disorder that tends to affect middle-age and elderly patients (usually older than 50 years). Onset of symptoms is usually rapid and includes fever, generalized fatigue, weight loss, and pain and stiffness associated with the shoulder girdle that may extend to involve other areas, including the pelvis. Laboratory tests invariably show signs of anemia and an elevated sedimentation rate usually exceeding 100 mm/hour (especially with temporal arteritis). Creatine phosphokinase levels are normal, ruling out muscle destruction. One-fourth to one-half of patients with polymyalgia rheumatica have temporal arteritis.

In many cases, temporal arteritis coexists with but usually develops after the onset of polymyalgia rheumatica. Symptoms of temporal arteritis (giant-cell arteritis) include unilateral headache, temporal area tenderness, visual disturbances, and jaw claudication. Women are more commonly affected than men. Whenever temporal arteritis is suspected, corticosteroids (60 mg/day of prednisone) should immediately be prescribed to prevent blindness, which is secondary to inflammation and occlusion of the ophthalmic arteries. Corticosteroids are also used to treat polymyalgia rheumatica, but in smaller doses (10 to 20 mg/day of prednisone) than that required for temporal arteritis. The diagnosis of polymyalgia rheumatica is usually based on clinical findings supported by the laboratory test; however, temporal arteritis is usually confirmed with a temporal artery biopsy. Treatment usually requires months of a slow, gradual taper of steroids while following the sedimentation rate. In some cases, medication may be needed for extended periods (up to 1 year); relapses requiring extended courses are not unusual.

Ferri F. *Ferri's Clinical Advisor, Instant Diagnosis and Treatment.* Philadelphia: Elsevier/Mosby; 2006:668.

129. Which of the following has been shown in multiple cohort studies to reduce the risk of colon cancer?
A) Folic acid
B) B complex vitamin
C) Aspirin
D) Vitamin C
E) Vitamin E

Answer and Discussion

The answer is C. Daily intake of aspirin has been demonstrated to decrease the risk of colorectal cancer in multiple cohort and case-control studies, although the benefit varies slightly among the studies. Considering the potential toxicity of aspirin, further information about which subgroups would benefit most from its regular use would be helpful.

Benamouzig R, Deyra J, Martin A. Daily soluble aspirin and prevention of colorectal adenoma recurrence: one-year results of the APACC trial. *Gastroenterology*. 2003;125:328–336.

130. Which of the following may prevent the development of Alzheimer's disease?
A) Ibuprofen
B) Folic acid
C) β—carotene
D) Aluminum exposure
E) Iron

Answer and Discussion

The answer is A. Observational studies suggest that the use of NSAIDs may prevent the development of Alzheimer's disease, but it is not clear if the benefit is a class effect or limited to specific agents. The role of aspirin has yet to be determined. There appears to be a consistent reduction in risk of Alzheimer's disease in patients who use NSAIDs, with greater benefit related to longer duration of use. Although aspirin also may have a protective effect, the evidence for this agent is not as evident as that for NSAIDs.

Etminan M, Gill S, Samii A. Effect of non-steroidal anti-inflammatory drugs on risk of Alzheimer's disease: systematic review and meta-analysis of observational studies. *BMJ.* 2003;327:128–131.

131. Which of the following statements about Charcot-Marie-Tooth syndrome is true?
A) Decreased pain, temperature, and vibratory sense are usually seen.
B) Symptoms include the development of a foot drop.
C) Symptoms are commonly noted at birth.
D) Hypertrophy of the distal leg muscles is common.
E) Hyperactive reflexes are noted.

Answer and Discussion

The answer is B. Charcot-Marie-Tooth syndrome (or peroneal muscular atrophy) is an inherited disorder, usually autosomal dominant, affecting the peripheral nervous system. Manifestations include weakness and atrophy of the peroneal and distal leg muscles. The condition affects motor and sensory nerves. Other features include impaired sensation and absent or hypoactive deep tendon reflexes. There are two types:

- *Type 1*: Usually occurs in middle childhood. Features include the development of a foot drop; decrease in pain, temperature, and vibratory sense; slow nerve conduction velocities; and loss of reflexes.
- *Type 2*: Usually occurs later in life and is slower in its clinical course than type 1. Nerve conduction velocities are usually normal. Patients with Charcot-Marie-Tooth syndrome typically present with abnormal high-stepped gait with frequent tripping or falling. Despite involvement with sensory nerves, complaints of limb pain and sensory disturbance are unusual. Treatment consists of braces to help prevent the associated foot drop. Surgery is reserved for those with severe foot deformities. Chemotherapeutic agents known to affect peripheral nerves should be used with great caution. Vincristine use should be avoided.

Kasper DL, Braunwald E, Fauci AS, et al., eds. *Harrison's principles of internal medicine,* 16th ed. New York: McGraw-Hill; 2005:2510.

132. Indications for pacemaker placement include which of the following?
A) Asymptomatic bradyarrhythmias
B) Mobitz II AV block
C) Atrial fibrillation
D) Atrial flutter
E) Mobitz I AV block

Answer and Discussion

The answer is B. The use of a permanent pacemaker is indicated if the patient suffers from symptomatic bradyarrhythmias, asymptomatic Mobitz II AV block, and complete heart block. First-degree AV block, thought to be a relatively benign arrhythmia, can be associated with severe symptoms that may benefit from permanent pacing. Specifically, some uncontrolled trials have shown a benefit from pacing in patients with a PR interval longer than 0.3 seconds. Type I second-degree AV block does not usually require permanent pacing, because progression to a higher degree AV block is not common. Permanent pacing is known to improve survival in patients with complete heart block, especially if they have had syncope. Single and dual chamber pacemakers are available and can be used depending on the patient's diagnosis. Typically, pacemakers are monitored on a regular basis by the patient's cardiologist with telephonic monitoring.

Kasper DL, Braunwald E, Fauci AS, et al., eds. *Harrison's principles of internal medicine,* 16th ed. New York: McGraw-Hill; 2005:1336–1356.

133. Which of the following statements about zidovudine (AZT) is true?
A) AZT is a macrolide antibiotic.
B) AZT inhibits cell wall synthesis.
C) AZT administration requires monitoring of complete blood cell counts (CBCs).
D) AZT is classified as an antifungal medication.
E) AZT does not prevent opportunistic infections in acquired immunodeficiency syndrome (AIDS) patients.

Answer and Discussion

The answer is C. AZT (Zidovudine) was the first drug approved for the treatment of HIV and AIDS. Also known as Retrovir, AZT is a thymidine analog that inhibits reverse transcriptase, an enzyme necessary for retroviral DNA synthesis, as well as viral replication. Side effects of the medication include suppression of blood elements, including erythrocytes, leukocytes (particularly granulocytes), and platelets. Because of this, frequent CBCs are necessary for monitoring; alterations in the dosage of the drug or its discontinuation may be necessary. The drug dramatically reduces perinatal transmission from HIV-infected mothers to their newborn. Combination therapy with other antiviral medications is superior to treatment with AZT alone for HIV individuals. Other side effects of the medication include headache, restlessness, malaise, dizziness, paresthesias, nausea, vomiting, and anorexia. Other drugs metabolized by the liver, including acetaminophen and TMP-SMX, may increase the risk of AZT toxicity.

Kasper DL, Braunwald E, Fauci AS, et al., eds. *Harrison's principles of internal medicine,* 16th ed. New York: McGraw-Hill; 2005:1124.

134. Which of the following medications is acceptable treatment for leishmaniasis?
A) Penicillin G
B) Tetracycline
C) Sodium antimony gluconate
D) Metronidazole
E) Acyclovir

Answer and Discussion

The answer is C. Leishmaniasis is a disease seen predominantly in Third-World countries and is transmitted by the bite of the sandfly. There are four types of this disease:

1. Visceral leishmaniasis (also known as *kala-azar* or *Leishmania donovani*) symptoms include cutaneous lesions, fever,

diarrhea, cough, lymphadenopathy, pancytopenia, cirrhosis, splenomegaly, superinfections, hyperpigmentation, and GI bleeding.

2. Old-World cutaneous leishmaniasis (*Leishmania tropica*, *Leishmania major*, and *Leishmania aethiopica*) is usually associated with a papule that develops into a necrotic lesion, followed by a hypopigmented scar on the face or legs.
3. New-World cutaneous leishmaniasis (*Leishmania braziliensis* or *Leishmania mexicana*) is associated with nodular or ulcerating lesions on the hands, face, or ears that usually resolve. Lesions associated with *L. braziliensis* may resolve or cause metastatic ulcers in the nasopharyngeal area months to years later.
4. Massive cutaneous leishmaniasis is associated with massive cutaneous lesions without involvement of the visceral organs.

Diagnosis of the condition is accomplished with biopsy of skin lesions. A leishmanin skin test can be used for diagnosis but is not widely available. Treatment is accomplished with the administration of sodium antimony gluconate, amphotericin B, or pentamidine. Itraconazole may become the drug of choice. Interferon (gamma) is used for refractive cases.

Ferri F. *Ferri's Clinical Advisor, Instant Diagnosis and Treatment.* Philadelphia: Elsevier/Mosby; 2006:477.

135. A 36-year-old construction worker is brought to the emergency room. He has been working in the sun all day and, on arrival, he exhibits hyperventilation, profuse sweating, subnormal body temperature, and hypotension. The most likely diagnosis is

A) heat stroke
B) hypothermia
C) heat exhaustion
D) thyroid storm
E) organophosphate poisoning

Answer and Discussion

The answer is C. Heat stroke is a medical emergency. Symptoms include headache, vertigo, fatigue, and increased body temperature (>40°C). Sweating is usually absent. The skin is hot and dry. Patients may exhibit bizarre and confused behavior, hallucinations, loss of consciousness, and seizures. Other manifestations include tachycardia and tachypnea; blood pressure is usually preserved. If circulatory collapse occurs, patients may suffer brain damage and even death. Patients should immediately be treated with cool water or wet dressings. Careful monitoring of body core temperature should be instituted to avoid conversion of hyperpyrexia to hypothermia. Once hospitalized, fluid replacement and further temperature management can be instituted. Complications include renal failure, cardiac failure, and the development of disseminated intravascular coagulopathy.

Heat exhaustion is different in that individuals affected usually exhibit hyperventilation, profuse sweating with substantial bodily fluid loss, and low blood pressure. Body temperature is usually normal and when elevated does not exceed 40°C. Mental status is usually normal, unlike in heat stroke. Treatment for heat exhaustion is similar to heat stroke and consists mainly of fluid resuscitation.

Beers MH, Porter RS, eds. *The Merck manual of diagnosis and therapy,* Merck Research Laboratories, 18th ed. Whitehouse Station, NJ: Merck & Co.; 2006:2608–2609.

> Heat exhaustion is different from heat stroke in that individuals affected usually exhibit hyperventilation, profuse sweating with substantial bodily fluid loss, and low blood pressure. Body temperature is usually normal and when elevated does not exceed 40°C. Mental status is usually normal, unlike in heat stroke.

136. Which of the following statements about diabetic retinopathy is true?

A) Proliferative retinopathy is associated with a poorer prognosis than nonproliferative retinopathy.
B) Nonproliferative retinopathy is associated with neovascularization.
C) Symptoms of retinopathy usually begin with eye pain.
D) Diabetics should have eye examinations every 3 years.
E) Unfortunately, there is no treatment for diabetic retinopathy.

Answer and Discussion

The answer is A. Diabetic retinopathy is the leading cause of blindness in middle-age Americans. The degree of retinopathy is highly correlated with the duration of the diabetes. The disease process is divided into the following:

- *Nonproliferative retinopathy*: characterized by dilated retinal veins, retinal hemorrhages, microaneurysms, retinal edema, and soft exudates (cotton-wool spots). Hard exudates are usually yellow in appearance and caused by chronic edema. Visual symptoms generally do not occur in the early stages of nonproliferative retinopathy.
- *Proliferative retinopathy*: associated with neovascularization and proliferation of blood vessels into the vitreous with resulting fibrosis and retinal detachment and hemorrhage.

Symptoms of diabetic retinopathy usually begin with a decrease in visual acuity. Diagnosis can be made with ophthalmologic examination and fluorescein angiography. Treatment involves panretinal laser coagulation and vitrectomy, as well as active management to control the diabetes and, if present, hypertension. The prognosis of proliferative retinopathy is worse than that of nonproliferative retinopathy. Diabetics should be encouraged to have yearly eye examinations.

Beers MH, Porter RS, eds. *The Merck manual of diagnosis and therapy,* Merck Research Laboratories, 18th ed. Whitehouse Station, NJ: Merck & Co.; 2006:918–919.

137. Which of the following findings characterize(s) aortic stenosis?

A) Lack of pressure gradient across the aortic valve
B) Angina, dyspnea, and syncope
C) Diastolic murmur that radiates to the axilla
D) Palpitations
E) Crescendo murmur with mid-systolic click

Answer and Discussion

The answer is B. Aortic stenosis occurs when there is obstruction in the blood flow through the aortic valve. Typically, there is a pressure gradient >10 mm Hg across the obstruction. The causes for aortic stenosis include previous rheumatic fever with associated damage to the valves, excessive calcification of the valves leading to narrowing, or congenital causes (e.g., bifid aortic valve). Men are more commonly affected than women. Cardiac output is usually maintained until the stenosis is severe. Once the condition becomes severe, symptoms may include the classic triad (i.e., angina, dyspnea, and syncope), especially with physical exertion. The classic symptoms of angina, exertional syncope, and dyspnea generally follow an extended latent period during which the patient is asymptomatic. The survival of patients with aortic stenosis is nearly normal until the onset of symptoms when survival rates decrease sharply. After the onset of symptoms, average survival is typically 5 years or less. Although the rate of progression of aortic stenosis is variable and difficult to predict, approximately 75% of patients with aortic stenosis die within 3 years after the onset of symptoms if the aortic valve is not replaced. Some patients with severe aortic stenosis remain asymptomatic, whereas others with moderate stenosis have symptoms attributable to the condition. The normal aortic valve area averages 2.5 cm^2, and there should normally be no gradient. A valve area of <0.8 cm^2 or a gradient of >50 mm Hg represents critical stenosis capable of causing symptoms or death. Severe cases can result in sudden death. Physical findings include a harsh systolic ejection murmur found at the left sternal border that radiates to the carotids, a palpable left ventricular heave, and delayed carotid pulse upstroke. Some patients may present with findings of CHF. Diagnosis is usually made with echocardiogram or cardiac catheterization. Severe cases should be referred for possible valve replacement. Those patients with severe aortic stenosis should avoid strenuous activity.

Shipton B, Wahba H. Valvular heart disease: review and update. *Am Fam Physician*. 2001;63:2201–2208.

138. Which of the following signs and symptoms are associated with Sjögren's syndrome?
A) Hepatomegaly, chronic rhinitis, and palmar erythema
B) Keratoconjunctivitis, parotid gland enlargement, and xerostomia
C) Confusion, tremors, and peripheral neuropathies
D) Polycythemia, leukocytosis, and negative rheumatoid factor
E) Hyperextensibility of joints, iriditis, and glossitis

Answer and Discussion

The answer is B. Sjögren's syndrome is a rare chronic inflammatory disorder that leads to dry mouth, dry eyes (keratoconjunctivitis sicca), dryness of other mucous membranes, and joint pain. Women are more commonly affected. The disease is often found in conjunction with autoimmune disorders such as scleroderma, rheumatoid arthritis, and lupus. The cause is unknown, but there has been a genetic link with the HLA-DR3 focus. Signs include keratoconjunctivitis, parotid gland enlargement, xerostomia, and loss of taste and smell. Other complications include alopecia, increased risk of pulmonary infections, pancreatitis, pericarditis, sensory neuropathies, interstitial nephritis, and renal tubular acidosis. Laboratory findings include positive rheumatoid factor (seen in 70% of affected patients), elevated ESR (70% of affected patients), anemia (33% of affected patients), and leukopenia and eosinophilia (25% of affected patients). Diagnosis is accomplished with the Schirmer test, which measures the quantity of tears secreted in 5 minutes in response to irritation from a filter paper strip placed under each lower eyelid. Many patients affected with Sjögren's are at increased risk for lymphoma and Waldenström's macroglobulinemia. Treatment is aimed at control of symptoms. In some cases, steroids and immunosuppressants may be used.

Beers MH, Porter RS, eds. *The Merck manual of diagnosis and therapy*, Merck Research Laboratories, 18th ed. Whitehouse Station, NJ: Merck & Co.; 2006:264–266.

139. Which of the following is the most appropriate medication for the treatment of hypertension in a diabetic patient?
A) β-Blocker
B) ACE inhibitor
C) Diuretic
D) Calcium-channel blocker
E) α-Blocker

Answer and Discussion

The answer is B. ACE inhibitors (e.g., captopril, enalapril, lisinopril, ramipril) function as afterload reducers by inhibiting the renin-angiotensin-aldosterone system. They have been shown to reduce mortality rates in patients with CHF. They are also widely used as a first-choice drug in the management of hypertension because of their favorable side effect profile. The mechanism of action involves the blockage of angiotensin I to angiotensin II, resulting in a decrease in aldosterone production, which leads to increased sodium and water excretion. Hemodynamic effects include decreased peripheral resistance, increased renal blood flow, and minimal effects on cardiac output and glomerular filtration rate. Adverse effects include headaches, nausea, dizziness, skin rashes, nonproductive irritative cough (10% to 20% of patients), acute renal failure in patients with renal artery stenosis, and angioneurotic edema. ACE inhibitors are generally not associated with depression, sedation, fatigue, or impotence. They can be useful in preserving renal function in patients with diabetes. Those patients with preexisting renal insufficiency or renal artery stenosis require close monitoring of renal function when ACE inhibitors are administered. Patients with CHF, diabetes, peripheral vascular disease, history of recent MI, hyperlipidemia, and renal insufficiency are good candidates for ACE inhibitors.

Kermani M, Dua A, Gradman AH. Underutilization and clinical benefits of angiotensin-converting enzyme inhibitors in patients with asymptomatic left ventricular dysfunction. *Am J Cardiol*. 2000;86:644–648.

Rakel RE, Bope ET. *Conn's Current Therapy 2005*. Philadelphia: Elsevier/Saunders; 2005:889, 36–37, 333–334, 833.

140. Which of the following factors is an absolute contraindication for the use of thrombolytics in the treatment of myocardial infarction?
A) Altered mental status
B) More than 4 hours has elapsed since the onset of the chest pain
C) Current menstruation
D) The patient has renal insufficiency
E) The patient has a history of diabetic retinopathy

Answer and Discussion

The answer is A. Every patient with an evolving myocardial infarction should be evaluated for thrombolytic therapy. Thrombolytic therapy reduces in-hospital and 1-year mortality by 25%. The criteria for an evolving myocardial infarction include the following:

- Thirty minutes of cardiogenic chest pain.
- At least 1 mm of ST elevation in at least two adjacent limbs or at least 2 mm elevation of precordial chest leads noted on ECG tracings.

- New left bundle branch block.
- Patients with complete bundle branch block and cardiogenic chest pain may also benefit from thrombolytics.

Patients with only ST segment depression do not benefit from thrombolytics, nor do patients with normal ECGs.

Medications such as tissue-type plasminogen activator (tPA), also known as alteplase, tenecteplase (TNK) and reteplase (rPA), and streptokinase, which are fibrin-specific agents, should be administered as soon as possible up to 12 hours after the onset of chest pain. Those who receive medication within the first 6 hours have the best outcome. Absolute contraindications to thrombolytics include recent surgery (within 4 weeks) or biopsy of a noncompressible site within 2 weeks, any history of hemorrhagic stroke, unclear mental status, the possibility of aortic dissection, active bleeding, pericarditis, prolonged (more than 10 minutes) of cardiopulmonary resuscitation, and antibodies to streptokinase or its use within the previous 12 months (in which case tissue-type plasminogen activator should be given). Relative contraindications include history of GI or GU hemorrhage within the past 6 months; trauma; history of cardiopulmonary resuscitation within the previous month; uncontrolled hypertension (systolic BP >180 mm Hg and diastolic BP >110 mm Hg); intracranial or systemic neoplasm; prior (nonhemorrhagic) stroke; pregnancy; or liver dysfunction. Minor hemorrhage, menstruation, and diabetic retinopathy are not contraindications to fibrinolytic therapy.

Kasper DL, Braunwald E, Fauci AS, et al., eds. *Harrison's principles of internal medicine,* 16th ed. New York: McGraw-Hill; 2005:1453–1454.

141. Which of the following tests is considered routine (recommended) in the initial evaluation of a patient with hypertension?

A) Chest x-ray
B) TSH
C) Uric acid level
D) 24-hour urine protein
E) ECG

Answer and Discussion

The answer is E. The initial evaluation of a patient with hypertension should include a thorough history and a number of tests, including the following:

Routine tests

- CBC
- Chemistry panel, including fasting, glucose, potassium, creatinine, and BUN
- Cholesterol panel (total cholesterol and HDL [LDL] cholesterol)
- 12-lead ECG
- Urinalysis

Optional tests

- Creatinine clearance
- 24-hour urinary protein
- Uric acid
- Glycosylated Hb
- TSH
- Limited echocardiography
- Chest x-ray

Hypertension exists when the diastolic blood pressure is consistently measured >90 mm Hg and a systolic blood pressure remains >140 mm Hg. Initial management should consist of sodium restriction, limitation of alcohol consumption, and a regular exercise program. Overweight patients should be counseled to lose weight. Other tests to assess kidney function, cardiac performance, or endocrine abnormalities (e.g., pheochromocytoma) are usually unnecessary. JNC 7 strongly recommends that physicians intervene with lifestyle modifications that can prevent or delay the onset of hypertension in patients. That recommendation takes on special importance in the definition of the new class of "prehypertension," those patients who have systolic pressures between 120 and 139 mm Hg or diastolic pressures between 80 and 89 mm Hg, who are at increased risk of bad outcomes and high risk for development of diagnosed hypertension. Furthermore, JNC 7 emphasizes that proper lifestyle intervention in hypertension should serve as the equivalent of one drug in a multidrug regimen.

Seventh Report of the Joint National Committee on Prevention, Detection, Evaluation and Treatment of High Blood Pressure (JNC 7) Express. National Heart, Lung, and Blood Institute. Bethesda, Md. 2003. *JAMA.* 2003;289:2560–2571.

142. A 62-year-old business executive with a history of migraines is noted to have hypertension; otherwise, he is healthy. Which of the following is the best medication for the treatment of his hypertension?

A) β-Blocker
B) Angiotensin-receptor blocker
C) α-Blocker
D) ACE inhibitor
E) Thiazide diuretic

Answer and Discussion

The answer is A. β-Blockers are used as first-line therapy for the treatment of uncomplicated hypertension. These agents decrease the heart rate and cardiac output. β1-Adrenergic receptors are located in the cardiac muscle, whereas β2-adrenergic receptors are located in the bronchial musculature. Adverse effects include exacerbation of bronchoconstriction in asthmatics because of β2-receptor blockade, bradycardia, left ventricular failure, nasal congestion, nightmares, Raynaud's phenomenon, fatigue, depression, cold extremities, and impotence. β-Blockers are also associated with elevated triglycerides and decreased HDL cholesterol; however, there is not enough effect on lipids to discourage their use in select cases. These agents are contraindicated in patients with poorly controlled diabetes, second- or third-degree heart block, or moderate to severe asthma; however, these agents have been shown to improve survival after myocardial infarction and in select patients with CHF. These agents have also been used for the treatment of "stage fright" and as migraine prophylaxis. β-Blockers should not be discontinued abruptly because of the risk of rebound hypertension.

Ko DT, Hebert PR, Coffey CS. Adverse effects of β-blocker therapy for patients with heart failure. A quantitative overview of randomized trials. *Arch Intern Med.* 2004;164:1389–1394.

Weir MR, Moser M. Diuretics and β-blockers: is there a risk for dyslipidemia? *Am Heart J.* 2000;139:174–184.

Salpeter SR, Ormiston TM, Salpeter EE. Cardioselective β-blockers in patients with reactive airway disease: a meta-analysis. *Ann Intern Med.* 2002;137:715–725.

Epstein PE. Fresh air and β-blockade [Editorial]. *Ann Intern Med.* 2002;137:766–767.

143. Which of the following combinations would be best utilized in the treatment of diastolic heart failure?
A) Calcium-channel blocker + α-blocker
B) β-blocker + diuretic
C) ACE inhibitor + α-blocker
D) Calcium-channel blocker + diuretic
E) Angiotensin-receptor blocker + calcium-channel blocker

Answer and Discussion

The answer is B. Diastolic heart failure is a major contributor of morbidity and mortality. The condition is defined as symptoms of heart failure in a patient with a normal left ventricular function. It is characterized by a stiff left ventricle with decreased compliance and impaired relaxation, which leads to increased end diastolic pressure. Signs and symptoms are similar to those of heart failure with systolic dysfunction. The diagnosis of diastolic heart failure is made with transthoracic echocardiography. Treatment of diastolic heart failure should include normalizing blood pressure, promoting regression of left ventricular hypertrophy, avoiding tachycardia, treating symptoms of congestion, and maintaining normal atrial contraction when possible. Diuretic therapy is the mainstay of treatment for preventing pulmonary congestion, while β blockers appear to be useful in preventing tachycardia and thereby prolonging left ventricular diastolic filling time. Angiotensin-converting enzyme inhibitors and angiotensin-receptor blockers may be beneficial in patients with diastolic dysfunction, especially those with hypertension.

Gutierriez C, Blanchard DG. Diastolic heart failure: challenges of diagnosis and treatment. *Am Fam Physician.* 2004;69:2609–2616.

144. A 58-year-old man presents to your office 4 weeks after being hospitalized for myocardial infarction. He is complaining of chest pain, fever, and multiple joint pain. Laboratory tests do not show an increase in cardiac enzymes. The most likely diagnosis is
A) Dressler's syndrome
B) costochondritis
C) Meigs' syndrome
D) recurrent myocardial infarction
E) pneumonia

Answer and Discussion

The answer is A. Dressler's syndrome, or postmyocardial infarction syndrome, occurs several days to several weeks after myocardial infarction. The condition is characterized by chest pain, fever, pericarditis with a pericardial friction rub, pericardial effusion, pleurisy, pleural effusions, and multiple joint pain. The cause is thought to be an autoimmune response to the damaged myocardial tissue and pericardium. The difference between Dressler's syndrome and recurrent myocardial infarction is difficult to determine; however, in Dressler's syndrome, there is minimal or no increase in cardiac enzymes. Treatment includes the use of aspirin, NSAIDs, and, in some cases, corticosteroids.

Beers MH, Porter RS, eds. *The Merck manual of diagnosis and therapy,* Merck Research Laboratories, 18th ed. Whitehouse Station, NJ: Merck & Co.; 2006:651–652, 732–737.

145. A patient transferred from an outlying hospital after being involved in a serious motor vehicle accident has a positive dipstick for hemoglobinuria, but erythrocytes are not noted on microscopic examination. The most likely diagnosis is
A) myocardial contusion
B) rhabdomyolysis
C) intravascular hemolysis
D) renal contusion
E) laceration of the spleen

Answer and Discussion

The answer is B. A positive urine dipstick for hemoglobin results from free hemoglobin or myoglobin in the urine. Free hemoglobin appears in the urine when there is intravascular hemolysis. Once haptoglobin becomes saturated, free hemoglobin spills into the urine. A common cause is a transfusion reaction. Myoglobinuria is associated with rhabdomyolysis and occurs when there is significant muscle injury with the release of myoglobin into the bloodstream. Causes include electrical shock or massive muscle trauma. Other causes may include toxin exposures, metabolic disorders, inflammatory conditions, and infection. Myoglobinuria causes a positive urine test for blood in the absence of urinary erythrocytes.

Beers MH, Porter RS, eds. *The Merck manual of diagnosis and therapy,* Merck Research Laboratories, 18th ed. Whitehouse Station, NJ: Merck & Co.; 2006:1930.

Myoglobinuria causes a positive urine test for blood in the absence of urinary erythrocytes.

146. Positive results for which of the following tests support the diagnosis of de Quervain's tenosynovitis?
A) Allen's test
B) Finkelstein's test
C) Lachman's test
D) Anterior–posterior drawer test
E) Phalen's test

Answer and Discussion

The answer is B. The abductor pollicis longus and the extensor pollicis brevis share a common protective sheath that can become inflamed, giving rise to de Quervain's tenosynovitis. Patients usually report pain with movement of the fibrous bands that make up the first dorsal compartment over the radial styloid. Paresthesia and pain that radiates distally into the thumb and dorsal part of the hand and index finger may occur. In most cases, the patient has a history of repetitive motions of the hand or thumb. A positive Finkelstein's test is the hallmark test finding: Pain occurs when a fist is made over the thumb and the wrist is placed in ulnar deviation. Long-standing inflammation may lead to calcification of the tendon and its sheath and is visible on a radiograph. Treatment options involve rest, anti-inflammatory agents, immobilization of the affected area with a thumb spica splint, and injection of the compartment with 0.5 mL of steroid and 1 mL of 1% lidocaine. The splint is to be worn for 3 weeks; surgery is rarely necessary but can be considered in refractive cases.

Rakel RE, Bope ET. *Conn's Current Therapy 2005.* Philadelphia: Elsevier/Saunders; 2005:1134.

147. Which of the following statements about testicular tumors is true?
A) Boys ages 10 to 15 years are most commonly affected.
B) African-American men are more commonly affected.

C) Seminomas are the most common type.
D) The prognosis is extremely poor.
E) Carcinoembryonic antigen levels are elevated.

Answer and Discussion

The answer is C. Testicular tumors are usually found in men between 20 and 35 years of age. They are relatively uncommon and tend to affect white men more than African-American men. Cryptorchidism is associated with a higher incidence of tumor formation. The tumors are categorized as seminomas (most common) or nonseminomatous germ cell tumors. Symptoms include painless swelling or enlargement of the testicle and testicular heaviness. Diagnosis is confirmed with testicular ultrasound examination. Tumor markers, including human chorionic gonadotropin and α-fetoprotein, may be elevated in affected patients. In most cases, treatment involves surgical removal of the testicle or radiation therapy. If diagnosed in the early stages, the prognosis is usually excellent; therefore, young men should perform monthly testicular self-examinations.

Kasper DL, Braunwald E, Fauci AS, et al., eds. *Harrison's principles of internal medicine,* 16th ed. New York: McGraw-Hill; 2005:550–552.

148. Olecranon bursitis is usually the result of
A) deposition of negative birefringent crystals in the bursa
B) repeated trauma to the elbow
C) autoimmune destruction of the joint leading to a reactive bursitis
D) referred pain from the wrist
E) staphylococcal infection

Answer and Discussion

The answer is B. Olecranon bursitis (also known as *miner's elbow*) is an inflammation that affects the olecranon bursa. The inflammation is usually caused by repeated trauma to the affected area, such as repeated weightbearing on the elbow. Patients usually report pain, discomfort, and swelling of the elbow area. In some cases, the bursa may harbor an infection, which may require antibiotic treatment; in most cases, there is no associated infection. Treatment involves anti-inflammatories, aspiration of the fluid, and, in some cases, steroid injection followed by the use of a pressure dressing to help prevent reaccumulation of fluid. Infection should be excluded before administering steroid medication. The avoidance of trauma to the elbow should also be emphasized for treatment. Surgery may be necessary for resistant and debilitating cases.

Chumbley EM, O'Conner FG, Nirschl RB. Evaluation of overuse elbow injuries. *Am Fam Physician.* 2000;61:691–700.

149. The most effective drug for the treatment of traveler's diarrhea is
A) metronidazole
B) tetracycline
C) ciprofloxacin
D) trimethoprim–sulfamethoxazole (TMP-SMX)
E) doxycycline

Answer and Discussion

The answer is C. Travel to Third-World countries can be complicated by traveler's diarrhea. The incidence ranges from 4% to >50%. The most common pathogens are enteropathogens (e.g., *E. coli*) in approximately 80% of cases; occasionally, viruses such as the Norwalk agent or rotavirus are causative. Traditionally, the problem was treated with TMP-SMX and bismuth subsalicylate (Pepto-Bismol). However, the quinolones (e.g., ciprofloxacin, levofloxacin, norfloxacin) are now the most effective drugs in the treatment of traveler's diarrhea. Loperamide (Imodium) can also be used if fever or bloody diarrhea is not present. The traveler should also take precautions by eating only freshly prepared foods that are adequately cooked, eating freshly peeled fruits, drinking only boiled or bottled water, and avoiding tap water and ice made from tap water (even in alcoholic drinks). Bismuth subsalicylate (Pepto-Bismol) is a helpful prophylaxis, but it must be taken four times daily (60 mL or 2 tablets). The use of prophylactic antibiotics is controversial, but, in most cases, is discouraged because of the risk of developing resistant organisms.

Kasper DL, Braunwald E, Fauci AS, et al., eds. *Harrison's principles of internal medicine,* 16th ed. New York: McGraw-Hill; 2005:727–728.

150. Which of the following statements about orthostatic hypotension is true?
A) It is a decrease in systolic blood pressure that occurs when moving from a standing to a sitting position.
B) It is commonly associated with a decrease in pulse rate.
C) In some cases, it is associated with antidepressant medications.
D) It is rarely associated with symptoms.
E) The condition results from volume overload.

Answer and Discussion

The answer is C. *Orthostatic hypotension* is defined as a decrease in systolic blood pressure of at least 20 mm Hg (systolic) and at least 10 mm Hg (diastolic) that occurs when moving from a supine to an upright position. Also, orthostatic tachycardia is defined as an increase in heart rate >27 bpm or to a level >108 bpm. Measurements of blood pressure and pulse rate should be taken after the individual has been in an upright position for 3 minutes. Causes of orthostatic hypotension include volume depletion, medications (e.g., tricyclic antidepressants, antihypertensive agents), and autonomic dysfunction (as seen in diabetic patients). Elderly patients are at increased risk, and syncope may result. Treatment involves volume replacement, discontinuation of offending pharmacologic medications, and slow positional changes.

Beers MH, Porter RS, eds. *The Merck manual of diagnosis and therapy,* Merck Research Laboratories, 18th ed. Whitehouse Station, NJ: Merck & Co.; 2006:581–584.

151. A 17-year-old woman arrives in the emergency room with carpal–pedal spasms and circumoral paresthesias. She was brought in by paramedics after she fainted at a rock concert. The most likely diagnosis is
A) cardiac arrhythmia
B) seizure disorder
C) hyperventilation
D) heat exhaustion
E) cocaine overdose

Answer and Discussion

The answer is C. Hyperventilation can lead to a significant respiratory alkalosis and is frequently the result of anxiety or extreme excitement. Other less common causes include drug effects, CNS dysfunction, alcohol withdrawal, asthma, heart failure, pulmonary embolus, exposure to high altitudes, intense exercise, and chronic pain. Symptoms include carpal–pedal spasms, circumoral and extremity paresthesias, light-headedness, giddiness, and sometimes syncope. Blood gases usually show low CO_2 (20 to 25 mm Hg) and elevated pH. Treatment can be accomplished by breathing into a paper bag. Other efforts should be directed at the treatment of anxiety or underlying contributing factors; relaxation training may be beneficial.

Beers MH, Porter RS, eds. *The Merck manual of diagnosis and therapy,* Merck Research Laboratories, 18th ed. Whitehouse Station, NJ: Merck & Co.; 2006:358–359.

152. Which of the following statements about herpes infections is true?
A) Type 1 is most commonly associated with genital infections.
B) Topical acyclovir is used for prophylaxis.
C) Recurrent outbreaks are usually more severe than an initial outbreak.
D) The rash usually consists of pustules, papules, and macules.
E) Multinucleated giant cells are seen with Tzanck smears.

Answer and Discussion

The answer is E. Herpes simplex infections are divided into type 1, which usually affects the oral mucosa, and type 2, which usually affects the genitals. The virus invades the nervous tissue and remains dormant in the skin or nerve ganglia. Symptoms include recurrent, clear vesicles that usually occur in clusters and are extremely painful; fever; arthralgias; and adenopathy. Initial attacks are usually more severe and longer in duration than repeated attacks. Before the appearance of the vesicles, the patient may report paresthesias or tingling at the site of the outbreak. Transmission occurs by direct contact and is usually sexually transmitted, particularly for type 2. Repeated attacks are usually precipitated by excessive sunlight exposure, menstruation, stress, and febrile illnesses. Laboratory tests include positive Tzanck smears (with the presence of multinucleated giant cells), cultures (gold standard for diagnosis), and rapid immunofluorescent antibody tests. The treatment of choice involves the use of topical and oral antiviral medication (acyclovir, valacyclovir, and famciclovir). Oral administration is more effective and should be begun at the initial onset of clinical symptoms. For severe cases, intravenous acyclovir may be used. In some cases, daily prophylactic oral therapy may be necessary.

Ferri F. *Ferri's Clinical Advisor, Instant Diagnosis and Treatment.* Philadelphia: Elsevier/Mosby; 2006:385–386.

153. A 42-year-old male presents with multiple pigmented skin lesions, ataxia, and decreased hearing. Other family members are similarly affected. The most likely diagnosis is
A) hemochromatosis
B) malignant melanoma
C) neurofibromatosis
D) Sturge–Weber syndrome
E) measles

Answer and Discussion

The answer is C. Neurofibromatosis (also known as von Recklinghausen's disease) is an autosomal-dominant disorder that is characterized by pigmented skin lesions (café-au-lait spots) and neuromas affecting the skin and nerves. As many as 33% of patients are asymptomatic. Symptomatic patients may have blindness, dizziness, ataxia, deafness secondary to acoustic neuromas, or other symptoms related to nerve compression from neuromas. The diagnosis of neurofibromatosis is supported by the detection of more than six pigmented lesions or one lesion larger than 1.5 cm. Asymptomatic patients do not require further therapy; however, those who exhibit symptoms may require surgery or radiation to remove offending neuromas. Genetic counseling is recommended.

Beers MH, Porter RS, eds. *The Merck manual of diagnosis and therapy,* Merck Research Laboratories, 18th ed. Whitehouse Station, NJ: Merck & Co.; 2006:2377–2379.

154. Guillain-Barré syndrome is most closely associated with
A) normal electromyogram (EMG) findings found late in the course
B) descending asymmetric paralysis
C) previous trauma
D) symptoms that usually begin in the lower extremities
E) low levels of protein in the cerebrospinal fluid (CSF)

Answer and Discussion

The answer is D. Guillain-Barré syndrome is an acute or subacute demyelinating polyradiculopathy that often follows an infection (two-thirds of patients recall a recent viral infection), vaccinations (rabies, influenza), malignancy (lymphomas), medications (streptokinase, captopril, danazol), or surgical procedure. Although it is believed to be associated with an immunologic response, the exact mechanism is unknown. The presenting complaint is usually weakness associated with the proximal muscles in a symmetric distribution that varies in severity. Paresthesias of the toes and fingers may also occur. The symptoms usually begin in the lower extremity and may progress to involve the arms and face (ascending symmetric paralysis). In severe cases, the respiratory muscles may be affected, and the patient may require mechanical ventilation. Sensory-related paresthesias are common. Other symptoms include tachycardia, hypotension, hypertension, diaphoresis, hyporeflexia, and loss of sphincter control. Laboratory findings include elevated protein levels and minimal lymphocytic pleocytosis in CSF samples, altered electromyelogram (EMG) findings, and evidence of demyelination on nerve biopsies. Treatment involving the use of plasmapheresis and intravenous Ig has been shown to be beneficial, particularly early in the course of the disease (i.e., within the first few days). Steroids have not been shown to be beneficial and may actually worsen the outcome. Most cases resolve spontaneously, but recovery may take months. Mortality is approximately 10%. Up to 20% of patients may be left with persisting deficits. Approximately 3% may develop relapses, sometimes years later.

Ferri F. *Ferri's Clinical Advisor, Instant Diagnosis and Treatment.* Philadelphia: Elsevier/Mosby; 2006:355.

The symptoms of Guillain-Barré syndrome usually begin in the lower extremities and may progress to involve the arms and face (ascending symmetric paralysis).

155. An obese, hypertensive woman is involved in a motor vehicle accident. Skull films show an enlarged sella turcica. Further questioning reveals that the patient has also complained of galactorrhea, and results of a recent prolactin test were abnormal. The most likely diagnosis is

A) Sheehan's syndrome
B) empty sella syndrome
C) subdural hematoma
D) subarachnoid hemorrhage
E) undetected pregnancy at 12 to 16 weeks' gestation

Answer and Discussion

The answer is B. Empty sella syndrome is a congenital abnormality that results in abnormal formation of the sella turcica, in which the hypothalamus and pituitary gland are found. In many cases, an enlarged sella turcica is seen by chance on a skull radiograph. Diagnosis is confirmed by a CT scan or MRI. Those affected are usually obese women who have hypertension and benign intracranial hypertension. In most cases, the individual is asymptomatic. However, patients may have persistent rhinorrhea or pituitary disorders, including tumors releasing growth hormone, ACTH, or prolactin. No treatment is required if empty sella syndrome is present without other abnormalities.

Beers MH, Porter RS, eds. *The Merck manual of diagnosis and therapy,* Merck Research Laboratories, 18th ed. Whitehouse Station, NJ: Merck & Co.; 2006:1179.

156. Which of the following medications would improve survival following a myocardial infarction?

A) Metoprolol
B) Hydrochlorothiazide
C) Warfarin
D) Nitroglycerin
E) Morphine

Answer and Discussion

The answer is A. β-Blockers reduce mortality during both acute and long-term management of myocardial infarction. Administration of intravenous β-blockers within 12 to 24 hours of infarction, followed by oral therapy, has been found to significantly reduce the mortality rate within the first week of infarction. The most marked reduction occurs in the first 2 days after infarction. Initiation of β-blocker therapy within days to weeks after infarction and continuation of therapy has been shown to reduce total mortality, nonfatal myocardial infarction and sudden death. This has been shown regardless of the patient's age or sex, infarct location, and initial heart rate, or the presence or absence of ventricular arrhythmias. The greatest benefit occurs in high-risk patients, including the elderly and those with large anterior infarctions, arrhythmias, or left ventricular dysfunction.

Kasper DL, Braunwald E, Fauci AS, et al., eds. *Harrison's principles of internal medicine,* 16th ed. New York: McGraw-Hill; 2005:1452, 1455.

157. A 72-year-old female presents to the emergency room with the acute onset of right-sided hemiplegia. She is conscious but confused and agitated. Blood pressure is measured at 210/110. She has no cardiac findings. Appropriate management at this time should be

A) the administration of IV labetatolol
B) oral administration of clonidine
C) additional dose of her calcium channel blocker
D) sublingual nifedipine
E) observation

Answer and Discussion

The answer is E. Unless systolic blood pressure >20 mm Hg or diastolic pressure >120 mm Hg (sustained on repeated measurement), elevated blood pressure should not be treated within the first days after ischemic stroke. The reason is that perfusion is directly linked to mean arterial pressure. Acute elevations in blood pressure are often transient, and spontaneous declines are common. Aggressive treatment of hypertension following acute ischemic stroke can convert vulnerable areas of the brain into an infarct. The two exceptions to this general recommendation are (1) after use of tissue plasminogen activator (tPA), blood pressure should be maintained below 185/110 mm Hg; and (2) in the presence of myocardial infarction, heart failure, or aortic dissection, elevated blood pressure should be treated aggressively. If antihypertensive therapy is necessary, agents that have a rapid onset and predictable response should be used.

Kasper DL, Braunwald E, Fauci AS, et al., eds. *Harrison's principles of internal medicine,* 16th ed. New York: McGraw-Hill; 2005:2373–2375.

158. Which of the following medications should be avoided in patients with hypertrophic obstructive cardiomyopathy?

A) Aspirin
B) Digoxin
C) Disopyramide
D) Acetaminophen
E) Atenolol

Answer and Discussion

The answer is B. Hypertrophic obstructive cardiomyopathy is an autosomal-dominant transmitted disorder that is characterized by an enlarged cardiac septum, which obstructs blood flow from the left ventricle. Symptoms include dizziness, light-headedness, palpitations, chest pain, dyspnea, or syncope with physical exertion. The most important complication of the disease is sudden death. The condition has an annual incidence of 4% to 6% in children and 2% of adults affected. Signs include pulses that are bifid and brisk in upstroke and a systolic-ejection-type murmur positioned along the left sternal border, which becomes louder with movements that decrease venous return (afterload), such as standing or Valsalva's maneuver. Movements that increase venous return (afterload), such as squatting, reduce the murmur. ECG usually shows evidence of left ventricular hypertrophy and septal Q waves in the lateral leads. Diagnosis is accomplished by echocardiogram. First-line treatment is accomplished with the use of β-blockers. Disopyramide (Norpace) may be used as an alternative. Verapamil has also been used frequently on an empiric basis especially in atrial fibrillation but its effect is unpredictable and acute hemodynamic collapse is described in patients with substantial gradients or severe diastolic dysfunction. Digoxin should be avoided. Because of the risk for sudden death, extreme physical exertion should be avoided.

Kasper DL, Braunwald E, Fauci AS, et al., eds. *Harrison's principles of internal medicine,* 16th ed. New York: McGraw-Hill; 2005:1410.

159. Which of the following statements regarding aminoglycosides is true?

A) Liver function should be followed closely during administration.
B) Volume of distribution is increased in obese patients.

C) Nephrotoxic effects can occur with administration.
D) Lupus-like syndrome can occur with prolonged use.
E) Respiratory depression is not associated with aminoglycosides.

Answer and Discussion

The answer is C. Toxicity associated with the use of aminoglycosides (e.g., gentamicin) includes ototoxicity with clinically apparent hearing loss (<1% of cases), tinnitus, and vertigo, as well as nephrotoxic effects (5% to 10% of adults who receive therapy for 10 to 14 days), including renal failure. Rarely, respiratory depression can occur. Drug levels should be followed after a steady state is achieved—every 3 to 5 days or more often if increases in serum creatinine are noted. Patients with decreased renal function may need an adjustment of medication based on their creatinine clearance. Some data suggest that once-daily administration may cause less nephrotoxicity. Aminoglycosides have low solubility in lipids; therefore, the volume of distribution is decreased in obese patients. Patients with trauma, burns, cancer, and postoperative septic shock have increased volumes of distribution. Neuromuscular depression from aminoglycosides is caused by reduced acetylcholine activity at postsynaptic membranes and can result in rare but severe respiratory depression. This can be largely avoided if the aminoglycoside is given intravenously over 30 minutes or by intramuscular injection. If respiratory depression does occur, it can be reversed by the administration of calcium.

Kasper DL, Braunwald E, Fauci AS, et al., eds. *Harrison's principles of internal medicine,* 16th ed. New York: McGraw-Hill; 2005:801–802.

160. Which of the following best describes migraine headaches?
A) Aura following the resolution of the headache
B) Recurrent headaches lasting less than 4 hours
C) Unilateral, throbbing headache
D) Bilateral band-like headache
E) Rhinitis with facial pain

Answer and Discussion

The answer is C. There are basically two types of migraine headaches: those with an aura (classic migraine) and those without an aura (common migraine). A classic migraine is characterized by recurrent attacks of a moderate to severe unilateral, throbbing headache that is usually preceded by visual prodrome, which may include scotomata, zigzag lines, photopsia, or visual distortions. Patients also report nausea, vomiting, photophobia, mood swings, food cravings, and heightened perception of smell. The unilateral "throbbing" headache may become generalized and usually lasts 4 to 72 hours. Patients usually report a positive family history. Migraines usually begin at 10 to 40 years of age and are more common in women. The pathophysiology is not fully understood. Whether vasodilation or vasoconstriction is a cause or an effect of the migraine is unclear.

Tryptans such as sumatriptan (Imitrex) that activate serotonin receptors (5-hydroxytryptamine) block neurogenic inflammation and can abort migraine pain in approximately 70% of patients. Additionally, vasoconstrictors, such as ergotamines, have also been used to treat migraines. Other medications used include NSAIDs and narcotic analgesics. Migraine attacks may be triggered by emotional or physical stress, lack of sleep, specific foods (e.g., chocolate, cheese), alcohol, oral contraceptives, or menstruation. Migraines usually disappear during pregnancy. Antiemetics and intravenous hydration may be needed if associated vomiting is severe. β-Blockers, low-dose amitriptyline, topiramate (Topamax) and other antiseizure medications, and calcium-channel blockers may be used for prophylaxis—particularly if patients have more than one migraine per week. Most patients experience a decrease in the number and intensity of headaches as they age. Common migraines are identical to classic migraines except the patient does not have an aura, and the headache may last longer.

Aukerman G, Knutson D, Miser WF. Management of acute migraine. *Am Fam Physician*. 2002;66:2123–2130, 2140–2141.

161. Which of the following can improve survival in patients with severe COPD?
A) Supplemental oxygen
B) Beta agonist
C) Inhaled corticosteroids
D) Smoking cessation
E) Pulse antibiotic therapy

Answer and Discussion

The answer is A. For patients with the diagnosis of severe COPD only the administration of supplemental oxygen has been shown to positively affect survival, reduce dyspnea, and reduce pulmonary artery pressure. B agonist and inhaled corticosteroids can lower the rate of exacerbations but have no direct effect on survival. Discontinuation of smoking can slow the decline in lung function but has no effect on survival. Pulse antibiotic therapy does not directly affect mortality.

Sin DD, McAlister FA, Man SF, et al. Contemporary management of chronic obstructive pulmonary disease: Scientific review. *JAMA*. 2003; 290(17):2301–2312.

162. Which of the following sequences represents how a typical anteroseptal myocardial infarction progresses on ECG?
A) Q-wave development, peaked T-waves, ST-segment elevation, T-wave inversion
B) T-wave inversion, Q-wave development, ST-segment elevation, peaked T-waves
C) Peaked T-waves, ST-segment elevation, Q-wave development, T-wave inversion
D) Peaked T waves, Q-wave development, ST-segment elevation, T-wave inversion
E) ST-segment elevation, T-wave inversion, Q-wave development, peaked T-waves

Answer and Discussion

The answer is C. The natural progression of ECG changes seen with myocardial infarction include peaked hyperacute T waves to ST-segment elevation, to Q-wave development, and to T-wave inversion. In anteroseptal infarction, ECG changes are usually noted in leads V1 through V3. Q waves indicate a transmural infarct.

Schroeder SA, Krupp MA, Tierney LM Jr, et al. *Current Medical Diagnosis and Treatment*. Norwalk, CT: Appleton & Lange; 1990:259.

163. The presence of a "bamboo spine" on spine radiographs, elevated erythrocyte sedimentation rate (ESR), and a positive test for HLA-B27 support the diagnosis of
A) multiple myeloma
B) Reiter's syndrome

C) ankylosing spondylitis
D) rheumatoid arthritis
E) Pott's disease

Answer and Discussion

The answer is C. Ankylosing spondylitis is an inflammatory condition that usually affects the axial skeleton of young men. The exact cause is not known. Symptoms include low-back pain or stiffness that radiates to the posterior thighs, decreased range of motion in the back or hips, and decreased range of motion of the chest wall. Sacroiliitis is usually one of the earliest manifestations. Other joints may be painful or swollen. Patients often report that the symptoms are worse with rest and improve with activity. Radiographs show periarticular destructive changes, destruction of the sacroiliac joint, development of syndesmophytes on the margins of the vertebral bodies, and bridging of osteophytes between the vertebral bodies, giving rise to the appearance of a "bamboo spine." Acute anterior uveitis (iritis) occurs in approximately 20% of these patients. Laboratory tests show an elevated ESR and a positive test for HLA-B27 antigen in approximately 90% of those affected. The course of the disease is variable. Some patients may have no symptoms or only mild stiffness, whereas others may experience chronic pain and significant disabilities. Most patients with ankylosing spondylitis can remain gainfully employed. Treatment includes the use of NSAIDs and physical therapy. Attacks of iritis are effectively managed with local glucocorticoids in conjunction with mydriatic agents. In severe cases, systemic steroids or immunosuppressive drugs may be used.

Kasper DL, Braunwald E, Fauci AS, et al., eds. *Harrison's principles of internal medicine,* 16th ed. New York: McGraw-Hill; 2005:1993.

164. Which of the following statements is a common feature of fibromyalgia?
A) Men are more commonly affected than women.
B) Alcohol abuse is commonly associated.
C) Joint inflammation and erythema
D) Aggravation of the condition with lack of sleep, trauma, or cold exposure
E) Normal autonomic and neuroendocrine regulation

Answer and Discussion

The answer is D. Fibromyalgia/fibromyositis is characterized by generalized pain, tenderness, and muscle stiffness. Pain at the point of tendon insertion ("trigger points") and surrounding soft tissue may also be present. Inflammation of joints is not characteristic. Although the etiology remains unclear, characteristic alterations in the pattern of sleep and changes in neuroendocrine transmitters such as serotonin, substance P, growth hormone, and cortisol suggest that dysregulation of the autonomic and neuroendocrine system appears to be the basis of the syndrome.

The condition may be aggravated by stress (both physical and mental), lack of sleep, trauma, exposure to cold, and sometimes infection. Primary fibromyalgia syndrome is more likely to affect young women who are tense, depressed, or anxious. Symptoms of stiffness and pain are usually diffuse and have an "achy" quality that comes on gradually. Localized symptoms tend to occur more abruptly. Other diseases (e.g., rheumatoid arthritis, hypothyroidism, polymyositis, polymyalgia rheumatica) must be excluded before the diagnosis is made. Myofascial pain syndrome is very similar to fibromyalgia/fibromyositis; however, the painful areas are usually regional, and men are as equally affected as women. In addition, fatigue is not a major finding. Treatment for fibromyalgia/fibromyositis includes low-dose tricyclic antidepressants (e.g., amitriptyline), acupuncture, and muscle relaxants (e.g., cyclobenzaprine). NSAIDS, although commonly used, have not been shown to be effective. Stress reduction counseling, exercise programs, and improved sleep habits can also be beneficial. American College of Rheumatology criteria for classification of fibromyalgia are as follows:

- Widespread pain for at least 3 months, defined as the presence of all of the following:
- Pain on the right and left sides of the body
- Pain above and below the waist (including shoulder and buttock pain)
- Pain in the axial skeleton (cervical, thoracic, or lumbar spine; anterior chest)
- Pain on palpation with a 4-kg force in 11 of the following 18 sites (9 bilateral sites, for a total of 18 sites):
  - Occiput: at the insertions of one or more of the following muscles: trapezius, sternocleidomastoid, splenius capitis, semispinalis capitis
  - Low cervical: at the anterior aspect of the interspaces between the transverse processes of C5–C7
  - Trapezius: at the midpoint of the upper border
  - Supraspinatus: above the scapular spine near the medial border
  - Second rib: just lateral to the second costochondral junctions
  - Lateral epicondyle: 2 cm distal to the lateral epicondyle
  - Gluteal: at the upper outer quadrant of the buttocks at the anterior edge of the gluteus maximus muscle
  - Greater trochanter: posterior to the greater trochanteric prominence
  - Knee: at the medial fat pad proximal to the joint line

Adapted with permission from Wolfe F, Smythe HA, Yunas MD, et al. The American College of Rheumatology 1990 criteria for the classification of fibromyalgia. Report of the Multicenter Criteria Committee. *Arthritis Rheum.* 1990;33:160–172.

Millea PJ, Holloway RL. Treating fibromyalgia. *Am Fam Physician.* 2000;62:1575–1582, 1587.

Myofascial pain syndrome is similar to fibromyalgia/fibromyositis; however, the painful areas are usually regional, and men are as equally affected as women.

165. A known HIV-positive patient presents to your office with a violaceous skin lesion. Further examination shows generalized lymphadenopathy. Microscopic examination of a skin punch biopsy shows spindle cells mixed with vascular tissue. The most likely diagnosis is
A) malignant melanoma
B) Kaposi's sarcoma
C) tinea corpora
D) cherry hemangioma
E) cryptococcal granuloma

Answer and Discussion

The answer is B. Kaposi's sarcoma is a malignant skin lesion that was once rare but is now seen more commonly in AIDS patients. The lesion is characterized histologically by spindle cells mixed with vascular tissue. Before the detection of AIDS, the disease was predominantly found in Eastern Europe, Italy, and equatorial Africa and affected mostly Italian or Jewish men. Symptoms include pink, violaceous, or red papules or plaques that affect any body surface and become widely disseminated with time and give rise to generalized lymphadenopathy. Serious cases can progress to visceral involvement. Treatment involves excision, cryotherapy, laser ablation, intralesional chemotherapy, external beam radiation, and the use of vincristine. Unfortunately, successful treatment and remission of Kaposi's sarcoma does not affect the overall survival of AIDS patients.

Rose LC. Recognizing neoplastic skin lesions. *Am Fam Physician.* 1998;58:873.

166. A 31-year-old woman presents with high fever, dysuria, flank pain, nausea, and vomiting. The most appropriate treatment is

A) hospitalization with administration of intravenous fluids and antibiotics
B) oral rehydration and oral antibiotics for 10 days
C) surgical consultation for exploratory laparotomy
D) extracorporeal shock wave lithotripsy
E) nothing given orally and nasogastric suction

Answer and Discussion

The answer is A. Acute pyelonephritis is an infection of the upper urinary tract. It affects the kidneys' collecting system and renal parenchyma. The most common causative agent is *E. coli*. Other causative agents include *Proteus, Pseudomonas, Enterobacter, Klebsiella, Staphylococcus*, and *Enterococcus*. Symptoms include lower abdominal pain, flank tenderness, fevers, chills, nausea, and vomiting. Physical findings include tenderness of the costovertebral angle and the abdomen. Laboratory findings include elevated white blood cell count, elevated ESR, pyuria, bacteriuria, hematuria, proteinuria, and possible white blood cell cast. Severe cases may cause bacteremia (20% of patients).

Treatment is accomplished with antibiotics—usually ampicillin and gentamicin—directed at gram-negative organisms, third-generation cephalosporins for inpatients, and TMP-SMX or fluoroquinolones for outpatients. Patients with mild to moderate symptoms can be managed as outpatients. Hospitalization is required if the patient has a high fever, dehydration, or other complicating medical conditions (e.g., pregnancy, diabetes). Duration of antibiotic therapy depends on clinical response but should be at least 10 to 14 days. Intravenous antibiotics should be continued until the patient is afebrile. Repeat cultures after treatment should be performed; if the patient has had repeated infections, further workup, including an intravenous pyelogram or voiding cystourethrogram, may be necessary.

Orenstein R, Wong ES. Urinary tract infections in adults. *Am Fam Physician.* 1999;59:1225–1234.

167. Which of the following is the medication of choice for the treatment of Legionnaire's disease?

A) Penicillin
B) Cefuroxime
C) Azithromycin
D) Gentamycin
E) Amphotericin

Answer and Discussion

The answer is C. Legionnaire's disease is caused by *Legionella pneumophila*. It was discovered after an outbreak in Philadelphia in 1976 that affected many American Legion members. The condition represents one of the atypical pneumonias that usually affects immunocompromised patients, diabetic patients, patients with renal disease, smokers, and patients with chronic lung disease. It also is a relatively common nosocomial infection. Most affected individuals are middle-aged or elderly men. Although the disease can strike healthy individuals, risk factors include immunosuppression, cigarette smoking, COPD, cardiac or renal disease, or diabetes. The *Legionella* bacteria are found in water supplies, air conditioners, showers, condensers, and aerosol nebulizers. Transmission occurs by inhalation of aerosolized bacteria. Symptoms include a nonproductive cough that becomes productive, high fevers with relative bradycardia, pleuritic chest pain, diarrhea, and a toxic appearance. Laboratory tests usually show a moderate leukocytosis (10,000 to 15,000 per mm^3), hyponatremia (50% of patients), hypophosphatemia, and elevated liver function tests. Sputum smears often show many polymorphonuclear neutrophils but do not show organisms. Chest radiographs show patchy infiltrates, which may progress to consolidations in the lobes. Pleural effusions are common. Diagnosis is achieved by culture, serologies, and direct and indirect antibody assays. The treatment of choice is typically oral erythromycin or similar macrolide antibiotic. More severe cases may require intravenous antibiotics and the addition of rifampin. Alternative medication includes clarithromycin, azithromycin, doxycycline, TMP-SMX, tetracycline, and ciprofloxacin.

Beers MH, Porter RS, eds. *The Merck manual of diagnosis and therapy*, Merck Research Laboratories, 18th ed. Whitehouse Station, NJ: Merck & Co.; 2006:1464.

168. Which of the following statements about babesiosis is true?

A) The disease is transmitted by fecal-oral contamination.
B) The disease is caused by a rickettsial organism.
C) Affected patients without spleens usually have a better prognosis.
D) Diagnosis is made with a peripheral blood smear.
E) Generalized paralysis occurs in those affected.

Answer and Discussion

The answer is D. Babesiosis is a tick-borne disease caused by *Babesia microti* and rarely affects humans. Most reported cases in the United States have been mild and were found on islands off the New York and Massachusetts coasts. Isolated cases have also been reported in Wisconsin, Georgia, and California. The disease is caused by a parasite that attacks the red blood cells. The symptoms of the disease resemble *Falciparum malaria* and include high fevers, hemolytic anemia, hemoglobinuria, jaundice, and renal failure. Those patients without spleens have a more severe course of symptoms. The diagnosis is obtained by observing the parasites (tetrad forms) in peripheral blood smears. Serologies can also be used for diagnosis. Treatment is usually unnecessary for those with intact spleens; however, for severe cases or cases that affect splenectomized patients, intravenous clindamycin and oral quinine are used for treatment.

Beers MH, Porter RS, eds. *The Merck manual of diagnosis and therapy*, Merck Research Laboratories, 18th ed. Whitehouse Station, NJ: Merck & Co.; 2006:1571–1572.

169. The drug of choice for cold-induced urticaria is

A) verapamil
B) cimetidine

C) diphenhydramine
D) cyproheptadine
E) hydroxyzine

Answer and Discussion

The answer is D. *Urticaria* is defined as an erythematous, pruritic rash that is often raised and occurs as discrete wheals and hives. The condition affects approximately 20% of the population. The rash involves the superficial layers of skin. The center of the wheal is usually pale, and the rash blanches with pressure. Involvement of the deeper layers is referred to as *angioedema*. The causes include allergen exposure; heat, cold, or sunlight exposure; and trauma. In many cases, a cause is never detected. The response is thought to be mediated by an IgE antibody. Those affected by cold may have cryoglobulins or cryofibrinogen, which become activated. In extreme cases, bronchoconstriction and anaphylaxis can occur. Unfortunately, an underlying cause is identified in only approximately 20% of cases. Treatment involves avoiding factors that trigger the response. Other treatment involves the use of antihistamine (H1) medications and histamine blockers (H2) such as cimetidine. Doxepin may also be beneficial. The drug of choice for cold-induced urticaria is cyproheptadine. Other causes of urticaria include medication use, malignancy, endocrinopathies, autoimmune diseases, insect bites, and infestations; psychogenic causes should also be investigated in complicated or persistent cases. Severe cases may require systemic steroids or the use of danazol.

Ferri F. *Ferri's Clinical Advisor, Instant Diagnosis and Treatment.* Philadelphia: Elsevier/Mosby; 2006:886.

170. In most situations, which of the following screening tests would be recommended for an otherwise healthy woman older than 50 years?
A) Chest radiograph
B) Mammogram
C) Treadmill exercise test
D) Urinalysis
E) CA 125 level

Answer and Discussion

The answer is B. Routine screening tests during general examinations should be focused according to the patient's age and gender. Annual mammograms should be performed for women older than 40 years. Chest radiographs (even for smokers), the treadmill exercise test, and urinalysis are not cost-effective for screening purposes. For cervical cancer screening, most organizations recommend a Papanicolaou test and pelvic examination at least every 3 years in patients between 20 (or when a woman first becomes sexually active) and 65 years of age. Annual fecal occult blood testing, or flexible sigmoidoscopy at 5 intervals or colonoscopy every 10 years are the standard recommendations for colorectal cancer screening in patients older than 50 years. Screening for prostate cancer remains an issue of debate. Some organizations recommend digital rectal examination and a serum prostate–specific antigen test for men older than 50 years, whereas others do not. In the absence of compelling evidence to indicate a high risk of endometrial cancer, lung cancer, oral cancer, and ovarian cancer, almost no medical organizations have developed cancer-screening guidelines for these types of cancer.

Beers MH, Porter RS, eds. *The Merck manual of diagnosis and therapy,* Merck Research Laboratories, 18th ed. Whitehouse Station, NJ: Merck & Co.; 2006:1150.

171. A 28-year-old man with no history of allergy to *Hymenoptera* stings presents to the emergency room after being stung by a yellow jacket. Other than local swelling at the site, he has no other symptoms. The most appropriate treatment involves
A) administration of epinephrine and antihistamine as well as hospitalization
B) ice therapy, administration of antihistamine, and observation at home
C) meat tenderizer sprinkled over the sting site, warm-water soaks, and aspirin
D) administration of steroids, epinephrine, intravenous hydration, and β2 agonist
E) immediate removal of the stinger using tweezers

Answer and Discussion

The answer is B. Stings by a *Hymenoptera* (e.g., bees, wasps, yellow jackets, hornets, and ants) may be fatal in a hypersensitive patient. Each year in the United States, more patients die of bee stings than of snakebites. Patients with a history of hypersensitivity may experience severe swelling at the site of the sting with the development of shock, often within minutes. Treatment should be immediate and includes application of ice to the sting site, administration of intramuscular epinephrine and oral antihistamine, and prompt transfer to the hospital. Removal of the stinger by tweezers is usually avoided because of the possibility of injecting further venom at the site. All patients with *Hymenoptera*-sting hypersensitivity should receive a prescription for an epinephrine kit and carry this with them whenever they are outdoors. Patients should also be counseled to receive hymenoptera desensitization immunotherapy. Individuals with no history of anaphylaxis may be treated by application of ice to the sting, administration of oral antihistamine, and observation at home. Large local reactions may be treated with glucocorticoids. Application of meat tenderizer containing papain is of no proven value.

Kasper DL, Braunwald E, Fauci AS, et al., eds. *Harrison's principles of internal medicine,* 16th ed. New York: McGraw-Hill; 2005:2605.

172. A 72-year-old farmer is admitted to the emergency room with symptoms of palpitations and shortness of breath. He denies chest pain. ECG findings show a rapid and irregular rhythm measured at 130 beats/minute. Appropriate treatment at this time includes
A) nifedipine
B) amiodorone
C) adenosine
D) diltiazem
E) flecainide

Answer and Discussion

The answer is D. Atrial fibrillation (AF) is the most common sustained arrhythmia. The following recommendations do not apply to patients with postoperative or post-MI AF, class IV heart failure, existing antiarrhythmic-drug therapy, or valvular disease. The majority of patients with newly detected AF should be managed with pharmacologic rate control (rather than rhythm control) plus ongoing anticoagulation therapy. (The expense and risk of antiarrhythmic drugs give rate control a slight advantage, despite equivalent efficacy.) Rhythm control is appropriate for specific subgroups, including patients with severe symptoms and those with a preference for this strategy. Recommended drugs for rate control are atenolol, metoprolol, diltiazem, and verapamil. Because digoxin is effective for rate control only at rest, it should be considered second-line therapy. Unless contraindicated, adjusted-dose warfarin should be used for ongoing anticoagulation therapy in AF patients with stroke risk factors. If a patient elects to undergo acute cardioversion to sinus rhythm, electrocardioversion and pharmacologic options are each appropriate. The most effective drugs are ibutilide, flecainide, dofetilide, propafenone, and amiodarone. Two anticoagulation strategies are appropriate for preventing thromboembolism: (1) 3 to 4 weeks of anticoagulation before and after cardioversion; and (2) early cardioversion guided by transesophageal echocardiography plus 3 weeks of anticoagulation after cardioversion. Most patients who undergo cardioversion should not receive long-term antiarrhythmic maintenance therapy. However, such therapy is indicated in some patients, based on symptoms and patient preference. The most effective maintenance drugs are amiodarone, disopyramide, propafenone, and sotalol.

Snow V, Weiss KB, LeFevre M. et al. Management of newly detected atrial fibrillation: A clinical practice guideline from the American Academy of Family Physicians and the American College of Physicians. *Ann Intern Med.* 2003; 139:1009–1017.

McNamara RL, Tarariz LJ, Segal JB, et al. Management of atrial fibrillation: Review of the evidence for the role of pharmacologic therapy, electrical cardioversion, and echocardiography. *Ann Intern Med.* 2003;139:1018–1033.

173. A 58-year-old secretary presents with asthenia and hyperpigmented changes on her elbows and inner cheek. She also has noted her blood pressure is low and she is dizzy when she stands. She has lost 10 pounds and has some nausea but no vomiting. A recent test for coccidioidomycosis was positive. Appropriate testing at this time includes

A) CT of the abdomen
B) esophagoduodenoscopy
C) glucose tolerance test
D) ACTH stimulation test
E) colonoscopy

Answer and Discussion

The answer is D. Addison's disease results from a progressive destruction of the adrenal glands, which must involve the majority of the glands before adrenal insufficiency appears. The adrenal is a frequent site for chronic granulomatous diseases, predominantly tuberculosis but also histoplasmosis, coccidioidomycosis, and cryptococcosis. Although infection with tuberculosis at one time was the most common cause of Addison's disease, now the most frequent cause is ideopathic atrophy, related to an autoimmune mechanism. Adrenocortical insufficiency caused by gradual adrenal destruction is characterized by a gradual onset of fatigability, weakness, anorexia, nausea and vomiting, weight loss, skin and mucous membrane pigmentation, hypotension, and in some cases hypoglycemia depending on the duration and degree of adrenal insufficiency. The manifestations vary from mild chronic fatigue to life threatening shock associated with acute destruction of the glands. Asthenia is the major presenting symptom. Early in the course it may be sporadic, occurring at times of stress. Late in the course the patient is continuously fatigued. Hyperpigmentation can occur. It commonly appears as a diffuse brown, tan, or bronze darkening of parts such as the elbows or creases of the hand and pigmented areas such as the areolae around the nipples. Bluish-black patches may appear on the mucous membranes. Some patients develop dark freckles and a persistent tan following sun exposure can occur. Hypotension with orthostasis is frequent, and blood pressure may be in the range of 80/50 mm Hg or less. Abnormalities of the gastrointestinal tract are often the presenting complaint. Symptoms include anorexia with weight loss to severe nausea, vomiting, diarrhea, and vague and sometimes severe abdominal pain. Patients may also exhibit personality changes, usually consisting of excessive irritability and restlessness. Axillary and pubic hair may be decreased in women due to loss of adrenal androgens. The diagnosis of adrenal insufficiency is made with the ACTH stimulation testing to assess adrenal reserve capacity for steroid production. The best screening test is the cortisol response 60 minutes after cosyntropin is given intramuscularly or intravenously. Cortisol levels should increase appropriately. If the response is abnormal, then primary and secondary adrenal insufficiency can be distinguished by measuring aldosterone levels from the same blood samples. In secondary, but not primary, adrenal insufficiency the aldosterone level is normal. In primary adrenal insufficiency, plasma ACTH and associated peptides are elevated because of loss of the usual cortisol-hypothalamic-pituitary feedback loop, whereas in secondary adrenal insufficiency, plasma ACTH values are low or "inappropriately" normal.

Kasper DL, Braunwald E, Fauci AS, et al., eds. *Harrison's principles of internal medicine,* 16th ed. New York: McGraw-Hill; 2005:2097–2099.

174. A 17-year-old surfer presents to your office complaining of an intensely pruritic, serpinginous type rash that has formed on the sole of his foot. The rash appears to be spreading and is forming bullae at the affected site. The most likely diagnosis is

A) tinea pedis
B) bathing suit dermatitis
C) leishmaniasis
D) ascariasis
E) cutaneous larva migrans

Answer and Discussion

The answer is E. Cutaneous larva migrans, also known as the *creeping eruption,* is a common, self-limited, parasitic infection seen in patients who live in warm climates or have recently traveled to tropical regions, particularly if they have been to beaches and shady areas. The most common infective agent is a dog and cat hookworm, *Ancylostoma caninum* and *Ancylostoma braziliense,* respectively. Familial outbreaks of cutaneous larva migrans have been noted where the infection began with the household pet. When the animal defecates, the hookworms are shed and the larvae are picked up by humans through breaks in the skin, hair follicles, and even through intact skin. The areas most often affected include the feet, hands, buttocks, thighs, and chest. The eruption begins as a pruritic lesion at the site of entry and progresses within a few hours into an inflamed papular or papulovesicular eruption. Serpinginous tracks left by the larvae's migration may also be seen. The eruption may spread up to 1 to 2 cm per day. Severe pruritus, vesicular and bullous lesions, local swelling, erosions, and folliculitis may be seen. Biopsy is generally not useful, and blood tests rarely show eosinophilia or elevated immunoglobulin E levels. Destructive therapies, such as cryotherapy, are often ineffective. Isolated cutaneous cases are treated with topical thiabendazole, especially when applied ahead of the advancing lesions. Because of the risk of systemic infection and the ease of oral treatment, some recommend routine systemic treatment with oral thiabendazole, albendazole, or ivermectin. Although thiabendazole has significant side effects that include nausea, vomiting, diarrhea, and dizziness, albendazole and ivermectin are reliable and have fewer adverse effects. Ivermectin may be given as a single dose with no known toxic side effects.

Loughrey MB, Irvine AD, Girdwood RW, et al. Cutaneous larva migrans: the case for routine oral treatment. *Br J Dermatol.* 1997;137:155–156.

Van den Enden E, Stevens A, Van Gompel A. Treatment of cutaneous larva migrans. *N Engl J Med.* 1998;339:1246–1247.

175. The most common cause of a community-acquired pneumonia in a 45-year-old otherwise healthy man is

A) *Streptococcus pneumoniae*
B) *Haemophilus influenzae*
C) *Mycoplasma pneumoniae*
D) *Legionella pneumoniae*
E) *Klebsiella pneumoniae*

Answer and Discussion

The answer is A. In young adults, causes for pneumonia include *Mycoplasma*, *Chlamydia pneumoniae* (formerly termed the *TWAR strain*), influenza, adenovirus, *Pneumocystis carinii* (in immunocompromised patients), and other community-acquired organisms including *Streptococcus, Haemophilus*, and, occasionally, *Legionella*. Pneumonia in adults with no underlying disease is usually caused by *S. pneumoniae*, representing more than 50% of community-acquired pneumonias that require hospitalization. Other causes in this patient group include *H. influenzae, Legionella, Mycoplasma* (more commonly seen in young adults), and influenza viruses. If the patient is older than 60 years and has other significant medical problems (e.g., diabetes, COPD, heart disease, alcoholism), the most common pathogens include the previously mentioned organisms as well as *Klebsiella, Enterobacteriaceae*, *Chlamydia*, and *S. aureus*. For patients with aspiration or nosocomial infections, the causative organisms include the previously mentioned organisms and the gram-negative organisms (including *Pseudomonas*) and anaerobes.

Ferri F. *Ferri's Clinical Advisor, Instant Diagnosis and Treatment.* Philadelphia: Elsevier/Mosby; 2006:652–660.

Pneumonia in adults with no underlying disease is usually caused by *Streptococcus pneumoniae*, representing more than 50% of community-acquired pneumonias that require hospitalization.

176. Which of the following factors is NOT associated with diabetic ketoacidosis?

A) Hyperglycemia
B) Acidosis
C) Dehydration
D) Hyperkalemia
E) Hyperosmolarity

Answer and Discussion

The answer is D. Diabetic ketoacidosis occurs in diabetics when a severe lack of insulin leads to (1) a breakdown of free fatty acids and (2) the production of acetoacetic acid, β-hydroxybutyric acid, and acetone, resulting in severe and life-threatening acidosis. The condition usually occurs in patients with type I diabetes mellitus and is often seen as the initial presentation. Triggering factors include infection, trauma, poor compliance with insulin administration, myocardial infarction, cerebrovascular accident, alcohol intoxication, or dehydration. Diabetic ketoacidosis is characterized by the following conditions:

- Hyperglycemia
- Acidosis
- Dehydration (secondary to osmotic diuresis)
- Hyperosmolarity
- Potassium loss

Symptoms include mental status changes, tachypnea, fruity breath (secondary to acetones), and nausea and vomiting with abdominal pain. In severe cases, coma may occur. Treatment involves the administration of insulin to lower glucose levels, fluid rehydration (usually >5 L), and replacement of potassium and other electrolyte losses. If the condition is severe, cardiovascular collapse may occur. Close follow-up with frequent monitoring of serum pH, electrolytes, and urine output is necessary during treatment. Further tests should be conducted to rule out infection as a precipitating cause. Unfortunately, the white blood cell count is not a reliable indicator for the presence of infection in those with diabetic ketoacidosis, because the stress of the illness often causes the white blood cell count to increase to 15,000 to 30,000 cells/μL.

Ferri F. *Ferri's Clinical Advisor, Instant Diagnosis and Treatment.* Philadelphia: Elsevier/Mosby; 2006:255–256.

177. Which of the following findings is consistent with the syndrome of inappropriate ADH secretion (SIADH)?

A) Hypernatremia
B) Hypertonic urine
C) Hypovolemia
D) Increased glomerular filtration rate
E) Hyperosmolality

Answer and Discussion

The answer is B. SIADH is defined as less than maximally dilute urine in the presence of plasma hypoosmolality and hyponatremia. The condition is associated with a number of disorders, including small cell carcinoma of the lung, Guillain-Barré syndrome, acute intermittent porphyria, other pulmonary disorders (e.g., pneumonia, tuberculosis), and neurologic disorders (e.g., meningitis, tumors, trauma, stroke). In many cases, the condition may be idiopathic. The cause is the inappropriate release of ADH with respect to the body's fluid osmolality. Findings include

- Hyponatremia and hypoosmolality of body fluids
- Normal glomerular filtration rate
- Urine hypertonicity (usually >300 mOsmol/kg) despite a subnormal plasma osmolality and serum sodium concentration
- Isovolemia or hypervolemia without the presence of edema
- Urinary sodium wasting that increases with salt loading

Symptoms include confusion, anorexia, lethargy, and muscle cramps. Treatment involves fluid restriction—often <1 L daily. More severe cases may require replacement of sodium and potassium deficits. Care should be taken not to replace deficits too quickly because of the risk of central pontine myelinolysis. Other treatments involve the long-term use of demeclocycline, which antagonizes the effect of ADH on the kidney and produces a nephrogenic diabetes insipidus and helps to correct hyponatremia.

Beers MH, Porter RS, eds. *The Merck manual of diagnosis and therapy*, Merck Research Laboratories, 18th ed. Whitehouse Station, NJ: Merck & Co.; 2006:1239,1240.

178. A 40-year-old woman complains of diffuse symmetric joint pain that is worse in the morning but improves as the day progresses. Examination shows inflammation of the proximal interphalangeal and metacarpophalangeal (MCP) joints. The most likely diagnosis is

A) Reiter's syndrome
B) Rheumatoid arthritis
C) polymyalgia rheumatica
D) lupus erythematosis
E) osteoarthritis

Answer and Discussion

The answer is B. Rheumatoid arthritis is a chronic, symmetric, and inflammatory condition that may involve multiple joints. Women are affected two to three times more often than are men, and family members of affected individuals are at increased risk. Onset is usually between the fourth and sixth decade, but may occur at any age. Synovial inflammation leads to the destruction of articular and periarticular structures and proliferation of the synovial tissue (termed *pannus*), all of which causes chronic joint pain. In 30% to 40% of patients, subcutaneous rheumatoid nodules may form at sites subject to trauma and are usually associated with more severe conditions. Patients often complain of multiple joint pain, low-grade fever, fatigue, weight loss, and depression. Symmetric swelling of the hands (especially the proximal interphalangeal and MCP joints), wrists, elbows, shoulder, neck, and ankles is typical; however, any joint may be affected. Patients usually report morning stiffness that involves the small joints of the hands. This stiffness improves as the day progresses. Carpal tunnel syndrome may also occur. Other manifestations, including vasculitis, pericarditis, and interstitial fibrosis, may be found in more severe cases. Laboratory findings include elevated ESR (90% of cases), mild anemia, and a positive rheumatoid factor (85% of cases). Radiographs show periarticular osteoporosis, joint-space narrowing, and joint erosion in more severe cases. However, no laboratory test, histologic finding, or radiographic feature confirms the diagnosis. Treatment consists of NSAIDs (first-line therapy), interarticular and systemic steroids, etanercept (Enbrel) (a tumor necrosis factor α-blocker), disease-modifying antirheumatic drugs, and antimalarials (primarily hydroxychloroquine, which requires eye examinations every 6 months because of the risk of vision loss), sulfasalazine, azathioprine, cyclosporine, and methotrexate with folate supplementation (which requires close monitoring of liver and renal function). Other agents (e.g., penicillamine, cyclophosphamide, gold compounds) are less widely used because of side effects. Traditional drug combinations for RA commonly include an NSAID, a disease-modifying antirheumatic drug, and short intermittent courses of oral corticosteroids. The use of etanercept and methotrexate has been effective and promising in the treatment of rheumatoid arthritis. Other associated conditions include Felty's syndrome (arthritis, splenomegaly, lymphadenopathy, anemia, neutropenia, and thrombocytopenia) and Sjögren's syndrome (arthritis; dry eyes and mucous membranes).

Ferri F. *Ferri's Clinical Advisor, Instant Diagnosis and Treatment.* Philadelphia: Elsevier/Mosby; 2006:88–89.

179. A high urinary sodium concentration in the presence of a low plasma osmolality is most closely associated with

A) syndrome of inappropriate antidiuretic hormone (SIADH)
B) third-degree burns
C) hyperglycemia
D) prolonged diarrhea
E) water overload

Answer and Discussion

The answer is A. Hyponatremia is a common electrolyte abnormality seen in patients. Common causes include medications (e.g., diuretics, SSRIs) and SIADH syndrome. Hyponatremia can be classified according to the volume status of the patient as hypovolemic, hypervolemic, or euvolemic. Hypervolemic hyponatremia may be caused by congestive heart failure, cirrhosis, and kidney disease. Distinguishing between euvolemia and hypovolemia can be determined by measurement of plasma osmolality. Hyponatremia with a high plasma osmolality is caused by hyperglycemia, whereas a normal plasma osmolality indicates pseudohyponatremia. The urinary sodium concentration helps in diagnosing patients with low plasma osmolality. High urinary sodium concentration in the presence of low plasma osmolality can be caused by renal disorders, endocrine deficiencies, reset osmostat syndrome, SIADH, and medications. Low urinary sodium concentration is caused by severe burns, gastrointestinal losses, and water overload. Management includes emergent treatment in patients with acute severe hyponatremia because of the risk of cerebral edema and hyponatremic encephalopathy. In patients with chronic hyponatremia, fluid restriction is the mainstay of treatment, with the use of demeclocycline in persistent cases. Rapid correction of hyponatremia should be avoided to reduce the risk of central pontine myelinolysis. Loop diuretics are useful in the treatment of edema in hyponatremic states and in chronic SIADH. In all cases, identifying the etiology of hyponatremia remains an important part of treatment.

Goh KP. Management of hyponatremia. *Am Fam Physician.* 2004;69:2387–2394.

180. When comparing Bell's palsy with a CNS lesion (e.g., stroke, tumor), the distinguishing feature of Bell's palsy is

A) involvement of the forehead muscles
B) involvement of the extremities
C) lack of involvement below the eyes
D) slurred speech

Answer and Discussion

The answer is A. Bell's palsy is characterized by a sudden onset of unilateral facial paralysis. It is thought to be the result of an infection (usually viral) affecting the facial nerve, which involves compression of the nerve within the temporal bone. Symptoms usually develop as pain behind the ear preceding the facial paralysis. In some cases, the patient cannot close the affected eye because of widening of the palpebral fissures. In 80% to 90% of cases, the physical findings resolve completely within weeks to months after onset; however, in some isolated cases, permanent deficits may occur. The distinguishing feature between Bell's palsy and CNS lesions (e.g., strokes, tumors) is that Bell's palsy involves the entire face (including muscles of the forehead), whereas CNS lesions tend to affect the face below the eyes and other areas including the arms and legs. Treatment involves the use of steroids, but they are somewhat controversial and are of questionable proven benefit. If the patient has difficulty closing the affected eye, it should be patched for protection against excessive drying.

Ferri F. *Ferri's Clinical Advisor, Instant Diagnosis and Treatment.* Philadelphia: Elsevier/Mosby; 2006:120.

181. A 30-year-old woman from Minneapolis presents to your office complaining of paresthesias, weakness, lack of coordination, and difficulty with gait. Her symptoms are worse after a hot shower. Examination of the cerebral spinal fluid shows oligoclonal bands of immunoglobulin G (IgG). The most likely diagnosis is

A) multiple sclerosis
B) Huntington's disease
C) Parkinson's disease
D) neurofibromatosis
E) amyotrophic lateral sclerosis (ALS)

Answer and Discussion

The answer is A. Multiple sclerosis is a slowly demyelinating disease that affects the CNS. It is characterized by remissions and exacerbations that are separated in time and involve different areas of the CNS. A second form identified is progressive. The cause is unknown but may be related to a combination of genetic factors and perhaps infection with a slow or latent virus. Women are affected more than men (2:1), and there appears to be a geographic predominance, with those in the northern United States affected more than those in the southern United States. The onset is usually between 20 and 40 years of age, and the geographic factor is present even if the individual relocates to a tropical climate (as long as they spent their first 15 years in the north). The pathology involves multiple plaques of demyelination that are found throughout the CNS. Symptoms include paresthesias, including Lhermitte's symptom (sensation of a momentary electrical current or shock when the neck is flexed), weakness, loss of coordination, or visual disturbances (monocular visual loss), initially followed by emotional lability, gait disturbances, and spasticity in more severe cases. Signs include optic neuritis, speech difficulties, cranial-nerve palsies, increased deep tendon reflexes, nystagmus, tremor, urinary incontinence, and impotence. Symptoms increase with exposure to heat. Diagnosis is usually made by the history, appearance of oligoclonal bands of IgG in the CSF, and MRI scans showing plaques of demyelination in the paraventricular white matter. Evoked potential nerve tests may also be abnormal. Treatment is usually supportive; however, steroids and immunosuppressive drugs have been used. Newer medications include interferon β-1b (Betaseron), interferon β-1a (Avonex), and glatiramer acetate (Copaxone), which are interferon-type medications used in the relapsing-remitting forms. In addition, antispasmodic drugs such as Baclofen have been used to treat the spasticity.

Johnson KP, Baringer JR. Current therapy of multiple sclerosis. *Hosp Pract.* 2001;36(4):21–22, 25–28; discussion 28–29.

Kasper DL, Braunwald E, Fauci AS, et al., eds. *Harrison's principles of internal medicine,* 16th ed. New York: McGraw-Hill; 2005:2461.

182. A 17-year-old boy is seen in the emergency room. He has miosis, bronchoconstriction, and diarrhea. He is also sweating, excessively salivating, and vomiting. His breath has a garlic odor. The most likely diagnosis is

A) alcohol overdose
B) organophosphate poisoning
C) cyanide ingestion
D) diabetic ketoacidosis
E) cocaine overdose

Answer and Discussion

The answer is B. Organophosphate insecticides are inhibitors of acetylcholinesterase and result in an accumulation of acetylcholine at the synaptic junction. Organophosphate poisoning is characterized by miosis, bronchoconstriction, sweating, salivation, headache, vomiting, diarrhea, muscle weakness, and convulsions. The patient's breath typically has a garlic odor. Treatment involves gastric lavage followed by activated charcoal or adequate cleansing if skin exposure occurs. Parasympathetic stimulation can be counteracted by the administration of atropine sulfate until symptoms disappear or until signs of atropine use occur (e.g., dilated pupils, dry mouth). Also, pralidoxime helps remove the organophosphate from the cholinesterase.

Kasper DL, Braunwald E, Fauci AS, et al., eds. *Harrison's principles of internal medicine,* 16th ed. New York: McGraw-Hill; 2005:226.

183. Which of the following statements about polycythemia vera is true?

A) It is a chronic myeloproliferative disorder that is associated with increased levels of hemoglobin (Hb) concentration and red blood cell mass (erythrocytosis).
B) It is associated with a neurodegenerative condition of the thalamus.
C) Physical examination usually shows decreased peripheral reflexes.
D) Leukopenia and thrombocytopenia are common.
E) The disease is associated with an increased life span of the red blood cell.

Answer and Discussion

The answer is A. Polycythemia vera is a rare, chronic myeloproliferative disorder that is associated with increased levels of hemoglobin concentration and increased red blood cell mass (erythrocytosis). The cause is unknown, and the condition is seen more commonly in men older than 60 years and in the Jewish population. The condition is associated with an increased production and turnover of red blood cells. As many as one-fourth of those affected develop a reduction in the red blood cell life span, an associated anemia, and sometimes myelofibrosis. Symptoms are associated with an increased viscosity and volume of blood and include headaches, visual disturbances, shortness of breath, weakness, and fatigue. Patients may also report generalized pruritus, particularly after bathing in warm water. Hepatosplenomegaly is common. Associated conditions include peptic ulcer disease, thrombosis, bone pain, renal lithiasis, and gout. The diagnosis should be considered when the hematocrit is >54% for men and >49% for women. Elevations in all three blood components (i.e., red blood cells, white blood cells, and platelets) are common. If the condition goes untreated, as many as 50% of those affected die within 1.5 years. Thrombosis is the most common cause of death, followed by complications of myeloid dysplasia, hemorrhage, and leukemia. With therapy, survival time is between 7 and 15 years. Treatment involves phlebotomy (especially for pregnant women and individuals younger than the age of 40 years) and, in some cases, myelosuppressive agents, including hydroxyurea. Hyperuricemia may also be treated with allopurinol.

Beers MH, Porter RS, eds. *The Merck manual of diagnosis and therapy,* Merck Research Laboratories, 18th ed. Whitehouse Station, NJ: Merck & Co., 2006:1102–1105.

184. Which of the following drugs is commonly used in the treatment of congestive heart failure (CHF) related to systolic dysfunction?
A) Verapamil
B) Diltiazem
C) Ramipril
D) Nifedipine
E) Isoproterenol

Answer and Discussion

The answer is C. The causes of CHF are numerous and include CAD (most common), dilated cardiomyopathy arising from toxins such as alcohol and doxorubicin, idiopathic causes, infection, and collagen vascular disorders. Other causes include hypertension, cardiac arrhythmias, cardiac valvular disorders, hypertrophic cardiomyopathy, and restrictive cardiomyopathies (caused by disorders such as amyloidosis, hemochromatosis, and sarcoidosis). CHF occurs when there is a decrease in cardiac contractility, which leads to decreased cardiac output that does not keep up with the body's physiologic demands. Initially, this inability to keep up with physiologic demands may only be seen with exercise. However, as the disease progresses, signs may also occur at a resting state. Symptoms include shortness of breath; paroxysmal nocturnal dyspnea, which awakens the patient and causes severe shortness of breath and diaphoresis, causing the patient to sit up for prolonged periods; orthopnea (dyspnea in the recumbent position); and peripheral swelling. Signs include jugular venous distention more than 4 cm elevated from the sternal angle with the patient's head elevated at a 45-degree angle, hepatomegaly, hepatojugular reflux, S3 heart sound, peripheral edema, and pulmonary rales (the most common finding).

Treatment consists of a low-sodium diet, diuretics, ACE inhibitors (ramipril, enalapril, lisinopril) or angiotensin II–receptor blockers (losartan, candesartan) if unable to tolerate ACE inhibitors, β-blockers (carvedilol, long-acting metoprolol succinate), digoxin (particularly in CHF complicated with atrial fibrillation), and other afterload-reducing medications (e.g., hydralazine, isosorbide dinitrate). Calcium-channel blockers, especially verapamil, should be avoided because of their negative inotropic effect on the heart; however, they are useful in cases of CHF caused by diastolic dysfunction and hypertrophic cardiomyopathy.

Ferri F. *Ferri's Clinical Advisor, Instant Diagnosis and Treatment.* Philadelphia: Elsevier/Mosby; 2006:211–213.

185. Which of the following statements about influenza is true?
A) Symptoms rarely include cough and coryza.
B) Influenza C is the most common cause of the epidemic flu.
C) Diagnosis requires acute and convalescent titers.
D) Immunization for healthy adults should begin at 65 years of age.
E) Neuroaminidase inhibitors can shorten the course of illness if given within the first 48 hours of the onset of symptoms.

Answer and Discussion

The answer is E. Influenza is an acute viral illness characterized by fever, cough, coryza, headache, myalgias, and fatigue. The usual symptoms last 3 to 7 days. On average, illnesses tend to cause 5 to 6 days of restricted activity, 3 to 4 days in bed, and 3 days lost from work or school. Residual symptoms (nonproductive cough, weakness) may last for several weeks. Epidemics usually occur in the winter months. The disease usually spreads through school-age children first. Those with underlying medical problems (e.g., diabetes, COPD, CHF, chronic renal disease, immunodeficiencies) are at higher risk. The causative agent is an RNA orthomyxovirus. There are three different types of influenza:

1. Influenza A is the most common cause of the flu.
2. Influenza B is usually caused by paramyxovirus, rhinovirus, or echovirus.
3. Influenza C is an endemic virus that occasionally causes mild respiratory disease.

Only types A and B cause epidemics.

Diagnosis is usually made clinically; however, rapid tests are now readily available. Treatment is usually symptomatic. In severe cases, antimembrane drugs [amantadine (Symmetrel) or rimantadine (Flumadine)] are used for influenza A (not influenza B), but are effective only if administered early in the course of the disease. Newer drugs (neuraminidase inhibitors) zanamivir (Relenza) and oseltamivir (Tamiflu), approved in 1999, work by inhibiting neuraminidase, a protein found on the surface of the virus that plays a role in the release of progeny virus from infected cells, and are effective for both influenza A and B. Zanamivir and oseltamivir shorten the duration of the influenzal febrile illness by 2 days and cause a reduction in viral titers within 2 days of administration, resulting in decreased transmission rate. Neuraminidase inhibitors appear to be more effective (compared to antimembrane drugs) for the treatment of influenza virus infection when given within 48 hours from the onset of symptoms. Unfortunately, however, antiviral agents are only slightly effective in preventing confirmed influenza or influenza-like illness. When given in the first few days of illness, the M2 ion blockers [amantadine (Symmetrel) and rimantadine (Flumadine)] and neuraminidase inhibitors [zanamivir (Relenza) and oseltamivir (Tamiflu)] reduce the duration of illness by approximately 1 day. Vaccination should begin at age 50 years and earlier in patients at high risk or with underlying medical problems. Young children should also receive vaccination.

Ferri F. *Ferri's Clinical Advisor, Instant Diagnosis and Treatment.* Philadelphia: Elsevier/Mosby; 2006:453–454.

> In severe cases, antimembrane drugs amantadine (Symmetrel) or rimantadine (Flumadine) are used for influenza A (not influenza B) but are only effective if administered early in the course of the disease.

186. Which of the following medications is the most appropriate to use in the emergent treatment of anaphylaxis?
A) Diphenhydramine
B) Isoproterenol
C) Epinephrine
D) Prednisone
E) Atropine

Answer and Discussion

The answer is C. Anaphylaxis may be caused by a variety of factors, including ingestion of certain foods, insect bites or stings, drugs, and contrast dyes. Symptoms include urticaria, angioedema, dyspnea, cough, hoarseness, wheezing, a sense of impending doom, abdominal pain, hypotension, and syncope. Death occurs in 3% of patients. The cause is a massive IgE-mediated response, which results in the release of large amounts of histamine from mast cells. Treatment must be prompt and includes

1. Securing the patient's airway
2. Administering intravenous fluids
3. Administering epinephrine, 0.2 to 0.5 mL of 1:1,000 subcutaneously, every 15 to 20 minutes, repeated three times if the patient is stable; if the patient is unstable, epinephrine should be administered intravenously

After the administration of epinephrine, diphenhydramine (H1-receptor blocker) should also be initiated; in severe reactions, cimetidine or ranitidine (H2-receptor blockers) should be initiated. All patients with anaphylaxis should be hospitalized and monitored for 24 hours. Corticosteroids have no role in the acute treatment of anaphylaxis but should be initiated to prevent a late-phase reaction. Bronchodilators such as albuterol and theophylline (if necessary) should also be used. Studies show that atopic individuals are not at increased risk for the development of IgE-mediated anaphylaxis as a result of drug reactions or insect stings.

Rakel RE, Bope ET. *Conn's Current Therapy 2005*. Philadelphia: Elsevier/Saunders; 2005:863–865.

187. Calcium supplementation appears to reduce the risk of which of the following conditions?

A) Ovarian cancer
B) Lung cancer
C) Breast cancer
D) Colon cancer
E) Prostate cancer

Answer and Discussion

The answer is D. Dietary calcium supplementation appears to reduce the risk of colon cancer in some studies. Combined evidence from two clinical trials of calcium supplementation lasting for several years revealed a reduced rate of recurrent colorectal adenoma. However, evidence is insufficient to recommend supplementation with dietary calcium for patients who have never had an adenoma. Although it would be beneficial to identify a simple, inexpensive, and safe dietary supplement to prevent colon cancer, comprehensive programs for healthy living are more likely to be effective. For prevention of colon cancer, the American Cancer Society recommends increasing the intensity and duration of physical activity; eating more vegetables and fruits; limiting intake of red meat; avoiding obesity; and avoiding excess alcohol consumption.

Weingarten MA, Zalmanovici A, Yaphe J. Dietary calcium supplementation for preventing colorectal cancer and adenomatous polyps. *Cochrane Database Syst Rev.* 2004;(3):CD003548.

Martinez ME, Willett WC. Calcium, vitamin D, and colorectal cancer: a review of the epidemiologic evidence. *Cancer Epidemiol Biomarkers Prev.* 1998;7:163–168.

Byers T, Nestle M, McTiernan A, et al. American Cancer Society guidelines on nutrition and physical activity for cancer prevention: reducing the risk of cancer with healthy food choices and physical activity. *CA Cancer J Clin.* 2002;52:92–119.

188. A 10-year-old boy is brought to the emergency room after suffering a bee sting on the hand. The patient complains of dizziness and shortness of breath. The appropriate course of action should be

A) to reassure patient and family and discharge patient with antihistamines
B) to intubate immediately, remove stinger with forceps, and monitor patient in an intensive care unit
C) to administer intravenous epinephrine, antihistamines, and fluids and observe closely
D) to provide ice therapy, sprinkle meat tenderizer on the sting site, and elevate the affected extremity
E) to prescribe an oral steroid taper, discharge the patient, and follow up with the child the following day in the office

Answer and Discussion

The answer is C. Bee stings are common, particularly in children. Each year, bee stings cause 3 to 4 times more deaths because of anaphylaxis than snakebites. The average person can safely tolerate 10 stings per lb of body weight; the average adult can withstand >1,000 stings, whereas 500 stings can kill a child. However, 1 sting can cause a fatal anaphylactic reaction in a hypersensitive person. Symptoms include local pain, swelling, and redness. In some patients, bee stings can lead to anaphylaxis with bronchoconstriction and shock. These patients require immediate attention with life-supporting measures and the administration of epinephrine. These patients should also be prescribed an epinephrine kit, which contains injectable epinephrine and diphenhydramine tablets, to carry with them whenever they are outdoors. For patients with mild reactions (local swelling and pain), ice should be applied, and the site should be gently rubbed to remove the stinger; the person removing the stinger should be careful not to pinch or grasp the stinger with forceps, because it may inject more venom at the site. Most symptoms increase over 24 to 48 hours but subside in 5 to 7 days. Antihistamines and anti-inflammatories may help to decrease reactions.

Beers MH, Porter RS, eds. *The Merck manual of diagnosis and therapy,* Merck Research Laboratories, 18th ed. Whitehouse Station, NJ: Merck & Co.; 2006:2639–2640.

189. Which of the following relationships between toxin exposure and symptoms is correct?

A) Vinyl chloride—behavioral changes
B) Mercury, lead, and pesticides—acroosteolysis
C) Iron, lithium, and lead—pulmonary fibrosis
D) Chromate and cocaine—nasal septal perforations

Answer and Discussion

The answer is D. Ingestion of toxins can cause a multitude of symptoms. However, there are specific symptoms particularly associated with specific toxins. The following are some toxins and their common identifiable symptoms:

- Mercury, lead, and pesticides—change of behavior
- Asbestos exposure—pulmonary fibrosis
- Vinyl chloride—acroosteolysis
- Chromate and cocaine—nasal septal perforations

Beers MH, Porter RS, eds. *The Merck manual of diagnosis and therapy,* Merck Research Laboratories, 18th ed. Whitehouse Station, NJ: Merck & Co.; 2006:2651–2695.

190. Side effects of 3-hydroxy-3-methylglutaryl coenzyme A (HMG CoA) reductase inhibitors include
A) chronic rhinitis
B) infertility
C) rhabdomyolysis
D) orthostatic hypotension
E) cataracts

Answer and Discussion

The answer is C. HMG CoA reductase inhibitors (also referred to as *statins*) are used for the treatment of moderate to severe hypercholesterolemia. The drugs (atorvastatin, pravastatin, cerivastatin, fluvastatin, lovastatin, simvastatin) inhibit HMG CoA reductase, the rate-limiting step in cholesterol production. Statin drugs decrease the patient's total and LDL cholesterol and increase the patient's HDL cholesterol. The drugs can cause elevation of liver function tests; therefore, serum transaminases should be performed before the initiation of treatment, and 12 weeks after initiation of therapy, or at increase of dose and periodically thereafter. Elevations more than three times the normal levels are an indication to discontinue the drug. Statin drugs should be used with caution in patients with underlying liver dysfunction and heavy alcohol use. Rhabdomyolysis with renal failure is also a potential side effect. Routine eye examinations for the detection of lens opacities are no longer recommended.

Rakel RE, Bope ET. *Conn's Current Therapy 2005*. Philadelphia: Elsevier/Saunders; 2005:407–408, 670, 692.

191. Which of the following statements about rheumatic fever (RF) is correct?
A) It is a complication of a group B streptococcal infection.
B) It most commonly affects the aortic valve.
C) It is most commonly seen in patients younger than 4 years.
D) Prophylaxis against recurrent attacks with monthly penicillin administration is indicated after an acute attack.
E) It usually follows a streptococcal skin infection.

Answer and Discussion

The answer is D. Rheumatic fever is an inflammatory complication of a group A streptococcal pharyngitis. In the early 1900s, it was not uncommon; however, since the advent of antibiotics, the condition is seen much less frequently. More virulent strains of streptococci appear to be returning to the United States, and the incidence may increase in the next few years. The condition continues to flourish in developing countries. Rheumatic fever can give rise to

- Migratory polyarthritis
- Chorea
- Carditis
- Subcutaneous nodules
- Erythema marginatum

Rheumatic fever affects mostly school-age children and is rare before age 4 years and after 18 years of age. The most dangerous lesion of rheumatic fever involves the cardiac valves. The mitral valve is most commonly affected, followed by the aortic valve. Diagnosis is made by fulfillment of the modified Jones criteria, which involves (1) one and preferably two of the five major manifestations listed previously in the presence of a recent streptococcal infection; and (2) minor manifestations such as fever, arthralgias, history of RF, elevated white blood cell count, an elevation in the ESR or C-reactive protein, and a prolonged PR interval. Treatment is directed toward the relief of pain and includes analgesics (e.g., aspirin) and, in some cases, steroids for carditis. Sedimentation rate is used to monitor treatment. Mild cases require treatment only with anti-inflammatories; however, patients with carditis should be treated with steroids continued for at least 1 week after the ESR normalizes—at that time steroids may be slowly tapered. Bed rest has no proven value in treatment. Physical restrictions to reduce or eliminate symptoms seem advisable only in patients with symptomatic heart failure. Antistreptococcal prophylaxis is indicated after an attack of RF to prevent recurrent attacks; monthly benzathine penicillin G or oral sulfadiazine is used and is usually continued until early adulthood (25 years of age); however, the duration of antistreptococcal prophylaxis is controversial.

Beers MH, Porter RS, eds. *The Merck manual of diagnosis and therapy*, Merck Research Laboratories, 18th ed. Whitehouse Station, NJ: Merck & Co.; 2006:2358–2363.

192. Gilbert's disease is associated with
A) overproduction of glucuronyl transferase
B) mild (benign) elevations of indirect (unconjugated) bilirubin
C) intravascular hemolysis
D) increased risk for liver disease

Answer and Discussion

The answer is B. Gilbert's disease is a persistent, lifelong condition that involves the deficiency of glucuronyl transferase. It affects as much as 5% of the population. There may be a familial component. Patients exhibit a persistent elevation in indirect (unconjugated) bilirubin. Stressful states and fasting may increase bilirubin levels. Patients do not exhibit symptoms, and there is no evidence of hemolysis. Gilbert's syndrome can be distinguished from hepatitis by normal liver function tests, absence of urinary bile, and predominantly unconjugated bilirubin fractionation. Hemolysis is differentiated by the absence of anemia or reticulocytosis. Liver histology is normal but biopsy is not needed for the diagnosis. No treatment is required, and no untoward effects are noted. Patients should be reassured that they do not have liver disease.

Beers MH, Porter RS, eds. *The Merck manual of diagnosis and therapy*, Merck Research Laboratories, 18th ed. Whitehouse Station, NJ: Merck & Co.; 2006:191, 195, 202.

193. Which of the following drugs used in the treatment of CHF has been shown to increase survival?
A) Digoxin
B) Furosemide
C) Hydralazine
D) Enalapril
E) Isosorbide dinitrate

Answer and Discussion

The answer is D. Medications for the treatment of CHF (related to systolic failure) include the following:

- *Diuretics*. Thiazide diuretics have been shown to be useful in decreasing fluid overload in patients with mild CHF by inhibiting sodium chloride reabsorption at the distal tubule; however, they are not usually effective in patients with advanced symptomatology. In moderate and severe cases, the loop diuretics (e.g., furosemide, bumetanide) are indicated; these agents inhibit solute resorption in the loop of Henle. Spironolactone (a potassium-sparing diuretic) can also be used in the treatment of CHF. Electrolytes should be monitored because of changes in serum potassium, as well as in sodium, magnesium, and calcium.

- *ACE inhibitors* (captopril, enalapril, lisinopril, ramipril). These medications serve as preload and afterload reducers by blocking (1) the production of angiotensin II, a potent vasoconstrictor, and (2) the release of aldosterone. ACE inhibitors are effective in the treatment of CHF and have been shown to increase survival in affected patients. Electrolytes should be monitored because of the possibility of hyperkalemia and renal insufficiency (especially in patients with renal artery stenosis). ACE inhibitors have also been shown to be beneficial in promoting renal blood flow in diabetes.
- *Angiotensin II–receptor blockers* (losartan, valsartan, candesartan) have similar effects to those of ACE inhibitors, although conclusive trials have not been reported regarding equal effectiveness.
- *Digoxin*. This medication has been shown to be effective in severe CHF and in CHF complicated by atrial fibrillation. Its mechanism of action involves the energy-dependent sodium–potassium pump, leading to increased intracellular calcium and a positive inotropic effect. Elderly patients and those taking other medication (e.g., quinidine, amiodarone) are at increased risk for toxicity and need close follow-up with monitoring of digoxin levels. Potassium levels should also be monitored closely; hypokalemia can precipitate arrhythmias in patients taking digoxin.
- *β-Blockers* (carvedilol, metoprololol) can reduce mortality in select patients—especially in patients with idiopathic dilated cardiomyopathy. With slower heart rates, diastolic function improves. Ventricular filling improves and the ejection fraction may improve over 6 to 12 months, giving rise to improved exercise capacity. Randomized control trials have shown significant reduction in all-cause mortality and cardiac events in patients taking carvedilol with mildly symptomatic CHF and an ejection fraction less than or equal to 35%.
- *Vasodilators* (e.g., hydralazine, isosorbide dinitrate) can be used if patients are unable to tolerate ACE inhibitors. They work by decreasing preload as a result of vasodilation.

Beers MH, Porter RS, eds. *The Merck manual of diagnosis and therapy,* Merck Research Laboratories, 18th ed. Whitehouse Station, NJ: Merck & Co.; 2006:652–665.

Ramahi TM. Beta blocker therapy for chronic heart failure. *Am Fam Physician.* 2000;62:2267–2274.

194. Which of the following statements regarding pneumococcal vaccination is true?
A) Immunosuppressed patients should not be immunized.
B) Indian populations are at high risk for complications and should be avoided.
C) Revaccination should occur every 10 years.
D) A one-time booster is given to patients over age 65 if they were vaccinated more than 5 years previously and they were over 65 at the time of their primary vaccination.
E) Sickle cell patients should be revaccinated every 5 years.

Answer and Discussion

The answer is D. Medical indications for pneumococcal vaccination include chronic disorders of the pulmonary system; cardiovascular diseases; diabetes mellitus; chronic liver diseases, including liver disease as a result of alcohol abuse (e.g., cirrhosis); chronic renal failure or nephrotic syndrome; functional or anatomic asplenia (e.g., sickle cell disease, splenectomy); immunosuppressive conditions (e.g., congenital immunodeficiency, HIV infection, leukemia, lymphoma, multiple myeloma, Hodgkin's disease, generalized malignancy, organ or bone marrow transplantation); chemotherapy with alkylating agents, antimetabolites, or long-term systemic corticosteroids; or cochlear implants. Geographic and other indications include Alaska Natives and certain American Indian populations. Other indications include residents of nursing homes and other long-term-care facilities. A one-time revaccination after 5 years is recommended for persons with chronic renal failure or nephrotic syndrome; functional or anatomic asplenia (e.g., sickle cell disease or splenectomy); immunosuppressive conditions (e.g., congenital immunodeficiency, HIV infection, leukemia, lymphoma, multiple myeloma, Hodgkin's disease, generalized malignancy, or organ or bone marrow transplantation); or chemotherapy with alkylating agents, antimetabolites, or long-term systemic corticosteroids. For persons older than 65 years, a one-time revaccination is recommended if they were vaccinated <5 years previously and were older than 65 years at the time of primary vaccination.

MMWR. Indications for pneumococcol vaccination. 2003;53 (MM43):1007.

195. A 24-year-old poorly controlled diabetic patient presents to your emergency room with ketoacidosis, fever, pain, and purulent drainage of the sinuses with black eschar formation affecting the nasal septum. The most likely diagnosis is
A) mucormycosis
B) cocaine use
C) chronic sinusitis
D) *Pseudomonas* infection
E) *Staphylococcus* infection

Answer and Discussion

The answer is A. Mucormycosis (phycomycosis) is a fungal infection that can be fulminant and lethal. It affects the nose, sinus, and orbit and is seen in patients with poorly controlled diabetes, diabetic ketoacidosis, or immunodeficiency. Symptoms include dull sinus pain; fever; orbital cellulitis; proptosis; nasal congestion and purulent or bloody nasal discharge; and gangrenous destruction of the nasal septum, orbits, or palate. In many cases, a black eschar is formed in the nasal area. If the fungus invades the cerebral vessels, then convulsions, blindness, and death can result. Diagnosis almost always involves biopsy. CT or MRI can help evaluate the extent of the disease. Treatment is accomplished with diabetic control, amphotericin B, and surgical débridement. The prognosis is poor, with up to a 50% mortality rate in disseminated cases.

Kasper DL, Braunwald E, Fauci AS, et al., eds. *Harrison's principles of internal medicine,* 16th ed. New York: McGraw-Hill; 2005:1190.

Mucormycosis affects the nose, sinus, and orbit and is seen in patients with poorly controlled diabetes, diabetic ketoacidosis, or immunodeficiency.

196. Pterygium is associated with
A) an increased risk of glaucoma
B) involvement of the pupillary area, which may require surgical excision if affected

C) improvement with the use of topical anesthetics
D) trauma to the retina
E) macular degeneration

Answer and Discussion

The answer is B. Pinguecula are hyaline, elastic nodules that appear yellow and affect both sides of the cornea but usually more on the nasal side. Occasionally they become inflamed and require treatment with topical steroids. However, in most cases no treatment is required. Pterygium is a fleshy, triangular growth of a pinguecula that involves the cornea. In some cases, it may involve the pupillary area and requires surgical removal. The causes include irritation from UV sunlight; allergens; and excessive drying, sandy, or windy conditions that cause chronic irritation. In most cases, treatment is supportive with topical vasoconstrictors, saline drops, and protection from sunlight. Surgery is reserved for more severe cases in which vision is compromised.

Stein HA, Slatt BJ, Stein RM. *The Ophthalmic Assistant, a Guide for Ophthalmic Medical Personnel.* St. Louis: Mosby; 2000:454.

197. Which of the following statements about Hodgkin's disease is true?
A) Lymphocyte-predominant disease has a better prognosis than mixed-cellularity type.
B) Lymphocyte-depleted Hodgkin's disease is the most common type.
C) Stages A and B are distinguished by the presence of metastatic disease to regional lymph nodes.
D) The disease most commonly affects patients between 40 and 50 years of age.
E) Treatment for stages 1A and 2A involves chemotherapy.

Answer and Discussion

The answer is A. Hodgkin's disease is a type of lymphoma that involves the presence of Reed-Sternberg cells. This type of cell is a large, abnormal macrophage-like cell with two prominent nuclei and surrounding halos that look like owl eyes. The disease has a bimodal distribution with a peak in individuals in their mid-20s and another peak in individuals older than 50 years. Symptoms include fever, weight loss, night sweats, and occasionally pain associated with involved lymph nodes with the ingestion of alcohol. Most patients affected present with painless lymphadenopathy in the neck. Metastasis is usually to local lymph nodes, with hematogenous spread late in the course of the disease. Chest radiographs may show asymmetric mediastinal lymphadenopathy (compared with sarcoidosis, which usually involves symmetric lymphadenopathy).The disease is classified into four different types:

1. Lymphocyte predominant
2. Nodular sclerosis (most common type)
3. Mixed cellularity
4. Lymphocyte depleted

Once the diagnosis is made, the disease is staged based on extent. Staging determines the modality of treatment:

Stage 1: one lymph node region involved
Stage 2: two areas of lymph nodes involved on the same side of the diaphragm
Stage 3: lymph node involvement on both sides of the diaphragm
Stage 4: disseminated disease with bone marrow or liver involvement

Further criteria involves stages of symptoms:

Stage A: lack of constitutional symptoms
Stage B: weight loss, fever, and night sweats are present

Treatment of stages 1A and 2A involves radiation. Stages 3B and 4 are treated with combination chemotherapy (i.e., the use of mechlorethamine vincristine [Oncovin], procarbazine, and prednisone). Treatment of stages 2B and 3A is controversial, but usually involves combined chemotherapy and radiotherapy. The prognosis is variable. Those with localized disease have excellent prognoses, whereas those with disseminated disease have poorer prognoses. In addition, those who have lymphocyte-predominant and nodular-sclerosing type fare better than those with mixed cellularity and lymphocyte-depleted forms.

Rakel RE, Bope ET. *Conn's Ccurrent Therapy 2005.* Philadelphia: Elsevier/Saunders; 2005:492–500.

198. Gamekeeper's thumb is associated with a sprain of the
A) extensor pollicis brevis tendon
B) extensor pollicis longus tendon
C) ulnar collateral ligament
D) flexor carpi ulnaris tendon
E) flexor retinaculum

Answer and Discussion

The answer is C. Gamekeeper's thumb (also known as *skier's thumb*) occurs when there is a sprain or traumatic rupture of the ulnar collateral ligament in the area of the thumb MCP joint. The injury occurs when there is hyperextension and hyperabduction of the thumb, usually as the result of a fall. The injury results in ulnar laxity of the MCP joint and often dorsal subluxation of the proximal thumb at the MCP joint. Patients often complain of weakness and pain when using the thumb to pinch and to perform activities such as opening car doors or jars or turning the key in a door lock. Other physical findings include swelling, erythema, ecchymosis, and tenderness over the MCP joint of the thumb on the ulnar side. As much as 95% of the injuries to the MCP joint occur on the ulnar side. Radiographs may show ulnar deviation of the proximal thumb and avulsion fracture of the ulnar collateral ligament at the base of the proximal phalanx. If the avulsed fragment is displaced more than 1 mm or involves more than 10% of the articular surface, surgery is indicated for repair. Also, if stress radiographs show laxity of the ulnar collateral ligament greater than 35 degrees on an anteroposterior radiograph, patients should be referred to an orthopedist. However, in less severe cases, immobilization in a thumb spica cast for 4 to 6 weeks is indicated.

Taylor RB, David AK, Johnson TA Jr, et al., eds. *Family medicine: principles and practice,* 5th ed. New York: Springer-Verlag; 1998:971–972.

199. Chronic alcohol consumption is associated with which of the following laboratory findings?
A) Increased high-density lipoprotein (HDL) cholesterol
B) Decreased aspartate transaminase
C) Decreased γ-glutamyl transferase
D) Increased testosterone
E) Microcytic anemia

Answer and Discussion

The answer is A. Fifteen percent of patients seen in family practice and 10% to 20% of patients in the hospital have an alcohol problem requiring at least minimal intervention. Chronic alcohol consumption can lead to a number of laboratory findings, including increased levels of HDL cholesterol; mild elevations of aspartate transaminase and, more specifically, γ-glutamyl transferase; megaloblastic anemia as a result of folate deficiency; thiamine deficiency; decreased serum calcium; and decreased testosterone levels. In most cases, cessation of alcohol consumption corrects the abnormal laboratory results, except in cases in which permanent damage has occurred. Screening for alcohol abuse may be accomplished quickly in the office setting with the CAGE questions. This acronym is used to remind the examiner of the following questions:

- Have you ever felt the need to **C**ut down on your drinking?
- Have you ever been **A**nnoyed by others' criticism of your drinking?
- Have you ever felt **G**uilty about your drinking?
- Have you ever had an "**E**ye opener" in the early morning?

A positive response to any of these questions should alert the examiner to ask more questions about the patient's alcohol consumption.

Ewing JA. Detecting alcoholism: the CAGE questionnaire. *JAMA.* 1984;252:1905–1907.

Rakel RE, Bope ET. *Conn's Current Therapy 2005.* Philadelphia: Elsevier/Saunders; 2005:1253, 1254.

200. A 55-year-old patient with a history of hypertriglyceridemia and severe abdominal pain with vomiting over the previous 6 hours is transferred from the emergency room to the hospital ward with the following laboratory findings:

- White blood cell count: 20,000
- Glucose: 295 mg/dL
- Aspartate aminotransferase: 333 IU/L
- Lactate dehydrogenase: 375 IU/L

The most likely diagnosis is
A) acute cholecystitis
B) acute pancreatitis
C) hepatitis
D) infectious mononucleosis
E) diabetic ketoacidosis

Answer and Discussion

The answer is B. Acute pancreatitis is caused by biliary tract disease, alcoholism, hyperlipidemia, hypercalcemia, hyperparathyroidism, trauma, medications (e.g., furosemide, valproic acid, sulfasalazine), infections, and structural abnormalities of the biliary tract. Symptoms include constant, boring, abdominal pain that radiates to the back; nausea; and repeated vomiting with a low-grade fever. Physical examination shows a distended rigid abdomen with positive peritoneal signs, tachycardia, tachypnea, and signs of dehydration and shock. Laboratory tests show an elevation in serum lipase (more sensitive) and amylase, elevated white blood cell count (12,000 to 20,000/mm^3), elevated liver function tests, increased bilirubin, hyperglycemia, and hypocalcemia. Chest radiographs may show pleural effusions. Abdominal films may show the presence of a sentinel loop (ileus of the transverse colon). Ultrasound or CT examination may show evidence of gallstones, dilation of the common bile duct, or edema of the pancreas. Pancreatitis associated with hemorrhage or necrosis of the pancreas has a mortality rate that approaches 50%. Hemorrhage is suspected if there is a grayish-blue discoloration of the back or flanks of the patient's body (Grey Turner's sign) or affecting the periumbilical area (Cullen's sign). Treatment involves bowel rest with nasogastric suction and fluid resuscitation with correction of electrolyte disturbances. Ranson's criteria are used to predict outcome at the time of admission:

- Older than 55 years
- White blood cell count >16,000/mm^3
- Serum glucose >200 mg/dL
- Lactate dehydrogenase >350 IU/L
- Aspartate aminotransferase level >250 IU/L

48 hours after admission:

- Greater than 10% decrease in hematocrit
- Elevation in BUN >5 mg/dL
- Serum calcium levels <8 mg/dL
- Base deficit >4 mEq/L
- Arterial PO_2 <60 mm Hg
- Greater than an estimated 6 L of fluid deposition in the body's interstitial spaces

If less than three signs are present at the time of admission, the mortality rate is <5%. The presence of three or more signs on admission has an associated mortality rate of 15% to 20%. If seven or more signs total are present, the mortality rate approaches 100%.

Beers MH, Porter RS, eds. *The Merck manual of diagnosis and therapy,* Merck Research Laboratories, 18th ed. Whitehouse Station, NJ: Merck & Co.; 2006:129–132.

201. A 40-year-old florist presents to your office complaining of a nontender nodule that formed on his hand, then enlarged, and finally ulcerated. In the days that followed, the patient developed similar nodules in the area of the axillary lymphatics. Otherwise he has had no other symptoms. The most likely diagnosis is
A) cat-scratch fever
B) sporotrichosis
C) tuberculosis
D) blastomycosis
E) histoplasmosis

Answer and Discussion

The answer is B. Sporotrichosis is a disease caused by inoculation of the plant *Sporothrix schenckii* when patients prick themselves with a thorn. The condition is associated with the formation of nodules, ulcers, and abscesses affecting the skin and lymphatic system. Farm workers and those who work around plants (i.e., florists, gardeners, nursery workers, and horticulturists) such as sphagnum moss, rosebushes, and barberry bushes are the most likely to be affected. Most patients present with a nontender nodule that forms on an arm or hand. The nodule enlarges, becomes erythematous (blush red), and finally ulcerates. In the following days, other nodules may form in the area of the draining lymphatics. Local pain and constitutional symptoms are usually absent. Other areas such as lungs, spleen, liver, kidney, genitalia, muscle, joints, and eyes may become involved. Diagnosis is usually achieved by culturing the organism from the nodules. Treatment is accomplished with itraconazole, extended courses of saturated solution of potassium iodide; in severe disseminated cases, intravenous amphotericin B or ketoconazole (less effective) is used.

Kasper DL, Braunwald E, Fauci AS, et al., eds. *Harrison's principles of internal medicine,* 16th ed. New York: McGraw-Hill; 2005:1193.

202. A hemodynamically unstable patient is noted to have supraventricular tachycardia. The most appropriate treatment is
A) electrical synchronized cardioversion
B) carotid massage
C) adenosine
D) verapamil
E) digoxin

Answer and Discussion

The answer is A. Supraventricular tachycardia is characterized by a rapid regular rhythm with a narrow QRS complex and abnormal P waves. The heart rate is usually 100 to 200 bpm. Some patients may be asymptomatic; others may experience chest pain, palpitations, and shortness of breath. Hemodynamically unstable patients with supraventricular tachycardia require immediate treatment with electrical synchronized cardioversion. For those patients who are stable, vagal stimulation can be attempted with carotid massage (but not in patients with previous cerebrovascular accidents or carotid bruits), Valsalva maneuvers, activation of the gag reflex, or placing a cold ice bag on the face. If these measures are unsuccessful, medication including adenosine, verapamil, diltiazem, or a β-blocker, can be used. Untreated supraventricular tachycardia may lead to heart failure.

Kasper DL, Braunwald E, Fauci AS, et al., eds. *Harrison's principles of internal medicine,* 16th ed. New York: McGraw-Hill; 2005:17.

203. The most common cause of tinnitus is
A) infection (otitis media)
B) chronic use of salicylates
C) sensorineural hearing loss
D) hypertension
E) acoustic neuroma

Answer and Discussion

The answer is C. Tinnitus is a common condition that is characterized by a ringing, roaring, rushing, buzzing, or whistling sound in the ears. The condition may be continuous or pulsatile with each heartbeat. In most cases, there is an associated hearing loss. In fact, the major cause of tinnitus is a sensorineural hearing loss. The list of associated conditions is extensive and includes obstruction of the canals, eustachian tube dysfunction, otosclerosis, Meniere's disease, aminoglycoside toxicity, chronic use of salicylates, anemia, hypertension, hypothyroidism, hyperlipidemia, noise-induced hearing loss, and tumors associated with the inner ear (e.g., acoustic neuroma). The evaluation of a patient with tinnitus includes an audiogram and CT scan or MRI of the head, with special emphasis given to the temporal area. Pulsatile tinnitus may require vascular studies to rule out aneurysm formation. Treatment depends on the diagnosis, but in most cases if the underlying disease is controlled, the tinnitus disappears. If no underlying disease process is present, background music or amplification may help to relieve symptoms.

Kasper DL, Braunwald E, Fauci AS, et al., eds. *Harrison's principles of internal medicine,* 16th ed. New York: McGraw-Hill; 2005:182–184.

204. A 65-year-old man is admitted to the hospital with complaints of shortness of breath. He has no prior medical care. The laboratory notifies you of a B-natriuretic peptide (BNP) value of 1500 pg/dL. You suspect the following diagnosis:
A) asthma exacerbation
B) COPD exacerbation
C) pulmonary embolism
D) deep venous thrombosis
E) congestive heart failure

Answer and Discussion

The answer is D. B-natriuretic peptide (BNP) is secreted by the heart's ventricles and is sensitive to changes in left ventricular function. Elevated levels are associated with elevated levels of end-diastolic pressure. BNP can be helpful in determining whether shortness of breath is due to cardiac versus a pulmonary etiology. A value $<$100 pg/mL is considered normal, whereas a value $>$400 pg/dL represents a $>$95% chance of congestive heart failure. Some pulmonary processes are associated with elevated BNP including lung cancer, cor pulmonale, and pulmonary embolism; however, elevations are usually not as high as seen in CHF. Decreased creatinine clearance is associated with higher levels of BNP.

Maisel AS, Zoorob R. B-type natriuretic peptide in congestive heart failure: diagnosis and management. *CME Bulletin.* 2004;3(3):1–10.

205. Which of the following toxin exposure–antidote associations is correct?
A) Cyanide–calcium carbonate
B) Ethylene glycol–ethanol and pyridoxine
C) Magnesium–amyl nitrite
D) Organic phosphates–epinephrine

Answer and Discussion

The answer is B. Toxin exposure is often treated by family physicians. The following are the drugs of choice for treating the associated toxin exposures:

Toxin	Treatment
Atropine	Physostigmine
Cyanide	Amyl nitrite
Magnesium	Calcium carbonate
Ethylene glycol	Ethanol and pyridoxine
Organic phosphates	Atropine

Beers MH, Porter RS, eds. *The Merck manual of diagnosis and therapy,* Merck Research Laboratories, 18th ed. Whitehouse Station, NJ: Merck & Co.; 2006:2652–2653.

206. Guttate psoriasis
A) are thick, scaly plaque-like lesions that are commonly identified as psoriasis
B) are not associated with respiratory illnesses
C) are not usually associated with skin creases
D) are insidious in their outbreak with large "bull's-eye" type lesions

Answer and Discussion

The answer is C. The condition of guttate psoriasis is characterized by numerous small, oval (teardrop-shaped) lesions that develop after an acute upper respiratory tract infection. These lesions are often not as scaly or as erythematous as the classic lesions of plaque-type psoriasis. Usually, guttate psoriasis must be differentiated from pityriasis rosea, another condition characterized by the sudden outbreak of red scaly lesions. Compared with pityriasis rosea, psoriatic lesions are thicker and scalier, and the lesions are not usually distributed along skin creases.

Pardasani AG, Feldman SR, Clark AR. Treatment of psoriasis: an algorthm-based approach for primary care physicians. *Am Fam Physician.* 2000;61:725–33, 736

The condition of guttate psoriasis is characterized by numerous small, oval (teardrop-shaped) lesions that develop after an acute upper respiratory tract infection.

207. In the treatment of external genital warts, it is important to
A) biopsy the visible lesions
B) aceto-white stain the areas to identify the affected lesions
C) obtain viral-typing of the lesions
D) remove visible warts

Answer and Discussion

The answer is D. Genital warts caused by human papillomavirus infection are frequently seen in primary care. Evidence-based treatment recommendations are limited, but treatment guidelines recently have changed. Biopsy, viral typing, aceto-white staining, and other diagnostic measures are not routinely required. The goal of treatment is removal of visible warts; some evidence exists that treatment reduces infectivity, but there is no evidence that treatment reduces the incidence of cervical and genital cancer. The choice of therapy is based on the number, size, site, and appearance of lesions, as well as patient preferences, cost, convenience, adverse effects, and clinician preference. Patient-applied therapy such as imiquimod cream or podofilox is increasingly recommended. Podofilox, imiquimod, surgical excision, and cryotherapy are the most convenient and effective options. Fluorouracil and interferon are no longer recommended for routine use.

Kodner CM, Nasraty S. Management of genital warts. *Am Fam Physician.* 2004;70:2335–2342, 2345–2346.

208. Silo filler's disease is caused by chronic inhalation of
A) carbon monoxide
B) nitrogen dioxide
C) nitrogen mustard
D) nitrous oxide
E) carbon dioxide

Answer and Discussion

The answer is B. Silo filler's disease is a pulmonary disease that is caused by the inhalation of nitrogen dioxide. Those affected are usually farmers who are exposed to the toxic gas, which is produced from moldy hay found in silos and grain bins. Because of the irritant effects, the gas can lead to the development of pulmonary edema, usually 10 to 12 hours after exposure to the gas. In severe cases, exposure can lead to bronchiolitis obliterans with associated respiratory failure and death. Symptoms include irritation to the mucous membranes and eyes, cough, hemoptysis, wheezing, nausea, vomiting, and dyspnea. Chest radiographs usually show alveolar infiltrates and pulmonary edema. Bacterial superinfections can occur and can lead to serious complications. Treatment usually involves bronchodilators, intravenous fluids, mechanical ventilation, and steroids. Chronic exposure may lead to chronic bronchitis.

Kasper DL, Braunwald E, Fauci AS, et al., eds. *Harrison's principles of internal medicine,* 16th ed. New York: McGraw-Hill; 2005:1522.

209. Which of the following is an effect of niacin use?
A) Increased LDL cholesterol
B) Increased triglyceride levels
C) Increased HDL cholesterol
D) Hypoglycemia
E) Decreased uric acid levels

Answer and Discussion

The answer is C. Niacin (nicotinic acid) is used to treat hyperlipidemia. It lowers LDL cholesterol and triglyceride levels and increases HDL cholesterol levels. It is the most effective drug for increasing HDLs. The medication is available without a prescription. Side effects include flushing, pruritus, hepatotoxicity, elevated glucose and uric acid levels, and GI irritation. Doses range from 500 mg/day to a maximum of 3 g/day. Aspirin taken approximately 45 minutes before the administration of niacin may help to decrease flushing episodes. Liver function tests should be periodically monitored when patients are taking the medication.

Beers MH, Porter RS, eds. *The Merck manual of diagnosis and therapy,* Merck Research Laboratories, 18th ed. Whitehouse Station, NJ: Merck & Co.; 2006:1308.

210. Which of the following tests is most sensitive for detecting maxillary sinusitis?
A) Plain radiographs
B) CT scan
C) Transillumination
D) Ultrasound
E) Tomograms

Answer and Discussion

The answer is B. Acute sinusitis is usually precipitated by an upper respiratory infection. Because sinusitis is rarely present without an associated inflammation of the nasal passageways, it is best referred to as *rhinosinusitis.* Rhinosinusitis occurs if there is insufficient draining of the sinus, which predisposes to development of purulent, infected fluid. In most cases, edematous sinus tissue is the cause of impaired drainage and the development of a bacterial infection. Typical pathogens include *S. pneumoniae, H. influenzae,* and other organisms such as *S. aureus* and *Moraxella catarrhalis.* Symptoms include purulent rhinorrhea, nasal congestion, impaired sense of smell, pain over the sinus area, and pressure behind the eyes, as well as pain associated with the upper dental area. Low-grade fevers may be present. In some cases, a dental infection or abscess may be the cause.

The diagnosis of acute rhinosinusitis is made primarily by a careful clinical history. Radiologic studies do not have a significant role in the diagnosis of acute rhinosinusitis. Although plain radiographs of the sinuses may show opacification, which supports the diagnosis, coronal CT scan of the sinuses is the most sensitive test for complicated cases. Cultures of nasal discharge are unreliable and are not useful in the diagnosis. Most cases of acute sinusitis have a viral cause and resolve within 2 weeks without antibiotic coverage. Antibiotics should be reserved for those with moderate to severe symptoms. When selecting an antibiotic, amoxicillin has better sinus penetration than ampicillin and is the medication of choice as a first-line drug. TMP-SMX is also effective as a first-line treatment. Duration of therapy is typically 10 to 14 days, although success can be achieved with shorter courses. The use of adjunctive treatments such as antihistamines has no proven benefit. Complications, although rare, include osteomyelitis, mucocele, and cavernous sinus thrombosis. Persistent epistaxis, pain, and recurrent sinusitis should alert the practitioner to the possibility of paranasal sinus cancer.

Ferri F. *Ferri's Clinical Advisor, Instant Diagnosis and Treatment.* Philadelphia: Elsevier/Mosby; 2006:782–783.

211. Which of the following statements best describes a case-control study?

A) It is an observational design-type study that begins with an outcome and then looks for common aspects among those who are affected.
B) It is a study that categorizes subjects into groups and observes outcomes.
C) It is a study that identifies outcomes and predictors of outcomes simultaneously.
D) It is a study that records information, activities, and observations but does not provide explanations.

Answer and Discussion

The answer is A. The following are types of studies encountered in the medical literature:

- *Case-control study:* This is an observational design–type study that begins with an outcome and then looks for common aspects among those who are affected.
- *Cohort study:* This is a prospective design study. Subjects with similar characteristics are categorized into groups and then researchers observe the outcome.
- *Cross-sectional study:* This is an observational design–type study that takes a subject group and identifies outcomes and their predictors simultaneously.
- *Clinical series study:* This is a descriptive-type study that records information, activities, and observations but provides no explanations. These studies usually lead to further explanatory-type studies.

Gehlbach SH. *Interpreting the Medical Literature: a Clinician's Guide.* New York: Collamore Press; 1981:18, 24, 30.

212. A 50-year-old man complains of gradual increasing shortness of breath, and evidence of honeycombing of pulmonary architecture is seen on a chest radiograph. Pulmonary function tests show both decreased vital and diffusing capacities as well as reduced total lung volumes with a normal forced expiratory volume in 1 second to forced vital capacity ratio. The most likely diagnosis is

A) chronic obstructive pulmonary disease (COPD)
B) tuberculosis
C) asthma
D) idiopathic pulmonary fibrosis
E) chronic pulmonary embolism

Answer and Discussion

The answer is D. Idiopathic pulmonary fibrosis, a form of interstitial lung disease, results when there is inflammation of the lung tissue with resulting fibrosis. A toxic exposure or antigenic response is thought to precipitate the inflammatory process. Affected patients may report a gradual, increasing shortness of breath; a dry cough; and generalized fatigue with lack of endurance with physical exercise. Physical examination shows bibasilar dry rales, clubbing, and, occasionally, cyanosis. In advanced disease, chest radiographs show honeycombing, and pulmonary function tests show a restrictive pattern with reduced vital capacity, diffusing capacity for carbon monoxide, and total lung volume. In addition, there is a normal or increased forced expiratory volume in 1 second to forced vital capacity ratio. Arterial blood gases may show mild hypoxemia, but hypercarbia is rare. The patient's ESR may be increased. Transthoracic or transbronchial biopsy is usually needed for a definitive diagnosis. The treatment of idiopathic pulmonary fibrosis is controversial because of a lack of understanding of the natural history of the disease. Only 10% to 15% of patients improve with corticosteroid therapy, and 26% of patients develop serious complications from the steroid therapy. Indicators of good response to steroid therapy include young age, female gender, ground-glass lesions on CT scan, and active inflammation on lung biopsy samples. Azathioprine, cyclophosphamide, and other cytotoxic drugs have been used as second-line agents or in combination with steroids as first-line therapy. Although the general prognosis was poor, combined treatment improved 3-year survival rates. Selected patients with idiopathic pulmonary fibrosis have been treated with lung transplantation.

Karnani NG, Reisfield GM, Wilson GR. Evaluation of chronic dyspnea. *Am Fam Physician.* 2005;71:1529–1537, 1538.

213. A 52-year-old man who is otherwise healthy is found to have a deep venous thrombosis (DVT) affecting his left lower extremity below the knee. Appropriate management includes

A) administration of clopidogrel (Plavix)
B) initiation of aspirin as an outpatient
C) observation
D) intravascular thrombolysis
E) administration of low-molecular-weight heparin as an outpatient

Answer and Discussion

The answer is C. DVT is a condition that involves thrombus formation, usually in the lower-extremity veins. Predisposing conditions include lack of activity; previous DVT; recent surgery; smoking; and hypercoagulable states, including antithrombin III deficiency, protein C or S deficiency, lupus, cancer, and estrogen use. Symptoms include pain and swelling, as well as erythema and warmth of the lower extremity. Physical examination may be normal, and a positive Homans' sign is not a reliable predictor for DVT. Diagnosis is usually made with Doppler ultrasound (duplex) studies, which is operator-dependent and does not detect thrombi below the knee very well. The gold standard test is contrast venography. A D-dimer is often elevated in patients with venous thrombosis. It is sensitive but not specific. Impedance plethysmography is highly sensitive for thrombi above the knee but less sensitive if the thrombosis is below the knee. Treatment for DVT above the knee involves intravenous heparin or low-molecular-weight heparin and oral warfarin. It is important to overlap heparin treatment with oral warfarin for at least 4 to 5 days because the full anticoagulant effect of warfarin is delayed. Warfarin should be continued for at least 3 to 6 months, although the optimal treatment time is controversial. Age and a history of thromboembolic events are strong risk factors for recurrence.

Treatment of DVT below the knee is controversial. Calf vein thrombosis should be either treated with anticoagulants or followed with serial Doppler studies to rule out propagation. DVT prophylaxis regimens depend on the level of risk:

- *Low risk*. Individuals who are at low risk include those who have major surgery requiring anesthesia for at least 30 minutes, immobilized patients, patients with myocardial infarction or CHF, and women after cesarean section. The prophylaxis is heparin at 5,000 U (given subcutaneously every 12 hours) and intermittent compressive devices (at least once per minute).
- *High risk*. Individuals who are at high risk include those who have pelvic or lower extremity surgery, including hip or knee replacement, or a previous DVT or pulmonary embolism. The prophylaxis is a combination of compression devices plus low-molecular weight heparin or warfarin.

The use of low-molecular-weight heparin is becoming more common in the treatment of DVT because it offers the advantages of having a more predictable anticoagulant effect, avoids the need for anticoagulation testing, and allows the patient to be treated at home. It is also associated with less antibody formation, a lower risk of heparin-induced thrombocytopenia, and a decreased overall mortality. Patients being treated at home must learn to give themselves subcutaneous injections and should have close follow-up. Warfarin therapy should be initiated on day 1 when using unfractionated or low-molecular-weight heparin. After 4 to 5 days and when the INR is greater than 2 for 2 consecutive days, the heparin therapy can be discontinued.

Patients who are at risk for bleeding may be candidates for inferior vena caval filter placement. There is little use in aggressive cancer workup in patients after an initial episode of DVT. A thorough history, physical examination, and age-appropriate cancer screening are adequate.

Kasper DL, Braunwald E, Fauci AS, et al., eds. *Harrison's principles of internal medicine,* 16th ed. New York: McGraw-Hill; 2005:1491–1492.

214. Which of the following statements is true regarding ulcerative colitis?

A) There is transmural involvement of the bowel wall.
B) There are skipped areas of inflammation that may have a cobblestone appearance on colonoscopy.
C) There is a smaller risk of developing intestinal cancer in comparison to Crohn's disease.
D) The area of involvement is localized to the colon and rectosigmoid area.
E) Aminosalicylic acid compounds are not effective in the treatment of ulcerative colitis.

Answer and Discussion

The answer is D. Ulcerative colitis is characterized by inflammation of the bowel that is limited to the mucosal surface and submucosa of the bowel wall (i.e., it is not transmural like Crohn's disease). The area of involvement is localized to the colon and rectosigmoid area in a continuous fashion; this is unlike Crohn's disease, which shows skipped areas of involvement. Symptoms include bloody diarrhea, abdominal pain, fever, and tenesmus. Complications include intestinal perforation, the development of toxic megacolon, and the development of cancer (which is more commonly seen in patients with ulcerative colitis than in those with Crohn's disease). Extracolonic involvement affects the skin, eyes, joints, and liver; however, the kidneys are not involved (as they are in Crohn's disease). Diagnosis is accomplished in the same manner as in Crohn's disease (i.e., colonoscopy or flexible sigmoidoscopy with biopsy or with x-ray contrast studies). Treatment of ulcerative colitis is similar to that for Crohn's disease; however, the oral forms of 5-aminosalicylic acid (e.g., sulfasalazine, olsalazine, mesalamine) are more effective in controlling recurrences and the severity of outbreaks in ulcerative colitis. Close follow-up is necessary for ulcerative colitis and Crohn's disease because of the increased risk of developing bowel cancer.

Ferri F. *Ferri's Clinical Advisor, Instant Diagnosis and Treatment.* Philadelphia: Elsevier/Mosby; 2006:879.

215. A 60-year-old man presents with pain, swelling, and redness of the first metatarsal phalangeal joint. His cardiologist recently prescribed hydrochlorothiazide for his hypertension. The most likely diagnosis is

A) podagra
B) degenerative joint disease
C) rheumatoid arthritis
D) osteomyelitis
E) Morton's neuroma

Answer and Discussion

The answer is A. Gout is a condition characterized by recurrent pain associated with peripheral joints. The cause is attributed to the development of monosodium urate crystals, which cause acute arthritis. Long-standing gout can lead to chronic, deforming arthritis. The greater the degree of hyperuricemia, the more likely is the development of gouty attacks. Most hyperuricemia is asymptomatic. Hyperuricemia may result from disorders of purine metabolism, which may be genetic or acquired. Disorders causing hyperuricemia include proliferative hematologic disorders, psoriasis, myxedema, parathyroid disorders, enzyme deficiencies, and renal disease; obesity and medications such as thiazide diuretics are also causative. Middle-age and elderly men are usually affected more frequently than women; however, menopause is associated with a sharp increase in incidence in women (especially in those using thiazides and those with renal impairment). Symptoms include severe, throbbing pain with redness and swelling that is usually monoarticular and affects the metatarsophalangeal joint of the great toe (podagra). However, other joints, including the ankle, knee, wrist, and elbow, may also be affected. Other symptoms include fever and malaise. Later attacks may become more frequent and affect multiple joints with resolution between attacks less complete. Precipitating factors include trauma, overindulgence of foods (processed meats), alcohol, surgery, fatigue, stress, infection, or the administration of medications (e.g., penicillin, insulin, thiazide diuretics). Diagnosis is usually made based on history and physical exam. Absolute confirmation involves joint aspiration with the detection of needle-shaped urate crystals that are negatively birefringent under a polarizing microscope. Asymptomatic treatment of hyperuricemia is generally not treated with medication. Treatment of gout involves the use of ice, rest, NSAIDs (e.g., indomethacin, naproxen, ibuprofen), colchicine (which may provide dramatic relief in the acute phase), and allopurinol (xanthine oxidase inhibitor) for patients who have chronically elevated uric acid levels after the acute attack has resolved (low-dose colchicine can also be used). In addition, uricosuric agents, including probenecid and sulfinpyrazone, may be helpful but should be used with caution in patients with renal problems. Prednisone may also be helpful in patients who cannot tolerate other medications. Transplantation recipients and those undergoing chemotherapy are usually protected with the use of allopurinol.

Ferri F. *Ferri's Clinical Advisor, Instant Diagnosis and Treatment.* Philadelphia: Elsevier/Mosby; 2006:350–351.

216. The use of proton pump inhibitors can result in
A) vitamin C deficiency
B) vitamin D deficiency
C) vitamin B_{12} deficiency
D) folate deficiency

Answer and Discussion

The answer is C. Vitamin B_{12} (cobalamin) deficiency is a common cause of macrocytic anemia and has been implicated in a host of neuropsychiatric conditions. The widespread use of gastric acid–blocking agents, which can lead to decreased vitamin B_{12} levels, may contribute to the development of vitamin B_{12} deficiency. Given the widespread use of these agents and the aging of the U.S. population, the actual prevalence of vitamin B_{12} deficiency may be even higher than statistics indicate. Vitamin B_{12} deficiency is associated with hematologic, neurologic, and psychiatric symptoms. Neurologic manifestations from vitamin B_{12} deficiency include paresthesias, peripheral neuropathy, and demyelination of the corticospinal tract and dorsal columns (subacute combined systems disease). Vitamin B_{12} deficiency also has been linked to psychiatric disorders, including impaired memory, irritability, depression, dementia and, rarely, psychosis. Dietary sources of vitamin B_{12} are primarily meats and dairy products. In a typical Western diet, a person obtains approximately 5 to 15 mcg of vitamin B_{12} daily, which is far greater than the recommended daily allowance of 2 mcg. Normally, individuals maintain a large vitamin B_{12} reserve, which can last 2 to 5 years even in the presence of severe malabsorption. However, nutritional deficiency can occur in specific populations. Elderly patients and chronic alcoholics are at especially high risk. The dietary restrictions of strict vegans make them another, less common at-risk population. The role of B_{12} deficiency in hyperhomocysteinemia and the promotion of atherosclerosis are under investigation. Diagnosis of vitamin B_{12} deficiency is based on measurement of serum vitamin B_{12} levels; however, about half of patients with subclinical disease have normal B_{12} levels. A more sensitive method of screening for vitamin B_{12} deficiency is measurement of serum methylmalonic acid and homocysteine levels, which are increased early in vitamin B_{12} deficiency. Use of the Schilling test for detection of pernicious anemia has been replaced for the most part by serologic testing for parietal cell and intrinsic factor antibodies. Contrary to prevailing medical practice, supplementation with oral vitamin B_{12} is a safe and effective treatment for the B_{12} deficiency state. Even when intrinsic factor is not present to aid in the absorption of vitamin B_{12} (pernicious anemia) or in other diseases that affect the usual absorption sites in the terminal ileum, oral therapy remains effective.

Oh RC, Brown DL. Vitamin B_{12} deficiency. *Am Fam Physician.* 2003;67:979–986, 993–994.

217. A 32-year-old man presents to your office. Approximately 5 days ago he was cleaning out his dark, undisturbed attic. That day he noticed an erythematous lesion with a clear center on his arm. Since then the lesion has necrosed in the center, giving rise to a crater-like eschar lesion. The most likely diagnosis is
A) Lyme disease
B) brown recluse spider bite
C) psittacosis
D) black widow spider bite
E) scorpion sting

Answer and Discussion

The answer is B. The brown recluse spider (violin spider) may be identified by a dark, violin-shaped design on its back. These spiders are usually found in dark areas, woodpiles, attics, and other undisturbed locations. The bite is initially mild (burning at site) and goes unnoticed, although some localized pain develops within 30 to 60 minutes. Within 1 to 4 hours, an erythematous, pruritic area with an ischemic pale center develops, giving the appearance of a bull's-eye target lesion. The central zone may progress to form a pustule that eventually fills with blood and ruptures; within 3 to 4 days, a crater-like lesion with necrosis develops. Large tissue defects may occur and include muscle. Healing usually requires extended periods; if large areas are involved, skin grafting may be necessary in some cases. Symptoms include headache, nausea and vomiting, low-grade fever, chills and sweats, generalized pruritus, malaise, arthralgias, severe pain (late in the course), and rash. Rare fatalities (none in the United States) have been reported with complications such as massive intravascular hemolysis with hemoglobinuria, renal failure, and disseminated intravascular coagulopathy. Treatment with dapsone has been recommended. Because dapsone can cause agranulocytosis and hemolytic anemia, which may be exaggerated in patients with G6PD deficiency, a G6PD test and CBC should be done before starting therapy. Systemic corticosteroids have shown no consistent or reliable benefit. Surgical débridement should be delayed until the area of necrosis is fully demarcated. Incision and suction is not recommended. Most bites require only local treatment. Ice therapy to the site may help reduce pain.

Beers MH, Porter RS, eds. *The Merck manual of diagnosis and therapy,* Merck Research Laboratories, 18th ed. Whitehouse Station, NJ: Merck & Co.; 2006:2648–2649.

218. A 60-year-old alcoholic man, currently being treated for gastritis, presents to the office with painful breasts that appear enlarged. The most likely cause is
A) breast cancer
B) excessive calcium carbonate ingestion
C) cimetidine use
D) trauma
E) prolactinoma

Answer and Discussion

The answer is C. Gynecomastia is a condition characterized by enlargement of the breasts in men. It occurs when there is hypertrophy of breast tissue beneath the areola. In young adolescents, it is a natural response to the body's hormones. During this time, the breast may be tender. Patients and their parents should be reassured this is a natural response and will eventually resolve (usually within 3 years). Gynecomastia in older males can result from medication use (e.g., cimetidine, INH, digitalis, phenothiazine, testosterone), substance abuse (e.g., alcohol; illegal drugs, including marijuana and heroin), endocrine disorders (e.g., hypogonadism, hyperthyroidism), Klinefelter's syndrome, liver disease, and neoplasm. The workup of gynecomastia should include a chest radiograph, β-human chorionic gonadotropin determination, luteinizing hormone, follicle-stimulating hormone, estrogen and testosterone levels, liver function tests, and thyroid function tests. Typically, the estrogen:testosterone ratio is high. If the human chorionic gonadotropin is elevated, then a testicular ultrasound should be performed to look for testicular tumor. Additionally, if the testes are small, a karyotype should be obtained to look for Klinefelter's syndrome. Other testing may be necessary, if indicated. Treatment involves correcting the underlying abnormality. If the condition does not resolve, suppressive medication or surgery may be indicated.

Kasper DL, Braunwald E, Fauci AS, et al., eds. *Harrison's principles of internal medicine,* 16th ed. New York: McGraw-Hill; 2005:2192.

Gynecomastia in older males can result from medication use (e.g., cimetidine, INH, digitalis, phenothiazine, testosterone), substance abuse (e.g., alcohol; illegal drugs, including marijuana and heroin), endocrine disorders (e.g., hypogonadism, hyperthyroidism), Klinefelter's syndrome, liver disease, and neoplasm.

219. Which of the following can distinguish atrial flutter from sinus tachycardia?
A) Carotid sinus massage
B) Administration of diltiazem
C) Administration of isoproterenol
D) Temporal artery massage
E) Administration of adenosine

Answer and Discussion

The answer is A. Atrial flutter is a regular, rapid cardiac rhythm characterized by an ectopic focus that gives rise to atrial rates from 280 to 350 impulses per minute. Usually, impulses are only transmitted to the ventricles every second, third, or fourth impulse. The heart rate is usually approximately 150 bpm. In many cases, atrial flutter is difficult to distinguish from sinus tachycardia; however, carotid sinus massage or Valsalva maneuvers may help distinguish the characteristic (sawtooth) flutter waves seen with atrial flutter. ECG shows flutter waves best in the inferior leads II, III, aVF, and in V1. RR interval may be regular, reflecting a fixed ratio AV block (2:1, 3:1), or may be variable, reflecting a Wenckebach periodicity. Limited data suggest that the risk of thromboembolism, although smaller than with atrial fibrillation, is increased, suggesting anticoagulation should be considered. Treatment consists of verapamil, diltiazem, β-blockers, or digoxin, which slows conduction through the AV node. Electric cardioversion (low energy) is indicated for patients who are unstable and show signs of CHF (e.g., pulmonary rales, hepatojugular reflux, distended neck veins).

Kasper DL, Braunwald E, Fauci AS, et al., eds. *Harrison's principles of internal medicine,* 16th ed. New York: McGraw-Hill; 2005:1344, 1347.

220. The drug of choice for the treatment of trigeminal neuralgia is
A) naproxen
B) prednisone
C) carbamazepine
D) valproic acid
E) phenobarbital

Answer and Discussion

The answer is C. Trigeminal neuralgia is a disorder that involves the trigeminal nucleus of the trigeminal nerve. This disorder is characterized by severe, unilateral, sharp, lancinating-type pain that occurs in the distribution of the trigeminal nerve. Most patients are of middle age or elderly. The symptoms usually occur in recurrent bouts and can be incapacitating. Women tend to be more frequently affected than men. Precipitating factors include touching the affected area and movement of the face (as with eating, talking, and brushing one's teeth), shaving, or feeling a cool breeze on the face. Patients afflicted with trigeminal neuralgia show no physical signs. If deficits are noted during neurologic examination, then alternative diagnosis, including masses impinging on the trigeminal nerve, demyelinating processes, or vascular malformation, should be considered. In most cases, the momentary bouts of pain become more and more frequent and remissions become shorter and shorter. A dull ache that is persistent between the episodes of severe stabbing pain may develop. Remissions may occur and last weeks or even months. The treatment of choice is carbamazepine, which requires monitoring of serial blood counts and liver function tests. Alternative medications include phenytoin and baclofen. Other treatments include injecting glycerol into the offending nerve, surgery to decompress nerve fibers from blood vessels and bony structures, and radiofrequency rhizotomy if medical therapy fails.

Ferri F. *Ferri's Clinical Advisor, Instant Diagnosis and Treatment.* Philadelphia: Elsevier/Mosby; 2006:865.

The treatment of choice for trigeminal neuralgia is carbamazepine, which requires monitoring of serial blood counts and liver function tests.

221. A 27-year-old woman reports a previous reaction to penicillin. She has had recurrent sinus and respiratory infections. Appropriate management would consist of
A) having the patient tested for penicillin allergies
B) using a cephalosporin if patient has had previous anaphylactoid response
C) administering amoxicillin instead of penicillin
D) administering diphenhydramine with penicillin
E) substituting imipenem for penicillin

Answer and Discussion

The answer is A. An allergy to penicillin is related to penicilloic acid—a breakdown product—and other degradation products that are involved in the metabolism of penicillin. All penicillins are cross-reactive and cross-sensitizing. As many as 25% of patients who report previous penicillin allergies have no reaction when given penicillin. Therefore, it is obvious that many patients are labeled with a penicillin allergy when, in fact, they can take penicillin safely. The incidence of penicillin allergy is approximately 1% to 4% of adults. Symptoms include characteristic anaphylactoid symptoms with shock and bronchoconstriction in type 1 hypersensitivity reactions. Other symptoms include rashes, oral lesions, fever, joint swelling, pruritus, and respiratory distress. Methicillin and nafcillin have caused interstitial nephritis with renal tubular acidosis. The decision to use penicillin in patients with previous reactions should be based on the severity of previous reactions. If the patient has had a severe anaphylactic reaction in the past, penicillins should be avoided. In addition, there is a 2% cross-reactivity between cephalosporins in patients with penicillin allergies; thus cephalosporins should be avoided in patients who have had an immediate reaction to penicillin. The same is true for imipenem. Skin tests that use penicilloyl–polylysine and undegraded penicillin may be used to detect patients who have true penicillin allergies.

Kasper DL, Braunwald E, Fauci AS, et al., eds. *Harrison's principles of internal medicine,* 16th ed. New York: McGraw-Hill; 2005:801, 1950.

222. Which of the following would best help to stop bleeding in a patient with von Willebrand's disease?
A) Fresh frozen plasma
B) Cryoprecipitate
C) Vitamin K
D) Platelets
E) Protamine sulfate

Answer and Discussion

The answer is B. von Willebrand's disease is an autosomal-dominant transmitted disorder that can lead to abnormal bleeding tendencies. Men and women are equally affected. It is the most common congenital bleeding disorder. The disease is due to a lack of production of von Willebrand factor (type 1) or when the von Willebrand factor is not synthesized properly and is nonfunctional (type 2). The result is a decreased ability of platelets to adhere to collagen. Symptoms include mild to moderate bleeding from small cuts, bruising, epistaxis, excessive menstrual blood loss, GI blood loss, and excessive bleeding during surgery. Laboratory results show an increased bleeding time with a slightly prolonged partial thromboplastin time (PTT) if factor VIII is below 25% to 30%. In most cases, the PT, PTT, and platelet count are normal. Definitive diagnosis for von Willebrand's disease type 1 is made by measuring the levels of (1) von Willebrand factor, (2) antibody response to von Willebrand's antigen, (3) factor VIII, and (4) ristocetin cofactor activity. In patients with type 1 disease, all four measurements are decreased; in patients with type 2 disease, electrophoresis studies may be needed for the diagnosis. Treatment involves the administration of cryoprecipitate, which replaces the von Willebrand factor and stops bleeding. A pasteurized intermediate-purity factor VIII concentrate contains large multimers of von Willebrand factor and is a safe (no HIV or hepatitis) alternative cryoprecipitate. Desmopressin acetate, a synthetic analog of vasopressin, stimulates the release of von Willebrand factor from endothelial cells and can be used in the treatment of mild type 1 disease (but not of type 2). Oral contraceptives can also increase the levels of factor VIII and may be beneficial for women with menorrhagia.

Kasper DL, Braunwald E, Fauci AS, et al., eds. *Harrison's principles of internal medicine,* 16th ed. New York: McGraw-Hill; 2005:340–341, 676.

223. Which of the following values is acceptable for a 65-year-old man who had a previous coronary artery bypass graft?
A) Total cholesterol of 215 mg/dL
B) HDL cholesterol of 32 mg/dL
C) LDL cholesterol of 68 mg/dL
D) Triglycerides of 228 mg/dL
E) Blood glucose of 130 mg/dL

Answer and Discussion

The answer is C. Guidelines have been published to help treat patients with hyperlipidemia. Total cholesterol levels should be kept <200 mg/dL, with HDL cholesterol (good cholesterol) >40 mg/dL. Further recommendations are divided into those for patients with CHD and those without CHD. CHD equivalents include peripheral arterial disease, abdominal aortic aneurysm, symptomatic carotid arterial disease and diabetes mellitus. For patients without CHD and fewer than two risk factors, LDL cholesterol should be kept <160 mg/dL. For those with two or more risk factors and no CAD, the goal is an LDL level <130 mg/dL. For patients who have CAD, the new recommendations give a goal for LDL cholesterol <100 mg/dL with <70 mg/dL as being optimal. Triglyceride levels are not as strongly associated with CAD but should be kept <150 mg/dL. Risk factors for CHD include the following:

- Age: men older than 45 years; women older than 55 years or with premature menopause without estrogen replacement
- Family history of premature CHD in first-degree relative
- Smoking
- Hypertension
- HDL cholesterol <35 mg/dL
- Diabetes
- Obesity
- History of cerebral or peripheral vascular disease

A negative risk factor includes an HDL cholesterol level higher than 60 mg/dL.

National Cholesterol Education Program. Third report of the expert panel on detection, evaluation, and treatment of high blood cholesterol in adults (Adult Treatment Panel III). Accessed online 6/5/06, at: http://www.nhlbi.nih.gov/guidelines/cholesterol/index.htm.

224. Which of the following statements about Still's murmur is true?
A) It is benign and resolves over time.
B) It is common in the elderly and results from decreased ventricular compliance.
C) It is associated with severe chronic aortic regurgitation.
D) It should always be assessed with an echocardiogram.
E) CHF is usually coexistent.

Answer and Discussion

The answer is A. Some murmurs are specific to certain cardiac conditions:

- *Austin Flint murmur* is associated with severe chronic aortic regurgitation and may be middiastolic or presystolic. The murmur occurs when there is backflow of blood from the aorta into the left ventricle and flow into the left ventricle from the left atrium. The regurgitant stream often prevents the full opening of the mitral valve, thus obstructing flow into the ventricle.
- *Still's murmur* affects children and is described as a humming or musical-sounding systolic murmur that is loudest at the left sternal border. It is a benign murmur. The murmur is usually heard in children 3 to 7 years of age and disappears before the onset of puberty.
- *Physiologic S_3 murmur* affects approximately 33% of children younger than 16 years who have a physiologic S3 heart sound that disappears before 30 years of age. The sound is best heard with the patient in the left lateral decubitus position, with the bell of the stethoscope over the point of maximal impulse. The sound is usually a low-frequency thud that occurs in early diastole.

Beers MH, Porter RS, eds. *The Merck manual of diagnosis and therapy,* Merck Research Laboratories, 18th ed. Whitehouse Station, NJ: Merck & Co.; 2006:575–579.

Still's murmur affects children and is described as a humming or musical-sounding systolic murmur that is loudest at the left sternal border. It is a benign murmur. The murmur is usually heard in children 3 to 7 years of age and disappears before the onset of puberty.

225. A hospitalized patient is receiving a blood transfusion. The floor nurse reports that the patient is flushed, is complaining of abdominal discomfort, and has a temperature of 101°F. The most appropriate management is to

A) give the patient acetaminophen and continue the transfusion at a slower rate
B) administer diphenhydramine and continue the transfusion
C) administer 100 mg of hydrocortisone intravenously and reduce the rate of the transfusion
D) stop the transfusion and increase intravenous fluids
E) administer intravenous ranitidine and order an abdominal series x-ray

Answer and Discussion

The answer is D. Many hemolytic transfusion reactions are caused by human error in the laboratory during the matching process or during the administration of blood. Symptoms may include anxiety, dyspnea, tachycardia, flushing, headache, chest or abdominal pain, nausea, vomiting, and shock with an acute decrease in blood pressure. In most cases, the severity of symptoms and the prognosis depend on the amount of transfusion, rate of delivery, degree of incompatibility, and overall health of the patient. The laboratory evaluation for hemolysis consists of measurements of serum haptoglobin, lactate dehydrogenase, and indirect bilirubin levels. The immune complexes that result in RBC lysis can cause renal dysfunction and failure. Treatment consists of stopping the transfusion as soon as possible, vigorous diuresis with furosemide or mannitol, and possible dialysis if renal failure occurs. With multiple transfusions, the patient may develop antibodies to white blood cell antigens, which cause febrile reactions that are manifested by chills and temperatures higher than 100.4°F. Using washed red blood cells helps prevent these reactions.

Kasper DL, Braunwald E, Fauci AS, et al., eds. *Harrison's principles of internal medicine,* 16th ed. New York: McGraw-Hill; 2005:665.

226. Which of the following statements regarding the reduction of stroke risk is true?

A) Vitamin E should be recommended to help reduce the risk of stroke.
B) Vitamin C has been shown to reduce the risk of stroke in multiple meta-analysis studies.
C) Dietary prevention of stroke should include increased intake of fruits and vegetables.
D) Risk factor modification has little impact on the risk for stroke.

Answer and Discussion

The answer is C. The use of vitamin E or vitamin C supplements is unlikely to reduce stroke risk in adult men with no history of cardiovascular disease or diabetes. Although some carotenoids may reduce stroke risk, there is insufficient evidence to recommend an increased intake of specific supplements. Dietary prevention of stroke should include increased intake of fruit and vegetables, as previous studies have suggested.

Ascherio A, Rimm EB, Hernan MA. Relation of consumption of vitamin E, vitamin C, and carotenoids to risk for stroke among men in the United States. *Ann Intern Med.* 1999;130:963–970.

227. A 24-year-old presents to your office with numbness noted in her feet bilaterally. She also complains of severe premenstrual syndrome (PMS) symptoms. The most likely cause for her symptoms related to her feet is

A) excessive use of ibuprofen
B) hysterical psychosis
C) folate deficiency
D) iron deficiency anemia
E) excessive vitamin B_6 intake

Answer and Discussion

The answer is E. Women frequently take large daily doses of vitamin B_6 for premenstrual syndrome (PMS), even though nutritional deficiency of this vitamin is rare. The recommended dietary allowance is about 2 mg/day; high intake has been associated with severe toxicity, including neuropathy. An intake of 200 mg/day may cause reversible damage, and an intake of 2,000 mg/day or greater is associated with peripheral neuropathy. In some European countries, the quantity of vitamin B_6 that may be purchased or prescribed has been restricted to reduce the risk of toxicity from excessive use.

Wyatt KM, Dimmock PW, Jones PW. Efficacy of vitamin B-6 in the treatment of premenstrual syndrome: systematic review. *BMJ.* 1999;318:1375–1381.

228. A 71-year-old presents to the emergency room with shortness of breath, hemoptysis, and chest pain. Further tests include an ECG with findings of right axis deviation, an S1-Q3-T3 pattern and right bundle branch block. The most likely diagnosis is

A) acute myocardial infarction
B) community-acquired pneumonia
C) bronchogenic carcinoma
D) pulmonary embolism
E) pericarditis

Answer and Discussion

The answer is D. A pulmonary embolism is a thrombus that lodges in the pulmonary vasculature and may give rise to a pulmonary infarction. In most cases, the thrombus forms in the leg or pelvic veins. The most dangerous thrombi form in the iliofemoral vein. Other causes of emboli include fat emboli after fractures and amniotic fluid emboli, which are rare. Risk factors for pulmonary embolism include malignancy, hereditary impaired coagulation, estrogen therapy, obesity, CHF, orthopedic or pelvic surgery, and prolonged anesthesia. Signs and symptoms include tachypnea, cough, hemoptysis, chest pain, fever, and cyanosis (in severe cases). Diagnosis is based on the clinical history and supportive tests, including a ventilation–perfusion scan and pulmonary arteriogram. Arterial blood tests show hypoxia (PO_2 <60 mm Hg), and ECG findings are nonspecific (T-wave abnormalities in the precordial leads and sinus tachycardia). In addition, right-axis deviation, an S1-Q3-T3 pattern, and a right bundle branch block may be observed. Further testing may include venous studies of the lower extremities to look for thrombus; however, >20% of patients may have no evidence of venous embolism. Chest radiographs are usually normal; however, a homogenous, wedge-shaped density based in the pleura and pointing to the hilum (Hampton's hump) is highly suggestive of pulmonary embolism. Treatment involves anticoagulation for 3 to 6 months with oral warfarin or thrombolytic therapy and embolectomy if the patient has hypotension and continuing hypoxemia while receiving high fractions of inspired oxygen. Thrombolytic therapy is not indicated for the routine treatment of patients with PE. A stepwise approach to the diagnosis of pulmonary embolus consists of a ventilation-perfusion scan. A high-probability ventilation-perfusion scan provides sufficient evidence for the initiation of treatment for PE. Likewise, a normal scan should be considered sufficient to exclude PE. Unfortunately, 50% to 70% of scans are indeterminate (low or intermediate probability). If the results show a high probability of PE, treatment with anticoagulants is indicated. If the ventilation–perfusion scan is normal, treatment is not indicated. If the lung scan shows intermediate or low probability of pulmonary embolus, a noninvasive leg test (ultrasound) for proximal DVT should be obtained. If the leg test is positive, then treatment is indicated. If the leg test is negative and suspicion is high, then a pulmonary angiogram or another ultrasound and D-dimer test can be repeated in 5 to 7 days. If the test is negative, the risk for pulmonary embolus is low. A spiral CT of the chest can also be used for rapid diagnosis.

Ramzi DW, Leeper KV. DVT and pulmonary embolism: Part I. Diagnosis. *Am Fam Physician.* 2004;69:2829–2836.

229. Which of the following statements about macular degeneration is true?

A) The wet form is usually more severe than the dry form.
B) Neovascularization is typically associated with drusen and the dry form.
C) It typically affects only peripheral vision.
D) The condition is more common in African-American individuals.
E) The condition is rarely progressive.

Answer and Discussion

The answer is A. Macular degeneration associated with aging is a leading cause of blindness in the elderly. The condition is more common in whites, appears to be hereditary, and is associated with atrophy or degeneration of the macular disc. There are basically two types: atrophic or dry and exudative or wet. Both types usually occur bilaterally and are progressive. The dry form usually progresses slowly and affects the outer retina, retinal pigment epithelium, choriocapillaries, and Bruch's membrane. The wet form of macular degeneration is more severe and progressive, usually affects the eyes sequentially, and is responsible for approximately 90% of blindness in those affected with macular degeneration. The wet form occurs when there is drusen (i.e., degeneration of the pigment epithelium and Bruch's membrane) and accumulation of serous fluid or blood in the retina that produces elevation of the retinal pigment membrane from Bruch's membrane. Neovascularization may then occur, giving rise to a subretinal neovascular membrane that causes permanent vision loss. There is no specific treatment for macular degeneration; however, laser photocoagulation may help stop neovascularization in select cases, and vision aids may help acuity. Macular degeneration affects central vision and does not affect peripheral vision.

Fine SL, Berger JW, Maguire MG. Age-related macular degeneration. *N Engl J Med.* 2000;342:483–491.

230. Hypersplenism is associated with all of the following EXCEPT

A) lymphoma
B) polycythemia vera
C) infectious mononucleosis
D) hereditary spherocytosis
E) congestive heart failure

Answer and Discussion

The answer is E. Hypersplenism is associated with a number of disorders that lead to a reduction in one or more blood constituents leading to leukopenia, thrombocytopenia, or a combination of both. Most cases of chronic hemolytic anemias are associated with splenomegaly. Causes of splenomegaly include lymphoma, leukemia, polycythemia vera, myelofibrosis, infectious mononucleosis, psittacosis, subacute bacterial endocarditis, tuberculosis, malaria, syphilis, kala-azar, brucellosis, sarcoidosis, amyloidosis, SLE, Felty's syndrome, hereditary spherocytosis, thalassemias, cirrhosis, Gaucher's disease, Niemann-Pick disease, Schüller-Christian disease, Letterer-Siwe disease, and thrombosis or compression of the portal or splenic veins. Patients may exhibit bleeding disorders, palpable splenomegaly, left-upper abdominal discomfort, or splenic bruits. Management usually involves treatment of the underlying disorder; elective splenectomy is reserved for refractory cases. Asplenic patients are at increased risk for infection secondary to encapsulated bacteria and should receive pneumococcal immunization.

Kasper DL, Braunwald E, Fauci AS, et al., eds. *Harrison's principles of internal medicine,* 16th ed. New York: McGraw-Hill; 2005:347.

231. Which of the following laboratory results best support the diagnosis of subclinical hypothyroidism?

A) Normal T4, low TSH
B) Normal T4, high TSH
C) Low T4, high TSH
D) Normal T4, normal TSH
E) Low T4, borderline low TSH

Answer and Discussion

The answer is B. The following are laboratory findings associated with thyroid dysfunction:

Diagnosis	Laboratory Findings
Overt hypothyroidism	Low T4, high sTSH
Subclinical hypothyroidism	Normal T4, high sTSH
Hypothyroidism secondary to hypopituitarism	Low T4, normal or borderline low sTSH
Euthyroid	Normal T4, normal sTSH
Subclinical hyperthyroidism	Normal T4, low sTSH

Beers MH, Porter RS, eds. *The Merck manual of diagnosis and therapy,* Merck Research Laboratories, 18th ed. Whitehouse Station, NJ: Merck & Co.; 2006:1192–1206.

232. The proportion of disease-free patients in whom a test result is negative is referred to as
A) the *p* value
B) sensitivity
C) specificity
D) reliability
E) variability

Answer and Discussion

The answer is C. *Specificity* is defined as the proportion of people who are not affected by a given disease and who also test negative for that disease. For example, the proportion of patients who do not have CAD and also test negative with a treadmill exercise test would be defined as the specificity. This specificity, as mentioned in the answer to question 234, is up to 95%. If this percentage is high, it is a highly specific test.

Mark DB. Chapter 2: Decision-making in clinical medicine. Available at Harrison's Online website (http://www.harrisonsonline.com). Accessed 6/4/06.

Specificity is defined as the proportion of people who are not affected by a given disease and who also test negative for that disease.

233. Inflammation and necrosis of the muscular tissue supplied by small- and medium-size arteries is known as
A) polyarteritis nodosa
B) pyoderma gangrenosum
C) polymyositis
D) giant cell arteritis
E) dermatomyositis

Answer and Discussion

The answer is A. Polyarteritis nodosa is a condition characterized by inflammation and necrosis of the muscular tissue supplied by small- and medium-size arteries. The cause is unknown but may be associated with an autoimmune response, medication (e.g., sulfonamides, iodide, thiazides, bismuth, penicillins), and infections. Involvement of the renal and visceral arteries is characteristic, but pulmonary arteries are usually spared. Affected individuals are usually between 40 and 50 years of age; men are more commonly affected. Symptoms include fever, abdominal pain, peripheral neuropathy, headaches, seizures, weakness, and weight loss. Those with renal involvement may show hypertension, edema, azotemia, and oligouria. Other symptoms include angina, nausea, vomiting, diarrhea, myalgias, and arthralgias. Palpable subcutaneous lesions that sometimes necrose may be found in the area of an affected artery. Laboratory studies show leukocytosis, proteinuria, microscopic hematuria, thrombocytosis, and an elevated ESR. Diagnosis is usually made with a biopsy of affected tissue, which shows necrotizing arteritis. Treatment involves avoidance of the offending agent and often long-term, high-dose steroid therapy and cyclophosphamide for severe cases and steroids alone for milder cases. The disease can be fatal if untreated.

Kasper DL, Braunwald E, Fauci AS, et al., eds. *Harrison's principles of internal medicine,* 16th ed. New York: McGraw-Hill; 2005:2007.

234. Which of the following symptoms is usually absent in a 5-year-old patient with streptococcal pharyngitis?
A) Rhinorrhea
B) Fever
C) Malaise
D) Abdominal discomfort
E) Sore throat

Answer and Discussion

The answer is A. *Streptococcus* pharyngitis is caused by group A β-hemolytic *streptococcus*. It is one of the most common childhood infections and accounts for up to 40% of exudative pharyngitis in children usually older than 3 years. Symptoms include sore throat, fever, malaise, and sometimes abdominal pain with nausea and vomiting (particularly in children). Rhinorrhea, a prominent cough, and hoarseness are typically not present in uncomplicated cases. Signs include erythema associated with the tonsillar pillars and associated exudates that may also involve the posterior pharynx, as well as tender cervical lymphadenopathy. Scarlet fever, which is characterized by an erythematous rash that blanches with pressure and has the appearance of fine sandpaper, may also be present with streptococcal pharyngitis. Diagnosis is made with a throat culture or a latex agglutination test, which is faster and widely available. The latex agglutination test ("rapid strep test") has a specificity of approximately 95%, with a sensitivity of approximately 76% to 87%; therefore, negative rapid *Streptococcus* tests should be sent for culture. Treatment of streptococcal pharyngitis usually does not shorten the course of the disease but does prevent complications, including the development of rheumatic fever. The treatment is 10 days of an appropriate antibiotic; penicillin (oral or intramuscular benzathine penicillin G) is usually used, and erythromycin is used if the patient is allergic to penicillin. Complications include the development of peritonsillar or retropharyngeal abscesses, cervical lymphadenitis, sinusitis, otitis, meningitis, endocarditis, and pneumonia. As much as 20% of the population may be an asymptomatic carrier of *Streptococcus*. In most cases, treatment should be limited to only those who are symptomatic, unless the carrier is transmitting the infection to others. Those who are asymptomatic carriers are not likely to develop complications such as rheumatic fever. Patients with streptococcal pharyngitis are considered contagious until they have been taking an antibiotic for 24 hours. Children should not go back to their daycare center or school until their temperature returns to normal and they have had at least 24 hours of antibiotic therapy. Group A β-hemolytic streptococci persist for up to 15 days on unrinsed toothbrushes and removable orthodontic appliances. The pathogens are not isolated from rinsed toothbrushes after 3 days. Instructing patients to rinse toothbrushes and removable orthodontic appliances thoroughly may help prevent recurrent infections. Transmission of group A β-hemolytic streptococci occurs principally through contact with respiratory secretions from an infected person. Although anecdotes are numerous and a few cases have been reported, family pets are rare reservoirs of group A β-hemolytic streptococci.

Hayes CS, Williamson H. Management of group A beta-hemolytic streptococcal pharyngitis. *Am Fam Physician.* 2001;63:1557–1564.

235. A 17-year-old girl presents to your office. She had an upper respiratory viral infection approximately 1 week before her visit. She now complains of severe vertigo. She has no other symptoms. The most likely diagnosis is
A) Meniere's disease
B) cholesteatoma

C) vestibular neuronitis
D) benign positional vertigo
E) acoustic neuroma

Answer and Discussion

The answer is C. Vestibular neuronitis is characterized by severe episodes of vertigo that may recur. The condition tends to affect young people and is thought to be secondary to a viral infection, which affects the eighth nerve. The first episode is usually associated with severe vertigo that lasts approximately 1 week, followed by spontaneous remission. Subsequent attacks may occur up to 18 months after the initial episode. In most cases, the subsequent attacks are less severe than the original attack. There is no loss of hearing or tinnitus, which is usually seen with Meniere's disease. The diagnosis is usually accomplished after other causes are eliminated. Severe cases can be treated with anticholinergic medication, antihistamines, antiemetics, steroids, and benzodiazepines. In most cases, symptoms are self-limited and resolve spontaneously. Vestibular neuronitis is a cause of peripheral vertigo. Symptoms associated with peripheral vertigo include tinnitus, nystagmus, and hearing loss; dysphagia, vomiting, and headache are more associated with a central cause of dizziness.

Beers MH, Porter RS, eds. *The Merck manual of diagnosis and therapy,* Merck Research Laboratories, 18th ed. Whitehouse Station, NJ: Merck & Co.; 2006:795.

236. The most common location for the development of Morton's neuroma is
A) the trigeminal nerve
B) interdigital nerves between the fourth and fifth metacarpal heads
C) interdigital nerves between the third and fourth metatarsal heads
D) the median nerve
E) the sural nerve

Answer and Discussion

The answer is C. Morton's neuroma is a common type of forefoot pain. The condition arises from entrapment of the common interdigital nerves between the metatarsal heads. This nerve entrapment leads to inflammation, edema, pain, and the formation of perineural fibrosis and demyelination, which causes a neuroma. The most common location for the neuroma is between the third and fourth metatarsal heads; they also commonly occur between the second and third metatarsal heads. Women are more commonly affected than men (5:1 ratio). Patients report pain, paresthesias, or occasionally a catching sensation in these locations, which may extend distally to the toes or proximally to the midfoot. Many patients report their symptoms are worse when wearing shoes. The distinguishing feature in the differential between metatarsalgia and Morton's neuroma is pain between the metatarsal heads. Radiographs are normal; however, MRIs may show the offending neuroma but are rarely necessary to make the diagnosis. Treatment involves NSAIDs, metatarsal footpads, wide shoes, and steroid injections (using a dorsal approach between the metatarsals); in severe cases, surgical excision of the neuroma is indicated, although persistent pain remains for approximately 33% of patients after surgery.

Tallia AF, Cardone DA. Diagnostic and therapeutic injection of the ankle and foot. *Am Fam Physician.* 2003;68:1356–1362.

237. Which of the following is associated with chronic fatigue syndrome?
A) Temporal artery tenderness
B) Minimal (less than 10%) impairment of normal activity
C) High incidence of associated psychiatric disorders
D) Muscle weakness
E) Recent EBV infection

Answer and Discussion

The answer is C. Fatigue is a common complaint heard in a family physician's office. As many as 25% of patients may complain of fatigue when asked. Broadly defined, the condition is described as long-standing severe fatigue without substantial muscle weakness and without proven psychologic or physical causes. More specifically defined, the syndrome consists of recurrent attacks of fatigue lasting at least 6 months, with 50% of impairment of activity and with other symptoms that include

- Exudative pharyngitis/sore throat
- Painful lymphadenopathy
- Headache
- Myalgias
- Low-grade fever/chills
- Generalized weakness
- Migratory arthralgias
- Neurologic complaints/poor concentration
- Sleep disturbance
- Abdominal pain

These symptoms may develop acutely. Typically, there are no signs of muscle weakness, arthritis, neuropathy, or organomegaly. Women are more often affected than men. The syndrome has not been proven to be associated with EBV; however, some believe it may be linked to a viral infection. Prior studies have shown that faulty blood pressure control may be linked to the development of chronic fatigue syndrome. There appears to be a high incidence of associated psychiatric disorders such as anxiety, depression, and somatization disorder. Although no placebo-controlled trials have supported the treatment antidepressants have shown some anecdotal benefits in those affected. Antiviral medication, immunologic treatments (steroids, immunoglobin, interferon), and vitamin therapy are used, but their effectiveness has not been proved. Psychological therapy may be beneficial. Patients should be encouraged to maintain a gradually increasing program of activity.

Craig T, Kakumanu S. Chronic fatigue syndrome: evaluation and treatment. *Am Fam Physician.* 2002;65:1083–1090, 1095.

238. Which of the following statements about PVCs is correct?
A) They are narrow electrocardiographic wave (QRS) complexes that are preceded by P waves.
B) In most cases, they disappear with exercise.
C) They are treated with type IC antiarrhythmics.
D) They may represent a risk for sudden death in healthy patients.
E) Caffeine use is not associated with PVCs.

Answer and Discussion

The answer is B. PVCs are abnormal ventricular beats that are characterized by wide QRS complexes, which are usually not preceded by P waves. In patients with normal hearts, PVCs usually disappear with exercise. If the patient remains asymptomatic and there is no organic heart disease, no further treatment is necessary. If PVCs are frequent, electrolyte abnormalities and heart disease should be excluded. Patients with frequent, repetitive, or multiform PVCs and underlying heart disease are at increased risk for sudden death because of cardiac arrhythmia (particularly ventricular fibrillation). Without underlying cardiac disease, bigeminy and trigeminy are considered benign rhythms. Treatment of PVCs is controversial but should be reserved for symptomatic patients. If MVP, hypertrophic obstructive cardiomyopathy, prolonged Q-T interval, left ventricular hypertrophy, or CAD is present, a trial of β blockers can be used. Types IA (quinidine, procainamide) and IB (lidocaine, mexiletine) antiarrhythmic agents may be used; however, they are associated with a high incidence of side effects and can make the arrhythmias worse. Type IC agents (flecainide, propafenone) should not be used because of their potential for increased mortality rates. Elimination of exogenous catecholamines, sympathomimetic amines, alcohol, and caffeine may decrease symptoms. In general, antiarrhythmic drug therapy is rarely necessary.

Beers MH, Porter RS, eds. *The Merck manual of diagnosis and therapy,* Merck Research Laboratories, 18th ed. Whitehouse Station, NJ: Merck & Co.; 2006:705.

239. Which of the following statements about lung cancer is true?

A) Squamous cell and small cell tumors are rarely associated with smoking.
B) Squamous cell tumors typically arise in central bronchi and may be diagnosed with sputum cytology.
C) Large cell tumors are common, arise centrally, and typically metastasize locally.
D) Small cell carcinoma is usually located peripherally and rarely metastasizes.
E) Yearly chest x-rays are recommended for smokers over age 50.

Answer and Discussion

The answer is B. Lung cancer caused by tobacco abuse is a significant health problem that accounts for approximately 150,000 deaths yearly in the United States. Most cases appear between 50 and 70 years of age. Unfortunately, at the time of diagnosis, only approximately 20% of patients have localized disease. The following are the most common types (typically the cancers are divided into small cell cancers and non-small cell cancers:

- *Squamous cell (epidermoid).* As much as 30% to 35% of lung cancers. One of the most common types seen in men, these tumors tend to arise from the central (larger) bronchi and are the most easily diagnosed with sputum cytology. Most of these tumors metastasize locally to the regional lymph nodes and are more localized at the time of diagnosis.
- *Large cell.* As much as 10% to 15% of lung cancers. Less common in incidence, these tumors usually metastasize through the bloodstream. Approximately 20% of patients may develop cavitary lesions. These tumors are usually located peripherally.
- *Adenocarcinoma.* As much as 25% to 35% of lung cancers. One of the more common types, these tumors are usually located peripherally and are usually advanced at the time of diagnosis. It spreads through the bloodstream and lymphatics. A subset of tumors referred to as *bronchoalveolar* is growing in incidence.
- *Small cell (oat cell).* Approximately 15% of lung cancers. This type also tends to occur centrally and is usually widespread at the time of diagnosis.

Chest radiographs for asymptomatic smokers may identify patients with early disease; however, routine screening with yearly chest radiographs is not recommended. In most cases, lung cancers are divided into small cell tumors and non-small cell tumors (which include squamous cell, large cell, and adenocarcinomas). Stage I or II non-small cell tumors can be treated with surgical resection; small cell tumors respond to chemotherapy and radiation therapy (cures are rare). Squamous cell tumors and small cell tumors are most often linked with cigarette smoking.

Beers MH, Porter RS, eds. *The Merck manual of diagnosis and therapy,* Merck Research Laboratories, 18th ed. Whitehouse Station, NJ: Merck & Co.; 2006:503–509.

240. Which of the following is a potentially severe complication of using warfarin that is unrelated to excessive bleeding?

A) Pancreatic neoplasm
B) Hepatitis
C) Skin necrosis
D) Peripheral neuropathy
E) Pulmonary fibrosis

Answer and Discussion

The answer is C. Warfarin is classified as an anticoagulant. Its mechanism of action is the inhibition of vitamin K–dependent clotting factors (i.e., factors II, VII, IX, and X). The medication is used in stroke prophylaxis for patients with prior neurologic events, atrial fibrillation, mechanical heart valves, or previous DVT or PE. Warfarin interacts with many medications, so concomitant use with other drugs should be monitored carefully. Most complications are related to bleeding; however, other side effects, including nausea, vomiting, fever, burning of the feet, and rashes, may occur. The most common complication unrelated to excessive bleeding is skin necrosis, which usually occurs within the first week of therapy. Some cases may be severe enough to require surgical débridement or even amputation. Patients treated with warfarin should have their PTs and INRs followed to ensure proper levels of anticoagulation.

Ansell J, Hirsh J, Poller L, et al. The pharmacology and management of the vitamin K antagonists: the Seventh ACCP Conference on Antithrombotic and Thrombolytic Therapy. *Chest.* 2004;126(3 suppl):204S–233S.

Warfarin's mechanism of action is the inhibition of vitamin K–dependent clotting factors (i.e., factors II, VII, IX, and X).

241. Which of the following is *not* in the diagnostic criteria for the presence of diabetes mellitus?

A) Random plasma glucose >200 mg/dL
B) Fasting plasma glucose of 140 mg/dL
C) Abnormal glucose tolerance test
D) Hemoglobin A1C (HbA_{1c}) of 7.5

Answer and Discussion

The answer is D. The diagnostic criteria for diabetes mellitus are (1) symptoms of diabetes mellitus plus a random plasma glucose concentration of at least 200 mg/dL (11.1 mmol/L); (2) a fasting plasma glucose level of 126 mg/dL (7.0 mmol/L) or higher; or (3) a 2-hour plasma glucose level of 200 mg/dL or more during an oral glucose tolerance test. However, the oral glucose tolerance test is time consuming and not usually used. Repeat testing on a different day is needed to confirm these findings. Although somewhat controversial the use of hemoglobin HbA_{1c} is not used in the diagnosis of diabetes mellitus.

Davidson MB, Schriger DL, Peters AL. Relationship between fasting plasma glucose and glycosylated hemoglobin. Potential for false-positive diagnoses of type 2 diabetes using new diagnostic criteria. *JAMA.* 1999;281:1203–1210.

American Diabetes Association. Report of the Expert Committee on the Diagnosis and Classification of Diabetes Mellitus. *Diabetes Care.* 1997;20:1183–1197.

242. Which of the following is indicated in the treatment of chronic congestive heart failure?

A) Atenolol
B) Metoprolol
C) Propanolol
D) Acebutolol
E) Timolol

Answer and Discussion

The answer is B. The U.S. Food and Drug Administration (FDA) has labeled only extended-release metoprolol succinate (Toprol XL) and carvedilol for the treatment of chronic heart failure. Metoprolol is β_1 selective, and carvedilol is nonselective. Extended-release metoprolol succinate can be started in a dosage of 25 mg/day in patients with New York Heart Association class II failure; in patients with more severe heart failure, the starting dosage should be 12.5 mg/day. The recommended starting dosage of carvedilol is 3.125 mg twice daily. The mortality benefits of metoprolol have been proven only for the extended-release form. A number of major trials have evaluated the mortality benefits of β-blockers in patients with chronic heart failure. The mortality benefit of β-blocker therapy in patients with chronic heart failure is clear. Studies continue to show less than ideal use of these medications in patients with chronic heart failure. Current expert guidelines recommend the use of β-blockers in all stable patients who have evidence of left ventricular systolic dysfunction (generally defined as an ejection fraction of less than 40%), unless there is a contraindication to their use.

Kukin ML. Beta-Blockers in chronic heart failure: considerations for selecting an agent. *Mayo Clin Proc.* 2002;77:1199–1206.

243. Which of the following would best help to prevent shin splints?

A) Change in running surfaces
B) Ice therapy
C) Running on inclined surfaces
D) More intensive training schedule
E) Stretching before exercise

Answer and Discussion

The answer is E. Shin splints (medial tibial stress syndrome) are a common condition caused by overuse of the lower extremity muscles. The condition is caused by a periosteitis of the tibia. They typically occur when an athlete's running surface (e.g., hills, inclines, stairs) is changed, when a different type of shoe is used, when an athlete's running style is altered, or when excessive training that does not allow adequate time for the muscles to recover is undertaken. Most affected athletes report pain over the lower tibial area that may be referred to the foot or knee. Any type of movement or exercise that works these muscle groups tends to make the pain worse. In addition to pain, mild diffuse swelling or redness may be noted over the tibia. The differential diagnosis includes stress fractures, exertional compartment syndrome, and tenosynovitis. Diagnosis is usually based on history and physical examination. In severe cases that are refractive to ice, rest, and NSAIDs, plain radiographs and perhaps a bone scan should be performed to rule out a stress fracture. If fractures are not noted, there may be diffuse increased uptake of technetium along the tibia in the area of the periosteum. If the patient is only mildly affected, exercise can be continued; however, more severe cases may require restriction of activity. When the pain and inflammation subsides, the athlete should be instructed in stretching exercises for the muscles of the lower extremity. If shin splints are recurrent, examination to rule out excessive pronation should be performed; if present, orthotics should be used to correct hyperpronation. It is now thought that medial tibial stress syndrome represents one end of a continuum of bony stress injury, with a focal stress fracture representing the other.

Sanderlin BW, Raspa RF. Common stress fractures. *Am Fam Physician.* 2003;68:1527–1532.

244. Which of the following is the treatment of choice for pyoderma gangrenosum?

A) Steroid therapy
B) Topical antibiotics
C) Oral antibiotics that treat methicillin-resistant *S. aureus*
D) Methotrexate
E) Plasmapheresis

Answer and Discussion

The answer is A. Pyoderma gangrenosum is a rapidly evolving and severely debilitating skin disease that is characterized by a painful hemorrhagic pustule that breaks down to form a chronic ulcer. The ulcer is associated with pus production, and there is usually a dusky red or purple halo around the ulcer. The cause of the lesions is unknown, but they tend to form at the sites of trauma (most commonly the legs). The borders of the lesions are usually irregular, and the lesions are boggy and usually quite painful. Although as many as 50% of cases have no associated underlying abnormality, other diseases associated with pyoderma gangrenosum include Crohn's disease, ulcerative colitis, leukemia, paraproteinemia, multiple myeloma, rheumatoid arthritis, hepatitis, and Behçet's disease. The diagnosis of pyoderma gangrenosum is usually made by the history and clinical findings. Laboratory tests show elevated ESR and leukocytosis. Treatment involves correction of underlying disease and the use of high-dose oral steroids or intravenous pulse steroid therapy. Additional findings in these patients include cutaneous anergy and benign monoclonal gammopathy.

Kasper DL, Braunwald E, Fauci AS, et al., eds. *Harrison's principles of internal medicine,* 16th ed. New York: McGraw-Hill; 2005:310–311.

245. Which of the following is acceptable treatment for *Helicobacter pylori* infection?

A) Bismuth, amoxicillin, metronidazole, and omeprazole
B) TMP-sulfamethoxazole, sucralfate, and metronidazole
C) Omeprazole, clindamycin, and sucralfate

D) Docusate, tetracycline, and metronidazole
E) Ranitidine, metronidazole, and ampicillin

Answer and Discussion

The answer is A. *Helicobacter pylori* is a bacteria found in the stomach that is present in > 80% of patients with duodenal ulcers and up to 60% of those with gastric ulcers. The prevalence of *H. pylori* in the United States is approximately 30%. The incidence appears to increase with increasing age. Most *H. pylori* colonization is asymptomatic. Diagnosis is accomplished by biopsy and histologic examination, the urea breath test for *H. pylori*, stool antigen test, or cultures of endoscopy-obtained samples. Serologic blood test can also be used to determine a history of *H. pylori* infection. To decrease the incidence of recurrent ulcers, *H. pylori* is treated with a 2-week regimen consisting of bismuth (Pepto-Bismol), tetracycline or amoxicillin, metronidazole, and omeprazole. Other regimens include clarithromycin. Treatment of nonulcer dyspepsia thought secondary to *H. pylori* is controversial.

Kasper DL, Braunwald E, Fauci AS, et al., eds. *Harrison's principles of internal medicine,* 16th ed. New York: McGraw-Hill; 2005:886–888.

246. Which of the following treatments is the treatment of choice for chronic allergic rhinitis?
A) Systemic antihistamines
B) Intranasal steroids
C) Topical decongestants
D) Cromolyn sodium
E) Bee pollen extract

Answer and Discussion

The answer is B. Allergic rhinitis is characterized by nasal congestion, clear rhinorrhea, mucosal thickening, and conjunctivitis with the absence of fever or sinus tenderness. Patients may exhibit a bluish discoloration below the eyelids ("allergic shiners") as a result of venous congestion. Constant nose rubbing is known as the "allergic salute" and can result in a crease across the bridge of the nose. Treatment involves avoiding the triggering factors such as pollens, molds, cigarette smoke, animal dander, and dust mites. Many patients report symptoms related to seasons (Spring, Summer, or Fall). The best treatment is the administration of intranasal steroids, which have few associated side effects. Other treatment options include montelukast (Singulair), azelastine (Astelin nasal spray) cromolyn sodium, ipratropium bromide, and second-generation (nonsedating) systemic antihistamines such as loratadine (Claritin), fexofenadine (Allegra), and cetirizine (Zyrtec). The chronic use of topical decongestants can lead to rebound congestion known as rhinitis medicamentosa and should be used only on a temporary basis (i.e., no more than 3 days). Immunotherapy may also be an alternative treatment for debilitating symptoms.

Ferri F. *Ferri's Clinical Advisor, Instant Diagnosis and Treatment.* Philadelphia: Elsevier/Mosby; 2006:742.

247. A 24-year-old intravenous drug abuser presents with fever, night sweats, chest pain, and arthralgias. On examination, painless erythematous lesions are noted on the palms of the hands; round, erythematous lesions with central clearing are noted in the retina; and splinter hemorrhages are noted on the fingernails. The most likely diagnosis is
A) HIV infection
B) bacterial endocarditis
C) syphilis
D) infectious hepatitis
E) Lyme disease

Answer and Discussion

The answer is B. Bacterial endocarditis is an infection of the endocardium and heart valves. It is characterized by fever, anemia, valvular dysfunction, cardiac murmurs, petechiae, emboli, and cardiac vegetations that may result in valve incompetence, abscesses, or aneurysms. The most serious complication is CHF. The aortic and mitral valves are the most commonly affected. Infections are usually caused by S. aureus or Streptococcus species (e.g., *Streptococcus viridans, S. pneumoniae*). Infections of prosthetic valves are of particular concern and usually require removal of the artificial valve. Splenomegaly is often seen in conjunction with endocarditis. Other symptoms include night sweats, malaise, weight loss, arthralgias, and chest pain. Painful erythematous nodules at the distal tips of the fingers are called *Osler's nodes.* Round, erythematous lesions with central clearing (Roth spots) can affect the retina. Painless erythematous lesions (Janeway lesions) can affect the palms or soles. Subungual "splinter hemorrhages" can affect the fingernails. Laboratory findings are usually nonspecific and may show anemia, reticulocytopenia, hypergammaglobulinemia, circulating immune complexes, and positive rheumatoid factor. The patient's ESR may be elevated. Urinalysis frequently shows proteinuria and microscopic hematuria.

Intravenous drug abuse is a major cause of endocarditis, which usually affects the right side (tricuspid valve) of the heart. If treated early, the prognosis is usually good. Echocardiography is the best diagnostic test for bacterial endocarditis. Transthoracic echocardiography detects vegetations in 50% of patients with endocarditis, whereas transesophageal echocardiography detects vegetations in >90% of cases. Blood cultures can determine the causative organism; however, 15% to 20% of patients with clinical endocarditis may test negative, usually as a result of recent antibiotic therapy.

Beers MH, Porter RS, eds. *The Merck manual of diagnosis and therapy,* Merck Research Laboratories, 18th ed. Whitehouse Station, NJ: Merck & Co.; 2006:724–731.

248. In diagnosing a pulmonary embolism (PE), which of the following tests is considered the "gold standard" test?
A) Ventilation/perfusion (V/Q) lung scan
B) Venous compression ultrasonography of the legs
C) Pulmonary angiography
D) Spiral computed tomography (CT) of the chest
E) D-dimer blood test

Answer and Discussion

The answer is C. Pulmonary embolism is potentially fatal, yet it's the determination of a PE that remains difficult because clinical features are often nonspecific, and available diagnostic tests have significant limitations. Pulmonary angiography is the accepted "gold standard" test, but it is invasive and difficult to interpret, and can give false-negative results. Many other tests have been developed and used in combination to assess the probability of pulmonary embolism in individual patients, including ventilation–perfusion (V/Q) lung scanning, venous compression ultrasonography of the legs, and contrast-enhanced spiral computed tomography (CT) of the chest. Initially, spiral CT was thought to have high sensitivity and specificity, but it is now known that the sensitivity is too low to reliably rule out pulmonary embolism without further testing. Nevertheless, the combination of spiral CT and leg compression ultrasonography might have sufficient sensitivity and specificity to safely exclude pulmonary embolism and avoid unnecessary anticoagulation in many patients. Experts advise that anticoagulant therapy can safely be withheld in patients with a low or intermediate probability of pulmonary embolism and negative spiral CT and ultrasonography. Anticoagulation can probably also be avoided in high-probability patients with negative testing if more advanced screening such as V/Q lung scan or pulmonary angiography also is negative.

Musset D, Parent F, Meyer G. Diagnostic strategy for patients with suspected pulmonary embolism: a prospective multicentre outcome study. *Lancet.* 2002;360:1914–1920.

249. Which of the following findings is associated with chronic myelocytic leukemia (CML)?

A) Leukopenia
B) Philadelphia chromosome
C) Elevated leukocyte alkaline phosphatase level
D) Thrombocytopenia
E) Decreased vitamin B_{12} levels

Answer and Discussion

The answer is B. CML is a clonal myeloproliferative disorder that results in the overproduction of granulocytes from the bone marrow, liver, and spleen. The average age of onset is approximately 45 years. In most cases, the CML clone has the potential to progress into an accelerated phase and final blast crisis but usually remains stable for years before transformation. Symptoms are usually nonspecific and include low-grade fever, weight loss, night sweats, fatigue, anorexia, and, in some cases, abdominal fullness secondary to splenomegaly. Physical examination may show significant splenomegaly and generalized lymphadenopathy (ominous signs). Laboratory findings include significant elevation in the white blood cell count (200,000 at the time of diagnosis) and thrombocytosis. Bone marrow studies show hypercellularity with a significant left shift and low leukocyte alkaline phosphatase value. Vitamin B_{12} levels and serum vitamin B_{12}–binding capacity are usually elevated as a result of increased granulocyte production of transcobalamin I, and there is almost always a Philadelphia chromosome (translocation of part of chromosome 9 to chromosome 22) present.

Treatment involves the use of chemotherapy medications such as hydroxyurea. In most cases, the patient may be kept asymptomatic for long periods while maintaining the white blood cell count at <50,000. True remission does not occur because of the persistence of the Philadelphia chromosome in the bone marrow. Median survival after the clinical onset is approximately 3 to 4 years. If a blast crisis occurs, the average survival is approximately 2 months but can be improved with adequate treatment. α-Interferon produces remission in 20% to 25%. Bone marrow transplantation has been shown to improve survival in select patients.

Beers MH, Porter RS, eds. *The Merck manual of diagnosis and therapy,* Merck Research Laboratories, 18th ed. Whitehouse Station, NJ: Merck & Co.; 2006:1113–1114.

250. The definition of chronic bronchitis is

A) a chronic productive cough of at least 3 months' duration that occurs for 2 consecutive years
B) a chronic productive cough that fails to respond to antibiotics
C) a condition associated with the destruction of lung tissue and the development of blebs
D) a chronic productive cough of at least 6 months' duration that occurs for 5 consecutive years
E) a reduction in lung compliance by 30% or more

Answer and Discussion

The answer is A. COPD is divided into two categories: chronic bronchitis ("blue bloaters") and emphysema ("pink puffers"). The basic underlying abnormality is an increased resistance to airflow during expiration. It is estimated that COPD develops in up to 15% of smokers.

Chronic bronchitis is a condition in which the patient has a chronic productive cough of at least 3 months' duration that occurs for at least 2 consecutive years. It is almost always caused by cigarette smoking, but also has been associated with pollution exposure and recurrent infections. Patients usually appear edematous, and diffuse rhonchi are heard on physical examination. There appears to be hypoxia with CO_2 retention early in the disease process. Lung compliance is usually normal, and the development of cor pulmonale is common. Infections are common in these patients. Chest radiographs may show increased markings, and blood tests may show an elevated hematocrit.

Emphysema is a condition associated with the destruction of lung tissue and the development of blebs (coalescence of alveoli). Emphysema is subclassified as follows:

- Panlobular, which is associated with an α1-antitrypsin deficiency
- Centrilobular, which is associated with smoking and chronic bronchitis

Patients tend to have a thin habitus and decreased breath sounds on physical examination. These patients usually do not exhibit hypoxia or CO_2 retention until late in the disease process. Diffusing capacity of the lungs is usually decreased; lung compliance is usually increased. Chest radiographs usually show decreased markings with hyperinflation and possibly bullae. Cor pulmonale usually does not develop until late in the disease course. Blood tests usually show a normal hematocrit. In most cases, chronic bronchitis and emphysema exist simultaneously; thus the term COPD.

Snow V, Lascher S, Mottur-Pilson C. The evidence base for management of acute exacerbations of COPD. Clinical practice guideline, part 1. *Chest.* 2001;119:1185–1189.

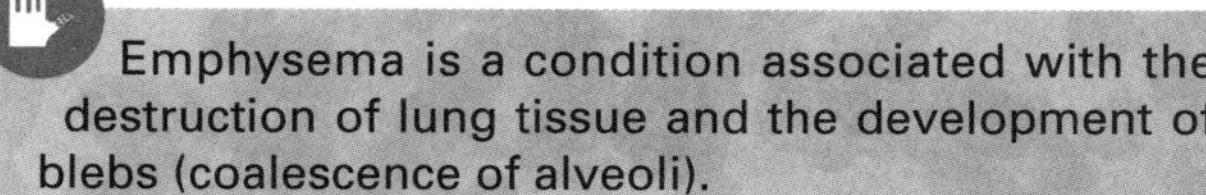
Emphysema is a condition associated with the destruction of lung tissue and the development of blebs (coalescence of alveoli).

251. A 72-year-old smoker with a positive history of severe degenerative arthritis, diabetes, and cardiovascular disease presents to your office complaining of bilateral leg pain that occurs after walking 200 yards. He reports that rest improves his symptoms. Which of the following would be appropriate?

A) Ankle/brachial indices
B) MRI of the lumbar spine
C) Ultrasonography of the lower extremities
D) Electromyogram of the lower extremities
E) Arteriogram of the lower extremities

Answer and Discussion

The answer is A. Claudication occurs when there is arterial insufficiency of the lower extremities. It usually occurs in the calf muscles, thighs, and buttocks and is bilateral and progressive. Symptoms include pain, fatigue or weakness associated with the lower legs that typically occurs after walking predictable distances, and, occasionally, impotence in men. If the pain or discomfort occurs with varying distances, a workup for other causes is necessary. Patients who experience significant restriction in their activities may be considered for surgery; however, their overall health status should be considered first. Many patients have underlying cardiovascular disease that may put them at surgical risk. Ankle/brachial indices (usually <0.90 with peripheral arterial disease) are the simplest method to estimate blood flow to the lower extremities. The use of arteriogram is not necessary unless the patient is considering surgery. Treatment involves

- Walking programs that gradually reduce the pain of claudication and promote adequate blood flow
- Pentoxifylline, a medication that promotes red blood cell flexibility to surpass obstructions
- Cessation of all tobacco products
- Surgery for severe cases unresponsive to medical therapy

Ischemic pain at rest usually affects the feet and toe area as opposed to the other proximal locations involved in claudication.

Beers MH, Porter RS, eds. *The Merck manual of diagnosis and therapy,* Merck Research Laboratories, 18th ed. Whitehouse Station, NJ: Merck & Co., 2006:462–469.

252. A 65-year-old man presents complaining of back pain and generalized fatigue. Laboratory findings include anemia with Rouleau formation, a monoclonal spike seen with serum protein electrophoresis, and hypercalcemia. Radiographs of the lumbar spine show lytic lesions. The most likely diagnosis is
A) metastatic prostate cancer
B) Paget's disease
C) osteitis fibrosa cystica
D) multiple myeloma
E) colon cancer

Answer and Discussion

The answer is D. Multiple myeloma is a malignancy associated with plasma cells and involves replacement of the bone marrow, bone destruction, and the formation of paraproteins that are found in the blood and urine. It is the most common primary malignancy that affects the spine. Affected patients are usually older than 60 years and present with anemia, bone pain, and an elevated sedimentation rate. Other manifestations include renal failure; spinal cord compression; or symptoms of hyperviscosity, including mucosal bleeding, vertigo, visual abnormalities, and alterations in mental status. Laboratory abnormalities include an anemia with Rouleau formation, abnormal serum and urine protein electrophoresis with a monoclonal spike in the β or γ region, hypercalcemia as a result of bone destruction, and radiographs showing lytic lesions associated with the skeletal bones (bone scans are inferior to conventional radiographs). Diagnosis is made by bone marrow biopsy showing more than 10% of plasma cells in the bone marrow. Treatment is aimed at palliation and involves chemotherapy and correction of hypercalcemia. Patients are at increased risk of infection caused by encapsulated organisms, such as *S. pneumoniae* and *H. influenzae,* because of impaired immune response. The median survival time is 3 to 5 years.

Ferri F. *Ferri's Clinical Advisor, Instant Diagnosis and Treatment.* Philadelphia: Elsevier/Mosby; 2006:541–542.

253. A true statement regarding the use of probiotics is
A) Probiotics should always be separated from antibiotics by a couple of hours.
B) Their use has not been shown to be useful.
C) Require a prescription for a licensed physician.
D) The microorganisms are heat-killed before packaging.

Answer and Discussion

The answer is A. Probiotics are living microorganisms used to colonize the intestine to prevent or treat disease. The most common probiotics are *Lactobacillus spp.* and *Saccharomyces spp.* Probiotics that contain species of *Lactobacillus* or *Saccharomyces* decrease the likelihood of diarrhea from antibiotics in children or adults. These products can be obtained over the counter. A typical dosage is 5 billion to 10 billion viable organisms administered three to four times a day. The probiotics should be separated from the antibiotics by a couple of hours.

Cremonini F, DiCaro S, Nista EC. Meta-analysis: the effect of probiotic administration on antibiotic-associated diarrhoea. *Aliment Pharmacol Ther.* 2002;16:1461–1467.

254. The anticoagulation effects associated with heparin therapy are best reversed with the use of
A) vitamin K
B) fresh frozen plasma
C) cryoprecipitate
D) protamine sulfate
E) platelet administration

Answer and Discussion

The answer is D. Heparin is an anticoagulant used to prevent thrombosis. Heparin works by binding to and activating antithrombin III, an extremely potent anticoagulant that prevents thrombin generation and fibrin formation. The drug is administered intravenously and subcutaneously. The major side effect is bleeding. If needed, protamine sulfate may be administered to rapidly reverse heparin's anticoagulant effect; in most cases, this measure is unnecessary and the discontinuation of heparin is adequate. Other complications include heparin-induced thrombocytopenia, which occurs in 10% of patients taking the medication. The thrombocytopenia can actually lead to a paradoxical arterial thrombosis, which can be life threatening. Discontinuation of the medication usually reverses the thrombocytopenia. When administering intravenous heparin, the PTT should be monitored. Any increase in heparin dose is usually detected 4 hours later (as noted with a prolonged PTT) and vice versa with decreased doses of heparin. The goal for anticoagulation is usually 1.5 to 2.0 times the normal value, but may depend on the individual case. Patients should not take aspirin while taking heparin; intramuscular injections should also be avoided. Chronic use of heparin may increase the risk of osteoporosis. Low-molecular-weight heparin is now available and is used for anticoagulation. PTT and thrombin times are minimally affected by typical therapeutic doses. Therefore, laboratory monitoring is not required.

Kasper DL, Braunwald E, Fauci AS, et al., eds. *Harrison's principles of internal medicine,* 16th ed. New York: McGraw-Hill; 2005:675, 688–689, 1564.

255. A 36-year-old runner presents with pain associated with the anterior heel. The patient reports his symptoms are worse on awakening and improve as the day progresses. The most likely diagnosis is
A) Achilles tendonitis
B) plantar fasciitis
C) calcaneal fracture
D) calcaneal bone spur
E) anterior talotibial impingement syndrome

Answer and Discussion

The answer is B. Plantar fasciitis is caused by inflammation or tearing (microtears) of the plantar fascia at the attachment site to the os calcis. It is a common complaint in runners. Symptoms include pain at the attachment of the plantar fascia at the calcaneus. The pain is usually worse in the morning on standing or standing after prolonged sitting. The pain may improve early in the day but usually worsens toward the end of the day and is relieved when the patient lies or sits down. Calcaneal spurs, visible on radiographs, may occur in chronic cases but are not responsible for evoking pain and discomfort. Treatment involves NSAIDs, stretching exercises (e.g., rolling a tennis ball under the foot), heel pads (Viscoheel), orthotics, rest, and ice therapy. In more severe cases that are refractory to these measures, iontophoresis, night splints, or steroid injection (0.5 mL of steroid and 1.0 mL of 1% lidocaine) can be used. In addition, surgery may be indicated for severe cases that are unresponsive to conservative therapy.

Young CC, Rutherford DS, Niedfeldt MW. Treatment of plantar fasciitis. *Am Fam Physician.* 2001;63:467–474, 477–478.

256. A 52-year-old man is seen for fevers and weight loss. A chest radiograph shows mediastinal lymphadenopathy. Laboratory findings show hypercalcemia, elevated alkaline phosphatase, and an elevated level of ACE. The most likely diagnosis is
A) small cell carcinoma of the lung
B) pulmonary tuberculosis
C) sarcoidosis
D) histoplasmosis
E) asbestosis

Answer and Discussion

The answer is C. Sarcoidosis is a systemic granulomatous disease that is characterized by noncaseating granulomas that may affect multiple organ systems. The condition occurs mainly in persons ages 20 to 40 years and is most common in Northern Europeans and African-Americans. Symptoms are variable and the etiology is unknown. Fever, weight loss, arthralgias, and erythema nodosum (more commonly seen in Europeans) are the usual initial presenting symptoms. Cough and dyspnea may be minimal or absent. Other manifestations include mediastinal lymphadenopathy seen on chest radiograph (hallmark finding in 90% of cases), hepatic granulomas, granulomatous uveitis, polyarthritis, cardiac symptoms (including angina, CHF, and conduction abnormalities), cranial-nerve palsies, and diabetes insipidus. Laboratory findings include leukopenia, hypercalcemia, hypercalciuria, and hypergammaglobulinemia (particularly in African-American patients). Other abnormalities include elevated uric acid (not usually associated with gout), elevated alkaline phosphatase, elevated gamma glutamyl transpeptidase, elevated levels of ACE, and pulmonary function tests showing restriction and impaired diffusing capacity. Diagnosis can be made with biopsy of peripheral lesions or fiberoptic bronchoscopy for central pulmonary lesions. Whole-body gallium scans can be used to show useful sites for biopsy and, in some cases, to follow disease progression. Serial pulmonary function tests are important for assessing disease progression and guiding treatment. The prognosis depends on the severity of the disease. Spontaneous improvement is common; however, significant disability can occur with multiorgan involvement. Pulmonary fibrosis is the leading cause of death. Treatment for symptomatic patients consists of corticosteroids, methotrexate, and other immunosuppressive medications if steroid therapy is not helpful.

Beers MH, Porter RS, eds. *The Merck manual of diagnosis and therapy,* Merck Research Laboratories, 18th ed. Whitehouse Station, NJ: Merck & Co.; 2006:462–469.

257. A cytomegalovirus infection has developed in a patient with AIDS. The most appropriate treatment is
A) ganciclovir
B) amphotericin B
C) amantadine
D) metronidazole
E) ciprofloxacin

Answer and Discussion

The answer is A. Cytomegalovirus is a viral infection that may occur congenitally or at any age. The severity of the infection varies. The virus is a variant of the herpes virus and is ubiquitous. Manifestations of the illness include fever, hepatitis, pneumonitis, and neurologic damage to brain tissue in the newborn (hearing losses or perinatal death in severe cases). The infection may be acquired in utero from an infected mother or by contact with infected secretions, including urine, saliva, breast milk, feces, blood, and semen. Patients with AIDS or immunocompromised conditions such as transplant patients and those living in institutions (such as nursing homes) or attending daycare centers are at increased risk. The infection is very common (as much as 90% of the population is affected) and in most cases is represented by mild symptoms. More severe cases can produce a mononucleosis-type illness, retinitis, or pneumonitis in adults. Congenital cytomegalovirus may include jaundice, hepatosplenomegaly, petechial rash, microcephaly, and cerebral calcifications. Diagnosis is achieved with the detection of the virus by immunofluorescence with monoclonal antibodies. Treatment is usually supportive; however, ganciclovir can be used in more severe cases and particularly in AIDS patients. Foscarnet sodium (Foscavir) is also effective, especially in ganciclovir-resistant cases.

Beers MH, Porter RS, eds. *The Merck manual of diagnosis and therapy,* Merck Research Laboratories, 18th ed. Whitehouse Station, NJ: Merck & Co.; 2006:1605–1606.

258. Which of the following ECG findings is associated with hypothermia?
A) J (Osborne) wave
B) Tachycardia
C) Atrioventricular dissociation
D) Atrial fibrillation
E) First-degree AV block

Answer and Discussion

The answer is A. Hypothermia is caused by prolonged exposure to a cold environment, causing the body's core temperature to fall below 35°C (or 95°F). Infants, the elderly, and those with altered mental status or debilitating illnesses are at increased risk. Others at increased risk include trauma and burn victims and those with malnutrition. Symptoms include shivering, decreased mental status with confusion, impaired coordination, drowsiness, bradycardia, and, in more severe cases, loss of the shivering reflex and coma. ECG tracings may show a characteristic J (Osborne) wave, a positive deflection after the QRS complex in the lateral leads. Death usually results from the progression of severe bradycardia to ventricular fibrillation. Treatment involves slow central body warming (over 2 to 3 hours to prevent shock) with warmed intravenous fluids, warmed oxygen, and warming blankets or warm baths. Life-sustaining measures should always be continued until the normal core body temperature is achieved.

Ferri F. *Ferri's Clinical Advisor, Instant Diagnosis and Treatment.* Philadelphia: Elsevier/Mosby; 2006:440.

259. Which of the following toxin–antidote associations is correct?

A) Organophosphates–atropine and pralidoxime
B) Carbon monoxide–nitrous oxide
C) Opioids–benzodiazepines
D) Methanol–isopropyl alcohol
E) Arsenic–flumazenil

Answer and Discussion

The answer is A. One of the common smells associated with poisonings is a garlic smell that may represent arsenic, dimethyl sulfoxide, organophosphates, and selenium toxicities. There is a cluster of symptoms that is associated with organophosphates represented by the acronym SLUDGE:

Salivation
Lacrimation
Urinary frequency
Defecation
Gastric hypersecretion
Emesis

The treatment for organophosphate poisoning is the concomitant use of atropine and pralidoxime. The treatment of choice for arsenic poisoning is penicillamine or dimercaprol. Sodium nitrite and sodium thiosulfate are antidotes for poisoning with cyanide amyl nitrate. Oxygen is used for carbon monoxide poisoning. Anticholinergic overdoses with medication such as atropine, scopolamine, and antihistamines are usually associated with symptoms in which the patient is described as "Dry as a bone, red as a beet, and mad as a hatter." Treatment involves the use of physostigmine as an antidote. Methanol overdoses are treated with ethanol, and opioid overdoses are treated with naloxone. Flumazenil (Romazicon) is used to treat benzodiazepine overdoses. Acetylcysteine is the treatment of choice for acetaminophen overdose.

Beers MH, Porter RS, eds. *The Merck manual of diagnosis and therapy,* Merck Research Laboratories, 18th ed. Whitehouse Station, NJ: Merck & Co.; 2006:2651–2695.

> The treatment for organophosphate poisoning is the concomitant use of atropine and pralidoxime.

260. A blood urea nitrogen (BUN):creatinine level greater than 20 is associated with

A) dehydration
B) renal stones
C) bladder outlet obstruction
D) hypercalcemia
E) renal artery stenosis

Answer and Discussion

The answer is A. Acute renal failure is divided into the following categories:

- *Prerenal.* This is due to inadequate renal perfusion. It can be caused by volume depletion (dehydration), cardiac or hepatic failure, and sepsis. Laboratory tests reveal a low urinary sodium (<20 mEq/L) and a high urine-to-plasma creatinine ratio (>20:1). The BUN to serum creatinine ratio is higher than 20.
- *Intrarenal.* This was previously known as acute tubular necrosis. Causes include ischemia, hypertension, vasculitis, metabolic disorders (e.g., hypercalcemia, hyperuricemia), toxins, x-ray dyes, myoglobinuria, and medications (e.g., aminoglycosides, penicillins, anesthetic agents). Laboratory tests show results similar to postrenal azotemia.
- *Postrenal.* This is usually caused by obstruction by renal calculi or bladder outlet obstruction (prostate enlargement). Laboratory tests show a high-urinary sodium (>40 mEq/L) and a low urine-to-plasma creatinine ratio (<20:1). The BUN to serum creatinine ratio is lower than 20.

Prerenal and postrenal causes for acute renal failure are potentially reversible. If caught early, some forms of intrarenal azotemia (e.g., drug effects, infections, hypertension) can be reversed.

Agrawal M, Swartz R. Acute renal failure. *Am Fam Physician.* 2000; 61:2077–2088.

261. Which of the following tests is used in the initial evaluation of persistent hemoptysis?

A) Fiberoptic bronchoscopy
B) Chest radiograph
C) Upper gastrointestinal (GI)
D) MRI of chest
E) CT scan of chest

Answer and Discussion

The answer is B. Hemoptysis is the presence of blood in the expectorate. Intrapulmonary causes include infections (e.g., bronchitis, pneumonia, tuberculous, fungal infections), neoplasm, bronchiectasis, pulmonary embolus, AV malformations, Goodpasture's disease, vasculitis, trauma, or the presence of a foreign body. Extrapulmonary causes include GI bleeding, CHF with pulmonary edema, severe mitral stenosis, epistaxis, or other conditions (including disseminated intravascular coagulation). Most cases are self-limited and require no additional workup; however, persistent or severe hemoptysis should be evaluated with sputum collection for Gram's stain and culture, cytology, acid-fast bacillus stains, CBC, PT, PTT, chest radiograph, and flexible bronchoscopy. If a lower respiratory tract source is suspected, the patient should undergo a chest x-ray first, and if a mass is noted, bronchoscopy should be performed. A high-resolution CT may be helpful in the diagnosis. It is important to distinguish between GI blood loss (which has a dark red color and acidic pH) and true hemoptysis, which is typically bright red in color and alkaline.

Kasper DL, Braunwald E, Fauci AS, et al., eds. *Harrison's principles of internal medicine,* 16th ed. New York: McGraw-Hill; 2005:207–209.

262. Thyroid replacement therapy can be assessed by measuring the patient's
A) T3 level
B) T4 level
C) TSH level
D) thyroid-releasing hormone level
E) none of the above

Answer and Discussion

The answer is C. Patients diagnosed with hypothyroidism should receive replacement therapy with levothyroxine. These patients can be monitored for effective replacement by evaluating their serum sTSH levels. A low-level TSH usually results from overreplacement, and adjustments should be made in the dose of medication; monitoring is repeated in 6 to 8 weeks. Underreplacement is represented by an increased TSH level and can be corrected by increasing the dose of thyroxine; monitoring is repeated in 6 to 8 weeks. Checking TSH levels earlier usually does not provide enough time for the levels to stabilize.

Rakel RE, Bope ET. *Conn's Current Therapy 2005.* Philadelphia: Elsevier/Saunders; 2005:761–762.

263. Which of the following statements is true regarding breast self-examination?
A) Multiple studies have shown benefit in breast self evaluation in the prevention of breast cancer.
B) The mortality risk of breast cancer is reduced by the practice of breast self-examination.
C) Breast self-examination may decrease overall mortality.
D) No benefit has been found with the use of breast self-examination.

Answer and Discussion

The answer is C. A large study conducted over 10 years demonstrates that a formal program of teaching breast self-examination has no effect on breast cancer mortality but may produce a small reduction in overall mortality.

Thomas DB, Gao DL, Ray RM. Randomized trial of breast self-examination in Shanghai: final results. *J Natl Cancer Inst.* 2002; 94:1445–1457.

264. Which of the following statements about ALS, or Lou Gehrig's disease, is true?
A) It is a progressive motor neuron disease that affects the corticospinal tracts.
B) The onset is usually before 20 years of age.
C) It typically destroys sensory function.
D) It may respond to high-dose steroid administration.
E) Dementia is common.

Answer and Discussion

The answer is A. ALS, or Lou Gehrig's disease, is a progressive motor neuron disease that affects the corticospinal tracts and/or the anterior horn cells and/or bulbar motor nuclei. Onset of the disease is usually after 40 years of age, and the disease is more common in men. Approximately 5% to 10% of cases are familial and are associated with an autosomal-dominant mode of transmission. The hands are usually affected first with cramps, followed by weakness. Other manifestations include atrophy, muscle fasciculations, spasticity, and increased reflex response. There is usually a combination of upper and lower motor neuron signs. Dysarthria and dysphagia may occur; however, extraocular muscles, sensory function, sexual function, and urinary continence are usually not affected. Dementia is usually not present. Late in the illness inappropriate, involuntary, and uncontrollable laughter or crying may occur. Diagnosis is usually made with EMG findings that correlate with the clinical presentation. Unfortunately, there is no treatment other than supportive care. Baclofen has been used to treat muscular spasticity and cramping. Death as a result of respiratory failure usually occurs within 5 years.

Beers MH, Porter RS, eds. *The Merck manual of diagnosis and therapy,* Merck Research Laboratories, 18th ed. Whitehouse Station, NJ: Merck & Co.; 2006:1897, 1899.

265. A 32-year-old man presents with recurrent oral and genital ulcers. He also has had arthralgias. Recently he was administered a tetanus vaccination and developed a sterile abscess at the site of the injection. The most likely diagnosis is
A) Behçet's disease
B) systemic herpes
C) syphilis
D) gonorrhea
E) Lyme disease

Answer and Discussion

The answer is A. Named after a famous Turkish dermatologist, Behçet's syndrome is an inflammatory disorder that may involve ocular, genital, articular, mucocutaneous, vascular, and CNS structures. Symptoms usually develop when patients are in their 30s. Men are more severely affected than women. Symptoms include episodic and recurrent oral and genital apthous type ulcers, uveitis, arthritis (usually affecting the knees and ankles), skin lesions, thrombophlebitis, and vasculitis. Signs include cranial-nerve palsies, seizures, mental disturbances, and spinal cord lesions. The disease is usually chronic and is characterized by remissions and exacerbations. The syndrome is usually benign; however, severe ocular involvement can lead to blindness. Steroids and immunosuppressive medication (interferon, azathioprine, cyclosporine) have been used for treatment, especially in cases of severe uveitis and CNS involvement. Other medications used in treatment include thalidomide, chlorambucil, and colchicine. The disease is more commonly seen in Japan and Korea, as well as the eastern Mediterranean countries. Sterile abscesses or pustules at the site of an injection are hallmark findings for the disease.

Kasper DL, Braunwald E, Fauci AS, et al., eds. *Harrison's principles of internal medicine,* 16th ed. New York: McGraw-Hill; 2005:2014.

266. The pneumococcal vaccine should be administered to healthy individuals at age
A) 50 years
B) 55 years
C) 60 years
D) 65 years
E) 70 years

Answer and Discussion

The answer is D. Adult immunizations include tetanus immunization, which should be given every 10 years. Pneumococcal immunization should be administered to those who are healthy and older than 65 years and those with other chronic or debilitating illnesses. The pneumococcal vaccine is typically a single, lifetime immunization; however, if the patient received their first dose before age 65 years and it has been more than 5 years they should receive a one-time booster. In addition, immunocompromised individuals or those with chronic underlying conditions should be considered for booster vaccination after 5 years. Influenza vaccination should be given yearly to those older than 50 years and those with underlying chronic illnesses. Patients born after 1956 should receive a booster measles vaccination, and those who have not had chickenpox (varicella) should receive the varicella vaccine. Adults who work in the health-care field or around body secretions or blood should receive the hepatitis B vaccination, which consists of three doses: one given at the initial visit, one 1 month later, and a booster 6 months later. In some cases, additional boosters may be necessary.

Centers for Disease Control and Prevention website. Summary of adolescent/adult immunization recommendations. Available at: http://www.cdc.gov/nip/recs/adult-schedule.pdf. Accessed 6/2/06.

267. A boy who plays Little League baseball presents with swelling over the lateral elbow and pain with valgus and varus stress while flexing and extending the elbow. The patient reports locking of the elbow. In addition, radiographs show the presence of loose bodies. The most likely diagnosis is

A) osteochondritis dissecans
B) chondromalacia
C) nursemaid's elbow
D) lateral epicondylitis

Answer and Discussion

The answer is A. Little leaguer's elbow is an overuse injury caused by compressive forces at the radiocapitellar joint and opposite pulling forces at the medial aspect of the elbow. These injuries usually occur in adolescents who use motions such as overhand pitching in sports such as baseball. The repetitive forces may lead to damage of the articular surface of the capitellum, ligamentous injury of the medial elbow, and ulnar nerve dysfunction. In severe cases, osteochondritis dissecans of the capitellum with the formation of loose bodies can occur and result in locking of the elbow joint. Other symptoms include pain and swelling over the lateral elbow and pain with valgus and varus stress while flexing and extending the elbow. For mild cases, treatment involves rest, ice, elevation, and NSAIDs. However, if there are signs of osteochondritis dissecans, orthopedic referral for possible surgical intervention is necessary.

Ferri F. *Ferri's Clinical Advisor, Instant Diagnosis and Treatment.* Philadelphia: Elsevier/Mosby; 2006:595.

268. Mitral valve prolapse (MVP) is associated with

A) elderly, obese men
B) diastolic click that disappears with Valsalva's maneuver
C) chest pain, dyspnea, and syncope
D) rheumatic heart disease
E) myxomatous transformation of the valve leaflet

Answer and Discussion

The answer is E. Mitral valve prolapse (MVP) (systolic-click syndrome, Barlow's syndrome, and floppy valve syndrome) is usually asymptomatic but may cause chest pain, palpitations, anxiety, dyspnea, or fatigue. The condition is common and associated with myxomatous transformation of the valve leaflet. MVP usually affects healthy, young (15 to 30 years of age), thin women. MVP is determined by the detection of a midsystolic click that is followed by a late systolic murmur and becomes louder with Valsalva's maneuver. A high-pitched late systolic crescendo–decrescendo murmur heard best at the apex may also be present. Presence of both murmur and click are not necessary for the diagnosis. In patients with MVP, cardiac arrhythmias, including PVCs, paroxysmal supraventricular tachycardia, and ventricular tachycardia, may cause palpitations and may need treatment (usually with β blockers).

Antibiotic prophylaxis for prevention of infective endocarditis during procedures that carry risk for bacteremia is recommended in most patients. Rarely, MVP may progress to mitral insufficiency because of rupture of the chordae tendineae and may require valve replacement.

Ferri F. *Ferri's Clinical Advisor, Instant Diagnosis and Treatment.* Philadelphia: Elsevier/Mosby; 2006:533, 1353.

> Mitral valve prolapse (MVP) is determined by the detection of a midsystolic click that is followed by a late systolic murmur and becomes louder with Valsalva's maneuver.

269. Which of the following statements about Peutz-Jeghers syndrome is true?

A) The condition is sex linked and usually skips a generation.
B) The condition involves the development of multiple polyps in the stomach and the small and large intestine that commonly show malignant change.
C) There is associated hyperpigmentation around the oral cavity, lips, soles of the feet, and dorsum of the hands.
D) The condition is associated with inflammatory bowel disease.
E) The condition is identified by elevation in carcinoembryonic antigen levels.

Answer and Discussion

The answer is C. Peutz-Jeghers syndrome is a familial autosomal-dominant condition that involves the development of multiple, benign, hamartomatous polyps in the stomach and in the small and large intestine. Malignant change has occurred but is rare. Those affected also have melanin-associated brownish-black hyperpigmentation around the oral cavity, lips, soles of the feet, and dorsum of the hands. The condition usually causes no problems except in severe cases in which abdominal pain, intestinal obstruction, or bleeding can occur. In these severe cases, surgery may be considered.

Beers MH, Porter RS, eds. *The Merck manual of diagnosis and therapy,* Merck Research Laboratories, 18th ed. Whitehouse Station, NJ: Merck & Co.; 2006:173, 1004, 1208.

270. Which of the following statements about angina pectoris is true?

A) It typically lasts 1 to 2 hours.
B) It may be associated with epigastric pain.
C) It causes predictable ECG changes.

D) It is typically associated with chest wall tenderness.
E) It rarely radiates to the neck, jaw, or left arm.

Answer and Discussion

The answer is B. Angina pectoris is typically described as substernal chest pain or pressure that may radiate to the neck, jaw, or left arm. Patients usually also experience shortness of breath, dizziness, nausea, and vomiting with diaphoresis. Symptoms are usually precipitated by physical exertion or stress and are relieved with rest. Episodes usually last 2 to 10 minutes and rarely last longer than 30 minutes. Atypical presentations include epigastric pain, indigestion, right-arm pain, light-headedness, nausea, or shortness of breath. These occurring alone are referred to as anginal equivalents. There are several types of angina:

- *Stable*: Intensity, character, and frequency of episodes are predictable; angina occurs in response to a known amount of exercise or stress.
- *Unstable*: Intensity, frequency, and duration are different and unpredictable; pain is precipitated by a lesser amount of exercise or the angina is longer in duration. Angina at rest or new-onset angina is unstable.
- *Variant*: Pain that may occur at rest and is secondary to spasm of the coronary arteries is variant angina.

Typically, the pain is relieved with the administration of sublingual nitroglycerin. ECG may show T-wave inversion or ST-segment depression, but in many cases is normal and should not be discounted if normal. Exercise stress testing can be used to determine coronary insufficiency. Treatment of angina is accomplished with the use of nitrates, β-blockers, and calcium-channel blockers.

Ferri F. *Ferri's Clinical Advisor, Instant Diagnosis and Treatment*. Philadelphia: Elsevier/Mosby; 2006:61–64.

271. Which of the following best describes Ludwig's angina?
A) Substernal chest pain that radiates to the right arm.
B) An infection involving the sublingual and submaxillary space.
C) Abdominal pain secondary to an enlarging abdominal aortic aneurysm.
D) A tonsillar infection that leads to chronic abscess formation.
E) Ischemic pain related to insufficient blood flow to an extremity.

Answer and Discussion

The answer is B. Ludwig's angina usually develops from a periodontal or dental infection and is one of the most common neck space infections. The condition is usually a rapidly developing, bilateral cellulitis that affects the sublingual and submaxillary space, without involvement of the lymph nodes or formation of abscesses. The infection usually rapidly arises from the second and third mandibular molars as a result of poor dental hygiene, tooth extraction, or trauma. Symptoms include edema and erythema of the upper neck (under the chin) and floor of the mouth, trismus, drooling, dysphonia, dysphagia, and dyspnea. Fever, chills, and tachycardia are usually present. Tongue displacement upward may also occur and threaten the airway. In severe cases, the condition may be fatal. Treatment includes protection of the airway in severe cases and intravenous antibiotics (e.g., penicillin, wide-spectrum cephalosporins) in high doses to cover anaerobic organisms (*Bacteroides*). Incision and drainage may be required.

Beers MH, Porter RS, eds. *The Merck manual of diagnosis and therapy*, Merck Research Laboratories, 18th ed. Whitehouse Station, NJ: Merck & Co.; 2006:824–825.

272. Vitamin A toxicity is associated with
A) peripheral neuropathy
B) renal stones
C) increased intracranial pressure and vomiting
D) night blindness
E) pulmonary fibrosis

Answer and Discussion

The answer is C. Excessive ingestion of vitamin A may cause acute or chronic toxicity. Acute toxicity especially in children may result from taking large doses (>100,000 μg or 300,000 IU). The condition is associated with increased intracranial pressure and vomiting, which may lead to death. After discontinuation, recovery is usually spontaneous, with no residual damage. Infants who are given 6,000 to 20,000 μg (20,000 to 60,000 IU)/day of water-soluble vitamin A may show evidence of toxicity within a few weeks. Birth defects have been reported in the children of women receiving 13-*cis*-retinoic acid (isotretinoin) for skin conditions during pregnancy. Megavitamin tablets containing vitamin A have occasionally induced acute toxicity when taken long term. Chronic toxicity usually affects older children and adults after doses of >33,000 μg (100,000 IU)/day have been taken for an extended course (i.e., months).

Beers MH, Porter RS, eds. *The Merck manual of diagnosis and therapy*, Merck Research Laboratories, 18th ed. Whitehouse Station, NJ: Merck & Co.; 2006:2684.

273. A 65-year-old female is undergoing a general examination. On your exam you note a fullness in the left adnexa. Which of the following conditions would be reassuring that the finding is benign?
A) A multi-loculated cyst noted on ultrasound
B) Elevated CA 125 level
C) Simple cyst measured at 2.5 cm
D) Elevated CEA level
E) All cysts in a postmenopausal female require surgical removal

Answer and Discussion

The answer is C. Adnexal masses are commonly encountered in women. In premenopausal women, physiologic follicular cysts and corpus luteum cysts are the most common adnexal masses. Ectopic pregnancy can occur and should be considered. Other causes for masses in this age group include endometriomas, polycystic ovaries, tubo-ovarian abscesses, and benign neoplasms. Malignant neoplasms become more frequent with increasing age. In postmenopausal women with adnexal masses, neoplasms must be considered, along with leiomyomas, ovarian fibromas and other lesions such as diverticular abscesses. Measurement of serum CA-125 is an appropriate test for assessing postmenopausal women with pelvic masses. Asymptomatic premenopausal patients with simple ovarian cysts <10 cm in diameter can be observed or placed on suppressive therapy with oral contraceptives. Postmenopausal women with simple cysts <3 cm in diameter may also be followed, provided the serum CA 125 level is not elevated and the patient has no signs or symptoms suggestive of malignancy. If the cyst is >3 cm or the CA 125 is elevated, further evaluation is necessary.

Drake J. Diagnosis and management of the adnexal mass. *Am Fam Physician*. 1998;57:2471.

274. Which of the following factors is associated with a cause of impotence?

A) Masturbation
B) Alcohol dependence
C) Nocturnal tumescence
D) Vacuum erection devices
E) Excessive testosterone levels

Answer and Discussion

The answer is B. Impotence (often referred to as *erectile dysfunction*) was for the most part attributed to psychogenic factors such as life stressors and performance anxiety. However, current studies show that up to 90% of men with erectile dysfunction have underlying organic pathology. Organic causes of impotence include diabetes, drug or alcohol dependency, vascular and neurogenic compromise, and medications (e.g., hypertension medications). Most causes are multifactorial in nature. Nocturnal tumescence studies have been advocated as a method to distinguish psychogenic versus organic impotence; however, there is no consensus on the use and validity of these studies. Most urologists now initiate diagnostic testing by injecting alprostadil (Caverject), with resultant increase in penile flow. The ability to obtain an erection with pharmacologic injection, for the most part, rules out significant vascular causes of impotence. Initial laboratory testing should include only basic tests (however, this is controversial); hormonal testing should be based on clinical suspicion. Many experts feel serum testosterone determination should only be obtained in cases of low sexual desire or abnormal physical findings. Serum prolactin measurements should be obtained only in patients with low sexual desire, gynecomastia, visual symptoms, and/or testosterone levels <4 ng/mL. Others advocate serum testosterone and prolactin levels for all those affected. If pituitary abnormalities are suspected, brain imaging to rule out pituitary tumors should be performed. Treatment may involve the use of phospodiesterase 5 inhibitors (PDE5) including oral sildenafil (Viagra), vardenafil (Levitra), and tadalafil (Cialis), testosterone patches or injections, penile injections (phentolamine, alprostadil), vacuum devices, or penile implants.

Rakel RE, Bope ET. *Conn's Current Therapy 2005*. Philadelphia: Elsevier/Saunders; 2005:818–822.

Miller TA. Diagnostic evaluation of erectile dysfunction. *Am Fam Physician*. 2000;61:95–104, 109–110.

275. Cephalosporins are contraindicated for which of the following groups?

A) Patients allergic to eggs
B) Patients who have had a mild rash as a result of penicillin administration
C) Patients with G6PD deficiency
D) Patients suspected of bacterial meningitis
E) None of the above

Answer and Discussion

The answer is E. Hypersensitivity reactions to cephalosporins may occur and include rash, urticaria, and, in severe cases, anaphylaxis. Because of the similar chemical structure, there is a small proportion (<2%) of patients with penicillin allergy who cross-react with cephalosporins. Therefore, cephalosporins should be avoided in patients with a history of an immediate reaction to penicillin. Cephalosporins are used in patients with a history of mild reactions to penicillins.

Kasper DL, Braunwald E, Fauci AS, et al., eds. *Harrison's principles of internal medicine,* 16th ed. New York: McGraw-Hill; 2005:801.

276. A 21-year-old man presents to your office complaining that his left testicle feels abnormal. On examination, the area adjacent to the left testicle feels like a "bag of worms" that gets larger with a Valsalva maneuver. The most likely diagnosis is

A) hydrocele
B) varicocele
C) left inguinal hernia
D) spermatocele
E) testicular cancer

Answer and Discussion

The answer is B. Varicoceles are a collection of veins (pampiniform plexus) usually associated with the left scrotum, which are separate from the testicle. They are found in up to 15% of adult men. On clinical examination, a varicocele feels like a bag of worms that becomes larger with a Valsalva maneuver. Some cases may be associated with decreased sperm counts and infertility. In these cases or if the patient has testicular pain or discomfort, surgical correction should be considered; otherwise, no further therapy is needed. Varicoceles are found most commonly on the left side, but up to 20% may be bilateral. Diagnosis should be made in a warm room by palpation of the spermatic cord with the patient in the standing position. Varicoceles are graded 1+ (palpable with Valsalva's maneuver only), 2+ (palpable), and 3+ (visible through the scrotal skin). An isolated right-sided varicocele or a lesion on either side that does not disappear when the patient assumes the supine position should prompt imaging of the retroperitoneum to evaluate for inferior vena caval or renal vein obstruction.

Kolettis PN. Evaluation of the subfertile man. *Am Fam Physician*. 2003;67:2165–2173.

> An isolated right-sided varicocele or a lesion on either side that does not disappear when the patient assumes the supine position should prompt imaging of the retroperitoneum to evaluate for inferior vena caval or renal vein obstruction.

277. Exposure to radon gas has been associated with the development of

A) renal cell carcinoma
B) pancreatic cancer
C) lung cancer
D) bladder cancer
E) esophageal cancer

Answer and Discussion

The answer is C. Radon gas exposure may be linked to the development of lung cancer. The highest amounts of radon exposure are associated with people who mine uranium. Radon found in the soil and in the water supply around homes represents a theoretic risk to inhabitants. Levels associated with excess lung cancer risk may be present in as many as 10% of houses in the United States. Concrete block foundations provide a better barrier against radon than do cinder block foundations. Adequate ventilation of the home is also important to minimize radon levels. According to the Environmental Protection Agency, the maximum limit for radon in homes is 4 pCi/L. Radon levels tend to be higher in the winter months when houses are more poorly ventilated. Radon levels <1.5 pCi/L are considered safe. When smokers reside in the affected household, the problem is potentially greater, because the molecular size of radon particles allows them to readily attach to smoke particles that are inhaled.

Viera AJ. Radon and lung cancer. *Am Fam Physician.* 2000; 62;950–951.

Kasper DL, Braunwald E, Fauci AS, et al., eds. *Harrison's principles of internal medicine,* 16th ed. New York: McGraw-Hill; 2005:1528.

278. A 28-year-old homosexual man presents to your office complaining of a nonproductive cough, shortness of breath, fever, and chills. A chest radiograph shows bilateral interstitial infiltrates. The best treatment is

A) oral azithromycin
B) intravenous penicillin
C) intravenous TMP-SMX
D) intravenous amphotericin
E) observation only

Answer and Discussion

The answer is C. *Pneumocystis jiroveci* (formerly *P. carinii*) is an opportunistic pulmonary infection that often affects patients with AIDS. As many as 30% of patients with AIDS present with this initial infection. Symptoms include a fever; dry, nonproductive cough; tachypnea; and hypoxia. Chest radiograph usually shows bilateral perihilar infiltrates; however, 20% to 30% may have a normal chest x-ray. ABGs show hypoxemia with an increase in the alveolar-arterial oxygen gradient. Diagnosis involves sputum collection followed by immunofluorescent tests. If the diagnosis is suspected and the sputum samples are negative, bronchoscopy may be necessary to collect adequate samples. Treatment involves TMP-SMX if the patient's PO_2 is <70 mm Hg for 21 days. Prednisone may also be added once tuberculosis is ruled out if the PaO_2 is <70 mm Hg. Prophylactic therapy should be initiated for all patients with a $CD4^+$ count <200 or a previous infection with *P. jiroveci.* Medications for patients with $CD4^+$ counts <200 include TMP/SMX, dapsone, or aerosolized pentamidine.

Beers MH, Porter RS, eds. *The Merck manual of diagnosis and therapy,* Merck Research Laboratories, 18th ed. Whitehouse Station, NJ: Merck & Co.; 2006:435–436.

279. Which of the following terms is used to describe a peripheral neuropathy with simultaneous or sequential involvement of individual, noncontiguous nerve trunks?

A) Polyneuropathy
B) Mononeuropathy
C) Mononeuropathy multiplex
D) Polyneuropathy simplex

Answer and Discussion

The answer is C. Peripheral neuropathies are classified into the following categories:

- Polyneuropathy, which affects peripheral nerves in a symmetrical bilateral distribution
- Mononeuropathy, which involves a single nerve
- Mononeuropathy multiplex, which is simultaneous or sequential involvement of individual noncontiguous nerve trunks

Symptoms include pain, paresthesias, numbness, burning, weakness, muscle atrophy, and loss of reflexes. Motor and sensory deficits may occur. Causes include diabetes and alcoholism, which usually lead to deficits in the distal extremities in a stocking-glove distribution; hereditary diseases (e.g., Charcot-Marie-Tooth syndrome); metabolic conditions (e.g., hypothyroidism, vitamin B_{12} deficiency); toxic disorders (e.g., INH administration, heavy metal ingestion, dapsone administration); inflammatory conditions (e.g., Guillain-Barré syndrome, diphtheria, sarcoidosis); and idiopathic disorders. Electromyographic studies are helpful in determining the extent of the deficit and for documenting progression or regression of the deficit. Treatment involves correction of the underlying cause. In severe cases, the use of tricyclic antidepressants can be used for chronic pain.

Kasper DL, Braunwald E, Fauci AS, et al., eds. *Harrison's principles of internal medicine,* 16th ed. New York: McGraw-Hill; 2005:2500–2508.

280. People who follow vegetarian diets should be counseled to

A) avoid the use of iron utensils
B) take a daily multivitamin
C) avoid the use of vitamin D
D) avoid calcium supplementation
E) none of the above

Answer and Discussion

The answer is B. The most common form of vegetarianism is ovolactovegetarianism, in which meat and fish are avoided, but eggs and dairy products are eaten. Vegetarian diets usually provide enough nutrition to satisfy most daily nutritional requirements. However, these diets are usually low in animal protein, iron, zinc, calcium, vitamin D, and vitamin B_{12}. In most cases, vegetarians should be counseled to take a multivitamin, which may help to satisfy the daily requirements that they may not achieve with their diets. The use of iron utensils when cooking can also help to maintain their iron requirements.

Beers MH, Porter RS, eds. *The Merck manual of diagnosis and therapy,* Merck Research Laboratories, 18th ed. Whitehouse Station, NJ: Merck & Co.; 2006:11.

281. Which of the following treatments should be used for a patient suspected of having Wernicke-Korsakoff syndrome?

A) Intravenous administration of glucose followed by administration of thiamine
B) Administration of folic acid followed by intravenous administration of dextrose
C) Administration of haloperidol with psychotherapy
D) Administration of thiamine followed by intravenous administration of dextrose
E) Lactated Ringer's solution with naloxone

Answer and Discussion

The answer is D. *Wernicke-Korsakoff syndrome* refers to the coexistence of Wernicke's encephalopathy and Korsakoff's psychosis. Wernicke's encephalopathy is characterized by gait ataxia, mental confusion, nystagmus, vomiting, fever, and ophthalmoplegia. The disease is primarily seen in alcoholics but can also occur in hyperemesis gravidarum or the use of vitamin-free nutrition (e.g., fad diets). The cause is thiamine deficiency (also known as *beriberi*). Wernicke's encephalopathy is a medical emergency and deserves prompt attention; otherwise, permanent brain damage or even death may occur. If Wernicke's encephalopathy is suspected, thiamine should always be administered before dextrose. Administration of glucose solution before thiamine administration may exhaust a patient's reserve of B vitamins and worsen his or her condition. Korsakoff's psychosis is also related to thiamine deficiency and may follow Wernicke's disease. Symptoms include retrograde amnesia, impaired learning ability, and confabulation. Treatment also involves the administration of thiamine.

Ferri F. *Ferri's Clinical Advisor, Instant Diagnosis and Treatment*. Philadelphia: Elsevier/Mosby; 2006:48, 468, 913.

282. Which of the following laboratory findings is *not* associated with Graves' disease?
A) Thyroid-stimulating antibodies
B) Increased TSH
C) Increased T4 level
D) Increased T3 level

Answer and Discussion

The answer is B. The following are thyroid conditions and their associated laboratory findings:

- Euthyroid sick syndrome: decreased serum T_3, increased reverse T_3, decreased total T_4, and normal serum TSH
- Primary thyroid gland failure (hypothyroidism): marked elevation of serum TSH with decreased serum T_3 and T_4 levels
- Thyrotoxicosis: increased T_4 and T_3
- T3 toxicosis: increased T_3 and normal T_4
- Graves' disease: increased T_4 and T_3, decreased TSH, and thyroid-stimulating antibodies present
- Plummer's disease (toxic multinodular goiter): increased T_3 and T_4, decreased TSH, thyroid-stimulating antibodies absent, and increased radioimmunoassay uptake in the hyperfunctioning nodule

Beers MH, Porter RS, eds. *The Merck manual of diagnosis and therapy*, Merck Research Laboratories, 18th ed. Whitehouse Station, NJ: Merck & Co.; 2006:1192–1206.

283. Benign positional vertigo is most easily confirmed by
A) orthostatic blood pressures
B) Dix-Hallpike maneuvers
C) cover–uncover test
D) MRI
E) cold–warm water calorics

Answer and Discussion

The answer is B. Benign positional vertigo is a condition characterized by severe episodes of vertigo that usually last less than 1 minute and are precipitated by certain head positions. The vertiginous symptoms are accompanied by nystagmus, and there is no tinnitus or hearing loss (as is seen in Meniere's disease). The diagnosis is usually based on the history and reproduction of symptoms by the Dix-Hallpike maneuver: The patient's head is turned to the side and the patient goes from a sitting to a lying position with the head positioned beneath the level of the bed. A positive response is noted when the patient reports vertigo and there is evidence of nystagmus. Most cases are self-limited, and repeating the position that causes the vertigo usually fatigues the vertiginous response. Vestibular-type exercises performed several times daily may help eliminate the symptoms, especially for younger patients. Labyrinthine sedatives are of little help for this condition. Canalith repositioning can also be attempted and is beneficial for select patients. If fatigability of symptoms does not occur, further workup may be indicated to rule out a central cause for the vertigo.

Froehling DA, Bowen JM, Mohr DN, et al. The canalith repositioning procedure for the treatment of benign paroxysmal positional vertigo: a randomized controlled trial. *Mayo Clin Proc*. 2000;75:695–700.

Kroenke K, Hoffman RM, Einstadter D. How common are various causes of dizziness? A critical review. *South Med J*. 2000;93:160–167.

Benign positional vertigo is a condition characterized by severe episodes of vertigo that usually last less than 1 minute and are precipitated by certain head positions. The vertiginous symptoms are accompanied by nystagmus, and there is no tinnitus or hearing loss (as is seen in Meniere's disease). The diagnosis is usually based on the history and reproduction of symptoms by the Dix-Hallpike maneuver.

284. A 72-year-old woman presents to your office with left-sided headaches, visual disturbances, low-grade fevers, generalized malaise, anorexia, and weight loss. Laboratory testing reveals a mild normocytic anemia, ESR of 120 mm/hour, and a mild leukocytosis. Appropriate management at this time consists of
A) MRI of the brain
B) colonoscopy
C) neurology referral
D) visual field testing
E) high-dose steroid therapy

Answer and Discussion

The answer is E. Temporal arteritis is an inflammatory disease that predominantly affects the temporal and occipital arteries, although other arteries of the aortic arch may be involved. Systemic symptoms include low-grade fever, malaise, weakness, anorexia, weight loss, painful joints, headaches in the temporal distribution, and visual disturbances. Most cases occur in patients older than 50 years, and women are more commonly affected than men. Although the cause is unknown, it is believed to be autoimmune in origin. Granulomatous inflammatory lesions involving the arteries are seen. The diagnosis is made by the clinical history and an elevated ESR (usually greater than 100 mm/hour). Leukocytosis and mild normochromic normocytic anemia are also usually seen. A biopsy of the temporal artery showing inflammation provides the definitive diagnosis. If left untreated, the major and most serious complication of temporal arteritis is blindness. If temporal arteritis is suspected, high doses of corticosteroids (at least 40 mg/day) should be initiated immediately to prevent blindness. Monitoring the patient's ESR can determine dose reduction of steroid therapy. Significant improvement is usually seen within 4 weeks of therapy. Extended therapy (up to 2 years) may be necessary to control the disease. Polymyalgia rheumatica occurs in 40% to 60% of patients with temporal arteritis.

Rakel RE, Bope ET. *Conn's Current Therapy 2005*. Philadelphia: Elsevier/Saunders; 2005:1144–1145.

285. Which of the following individuals is not a candidate for 23-valent pneumococcal vaccination (Pneumovax)?
A) A 48-year-old smoker with COPD
B) A 37-year-old African-American woman with sickle cell anemia
C) A healthy 75-year-old individual
D) A 15 month old with asthma
E) A 28-year-old man with cystic fibrosis

Answer and Discussion

The answer is D. The pneumococcal vaccination (Pneumovax) contains the purified polysaccharide antigens from 23 of the most common strains of *S. pneumoniae*. These serotypes consist of approximately 90% of the different subtypes that cause pneumococcal pneumonia. In most individuals, it takes approximately 2 weeks before antibodies are formed. Those recommended to receive the vaccination include the following:

Adults

- Immunocompetent adults who are at increased risk of pneumococcal disease or its complications because of chronic illnesses (e.g., cardiovascular disease, pulmonary disease, diabetes mellitus, alcoholism, cirrhosis, or CSF leaks) or who are 65 years old or older.
- Immunocompromised adults at increased risk of pneumococcal disease or its complications (e.g., persons with splenic dysfunction or anatomic asplenia, Hodgkin's disease, lymphoma, multiple myeloma, chronic renal failure, nephrotic syndrome, or conditions such as organ transplantation associated with immunosuppression).
- Adults with asymptomatic or symptomatic HIV infection.

Children

- Children 2 years of age or older with chronic illnesses specifically associated with increased risk of pneumococcal disease or its complications [e.g., anatomic or functional asplenia (including sickle cell disease), nephrotic syndrome, CSF leaks, and conditions associated with immunosuppression].
- Children 2 years of age or older with asymptomatic or symptomatic HIV infection.
- The currently available 23-valent vaccine is not indicated for patients having only recurrent upper respiratory tract disease, including otitis media and sinusitis.

Special Groups

- Persons living in special environments or social settings with an identified increased risk of pneumococcal disease or its complications (e.g., certain Native American populations).

The vaccine is routinely given as a one-time dose; administer if previous vaccination history is unknown. A one-time revaccination is recommended 5 years later for persons at highest risk of fatal pneumococcal infection or rapid antibody loss (e.g., renal disease) and for persons age 65 years and older if the first dose was given prior to age 65 and 5 years or more have elapsed since the prior dose.

Side effects of the vaccination include erythema and pain at the site of injection (50% of patients), fever, and myalgia; rare cases of anaphylaxis (5:1,000,000) have been reported. Safety and effectiveness in children younger than 2 years have not been established.

In 2000, a 7-valent pneumococcal conjugate vaccine (Prevnar) was approved for young children. When initiated during infancy, the four-dose vaccination schedule is set at 2, 4, 6, and 12 to 15 months of age. Adverse reactions are minimal. Efficacy is reported to be 94%.

Centers for Disease Control and Prevention website. Recommendations of the Immunization Practices Advisory Committee Pneumococcal Polysaccharide Vaccine. Available at: http://cdc.gov, accessed 6/2/06.

Zimmerman RK. Pneumococcal conjugate vaccine for young children. *Am Fam Physician*. 2001;63:2003–2004.

286. Which of the following statements regarding enoxaparin (Lovenox) is true?
A) It use has not been shown to be cost effective in an outpatient setting.
B) The medication does not require laboratory monitoring.
C) The incidence of thrombocytopenia is the same as with heparin.
D) It must be given through an intravenous route.
E) It is safe to use in renal failure patients.

Answer and Discussion

The answer is B. Enoxaparin (Lovenox) was the first LMW heparin approved by the U.S. FDA for the treatment of DVT in a dosage of 1 mg/kg twice daily or 1.5 mg once daily. Low-molecular-weight (LMW) heparin offers distinct advantages over unfractionated heparin: It can be administered subcutaneously once or twice daily, it has a longer biologic half-life, dosing is fixed, and laboratory monitoring is not required. In addition, thrombocytopenia appears to be less likely. In patients with DVT, subcutaneous administration of heparin is as effective as continuous infusion of unfractionated heparin in preventing complications and reducing the risk of recurrence. Outpatient management of DVT using LMW heparin for short-term anticoagulation until warfarin is at a therapeutic level is considered safe and cost-effective. Candidates for outpatient therapy must be hemodynamically stable, without renal failure, and not at high risk for bleeding. Additionally, they must have an appropriate supportive home environment, and be capable of daily monitoring until the INR is therapeutic. LMW heparin is typically given in combination with warfarin for 4 to 5 days. Simultaneous initiation of warfarin and unfractionated heparin or LMW heparin has not been associated with adverse outcomes. Dalteparin (Fragmin), another LMW heparin, is approved only for prophylaxis of DVT. The FDA has also approved the use of tinzaparin (Innohep) for the treatment of DVT.

Ramzi DW, Leeper KV. DVT and pulmonary embolism: part II. diagnosis. *Am Fam Physician*. 2004;69:2841–2848.

287. A 59-year-old man presents to your office with complaints of vasomotor rhinitis with only symptoms of rhinorrhea. Appropriate treatment would be
A) topical corticosteroid
B) topical anticholinergic
C) topical antihistamine
D) oral antihistamine
E) topical decongestant

Answer and Discussion

The answer is B. Vasomotor rhinitis is manifested by a combination of symptoms that includes nasal obstruction and rhinorrhea.

Vasomotor rhinitis is a usually a diagnosis of exclusion. According to a 2002 evidence-based report published by the Agency for Healthcare Research and Quality (AHRQ), treatment involves avoiding known environmental triggers such as odors (e.g., cigarette smoke, perfumes, bleach, formaldehyde, newspaper or other inks); auto emission fumes; light stimuli; temperature changes; and hot or spicy foods. A stepwise pharmacologic approach includes an initial treatment based on the patient's major symptom. If the presenting symptom is solely rhinorrhea, a topical anticholinergic [ipratropium (Atrovent)] is considered the initial step. If nasal congestion and obstruction are present, a topical corticosteroids is recommended. If the patient presents with the full spectrum of symptoms including rhinorrhea with sneezing, postnasal drip, and congestion, a topical antihistamine [azelastine (Astelin)] may be utilized. After an adequate trial period, changes and additions should be made if the response is inadequate. Exercise is beneficial for overall health and may be a useful treatment addition because it produces decreased airway resistance and assists natural nasal decongestion. The effect of exercise on nasal decongestion is short-lived, but it has numerous other benefits and can be repeated. Traditional oral antihistamines have no established beneficial effect in patients with vasomotor rhinitis and may be associated with sedation. Newer, less-sedating antihistamines also have no proven effectiveness for vasomotor rhinitis, and their use may delay proper treatment while incurring significant cost. The empiric use of the topical decongestant ephedrine on a chronic basis can result in tolerance and development of rhinitis medicamentosa.

Wheeler PW, Wheeler SF. Vasomotor rhinitis. *Am Fam Physician.* 2005;72:1057–1062.

288. Postpolio syndrome typically occurs
A) immediately after the primary infection
B) 3 to 6 months after the initial infection
C) 2 to 3 years after the initial infection
D) 5 to 10 years after the initial infection
E) 15 to 30 years after the initial infection

Answer and Discussion

The answer is E. Postpolio syndrome is a constellation of symptoms that affects patients previously infected with the poliovirus. Typically, symptoms occur 15 to 30 years after the initial infection and include progressive generalized weakness, muscle pain, cramps, fasciculations, and atrophy. Other findings include cold, cyanotic extremities that have adequate pulses, and diffuse joint pain. Typically, the areas that were affected during the original infection are the same areas affected with the postpolio syndrome. In most, new symptoms are not due to progression of remote polio but to a superimposed second condition such as diabetes, disk herniation, or degenerative joint disease. Treatment is supportive and involves rest.

Kasper DL, Braunwald E, Fauci AS, et al., eds. *Harrison's principles of internal medicine,* 16th ed. New York: McGraw-Hill; 2005:1144.

289. Clubbing is thought to be a result of
A) chronic hypercarbia
B) chronic hypoxemia
C) excess nitrogen production
D) malignancy
E) protein storage disease

Answer and Discussion

The answer is B. Clubbing has interested physicians for years. The cause is thought to be related to chronic hypoxemia. The condition is evident when the patient has an enlargement and softness of the nail beds and a reduction in the angle between the nail and the distal phalanx. The ratio of the anteroposterior diameter of the finger at the nail bed to that at the distal interphalangeal joint is a simple measurement of finger clubbing. If the ratio is more than 1, clubbing is present. Causes include pulmonary processes such as bronchogenic carcinoma, chronic pulmonary tuberculosis, COPD, and bronchiectasis; cyanotic congenital heart disease; subacute bacterial endocarditis; inflammatory bowel disease; and biliary cirrhosis. Clinical evidence of clubbing should be further evaluated with a chest radiograph because of the possibility of underlying lung disease.

Beers MH, Porter RS, eds. *The Merck manual of diagnosis and therapy,* Merck Research Laboratories, 18th ed. Whitehouse Station, NJ: Merck & Co.; 2006:259, 354.

290. Which of the following statements about myasthenia gravis is true?
A) Symptoms usually improve with administration of norepinephrine-inhibiting medications.
B) Symptoms include ptosis, diplopia, dysarthria, dysphagia, and proximal muscle weakness of the limbs.
C) Symptoms are aggravated by the administration of edrophonium.
D) Symptoms rarely fluctuate and usually spare the facial nerves.

Answer and Discussion

The answer is B. Myasthenia gravis is a neuromuscular transmission disorder. It may occur at any age and may be associated with thymic tumors, thyrotoxicosis, lupus, or rheumatoid arthritis. It is more commonly seen in young women and appears to be linked to the HLA-DR3 genetic focus. If the patient is an elderly man, there is often an associated thymoma. Episodic muscle weakness is a symptom that often fluctuates in intensity, particularly in muscles associated with the cranial nerves; this includes ptosis, diplopia, dysarthria, dysphagia, and proximal muscle weakness in the limbs. These symptoms improve when cholinesterase-inhibiting medication is administered. Sensory function and deep tendon reflexes are unaffected. The disease is thought to be associated with an autoimmune-mediated attack on the postsynaptic acetylcholine-receptor sites, which prevents neurosynaptic transmission.

Diagnosis is usually confirmed by the edrophonium (Tensilon) test, which involves administration of an anticholinesterase medication. This test can help distinguish between a myasthenic and a cholinergic crisis. The patient is given 2 mg of edrophonium intravenously. If the patient's symptoms improve, the diagnosis of myasthenia gravis is confirmed. If symptoms become worse, a cholinergic crisis should be suspected. Because of the potential for respiratory arrest, atropine must be available as an antidote. Other findings that support the diagnosis of myasthenia gravis include the detection of acetylcholine-receptor antibodies in the patient's serum and the detection of thymomas by chest CT scans. Treatment is accomplished with the use of anticholinesterase medications (e.g., pyridostigmine, neostigmine), thymectomy, corticosteroids, immunosuppressive agents, and plasmapheresis.

Kasper DL, Braunwald E, Fauci AS, et al., eds. *Harrison's principles of internal medicine,* 16th ed. New York: McGraw-Hill; 2005:2518.

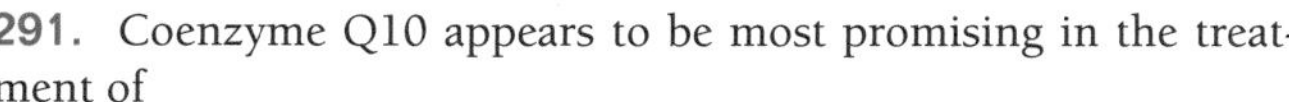

291. Coenzyme Q10 appears to be most promising in the treatment of

A) Parkinson's disease
B) diabetes mellitus
C) congestive heart failure
D) hyperthyroidism

Answer and Discussion

The answer is A. Coenzyme Q10 is a supplement used in the treatment of a variety of medical conditions primarily related to low cellular energy metabolism and oxidative injury. Coenzyme Q10 appears most promising for neurodegenerative disorders such as Parkinson's disease and certain encephalomyopathies for which coenzyme Q10 has been used. Results in other areas of research, including treatment of congestive heart failure and diabetes, appear to be contradictory or need further clarification before proceeding with recommendations. Coenzyme Q10 appears to be a safe supplement with minimal side effects (e.g., gastrointestinal) and low drug interaction potential.

Shults CW, Oakes D, Kieburtz K, et al. Effects of coenzyme Q10 in early Parkinson disease: evidence of slowing of the functional decline. *Arch Neurol.* 2002;59:1541–1550.

292. A 60-year-old woman presents with complaints of diffuse proximal muscle pain, low-grade fevers, and generalized fatigue. Laboratory findings include an elevated ESR and mild anemia. The most likely diagnosis is

A) influenza
B) dermatomyositis
C) polymyalgia rheumatica
D) systemic lupus erythematosis
E) rheumatoid arthritis

Answer and Discussion

The answer is C. Polymyalgia rheumatica is an inflammatory disease characterized by pain and stiffness associated with the proximal muscle groups. The condition is more common in women and usually occurs in patients older than 50 years. As many as 25% of patients may have associated giant cell arteritis, which can lead to blindness if not treated immediately with steroids. Symptoms include symmetric pain and morning stiffness associated with the proximal muscles such as the neck, shoulders, and hips. Patients may also report fever, generalized fatigue, anorexia, and weight loss. Laboratory findings include an elevated ESR (usually >50 mm/hour and often >100 mm/hour) and anemia of chronic disease. The physical examination is unremarkable with no evidence of synovitis or true muscle weakness. Diagnosis is made based on the clinical findings and confirmed with response to therapy. Treatment involves the use of orally administered corticosteroids (prednisone 10 to 20 mg/day); usually the patient responds immediately. Once the ESR returns to normal and the patient's symptoms are improved, the steroids may be slowly tapered. In some cases, it may take months to years to completely taper the medication.

Ferri F. *Ferri's Clinical Advisor, Instant Diagnosis and Treatment.* Philadelphia: Elsevier/Mosby; 2006:668.

293. Which of the following statements best describes the rash associated with Rocky Mountain spotted fever?

A) It usually develops first on the extremities and spreads centrally.
B) It usually develops first on the trunk and spreads to the extremities.
C) It typically affects only the face.
D) It appears as bull's-eye lesions with central clearing.
E) The lesions are erythematous, raised papules that are intensely pruritic.

Answer and Discussion

The answer is A. The causative agent of Rocky Mountain spotted fever is *Rickettsia rickettsii,* which is transmitted by the bite of the wood tick. The disease is usually found in the southern United States and is more commonly seen during the summer months. Symptoms include a flu-like prodrome that is followed by fevers, headaches, generalized myalgias, and, occasionally, delirium, seizures, and coma. In most cases, a rash develops on the wrist and ankles, sparing the face, and spreads centrally after the first few days of the fever. The rash, initially erythematous and macular, often becomes petechial. Laboratory findings include anemia, thrombocytopenia, leukocytopenia, proteinuria, and hematuria. Treatment involves the use of doxycycline, tetracycline, chloramphenicol, or rifampin. Mortality rates for the elderly can approach 70%, whereas mortality rates for children are less than 20%.

Kasper DL, Braunwald E, Fauci AS, et al., eds. *Harrison's principles of internal medicine,* 16th ed. New York: McGraw-Hill; 2005:999.

> In most cases of Rocky Mountain Spotted Fever, a rash develops on the wrist and ankles, sparing the face, and spreads centrally after the first few days of the fever. The rash, initially erythematous and macular, often becomes petechial.

294. Which of the following is associated with pseudogout?

A) Calcium pyrophosphate crystal deposition in the large joints
B) Lack of response with the use of colchicine
C) High uric acid levels
D) Lack of response with the use of anti-inflammatory medication
E) Negative birefringence seen with polarized microscopy

Answer and Discussion

The answer is A. Pseudogout is a condition that results from the deposition of calcium pyrophosphate crystals in the large joints (principally the knees) and leads to a reactive synovitis. Affected patients are usually older than 60 years. Men and women are affected equally, except in some studies that show women are more affected than men. Pseudogout is associated with trauma, surgery, amyloidosis, hemochromatosis, and hyperparathyroidism. Diagnosis is made by joint aspiration and examination of the fluid under a polarized microscope. Calcium pyrophosphate exhibits a positive birefringence in contrast to a negative birefringence seen with urate crystals in gout. Laboratory tests do not show elevated uric acid levels. Radiographs of the affected joints usually show degenerative changes and calcification of the surrounding cartilaginous structures. Treatment involves the use of anti-inflammatory agents and colchicine. Intra-articular steroid injection is occasionally helpful in resistant cases.

Chokkalingam S, Velazquez C, Mody A, et al. Diagnosing acute monoarthritis in adults: a practical approach for the family physician. *Am Fam Physician.* 2003;68:83–90.

295. Diabetic foot ulcers
A) are typically polymicrobial
B) rarely become infected
C) require topical antibiotics
D) should not be débrided because of the risk of bacteremia

Answer and Discussion

The answer is A. Foot ulcers in diabetic patients result from a diminished sensation associated with peripheral neuropathy and peripheral vascular disease (which is also usually present). Persistent pressure from ill-fitting shoes or skin cracking secondary to tinea pedis may predispose the patient's feet to infection. Diabetics who smoke should be encouraged to stop, and alcohol use should be discouraged. Infections associated with the feet are usually caused by *Staphylococcus, Streptococcus,* anaerobes, and gram-negative organisms. Aerobic and anaerobic cultures should be taken when signs of infection, such as purulence or inflammation, are present. Cultures are best taken from purulent drainage or curetted material from the ulcer base. Because all ulcers are contaminated, culture of noninfected wounds is generally not recommended. Polymicrobial infections predominate in severe diabetic foot infections and include a variety of aerobic gram-positive cocci, gram-negative rods, and anaerobes. Treatment involves débridement of nonvital and necrotic tissue, as well as oral or intravenous antibiotics. In severe cases, amputation may be necessary. Topical antibiotics are of little help and may delay healing. Osteomyelitis should always be considered in severe and persistent cases. Periodic examinations and treatment by a podiatrist are recommended.

Frykberg RG. Diabetic foot ulcers: pathogenesis and management. *Am Fam Physician.* 2002;66:1655–1662.

296. A 16-year-old girl presents to the office complaining of throat pain, difficulty swallowing, and trismus. Physical examination shows erythema and enlargement of the left tonsillar pillar. In addition, the patient holds her head to the left side and has muffled speech. The most likely diagnosis is
A) peritonsillar abscess
B) streptococcal pharyngitis
C) tonsillar cancer
D) epiglottitis
E) retropharyngeal abscess

Answer and Discussion

The answer is A. Peritonsillar abscess (also known as *quinsy*) is the most common ear, nose, and throat abscess. It is seen most commonly in teenagers and young adults and is rare in children under the age of 5 years. The condition occurs when an abscess develops between the tonsil and the superior constrictor muscle. Symptoms include worsening throat pain, muffled speech (hot-potato voice), trismus, and difficulty swallowing. The patient often holds his or her head toward the side that the abscess affects. If the abscess is large, airway compromise may occur. Ultrasound or CT scanning can help distinguish between cellulitis and abscess formation. Treatment of peritonsillar abscess is accomplished by lancing a fluctuant area, if present, with an 18-gauge needle (making certain not to go deeper than 1 cm where the internal carotid artery passes) and prescribing penicillin-containing antibiotics. The fluid should be cultured before initiation of antibiotics. Common infecting organisms include group A *Streptococcus* and anaerobes. Recurrent episodes necessitate tonsillectomy.

Ferri F. *Ferri's Clinical Advisor, Instant Diagnosis and Treatment.* Philadelphia: Elsevier/Mosby; 2006:978.

297. What is the threshold body mass index (BMI) for obesity?
A) 25
B) 27
C) 30
D) 35
E) 40

Answer and Discussion

The answer is C. The BMI is an approximate measure of body fat. It is based on height and weight. A BMI between 19 and 25 is considered normal. If a patient's BMI is 25 to 29.9, that individual is considered to be overweight. A person is categorized as obese if his or her BMI is 30 or higher.

Kasper DL, Braunwald E, Fauci AS, et al., eds. *Harrison's principles of internal medicine,* 16th ed. New York: McGraw-Hill; 2005:402, 422.

298. The mother of a 4-year-old calls to report that her child was bitten by a pet hamster. Which of the following is the appropriate management?
A) Human diploid cell vaccine
B) Rabies immune globulin
C) Reassurance to the mother with no further treatment
D) Immediate sacrifice of the hamster for pathologic evaluation
E) Hospitalization and close observation of the child for abnormal behavior

Answer and Discussion

The answer is C. Rabies is an infectious viral infection that is often transmitted by the bite of an infected animal or, rarely, by exposure of mucous membranes and saliva with a skin abrasion. The rabies virus affects the CNS, and the presence of intracytoplasmic Negri bodies seen microscopically is pathognomonic for the infection. Symptoms affecting humans include depression, difficulty with concentration, malaise, fever, extreme restlessness with excessive salivation, painful laryngeal and pharyngeal muscle spasms, and convulsions. Although patients often experience extreme thirst, they are hydrophobic, because drinking can often precipitate pharyngeal spasms. Death usually occurs secondary to exhaustion and asphyxia with generalized paralysis. The disease is usually found in wild animals such as skunks, foxes, coyotes, raccoons, bobcats, and bats, but is also seen in domestic dogs and cats. Other animals affected include livestock. Treatment of those bitten includes confining the animal that bit the patient for at least 10 days to look for abnormal behavior. If no changes are seen, the patient usually does not need treatment. Animals with abnormal behavior should be sacrificed and examined pathologically for rabies infection. If the animal cannot be caught or if the animal exhibits abnormal behavior and has evidence of rabies infection, the patient should be treated with human diploid cell vaccine or rabies vaccine, adsorbed: 1 mL administered intramuscularly at the time of presentation and then at days 3, 7, 14, and 28 for a total of five doses. Rabies vaccine (adsorbed) should not be given intradermally. Also, to bridge the gap of time it takes for the patient to develop antibodies to the rabies vaccine, 20 IU/kg of rabies immune globulin is given, with much of the dose administered at the site of the bite and the rest administered at a distant site from vaccine inoculation intramuscularly. In most cases, the wound should not be sutured. If rabies does develop, aggressive symptomatic treatment is required. The prognosis is not universally fatal, but there is significant mortality associated with rabies. Prophylaxis for rabies should be considered for high-risk populations such as veterinarians, animal handlers, technicians in laboratories in which rabies is present, and travelers spending a month or more in countries in which rabies is common. Bites of rodents such as squirrels, opossums, rats, mice, guinea pigs, gerbils, hamsters, rabbits, and hares rarely, if ever, require rabies prophylaxis.

Ferri F. *Ferri's Clinical Advisor, Instant Diagnosis and Treatment.* Philadelphia: Elsevier/Mosby; 2006:713.

299. A 65-year-old man complains of gynecomastia and galactorrhea with erectile dysfunction. The most likely diagnosis is
A) breast cancer
B) testicular cancer
C) prolactinoma
D) adrenal adenoma
E) diabetes mellitus

Answer and Discussion

The answer is C. Prolactinomas are the most common functioning, secreting pituitary tumors. Galactorrhea, oligomenorrhea, primary and secondary amenorrhea, and infertility are seen in women with prolactinomas. Men may experience impotence, infertility, and, less commonly, gynecomastia and/or galactorrhea. Prolactin levels >300 μg/L usually indicate a pituitary adenoma. Patients with hypogonadism, impotence, or galactorrhea may have abnormal prolactin levels associated with prolactinomas. Some medications, including oral contraceptives, phenothiazines, tricyclic antidepressants, antihypertensives (e.g., α-methyldopa), and opioid-type medications, may increase prolactin levels. Other causes for hyperprolactinemia include nipple stimulation, pregnancy, stress, sexual intercourse, sleep, hypoglycemia, hypothyroidism, sarcoidosis, paraneoplastic syndromes (bronchogenic carcinoma and hypernephroma), and chronic renal failure. Treatment (controversial) for larger tumors involves the use of bromocriptine (dopamine agonist), which lowers the serum prolactin level. If residual tumor remains, surgery or radiotherapy may be necessary. With small tumors, close observation may be instituted if the patient is asymptomatic.

Beers MH, Porter RS, eds. *The Merck manual of diagnosis and therapy,* Merck Research Laboratories, 18th ed. Whitehouse Station, NJ: Merck & Co.; 2006:1187–1189.

300. Which of the following statements about clonidine is true?
A) Rapid withdrawal may precipitate a hypertensive crisis.
B) It is classified as an ACE inhibitor.
C) Concomitant use with β-blockers decreases the risk of hypertensive crisis when both medications are discontinued.
D) The mechanism of action involves the increased release of renin and α-receptor activation.
E) Use of the drug can exacerbate restless legs syndrome.

Answer and Discussion

The answer is A. Clonidine is a second-line drug used in the treatment of hypertension, restless legs syndrome, nicotine withdrawal, prophylaxis for vascular headaches, and opiate withdrawal. Clonidine works by decreasing vascular resistance through α-receptor blockade and inhibiting renin release. Rapid withdrawal of the medication may precipitate a hypertensive crisis, which can be life threatening. Symptoms of hypertensive crisis include tachycardia, diaphoresis, headache, nervousness, and abdominal pain. Concomitant use with β-blockers may also increase the risk of hypertensive crisis when both medications are discontinued.

Beers MH, Porter RS, eds. *The Merck manual of diagnosis and therapy,* Merck Research Laboratories, 18th ed. Whitehouse Station, NJ: Merck & Co.; 2006:614, 1699.

301. A 62-year-old woman presents complaining of joint pain, polyuria, polydipsia, and generalized fatigue. The woman reports a history of recurrent kidney stones and depression. Radiographs show osteopenia and subperiosteal resorption on the phalanges. Which of the following blood tests may best help determine the cause of her symptoms?
A) ACE level
B) Parathyroid hormone level
C) Antinuclear antibody (ANA) test
D) Sedimentation rate (ESR)
E) Bone densitometry

Answer and Discussion

The answer is B. Primary hyperparathyroidism is a disorder caused by excessive secretion of parathyroid hormone. Findings include hypercalcemia (ionized), hypophosphatemia (hyperphosphatemia suggests secondary hyperparathyroidism), an excessive bone loss leading to cystic bone lesions, and osteitis fibrosa cystica. Most patients are asymptomatic; however, some may present with renal lithiasis, joint or back pain, polyuria and polydipsia, constipation, and fatigue. It is the most common cause of hypercalcemia in the general population. Familial cases are often related to endocrine tumors. The condition is more common in women and in patients older than 50 years. It also occurs in high frequency three or more decades after neck irradiation. It is usually caused by an adenoma of the parathyroid (90% of cases); carcinoma is rare (3% of cases). Radiographs may show subperiosteal resorption of the phalanges and osteopenia. Treatment usually involves surgical exploration and removal of parathyroid adenoma. For patients with mild, asymptomatic primary hyperparathyroidism the recommendations for surgery are controversial.

Beers MH, Porter RS, eds. *The Merck manual of diagnosis and therapy,* Merck Research Laboratories, 18th ed. Whitehouse Station, NJ: Merck & Co.; 2006:1254–1255.

302. The most common cause of chronic cough is
A) postnasal drip
B) bronchiectasis
C) gastroesophageal reflux
D) asthma
E) ACE inhibitors

Answer and Discussion

The answer is A. Coughing is part of the body's infection protective system and helps remove particles and material from the airway. In some cases, the patient may experience a chronic cough that can be attributed to a number of different problems, including postnasal drip (most common cause), gastroesophageal reflux, and bronchoconstriction as seen in cough-variant asthma patients. Other common associated conditions include the use of ACE inhibitors, chronic bronchitis seen in smokers, and bronchiectasis. Treatment involves eliminating the underlying cause. Treatment of conditions, such as asthma and COPD, may involve the use of bronchodilators (β agonist or theophylline), cromolyn sodium, and inhaled steroids; the treatment of postnasal drip may involve the use of antihistamines and topical nasal steroids. Patients should be informed that it may take 8 to 12 weeks before their cough improves when using inhaled steroids. Treatment of gastroesophageal reflux involves the use of antacids, H_2-receptor blockers, and proton pump inhibitors. Eliminating a cough caused by ACE inhibitors usually takes several days before improvement is seen. Unfortunately, it is more difficult to treat patients with chronic bronchitis. The use of antibiotics with the absence of supporting symptoms suggestive of infection is not useful and should be avoided. Mucolytics have not been shown to be beneficial.

Holmes RL, Fadden CT. Evaluation of the patient with chronic cough. *Am Fam Physician.* 2004;69:2159–2166, 2169.

303. A 26-year-old single man presents to your office complaining of a painless ulcer that formed on his penis approximately 3 months ago. The ulcer healed, but an erythematous rash on the palms and soles of his feet has recently developed. He also reports generalized fatigue, malaise, fever, headache, and arthralgias. The most likely diagnosis is

A) gonorrhea
B) chancroid
C) syphilis
D) Reiter's syndrome
E) Lyme disease

Answer and Discussion

The answer is C. Syphilis, also known as *lues,* is a disease caused by the spirochete *Treponema pallidum.* The disease is characterized by differing clinical stages that may affect multiple organ systems and is transmitted primarily by sexual contact. The usual incubation period is approximately 4 to 5 weeks. The following are the different stages associated with the disease:

- Primary syphilis is the initial stage of syphilis and is marked by the appearance of a chancre, which is a papule that ruptures and develops into a painless ulcer. In most cases, the ulcer heals in 4 to 6 weeks. Chancres occur on the penis; vulva; cervix; anus; and also the lips, tongue, oral mucosa, fingers, and other body parts. In addition to the ulcer, there may be associated lymphadenopathy but usually no other symptoms.
- Secondary syphilis is the second stage of syphilis and is characterized by cutaneous rashes that usually affect the volar surfaces of extremities, such as the palms of the hands and soles of the feet. They appear 6 to 12 weeks after the initial infection and are usually circular macules, papules, or pustules that are not pruritic. Other areas can be affected, and uveitis, periostitis, hepatitis, meningitis, and glomerulitis can occur. Additional symptoms include flu-like symptoms such as generalized fatigue, anorexia, malaise, fever, headache, anemia, lymphadenopathy, and arthralgias. Mucous membranes often become ulcerated and form circular ulcerated lesions. The secondary stage may last up to 1 year.
- Latent syphilis is characterized by the resolution of the rashes seen during the secondary stage and may last for many years after the initial infection. During this period, the patient is usually completely asymptomatic but has a positive treponemal antibody test.
- Late or tertiary syphilis occurs 10 or more years after the initial infection and is characterized by benign tertiary syphilis involving the skin and giving rise to gummas (granulomatous lesions that lead to fibrosis, necrosis, and scarring), cardiovascular syphilis (giving rise to thoracic aortic aneurysms and aortic insufficiency), and neurosyphilis (causing a multitude of neurologic disorders including headaches, insomnia, blurred vision, confusion, seizures, and decreased motor function with paralysis). Tabes dorsalis presents as symptoms and signs of demyelination of the posterior columns, dorsal roots, and dorsal root ganglia. Symptoms include an ataxic wide-based gait, paresthesias, bladder dysfunction, impotence, areflexia, and loss of pain, temperature, and position sensation.

Screening tests for syphilis include a VDRL test and the rapid plasma reagin test. If positive, a confirming fluorescent treponemal antibody–absorption test should be performed. In addition, microscopic examination of fluid taken from lesions can be examined with darkfield microscopy to look for spirochetes. The treatment of choice is penicillin given in the long-acting benzathine form intramuscularly. In many cases, there is a reaction to treatment after 6 to 12 hours called the Jarisch-Herxheimer reaction; symptoms include fatigue, headaches, low-grade fever, sweating, and more severe reactions, including seizures in patients with neurologic involvement. It is important to distinguish these reactions from allergic reactions to penicillin. A repeated VDRL or rapid plasma reagin can be assessed to ensure adequate treatment. In most cases, they become negative 1 year after treatment. Sexual contacts should also be treated appropriately. Any patient suspected of having syphilis more than 1 year should have a CSF examination.

Kasper DL, Braunwald E, Fauci AS, et al., eds. *Harrison's principles of internal medicine,* 16th ed. New York: McGraw-Hill; 2005:977.

Screening tests for syphilis include a VDRL test and the rapid plasma reagin test. If positive, a confirming fluorescent treponemal antibody–absorption test should be performed.

304. An 18-year-old hiker presents with an erythematous, maculopapular rash that began on the palms and feet and now has spread to involve the trunk area. He complains of low back pain, fever, and headaches. Laboratory evaluation shows hyponatremia and thrombocytopenia. The most likely diagnosis is

A) Lyme disease
B) Rocky Mountain spotted fever
C) infectious mononucleosis
D) poison ivy
E) tularemia

Answer and Discussion

The answer is B. Rocky Mountain spotted fever is caused by *Rickettsia rickettsii* and is the most common rickettsial disease in the United States. The wood tick (*Dermacentor andersoni*) is the principal vector in the western United States, whereas the dog tick (*Dermacentor variabilis*) is the most common vector in the eastern and southern United States. Transmission from person to person is not thought to occur. The incidence of Rocky Mountain spotted fever is highest in children 5 to 9 years of age. A tick bite is recalled by only 50% to 70% of patients. The onset of symptoms of Rocky

Mountain spotted fever usually begins 5 to 7 days after inoculation. Common symptoms include generalized malaise, myalgias (especially in the back and leg muscles), fever, frontal headaches, nausea, and vomiting. Other symptoms may include nonproductive cough, sore throat, pleuritic chest pain, and abdominal pain. The classic presenting symptoms include sudden onset of headache, fever, and chills accompanied by an exanthem appearing within the first few days of symptoms. Initially, lesions appear on the palms, soles, wrists, ankles, and forearms. The lesions are pink and macular and fade with applied pressure. The rash then extends to the axilla, buttocks, trunk, neck, and face, becoming maculopapular and then petechial. The lesions may then coalesce to form large areas of ecchymosis and ulceration. Respiratory and circulatory failure, as well as neurologic compromise, may occur. Patients with glucose-6-phosphate dehydrogenase (G6PD) deficiency are at especially high risk for complications and poor outcomes. Diagnosis is based primarily on clinical signs and symptoms. If a rash is present, the use of skin biopsy and immunofluorescent staining for *Rickettsia* is highly specific, although with only slightly more than 60% sensitivity. Laboratory testing is of limited usefulness but may include thrombocytopenia and hyponatremia. Elevation of specific enzyme-linked immunosorbent assay (ELISA) and latex agglutination titers usually is delayed until the convalescence period. Fever and headache during peak months of tick exposure in endemic areas should suggest Rocky Mountain spotted fever. Rash, thrombocytopenia, and hyponatremia make immediate treatment imperative. Antimicrobial agents for the treatment of Rocky Mountain spotted fever include tetracycline, doxycycline (Vibramycin), and chloramphenicol (Chloromycetin) for a minimum of 7 days. Fluoroquinolones also may be effective, but are not recommended for routine use in patients with Rocky Mountain spotted fever because of a lack of evidence. For optimal effect, it is critical to treat patients early in the course of their illness. Treatment should not be delayed until laboratory confirmation is obtained.

Bratton RL, Corey GR. Tick-borne disease. *Am Fam Physician.* 2005;72:1057–1062.

305. A 16-year-old surfer presents with an erythematous, maculopapular rash that was noted in the area of his bathing suit. Initial treatment includes

A) cryotherapy
B) clotrimazole cream
C) ice packs
D) application of vinegar
E) zinc oxide

Answer and Discussion

The answer is D. Swimmers or surfers with seabather's eruption present with an urticarial maculopapular rash on areas of the body that were covered by the swimsuit. The rash may appear while the bather is in the water or up to 1.5 days later. The rash may last for 2 to 28 days; most reactions resolve within 1 to 2 weeks. Systemic symptoms include fever, nausea, vomiting, and headache and are more likely to affect children. Initial treatment involves the topical application of heat or vinegar. Further treatment is symptomatic and may include topical corticosteroids, oral antihistamines, and oral steroids. Twice-daily application of thiabendazole (Mintezol) can be beneficial. The swimsuit should be cleaned thoroughly because larvae can persist and re-envenomate.

Zoltan TB, Taylor KS, Achar SA. Health issues for surfers. *Am Fam Physician.* 2005;71:2313–2317.

306. Which of the following medications should generally be avoided in diabetic nephropathy?

A) Lisinopril
B) Nifedipine
C) Losartan
D) Terazocin
E) Hydrochlorothiazide

Answer and Discussion

The answer is B. Diabetic nephropathy is a complication of long-standing, poorly controlled diabetes. It is more commonly seen in patients with insulin-dependent diabetes or coexisting, poorly controlled hypertension. Almost all diabetic patients develop glomerulosclerosis, but only approximately 35% develop nephropathy. In most cases, these findings develop 15 to 20 years after the diagnosis of diabetes. Diabetic nephropathy is the most common cause of end-stage renal disease in the United States. Diagnosis is made by the detection of proteinuria, decreased creatinine clearance, and, in some cases, the development of hypertension. ACE inhibitors (e.g., lisinopril, enalapril) and angiotensinreceptor blockers (ARBs) such as losartan and candesartan have been shown to be beneficial (renoprotective) for patients with diabetes. Dietary measures, including the restriction of protein, sodium, phosphorous, and potassium, may be necessary if the creatinine clearance is <20 mL/minute. In severe cases, dialysis may be instituted.

American Diabetes Association. Standards of medical care in diabetes. *Diabetes Care.* 2004;27(suppl 1): S15–S35.

307. Which of the following conditions is NOT associated with smoking?

A) Peptic ulcer disease
B) Depression
C) Children of smokers are at increased risk for otitis media
D) Osteoporosis
E) Cervical cancer

Answer and Discussion

The answer is B. Smoking is the largest single health risk in the United States and other developed countries. Smokers are at significant risk for multiple lung diseases, particularly lung cancer. Other cancers that occur more frequently in smokers include laryngeal cancer, pancreatic cancer, cervical cancer, bladder cancer, and leukemia. Other diseases linked with smoking include coronary atherosclerosis, peptic ulcer disease, and osteoporosis. In addition, smoking increases free fatty acids, very-low-density lipoprotein cholesterol, and serum glucose. Smoking decreases HDL cholesterol. Children of parents who smoke tend to have more respiratory illnesses, including otitis media, and are more likely to smoke than children of nonsmoking parents. Secondhand smoke has been declared harmful and can increase the risk of lung cancer. Therefore, at each office visit, physicians should strongly encourage patients who smoke to stop.

Beers MH, Porter RS, eds. *The Merck manual of diagnosis and therapy,* Merck Research Laboratories, 18th ed. Whitehouse Station, NJ: Merck & Co.; 2006:2733–2736.

308. Which of the following infections causes tabes dorsalis?

A) Gonorrhea
B) Tuberculosis
C) Syphilis

D) Bacterial meningitis
E) ALS

Answer and Discussion

The answer is C. Tabes dorsalis is the result of syphilitic lesions that affect the posterior columns of the spinal cord. Symptoms include the insidious onset of pain, loss of sensation, proprioception and vibratory sense, loss of reflexes, and ataxia. The main symptom is an insidious, sharp, stabbing pain that is periodic and recurrent and affects the lower extremities. Over time, the patient may experience increasing difficulty with gait, particularly in poorly illuminated areas. Paresthesias and loss of sensation are commonly associated with the soles of the feet. Other findings include a thin appearance with sad- or depressed-appearing facies, Argyll Robertson pupils (react poorly to light but well to accommodation), positive Romberg's sign, loss of reflexes in the lower extremities, bladder disturbances, and visible ataxia. Acute abdominal pain with vomiting (visceral crisis) can occur in 15% to 30%. In tabes dorsalis, the rapid plasma reagin and VDRL tests may not be positive; however, the fluorescent treponemal antibody absorption test is usually positive. Treatment involves the administration of a prolonged course of high-dose penicillin to treat syphilis. Pain medications along with chlorpromazine and carbamazepine may be helpful for the control of pain. Unfortunately, tabes dorsalis often progresses despite treatment.

Kasper DL, Braunwald E, Fauci AS, et al., eds. *Harrison's principles of internal medicine,* 16th ed. New York: McGraw-Hill; 2005:83, 980, 2446.

309. A 21-year-old otherwise healthy woman is seen in your office with a recent purified protein derivative tuberculin skin test that is positive. The woman has never had a positive test before. A chest radiograph is negative, and there are no signs of disease. The most appropriate treatment is

A) reassurance
B) isoniazid (INH) and rifampin for 6 months
C) INH for 6 months
D) INH, rifampin, and streptomycin (or ethambutol) for 12 months
E) streptomycin for 6 months

Answer and Discussion

The answer is C. Tuberculosis is caused by *Mycobacterium tuberculosis*, a nonmotile acid-fast rod that is spread primarily by inhalation. The organism can affect many different systems but usually affects the lungs. There has been a recent increase in incidence, particularly in the immunocompromised and elderly populations. Symptoms include fever, fatigue, weight loss, a productive cough, dyspnea, and, occasionally, hemoptysis. Diagnosis is usually accomplished with a chest radiograph, which shows apical infiltrates and mediastinal lymphadenopathy, and microscopic examination of sputum, which shows acid-fast rods. A definitive diagnosis is achieved with a culture of early morning sputum growing *M. tuberculosis.* A Mantoux tuberculin skin test using purified protein derivative injected intradermally is also used to support the diagnosis. In most cases, an area of induration >10 mm (with risk factors), 15 mm (without risk factors), or 5 mm (in HIV patients) 48 hours after administration is a positive response. A negative response does not exclude the diagnosis. A calcified focus of infection seen on chest radiograph is referred to as a *Ghon complex.*

Treatment for active disease is accomplished with INH, rifampin, and pyrazinamide. In some cases, a fourth drug (e.g., streptomycin or ethambutol) is necessary. Most treatment regimens require extended courses lasting at least 6 to 9 months. Patients younger than 35 years who have a positive skin test but no evidence of disease (including a negative chest radiograph) are usually treated with INH for 6 to 9 months. Immunocompromised patients may require longer treatment times. Older patients are at risk for INH's side effects, including liver toxicity, and are generally not given prophylactic therapy. In addition, compliance is a critical factor in ensuring adequate treatment, particularly for the elderly. Other sites affected by tuberculosis include the kidneys, pericardium, and spine. All patients with a new diagnosis of tuberculosis should be tested for HIV (and vice versa).

Jerant AF, Bannon M, Rittenhouse S. Identification and management of tuberculosis. *Am Fam Physician.* 2000;61:2667–2678, 2681–2682.

310. A 32-year-old woman reports frequent bouts of constipation alternating with diarrhea. She frequently experiences abdominal discomfort, which is relieved with bowel movements. Stress tends to aggravate her symptoms. The most appropriate treatment includes

A) steroid enemas
B) mesalamine enemas
C) fiber supplement
D) metoclopramide
E) none of the above

Answer and Discussion

The answer is C. Irritable bowel syndrome is characterized by bouts of recurrent and intermittent diarrhea and constipation that tend to be aggravated by stress or anxiety. It begins before 50 years of age (median age is 35 years) and affects women more frequently than men. Symptoms include abdominal pain and distention that are relieved with bowel movements, which are often mixed with mucus, bloating, nausea, flatulence, the sensation of incomplete voiding, and, occasionally, pelvic or back pain. The diagnosis is made by excluding organic causes for the symptoms. The workup includes stool cultures, examination of stool for occult blood, CBC, flexible sigmoidoscopy, and barium enema, all of which are found to be normal. Colonoscopy is usually unnecessary, unless other studies are abnormal. Treatment involves stress reduction, reassurance to the patient, and maintenance of a high-fiber diet that avoids triggering foods. Fiber supplements, such as psyllium (Metamucil), are often helpful. Antidiarrheal medication and antispasmodics may be necessary in some patients. Irritable bowel syndrome is a benign disease that has no anatomic abnormality or inflammatory component. Symptoms associated with organic disease that are not associated with irritable bowel syndrome include abdominal pain that interrupts sleep, nocturnal diarrhea, visible or occult blood found in the stool, fever, and weight loss.

Kasper DL, Braunwald E, Fauci AS, et al., eds. *Harrison's principles of internal medicine,* 16th ed. New York: McGraw-Hill; 2005:1789.

311. Which of the following statements about treadmill exercise testing is true?

A) Women have a low incidence of false-positive results.
B) It is recommended for patients who experience angina at rest to document ECG changes.
C) It is contraindicated in patients with moderate to severe aortic stenosis.

D) The appearance of a bundle branch block on ECG represents no concern.
E) A positive result requires >3 mm of ST-segment depression.

Answer and Discussion

The answer is C. Exercise stress testing is used to evaluate chest pain in patients with suspected cardiovascular disease. The sensitivity ranges from 56% to 81%, and the specificity ranges from 72% to 96%. With this in mind, the exercise stress test has relatively low sensitivity and specificity. Because of this, a patient with a high pretest likelihood of ischemic heart disease still has a high probability of developing significant disease even in the face of a normal (negative test). Furthermore, a patient with a low probability of ischemic heart disease still has a low chance of significant disease even if the test is positive. The optimal use of diagnostic testing is for those patients with moderate pretest probabilities. Women tend to have a higher incidence of false-positive results. There are two basic protocols: the Bruce protocol and the Ellestad protocol. In the standard exercise stress test (Bruce protocol), the patient is asked to exercise for 3-minute intervals on a motorized treadmill device while being monitored for the following: heart rate and blood pressure response to exercise, symptoms during the test, ECG response (specifically ST segment displacement), dysrhythmias, and exercise capacity. A positive test is defined as a ST segment depression of at least 1 mm below baseline. Contraindications to exercise stress testing include the following:

- Recent myocardial infarction within the preceding 4 to 6 weeks [except for a submaximal exercise stress test (65% of predicted maximum heart rate) that is often performed before hospital discharge for patients with a recent myocardial infarction]
- Angina at rest
- Rapid ventricular or atrial arrhythmias
- High-grade AV block or bradyarrhythmias
- Uncompensated CHF
- Recent acute illness (noncardiac in origin)
- Moderate to severe aortic stenosis
- Uncontrolled blood pressure (systolic >200 or diastolic >110 mm Hg before onset of exercise)
- Active myocarditis/pericarditis
- Acute pulmonary embolism
- Systemic illness
- Noncompliant patient

Criteria for stopping an exercise stress test include:

- Predicted heart rate is achieved
- Patient complains of excessive fatigue, claudication, or dyspnea
- PVCs that increase in frequency or ventricular tachycardia
- High-grade AV block appears on ECG
- Significant ST changes seen on ECG (>3 mm depression)
- Severe angina
- Systolic blood pressure >220 or diastolic blood pressure >120 during exercise or a decrease in systolic blood pressure with exercise
- Appearance of a bundle branch block
- Equipment malfunction or technical failure

The following are considered to be parameters associated with poor prognosis or increased disease severity: failure to complete stage 2 of a Bruce protocol, failure to achieve a heart rate >120 bpm (off β-blockers), onset of ST-segment depression at a heart rate of <120 bpm, ST-segment depression more than 2 mm, ST-segment depression lasting >6 minutes into recovery, ST-segment depression in multiple leads, poor systolic blood pressure response to exercise, ST-segment elevation, angina with exercise, and exercise-induced ventricular tachycardia.

Beers MH, Porter RS, eds. *The Merck manual of diagnosis and therapy,* Merck Research Laboratories, 18th ed. Whitehouse Station, NJ: Merck & Co.; 2006:602.

Lee TH, Boucher CA, Noninvasive tests in patients with stable coronary artery disease. *N Engl J Med.* 2001;344:1840–1845.

312. Anemia of chronic disease is associated with which of the following?
A) Macrocytic, normochromic anemia
B) Increased serum ferritin
C) Increased TIBC
D) High serum iron level
E) Hemoglobin of 5 to 8 mg/dL

Answer and Discussion

The answer is B. Anemia of chronic disease can be caused by

- Chronic infections, such as osteomyelitis and subacute bacterial endocarditis
- Chronic disorders, including rheumatoid arthritis, lupus, renal failure, sarcoidosis, and polymyalgia rheumatica
- Other disorders, including neoplasm, liver disorders, and hypothyroidism

Symptoms include typical complaints associated with anemia such as generalized fatigue, malaise, decreased mentation, and those symptoms associated with the primary disorder. Laboratory tests show a mild, normocytic normochromic anemia with an Hb at approximately 10 mg/dL. Microcytic indices are also possible. Serum ferritin is also usually increased, with a low TIBC and low serum-iron level. The only therapy is treatment of the underlying disorder. The administration of iron, folic acid, or vitamin B_{12} is ineffective. Transfusion should only be considered in advanced cases in patients with severe symptoms.

Kasper DL, Braunwald E, Fauci AS, et al., eds. *Harrison's principles of internal medicine,* 16th ed. New York: McGraw-Hill; 2005:334.

313. Which of the following would be best in the short- and long-term treatment of back pain?
A) Regular physical activity
B) Back supports
C) Work site modification
D) Back education school

Answer and Discussion

The answer is A. U.S. Preventive Services Task Force (USPSTF) recommendations on low back pain include the following: Although exercise has not been shown to prevent low back pain, regular physical activity has other proven health benefits, including prevention of cardiovascular disease, hypertension, type 2 diabetes, obesity, and osteoporosis. Neither lumbar supports nor back belts appear to be effective in reducing the incidence of low back pain. Work site modifications, including educational interventions, have some short-term benefit in reducing the incidence of low back pain. However, their applicability to the primary care setting is unknown. Back (educational) schools may prevent further back injury for persons with recurrent or chronic low back pain, but their long-term effectiveness has not been well studied.

Krishnaraj R. Primary care interventions to prevent low back pain: a brief evidence update for the U.S. Preventive Services Task Force. Agency for Healthcare Research and Quality, 2003. Accessed online September 17, 2005, at: http://www.ahrq.gov/clinic/uspstf/uspsback.htm.

Neither lumbar supports nor back belts appear to be effective in reducing the incidence of low back pain.

314. A 75-year-old presents with a painful erythematous and vesicular rash that is developing on the forehead in the periorbital area. The rash began yesterday. The patient has had some generalized myalgias and low-grade fevers. Appropriate management at this time includes

A) antiviral medication and follow up in 3 to 5 days
B) antibiotics plus antiviral medications and follow up in 3 to 5 days
C) reassurance
D) hospitalization with IV antibiotics
E) antiviral medication and ophthalmology referral

Answer and Discussion

The answer is E. The most common complication of herpes zoster is postherpetic neuralgia (i.e., pain along cutaneous, dermatomal nerves persisting >30 days after the lesions have healed). The incidence of postherpetic neuralgia increases with age and is not commonly seen in patients younger than 60 years. Herpes zoster lesions can become secondarily infected with staphylococci or streptococci, and cellulitis may develop. Herpes zoster involving the ophthalmic division of the trigeminal nerve can lead to ocular complications and visual loss. In these cases immediate referral to an ophthalmologist is recommended. Other less common complications include motor paresis and encephalitis.

Mouncey AL, Matthew LG, Slawson DC. Herpes zoster and postherpetic neuralgia: prevention and management. *Am Fam Physician.* 2005;72:1075–1080.

315. Addison's disease (primary adrenal insufficiency) is associated with

A) increased adrenocorticotropic hormone (ACTH) production
B) decreased ACTH production
C) increased urine 17-hydroxysteroids and 17-ketosteroids
D) hypernatremia
E) hypothalamic dysfunction

Answer and Discussion

The answer is A. Primary adrenal insufficiency (Addison's disease) is a condition resulting from adrenocortical insufficiency. Secondary adrenal insufficiency is secondary to a lack of ACTH production from the pituitary gland. The primary disease results in electrolyte disturbances, such as hyponatremia, hyperkalemia, low bicarbonate, and elevated BUN. The plasma renin and ACTH are increased with primary adrenal insufficiency. Other laboratory findings include moderate neutropenia, lymphocytosis, eosinophilia, low plasma cortisol, decreased urine 17-hydroxysteroids, and decreased 17-ketosteroids. There is also a failure of plasma cortisol to rise after administration of ACTH (corticotropin). Symptoms include weakness, fatigue, anorexia with nausea, vomiting, and diarrhea. Physical findings include hypoglycemia; sparse axillary hair; and increased pigmentation of the gingival mucosa, nipples, labia, and linea alba. Treatment involves the replacement of glucocorticoids and mineralocorticoids. Symptoms of adrenal crisis include severe abdominal pain, generalized muscle weakness, hypotension, and shock. Severe cases may result in death.

Beers MH, Porter RS, eds. *The Merck manual of diagnosis and therapy,* Merck Research Laboratories, 18th ed. Whitehouse Station, NJ: Merck & Co.; 2006:1207–1210.

316. Which of the following tests is the most appropriate to diagnose carbon monoxide poisoning?

A) Arterial blood gas
B) Chest radiograph
C) Carboxyhemoglobin levels
D) CBC
E) Lactic acid levels

Answer and Discussion

The answer is C. Carbon monoxide poisoning is a dangerous but relatively common occurrence. It usually occurs during the winter months in cold regions of the United States. The affinity of CO for hemoglobin is 240 times greater than that of oxygen; it shifts the oxygen dissociation curve to the left, which impairs hemoglobin release of oxygen to tissues and inhibits the cytochrome oxidase system. Symptoms include headache, confusion, fatigue, and nausea; in more severe cases, seizures, rhabdomyolysis, Parkinsonian-type symptoms, coma, and death may occur. In many cases, the initial symptoms are attributed to a flu-like illness, and CO poisoning is overlooked. The diagnosis is usually made by obtaining a history of exposure (usually a fuel oil furnace or exhaust fumes in a poorly ventilated enclosure) and laboratory testing, which shows elevated carboxyhemoglobin levels. Treatment involves the use of 100% oxygen and, in severe cases, hyperbaric oxygen. Prolonged exposures usually have a worse prognosis. Patients with CO poisoning necessitating treatment need follow-up neuropsychiatric examinations.

Kasper DL, Braunwald E, Fauci AS, et al., eds. *Harrison's principles of internal medicine,* 16th ed. New York: McGraw-Hill; 2005:1634–1635.

317. Barrett's esophagus is associated with

A) overuse of proton pump inhibitors
B) tracheoesophageal fistula
C) trauma associated with prior esophagogastroduodenoscopy
D) transformation of columnar epithelium to squamous epithelium
E) adenocarcinoma of the esophagus

Answer and Discussion

The answer is E. Barrett's esophagus is the result of chronic gastroesophageal reflux. The condition causes metaplasia and transformation of squamous to columnar epithelium in the areas affected. Patients usually report symptoms of pyrosis and, occasionally, dysphagia if strictures develop. Men are more commonly affected than women. The diagnosis is made with esophagoscopy and biopsy of suspected areas. Treatment is accomplished with H_2-blockers and proton pump inhibitors. Proton pump inhibitors strongly inhibit gastric acid secretion. They act by irreversibly inhibiting the H^+–K^+ adenosine triphosphatase pump of the parietal cell. By blocking the final common pathway of gastric acid secretion, the proton pump inhibitors provide a greater degree and duration of gastric acid suppression compared with H_2-receptor blockers. Clinical trials have clearly shown that the proton pump inhibitors provide better symptom control, esophageal healing, and maintenance of remission than H_2-receptor blockers or prokinetic agents. Long-term use of proton pump inhibitors in humans has not been associated with an increased risk of gastric carcinoma, although this was initially a concern. Prolonged use of the drugs has been associated with gastric atrophy; however, atrophy is more likely to be a problem in patients infected with *H. pylori*. The proton pump inhibitors are fairly well tolerated. The most common side effects are nausea, diarrhea, constipation, headache, and skin rash. Proton pump inhibitors are more expensive than standard-dose H_2-receptor blockers or prokinetic agents. However, when prescribed appropriately to patients with severe symptoms or refractory disease, the proton pump inhibitors are more cost-effective because of their higher healing and remission rates and the consequent prevention of complications. Occasionally, severe cases of Barrett's esophagitis are treated with surgery. Because of a 10% increased risk for the development of adenocarcinoma in the affected areas, follow-up with endoscopy every 3 to 5 years is indicated, although screening endoscopy time frames are controversial. Treatment of gastroesophageal reflux disease associated with Barrett's esophagus has not been shown to eliminate the metaplasia of that condition or the risk of malignancy. Consequently, patients with Barrett's esophagus require periodic endoscopic biopsy to assess esophageal tissue for malignant changes.

Shalauta MD, Saad R. Barrett's esophagus. *Am Fam Physician.* 2004;69:2113–2118, 2120.

318. Type I diabetes mellitus is associated with

A) hypersensitivity to glucose
B) overproduction of glucagon
C) lack of insulin production by the pancreas
D) tissue resistance to insulin
E) excessive growth hormone secretion

Answer and Discussion

The answer is C. Diabetes mellitus type I (juvenile diabetes) tends to occur in individuals younger than 30 years. The cause is complete failure of the beta islet cells in the pancreas to produce insulin. A genetic predisposition and perhaps a viral or autoimmune reaction that destroys the insulin-producing beta cells are believed to be the cause. The incidence among school children is reported to be 1 in 500. Symptoms include polydipsia, polyphagia, polyuria, dry mouth, nausea, vomiting and abdominal pain, weight loss, and fatigue. In severe cases, the patient may present in diabetic ketoacidosis with stupor, coma, dehydration, labored Kussmaul-type respirations, abdominal distention, and pain. The treatment is aggressive fluid and electrolyte replacement along with exogenous insulin administration. Diabetic complications include retinopathy, nephropathy, macrovascular disease, and diabetic foot ulcers. Judicious control of glucose may help to prevent these complications. Typically, patients require 0.5 to 1.0 U/kg/day of insulin. This daily dose is divided as follows:

- *Morning dose.* Two-thirds of the total daily dose is administered in the morning. The morning dose is composed of two-thirds intermediate-acting insulin and one-third short-acting regular insulin.
- *Evening dose.* One-third of the total daily dose is administered in the evening; 50% is short-acting regular insulin, which the patient takes before the evening meal, and 50% is intermediate-acting insulin, which the patient takes at bedtime.

Kasper DL, Braunwald E, Fauci AS, et al., eds. *Harrison's principles of internal medicine,* 16th ed. New York: McGraw-Hill; 2005:2174.

319. Which of the following is a common ophthalmologic finding in patients with HIV infection?

A) Retinal tears
B) Cataracts
C) Retinitis
D) Glaucoma
E) Conjunctivitis

Answer and Discussion

The answer is C. HIV syndrome can affect many different organ systems. Ophthalmologic findings include toxoplasmic and cytomegalovirus retinitis, herpes infections, syphilis, and pneumocystic infections of the eye. The most common ophthalmologic finding is cotton-wool spots caused by retinal ischemia secondary to microvascular disease. All patients with HIV should undergo complete eye examinations to rule out associated conditions.

Kasper DL, Braunwald E, Fauci AS, et al., eds. *Harrison's principles of internal medicine,* 16th ed. New York: McGraw-Hill; 2005:1119.

320. Which of the following statements is true regarding insulin injections?

A) Absorption from the buttock is rapid and can be used as a site just before eating.
B) Rotation of injections to different zones of the body can cause wide variations in serum glucose levels.
C) Injection in the arm often leads to exercise-induced hypoglycemia.
D) The thigh is the best site for reliable and predictable absorption.

Answer and Discussion

The answer is B. The abdomen is the best site for insulin administration, because the insulin is more reliably and predictably absorbed. Injection in exercised areas (e.g., the thigh) may lead to development of exercise-induced hypoglycemia. However, insulin injection at the arm does not cause as much exercise-induced hypoglycemia and thus can be used as an alternative injection site. Absorption from the buttocks is the slowest and is a good site to use at bedtime to avoid nocturnal hypoglycemia. Rotation of injection sites can lead to erratic absorption of insulin with wide variations in serum glucose levels. Thus, injection sites should remain within the same zone (abdomen, arm, or buttock) but rotated at different sites within the zones to prevent lipohypertrophy.

Green GB, Harris IS, et al. *The Washington Manual of Medical Therapeutics,* 31st ed. Lippincott Williams & Wilkins; 2004:474.

321. The treatment of choice for adult respiratory distress syndrome (ARDS) is

A) loop diuretics
B) corticosteroids
C) positive end-expiratory pressure

D) β2 agonist
E) high-dose immunosuppressive drugs

Answer and Discussion

The answer is C. Acute Respiratory Distress Syndrome (ARDS) is characterized by respiratory distress that may be caused by different insults, including trauma, near-drowning, aspiration, pneumonia, sepsis, and multiple blood transfusions. The predominate medical risk factor for ARDS is sepsis, particularly from an abdominal source. The mechanism of injury involves damage of capillary endothelial cells and alveolar epithelial cells, which leads to pulmonary edema with decreased pulmonary compliance and decreased functional residual capacity. Symptoms include rapid onset of dyspnea usually 12 to 48 hours after the insult, with wheezing and intercostal retractions. Laboratory tests show hypoxemia that responds poorly to oxygen administration, requiring frequent monitoring of arterial blood gases. Radiographs show diffuse or patchy alveolar and interstitial infiltrates without cardiomegaly or pulmonary vascular redistribution. Treatment involves mechanical ventilation with the use of low volume ventilation with positive end-expiratory pressure (PEEP). Fluids should be minimized. Patients are usually paralyzed with pancuronium. Antibiotics are unnecessary, but nosocomial infections may develop. Most patients with the development of ARDS also have multiple organ failure, which is the major cause of death. Mortality rates approach 50%.

Mortelliti MP, Manning HL. Acute respiratory distress syndrome. *Am Fam Physician.* 2002;65:1823–1830.

The predominate medical risk factor for ARDS is sepsis, particularly from an abdominal source.

322. Which of the following is associated with rebound hypertension?
A) Oral contraceptives
B) Hyperthyroidism
C) Excessive alcohol consumption
D) Abrupt withdrawal of β-blockers
E) Pheochromocytoma

Answer and Discussion

The answer is D. Causes for secondary hypertension are numerous and include the use of oral contraceptives, excessive alcohol consumption, disorders of the renal parenchyma associated with malfunction of the renin-aldosterone system, Cushing's syndrome, pheochromocytoma, primary aldosteronism, hyperthyroidism, myxedema, renal vascular disease, and coarctation of the aorta. In many cases, blood pressure may be difficult to control. Physical examination may reveal abdominal bruits, suggestive of renovascular hypertension, or other findings suggestive of contributing disease. Adequate treatment is necessary to prevent the long-term detrimental effects of hypertension. Abrupt discontinuation of β blockers is associated with rebound hypertension.

Seventh Report of the Joint National Committee on Prevention, Detection, Evaluation and Treatment of High Blood Pressure (JNC 7) Express. National Heart, Lung, and Blood Institute. Bethesda, Md. 2003. *JAMA.* 2003;289:2560–2571.

323. A 27-year-old patient with asthma presents to your office complaining of shortness of breath with wheezing. Which of the following medications is indicated in the initial treatment of this patient?
A) Salmeterol
B) Albuterol
C) Cromolyn sodium
D) Ipratropium bromide
E) Theophylline

Answer and Discussion

The answer is B. Asthma is a reversible obstructive lung disorder that is characterized by reactive airways. The condition is thought to be inherited; however, some individuals may be affected without a family history. Many factors may precipitate an attack, including infections, smoke, cold weather, exercise, toxic fumes, and stress. Symptoms include wheezing, shortness of breath, tachypnea, cough (particularly in children), and tightness or pressure in the chest. The mainstay of acute treatment (rescue therapy) is an inhalant form of a β2-adrenergic agonist, such as albuterol. Inhaled corticosteroids and salmeterol (a long-acting β2-adrenergic agonist) are used in chronic therapy. For patients who have more severe asthmatic attacks, short courses of oral corticosteroids may be necessary, particularly with upper respiratory infections. Theophylline, once readily prescribed, is used less frequently, and its benefits are controversial. Cromolyn sodium, a mast cell stabilizer, and ipratropium bromide, an anticholinergic medication, and the leukotriene modifiers can be used for chronic asthmatic conditions. Pulmonary function tests in patients affected with asthma usually show a normal or decreased vital capacity, decreased forced expiratory volume in 1 second, increased residual volume, increased total lung capacity, and a positive response to inhaled bronchodilators. In children, rescue β2-adrenergic agonists are the treatment of choice for mild intermittent asthma.

Beers MH, Porter RS, eds. *The Merck manual of diagnosis and therapy,* Merck Research Laboratories, 18th ed. Whitehouse Station, NJ: Merck & Co.; 2006:381–398.

324. A 22-year-old sexually active female presents with a 24-hour history of dysuria. She is otherwise healthy and has no other symptoms. Appropriate management includes
A) urine culture followed by antibiotics until culture result is determined
B) dipstick urinalysis followed by antibiotic coverage if positive
C) continued observation
D) midstream urinalysis followed by microscopic evaluation and treatment if positive

Answer and Discussion

The answer is B. Sexually active young women are at an increased risk to develop urinary tract infections. Their likelihood to develop UTIs is related to their anatomy (short urethra) and certain behavioral factors, including delays in micturition, sexual activity, and the use of diaphragms and spermicides (both of which increase the colonization of the periurethral area with coliform bacteria). Most UTIs in this group are uncomplicated and are rarely associated with functional or anatomic abnormalities. Extensive diagnostic work-ups are not necessary in young women presenting with an uncomplicated episode of cystitis. The diagnosis of UTI was once based on a quantitative urine culture yielding > 100,000 colony-forming units (CFU) of bacteria per milliliter of urine. However, CFU counts below this level (low-coliform-count infections) have been associated with cystitis in symptomatic women. Therefore, urine cultures are no longer recommended as part of the routine work-up of these patients. Instead, patients should undergo an abbreviated laboratory work-up in which the presence of pyuria is confirmed by traditional urinalysis or a dipstick test for leukocyte esterase. A positive leukocyte esterase test has a reported sensitivity of 75% to 90% in detecting pyuria associated with a UTI. The dipstick test for nitrite is used as a surrogate marker for bacteriuria. It should be noted that not all uropathogens reduce nitrates to nitrite; *Enterococcus, S. saprophyticus,* and *Acinetobacter* species do not, and therefore give false-negative results. Treatment options for uncomplicated cystitis include 3- or 7-day courses of antibiotics. Three-day regimens offer the optimal combination of convenience, low cost, and efficacy comparable to that of 7-day or longer regimens but with fewer side effects. When considering cost and efficacy, trimethoprim–sulfamethoxazole remains the antibiotic of choice in the treatment of uncomplicated UTIs in young women. The use of fluoroquinolones as first-line therapy for uncomplicated UTIs should be avoided, except in patients who cannot tolerate sulfonamides or trimethoprim, who have a high frequency of antibiotic resistance because of recent antibiotic treatment, or who reside in an area in which significant resistance to trimethoprim–sulfamethoxazole has been noted. A 7-day antibiotic course should be considered in pregnant women, diabetic women, and women who have had symptoms for more than 1 week and thus are at higher risk for pyelonephritis because of the delay in treatment.

Orenstein R, Wong ES. Urinary tract infections in adults. *Am Fam Physician.* 1999;59:1225.

325. Shy-Drager syndrome is associated with
A) peripheral neuropathies
B) autonomic instability
C) bilateral foot drop
D) tearing and excessive salivation
E) emotional lability

Answer and Discussion

The answer is B. Patients with Shy-Drager syndrome have plasma norepinephrine levels that do not increase on standing. In this condition there is widespread autonomic dysfunction in addition to failure of arteriolar and venous vasoconstriction; loss of sweating; bowel, bladder, and stomach atony; impotence; decreased salivation and tearing; mydriasis; and impaired visual accommodation. Paradoxically, blood pressure may be elevated in the supine position, even when severe postural hypotension is present, because of loss of parasympathetic, as well as sympathetic, regulation of the cardiovascular system. Orthostatic hypotension is accentuated in the early morning due to overnight natriuresis and may also be more prominent postprandially and after exercise. In Shy-Drager syndrome, bulbar dysfunction and laryngeal stridor may be fatal. Occasionally, the physical and pathologic findings are those of Parkinson's disease plus involvement of the intermediolateral cell columns of the spinal cord. Treatment includes intravascular volume expansion with fludrocortisone, salt supplementation, application of constrictive garments to the lower body (including the abdomen), and α adrenoreceptor stimulation with ephedrine. Keeping the head raised during sleep may reduce morning orthostatic hypotension. Metoclopramide, parenteral dihydroergotamine, and indomethacin are effective in some patients. Metoclopramide may exacerbate parkinsonian symptoms in some, and long-term use may lead to tardive dyskinesia, dystonia, or akathisia.

Beers MH, Porter RS, eds. *The Merck manual of diagnosis and therapy,* Merck Research Laboratories, 18th ed. Whitehouse Station, NJ: Merck & Co.; 2006:1768–1769.

326. Which of the following statements about use of ticlopidine is true?
A) The drug inhibits von Willebrand factor.
B) Side effects include peripheral neuropathy and tremor.
C) Liver function tests and blood counts should be monitored initially.
D) The drug is associated with gastric ulceration.
E) The drug inhibits vitamin K–dependent clotting factors.

Answer and Discussion

The answer is C. Ticlopidine (Ticlid) and clopidogrel (Plavix) are used as an alternative to aspirin when selecting an anticoagulant for stroke prophylaxis. Ticlopidine works by inhibiting platelet aggregation by blocking adenosine diphosphate–induced aggregation. Major side effects include diarrhea, nausea, dyspepsia, rash, an abnormal liver function test, and severe neutropenia and thrombocytopenia. Most side effects, including blood dyscrasias, occur within the first 3 months. Blood tests, including CBCs and liver function tests, should be monitored every 2 weeks for the first 3 months of drug therapy. Abnormalities may necessitate the discontinuation of the medication. Unlike aspirin, ticlopidine is not associated with gastric ulceration. Because of safety and tolerance issues associated with ticlopidine, clopidogrel is the more widely used second-line antiplatelet agent. Neutropenia, rash, diarrhea, and thrombotic thrombocytopenic purpura (TTP) occur less frequently with clopidogrel than with ticlopidine. The incidence of ticlopidine-related TTP is estimated to be 1 case per 1,600 to 5,000 patients treated. Although clopidogrel and aspirin have similar safety profiles, there have been rare reports of clopidogrel-related TTP, with the majority of cases occurring within 2 weeks of initiation of the drug.

Solenski NJ. Transient ischemic attacks. *Am Fam Physician.* 2004;69:1681–1688.

327. Which of the following positive test results supports the diagnosis of Raynaud's phenomenon?
A) Allen's test
B) Finkelstein's test
C) Phalen's test
D) Reverse Phalen's test

Answer and Discussion

The answer is A. Raynaud's phenomenon is secondary to spasm of the arterioles that usually supply the hands but can also affect the nose and other appendages. It is usually idiopathic (termed *Raynaud's disease*), but has been associated with emotional stress, connective tissue diseases (e.g., lupus, rheumatoid arthritis, scleroderma), arterial obstructive diseases, medications (e.g., ergots, β-blockers, clonidine, methysergide), and endocrine disorders. Idiopathic Raynaud's phenomenon occurs more frequently in women and frequently occurs in patients with migraines or variant angina. Symptoms include blanching, cyanosis, and paresthesias that affect the distal extremities. Diagnosis can be determined by performing Allen's test. The radial and ulnar arteries are occluded by the examiner while the patient makes a fist. The hand is then opened, and one side of the wrist is released. Blood flow to the hand should be detected by color, which is restored to the hand. If the hand remains pale and cyanotic with either of the two sides, Raynaud's phenomenon should be suspected. During asymptomatic periods the examination is entirely normal. Treatment for mild to moderate cases should only involve avoiding triggering factors (e.g., cold, stress, nicotine, previously listed medications). The medication of choice for the treatment of severe Raynaud's phenomenon includes the calcium channel blockers nifedipine and diltiazem. Other medications include reserpine, phenoxybenzamine, methyldopa, terazosin, doxazosin, and prazosin. Surgical treatment for resistant, severe cases involves sympathectomy.

Kasper DL, Braunwald E, Fauci AS, et al., eds. *Harrison's principles of internal medicine,* 16th ed. New York: McGraw-Hill; 2005:1489–1490.

328. Which of the following statements about the diagnosis of systemic lupus erythematosis (SLE) is true?
A) The ANA test is specific.
B) The LE prep test is a confirmatory test.
C) The LE prep test should be used as a screening test.
D) The anti-double-stranded DNA test is a confirmatory test.

Answer and Discussion

The answer is D. Systemic lupus erythematosis (SLE) is an autoimmune disorder affecting all major organ systems. Symptoms wax and wane and include diffuse joint pain, facial rashes (butterfly distribution), cardiac involvement (including pericarditis, myocarditis, and endocarditis), renal involvement (proteinuria, hypertension, and uremia), pulmonary involvement (pleuritis, pleural effusions), CNS findings (depression, transient ischemic attacks, strokes, chorea, and psychosis), and vasculitis. GI involvement is less common. Women are more commonly affected than men. Laboratory findings include a positive fluorescent ANA screening test, which is sensitive but not specific. The anti-double-stranded DNA is a confirmatory test that is specific but not sensitive. Because of the high rate of false-positive ANA titers, testing for SLE with an ANA titer or other autoantibody test is not recommended in patients with isolated myalgias or arthralgias in the absence of these specific clinical signs. Under most circumstances, a persistently negative ANA titer (<1:40) can be assumed to rule out SLE. A normal-range ANA titer in the setting of organ system involvement that suggests SLE should prompt an evaluation for alternative diagnoses. If no other cause is identified, the diagnosis of ANA-negative SLE and consultation with a rheumatologist should be considered. If patients with a normal ANA titer develop new clinical features that are consistent with SLE, ANA testing should be repeated. According to a guideline from the College of American Pathologists (CAP), no further laboratory tests are necessary in patients who meet diagnostic criteria for SLE and also have a positive ANA test result. Testing for antibody to double-stranded DNA antigen (anti-dsDNA) and antibody to Sm nuclear antigen (anti-Sm) may be helpful in patients who have a positive ANA test but do not meet full criteria for the diagnosis of SLE. Anti-dsDNA and anti-Sm, particularly in high titers, have high specificity for SLE, although their sensitivity is low. Therefore, a positive result helps to establish the diagnosis of the disease, but a negative result does not rule it out. The CAP guideline recommends against testing for other autoantibodies in ANA-positive patients, because there is little evidence that these tests are of benefit. Treatment involves the use of local or systemic steroids, antimalarials, and other immunosuppressive agents. The major challenge for physicians managing patients with SLE is to treat the active phase without allowing the treatment itself to cause long-term damage. This intent has led to a major change in treatment approach, with the goal of limiting corticosteroid exposure, if possible. As a result, physicians are now less reluctant to turn to immunosuppressive drugs such as azathioprine (Imuran) or cyclophosphamide (Cytoxan). Treatment for active SLE differs depending on the organ systems involved and disease severity. Current treatment often includes a combination of drugs.

Gill JM, Quisel AM, Rocca PV, et al. Diagnosis of systemic lupus erythematosis. *Am Fam Physician.* 2003;68:2179–2186.

329. Recurrent vertigo, tinnitus, and hearing loss are hallmark findings of
A) Meniere's disease
B) cholesteatoma
C) vestibular neuronitis
D) benign positional vertigo
E) acoustic neuroma

Answer and Discussion

The answer is A. Meniere's disease is a peripheral cause of vertigo. Symptoms include the hallmark findings of recurrent vertigo, tinnitus, and hearing loss. The cause is thought to arise from endolymphatic hydrops. In most cases, the vertigo lasts for several hours, up to an entire day. Although at first hearing may be little affected, over time it deteriorates. Tinnitus is usually constant and may become worse during the acute attacks. Vertigo may be severe and accompanied by nausea and vomiting. Treatment consists of salt restriction (i.e., no more than 2 g/day) and the use of hydrochlorothiazide, anticholinergics, antihistamines, and antiemetics. Resistant cases may require referral to an ear-nose-throat specialist.

Labuguen RH. Initial evaluation of vertigo. *Am Fam Physician.* 2006;73:244–251, 254

330. Primary hypothyroidism is associated with a deficiency of
A) T4
B) TSH
C) thyroid-releasing hormone
D) thyroid-stimulating antibodies
E) none of the above

Answer and Discussion

The answer is A. There are basically two types of hypothyroidism:

1. Primary hypothyroidism (most common form), which is a deficiency of T4 that is caused by thyroid gland disease.
2. Secondary hypothyroidism, which is associated with a deficiency in TSH from the pituitary gland or deficient thyroid-releasing hormone by the hypothalamus.

Hypothyroidism is seen more commonly in patients older than 55 years and in women. The most common form occurs as a result of Hashimoto's thyroiditis followed by post-therapeutic hypothyroidism, especially after radioactive iodine therapy or surgery for hyperthyroidism. Symptoms include fatigue, weakness, cold intolerance, constipation, hair loss, menorrhagia, carpal tunnel syndrome, dry skin, nonpitting edema (also referred to as *myxedema*) caused by deposition of mucopolysaccharides, weight gain, memory impairment, depression, hoarseness, delayed relaxation of reflexes, altered mental status, and bradycardia. A low free T4 with a high TSH is seen in primary hypothyroidism, whereas a low free T4 with a low TSH is indicative of secondary or tertiary hypothyroidism. In congenital hypothyroidism, the deficiency of thyroid hormone is severe and symptoms usually develop in the early weeks of life. Affected infants may show hypotonia and developmental delay. In the United States, mandatory newborn routine testing includes tests to rule out hypothyroidism, which has made the complications of neonatal hypothyroidism rare. Mental retardation may occur if infants are not identified and treated.

Beers MH, Porter RS, eds. *The Merck manual of diagnosis and therapy,* Merck Research Laboratories, 18th ed. Whitehouse Station, NJ: Merck & Co.; 2006:1200–1203.

331. Which of the following statements about Osler-Weber-Rendu disease is true?

A) The condition is not associated with hereditary transmission.
B) It is associated with telangiectasia lesions of the face, lips, nasal and oral mucosa, and GI mucosa.
C) The pulmonary system is unaffected.
D) Treatment involves high-dose prednisone.
E) Laboratory studies show pernicious anemia.

Answer and Discussion

The answer is B. Osler-Weber-Rendu disease (also known as *hereditary hemorrhagic telangiectasia*) is a hereditary disorder that is associated with telangiectasia lesions on the face, lips, nasal and oral mucosa, and GI mucosa. The mode of transmission is autosomal dominant. The condition can lead to significant GI hemorrhage or epistaxis. Some patients may have pulmonary arteriovenous malformations and may experience hemoptysis or dyspnea. Cerebral or spinal arteriovenous malformations may cause subarachnoid hemorrhage, seizures, or paraplegia. Laboratory findings may indicate an iron deficiency anemia. Treatment is nonspecific and involves topical hemostatics and laser ablation of accessible lesions. In severe cases, blood transfusions may be necessary. Iron supplementation is also recommended.

Beers MH, Porter RS, eds. *The Merck manual of diagnosis and therapy,* Merck Research Laboratories, 18th ed. Whitehouse Station, NJ: Merck & Co.; 2006:1089.

> Osler-Weber-Rendu (also known as hereditary hemorrhagic telangiectasia) is a hereditary disorder that is associated with telangiectasia lesions on the face, lips, nasal and oral mucosa, and GI mucosa.

332. B-type natriuretic peptide (BNP) is used in the diagnosis of

A) pulmonary embolism
B) congestive heart failure
C) type 1 diabetes mellitus
D) asthma
E) amyloidosis

Answer and Discussion

The answer is B. B-type natriuretic peptide (BNP) has shown sensitivity and specificity in the diagnosis of heart failure. This peptide is released by ventricular myocytes when heart failure causes increased wall stretch. It is a simple and rapid test that reliably predicts the presence or absence of left ventricular dysfunction on an echocardiogram. A BNP level of 100 pg/mL or below is unlikely to support the diagnosis of congestive heart failure, and an elevation >400 to 500 pg/mL is indication that heart failure is likely present. Intermediate values require physicians to rely on other standard evaluation measures to decide whether heart failure was present.

Mueller C, Scholer A, Laule-Kilian K. Use of B-type natriuretic peptide in the evaluation and management of acute dyspnea. *N Engl J Med.* 2004;350:647–654.

333. Which of the following are rich in omega-3 fatty acids?

A) Legumes
B) Vegetable oils
C) Fish
D) Meats
E) Tomatoes

Answer and Discussion

The answer is C. Omega-3 fatty acids have been shown to reduce the risk of mortality in patients with known coronary heart disease. Fish, including salmon and tuna, and fish oil are rich sources of the omega-3 fatty acids eicosapentaenoic acid and docosahexaenoic acid. Flaxseed, canola oil, and walnuts are also good dietary sources of omega-3 fatty acids. The omega-3 fatty acids are antithrombotic and anti-inflammatory. In contrast, omega-6 fatty acids, which are present in most seeds, vegetable oils, and meat, are prothrombotic and proinflammatory. Omega-3 fatty acids also are used to treat hyperlipidemia, hypertension, and rheumatoid arthritis. There appears to be no significant drug interactions with omega-3 fatty acids. The American Heart Association recommends consumption of two servings of fish per week for persons with no history of coronary heart disease and at least one serving of fish daily for those with known coronary heart disease. Approximately 1 g/day of omega-3 fatty acid is recommended for cardioprotection. Higher dosages of omega-3 fatty acids are required to reduce elevated triglyceride levels (2 g to 4 g per day) and to reduce morning stiffness and the number of tender joints in patients with rheumatoid arthritis (at least 3 g/day). Modest decreases in blood pressure occur with significantly higher dosages of omega-3 fatty acids.

Covington MG. Omega-3 fatty acids. *Am Fam Physician.* 2004;70:133–140.

334. Which of the following conditions is often the first sign of amyloidosis?

A) Proteinuria
B) CHF
C) Cardiac arrhythmias
D) Rheumatoid arthritis
E) Night blindness

Answer and Discussion

The answer is A. Amyloidosis is a condition characterized by excessive protein deposition in tissues, which interferes with normal organ functioning. Common forms include the following:

- Primary idiopathic amyloidosis, or that associated with multiple myeloma. This condition is also referred to with the designation *AL,* which denotes amyloidosis involving Ig light chains. Fewer than 20% of patients with AL have myeloma. Approximately 15% to 20% of patients with myeloma have amyloidosis. AL is a systemic disease that has the capability of affecting multiple organ systems.

- Secondary amyloidosis (designated *AA*, reactive or acquired amyloidosis) is associated with chronic inflammatory diseases such as tuberculosis, osteomyelitis, and leprosy. It more commonly affects the liver, spleen, kidneys, adrenal glands, and lymph nodes. Vascular involvement may be widespread. Effective treatment of the underlying chronic inflammatory disease has reduced the incidence in developed countries.

Diagnosis is usually accomplished after the point of irreversible organ damage and involves biopsy of the abdominal fat or rectal mucosa. Tissue is then examined under a polarizing microscope using Congo red stain to look for a characteristic green birefringence of amyloid. Proteinuria is often the first symptom associated with systemic amyloidosis, particularly the AA and AL types. Nephrotic syndrome may be severe and lead to renal failure. Myocardial amyloidosis–causing arrhythmias and CHF are two common forms of death in those affected with amyloidosis. Generalized amyloidosis is usually a slowly progressive disease that leads to death in several years, but, in some instances, prognosis is improving. The most effective form of treatment (for the AL form) is stem-cell transplantation and immunosuppressive drugs (melphalan). Cardiac transplantation has also been used.

Kasper DL, Braunwald E, Fauci AS, et al., eds. *Harrison's principles of internal medicine,* 16th ed. New York: McGraw-Hill; 2005:2024.

335. Which of the following statements is true regarding acyclovir?

A) The medication is not effective for the treatment of herpes zoster.
B) The drug effectively prevents the transmission of herpes from those affected.
C) Topical acyclovir is less effective than oral acyclovir.
D) The medication is most effective after the onset of vesicles.
E) Seizures are not associated with the use of acyclovir.

Answer and Discussion

The answer is C. Acyclovir is a purine compound used as an antiviral agent against the herpes virus. The medication is incorporated into the viral DNA and inhibits DNA polymerase, thus preventing replication of the virus. The medication is used for genital and oral herpes, as well as the herpes zoster infection. Immunocompromised patients infected with the varicella virus may also benefit from acyclovir. The medication should be used with caution in patients with underlying renal disease or dehydration. Adverse reactions include headache, encephalopathic signs (e.g., lethargy, obtundation, hallucinations, seizures), hypotension, rash, pruritus, nausea, vomiting, diarrhea, renal dysfunction, and arthralgias. The patient must be informed that the medication helps decrease the number and severity of occurrences but does not cure the virus. The best response is achieved when the medication is taken at the first symptoms of an outbreak of the virus. Patients should also be counseled that there is risk of herpes transmission even when there is no visible evidence of the virus. Topical use of acyclovir may help but is less effective than oral medication.

Emmert DH. Treatment of common cutaneous herpes simplex viral infections. *Am Fam Physician.* 2000;61:1697–1704, 1705–1706, 1708.

336. Which of the following tests is used to detect hepatitis B infection during the "window period"?

A) Hepatitis B surface antigen
B) Hepatitis B surface antibody
C) Hepatitis B core antibody (IgM)
D) Hepatitis B e antigen
E) Hepatitis B antibody to the delta agent

Answer and Discussion

The answer is C. The following are specific tests used when assessing a patient infected with hepatitis B virus:

- *Hepatitis B surface antigen (Australian antigen).* This test detects the surface antigen of the hepatitis B virus. It is usually detected 1 to 4 months after exposure to the virus. Its presence represents infection with the virus. In approximately 10% of cases, this test remains positive and no antibodies are formed. This state denotes the chronic carrier state.
- *Hepatitis B antibody.* This test detects the presence of antibodies to the hepatitis B surface antigens. It usually occurs 5 months after exposure to the virus and persists for life. Its presence represents past infection and relative immunity to hepatitis B. It can also be used to check for antibodies after immunization for the hepatitis B virus.
- *Hepatitis B core antibody IgM and IgG.* Anti–hepatitis B core antibody IgM is useful when trying to determine infection with the virus during the "window period" (i.e., the time between the disappearance of the surface antigen and the development of the antibody). Its presence indicates a current infection with hepatitis B. Anti–hepatitis B core antibody IgG indicates a previous hepatitis B infection, and its presence remains indefinitely.
- *Hepatitis B e antigen.* The presence of the e antigen indicates that the blood is highly infectious. It is associated with more severe cases and the development of the chronic carrier state. Its persistence for longer than 8 weeks indicates that a chronic carrier state has developed. In 90% of cases, hepatitis B e antigen–positive mothers infect their fetuses.
- *Hepatitis B antibody to the delta agent.* Conversion from the hepatitis B e antigen to the anti–hepatitis B e indicates a lower infectivity rate and improvement in the patient's liver function status. It usually reflects a benign outcome.

Beers MH, Porter RS, eds. *The Merck manual of diagnosis and therapy,* Merck Research Laboratories, 18th ed. Whitehouse Station, NJ: Merck & Co.; 2006:219–230.

337. In which of the following clinical situations is digoxin best used?

A) CHF in the setting of diastolic dysfunction
B) Idiopathic hypertrophic subaortic stenosis
C) Recent myocardial infarction with CHF
D) Supraventricular arrhythmia with the development of CHF
E) Emergent treatment of ventricular fibrillation

Answer and Discussion

The answer is D. The use of cardiac glycosides, such as digoxin, is not disputed and is generally recommended if there is a supraventricular arrhythmia present, such as atrial fibrillation in the presence of CHF. Digoxin is also used in cases of CHF in which the heart is dilated and the systolic function is significantly impaired. In patients with normal systolic function but with decreased ventricular compliance (diastolic dysfunction) that gives rise to CHF, the use of digoxin is not recommended. Digoxin should also not be used in patients with idiopathic, hypertrophic, subaortic stenosis; the medication is also usually withheld in patients with an acute myocardial infarction and CHF, unless diuretics and vasodilators fail to improve cardiac failure. Other agents, including ACE inhibitors, β blockers, and spironolactone, are being used increasingly to prolong life in patients with heart failure. Although digoxin has been used to treat heart failure for >200 years, its role in patients with CHF and sinus rhythm is still debatable. Since the mid-1990s, digoxin has received renewed attention because of recognition of its neurohormonal effect and the successful use of lower dosages. In recent trials, digoxin has been shown to reduce morbidity associated with CHF but to have no demonstrable effect on survival. The goal of digoxin therapy in patients with CHF is to improve quality of life by reducing symptoms and preventing hospitalizations.

Haji SA, Movahed A. Update on digoxin therapy in congestive heart failure. *Am Fam Physician.* 2000;62:409–416.

338. Which of the following conditions is a cardiovascular contraindication to vigorous exercise?
A) Myocardial infarction that occurred 1 year ago
B) Compensated CHF
C) Myocarditis occurring 1 month ago
D) Mild aortic stenosis
E) Pulmonary embolism that occurred 6 months ago

Answer and Discussion

The answer is C. Cardiovascular contraindications to vigorous exercise include the following:

- Recent (within 6 to 8 weeks) acute myocardial infarction
- Cardiac arrhythmia that compromises cardiac function
- Uncompensated CHF
- Severe aortic stenosis
- Unpaced third-degree heart block
- Severe idiopathic hypertrophic subaortic stenosis
- Episode of myocarditis within the past year
- Cardiomyopathy
- Aortic dissection
- Recent (within 6 to 8 weeks) pulmonary embolism or thrombophlebitis

An exercise program should be a gradual increase of activity that keeps the heart rate in the desired range (220 bpm—patient's age × 75% to 90%) for 30 minutes performed at least 5 times weekly. Select patients may benefit from cardiac stress testing before the onset of vigorous exercise.

Murphy JG. *Mayo Clinic Cardiology Review,* 2nd ed. Philadelphia: Lippincott Williams & Wilkins; 2000:244.

339. The treatment of choice for cryptococcal meningeal infection is
A) amphotericin B and flucytosine
B) metronidazole
C) acyclovir
D) amantadine
E) penicillin G

Answer and Discussion

The answer is A. Cryptococcus is an infection caused by the fungus *Cryptococcus neoformans* that usually involves the lungs with spread to the meninges and occasionally to other sites, including the kidneys, bones, and skin. The disease is found worldwide and tends to affect immunodeficient patients with lymphoma and AIDS or those chronically taking steroids. Symptoms include headaches (usually the first symptom), blurred vision, and mental status changes seen with meningeal involvement. In addition, the patient usually reports a persistent cough, which reflects pulmonary involvement. The disease is acquired by respiratory transmission. Skin lesions and the development of osteomyelitis are infrequent; however, as many as 33% of patients with meningeal involvement also have renal involvement. Laboratory tests show CSF with an increased protein, a white cell count that is mostly lymphocytes, and a decreased glucose level with meningeal involvement. Culture of sputum, blood, urine, or other areas of involvement is diagnostic. The diagnosis is also supported with the evidence of budding yeast seen with India ink preparation. The treatment of choice for cryptococcal meningitis is the administration of intravenous amphotericin B and oral flucytosine until lumbar cultures are clear, followed by lifelong prophylaxis with amphotericin, fluconazole, or ketoconazole. Nonprogressive pulmonary cryptococcus may not require treatment in patients who are not immunocompromised.

Beers MH, Porter RS, eds. *The Merck manual of diagnosis and therapy,* Merck Research Laboratories, 18th ed. Whitehouse Station, NJ: Merck & Co.; 2006:1566–1567.

340. A 28-year-old active runner presents to your office complaining of lateral knee and hip pain. The patient reports she has been training intensely for an upcoming marathon. On physical examination, tenderness of the lateral portion of the thigh and a prominent lateral epicondyle are noted. The most likely diagnosis is
A) patellofemoral syndrome
B) ITB syndrome
C) tibial plateau fracture
D) pes anserine bursitis
E) stress fracture

Answer and Discussion

The answer is B. Iliotibial band (ITB) syndrome is characterized by lateral knee pain and, occasionally, lateral hip pain. The pain is caused by inflammation of the distal portion of the ITB band or at the point in which the ITB crosses the lateral femoral epicondyle. Runners, hammer throwers, and racket sport enthusiasts are those usually affected. The condition usually affects runners when there is an increase in the running distance, increased speed or hill running, change in running surface, or consistent running on a banked surface. These activities lead to increased friction of the ITB and cause inflammation. Associated conditions include genu valgum, prominent lateral epicondyle, trochanteric bursitis, leg-length discrepancy, excessive foot pronation, and quadriceps weakness. Testing may show an excessively tight ITB or gluteus maximus. Treatment involves relative rest, anti-inflammatory medication, ice massage, and electronic galvanic stimulation. Prevention is aimed at proper stretching techniques (e.g., quadriceps strengthening) and measures to correct underlying abnormalities (e.g., excessive pronation).

Sullivan JA, Anderson SJ, eds. *Care of the young athlete.* American Academy of Pediatrics. Rosemont, Il: American Academy of Orthopaedic Surgeons; 2000:374.

341. Which of the following statements about the use of digoxin is true?

A) It is contraindicated in the treatment of CHF and supraventricular tachyarrhythmias.
B) It decreases conduction through the AV node.
C) It can be associated with hepatic failure.
D) Hyponatremia can increase the heart's sensitivity to the medication, leading to cardiac arrhythmias.
E) Patients with a history of Cushing's disease are more sensitive to the effects of digoxin.

Answer and Discussion

The answer is B. Digoxin is classified as a cardiac glycoside. It is used in the treatment of CHF and in supraventricular tachyarrhythmias. In previous trials, digoxin has been shown to reduce morbidity associated with congestive heart failure but to have no demonstrable effect on survival. The goal of digoxin therapy in patients with congestive heart failure is to improve quality of life by reducing symptoms and preventing hospitalizations. The mechanism of action involves positive inotropic activity, which increases the contractility of the cardiac muscle. It also has a negative chronotropic effect, which depresses the sinoatrial node and decreases conduction through the AV node. The drug is distributed widely throughout the body, and approximately 20% to 30% is bound to plasma proteins. The drug is excreted by the kidneys; therefore, drug levels of patients who are elderly or who have renal insufficiency must be monitored closely and the dosage adjusted. Patients with a history of hypothyroidism are also more sensitive to digoxin's effects. Hepatic failure is not associated with digoxin toxicity, because only approximately 10% of the drug goes through enterohepatic recirculation. Potassium levels should also be monitored carefully when administering digoxin. Hypokalemia can increase the heart's sensitivity to the medication and lead to toxicity. Digoxin toxicity is manifested by cardiac arrhythmias, nausea, vomiting, and yellow-green halos around visual images or lights. In severe cases of toxicity, the drug should be withheld and digoxin-specific antibody fragments (Digibind) can be given. Digibind binds the digoxin and allows rapid excretion.

Haji SA, Movahed A. Update on digoxin therapy in congestive heart failure. *Am Fam Physician.* 2000;62:409–416.

> Digoxin toxicity is manifested by cardiac arrhythmias, nausea, vomiting, and yellow-green halos around visual images or lights.

342. Which of the following statements about rapid streptococcal screening tests (enzyme immunoassays) is true?

A) Their accuracy is generally unreliable.
B) They are less accurate than latex agglutination tests.
C) They are expensive and difficult to perform.
D) They are rarely used when compared to cultures.
E) They may be avoided if the criteria for strep pharyngitis is met.

Answer and Discussion

The answer is E. Rapid *Streptococcus* screen tests are quick, easy to perform, and approximately as accurate as the latex agglutination tests. Their sensitivity approaches 80%, whereas their specificity is 85% to 100%; thus, a positive test is fairly predictive of a streptococcal infection and a culture is unnecessary. If negative, cultures can be performed to confirm the results. In adults, many experts are recommending that treatment can be started or avoided without a strep test. The criteria include: history of fever, tonsillar exudates, absence of cough, and tender anterior cervical lymphadenopathy. Patients who have 0 or only 1 criterion are unlikely to have strep pharyngitis and do not need to be tested. Patients who have 2 criteria can be tested. Those with 3 or 4 criteria can be tested or treated empirically.

Sheeler RD, Houston MS, Radke S. Accuracy of rapid strep testing in patients who have had recent streptococcal pharyngitis. *J Am Board Fam Pract.* 2002;15:261–265.

Beers MH, Porter RS, eds. *The Merck manual of diagnosis and therapy,* Merck Research Laboratories, 18th ed. Whitehouse Station, NJ: Merck & Co.; 2006:826.

343. The treatment of choice for mucormycosis is

A) amphotericin
B) ketoconazole
C) clotrimazole
D) miconazole

Answer and Discussion

The answer is A. Mucormycosis infections are usually fulminant and can be fatal. Necrotic lesions usually appear on the nasal mucosa or sometimes the palate. Vascular invasion by hyphae leads to progressive tissue necrosis that may involve the nasal septum, palate, and bones surrounding the orbit or sinuses. Findings include pain, fever, orbital cellulitis, proptosis, purulent nasal discharge, and mucosal necrosis. Extension of the infection to involve the brain can cause cavernous sinus thrombosis, convulsions, aphasia, or hemiplegia. Patients with diabetic ketoacidosis are most commonly affected, but opportunistic infections may also develop in chronic renal disease or with immunosuppression, particularly with neutropenia or high-dose corticosteroid therapy. Pulmonary infections resemble invasive aspergillosis. Diagnosis requires a high index of suspicion and careful examination of tissue samples for large nonseptate hyphae with irregular diameters and branching patterns, because much of the necrotic debris contains no organisms. Cultures usually are negative, even when hyphae are clearly visible in tissues. CT scans and x-rays often underestimate or miss significant bone destruction. Effective antifungal therapy requires that diabetes be controlled or, if at all possible, immunosuppression reversed. IV amphotericin B must be used, because azoles are ineffective. Surgical debridement of necrotic tissue may be indicated, because amphotericin B cannot penetrate into these avascular areas to clear remaining organisms.

Beers MH, Porter RS, eds. *The Merck manual of diagnosis and therapy,* Merck Research Laboratories, 18th ed. Whitehouse Station, NJ: Merck & Co.; 2006:1534.

344. Cardiac troponins may remain elevated up to

A) 24 hours
B) 48 hours
C) 72 hours
D) 1 week
E) 2 weeks

Answer and Discussion

The answer is E. The term *acute coronary syndrome* refers to a range of thrombotic coronary artery diseases, including unstable angina and both ST-segment elevation and non-ST-segment elevation myocardial infarction. Symptoms of acute coronary syndrome include chest pain, referred pain, nausea, vomiting, dyspnea, diaphoresis, and lightheadedness. Pain may be referred to the arms, the jaw, the neck, the back, or even the abdomen. Pain radiating to the shoulder, left arm, or both arms increases the likelihood of acute coronary syndrome. Typical angina is described as pain that is substernal, occurs on exertion, and is relieved with rest. Diagnosis utilizes an electrocardiogram and a review for signs and symptoms of cardiac ischemia. In acute coronary syndrome, common electrocardiographic abnormalities include T-wave tenting or inversion, ST-segment elevation or depression (including J-point elevation in multiple leads), and pathologic Q waves. Most high-risk patients should be hospitalized. Intermediate-risk patients should undergo further evaluation, often in a chest pain unit. Many low-risk patients can be discharged with appropriate follow-up. Troponin T or I generally is the most sensitive determinant of acute coronary syndrome, although the MB isoenzyme of creatine kinase also is used. Troponins (T, I, C) are found in striated and cardiac muscle. They are the preferred markers for the diagnosis of myocardial injury. Troponin T and I have similar sensitivity and specificity for the detection of myocardial injury. Unlike troponin I levels, troponin T levels may be elevated in patients with renal disease, polymyositis, or dermatomyositis. The cardiac troponins typically are measured at emergency department admission and repeated in 6 to 12 hours. Patients with a normal CK-MB level but elevated troponin levels are considered to have sustained minor myocardial damage or microinfarction or cardiac strain, whereas patients with elevations of both CK-MB and troponins are considered to have had acute myocardial infarction. The cardiac troponins may remain elevated up to 2 weeks after symptom onset, which makes them useful as late markers of recent acute myocardial infarction. An elevated troponin T or I level is helpful in identifying patients at increased risk for death or the development of acute myocardial infarction. Increased risk is related quantitatively to the serum troponin level.

Achar SA, Kundu S, Norcross WA. Diagnosis of acute coronary syndrome. *Am Fam Physician.* 2005;72:119–126.

345. A 45-year-old carpenter has a history of hepatitis C. He is returning for a check up and is doing well without complaints. You should make the following recommendation:

A) Ibuprofen is considered safe.
B) Even low-dose acetaminophen should be avoided.
C) Vaccination for hepatitis A and B is recommended.
D) Milk thistle should be avoided.
E) Mild to moderate alcohol use has little detrimental effect.

Answer and Discussion

The answer is C. Hepatitis C virus infection is the most frequent cause of chronic liver disease and the most common reason for liver transplantation. Chronic liver disease is the tenth leading cause of death in the United States. Preventive care can significantly reduce the progression of liver disease. Because alcohol in the setting of hepatitis C can increase the development of cirrhosis, patients with hepatitis C infection should abstain from alcohol use. Because associated infections with hepatitis A or B virus can lead to liver failure, vaccination of both is recommended. Medications that are potentially hepatotoxic should be avoided or used with caution in patients with chronic liver disease. In general, NSAIDs should be avoided; acetaminophen in a dosage below 2 g/day is a safer alternative. Many herbal remedies are potentially hepatotoxic and should also be avoided. Milk thistle can be used safely in patients who have chronic liver disease and may be beneficial. Weight reduction and exercise can improve liver function in patients with fatty infiltration of the liver.

Riley TR III, Bhatti AM. Preventive strategies in chronic liver disease: Part I. Alcohol, vaccines, toxic medications and supplements, diet and exercise. *Am Fam Physician.* 2001; 64:1555–1560.

346. Which of the following statements concerning the use of metformin is true?

A) The drug is an oral sulfonylurea.
B) Weight gain is common with its use.
C) The most common side effect is headache.
D) Patients using metformin must have periodic liver function tests.
E) The most serious side effect is lactic acidosis.

Answer and Discussion

The answer is E. Metformin belongs to the class of drugs referred to as *biguanides.* Metformin decreases hepatic glucose production by inhibiting gluconeogenesis. The drug also decreases insulin production as a result of decreasing insulin resistance. Metformin decreases plasma triglycerides and LDL cholesterol and increases HDL cholesterol. Hypoglycemia does not occur with metformin monotherapy, and, in contrast to other hypoglycemic agents, weight is not gained and even may be lost with its use. The most common side effects are GI irritation, abdominal cramps, and diarrhea. Patients with inflammatory bowel disease and peptic ulcer disease are not good candidates for metformin therapy. The most severe side effect is lactic acidosis, which can be fatal. Metformin is contraindicated in men with a serum creatine greater than 1.5 mg/dL, or greater than 1.4 mg/dL in women, in patients receiving intravenous radiographic iodinated contrast media, acute myocardial infarction, CHF, and any ischemic condition.

Rakel RE, Bope ET. *Conn's Current Therapy 2005.* Philadelphia: Elsevier/Saunders; 2005:665, 666.

347. A 28-year-old man presents to your office complaining of pain in the perirectal area for the last week. Examination shows an area of tenderness, redness, and induration just superior to the anus in the gluteal cleft. The area is warm and fluctuant. The area is otherwise unremarkable. The most appropriate management is

A) warm sitz baths
B) oral antibiotics and warm sitz baths as an outpatient
C) high-dose, intravenous antibiotics as an inpatient
D) topical steroids applied to the rectal area
E) surgical incision and drainage

Answer and Discussion

The answer is E. Pilonidal disease often affects young, white, hirsute males. The disease is related to acute abscesses or chronic draining sinuses that form in the sacrococcygeal region. These sinuses or pits may form a cavity often containing hair. The lesion is often painless unless it becomes infected. Treatment involves incision and drainage and removal of communicating sinus tracts. In many cases, antibiotics are not necessary.

Beers MH, Porter RS, eds. *The Merck manual of diagnosis and therapy,* Merck Research Laboratories, 18th ed. Whitehouse Station, NJ: Merck & Co.; 2006:166.

348. The drug of choice for treatment of severe coccidioidomycosis ("valley fever") is
A) ceftriaxone
B) tetracyline
C) ciprofloxacin
D) mefloquin
E) amphotericin

Answer and Discussion

The answer is E. Coccidioidomycosis ("valley fever") is an infection that is usually asymptomatic. In some cases, nonspecific respiratory symptoms resembling influenza or acute bronchitis occur. Less frequently, acute pneumonia or pleural effusion can develop. Symptoms include fever, cough, chest pain, chills, sputum production, sore throat, and hemoptysis. Physical signs may be absent or limited to scattered rales with or without areas of dullness to percussion over lung fields. Leukocytosis and, in some cases, eosinophilia is seen. Other symptoms include arthritis, conjunctivitis, erythema nodosum, or erythema multiforme. Primary pulmonary lesions sometimes resolve, leaving nodular coin lesions that may be confused with neoplasms and tuberculosis or other granulomatous infections. In some cases, cavitary lesions develop that may vary in size over time and often appear thin-walled. Although dissemination does not occur from these residual areas, a small percentage of these cavities fail to heal. Hemoptysis or the threat of rupture into the pleural space may occasionally require surgery. Treatment for mild primary coccidioidomycosis is unnecessary in low-risk patients. Mild to moderate nonmeningeal extrapulmonary involvement should be treated with fluconazole or itraconazole. IV amphotericin B or fluconazole is preferable for severely ill patients. As with histoplasmosis, patients with AIDS-associated coccidioidomycosis require maintenance therapy to prevent relapse. Treatment for meningeal coccidioidomycosis must be continued for many months, probably lifelong. Surgical removal of involved bone may be necessary to cure osteomyelitis.

Beers MH, Porter RS, eds. *The Merck manual of diagnosis and therapy,* Merck Research Laboratories, 18th ed. Whitehouse Station, NJ: Merck & Co.; 2006:1530–1531.

349. A 65-year-old woman with a seizure disorder controlled with phenytoin presents to your office complaining of muscle cramps, dry skin, and depression. Examination shows carpal pedal spasms after application of a blood pressure cuff. The most likely diagnosis is
A) hypothyroidism
B) hyperventilation with panic attacks
C) hyperkalemia
D) hypocalcemia
E) hyponatremia

Answer and Discussion

The answer is D. Hypocalcemia is defined as a decrease in total plasma calcium concentration <8.8 mg/dL in the presence of normal plasma protein concentration. Causes include hypoparathyroidism; vitamin D deficiency; renal tubular disease; magnesium depletion; acute pancreatitis; hypoproteinemia; septic shock; hyperphosphatemia; and drugs, including phenytoin, phenobarbital, and rifampin. Most patients are asymptomatic. Symptoms, when present, include muscle cramps involving the legs and back, mental status changes, dry skin, depression, and psychosis. Papilledema may occasionally occur, and cataracts may develop after prolonged hypocalcemia. Severe hypocalcemia (<7 mg/dL) may cause tetany, laryngospasm, or generalized seizures. With hypocalcemia giving rise to latent tetany, the patient may exhibit a positive Chvostek's sign (involuntary twitching of the facial muscles caused by a light tapping of the facial nerve just anterior to the exterior auditory meatus) or a positive Trousseau's sign (carpopedal spasm caused by reduction of the blood supply to the hand with a blood pressure cuff inflated to 20 mm Hg above the systolic BP applied to the forearm after 3 minutes). Hypocalcemia can cause heart block and arrhythmias. ECG changes show prolongation of the QTc and ST intervals. T-wave peaking or inversion can also occur. Severe hypocalcemic tetany is treated initially with intravenous infusion of calcium salts (calcium gluconate). In chronic hypocalcemia, oral calcium and vitamin D supplements are usually sufficient. Treatment of hypocalcemia in patients with renal failure must be combined with dietary phosphate restriction and phosphate-binding agents such as calcium carbonate to prevent hyperphosphatemia and metastatic calcification.

Beers MH, Porter RS, eds. *The Merck manual of diagnosis and therapy,* Merck Research Laboratories, 18th ed. Whitehouse Station, NJ: Merck & Co.; 2006:1250–1254.

350. Shy-Drager syndrome is best characterized by
A) autonomic dysfunction
B) unilateral foot drop
C) peripheral neuropathy
D) proximal muscle weakness
E) muscle atrophy

Answer and Discussion

The answer is A. Shy-Drager syndrome affects multiple organ systems and causes neurologic damage, including autonomic dysfunction with cerebellar ataxia, Parkinsonism, corticospinal, and corticobulbar tract dysfunction. Patients may experience orthostatic hypotension, impotence, urinary retention, fecal incontinence, decreased sweating, iris atrophy, and decreased tearing and salivation. Treatment consists of intravascular volume expansion with the administration of fludrocortisone, application of constrictive garments to the lower extremities, and the administration of an α-adrenoreceptor stimulator midodrine. Bulbar dysfunction and laryngeal stridor can be fatal if not treated.

Beers MH, Porter RS, eds. *The Merck manual of diagnosis and therapy,* Merck Research Laboratories, 18th ed. Whitehouse Station, NJ: Merck & Co.; 2006:1768.

> Treatment of Shy-Drager syndrome consists of intravascular volume expansion with the administration of fludrocortisone, application of constrictive garments to the lower extremities, and the administration of an alpha-adrenoreceptor stimulator midodrine.

351. A 24-year-old yard maintenance worker is bitten by a venomous snake. Which of the following is considered acceptable treatment?
A) Arterial tourniquet
B) Application of ice
C) Wound incision and forced bleeding

D) Lymphatic tourniquet
E) None of the above

Answer and Discussion

The answer is D. Poisonous snakebites, although rare, are a potentially life-threatening emergency in the United States. Rattlesnakes are responsible for most snakebites and related fatalities. Venomous snakes in the United States can be classified as having hemotoxic or neurotoxic venom. Associated signs and symptoms ranging from fang marks, with or without local pain and swelling, to life-threatening coagulopathy, renal failure, and shock are seen. First-aid techniques such as arterial tourniquets, application of ice, and wound incisions are ineffective and can be harmful; however, suction with a venom extractor within the first 5 minutes after the bite may be useful. Conservative measures, such as immobilization and lymphatic constriction bands, are now advocated until emergency care can be administered. Equine-derived antivenin is considered the standard of care; however, a promising new treatment is sheep-derived antigen binding fragment ovine (CroFab), which is much less allergenic. Surgical intervention with fasciotomy is now reserved for rare cases. Snakebite prevention should be taught to patients.

Juckett G, Hancox JG. Venomous snakebites in the United States: management review and update. *Am Fam Physician.* 2002;65:1367–1374.

352. Which of the following statements is true regarding low-carbohydrate diets?
A) They may be more effective than low-fat diets in helping patients lose weight in the short term.
B) They cause adverse changes in lipid values.
C) They are often effective years after initiation.
D) They invariably lead to longer healthier lives.

Answer and Discussion

The answer is A. A low-carbohydrate diet can help patients lose more weight in the short term than a conventional low-fat diet. Although a low-carbohydrate diet does not cause adverse changes in lipid levels, it may not help patients live longer, better lives, which is the goal of diet therapy. There appears to be a diminishing benefit after 12 months.

Samaha FF, Iqbal N, Seshadri R. A low-carbohydrate as compared with a low-fat diet in severe obesity. *N Engl J Med.* 2003;348:2074–2081.

Foster GD, Wyatt HR, Hill J. A randomized trial of a low-carbohydrate diet for obesity. *N Engl J Med.* 2003;348:2082–2090.

353. A 42-year-old indigent patient is found to have secondary syphilis and treatment is started. Two hours after his first dose of antibiotics, the patient is noted to have low-grade fever, chills, myalgias, headache, tachypnea, and tachycardia. Appropriate management at this point consists of
A) stopping all antibiotics
B) ordering ECG, chest x-ray, blood cultures, and urinalysis
C) starting intravenous dexamethasone
D) administering acetaminophen for symptomatic treatment
E) administering diphenhydramine and epinephrine

Answer and Discussion

The answer is D. The Jarisch-Herxheimer reaction is usually a mild reaction consisting of acute, transient fever (low grade), chills, myalgias, headache, tachycardia, increased respiratory rate, increased circulating neutrophil count (average total white blood cell count, 12,500/μL), and vasodilation with mild hypotension that may follow the initiation of treatment for syphilis or other spirochete-related illness. This reaction occurs in approximately 50% of patients with primary syphilis, 90% of those with secondary syphilis, and 25% of those with early latent syphilis. The onset comes within 2 hours of treatment, the temperature peaks at approximately 6 to 8 hours, and defervescence takes place within 12 to 24 hours. The reaction is more delayed in neurosyphilis, with fever peaking after 12 to 14 hours. In patients with secondary syphilis, erythema and edema of the mucocutaneous lesions increase; occasionally, subclinical or early mucocutaneous lesions may first become apparent during the reaction. The pathogenesis of this reaction is undefined, although recent studies have demonstrated the induction of inflammatory mediators such as tumor necrosis factors by treponemal lipoproteins. Patients should be warned to expect such symptoms, which can be managed by symptomatic treatment. Adjunctive steroid and anti-inflammatory therapy has not been shown to prevent the Jarisch-Herxheimer reaction in syphilis and is not recommended for this transient reaction.

Lukehart SA. Chapter 153: Syphilis. Available at Harrison's Online website (http://www.harrisonsonline.com). Accessed 6/1/06.

The Jarisch-Herxheimer reaction is usually a mild reaction consisting of acute, transient fever (low grade), chills, myalgias, headache, tachycardia, increased respiratory rate, increased circulating neutrophil count (average total white blood cell count, 12,500/μL), and vasodilation with mild hypotension that may follow the initiation of treatment for syphilis or other spirochete-related illness.

354. You are covering the local high school football game on Friday night. An 18-year-old star running back goes down on the field after a hard tackle. When you arrive at his side, he is holding his knee. He describes a "pop" followed by severe pain. Which of the following would be most helpful in the initial diagnosis?
A) Ability to walk
B) Lachman's test
C) Anterior drawer test
D) CT of the knee
E) Arthrogram of the knee

Answer and Discussion

The answer is B. ACL injuries typically present after a noncontact deceleration, a "cutting" movement or hyperextension, often accompanied by a "pop," with the inability to continue sports participation and associated knee instability. In all cases of knee injury it should be determined how quickly swelling occurred after the injury. If an effusion evolved within 4 hours of injury, there is a high likelihood of major osseous, ligamentous, or meniscal injury. The ACL is particularly prone to injury. Physical findings include effusion, positive ACL tests, and chronic quadriceps atrophy. The Lachman's test is performed with the knee in 20 degrees of flexion. The tibia is pulled anteriorly on a secured femur. A positive test result is indicated by increased tibial movement compared with the unaffected knee. The quality of the end point should also be noted;

a soft end point indicates an ACL tear. The anterior drawer test (although much less specific) is performed with the knee in 90 degrees of flexion. Similar to the Lachman's test, the tibia is drawn anteriorly, and asymmetric movement is an indicator of ACL injury. The most specific test for ACL disruption is the pivot shift test, but this test is often difficult to perform because of patient guarding and apprehension. Radiographs should be obtained in patients with suspected ACL injuries to rule out associated intra-articular fractures and possibly determine the presence of a marginal avulsion fracture off the lateral tibial plateau (Segond fracture), which helps confirm the diagnosis. MRI is not necessary to diagnose ACL disruption but is often used and may be helpful in diagnosing associated meniscal pathology. Treatment involves rehabilitation with physical therapy and, in some cases, surgical repair.

Johnson MW. Acute knee effusion: a systematic approach to diagnosis. *Am Fam Physician.* 2000;61:2391–2400.

355. A 78-year-old retired carpenter presents to your office complaining of gradually increasing right-sided shoulder pain. The patient reports he is unable to sleep on his right side and has a difficult time raising the right arm. Physical examination shows his shoulder's range of motion is significantly restricted. X-rays of the shoulder show osteopenia of the humeral head. The most likely diagnosis is

A) biceps muscle tear
B) adhesive capsulitis
C) multiple myeloma
D) subacromial bursitis
E) osteoporosis

Answer and Discussion

The answer is B. Adhesive capsulitis, or frozen shoulder, results from thickening and contraction of the capsule around the glenohumeral joint and causes loss of motion and pain. Frozen shoulder classically consists of shoulder pain that is slow in onset and presents without any radiographic abnormalities. Usually the discomfort is localized near the deltoid insertion, the patient is unable to sleep on the affected side, and glenohumeral elevation and external rotation are restricted. Frozen shoulder most often occurs as a result of immobility after a shoulder injury. An autoimmune cause of frozen shoulder has been proposed. The diagnosis is usually made clinically, and physicians should always be concerned about a possible underlying rotator cuff tear. Radiographs often appear normal, although osteopenia of the humeral head may be noted as a result of disuse. Arthrography demonstrates generalized constriction of the joint capsule, with loss of the normal axillary and subscapularis spaces. The capsule can be dilated during arthrography, converting the procedure from a diagnostic to a therapeutic one. A carefully designed treatment plan for patients with frozen shoulder may include physical therapy, pain medication such as NSAIDs, and, occasionally, intra-articular corticosteroid injection. Surgical referral may be indicated after conservative treatment has failed, although the exact timing of surgery should be decided on an individual basis.

Woodward TW, Best TM. The painful shoulder: Part II. Acute and chronic disorders. *Am Fam Physician.* 2000;61:3291–3300.

356. During one rescuer CPR the ventilation/compression ratio should be

A) 1:1
B) 1:5
C) 1:10
D) 2:10
E) 2:30

Answer and Discussion

The answer is E. The new algorithm for adult basic life support recommends the following sequence when a rescuer finds an unresponsive person:

1. Call for help and an AED (if available).
2. Open the adult's airway, check for breathing, and give two breaths if he or she is not breathing.
3. Start cycles of 30 compressions and two breaths (100 compressions/minute).
4. On arrival of a defibrillator or AED, check for a shockable rhythm (ventricular fibrillation or tachycardia).
5. Give one shock (if indicated), then resume CPR for another five cycles; if no shock is indicated, continue another five cycles of CPR before rechecking the rhythm.

Health-care professionals are to check for a pulse after the initial breaths (step 2) and continue with one rescue breath every 5 or 6 seconds if there is a pulse, but this step is not recommended for lay rescuers.

American Heart Association. 2005 American Heart Association guidelines for cardiopulmonary resuscitation and emergency cardiovascular care. *Circulation.* 2005;112(24 suppl): IV1–203.

357. Of the following supplements, which has been associated with an increased risk of lung cancer in smokers?

A) Folic acid
B) β Carotene
C) Ginseng
D) Vitamin E
E) Saw palmetto

Answer and Discussion

The answer is B. Many carotenoids are known, but their functions are not yet understood. β Carotene is a vitamin A precursor carried in plasma and LDL. It reduces oxidized LDL uptake but does not prevent LDL oxidation. Sources of dietary carotenoids include fruits, yellow-orange vegetables (e.g., carrots, squash, and sweet potatoes), and deep-green vegetables (e.g., spinach and broccoli). No recommended daily allowance has been established for carotenoids. Research supports the benefit of a carotenoid-rich diet, but not β carotene supplementation. The Beta-Carotene and Retinol Efficacy Trial combined β carotene and retinol supplementation in 18,314 smokers and patients with asbestos exposure. However, the study was terminated prematurely because of a significant increase in lung cancer mortality and a nonsignificant increase in CHD mortality. In 12 years of β carotene supplementation in 22,071 male physicians, no significant beneficial effects on CHD mortality, nonfatal myocardial infarction, or stroke were found. In addition, no interactive effect with cigarette smoking (i.e., no harm or benefit) was demonstrated. A nonsignificant reduction in CHD events occurred in the groups who had clinical evidence of atherosclerosis.

Forman D, Altman D. Vitamins to prevent cancer: supplementary problems [Editorial]. *Lancet.* 2004;364:1193–1194.

358. A urine culture grows more than 100,000 colony-forming units. The patient is asymptomatic. For which of the following patients is treatment indicated?

A) 94-year-old nursing home resident
B) 72-year-old business executive
C) 68-year-old with a history of breast cancer
D) 78-year-old scheduled for cataract surgery
E) 28-year-old pregnant woman at 38 weeks' gestation

Answer and Discussion

The answer is E. Asymptomatic bacteriuria is defined as the presence of >100,000 colony-forming units/mL of voided urine in persons with no symptoms of urinary tract infection. The largest patient population at risk for asymptomatic bacteriuria is the elderly (particularly women). Up to 40% of elderly men and women may have bacteriuria without symptoms. Although early studies noted an association between bacteriuria and excess mortality, more recent studies have failed to demonstrate any such link. Aggressively screening elderly persons for asymptomatic bacteriuria and subsequent treatment of the infection has not been found to reduce infectious complications or mortality. Consequently, this approach is currently not recommended. Three groups of patients with asymptomatic bacteriuria have been shown to benefit from treatment: (1) pregnant women, (2) patients with renal transplants, and (3) patients who are about to undergo genitourinary tract procedures. Between 2% and 10% of pregnancies are complicated by urinary tract infections; if left untreated, 25% to 30% of these women develop pyelonephritis. Pregnancies that are complicated by pyelonephritis have been associated with low-birth-weight infants and prematurity. Thus, pregnant women should be screened for bacteriuria by urine culture at 12 to 16 weeks of gestation. The presence of 100,000 colony-forming units of bacteria per milliliter of urine is considered significant. Pregnant women with asymptomatic bacteriuria should be treated with a 3- to 7-day course of antibiotics, and the urine should subsequently be cultured to ensure cure and the avoidance of relapse.

Orenstein R, Wong ES. Urinary tract infections in adults. *Am Fam Physician.* 1999;59(5):1235.

Beers MH, Porter RS, eds. *The Merck manual of diagnosis and therapy,* Merck Research Laboratories, 18th ed. Whitehouse Station, NJ: Merck & Co.; 2006:317–318.

359. Which of the following statements is true regarding orolabial herpes?

A) Highest rate of infection occurs in adolescent children.
B) Lesions are usually painless vesicles that form on the tongue, palate, and gingival area.
C) Topical acyclovir is the drug of choice.
D) Recurrent infections are less severe and shorter in duration.
E) Pain associated with lesions typically lasts 2 to 3 weeks.

Answer and Discussion

The answer is D. Orolabial herpes (gingivostomatitis) is the most prevalent form of mucocutaneous herpes infection; 35% to 60% of White persons in the United States show serologic evidence of having been infected by herpes simplex virus (HSV)-1. African-American persons and persons from low-economic populations are infected earlier in life. Overall, the highest rate of infection occurs during the preschool years. Female gender, history of sexually transmitted diseases, and multiple sexual partners have also been identified as risk factors for HSV-1 infection. Primary herpetic gingivostomatitis usually affects children under the age of 5 years. It typically takes the form of painful vesicles and ulcerative erosions on the tongue, palate, gingiva, buccal mucosa, and lips. Edema, halitosis, and drooling may be present, and tender submandibular or cervical lymphadenopathy is not uncommon. Hospitalization may be necessary when pain prevents eating or fluid intake. Systemic symptoms are often present, including fever [38.4° to 40°C (101° to 104°F)], malaise, and myalgia. The pharyngitis and flu-like symptoms are difficult to distinguish from mononucleosis in older patients. The duration of the illness is 2 to 3 weeks, and oral shedding of the virus may continue for as long as 23 days. Recurrences typically occur 2 or 3 times per year. The duration is shorter and the discomfort less severe than in primary infections; the lesions are often single and more localized, and the vesicles heal completely by 8 to 10 days. Pain diminishes quickly in 4 to 5 days. UV radiation predictably triggers recurrence of orolabial HSV-1, an effect that, for unknown reasons, is not fully suppressed by acyclovir. Pharmacologic intervention is therefore more difficult in patients with orolabial infection.

Topical medication for HSV infection is generally not highly effective. In the treatment of primary orolabial herpes, oral acyclovir or valcyclovir can reduce the severity and duration of the outbreak. Standard analgesic therapy with acetaminophen or ibuprofen, careful monitoring of hydration status, and aggressive early rehydration therapy are usually sufficient to avoid hospitalization. Although long-term suppression of orolabial herpes has not been addressed by clinical trials, episodic prophylaxis has been studied because of the predictable trigger effect of UV radiation. Short-term prophylactic therapy with acyclovir may be desirable in some patients who anticipate intense exposure to UV light (e.g., skiers or those who work outdoors), although the clinical effect may vary. Early treatment of recurrent orolabial HSV infection with high doses of antiviral medication has been found to markedly decrease the size and duration of lesions.

Emmert EH. Treatment of common cutaneous herpes simplex infections. *Am Fam Physician.* 2000;61:1697–1704, 1705–1706, 1708.

360. Vegan diets differ from vegetarian diets in that

A) vegetarian diets can lead to iron deficiency
B) vegans avoid all animal products in their diets
C) vegan diets allow for consumption of eggs and their products
D) vegetarians rarely satisfy nutritional needs

Answer and Discussion

The answer is B. Vegetarian diets differ according to the degree of avoidance of foods of animal origin. According to the traditional definition, a vegetarian diet consists primarily of cereals, fruits, vegetables, legumes, and nuts; animal foods, including milk, dairy products, and eggs are generally excluded. Several less restrictive vegetarian diets may include animal flesh, eggs, or milk and dairy products. Vegan diets are more rigid in that all animal products, including eggs, milk, and milk products, are excluded from the diet. Some vegans do not use honey and may refrain from using animal products such as leather or wool. They also may avoid foods that are processed or not organically grown. Vegetarian diets usually satisfy nutritional needs for growth and development if they are carefully planned with attention to the following possible limiting nutrients: energy, protein, iron, zinc, calcium, vitamin D, vitamin B_{12} (cyanocobalamin), and dietary fiber.

Johnston PK. Vegetarians among us: Implications for health professionals. *Top Clin Nutr.* 1995;10:1.

Vegan diets are more rigid than vegetarian diets in that all animal products, including eggs, milk, and milk products, are excluded from the diet.

361. In assessing the risk of coronary artery disease (CAD), a diet with high levels of __________ would increase the patient's risk.
A) trans-fatty acids
B) polyunsaturated fatty acids
C) monounsaturated fatty acids
D) polysaccharides

Answer and Discussion

The answer is A. Diet plays an important role in the risk of coronary heart disease (CHD). Higher cholesterol levels show a consistent relationship with the incidence of CHD. The type of fat consumed appears to be more important than the amount of total fat. Based on current knowledge, trans-fatty acids increase risk of CHD, while polyunsaturated fat and monounsaturated fat decrease risk. Additionally, an increase in carbohydrates tends to reduce the serum level of high-density lipoprotein (HDL) cholesterol in addition to total and low-density lipoprotein (LDL) cholesterol. Thus, the reduction in CHD risk may be less than predicted by the effect of saturated fat alone on cholesterol levels. Diets with a high glycemic load also decrease the serum HDL concentration. The major sources of trans-fats include margarines and partially hydrogenated vegetable fats. These fats are present in many manufactured foods (e.g., store-bought bread and cookies). Another major source is oils that are maintained at high temperatures for a sustained period of time, such as in fast food restaurants where oils are used to fry meat and potatoes.

Trans fatty acids and coronary heart disease risk. Report of the expert panel on trans fatty acids and coronary heart disease. *Am J Clin Nutr.* 1995;62:655S.

Hooper L, Summerbell CD, Higgins JP, et al. Reduced or modified dietary fat for preventing cardiovascular disease (Cochrane Review). *Cochrane Database Syst Rev.* 2001;3:CD002137.

362. A 40-year-old woman who is otherwise healthy presents to your office complaining of a lump in her neck. On examination, she is found to have a firm 2-cm nodule associated with the left lobe of the thyroid gland. Appropriate management at this time includes
A) ultrasound of the thyroid
B) thyroid uptake scan
C) fine-needle aspiration
D) radiation ablation
E) surgical excision

Answer and Discussion

The answer is C. Thyroid nodules are frequently encountered by family physicians. The majority of these are benign; however, children and the elderly have a higher incidence of malignancy. Previous studies have found that the prevalence of thyroid carcinoma was similar (i.e., approximately 5%) in palpable and nonpalpable nodules. Nearly all single thyroid nodules should be evaluated with needle aspiration biopsy. Ultrasonographically guided fine-needle aspiration biopsy of thyroid nodules should be performed if the patient has a history of radiation to the head, neck, or upper chest or a family history of thyroid carcinoma; the diameter of the nodule is 1.0 cm or greater; or suspicious ultrasonographic characteristics are present. In the absence of these findings, follow-up every 6 to 12 months is appropriate, because most occult carcinomas are papillary and rarely aggressive. Calcifications associated with thyroid nodules suggest the presence of psammoma bodies, which are associated with papillary carcinoma. TSH-suppressive therapy for benign solitary thyroid nodules is controversial. The effectiveness of such therapy in reducing nodule size is uncertain. Suppressive therapy is more appropriate for younger patients. Older patients may experience a decrease in bone mineral density or increase the risk of atrial fibrillation and cardiac hypertrophy.

Welker MJ, Orlov D. Thyroid nodules. *Am Fam Physician.* 2003;67:559–566, 573–574.

363. Which of the following effects is associated with selective estrogen receptor modulators?
A) Estrogen-like effects on endometrium
B) Estrogen-like effects on lipids
C) Estrogen antagonistic effects on bone
D) Estrogen-like effects on the breast
E) Decreased risk of thromboembolic events

Answer and Discussion

The answer is B. Raloxifene (Evista) is a selective estrogen receptor modulator that produces estrogen-agonistic effects on bone and lipid metabolism and estrogen-antagonistic effects on uterine endometrium and breast tissue. Because of its tissue selectivity, raloxifene may have fewer side effects than are typically observed with estrogen therapy. The most common adverse effects of raloxifene are hot flushes and leg cramps. The drug is also associated with an increased risk of thromboembolic events. The beneficial estrogenic activities of raloxifene include a lowering of total and LDL cholesterol levels and an augmentation of bone mineral density. Raloxifene has been labeled by the U.S. FDA for the prevention of osteoporosis. Studies are also being conducted to determine its impact on breast and endometrial cancer reduction.

Selective estrogen receptor modulators. Washington, D.C.: American College of Obstetricians and Gynecologists, 2002. Accessed online May 27, 2005, at: http://www.ngc.gov/summary/summary.aspx?ss=15&doc_id=3987.

364. A 68-year-old retired fisherman presents to your office complaining of a lesion that developed on the dorsal aspect of his hand over the last few months. Inspection of the lesion shows a dome-shaped lesion measuring 2 cm in diameter. The volcano-shaped lesion has a protruding mass of keratin. The most likely diagnosis is
A) basal cell carcinoma
B) keratoacanthoma
C) sebaceous cyst
D) malignant melanoma
E) dermatofibroma

Answer and Discussion

The answer is B. Keratoacanthoma appears as a skin-colored or pink smooth lesion that becomes dome-shaped during a period of very rapid growth. Onset is rapid; usually within 1 to 2 months the lesion reaches its full size. Common sites include the face, dorsum of the hands, and forearms. When mature, it is volcano-shaped, with protruding masses of keratin resembling lava. Classic keratoacanthoma is not malignant and regresses spontaneously, but atypical lesions may actually be squamous cell carcinoma. Many dermatopathologists include keratoacanthoma in the spectrum of squamous cell carcinoma. Total excision is the preferred treatment for most solitary keratoacanthomas. For smaller lesions, electrodesiccation and curettage or blunt dissection is sufficient. Mohs' surgery can be used in difficult areas, especially around the nose and ears. Alternative therapies include oral isotretinoin, topical (Effudex) and intralesional (Adrucil) fluorouracil, intralesional methotrexate (Rheumatrex), and intralesional 5-interferon alfa-2a (Roferon-A). Radiotherapy is an option for patients with recurrence or larger lesions.

Luba MC, Bangs SA, Mohler AM, et al. Common benign skin tumors. *Am Fam Physician*. 2003;67:729–738.

365. In a placebo-controlled trial involving 100 patients, 30 died during the study period (10 receiving active drug and 20 receiving placebo), giving a mortality of 20% with active drug versus 40% with placebo. The number needed to treat (NNT) is
A) 5
B) 10
C) 25
D) 50
E) 100

Answer and Discussion

The answer is A. The benefit of an intervention can be expressed by the "number needed to treat" (NNT). NNT is the reciprocal of the absolute risk reduction (the absolute adverse event rate for placebo minus the absolute adverse event rate for treated patients). From a practical standpoint, an NNT interpretation can be shown by the following statement: "This study suggests that I would have to treat five patients with a drug to prevent one death." As an example, consider a placebo-controlled trial involving 100 patients. Thirty patients died during the study period (10 receiving active drug and 20 receiving placebo), giving a mortality rate of 20% with active drug [10 divided by (10 + 40)], versus 40% [20 divided by (20 + 30)] with placebo. The difference between these two rates, the "risk difference," is used to calculate NNT.

40% minus 20% = 20% = 0.2
1 divided by 0.2 = 5

Thus, this study suggests that only five patients need to be treated with the drug (compared with placebo) to prevent one death.

Bonis PAL. Glossary of common biostatistical and epidemiological terms. Accessed from Up to Date 9/19/2005 at http://uptodateonline.com.

366. The test of choice for screening for hereditary hemochromatosis is
A) aspartate aminotransferase (AST)
B) serum ferritin
C) transferrin saturation
D) total iron
E) total iron binding capacity

Answer and Discussion

The answer is C. Initial screening of individuals with suspected iron overload and those over the age of 20 years who are first-degree relatives of known cases of hereditary hemochromatosis should be done by measurement of transferrin saturation after an overnight fast. Simultaneous serum ferritin determination increases the predictive accuracy for diagnosis of iron overload. Transferrin saturation is also the test of choice for screening the general adult population for iron overload states.

Tavill AS. AASLD guideline: diagnosis and management of hemochromatosis. *Hepatology*. 2001;33:1321.

367. Mad cow disease (bovine spongiform encephalopathy [BSE]) has symptoms similar to which of the following conditions?
A) Lyme disease
B) Syphilis
C) Chronic fatigue syndrome
D) Malaria
E) Creutzfeldt-Jakob disease

Answer and Discussion

The answer is E. The FDA Center for Veterinary Medicine is responsible for protection against animal feed that can affect the safety of derived human food. In recent years, the spread of BSE, the so-called mad cow disease, in foreign countries has prompted the Center for Veterinary Medicine to place restrictions on the production of several types of feed. The action was based on research indicating that BSE is transferred among cows through feed made from the rendered carcasses of cattle that contain a prion that has been linked to BSE. The seriousness of the problem was magnified by the emergence in the United Kingdom of the human illness "new-variant Creutzfeldt-Jakob disease," which gave rise to a theory that BSE can be transferred to humans. Because of the potential risk of transmission, the Center for Veterinary Medicine has banned the use of mammalian tissues such as meat, bone meal, meat byproducts, and cooked bone marrow in feed for cattle and other ruminant animals. The implementation of the ban is verified through intensive inspection of rendering plants and feed manufacturers.

U.S. Food and Drug Administration. A proposed framework for evaluating and assuring the human safety of the microbial effects of antimicrobial new animal drugs intended for use in food-producing animals. Center for Veterinary Medicine. Available at: http://www.fda.gov/cvm. Accessed June 22, 2000.

368. Charcot foot is most commonly seen in patients with
A) gonorrhea
B) primary syphilis
C) rheumatoid arthritis
D) diabetes mellitus
E) neurofibromatosis

Answer and Discussion

The answer is D. First described in patients with tertiary syphilis, Charcot foot is now seen mostly in patients with diabetes mellitus. It is a condition of acute or gradual onset and, in its most severe form, causes significant disruption of the bony architecture of the foot. It often results in foot deformities and causes abnormal pressure distribution on the plantar surface, foot ulcers, and, in some cases, requires amputation. The exact pathogenesis is unknown, but underlying sensory neuropathy is nearly universal. Arteriovenous shunting due to autonomic neuropathy is also thought to play a role. Repeated unrecognized microtrauma or an identifiable injury may be the inciting factors of Charcot foot. Approximately 50% of patients with Charcot foot remember a precipitating event such as a slip or a trip, or they may have had unrelated surgery on the foot as an antecedent event. In approximately 25% of patients, a similar problem ultimately develops on the other foot. Clinical findings in patients with an acute Charcot process include warmth, erythema, and swelling, and the disease is often thought to be cellulitis. Pain and tenderness are usually absent because of sensory neuropathy, which is universal and is probably a component of the basic pathogenesis of the Charcot foot. However, because patients with Charcot foot may have some pain if the sensory loss is not complete, the presence of pain does not totally exclude the diagnosis. Such pain is always much less than would be expected for the severity of the clinical and/or radiographic findings. Although cellulitis should be considered in any patient with diabetes, missing the diagnosis of Charcot foot can be serious, because failure to initiate proper treatment of the Charcot foot can lead to total loss of function. Inappropriate treatment with antimicrobial therapy and even incision and drainage can lead to unnecessary complications. Minimal pain or the absence of pain (characteristic of a Charcot fracture) can lead patients and physicians to ignore this serious disease. The initial radiographic findings can be normal, making the diagnosis difficult, but if a Charcot foot is strongly suspected from the clinical presentation, treatment should be initiated and serial radiographs should be taken. The proper treatment for a hot, swollen foot in a patient with sensory neuropathy is immobilization. Most cases of Charcot foot can be treated nonsurgically with pressure-relieving methods such as total contact casting (TCC), which is considered to be the gold standard of treatment.

Sommer TC, Lee TH. Charcot foot: the diagnostic dilemma. *Am Fam Physician.* 2001;64:1591–1598.

While cellulitis should be considered in any patient with diabetes, missing the diagnosis of Charcot foot can be serious, because failure to initiate proper treatment of the Charcot foot can lead to total loss of function.

369. A 38-year-old describes severe rectal pain associated with pallor, diaphoresis, and tachycardia that lasts for only a few minutes. The pains occur mostly at night and are described as spasms. The most likely diagnosis is

A) thrombosed hemorrhoids
B) irritable bowel syndrome
C) ulcerative colitis
D) gay bowel syndrome
E) proctalgia fugax

Answer and Discussion

The answer is E. Proctalgia fugax is a unique anal pain. Patients with proctalgia fugax experience severe episodes of spasm-like pain that often occur at night. Proctalgia fugax may only occur once a year, or may be sporadic in waves of three or four times per week. Each episode lasts only minutes, but the pain is severe and may be accompanied by sweating, pallor, and tachycardia. Patients experience urgency to defecate, yet pass no stool. No specific etiology has been found, but proctalgia fugax may be associated with spastic contractions of the rectum or the muscular pelvic floor in irritable bowel syndrome. Other unproven associations are food allergies, especially to artificial sweeteners or caffeine. Reassurance that the condition is benign may be helpful, but little can be done to treat proctalgia fugax. Medications are not helpful, because the episode is likely to be over before the drugs become active. Sitting in a tub of hot water or, alternatively, applying ice may provide symptomatic relief. A low dose of diazepam (Valium) at bedtime may be beneficial in cases of frequent and disabling proctalgia fugax.

Pfenninger JL, Zainea GG. Common anorectal conditions: Part I. Symptoms and complaints. *Am Fam Physician.* 2001; 63:2391–2398.

370. The procedure of choice for detecting osteomyelitis in diabetic foot ulcers is

A) plain films
B) CT scan
C) MRI
D) technetium bone scan
E) indium scan

Answer and Discussion

The answer is C. Although plain films of the feet are usually ordered initially, magnetic resonance imaging (MRI) is the imaging procedure of choice for osteomyelitis in diabetic foot ulcers. The following values for sensitivity and specificity were obtained in a study in which 19 patients with diabetic foot infection underwent all four of the following imaging studies; 9 had osteomyelitis on bone biopsy: MRI (88% and 100%), plain radiography (22% and 94%), technetium bone scan (50% and 50%), and indium scan (33% and 69%). MRI can show abnormal bone marrow signal, soft tissue masses, and cortical destruction characteristic of osteomyelitis. Unlike plain films, MRI can detect these changes early (within days) in infection. MRI also provides the anatomic detail, necessary when surgical debridement is required.

Croll SD, Nicholas GG, Osborne MA, et al. Role of magnetic resonance imaging in the diagnosis of osteomyelitis in diabetic foot infections. *J Vasc Surg.* 1996;24:266.

Beers MH, Porter RS, eds. *The Merck manual of diagnosis and therapy,* Merck Research Laboratories, 18th ed. Whitehouse Station, NJ: Merck & Co.; 2006:317–318.

371. The *BRCA* genetic locus has been linked with all of following cancers *except*

A) breast cancer
B) ovarian cancer
C) prostate cancer
D) colon cancer
E) gastric cancer

Answer and Discussion

The answer is E. Discovered in the 1980s, *BRCA1* is a gene on chromosome 17 that is known to be involved in tumor suppression. A woman with certain known mutations in *BRCA1* has an increased risk for breast cancer and ovarian cancer. There is a higher risk in Ashkenazi Jewish women (most Jewish people in the United States are of this Eastern European origin). *BRCA2* is another susceptibility gene for breast cancer and is found on chromosome 13. Mutations in *BRCA2* confer an elevated breast cancer risk similar to that occurring with *BRCA1* mutations. As with *BRCA1*, *BRCA2* mutations are also found in a higher percentage of

Ashkenazi Jewish women. Mutations in *BRCA1* and *BRCA2* are associated with early-onset breast cancer. As many as one-third of women under age 29 years with breast cancer carry a *BRCA1* or -2 mutation, but only 2% of women ages 70 to 79 years with breast cancer carry such a mutation. Genetic studies in high-risk families suggest that *BRCA1* and -2 mutations may account for 50% of inherited breast and ovarian cancers and are also associated with an increase in prostate and colon cancers. A task force organized by the National Institutes of Health and the National Human Genome Research Institute proposed recommendations for monitoring known carriers of *BRCA1* and -2 mutations. The consensus panel acknowledged the lack of proven benefit for early screening, but suggested that known carriers should begin performing monthly breast self-examinations at age 18 years and should begin having annual clinical examinations at age 25 years. Annual mammography was also recommended beginning at age 25 years. The panel noted that "insufficient evidence [exists] to recommend for or against prophylactic mastectomy." Even this invasive procedure does not appear to provide definitive treatment, as cases have been reported of breast cancer occurring after bilateral mastectomies. Women who have a family history of breast cancer under age 50 years, two first-degree relatives with the disease, a male relative with breast cancer, or ovarian cancer in relatives under age 50 years are at increased risk for carrying a *BRCA1* or -2 mutation. These women should be offered genetic counseling. Currently, the U.S. Preventive Services Task Force (USPSTF) recommends against routine referral for genetic counseling or routine breast cancer susceptibility gene (*BRCA*) testing for women whose family history is *not* associated with an increased risk for deleterious mutations in breast cancer susceptibility gene 1 (*BRCA1*) or breast cancer susceptibility gene 2 (*BRCA2*). Additionally, the USPSTF recommends that women whose family history is associated with an increased risk for deleterious mutations in *BRCA1* or *BRCA2* genes be referred for genetic counseling and evaluation for *BRCA* testing.

Burke W, Daly M, Garber J, et al. Recommendations for follow-up care of individuals with an inherited predisposition to cancer. II. BRCA1 and BRCA2. Cancer Genetics Studies Consortium. *JAMA*. 1997;277:997–1003.

U.S. Preventive Services Task Force (USPSTF). Genetic risk assessment and *BRCA* mutation testing for breast and ovarian cancer susceptibility. *Ann Intern Med*. 2005;143:355–361.

372. Which of the following statements regarding hepatitis C is correct?

A) Most patients are symptomatic with development of the disease.
B) The course of the disease shows no variability and is progressive.
C) Most patients develop chronic hepatitis.
D) The disease is not transferred through sexual contact.
E) Immune globulin is effective for post-exposure prophylaxis.

Answer and Discussion

The answer is C. Hepatitis C virus is the most common chronic blood-borne infection in the United States. The hepatitis C virus (HCV), identified in 1988 through molecular biologic techniques, is an enveloped RNA virus that is classified as a separate genus in the Flaviviridae family. The incubation period for newly acquired (acute) HCV infection ranges from 2 weeks to 6 months, with an average incubation period of 6 to 7 weeks. However, viral replication can be detected as early as 1 week after exposure. Of patients with acute HCV infection, 60% to 70% are asymptomatic; 20% to 30% have jaundice; and 10% to 20% have nonspecific symptoms such as loss of appetite, fatigue, and abdominal pain. The course of acute hepatitis C is variable, although its most characteristic feature is fluctuating, polyphasic ALT patterns. Normalization of ALT levels, which may occur, suggests full recovery, but is frequently followed by ALT elevations, indicating chronic liver disease. Most patients with acute HCV infection develop persistent infection; chronic hepatitis develops in an average of 70% of infected patients. No clinical features of the acute disease or risk factors for infection, including a history of percutaneous exposures, have been found to be predictive of chronicity. HCV is a blood-borne virus that is most efficiently transmitted through large or repeated percutaneous exposures to blood, such as transfusions or transplants from infected donors, inadvertent contamination of supplies shared among patients undergoing chronic hemodialysis, or sharing of equipment among injection drug users. Transmission of HCV may also occur through high-risk sex, perinatal exposure, percutaneous exposures in the health-care setting, or exposure to an infected household contact. The diagnosis of HCV infection can also be made through detection of HCV RNA using reverse transcriptase-polymerase chain reaction techniques. HCV RNA can be detected within 1 to 2 weeks after exposure to the virus, weeks before the onset of ALT elevations or the appearance of anti-HCV. In some patients, the detection of HCV RNA may be the only evidence of HCV infection. No tests are available to differentiate acute, chronic, and resolved infections, and the diagnosis of chronic hepatitis C is usually based on the presence of elevated ALT values in patients who are positive for anti-HCV. For anti-HCV-positive patients with a normal ALT value, the presence of ongoing liver inflammation should be assessed by monitoring serum ALT values several times over 6 to 12 months because abnormalities may be present only intermittently in patients with chronic hepatitis C. There is no vaccine to prevent HCV infection, and immune globulin is not effective for postexposure prophylaxis. A recent National Institutes of Health consensus conference recommended that all patients who have bridging hepatic fibrosis and moderate inflammation together with detectable viremia should receive treatment with pegylated interferon and ribavirin. These medications are very expensive and have significant side effects. Hematologic toxicities include anemia and leukopenia. These can be managed with close monitoring, use of growth factors, or dose reductions. Depression also can be caused or exacerbated by these medicines and may require treatment with a selective serotonin reuptake inhibitor, co-management with psychiatry, or cessation of pegylated interferon and ribavirin treatment. Contraception is imperative because ribavirin is highly teratogenic. Influenza-like symptoms of fatigue, nausea, and mild fevers can be helped by patient education and support including frequent office visits.

Moyer LA, Mast EE, Alter MJ. Hepatitis C: Parts I and II. Routine serologic testing and diagnosis, prevention counseling, and medical evaluation. *Am Fam Physician*. 1998;59:79–92.

Ward RP, Kugelmas M. Using pegylated interferon and ribavirin to treat patients with chronic hepatitis C. *Am Fam Physician*. 2005;72:655–662.

373. The most common cause of bacterial conjunctivitis in American adults is

A) *Streptococcus pneumoniae*
B) *Haemophilus influenzae*

C) *Chlamydia trachomatis*
D) *Staphylococcus aureus*
E) *Klebsiella*

Answer and Discussion

The answer is D. The conjunctiva is a thin, translucent, relatively elastic tissue layer with bulbar (outer aspect of the globe) and palpebral (inside of the eyelid) portions. Underneath the conjunctiva lie the episclera, sclera, and uveal tissue layers. Conjunctivitis is the most common cause of red eye. Most frequently, acute conjunctivitis is caused by a bacterial or viral infection. Sexually transmitted diseases such as chlamydia and gonorrhea are less common causes of conjunctivitis. Ocular allergy is one of the major causes of chronic conjunctivitis. Blepharitis (inflammation of the eyelid margin), dry eye, and the prolonged use of ophthalmic medications, contact lenses, and ophthalmic solutions are also frequent causes of chronic conjunctival inflammation. Adenovirus is by far the most common cause of viral conjunctivitis, although other viruses can also cause the condition. Viral conjunctivitis often occurs in community epidemics, with the virus transmitted in schools, workplaces, and physicians' offices. The usual modes of transmission are contaminated fingers, medical instruments, and swimming pool water. Patients with viral conjunctivitis typically present with an acutely red eye, watery discharge, conjunctival swelling, a tender preauricular node, and, in some cases, photophobia and a foreign-body sensation. Both eyes may be affected simultaneously, or the second eye may become involved a few days after the first eye. Some patients have an associated upper respiratory tract infection. Patients should be instructed to avoid direct contact with other persons for at least 1 week after the onset of symptoms. Treatment is supportive. Cold compresses and topical vasoconstrictors may provide symptomatic relief. Topical antibiotics are rarely necessary, because secondary bacterial infection is uncommon. The three most common pathogens in bacterial conjunctivitis are *S. pneumoniae, H. influenzae,* and *S. aureus*. Infections with *S. pneumoniae* and *H. influenzae* are more common in children, whereas *S. aureus* most frequently affects adults. Newer childhood immunizations for *H. influenzae* and *S. pneumoniae* further decrease the incidence of these causative organisms. Treatment requires good eyelid hygiene and the application of topical antibiotics. Empiric treatment with a topical medication is a safe and cost-effective approach in most patients with clinically mild acute bacterial conjunctivitis. Allergic conjunctivitis is distinguished by severe itching and allergen exposure. This condition is generally treated with topical antihistamines, mast-cell stabilizers, or anti-inflammatory agents. Pain and photophobia are not typical features of a primary conjunctival inflammatory process. If these features are present, the physician should consider more serious underlying ocular or orbital disease processes, including uveitis, keratitis, acute glaucoma, and orbital cellulitis. Similarly, blurred vision that fails to clear with a blink is rarely associated with conjunctivitis. Patients with pain, photophobia, or blurred vision should be referred to an ophthalmologist.

Morrow GL, Abbott RL. Conjunctivitis. *Am Fam Physician.* 1998; 57:735.

Beers MH, Porter RS, eds. *The Merck manual of diagnosis and therapy,* Merck Research Laboratories, 18th ed. Whitehouse Station, NJ: Merck & Co.; 2006:889–894.

374. β- Blockers
A) are not associated with depression
B) are not associated with fatigue
C) do not produce sexual related side effects
D) have been found to have significant side effects that limit their use

Answer and Discussion

The answer is A. Depression, fatigue, and sexual dysfunction are commonly cited side effects of β-blockers, and may represent reasons why use of β-blockers is lower than expected for some approved indications. However, these associations are primarily based on flawed studies. Thus, although beta blockers appear to cause small increases in the risk of fatigue and sexual dysfunction, the risk is much lower than previously thought, and beta blockers should not be withheld based on concerns about developing these adverse effects. Additionally, there was no significant increased risk of reported depressive symptoms when taking β-blockers.

Ko DT, Hebert PR, Coffey CS, et al. Beta-blocker therapy and symptoms of depression, fatigue, and sexual dysfunction. *JAMA.* 2002;288:351.

375. Which of the following drugs is a leukotriene antagonist/inhibitor?
A) Theophylline
B) Prednisone
C) Salmeterol
D) Terbutaline
E) Zafirlukast

Answer and Discussion

The answer is E. Medications used in the treatment of asthma are divided into long-term control medications that are taken regularly and quick-relief (rescue) medications that are taken as needed to relieve bronchoconstriction rapidly. Long-term control medications include anti-inflammatory agents [i.e., corticosteroids, cromolyn sodium (Intal), nedocromil (Tilade), and leukotriene modifiers] and long-acting bronchodilators. Quick-relief medications include short-acting β2 agonists, anticholinergics, and systemic corticosteroids. Patients with persistent asthma require treatment with long-term control and quick-relief medications. Corticosteroids remain the most potent and effective anti-inflammatory agents available for the management of asthma. They are useful in treating all types of persistent asthma in patients of all ages. For long-term use, inhaled steroids are preferred over oral steroids, because the inhaled agents have fewer systemic side effects. Oral steroid therapy for long-term control is usually used only to treat refractory, severe, persistent asthma. Cromolyn and nedocromil are very safe agents with a mild to moderate anti-inflammatory effect. Both drugs inhibit the early- and late-phase asthmatic response to allergens and exercise. Nedocromil appears to be more effective than cromolyn in inhibiting bronchospasm induced by exercise, cold air, and provocative testing. Because of their excellent safety profiles, cromolyn and nedocromil are good initial long-term control medications in children and pregnant women with mild persistent asthma. Salmeterol (Serevent) is a long-acting β2 agonist. Its mechanism of action and side effect profile are similar to those of other β2 agonists. Unlike the short-acting agents, salmeterol is not intended for use as a quick-relief agent. It should not be used as a single agent for long-term control but instead should be used in combination with inhaled corticosteroids or other anti-inflammatory agents. Newer recommendations suggest limitation of its use in favor of inhaled corticosteroids. Albuterol (Proventil Repetabs, Volmax) is available as an oral, extended-release tablet for the long-term control of asthma. Like salmeterol, this long-acting β2 agonist is not intended to be used as a rescue medication. It is an alternative to sustained-release theophylline or inhaled salmeterol, especially in patients who have nocturnal asthma despite treatment with high-dose anti-inflammatory agents. Theophylline, once the mainstay of asthma treatment, is now considered a second- or third-line agent because of its adverse effect profile and potential interactions with many drugs. Furthermore, serum theophylline levels have to be monitored during treatment. In addition to its well-known bronchodilator effects, theophylline has anti-inflammatory activity. Currently, theophylline therapy is generally reserved for use in patients who exhibit nocturnal asthma symptoms that are not controlled with high-dose anti-inflammatory medications. Zafirlukast (Accolate) and zileuton (Zyflo) are two new drugs that antagonize the action of leukotrienes at their receptor (zafirlukast) or inhibit the lipoxygenase pathway (zileuton). Both drugs are approved for the management of chronic asthma in adults and in children older than 12 years. Zafirlukast and zileuton have numerous drug interactions. Short-acting inhaled β2 agonists are the agents of choice for relieving bronchospasms and preventing exercise-induced bronchospasms. Selective β2 agonists, including albuterol, bitolterol (Tornalate), metaproterenol (Alupent), pirbuterol (Maxair), and terbutaline (Brethaire), are preferred to nonselective β agonists such as epinephrine, ephedrine, and isoproterenol (Isuprel), because the selective agents have fewer cardiovascular side effects and a longer duration of action. Inhaled β2 agonists have a rapid onset of action. Short-term systemic corticosteroid therapy is useful for gaining initial control of asthma and for treating moderate to severe asthma exacerbations. The intravenous administration of systemic corticosteroids offers no advantage over oral administration when GI absorption is not impaired. Ipratropium (Atrovent) is a quaternary atropine derivative that inhibits vagal-mediated bronchoconstriction. It may be useful as an adjunct to inhaled β2 agonists in patients who have severe asthma exacerbations or who cannot tolerate β2 agonists.

Gross KM, Ponte CD. New strategies in the medical management of asthma. *Am Fam Physician*. 1998;58:89.

376. The most common primary cancer of the bone in adults is
A) multiple myeloma
B) osteosarcoma
C) osteoid osteoma
D) osteitis fibrosa cystica
E) metastatic prostate cancer

Answer and Discussion

The answer is A. Multiple myeloma is the malignant proliferation of plasma cells involving more than 10% of the bone marrow. Multiple myeloma is the most common primary cancer of the bones in adults. The median age at diagnosis of multiple myeloma is 62 years. Only 2% to 3% of cases are reported in patients younger than 30 years. African Americans in the United States are twice as likely to develop multiple myeloma as Whites.

The multiple myeloma cell produces monoclonal immunoglobulins that may be identified on serum or urine protein electrophoresis. Bone pain related to multiple lytic lesions is the most common clinical presentation. However, up to 30% of patients are diagnosed incidentally while being evaluated for unrelated problems, and one-third of patients are diagnosed after a pathologic fracture, commonly of the axial skeleton. Multiple myeloma must be differentiated from other causes of monoclonal gammopathy, including monoclonal gammopathy of undetermined significance, heavy chain disease, plasmacytoma, and Waldenstrom macroglobulinemia. Routine laboratory workup may show pancytopenia, abnormal coagulation, hypercalcemia, azotemia, elevated alkaline phosphatase and ESR, and hypoalbuminemia. Examination may reveal proteinuria, hypercalciuria, or both. Urine dipstick tests may not indicate the presence of Bence Jones proteinuria. All patients with suspected multiple myeloma require a 24-hour urinalysis by protein electrophoresis to determine the presence of Bence Jones proteinuria and kappa or lambda light chains. Serum protein electrophoresis identifies an M protein as a narrow peak or "spike" in the γ, β, or α2 regions of the densitometer tracing. Chemotherapy with melphalan and prednisone is the standard treatment for multiple myeloma. Other treatment modalities include polychemotherapy (thalidomide, immunomodulatory drugs, proteasome inhibitors) and bone marrow transplantation. Only 50% to 60% of patients respond to therapy. The aggregate median survival for all stages of multiple myeloma is 3 to 5 years.

George ED, Sadovsky R. Multiple myeloma: recognition and management. *Am Fam Physician*. 1999;59:1890.

377. A 21-year-old returns from a camping trip early complaining of a dull numbness affecting his upper left extremity. He recalls a sharp pinprick sensation before the development of symptoms. The patient now describes a cramping pain and muscle rigidity of the back and chest area. A red, indurated area is found on the distal left arm. The patient has profuse sweating, nausea, vomiting, and shortness of breath. The likely diagnosis is
A) Lyme disease
B) tick paralysis
C) malaria
D) black widow spider envenomation
E) Rocky Mountain spotted fever

Answer and Discussion

The answer is D. Black widow spider bites are associated with a sharp, pinprick-like pain, followed by a dull, sometimes numbing pain in the affected extremity and by cramping pain and muscular rigidity in the abdomen or the shoulders, back, and chest. Associated manifestations may include severe abdominal pain, restlessness, anxiety, sweating, headache, dizziness, ptosis, eyelid edema, rash and pruritus, respiratory distress, nausea, vomiting, salivation, weakness, and increased skin temperature over the affected area. Blood pressure and CSF pressure are usually elevated in more severe cases in adults. An ice cube may be placed over a black widow spider bite to reduce pain. Patients younger than 16 years or older than 60 years, those with hypertensive cardiovascular disease, or those with symptoms and signs of severe envenomation should be hospitalized and, when symptomatic treatment is unsuccessful, should be given antivenin. Antivenin must be given within 30 minutes and the manufacturer recommends skin testing prior to administration (however, skin testing does not always predict anaphylaxis). Children may require respiratory assistance. Vital signs should be checked frequently during the 12 hours after the bite. In the elderly, acute hypertension may require treatment. For muscle pain and spasms, intravenous calcium gluconate may be given slowly and requires cardiac monitoring. Several doses at 4-hour intervals may be necessary.

Beers MH, Porter RS, eds. *The Merck manual of diagnosis and therapy,* Merck Research Laboratories, 18th ed. Whitehouse Station, NJ: Merck & Co.; 2006:2649.

378. A 75-year-old man presents to your office complaining of flashes of light and blurred vision. He reports no pain. In-office examination reveals no findings other than decreased visual acuity. Appropriate management consists of

A) patching of the affected eye
B) course of oral steroids
C) ultrasound of the carotids
D) initiation of aspirin therapy
E) immediate ophthalmology referral

Answer and Discussion

The answer is E. Retinal detachment can occur as the result of a retinal tear (occurs more frequently in myopia, after cataract surgery, or after ocular trauma), by detachment without a tear as a result of vitreal traction (seen in proliferative retinopathy of diabetes or sickle cell disease), or by transudation of fluid into the subretinal space (e.g., severe uveitis or primary or metastatic choroidal tumors). Retinal detachment is painless. Early symptoms may include dark or irregular vitreous floaters, flashes of light, or blurred vision. As the detachment progresses, the patient notices a curtain or veil in the field of vision. If the macula is involved, central visual acuity is significantly affected. Direct ophthalmoscopy may show retinal irregularities and a retinal elevation with darkened blood vessels. Indirect ophthalmoscopy, including scleral depression, is necessary for detecting peripheral breaks and detachment. If a vitreous hemorrhage obscures the retina, especially in myopia, postcataract extraction, or eye injury, retinal detachment should be suspected and B-scan ultrasonography performed. Although often localized, retinal detachments due to retinal tears can expand to involve the entire retina if not treated promptly. Any patient with a suspected or established retinal detachment should be seen urgently by an ophthalmologist.

Beers MH, Porter RS, eds. *The Merck manual of diagnosis and therapy.* Merck Research Laboratories, 18th ed. Whitehouse Station, NJ: Merck & Co.; 2006:919–920.

> Retinal detachment is painless. Early symptoms may include dark or irregular vitreous floaters, flashes of light, or blurred vision. As the detachment progresses, the patient notices a curtain or veil in the field of vision.

379. Which of the following statements concerning diarrhea in the United States is true?

A) Diarrhea is defined as frequent stools with >30% of stool mass in liquid.
B) Traveler's diarrhea is caused by a virus in most cases.
C) Pathogens are not identifiable in more than 50% of cases of diarrhea.
D) The goal of treatment is eradication of the causative agent.
E) Resistance to antimicrobial agents is not a concern with treatment of diarrhea.

Answer and Discussion

The answer is C. *Diarrhea* is defined as watery or liquid stools, usually with increases in daily frequency and in total stool weight (e.g., >300 g/day). In Western countries, stool amounts are typically 100 to 300 g/day in healthy adults. Infants typically produce 10g/kg/day. The pathogens that commonly cause sporadic diarrhea in adults in developed countries are *Campylobacter, Salmonella,* and *Shigella* species; *E. coli; Yersinia* species; protozoa; and viruses. However, pathogens are not identifiable in more than one-half of cases. Traveler's diarrhea is caused by bacteria in approximately 80% of patients. Common pathogens are enterogenic *E. coli, Salmonella, Shigella, Campylobacter, Vibrio, Yersinia,* and *Aeromonas* species. Death from diarrhea is rare, but infants, elderly patients, and those in long-term care facilities are at greater risk. The goals of treatment include reducing the infectious period, length of illness, risk of transmission to others, risk of dehydration, and rates of severe illness. Empiric treatment of traveler's diarrhea shortened the length of illness, although it was occasionally associated with prolonged presence of the causative pathogen in the stool and the development of resistant strains. Empiric treatment of community-acquired diarrhea with ciprofloxacin shortened the length of illness by 1 to 2 days. Development of resistant strains occurred with the use of some antibiotics but not with others. Adverse effects were similar to those noted for traveler's diarrhea.

de Bruyn G. Infectious disease: diarrhea. *West J Med.* 2000; 172:409–412.

Herbert ME. Medical myths. Measuring white blood cells in the stools is useful in the management of acute diarrhea. *West J Med.* 2000;172:414.

380. A 25-year-old HIV patient presents with pain associated with his gums. He has also noted bleeding of his gums when he brushes his teeth. The most likely severe complication of this condition is

A) necrotizing ulcerative gingivitis
B) plaque deposition
C) dental caries
D) glossitis
E) bacterial endocarditis

Answer and Discussion

The answer is A. HIV-infected persons may present with various periodontal diseases, from mild inflammation (HIV gingivitis) to localized acute necrotizing ulcerative gingivitis and from localized periodontitis to necrotizing stomatitis. Patients with HIV gingivitis present with a bright erythematous line along the gingival margin and complain of spontaneous bleeding. In acute necrotizing ulcerative gingivitis, the gingiva appears erythematous, with ulcerations of the papillae that become tender and bleed when teeth are brushed. Rapid bone and soft tissue loss and loosening teeth are characteristic of HIV periodontitis. Patients complain of "deep" pain, and the condition can rapidly progress to large areas of necrotizing stomatitis. Patients affected with HIV gingivitis should be referred to an oral surgeon for débridement, scaling, and curettage of the involved areas. This treatment is followed by administration of metronidazole (Flagyl), irrigation with povidone iodine, and daily mouth rinsing with chlorhexidine gluconate (Peridex). Because it may potentiate peripheral neuropathy, metronidazole should not be given to patients taking didanosine (Videx) or zalcitabine (Hivid). In these patients clindamycin (Cleocin) or amoxicillin may be used.

Moazzez AH, Alvi A. Head and neck manifestations of AIDS in adults. *Am Fam Physician.* 1998;57:1813.

381. Which of the following medications would be most effective to treat postmenopausal flushing?

A) Venlafaxine
B) Amitryptyline
C) Green tea

D) Trazadone
E) Propanolol

Answer and Discussion

The answer is A. The selective serotonin reuptake inhibitors (SSRIs) including paroxetine (Paxil) and venlafaxine (Effexor) have been used to relieve the symptoms of vasomotor instability (hot flushes) associated with menopause and are considered first line therapy in women who are not taking estrogen. Their efficacy has been demonstrated in a number of randomized trials.

Loprinzi CL, Kugler JW, Sloan JA, et al. Venlafaxine in management of hot flashes in survivors of breast cancer: a randomised controlled trial. *Lancet*. 2000;356:2059.

Stearns V, Beebe KL, Iyengar M, et al. E. Paroxetine controlled release in the treatment of menopausal hot flashes: a randomized controlled trial. *JAMA*. 2003;289:2827.

382. Patients with antithrombin deficiency are at increased risk for
A) myelodysplasia
B) thrombosis
C) multiple myeloma
D) vitamin K deficiency
E) bleeding complications while taking warfarin

Answer and Discussion

The answer is B. Antithrombin is a protein that inhibits thrombin and factors Xa, IXa, and XIa. Deficiency of plasma antithrombin is inherited in an autosomal-dominant fashion with a prevalence of approximately 0.2% to 0.4%; approximately one-half of these persons experience venous thrombotic episodes. Acquired deficiencies in antithrombin levels are observed in patients with acute thrombosis, disseminated intravascular coagulation, liver disease, or nephrotic syndrome and during heparin therapy, estrogen therapy (including contraceptive use), or L-asparaginase therapy. Homozygous deficiency is usually lethal to the fetus in utero. Laboratory screening involves quantification of plasma inhibition of thrombin in the presence of heparin. Oral anticoagulation with warfarin is highly effective prophylaxis for patients who have experienced or are at risk of thrombosis.

Beers MH, Porter RS, eds. *The Merck manual of diagnosis and therapy,* Merck Research Laboratories, 18th ed. Whitehouse Station, NJ: Merck & Co.; 2006:1082.

383. An essential tremor most commonly affects the
A) head
B) voice
C) tongue
D) legs
E) hands

Answer and Discussion

The answer is E. Tremor is a symptom of many disorders, including Parkinson's disease, essential tremor, orthostatic tremor, cerebellar disease, peripheral neuropathy, and alcohol withdrawal. Tremors may be classified as postural, rest, or action tremors. Symptomatic treatment is directed to the tremor type:

- *Parkinson's tremor.* The tremor in Parkinson's disease occurs at rest and is characterized by a frequency of 4 to 6 Hz and medium amplitude. It is classically referred to as a *pill rolling* tremor of the hands, but can also affect the head, trunk, jaw, and lips. Combination therapy with carbidopa and levodopa is commonly used for Parkinsonian tremor.
- *Essential tremor.* Essential tremor is the most common movement disorder. Its onset occurs anywhere between the second and sixth decades of life and its prevalence increases with age. The tremor is usually bilateral. The tremor is minimal or absent at rest. The tremor is slowly progressive over a period of years, and the specific pathophysiology of essential tremor remains unknown. Essential tremor occurs sporadically or can be inherited (in 50% of patients, inheritance is autosomal dominant). It most commonly affects the hands, but can also affect the head, voice, tongue, and legs. In many cases, essential tremor is alleviated by small amounts of alcohol, an effect not found in Parkinson's disease. Essential tremor may be amenable to propranolol or primidone.
- *Other tremors.* Propranolol may be useful in treating alcohol withdrawal tremor, and INH may control the cerebellar tremor associated with multiple sclerosis. Clonazepam may relieve orthostatic tremor. Other agents are also available for the treatment of tremor. When medical therapy fails to control the tremor, surgical options such as thalamotomy, pallidotomy, and thalamic stimulation should be considered in severe cases. Thalamic stimulation, the most recent of these surgical approaches, offers the advantage over ablative procedures of alleviating tremor without the creation of a permanent lesion.

Charles PD, Esper GJ, Davis TL, et al. Classification of tremor and update on treatment. *Am Fam Physician.* 1999;59: 1565–1572.

384. Which of the following statements is true regarding firearm-related injuries?
A) The incidence has risen significantly over the last few years.
B) Most of the nonfatal injuries occurring in adult men ages 15 to 44 years were inflicted by others.
C) The rates for African-American and Hispanic individuals have decreased.
D) Law enforcement practices have not affected the incidence.
E) Increases in the cocaine market have attributed to increases in firearm injuries.

Answer and Discussion

The answer is C. The overall annual rates of nonfatal and fatal firearm-related injuries in the United States declined consistently from 1993 to 1997. The annual nonfatal rate decreased by 40.8%. The annual mortality rate also declined by 21.1%. The declines in the rates of nonfatal and fatal firearm-related injury were generally consistent across all population subgroups. The decreases in the rates of nonfatal and fatal injuries were similar in men and women. Declines in fatality rates in African Americans and Hispanics were similar and were both greater than the decline in non-Hispanic Whites. In the rates of nonfatal injury, no consistent pattern was seen in the estimated decline across age groups, but, in the rates of fatal injury, age and percentage change were inversely related. Most of the nonfatal injuries occurred among men 15 to 44 years of age; were self-inflicted; and were associated with hunting, target shooting, and routine gun handling.

Numerous factors may have contributed to the decline in the rates of nonfatal and fatal assaultive firearm-related injury. These factors include: improvements in economic conditions; the aging of the population; the decline in the "crack" cocaine market; changes in legislation, sentencing guidelines, and law-enforcement practices; and improvements associated with violence prevention programs.

American Academy of Family Physicians website. Morbidity and mortality related to firearm injuries. Available at: http://www.aafp.org/afp/20000401/clinical.html#5. Accessed 11/28/06.

Morbidity and Mortality Weekly Report website. Available at http://www.cdc.gov/mmwr/mmwr_wk.html. Accessed 11/28/06.

385. The Health Insurance Portability and Accountability Act (HIPAA) has recently been updated and calls for

A) mandatory health insurance for all people who earn less than $12,000/year
B) stringent codes for the uniform transfer of medically related data
C) health maintenance organizations to allow more diagnostic testing of patients and less scrutiny of physicians
D) all Americans to invest in a medical savings account
E) improved access of third parties to patients' medical records

Answer and Discussion

The answer is B. The HIPAA of 1996 (also known as the *Kassenbaum-Kennedy legislation*) has recently been implemented. HIPAA was signed into law in 1996, and includes the "portability" aspect of the law (which protects the ability of people with current or preexisting medical conditions to get health insurance) and the "accountability" aspects of the law (which include enforcement). Its multiple provisions include strict codes for the uniform transfer of electronic data, including billing and other routine exchanges, and new patient rights regarding personal health information, including the right to access this information and to limit its disclosure. Also outlined are specific physical, procedural, and technological security protections all health-care organizations must take to ensure the confidentiality of patients' medical information. The purpose of HIPAA is to improve the portability of health insurance coverage in the group and individual markets, focus on health-care fraud and abuse, promote the use of medical savings accounts, improve access to long-term care services and coverage, and simplify the administration of health insurance. The U.S. Department of Health and Human Services is developing new standards for the electronic transmission of health records and financial transactions, identifiers for individuals, health plans, employers and providers, code sets and classification systems, and security standards and safeguards. Once the standards are developed and implemented, failure to comply will result in fines and/or imprisonment. Every medical practice in the United States must comply with these regulations, including transaction standards (i.e., the rules standardizing electronic data exchange of health-related information).

Kibbe DC. What you need to know about HIPAA now. *Fam Pract Manag.* 2001;8(3):43.

> The purpose of HIPAA is to improve the portability of health insurance coverage in the group and individual markets, focus on health care fraud and abuse, promote the use of medical savings accounts, improve access to long-term care services and coverage, and simplify the administration of health insurance.

386. The drug of choice for the treatment of chronic opioid dependence is

A) naloxone
B) bupropion
C) disulfiram (Antabuse)
D) methadone
E) diazepam

Answer and Discussion

The answer is D. Opioid dependence is a chronic, often relapsing, disorder that can be very challenging to treat. Between 500,000 and 1,000,000 Americans are believed to be opioid dependent at any point in time. Opioid-related disorders are more prevalent in men than in women by a ratio of up to 4:1. Opioid dependency is often linked to a history of drug-related criminal activity, antisocial personality disorder, and coexisting mood disorders, especially depression. Methadone is effective in reducing illicit narcotic use, retaining patients in treatment, and decreasing illegal drug use. Ongoing methadone maintenance decreases the risk of contracting and transmitting HIV, hepatitis B virus, and HCV and is considered a cost-effective intervention. Long-term methadone maintenance is more successful in averting relapse than shorter-term treatment. The goals of early treatment with methadone are to decrease withdrawal symptoms, diminish opioid craving, and arrive at a tolerance threshold, while preventing euphoria and sedation from overmedication. Detoxification is indicated when a patient demonstrates consistent, long-term abstinence and possesses adequate supportive resources (e.g., productive use of time, a stable home life). Patient acceptance of community resources for opiate addicts such as Narcotics Anonymous is a good prognostic sign. Narcotics Anonymous is also a useful tool in relapse prevention.

Krambeer LL, McNelly WV, Gabrielli WF, et al. Methadone therapy for opioid dependence. *Am Fam Physician.* 2001;63: 2404–2410.

387. The use of anti-obesity medication is acceptable when the body mass index (BMI) is

A) >10 kg/m^2
B) >20 kg/m^2
C) >30 kg/m^2
D) greater than the normal weight of the individual
E) more than the calculated fat percentage of the patient

Answer and Discussion

The answer is C. Obesity is epidemic in the United States and other industrialized nations. Obesity is defined as a BMI (BMI = weight in kg divided by height in m^2) of 30 kg/m^2 or more. There are three classes of severity:

- Class I (BMI of 30.0 to 34.9 kg/m^2)
- Class II (BMI of 35.0 to 39.9 kg/m^2)
- Class III (BMI of 40.0 kg/m^2 or higher).

The age-adjusted prevalence rates of classes I, II, and III obesity in American adults are estimated to be 14.4%, 5.2%, and 2.9%, respectively. These estimates represent a substantial increase in the prevalence of all three obesity classes since the mid-1990s. Although behavior modification strategies are helpful for most obese patients, they do not guarantee long-term weight-loss maintenance. Without ongoing management, most or all of the weight patients lose can be regained within 3 to 5 years. This limitation contributes to the active development of pharmacologic approaches to obesity. Current guidelines consider pharmacotherapy to be an adjunct to lifestyle modification programs and are targeted toward at-risk patients (patients with a BMI of 30 or greater or a BMI of 27 or greater combined with medical comorbidities such as hypertension or insulin resistance).

- *Noradrenergic drugs.* One class of weight-loss medications is the noradrenergic drugs that affect weight loss by suppressing one's appetite. Some noradrenergic agents include phentermine resin (Ionamin), mazindol (Sanorex), phenylpropanolamine (Dexatrim, recently removed from the market), phendimetrazine (Plegine), and diethylpropion (Tenuate). When combined with dietary programs, these drugs produced modest short-term net weight losses compared with dietary changes and placebo. The FDA has not labeled any of these drugs for long-term treatment of obesity.
- *Orlistat.* Orlistat (Xenical) is an intestinal lipase inhibitor that has been approved by the FDA for long-term use. After 12 weeks of treatment with orlistat (360 mg/day), patients showed weight losses of up to 5 kg (11 lb), compared with 2- to 3-kg losses (4.4 to 6.6 lb) among patients in the placebo group. Weight losses appear to be dosage dependent, with lower dosages producing smaller weight losses. Flatus, oily stools, and diarrhea are common but usually resolve during the second year of treatment. Vitamin deficiencies can occur with its use, and a vitamin supplement is recommended.
- *Sibutramine.* Sibutramine (Meridia), which has been approved by the FDA for long-term treatment of obesity, is a centrally acting, specific reuptake inhibitor of norepinephrine and serotonin, thus having satiating and potential thermogenic effects. Several clinical studies of 12 to 52 weeks' duration showed weight losses of 4.7 to 7.6 kg (10.3 to 16.7 lb) in patients receiving sibutramine. Weight losses were dosage dependent and tended to plateau by the twenty-fourth week. Efficacy of sibutramine at 1 year has also been established. Patients taking 5-, 10-, and 15-mg daily dosages experienced dosage-related weight loss for up to 12 weeks, and all dosages were well tolerated. Common adverse effects are headache, dry mouth, insomnia, and constipation. The most common serious side effect is hypertension. Sibutramine should not be used with SSRIs and in patients with cardiovascular disorders, particularly poorly controlled hypertension.

Because of the inherent difficulties in treating obesity, physicians should attempt to develop continuous care programs emphasizing lifestyle modifications such as enduring changes in dietary and activity habits. Patients using behavior modification strategies to make these changes are more likely to succeed in long-term weight maintenance. Weight loss related to drug treatment is modest (5% to 10%) and occurs in the first 6 months. Medication appears to be more effective at maintaining weight loss.

Poston WSC, Foreyt JP. Successful management of the obese patient. *Am Fam Physician.* 2000;61:3615–3622.

388. Which of the following statements regarding onychomycosis is true?

A) The infection is caused by *Trichophyton rubrum.*
B) Fungi are responsible for 90% of nail dystrophies.
C) Ciclopirox (Penlac) is very effective for the treatment of onychomycosis.
D) Griseofulvin and ketoconazole are first-line medications for the treatment of onychomycosis.
E) Periodic testing of renal function is indicated with the use of antifungal medication.

Answer and Discussion

The answer is A. Onychomycosis (*tinea unguium*) is a fungal infection of the nail bed, matrix, or plate. Toenails are affected more often than fingernails. The infection is usually caused by *T. rubrum*, which invades the nail bed and the underside of the nail plate beginning at the hyponychium and then migrating proximally through the underlying nail matrix. Because fungi are responsible for only approximately one-half of nail dystrophies, the diagnosis of onychomycosis may need to be confirmed by potassium hydroxide preparation, culture, or histology. Psoriasis, lichen planus, contact dermatitis, trauma, nail-bed tumor, and yellow nail syndrome may be mistakenly diagnosed as onychomycosis. The FDA has approved ciclopirox (Penlac) nail lacquer for the treatment of mild to moderate onychomycosis caused by *T. rubrum* without involvement of the lunula. Although safe and relatively inexpensive, ciclopirox therapy is seldom effective. Triazole and allylamine antifungal drugs have largely replaced griseofulvin and ketoconazole as first-line medications in the treatment of onychomycosis. These agents offer shorter treatment courses, higher cure rates, and fewer relapses. Of the newer drugs, terbinafine (Lamisil), itraconazole (Sporanox), and fluconazole (Diflucan) are the most widely used. Liver enzyme monitoring is recommended before continuous medication therapy is initiated and every 4 to 6 weeks during treatment. Onychomycosis is expensive to treat. Costs include medications, procedures, laboratory tests, and health-care providers' time, as well as expenses associated with the management of adverse drug effects and treatment failures.

Rodgers P, Bassler M. Treating onychomycosis. *Am Fam Physician.* 2001;63:663–672, 677–678.

389. A 31-year-old man who enjoys scuba diving presents to your office after a dive complaining of severe back pain, loss of sensation around the trunk, and numbness of the legs. Appropriate management consists of

A) administration of acetazolamide
B) furosemide (Lasix) and fluid restriction
C) NSAIDs and narcotic pain medication
D) intravenous steroids
E) transfer to a facility with a recompression chamber

Answer and Discussion

The answer is E. Recreational scuba diving, which is defined as pleasure diving without mandatory decompression to a maximum depth of 130 feet, has become a popular activity since the mid-1980s. Although divers are concentrated along coastal regions, many others dive in inland lakes, streams, quarries and reservoirs, or fly to distant dive sites. Physicians practicing almost anywhere in the United States may see a patient with a dive-related injury or complaint. Injuries related to diving are usually mild and include ear-related complaints. Barotrauma to the middle or inner ear can occur during the descent or ascent phases of the dive and may cause vertigo and other neurologic symptoms. Middle-ear barotrauma of descent is the most common type of diving injury and may involve hemorrhage and rupture of the tympanic membrane. Symptoms include the acute onset of pain, vertigo, and conductive hearing loss. In severe cases (usually during ascent), increased pressure in the middle ear can cause reversible weakness of the facial nerve and Bell's palsy (facial baroparesis). The most severe illness related to diving is decompression illness (the "bends"). Neurologic decompression sickness can present with a wide spectrum of symptoms. A prodrome of malaise, fatigue, anorexia, and headache is common. The most severe presentation is partial myelopathy referable to the thoracic spinal cord. Patients complain of paresthesias and sensory loss in the trunk and extremities, a tingling or constricting sensation around the thorax, ascending leg weakness ranging from mild to severe, pain in the lower back or pelvis, and loss of bowel and/or bladder control. The neurologic examination often reveals monoparesis or paraparesis, a sensory level, and sphincter disturbances. However, neurologic examination also may be normal. The diagnosis of neurologic decompression sickness is clinical and should be suspected in any patient with a recent history of diving who has a consistent presentation. Flying shortly after a dive can precipitate symptoms. The initial management of neurologic decompression sickness requires transport to a recompression facility. The majority of recreational divers with neurologic decompression sickness have an excellent recovery after prompt recompression therapy.

Newton HB. Neurologic complications of scuba diving. *Am Fam Physician.* 2001;63:2211–2218, 2225–2226.

390. Which of the following may increase the risk of lung cancer in smokers?
A) Vitamin C
B) Vitamin E
C) Folate
D) β-Carotene
E) Vitamin D

Answer and Discussion

The answer is D. Research studies suggest that, although once thought to be protective against the development of malignancy, β-carotene actually increased the risk of lung cancer in smokers. The ATBC (Alpha-Tocopherol, Beta-Carotene) cancer prevention trial involved almost 30,000 male cigarette smokers in Finland; the patients given supplemental β-carotene for 5 to 8 years had an 18% increase in the incidence of lung cancer. The excess risk appeared to decline once supplements were discontinued.

The Alpha-Tocopherol Beta Carotene Cancer Prevention Study Group. The effect of vitamin E and beta carotene on the incidence of lung cancer and other cancers in male smokers. *N Engl J Med.* 1994;330:1029.

Research studies suggest that, although once thought to be protective against the development of malignancy, beta-carotene actually increased the risk of lung cancer in smokers.

Chapter 2

Pediatrics

Questions

Each of the following questions or incomplete statements is followed by suggested answers or completions. Select the ONE BEST ANSWER in each case.

1. A 14-year-old boy presents to your office with a mildly pruritic rash that involves his chest and back. He reports it began with a single lesion on his back, but now has spread to involve his entire back and chest. You note on your examination the presence of multiple secondary lesions that appear to follow cleavage lines. The most likely diagnosis is

A) *Herpes zoster*
B) *Pityriasis rosea*
C) *Tinea versicolor*
D) *Varicella*
E) *Rhus* dermatitis

Answer and Discussion

The answer is B. Pityriasis rosea is a common, acute exanthem of uncertain etiology. Viral and bacterial causes have been sought, but exact causes have not yet been identified. Pityriasis rosea typically affects children and young adults. It is characterized by an initial herald patch, followed by the development of a diffuse papulosquamous rash. The herald patch often is misdiagnosed as eczema. Pityriasis rosea is difficult to identify until the appearance of characteristic smaller secondary lesions that follow Langer's lines (cleavage lines) in a "Christmas tree–like pattern." Several medications can cause a rash similar to pityriasis rosea, and several diseases, including secondary syphilis, should be included in the differential diagnosis. One small controlled trial reported faster clearing of the exanthem with the use of erythromycin, but the mechanism of effect is unknown. Resolution of the rash may be hastened by ultraviolet light therapy, but not without the risk of hyperpigmentation. Topical or systemic steroids and antihistamines often are used to relieve itching.

Stulberg DL, Wolfrey J. Pityriasis rosea. *Am Fam Physician.* 2004;69:87–92, 94.

Pityriasis rosea is characterized by an initial herald patch, followed by the development of a diffuse papulosquamous rash.

2. What is the most common cause of nephritic syndrome in a 4 year old?

A) Trauma
B) Recent strep infection
C) Dehydration
D) Nonsteroidal anti-inflammatories (NSAIDs)
E) Varicella infection

Answer and Discussion

The answer is B. Poststreptococcal glomerulonephritis is the leading cause of acute nephritic syndrome. The condition is most frequently encountered in children between 2 and 6 years of age with a recent history of pharyngitis. It is rare in children younger than 2 and adults older than 40. The incidence of poststreptococcal glomerulonephritis appears to be decreasing. The condition typically develops approximately 10 days after pharyngitis or 2 weeks after a skin infection with a nephritogenic strain of group A hemolytic *Streptococcus.* It has not been determined whether antibiotic treatment of the primary skin infection affords protection from the development of poststreptococcal glomerulonephritis. The classic presentation of poststreptococcal glomerulonephritis is a nephritic syndrome with oliguric acute renal failure. Most patients have milder disease, and subclinical cases are common. Patients with severe disease experience gross hematuria characterized by red or smoky urine, headache, and generalized symptoms such as anorexia, nausea, vomiting, and malaise. Inflammation of the renal capsule can lead to flank or back pain. Physical examination may show hypervolemia, edema, or hypertension. Acute poststreptococcal glomerulonephritis usually is diagnosed on clinical and serologic grounds without the need for biopsy, especially in children with a typical history. The overall prognosis in classic poststreptococcal acute proliferative glomerulonephritis is good. Most patients recover spontaneously and return to baseline renal function within 3 to 4 weeks with no long-term complications.

Hahn RG, Knox LM, Forman TA. Evaluation of poststreptococcal illness. *Am Fam Physician.* 2005;71:1949–1954.

3. At what age do children normally articulate most words and know basic colors?

A) 3 years
B) 4 years
C) 5 years
D) 6 years
E) 7 years

Answer and Discussion

The answer is B. Motor development during the preschool years results in children running, jumping, and climbing. Children learn to balance on one foot and hop. Vocabulary continues to develop rapidly with the mastery of hundreds of words. Language development proceeds with multiword sentences, the use of pronouns, and the gradual improvement in articulation skills. Children normally master the concept of numbers 1, 2, and 3 by 3 1/2 years. Four-year-old children should know basic colors and clearly articulate most words.

Hay WW Jr, Levin MJ, Sondheimer JM, et al., eds. *Current pediatric diagnosis & treatment,* 18th ed. New York: McGraw-Hill; 2007:74–79.

4. At what age is it necessary to perform orchiopexy in a child affected with cryptorchism?
A) 12–24 months
B) 36–48 months
C) 5 years
D) 7 years
E) orchioplexy is not necessary

Answer and Discussion

The answer is A. Either one or both testes may be absent from the scrotum at birth in about one in five premature or low-birth-weight male infants and in 3% to 6% at full term infants. Cryptorchism is found in 1% to 2% of males after 1 year of age but can be confused with retractile testes that is associated with a strong cremasteric reflex, which requires no treatment. Cryptorchism should be corrected before age 12 to 24 months in an attempt to reduce the risk of infertility, which occurs in up to 75% of males with bilateral cryptorchism and in 50% of men with unilateral cryptorchism. It is not clear, however, whether such early orchiopexy improves ultimate fertility. Some patients have underlying hypogonadism. Cryptorchism is also associated with testicular carcinoma mainly in the undescended testicle and particularly with intra-abdominal malposition; however, up to 10% of cancers can occur on the unaffected side.

Hay WW Jr, Levin MJ, Sondheimer JM, et al., eds. *Current pediatric diagnosis & treatment,* 18th ed. New York: McGraw-Hill; 2007:967.

5. A 5 year old presents to your office complaining of scrotal pain and you note swelling of the left testis. Appropriate management at this time includes
A) continued observation
B) elevation of the scrotum and ice therapy
C) ultrasound evaluation
D) doppler stethoscope evaluation
E) CT scan of the pelvis

Answer and Discussion

The answer is C. Testicular torsion should be suspected in patients who complain of acute scrotal pain and swelling. Torsion of the testis is a surgical emergency because the likelihood of testicular damage increases as the duration of torsion increases. Associated conditions that may resemble testicular torsion, such as torsion of a testicular appendage, epididymitis, trauma, hernia, hydrocele, varicocele, and Henoch-Schönlein purpura, in general do not require immediate surgical intervention. Testicular torsion is most common in neonates and postpubertal boys, although it can occur in males of any age. Henoch-Schönlein purpura and torsion of a testicular appendage typically occur in prepubertal boys, whereas epididymitis most often develops in postpubertal boys. The cause of an acute scrotum can usually be made based on a careful history, a thorough physical examination and appropriate diagnostic tests. The onset, character, and severity of symptoms must be determined. The physical examination should include inspection and palpation of the abdomen, testis, epididymis, scrotum, and inguinal region. Urinalysis should always be performed. Scrotal imaging with Doppler color flow ultrasound is necessary when the diagnosis remains unclear. Once the correct diagnosis is established, prompt surgical evaluation should be performed.

Galejs LE, Kass EJ. Diagnosis and treatment of the acute scrotum. *Am Fam Physician.* 1999;59(4):817.

6. Which of the following statements is true regarding head lice infestations?
A) Females are more likely affected.
B) Retreatment with pyrethrin is rarely needed.
C) Head lice can live off the body up to 1 week.
D) Low socioeconomic children are more likely affected.
E) Dogs are a common vector for head lice.

Answer and Discussion

The answer is A. Head lice are thought to be the most common type and are developing resistance to commonly used pediculicides. Every year, between 6 million and 12 million people in the United States, primarily children 3 to 10 years of age, are infested with head lice. Girls are at greater risk because they have more frequent head-to-head contact. Head lice affect people of all socioeconomic status. Head lice are obligate parasites that live on human skin and survive on human blood. No other animal is affected. Head lice die if they are away from the host head for more than 2 days. Lice are wingless and cannot jump, but they climb quickly from hair to hair when the hair is dry. Lice move slowly on wet hair and can be removed more easily with a gloved hand or a fine-toothed comb. The adult female louse lays 7 to 10 eggs daily that attach to human hair with a gluelike, water-soluble substance. By 7 to 10 days, a nymph emerges from the egg and is close enough to the scalp to obtain its first meal of blood. Adult lice, after the 7- to 10-day period of molting stages, live about 30 days. Infested people usually have no more than 10 to 12 live head lice at a time, but can harbor hundreds of eggs and nits. Those affected describe itching and a sensation of "something crawling on my head." Scratching may cause excoriations and secondary infection. Most infestations are asymptomatic. Prior to treatment, live lice can be identified under a magnifying glass, which is best done when the hair is wet. After infestation is confirmed, treatment consists of application of a pediculicidal agent to the hair, followed by mechanical removal. The hair should not be washed for 2 to 3 days after the pediculicide is applied. Thorough physical removal of lice and nits with a sturdy, fine-tooth comb is recommended for several days after application because no pediculicide guarantees total eradication of lice. First-line topical agents containing pyrethrins or permethrin are available over the counter and are relatively non-toxic. Retreatment is advised 7 to 10 days after the first application of pyrethrins. Because permethrin remains active for a longer period, retreatment generally is not necessary. Permethrin 5% cream is available by prescription for use in resistant cases. Alternative agents include lindane or malathion. Lindane has been shown to have limited success and is systemically absorbed, so its use is now considered second-line. Malathion was recently labeled by the U.S. Food and Drug Administration (FDA) for the treatment of head lice and is available in a lotion that is left on the head for 8 to 12 hours. Oral agents include ivermectin and trimethoprim–sulfamethoxizole. Resistance is possible with any treatment because of reduced susceptibility or incorrect use of the medication.

All household members with active infestation should be treated simultaneously. For children younger than 2 years, there is no recommended pediculicide; therefore, treatment consists of manual removal only. Lice that remain active 8 to 12 hours after treatment may require an alternative agent. Itching may persist for up to 10 days after successful treatment and should not be mistaken for treatment failure. The Centers for Disease Control and Prevention recommend that all clothing and bedding in contact with the infested person during the 2 days before application of the pediculicide be laundered in hot water and machine dried using a hot dry cycle. All nonwashable items should be quarantined in a plastic bag for 2 weeks. Combs and brushes should be disinfected with hot water or alcohol.

Mazurek CM, Lee NP. How to manage head lice. *West J Med.* 2000;172:342–345.

7. A 4 year old presents with short stature. Further evaluation confirms a delayed bone age. The most likely diagnosis is
A) hypothyroidism
B) cartilage defects
C) growth plate disorder
D) genetic influence of the parents

Answer and Discussion

The answer is A. Short stature may affect children as a result of intrinsic growth defects or because of acquired extrinsic factors that impair growth. In general, delayed bone age in a child with short stature is suggestive of a hormonal or systemic disorder, whereas normal bone age in a short child is more likely to be caused by a genetic cartilage disorder or growth plate disorder.

Kasper DL, Braunwald E, Fauci AS, et al., eds. *Harrison's principles of internal medicine,* 16th ed. New York: McGraw-Hill; 2005:2088, 2216.

8. An 8 year old is seen in the emergency room secondary to abdominal pain. Further evaluation confirms the presence of intussusception. The most likely precipitating cause is
A) colon polyp
B) Meckel's diverticulum
C) lymphoma
D) parasite infection
E) foreign body

Answer and Discussion

The answer is C. Intussusception is the most common cause of intestinal obstruction in the first 2 years of life. It is more common in males than in females. In most cases (85%) the cause is not apparent. Associated conditions that can result in intussusception include polyps, Meckel's diverticulum, Henoch–Schönlein purpura, lymphoma, lipoma, parasites, foreign bodies, and viral enteritis with hypertrophy of Peyer patches. Intussusception of the small intestine occurs in patients with celiac disease and cystic fibrosis—related to the bulk of stool in the terminal ileum. Henoch–Schönlein purpura may also cause isolated small-bowel intussusception. In children older than 6 years, lymphoma is the most common cause. Intermittent small-bowel intussusception is a rare cause of recurrent abdominal pain.

Hay WW Jr, Levin MJ, Sondheimer JM, et al., eds. *Current pediatric diagnosis & treatment,* 18th ed. New York: McGraw-Hill; 2007:616–617.

9. The initial treatment of choice for symptomatic labial adhesions is
A) testosterone cream
B) estrogen cream
C) GnRH antagonist
D) hydrocortisone cream
E) surgical separation

Answer and Discussion

The answer is B. Labial adhesions are common in prepubertal females. The cause is thought related to low levels of circulating estrogen. Most women with small areas of labial adhesions are asymptomatic. However, interference with urination or accumulation of urine behind the adhesion can lead to discomfort and symptoms. Dysuria and recurrent vulvar and vaginal infections are associated symptoms. In rare situations urinary retention may occur. Asymptomatic labial fusion usually does not require treatment. Symptomatic adhesions may be treated with a short course of estrogen cream applied twice daily for 7 to 10 days; this may separate the labia. A new alternative treatment is to use estrogen transdermal patches in close proximity to the labia. When medical treatment fails or if severe urinary symptoms exist, surgical separation of the labia is indicated. This can be done as an office procedure using 1% to 2% topical xylocaine gel. Because of inadequate levels of estrogen, recurrences of labial adhesion are common until puberty. Following puberty, the condition usually resolves spontaneously. Improved hygiene and removal of vulvar irritants may help prevent recurrences.

DeCherney AH, Nathan L. *Current Obstetric & Gynecologic Diagnosis and Treatment,* 9th ed. New York: McGraw-Hill; 2003:67.

10. Which of the following statements is true regarding iron deficiency in childhood?
A) Iron deficiency commonly occurs in term infants <6 months.
B) Ingestion of cow's milk can result in iron overload.
C) Iron deficiency rarely leads to complications.
D) Pica is associated with iron deficiency.
E) Mild iron deficiency typically leads to symptoms of pallor, fatigue, and delayed motor development.

Answer and Discussion

The answer is D. The incidence of iron deficiency in children has decreased substantially due to improved nutrition and the increased availability of iron-fortified infant formulas and cereals. Normal-term infants are born with sufficient iron stores to prevent iron deficiency for the first 4 to 5 months of life. Thereafter, sufficient iron needs to be absorbed to maintain the needs of rapid growth. For this reason, nutritional iron deficiency is most common between 6 and 24 months of life. A deficiency earlier than age 6 months may occur if iron stores at birth are reduced by prematurity, small birth weight, neonatal anemia, or perinatal blood loss or if there is subsequent iron loss due to hemorrhage. Iron-deficient children older than age 24 months should be evaluated for blood loss. Iron deficiency, in addition to causing anemia, has adverse effects on multiple organ systems. Symptoms and signs vary with the severity of the deficiency. Mild iron deficiency is usually asymptomatic. In infants with more severe iron deficiency, pallor, fatigue, irritability, and delayed motor development are common. Children whose iron deficiency is due in part to ingestion of unfortified cow's milk may be fat and flabby, with poor muscle tone. A history of pica is common.

Hay WW Jr, Levin MJ, Sondheimer JM, et al., eds. *Current pediatric diagnosis & treatment,* 18th ed. New York: McGraw-Hill; 2007:837–838.

A history of pica is common in iron deficiency anemia.

11. In treating acute sinusitis in children, which of the following sinuses is unlikely to be infected in a 6 year old?
A) Frontal
B) Maxillary
C) Ethmoidal
D) Sphenoidal
E) Sinusitis does not occur in children younger than 8.

Answer and Discussion

The answer is A. Acute bacterial infection of the sinuses that lasts <30 days and completely resolves is called *acute bacterial sinusitis.* The maxillary and ethmoidal sinuse most commonly involved when mucociliary function and drainage are impaired by a URI or allergic rhinitis. Both the ethmoid and maxillary sinuses are present at birth, forming in the third to fourth gestational month. The sphenoid sinuses pneumatize as an extension of a posterior ethmoid cell by age 5 years, and the frontal sinuses form from an anterior ethmoid cell appearing about age 7 to 8 years. Frontal sinusitis is unusual before age 10 years.

Hay WW Jr, Levin MJ, Sondheimer JM, et al., eds. *Current pediatric diagnosis & treatment,* 18th ed. New York: McGraw-Hill; 2007:476–478.

12. Which of the following statements regarding attention-deficit/hyperactivity disorder is true?
A) Specific biologic markers are used in the diagnosis.
B) The Conner's ADHD Index is a checklist that helps identify children affected with ADHD.
C) Stimulant medications rarely benefit children with ADHD.
D) Symptoms of ADHD typically progress over time.
E) Drug therapy combined with psychosocial therapy is universally better than medication alone.

Answer and Discussion

The answer is B. Attention-deficit/hyperactivity disorder (ADHD) is manifest by inappropriate-for-age hyperactivity, impulsivity, and lack of attention. ADHD cannot be easily diagnosed by a specific test or biologic marker, and some are unclear if the disorder is a truly pathologic condition or just one end of the behavioral spectrum. ADHD is more frequently diagnosed in children with behavioral difficulties and academic underachievement. The prevalence of ADHD is between 6.8% and 10.3%, with boys affected threefold more often than girls. Associated psychiatric conditions, including oppositional–defiant disorder, conduct disorder, depressive disorder, and anxiety disorders, are common. The Conners' ADHD Index and symptom scales from the *Diagnostic and Statistical Manual of Mental Disorders,* 4th ed. (DSM-IV), are ADHD-specific checklists and have a high sensitivity for identification of children with the disorder. Reviews of the pharmacologic management of ADHD with methylphenidate hydrochloride (Ritalin, Concerta), dextroamphetamine sulfate (Adderall, Dexedrine), and pemoline (Cylert) show these drugs to be generally effective for most children affected. Nonpharmacologic treatments that may have some beneficial effect on behavior and academic performance are behavioral modification and intensive contingency management therapy. Combining drug therapy with psychosocial therapy shows no clear advantage when compared to drug therapy alone. However, the addition of behavioral therapies to medication may have some benefit, including reduction of anxiety and improvement in social skills. The symptoms of ADHD tend to decrease over the long-term, but may continue into adolescence and adulthood. The most common treatment is stimulant medication.

Guevara JP. Attention deficit hyperactivity disorder. *West J Med.* 2001;175:189–192.

Hunt RD, Paquin A, Payton K. An update on assessment and treatment of complex attention-deficit hyperactivity disorder. *Pediatr Ann.* 2001;30(3):162–172.

13. A 12-year-old obese boy presents to your office complaining of bilateral leg pain that occurs only at night. His mother denies any pain during the day and reports he has not had a limp. The most likely diagnosis is
A) slipped capital femoral epiphysis
B) Legg-Calve-Perthes disease
C) Osgood Schlatter's disease
D) patellofemoral syndrome
E) "growing pains"

Answer and Discussion

The answer is E. A diagnosis of "growing pains" must meet three criteria: (1) the leg pain is bilateral; (2) the pain occurs only at night; and (3) the patient has no limp, pain, or symptoms during the day. To inaccurately diagnose a limping child with growing pains can be dangerous, as the physician risks missing the underlying pathology. However, if a child does fit the criteria for growing pains, the parents should be reassured that this is a benign, self-limited process that occurs for unknown reasons.

Leet AI, Skaggs DL. Evaluation of the acutely limping child. *Am Fam Physician.* 2000;61:1011–1018.

14. The gold standard for diagnosing peritonsillar abscess is
A) lateral plain films
B) ultrasound
C) CT scan
D) MRI evaluation
E) needle aspiration

Answer and Discussion

The answer is E. Peritonsillar abscess is most common in persons 20 to 40 years of age. Young children are seldom affected unless they are immunocompromised, but the infection can cause significant airway obstruction in children. The infection affects males and females equally. Chronic tonsillitis or multiple trials of oral antibiotics for acute tonsillitis may predispose persons to the development of a peritonsillar abscess. The presenting symptoms include fever, throat pain, and trismus. Ultrasonography and computed tomographic scanning are useful in confirming a diagnosis. Needle aspiration remains the gold standard for diagnosis and treatment of peritonsillar abscess. After performing aspiration, appropriate antibiotic therapy (including penicillin, clindamycin, cephalosporins, or metronidazole) must be initiated. In advanced cases, incision and drainage or immediate tonsillectomy may be required. *Streptococcus pyogenes* (group A β-hemolytic *Streptococcus*) is the most common aerobic organism associated with peritonsillar abscess. The most common anaerobic organism is *Fusobacterium*. For most abscesses, a mixed group of both aerobic and anaerobic organisms cause the infection.

Steyer TE. Peritonsillar abscess: diagnosis and treatment. *Am Fam Physician*. 2002;65:93–96.

15. A 12-year-old boy is brought in to your office by his mother and father. The child has been experiencing swelling of his joints, fevers, and a rash. An examination reveals hepatosplenomegaly and lymphadenopathy. Laboratory evaluation shows anemia, leukocytosis, and thrombocytosis. You suspect juvenile rheumatoid arthritis. Which of the following medications would be first-line treatment?

A) Acetaminophen
B) Ibuprofen
C) Codeine
D) Methotrexate
E) Prednisone

Answer and Discussion

The answer is B. Juvenile rheumatoid arthritis (JRA), formerly known as Still's disease, is a diverse group of diseases that is clinically distinct from adult rheumatoid arthritis. Most children with JRA have long remissions without loss of function or significant residual deformity. There are no specific laboratory tests to diagnose JRA. One must exclude other causes for arthritis, including reactive arthritis from extra-articular infection, septic arthritis, neoplastic disorders, endocrine disorders (e.g., thyroid disease, type 1 diabetes mellitus), degenerative or mechanical disorders, or idiopathic pediatric joint pain. Diagnosis of JRA requires signs of inflammation rather than simply arthralgias persisting for more than 6 weeks, with onset before age 16 years. JRA has three major subtypes: pauciarticular (40% to 50%), polyarticular (25% to 40%), and systemic (10% to 20%). Each type has different clinical presentations and courses, and treatment is determined by differentiating among the various types. Pauciarticular JRA involves four or fewer joints, usually large joints asymmetrically. Early-onset pauciarticular JRA affects mostly girls younger than 4 years and has a 30% risk of chronic iridocyclitis and a 10% risk of ocular damage. Late-onset pauciarticular JRA affects mostly boys older than 8 years; many of whom later develop spondyloarthropathies; 10% develop iridocyclitis. Slit-lamp ophthalmic examinations are recommended. Polyarticular JRA is defined as arthritis in five or more joints; patients are either RF positive or RF negative. RF-positive patients usually are girls age 8 years or older, have symmetric small-joint arthritis, and have a worse prognosis than do RF-negative patients. Systemic-onset JRA is characterized by high intermittent fevers (>102°F), rash, hepatosplenomegaly, lymphadenopathy, arthralgias, pericarditis, pleuritis, and growth delay. Anemia, leukocytosis, and thrombocytosis are common laboratory findings. Extra-articular symptoms are usually mild and self-limited. Boys and girls are equally affected. NSAIDs are the first-line treatment for JRA. Clinical improvement may not be seen for up to 1 month. Methotrexate is often used with NSAIDs, particularly for systemic and polyarticular JRA. Corticosteroids are used orally for severe, life-threatening, systemic JRA and intra-articularly for pauciarticular JRA. Most children with JRA require a great deal of physical as well as psychologic support. Physical and occupational therapy is important because children often stop using painful joints, adding to disability.

Rakel R. *Textbook of Family Practice*, 6th ed. Philadelphia: WB Saunders; 2002:990.

16. An asthmatic 8 year old is complaining of wheezing and shortness of breath in your office. An albuterol nebulizer treatment is given, and the child's PEFR is measured at 75%. The appropriate next step would be

A) add an oral steroid
B) add theophylline
C) add ipratropium
D) administer epinephrine
E) intubate the child

Answer and Discussion

The answer is A. Early treatment of asthma exacerbations is important to prevent progression to severe disease. First-line treatment should be with a short-acting inhaled β_2-agonist such as albuterol; 2 to 4 puffs from a metered-dose inhaler can be given every 20 minutes up to three times, or a single treatment can be given by nebulizer. If the response is acceptable as assessed by sustained symptom relief or improvement in PEFR to over 80% of the child's best, the short-acting β_2-agonist can be continued every 3 to 4 hours for 24 to 48 hours. For patients taking inhaled corticosteroids, the dose may be doubled for 7 to 10 days. If the child does not completely improve from the initial therapy, with PEFR between 50% and 80%, the β_2-agonist should be continued, and an oral corticosteroid should be added. If the child experiences marked distress or if PEFR persists under 50%, the patient should repeat the β_2-agonist immediately. Further emergent treatment may be necessary.

Hay WW Jr, Levin MJ, Sondheimer JM, et al., eds. *Current pediatric diagnosis & treatment,* 18th ed. New York: McGraw-Hill; 2007:1058–1059.

17. An 18-month-old female presents to your office with her mother. A urinary tract infection is discovered. Appropriate treatment at this time including antibiotic coverage includes

A) intravenous pyelogram
B) cystoscopy
C) renal ultrasound and voiding cysturethrography (VCUG)
D) observation with no further testing

Answer and Discussion

The answer is C. Practice guidelines from the American Academy of Pediatrics recommend renal ultrasonography and voiding cystourethrography (VCUG) in all children two months to two years of age with a documented first urinary tract infection (UTI). After age two some controversy exists. Some authorities recommend postponing workup for the first UTI in females.

Hoberman A, Charron M, Hickey RW. Imaging studies after a first febrile urinary tract infection in young children. *N Engl J Med.* 2003;348:195–202.

> Practice guidelines from the American Academy of Pediatrics recommend renal ultrasonography and voiding cystourethrography (VCUG) in all children two months to two years of age with a documented first urinary tract infection (UTI).

18. Which of the following statements is true regarding child safety seats?

A) Newborn infants should face forward in the back seat of cars.
B) A child outgrows a forward facing seat when their shoulders extend beyond the back of the seat.

C) Once a child is >40 lbs it is important to make sure the harness of the child seat is used.
D) Low-back booster seats are safe to use in children >40 lbs.
E) To sit with a standard seat belt the child's weight should be at least 81 lbs.

Answer and Discussion

The answer is E. Motor vehicle crashes continue to be the leading cause of death in children 1 to 14 years of age. Properly used child safety seats significantly reduce child morbidity and mortality. Although many parents know child safety seats are important, >80% of seats are misused. Children should sit in the back seat. The rear-facing position should be used until the child is 1 year of age and weighs 20 lbs (9 kg). Forward-facing child seats face forward and are for children heavier than 20 lbs and older than 1 year. A child outgrows this seat when the ears are above the back of the seat or when the child passes the height or weight limit of the seat (usually 40 lbs). High-back booster seats face forward and have removable harnesses. They are meant for use with children heavier than 20 to 30 lbs (9 to 13.5 kg), depending on the manufacturer, and older than 1 year. The high back protects the head and neck in a rear-end collision. The harness should be used until the child exceeds the weight limit of the harness system (usually 40 lbs). Once the child is heavier than 40 lbs, the harness is removed, and the seat is used to position the vehicle seat belt correctly (over the midclavicle and midchest, and tight over the upper thighs. High-back belt-positioning booster seats boost the child up so that the vehicle seat belt fits correctly. They can only be used with a shoulder-lap belt system. High-back booster seats are for use with children heavier than 40 lbs and can be used until the child fits properly in the vehicle seat belt system. Because safer restraint systems are available for children weighing more than 40 lbs, the use of low-back booster seats is not recommended. To properly fit a child in a standard car seat belt, three elements must be present: (1) the child's legs should bend over the edge of the auto seat with the buttocks against the seat back; (2) the shoulder portion of the belt should be over the midclavicle and center of the chest; and (3) the lap belt should be tight over the upper thighs or the pelvis. A child should have a sitting height of 29 in. (74 cm) to have a proper seat belt fit. This sitting height roughly correlates to a standing height of 58 in. (147 cm) and a weight of 81 lbs (36.5 kg). Increased education of parents regarding proper use of child safety seats can protect children from potentially fatal crash forces. Parents may also be educated about community resources and the several types of child safety seats.

Biagioli F. Proper use of child safety seats. *Am Fam Physician.* 2002;65:2085–2090.

19. Which of the following findings is *not* associated with rotavirus infections?
A) Metabolic acidosis
B) Hypernatremia
C) WBCs noted in the stool
D) Normal WBC count
E) Lactic acidosis

Answer and Discussion

The answer is C. Vomiting is the first manifestation of rotavirus in the majority of patients, followed within 24 hours by low-grade fever and repeated bouts of watery diarrhea. Diarrhea usually lasts 4 to 8 days but can last longer in young infants or immunocompromised patients. The white blood cell count is rarely elevated. As patients become dehydrated from unreplaced fecal water loss, they may become hypernatremic. The stool does not contain blood or white cells. Metabolic acidosis results from bicarbonate loss in the stool, ketosis from poor intake, and lactic acidemia from hypotension and hypoperfusion. Replacement of fluid and electrolyte deficits and ongoing losses is critical, especially in small infants. The use of oral rehydration fluid is appropriate in most cases. The use of clear liquids or hypocaloric (dilute formula) diets for more than 48 hours is not advisable in uncomplicated viral gastroenteritis because starvation depresses digestive function and prolongs diarrhea. Intestinal lactase levels are reduced during rotavirus infection. Brief use of a lactose-free diet is associated with a shorter period of diarrhea but is not critical to successful recovery in most healthy infants. Reduced fat intake during recovery may reduce nausea and vomiting. Antidiarrheal medications are not effective and can be dangerous (loperamide, tincture of opium, diphenoxylate with atropine). Bismuth subsalicylate preparations may reduce stool volume but are not necessary for recovery. Specific identification of rotavirus is not required in every case, especially in outbreaks. Rotavirus antigens can be identified in stool. False positives (which may actually be nonpathogenic rotavirus) are seen in neonates. Some immunity is imparted by the first episode of rotavirus infection. Repeat infections occur but are usually less severe. Prevention of rotavirus is mainly by good hygiene and prevention of fecal–oral contamination. In July 1999, the American Academy of Pediatrics recommended suspending the use of oral rotavirus vaccine in the United States because of its association with intussusception in the first 3 weeks following vaccine administration. Recently, newer vaccines have been developed with an improved safety record.

Hay WW Jr, Levin MJ, Sondheimer JM, et al., eds. *Current pediatric diagnosis & treatment,* 18th ed. New York: McGraw-Hill; 2007:619–621.

20. Which of the following is not associated with early sexual activity?
A) Academic deficiencies
B) Repeat pregnancies
C) Sex education classes
D) Increased STDs
E) Low socioeconomic status

Answer and Discussion

The answer is C. Early sexual activity can have a substantial negative impact on adolescents. Currently in the United States, more than 900,000 teenagers become pregnant each year. Those who give birth tend to have more academic deficiencies, poorer socioeconomic outcomes, and repeat pregnancies, and they are more likely to be single parents. In addition, adolescents who engage in early sexual activity expose themselves to sexually transmitted diseases (STDs). Of all STD cases reported in the United States, more than two thirds occur in adolescents and young adults. Prevention strategies should be established to reduce early sexual activity in adolescents.

Lonczak HS, Abbott RD, Hawkins JD. Effects of the Seattle Social Development Project on sexual behavior, pregnancy, birth, and sexually transmitted disease outcomes by age 21 years. *Arch Pediatr Adolesc Med.* 2002;156:438–447.

21. When evaluating febrile seizures, when is a lumbar puncture indicated?
A) If the seizure is generalized
B) If the seizure lasts 15 minutes

C) If there is a second seizure within 24 hours
D) If the seizure is associated with a recent vaccination
E) All children affected with a febrile seizure should have a lumbar puncture.

Answer and Discussion

The answer is C. The majority of seizures in children <5 years are febrile type seizures, and children with a positive family history have a higher incidence. A febrile seizure is defined as any seizure occurring in a child who is 6 months to 5 years of age accompanied by a current or recent fever [at least 38°C (100.4°F)] and without previous seizure or neurologic events. Febrile seizures are typically categorized as simple or complex. Simple febrile seizures are characteristically generalized, usually last <15 minutes, and occur only once in a 24-hour period. Complex febrile seizures may have focal features, last >15 minutes, and recur within a 24-hour period. Viral infections are often present with febrile seizures, with human herpes virus 6 and 7 and influenza A and B being important causes. There also is a significant increased risk of febrile seizures within 24 hours of receiving vaccination for diphtheria and tetanus toxoids and whole-cell pertussis, and within 8 to 14 days of receiving a measles, mumps, and rubella (MMR) vaccination. The risk of recurrent febrile seizures is increased in patients whose initial febrile seizure occurred at <12 months of age, patients with a lower rectal temperature at first seizure [<40°C (104°F)], patients with shorter duration of fever before their first seizure (<24 hours), patients with a family history of febrile seizures, and patients with complex features with the first febrile seizure. The risk of development of epilepsy is slightly higher among persons having simple febrile seizures but is significantly increased among those who have one or more complex febrile seizures. Initial evaluation of children with febrile seizure includes airway and circulatory support, ideally with noninvasive measures until the postictal state resolves. A thorough medical history that includes past seizures and other neurologic conditions, exposure to medications or toxins, allergies, or trauma may point to a specific seizure cause. Treatment with antipyretics is rarely necessary in the typical seizure case. Patients with seizures that last longer than 5 minutes should receive benzodiazepines to control the seizure. After the seizure ends, the physician should conduct a mental status examination and a physical evaluation. Routine laboratory studies include only a blood glucose test; an electrolyte test may be appropriate if a metabolic abnormality is being considered. In most cases no further work-up is necessary, but lumbar puncture is indicated in patients with suspected meningitis. A lumbar puncture should be considered in children younger than 18 months who have a febrile seizure with the following: (1) a history of irritability, decreased feeding, or lethargy; (2) an abnormal appearance or mental state on initial observation after the postictal period; (3) any physical examination evidence of meningitis; (4) any complex features; (5) any slow postictal clearing of mentation; or (6) pretreatment with antibiotics. Neuroimaging only is appropriate in patients at risk of cerebral abscess, in those who have clinical evidence of increased intracranial pressure, in patients who have evidence of trauma, or in patients who have status epilepticus or have had a complex seizure. Children with simple febrile seizures can be cared for at home after providing parental education and making plans to follow up with the family. Routine prophylaxis using phenobarbital, valproic acid, oral diazepam, or antipyretics is controversial and usually not indicated.

Warden CR, Zibulewsky J, Mace S. Evaluation and management of febrile seizures in the out-of-hospital and emergency department settings. *Ann Emerg Med.* 2003;41:215–222.

22. Which of the following statements is true regarding sexual development in females?
A) The average age of menarche is earlier than it was 75 years ago.
B) African American girls usually experience menarche at an older age.
C) Breast development is usually the last physical characteristic to develop.
D) Girls who mature earlier are typically taller than girls who develop late.
E) The height spurt correlates more with pubic hair development than with breast development.

Answer and Discussion

The answer is A. Teenagers are entering puberty at earlier ages during the 20th century because of various factors, including better nutrition and improved socioeconomic conditions. In the United States, the average age at menarche is 12.16 years in African American girls and 12.88 in White girls. However, menarche may be delayed until age 16 years or may begin as early as age 10. The first objective sign of puberty in girls is the beginning of the height spurt. This is followed by development of breast buds between ages 8 and 11 years. Although breast development usually precedes the growth of pubic hair, in some girls the sequence may be reversed. Among girls, the growth spurt starts at about age 9 years and reaches a peak at age 11.5 years. The spurt usually ends by age 14 years. Girls who mature early reach their peak height velocity sooner and attain their final height earlier. Girls who mature late attain a greater ultimate height because of the longer period of growth before the growth spurt. Final height is related to skeletal age at onset of puberty as well as genetic factors. The height spurt correlates more closely with breast developmental stages than with pubic hair stages.

Hay WW Jr, Levin MJ, Sondheimer JM, et al., eds. Deterding RR. *Current pediatric diagnosis & treatment,* 18th ed. New York: McGraw-Hill; 2007:112–113.

23. Which of the following blood tests may be helpful in determining a recent strep infection in a patient that has a possible poststreptococcal complication?
A) erythrocyte sedimentation rate
B) C-reactive protein
C) complete blood count
D) antistreptolysin O titer

Answer and Discussion

The answer is D. Group A beta-hemolytic streptococcal pharyngitis, scarlet fever, and in rare cases asymptomatic carrier states are associated with poststreptococcal complications. Children are most commonly affected in streptococcal pharyngitis, acute rheumatic fever, pediatric autoimmune neuropsychiatric disorders associated with streptococcal infection, and poststreptococcal glomerulonephritis. The hallmarks of rheumatic fever include arthritis, carditis, cutaneous disease, chorea, and subsequent acquired valvular disease. Pediatric autoimmune neuropsychiatric disorders include a subgroup of illnesses involving the basal ganglia in children with obsessive-compulsive disorders, tic disorders, dystonia, chorea encephalitis, and dystonic choreoathetosis. Poststreptococcal glomerulonephritis occurs most frequently in children between 2 and 6 years of age with a recent history of pharyngitis and a rash during the winter months. The clinical examination of a patient with possible poststreptococcal complications should include an evaluation for signs of inflammation (i.e., complete blood count, erythrocyte sedimentation rate, C-reactive protein) and evidence of a preceding streptococcal infection. Antistreptolysin O titers should be obtained to confirm a recent invasive streptococcal infection. Other important antibody markers include antihyaluronidase, antideoxyribonuclease B, and antistreptokinase antibodies.

Hahn RG, Knox LM, Forman TA. Evaluation of poststreptococcal illness. *Am Fam Physician*. 2005;71:1949–1954.

24. A 13-year-old girl is brought to your office by her mother. The child has experienced a recent sore throat with fevers, and now is complaining of bilateral knee pain. Laboratory evaluation shows an elevated sedimentation rate. The most likely diagnosis is

A) juvenile rheumatoid arthritis
B) acute rheumatic fever
C) Lyme disease
D) Osgood Schlatter disease
E) patellofemoral syndrome

Answer and Discussion

The answer is B. Rheumatic fever is complication of acute group A streptococcal pharyngitis that presents as an acute systemic febrile illness. Associated findings include a migratory arthritis involving the large joints, signs and symptoms of carditis and valvulitis, the erythema marginatum rash, subcutaneous nodules, and choreoathetotic movements of Sydenham's chorea. Damage to the cardiac valves may be chronic and progressive, resulting in significant cardiac dysfunction. Although the Modified Jones Criteria help with the clinical diagnosis, no specific symptoms, clinical signs, or laboratory tests are pathognomonic for rheumatic fever. Additionally, not all patients with rheumatic fever fulfill the Modified Jones Criteria. The criteria consist of major manifestations that include carditis, erythema marginatum, polyarthritis, subcutaneous nodules, and Sydenham's chorea. Minor manifestations include clinical (e.g., arthralgia, fever) and laboratory (e.g., elevated C-reactive protein and erythrocyte sedimentation rate, prolonged PR interval on electrocardiograph) findings. A diagnosis of rheumatic fever is supported by evidence of preceding group A streptococcal infection (i.e., positive throat culture or rapid streptoccocal antigen test, elevated or rising antistreptolysin titer), and the presence of two major manifestations or of one major and two minor manifestations. Arthritis is the most frequent and least specific manifestation of rheumatic fever. It usually affects the large joints and may be the first sign of illness. The lower extremities generally are affected first, followed by the upper extremities. Joint involvement occurs early in the illness and is more common and severe in younger patients. The arthritis may be painful, but it is transient; the inflammation lasts about 2 to 3 days in each joint and 2 to 3 weeks total. Radiographic evaluation can show slight joint effusions but usually the results are normal. The arthritis is self-limited, resolves without complications, and is treated with salicylates and nonsteroidal anti-inflammatory drugs (NSAIDs). Carditis associated with rheumatic fever presents as pericarditis, myocarditis, and most commonly, endocarditis. Pericarditis can present with chest discomfort, pleuritic chest pain, pericardial friction rubs, and distant heart sounds. Myocarditis is rare in isolation and can present with signs and symptoms of heart failure. Endocarditis may be asymptomatic or present with a new heart murmur. Cardiac murmurs do not always indicate valvular involvement, and they may be transient. If valvular disease occurs, it is most likely in the mitral, aortic, tricuspid, or pulmonary valve, in that order. Electrocardiograph and echocardiogam abnormalities may be present in about one third of patients with carditis. Rheumatic heart disease is an important long-term consequence of rheumatic fever and is the major cause of acquired valvular disease internationally. Rheumatic heart disease typically occurs 10 to 20 years after the original rheumatic fever episode. Significant mitral stenosis can occur and require surgery. Sydenham's chorea is characterized by involuntary movements, muscular weakness, and emotional disturbances. It usually is more marked on one side of the body than the other, and may be completely unilateral. Atypical behavior such as crying and restlessness are seen and, in rare cases, features of a psychosis may be noted. There is no sensory loss or involvement of the pyramidal tracts. Sydenham's chorea is typically self-limited and occurs in <5 % of those affected. The condition typically lasts 2 to 3 months. Antistreptococcal prophylaxis should be maintained continuously after an attack of acute rheumatic fever or chorea to prevent recurrences.

Hahn RG, Knox LM, Forman TA. Evaluation of poststreptococcal illness. *Am Fam Physician*. 2005;71:1949–1954.

25. A child presents to the emergency room with abdominal pain. An abdominal series shows a "bird's beak" sign. The most likely diagnosis is

A) intussusception
B) volvulus
C) pyloric stenosis
D) malrotation
E) acute appendicitis

Answer and Discussion

The answer is B. Sigmoid volvulus is a rare problem seen in children and adolescents. Volvulus occurs when a floppy sigmoid loop rotates around its base, producing arterial and venous obstruction of the affected segment, followed by rapid distention of the closed loop. Because the consequences can be life-threatening, sigmoid volvulus should be included in the differential diagnosis of acute and recurrent episodes of abdominal pain or bowel obstruction in children, especially if colonic dilation is seen on radiographs. Boys are more commonly affected than girls. Symptoms can be either acute or recurrent. The most common symptoms are abdominal pain that is relieved by passage of stool or flatus, abdominal distention, and vomiting. Radiographic evaluation often reveals colonic dilation. Barium enema often confirms or suggests the diagnosis, and should be performed under fluoroscopic control; a "twisted-taper" or "bird's-beak" appearance of the affected colon is characteristic. The most common associated conditions include Hirschsprung's disease and imperforate anus. Although sigmoid volvulus can resolve spontaneously, nonoperative management begins with fluid resuscitation and antibiotics, followed by barium enema detorsion of the sigmoid. Other nonoperative modalities include proctosigmoidoscopy and decompression by rectal tube. Operative management most commonly consists of sigmoidectomy.

Salas S, Angel CA, Salas N. Sigmoid volvulus in children and adolescents. *J Am Coll Surg.* 2000;190:717–723.

Barium enema often confirms or suggests the diagnosis of a sigmoid volvulus, and should be performed under fluoroscopic control; a "twisted-taper" or "bird's-beak" appearance of the affected colon is characteristic.

26. The drug of choice for otitis media is

A) azithromycin
B) amoxicillin
C) cefuroxime
D) amoxicillin–clavulanate
E) ceftriaxone

Answer and Discussion

The answer is B. Antibiotic resistance is growing among the organisms that commonly cause acute otitis media. Associated risk factors for resistant pathogens include recent antibiotic treatment, children in day care facilities, infections occurring in the winter, and acute otitis media in children <2 years of age. Amoxicillin remains the antibiotic of first choice, although a higher dosage (80 mg/kg/day) is recommended to ensure adequate eradication of resistant *Streptococcus pneumoniae*. Oral cefuroxime (Ceftin) or amoxicillin–clavulanate (Augmentin) and intramuscular ceftriaxone (Rocephin) are suggested second-line choices for treatment failure. Compliance with antibiotic regimens is enhanced by selecting medications that require less frequent dosing (such as one or two times a day) and by prescribing shorter (5 days or less) treatment courses. Selective use of tympanocentesis if the patient does not respond to empiric therapy can help confirm the diagnosis and guide effective therapy.

Pichichero ME. Acute otitis media: Part II. Treatment in an era of increasing antibiotic resistance. *Am Fam Physician.* 2000;61:2410–2416.

27. Which of the following is a contraindication to influenza vaccine?

A) Allergy to eggs
B) Recent strep infection
C) Allergy to aluminum
D) Age <6 years

Answer and Discussion

The answer is A. Influenza vaccine (Fluzone, Fluvirin) should optimally be given in October and November, but can be given throughout the influenza season. Unvaccinated children younger than 9 years should be given 2 doses at least 1 month apart. Children ages 6 to 35 months are given 0.25 mL IM, whereas children ages 3 years and older are given 0.5 mL IM. (Fluvirin is indicated for use in only children ages 4 years and older.) Because vaccine viruses are first grown in eggs, the vaccine is contraindicated in persons with a history of allergy to eggs or egg products. It is also contraindicated in persons known to be sensitive to thimerosal. The FDA has approved a live attenuated influenza vaccine that is administered nasally (FluMist). It is to be used in healthy children ages 5 to 17 years and adults ages 18 to 49 years. Its safety in asthmatic individuals has not been established, and it is not currently recommended for use in patients with high-risk conditions, such as chronic cardiovascular, pulmonary, renal, or metabolic disorders, and in pregnant women. It is contraindicated in persons with a history of allergic reactions to any vaccine component, including eggs and children receiving chronic aspirin therapy or who are immunosuppressed.

Obtained from AAFP website: http://www.aafp.org/x22166.xml. Accessed 11/02/05.

28. Which of the following statements regarding immunizations is true?

A) Measles–mumps–rubella (MMR) vaccine can cause autism.
B) Hepatitis B vaccine can lead to multiple sclerosis.
C) Children with egg allergies may be given MMR vaccine.
D) Children with a prior local reaction to neomycin should avoid the varicella vaccine.

Answer and Discussion

The answer is C. Controversy has risen about the safety of some vaccines because of rare but serious adverse effects that have been attributed to them. Pain, swelling, and redness at the injection site are common local reactions to vaccines. Fever and irritability may occur after some immunizations. Currently, no substantial evidence links MMR vaccine to autism or hepatitis B vaccine to multiple sclerosis. Thimerosal is being eliminated from routine childhood vaccines because of concerns that multiple immunizations with vaccines containing this preservative could exceed recommended mercury exposures. Children with a history of egg allergy may be given MMR vaccine, even though it is derived from chick embryo fibroblast tissue culture. However, influenza vaccine should not be given to a person with a history of egg allergy. Traces of antibiotics such as neomycin, which is present in varicella (chickenpox), trivalent inactivated poliovirus (IPV), and MMR vaccines, have been considered possible causes of adverse reactions. A history of anaphylactic reaction to neomycin is a contraindication to future immunization, whereas a local reaction is not.

Kimmel SR. Vaccine adverse events: separating myth from reality. *Am Fam Physician.* 2002;66:2113–2120.

29. Which of the following statements regarding pertussis is true?

A) Whole cell vaccine has been shown to be safer than acellular vaccine.
B) The incidence of pertussis is decreasing.
C) Those vaccinated against pertussis have no risk of contracting the disease.
D) Use of DTaP in adolescents is contraindicated.
E) Acellular pertussis vaccine is indicated throughout the primary vaccination series.

Answer and Discussion

The answer is E. The annual number of pertussis cases in the United States has increased since the 1980s. Pertussis is highly contagious, affecting the majority of susceptible household contacts with epidemics occurring in the United States every 3 to 5 years. Children younger than 6 months account for the majority of pertussis hospitalizations, but children ages 10 to 19 years and adults 20 years and older account for increasing numbers of pertussis cases. Acellular pertussis vaccines combined with diphtheria tetanus (DT) are recommended for U.S. children younger than 7 years who do not have a contraindication to vaccination. These vaccines are immunogenic and produce fewer adverse local and systemic reactions than whole-cell pertussis vaccines (DTwP). The same brand of DTaP vaccine should be used throughout the primary vaccination series whenever possible, because there are few data on safety or efficacy when different formulations are interchanged. If the previously used vaccine is not known or is unavailable, any DTaP vaccine licensed for use in the primary series may be given to complete the series. Additionally, an increasing number of pertussis outbreaks have occurred in populations with a high rate of vaccination. The presentation of pertussis is less severe in vaccinated persons than it is in unvaccinated persons, leading to likely underestimation and misdiagnosis of cases. Use of DTaP results in antibody levels to tetanus, diphtheria, and pertussis in adolescents and adults. It is likely that recommendations soon will be made for its use in these groups.

Tozzi AE, Rava L, Ciofi Degli Atti ML. Clinical presentation of pertussis in unvaccinated and vaccinated children in the first six years of life. *Pediatrics.* 2003;112:1069–1075.

30. A child is born at 34 weeks gestation and now presents to your office for a hospital follow-up visit. What advice do you provide the mother regarding health maintenance?

A) Vaccinations should be delayed until the child is 2 months old based on the anticipated due date.
B) Hepatitis B should be delayed until the child is 1 month of age.
C) Vitamin supplements are contraindicated in breast-fed infants.
D) Supplemental iron is not recommended.
E) Adjustments are not necessary when monitoring growth and development in premature infants.

Answer and Discussion

The answer is B. If an infant weights <2 kg at birth and the mother is antigen-negative, this infant should delay the first dose of hepatitis B vaccine until they have reached the chronological age of 1 month. If the mother is antigen-positive or if her antigen status is not known, the child should receive the first dose of hepatitis vaccine plus HBIG within 12 hours of birth, regardless of the infant's birth weight. If these infants weigh <2 kg at birth, this initial dose should not be counted toward completion of the hepatitis B vaccine series, and three additional doses should be administered beginning when the infant is 1 month of age.

Accessed from the CDC.gov website http://www.cdc.gov/nip/recs/contraindications.htm on 6/17/06.

31. Bottle-feeding at bedtime can result in

A) increased risk for aspiration
B) dental caries
C) oral candidiasis
D) nasal polyps
E) development of hiatal hernia

Answer and Discussion

The answer is B. Baby-bottle tooth decay can occur after a child repeatedly falls asleep with a bottle in his or her mouth. It is more commonly seen in lower socioeconomic groups and can lead to major dental problems with the development of caries. Prevention should be aimed at educating the parents about this problem so that they can avoid bottle-feeding at bedtime.

Behrman RE, Kliegman RM, Jenson HB. *Nelson Textbook of Pediatrics,* 17th ed. Philadelphia: WB Saunders; 2004:1210.

32. Which of the following is true concerning DTaP vaccination?

A) The vaccine is routinely administered at 4, 6, and 12 months and again at 5 years of age.
B) The whole cell form is indicated for those who are immunocompromised.
C) The oral form is an inactivated vaccine.
D) Development of pertussis has been linked to the whole cell form.
E) The acellular form is recommended for routine vaccination of all infants.

Answer and Discussion

The answer is E. Current recommendations for the diphtheria, pertussis, and tetanus immunization of young children state that DTaP is usually given at 2, 4, 6, and 12 to 15 months, with an additional dose at 4 to 6 years. The acellular pertussis form is preferred for all doses to help reduce the occurrence of side effects. Tetanus toxoid, reduced diphtheria toxoid, and acellular pertussis vaccine (Tdap adolescent preparation) is recommended at age 11 to 12 years for those who have completed the recommended childhood DTP/DTaP vaccination series and have not received a tetanus and diphtheria toxoid (Td) booster dose. Adolescents aged 13 to 18 years who missed the 11 to 12 year Td/Tdap booster dose should also receive a single dose of Tdap if they completed the recommended childhood DTP/DTaP vaccination series. Subsequent boosters are recommended every 10 years. Contraindications to the DPT vaccine include the following:

1. Previous anaphylaxis to the vaccine
2. Moderate or severe illness
3. Previous encephalopathy within 7 days after DPT injection
4. Progressive neurologic problem that is undiagnosed
5. Fever higher than 105°F after previous DPT
6. Continuous crying lasting 3 hours or more after previous DPT
7. Seizure within 3 days after previous DPT
8. Previous collapse, limp, or pale episode with previous DPT

Items 5 through 8 are relative contraindications and should be evaluated individually. The DTaP immunization should be given intramuscularly. A combined vaccine with DPT and Hib (Tetramune), which can be given at 2, 4, 6, and 12 to 15 months, is available.

Accessed from *The Red Book* online at http://aapredbook on 6/17/06.

33. Which of the following vaccines is no longer recommended for routine vaccination in children?

A) Live oral polio vaccine
B) Inactivated injectable polio vaccine
C) DTaP (diphtheria, tetanus, acellular pertussis)
D) Hemophilus influenza
E) Hepatitis B

Answer and Discussion

The answer is A. Sabin's [oral poliovirus vaccine (OPV)] vaccine for poliomyelitis prevention is an oral, live, attenuated, trivalent vaccine that was given at 2, 4, and 18 months, and 5 years. Because of cases of the risk associated with the live vaccine it is no longer used. In its place the injectable (Salk) vaccine, referred to as *inactivated poliovirus vaccine*, should be administered. The inactivated poliovirus vaccine has now been recommended for routine immunization in all infants because of the risk of developing polio from the live attenuated Sabin's vaccine. The schedule is the same for inactivated poliovirus vaccine.

Accessed from *The Red Book* online at http://aapredbook on 6/17/06.

34. Infant formula typically contains
A) 1 calorie/ounce
B) 10 calories/ounce
C) 20 calories/ounce
D) 50 calories/ounce
E) 100 calories/ounce

Answer and Discussion

The answer is C. Commonly, formula preparations provide 20 calories/ounce. Formulas exist as cow's milk–based, soy-based, and casein-based preparations. Cow's milk–based formula is the preferred, non-breast-milk preparation for otherwise healthy term infants who do not breast-feed or for whom breast-feeding has been terminated prior to 1 year of age. Cow's milk–based formula closely resembles human breast milk and is composed of 20% whey and 80% casein with 50% more protein/dL than breast milk, as well as iron, linoleic acid, carnitine, taurine, and nucleotides. Approximately 32 ounces meets 100% of the recommended daily allowance (RDA) for calories, vitamins, and minerals. These formula preparations are diluted to a standard 20 calories/ounce and are typically whey-dominant protein preparations with vegetable oils and lactose. There are also multiple lactose-free preparations. Most standard formula preparations do not meet the RDA for fluoride, and exclusively formula-fed infants may require 0.25 mg/day of supplemental fluoride.

Hay WW Jr, Levin MJ, Sondheimer JM, et al., eds. *Current pediatric diagnosis & treatment,* 18th ed. New York: McGraw-Hill; 2007:301–303.

35. Which of the following is a risk factor for the development of otitis media in children?
A) Low birth weight
B) Premature birth
C) Family history of allergies/asthma
D) African American descent
E) Pacifier use

Answer and Discussion

The answer is E. Otitis media usually results as a complication of an upper respiratory (viral) infection. It is particularly common in children between 6 months and 3 years of age. The most common etiologic agents include *Streptococcus pneumoniae, Haemophilus influenzae*, and *Moraxella (Branhamella) catarrhalis*. In newborns, *Escherichia coli* and *Staphylococcus aureus* are major causes. Viral causes include respiratory syncitial virus (RSV), parainfluenza virus, influenza virus, enteroviruses, and adenoviruses. Risk factors include attending daycare at or before 2 months of age, in daycare >30 hours/week; bottle-feeding; exposure to cigarette smoke; pacifier use; and Polynesian, Native American, or Alaskan/Canadian Eskimo descent. Low birth weight, young gestational age, and a family history of allergies or asthma are not significantly associated with an increased risk of acute otitis media.

Symptoms include earache, nausea, vomiting, diarrhea, hearing loss, and otorrhea. Fever may be present, but it may be absent in as many as 33% of those affected. Signs include bulging of the tympanic membrane with loss of the light reflex and normal landmarks as well as tympanic membrane immobility. Perforation and vestibular dysfunction may also occur. Diagnosis is based on clinical findings and requires the presence of fluid under pressure in the middle ear plus one sign of acute local or systemic illness. Eardrum motion is best assessed by looking at the pars flaccida in the superior part of the drum. A red drum with normal mobility is common in crying children and is not diagnostic of acute bacterial infection. The drug of choice for treatment is amoxicillin in patients who are not at increased risk of being infected with a drug-resistant organism. Complications include mastoiditis, labyrinthitis, conductive and sensory neural hearing loss, and meningitis.

Semchenko A, Baroody F, Culpepper L. Management of acute sinusitis and acute otitis media. *Am Fam Physician.* Monograph No. 1, 2001:4.

Risk factors for otitis media include attending daycare at or before 2 months of age, in daycare more than 30 hours/week, bottle-feeding, exposure to cigarette smoke, pacifier use, Polynesian descent, Native American descent, and Alaskan and Canadian Eskimo descent.

36. Elevations in blood lead levels can result in
A) decline in IQs
B) development of personality disorders
C) hyperactivity disorder
D) clear cell carcinoma of the vagina
E) visual deficits

Answer and Discussion

The answer is A. A significant number of preschool-age children in the United States have blood lead levels >10 μg/dL (0.50 μmol/L), and these levels have been associated with a decline in IQ. The Centers for Disease Control and Prevention (CDC) advocates the use of a screening questionnaire to identify lead exposure or toxicity in all children. Efforts to remove lead from gasoline and paint have led to a reduction of blood lead levels in children. Secondary prevention through lead paint removal is effective in homes that have a high lead burden. Children with lead levels of 45 to 69 μg/dL (2.15 to 3.35 μmol/L) should receive chelation therapy using succimer (DMSA) or edetate calcium disodium (CaNa2EDTA). Use of both CaNa2EDTA and dimercaprol (BAL in oil) is indicated in children with blood lead levels higher than 70 μg/dL (3.40 μmol/L).

Ellis MR, Kane KY. Lightening the lead load in children. *Am Fam Physician.* 2000;62:545–554, 559–560.

37. A 14-year-old boy presents to your office complaining of pain in his left leg. Radiographs of the area show an aneurysmal bone cyst associated with the metaphysis and periosteal elevation of the mid tibia. The most appropriate management includes
A) leg casting for 6 to 8 weeks
B) nonsteroidal anti-inflammatory drugs (NSAIDs) and reassurance
C) administration of growth hormone
D) technetium bone scan
E) orthopedic surgery referral

Answer and Discussion

The answer is E. Unicameral bone cysts (simple bone cysts) usually affect the metaphysis in long bones of pediatric patients (predominantly the femur, humerus). Most are asymptomatic and come to the attention of the patient, parents, and physician when a fracture occurs in the area of the bone cyst. Most small cysts heal without difficulty; a larger cyst may require surgery that involves removal of the cyst and bone grafting. Most patients recover without permanent disability. An aneurysmal bone cyst is a cyst that occasionally grows larger; these cysts usually occur before 20 years of age. Areas of involvement include expansion beyond the metaphyseal cartilage of the long bones. Patients may report pain and swelling in the region of the cyst. Radiographs may show well-circumscribed areas of rarefaction with periosteal elevation. Treatment usually involves surgery to remove the cyst. Occasionally, radiation therapy is used for vertebral lesions that threaten the spinal cord if surgery is contraindicated; however, postradiation sarcomas can occur. The prognosis for unicameral and aneurysmal bone cysts after treatment is excellent.

Behrman RE, Kliegman RM, Jenson HB. *Nelson Textbook of Pediatrics,* 17th ed. Philadelphia: WB Saunders; 2004: 1721–1722.

38. The definition of *amblyopia* is
A) congenital cataracts noted at birth
B) retinal detachment seen in premature children
C) irregular pupillary size
D) increased distance between the medial and lateral canthus
E) subnormal visual acuity in one or both eyes despite correction of refractive error

Answer and Discussion

The answer is E. Amblyopia is subnormal visual acuity in one or both eyes despite correction of refractive error. It results when the child suppresses the vision in one eye to avoid diplopia. Organic disease may be present but is insufficient to explain the level of vision. Normal visual development requires that a focused image form in each eye that can be fused (superimposed and integrated) by the brain into a single image. Any problem that interferes with a focused, fusible image during the first 8 to 10 years of life is capable of causing amblyopia. The most common causes of amblyopia include strabismus (misalignment of the eyes, images that are not fusible), anisometropia (unequal refractive components of eyes, images are not focused simultaneously), and deprivation (cataract, ptosis, corneal scar). Visual screening can usually detect early cases of amblyopia. If suspected, the child should be referred for ophthalmologic evaluation. Children at greatest risk for the development of amblyopia are younger than 2 to 3 years of age, and those younger than 6 months of age are at the highest risk. The key to successful outcome is early detection and treatment, which includes correction of refraction error or removal of cataract, as well as forced use of the amblyopic eye by patching the better eye. The earlier the diagnosis is made, the better the prognosis.

Beers MH, Porter RS, eds. *The Merck manual of diagnosis and therapy,* Merck Research Laboratories, 18th ed. Whitehouse Station, NJ: Merck & Co.; 2006:2445.

39. Leukocoria is most likely associated with
A) pregnancy
B) infection
C) retinoblastoma
D) leukemia
E) pyuria

Answer and Discussion

The answer is C. An abnormal pupillary light reflex (called *leukocoria* if the pupil appears white) may indicate a disorder anywhere within the eye. Associated disorders include corneal opacity, blood (hyphema) or other material in the anterior chamber, cataract, vitreous opacity or retinal disease. The most serious diagnosis is retinoblastoma, a malignancy that is thought to arise from retinal germ cells. Because it may be hereditary, a family history of retinoblastoma or of enucleation is of special concern. Although retinoblastoma is almost uniformly fatal without treatment, the cure rate is better than 90% when the condition is promptly recognized and treated, and many children can be effectively treated without enucleation.

Simon JW, Kaw P. Commonly missed diagnoses in the childhood eye examination. *Am Fam Physician.* 2001;64:623–628.

40. Which of the following statements is true regarding hyperbilirubinemia?
A) Physiologic jaundice is rare in newborns.
B) Switching from formula feeding to breast-feeding may help decrease bilirubin levels.
C) Coombs' testing offers little information in the workup of hyperbilirubinemia.
D) For the condition of kernicterus to occur in premature infants the level of bilirubin must be higher than in term newborns.
E) Complications of kernicterus include hearing loss, seizures, and mental retardation.

Answer and Discussion

The answer is E. Kernicterus occurs when the serum unconjugated (indirect) bilirubin becomes dangerously elevated (usually >25 mg/dL) in newborns. Symptoms include poor feeding, flaccidity, apnea, opisthotonos, and seizures; in severe cases, death may occur. Children who do survive may suffer hearing loss, seizures, and mental retardation. Risk factors include prematurity, blood incompatibilities, infection, and acidosis. Physiologic jaundice is the most common form of jaundice, and occurs in up to 50% of newborns. The condition is benign and usually resolves in 1 week. Most bilirubin levels peak in 3 to 5 days. The workup of a child with hyperbilirubinemia should include the following:

- Careful history to detect risk factors and physical examination to rule out petechiae, hepatosplenomegaly, bruising, and signs of infection
- Measurement of bilirubin levels
- Complete blood cell count, reticulocyte count, and peripheral blood smear
- Coombs' test
- Typing of mother's and infant's blood
- Thyroid function tests

Treatment for hyperbilirubinemia of newborns includes the following:

- Increasing formula feedings for the infant will increase GI motility and frequency of stools, thereby minimizing the enterohepatic circulation of bilirubin.
- Increasing frequency of breastfeeding. If the bilirubin continues to rise, switch from breast-feeding to formula for a few

days until the bilirubin is <15 mg/dL (the mother should continue with breast pumping during this time)
- Phototherapy, which helps degrade unconjugated bilirubin
- Exchange transfusion for severe cases of persistent hyperbilirubinemia (usually >20 mg/dL) or hemolysis with anemia

In premature infants, kernicterus may occur with lower bilirubin levels.

Beers MH, Porter RS, eds. *The Merck manual of diagnosis and therapy,* Merck Research Laboratories, 18th ed. Whitehouse Station, NJ: Merck & Co.; 2006:2275–2279.

41. Preterm breast milk
A) has the same components as breast milk produced at term
B) persists for 1 week before the composition approaches that of term infant breast milk
C) contains lower concentrations of important electrolytes and immunoglobulins
D) typically requires fortification with human milk fortifiers
E) contains excessive amounts of calcium

Answer and Discussion

The answer is D. The composition of breast milk in mothers of preterm infants is different from that of term infants. This difference persists for approximately 4 weeks before the composition approaches that of term infant breast milk. The difference in preterm milk composition reflects the increased nutrient demands of preterm infants. Preterm breast milk contains higher concentrations of total and bound nitrogen, immunoglobulins, sodium, iron, chloride, and medium-chain fatty acids. However, it may not contain sufficient amounts of phosphorus, calcium, copper, and zinc. Preterm infants are more likely to require fortification with human milk fortifiers (HMF) to correct these deficiencies.

Hay WW Jr, Levin MJ, Sondheimer JM, et al., eds. *Current pediatric diagnosis & treatment,* 18th ed. New York: McGraw-Hill; 2007:302.

42. A 12-year-old boy presents to your office complaining of gradual, increasing hip pain that radiates to the thigh and knee. Physical examination shows an obese boy with pain associated with hip abduction and adduction. Radiographs show evidence of acetabular dysplasia. The most likely diagnosis is
A) congenital dislocation of the hip
B) Osgood-Schlatter disease
C) slipped capital femoral epiphyses
D) sacral insufficiency fracture
E) transient synovitis of the hip

Answer and Discussion

The answer is C. Slipped capital femoral epiphyses are usually seen in overweight boys between 11 and 14 years of age. The condition occurs when the femoral head slips posteriorly and inferiorly, exposing the anterior and superior aspects of the metaphysis of the femoral neck. When the condition occurs before puberty, an underlying endocrine disorder (hypothyroidism, growth hormone deficiency) should be suspected. Symptoms, including pain and a limp, are usually gradual in onset and usually involve the hips or are referred to the thigh or knee. The condition is bilateral in 20% of cases. Radiographs should be performed, including frog-leg views. Findings include abnormalities with the femoral head, including acetabular dysplasia. Treatment involves orthopedic referral with surgical pinning. Complications include avascular necrosis of the hip and erosion of cartilage.

Behrman RE, Kliegman RM, Jenson HB. *Nelson Textbook of Pediatrics,* 17th ed. Philadelphia: WB Saunders; 2004: 2278–2279.

43. A 4 year old is brought to your office. The parent complains that the child's hair is falling out. Closer inspection shows the hair shafts are broken just above the scalp. There are scaly, pruritic, mildly inflamed gray patches, and scrapings of the area show the presence of hyphae. The treatment of choice is
A) topical antifungals
B) oral antifungals
C) topical hydrocortisone cream
D) permethrin cream
E) shave the hair off at the scalp and let it regrow

Answer and Discussion

The answer is B. Tinea capitis is a fungal infection of the scalp that usually affects infants and young children. It is contagious and may become epidemic. It is caused by fungi including *Trichophyton*, *Microsporum*, and *Epidermophyton*. Lesions of the scalp usually cause scaly, gray patches that are pruritic. Multiple areas of hair loss may occur with hair shafts broken just above the scalp. Microscopic examination of scrapings after treatment with 10% potassium hydroxide reveals fungal hyphae. Hair examined with black light fluorescences show a greenish-yellow color in cases of microsporosis. Treatment for most tinea infections involves the use of topical antifungals but is not sufficient for tinea capitus, which requires oral administration of griseofulvin or ketoconazole. Severely inflamed lesions benefit from systemic or intralesional steroids. Until tinea capitis is cured, an imidazole or ciclopirox cream should be applied to the scalp to prevent spread, especially to other children, and selenium sulfide 2.5% shampoo should be used daily. Children can attend school during treatment, and the risk of transmission is low.

Beers MH, Porter RS, eds. *The Merck manual of diagnosis and therapy,* Merck Research Laboratories, 18th ed. Whitehouse Station, NJ: Merck & Co.; 2006:988–992.

44. An 18-year-old high school student presents with a painless mass in his neck. He also reports a slight cough over the last 6 weeks. Additionally, he reports some fatigue and generalized pruritus. The most likely diagnosis is
A) infectious mononucleosis
B) brachial cleft cyst
C) *Streptococcus* pharyngitis
D) Lyme disease
E) Hodgkin's disease

Answer and Discussion

The answer is E. The incidence of Hodgkin's disease increases throughout childhood and peaks in the late teens. The most common presenting complaint is a painless mass in the neck. Other presentations include a persistent cough secondary to a mediastinal mass or, less commonly, splenomegaly or enlarged axillary or inguinal lymph nodes. About one third of children with Hodgkin's disease present with constitutional symptoms. These symptoms may include intermittent fever, night sweats, and weight loss. These are referred to as "B" symptoms. The "A" designation refers to the absence of these symptoms. Other symptoms include anorexia, fatigue, and pruritus. Any persistent painless mass (especially a neck mass) that does not respond to antibiotics should be evaluated. This investigation should include a lymph node biopsy. Because of sampling errors and difficulties in obtaining an accurate diagnosis, excisional biopsy (rather than needle biopsy) of enlarged lymph nodes should be performed. A persistent cough, especially in the presence of any "B" symptoms, should be investigated. As part of this evaluation, a chest radiograph should be obtained. It is also important to investigate "B" symptoms associated with any lymphadenopathy or splenomegaly. Laboratory tests can often be helpful in confirming the diagnosis. Although nonspecific, elevations in the erythrocyte sedimentation rate, lactate dehydrogenase level, and ferritin level are suspicious findings in children with other signs or symptoms of Hodgkin's disease. Infrequently, the CBC reveals abnormalities, including anemia and eosinophilia.

Hay WW Jr, Levin MJ, Sondheimer JM, et al., eds. *Current pediatric diagnosis & treatment,* 18th ed. New York: McGraw-Hill; 2007:896–898.

The incidence of Hodgkin's disease increases throughout childhood and peaks in the late teens. The most common presenting complaint is a painless mass in the neck.

45. The condition of facial acne is associated with
A) ingestion of fatty foods
B) presence of *Propionibacterium acnes*
C) consumption of chocolate
D) presence of *Staphylococcus aureus*
E) poor hygiene

Answer and Discussion

The answer is B. Acne is one of the most common presenting complaints in a family physician's office. Adolescent patients between 12 and 25 years of age are the most commonly affected. The condition results when keratinization blocks follicular canals. Increased sebum production occurs, and bacterial proliferation causes inflammation. Increased androgen production is often related to the development of acne. The plugged pilosebaceous unit is referred to as a "whitehead" if the lesion is a closed comedone, or a "blackhead" if the comedone is open. The most common infecting bacterium is *Propionibacterium acnes*, which proliferates and releases chemotactic factors that attract leukocytes. The diagnosis of acne is made by observing characteristic lesions on the face, back, shoulders, and chest. Treatment involves washing with mild soaps on a regular basis; application of benzoyl peroxide; topical tretinoin (Retin-A); or topical antibiotics such as erythromycin, clindamycin, tetracycline, or meclocycline. Oral antibiotics may be necessary for more severe cases. Severe nodulocystic acne that fails to respond to the previously mentioned measures may be treated with oral isotretinoin (Accutane). Close monitoring of liver function tests, triglyceride levels, and complete blood cell counts are required. In addition, the drug has many other side effects (i.e., xerosis, epistaxis, myalgias, and arthralgias) and is highly teratogenic. Patients should be aware that acne is not a disease of hygiene. They should not try to scrub the lesions away, and they should not use alcohol-based astringents that can dry and irritate their skin. Patients should be instructed to wash their face twice a day with a mild soap and water. Patients should also be informed that acne has no relationship to diet (e.g., chocolate, pizza, soda). Many think acne is caused by stress, but no studies support this association. It may be that the acne itself causes stress, not vice versa. Cosmetics have long been blamed for the development of acne lesions. Although the causal relationship between cosmetics and acne may be overstated, patients should be directed to use oil-free, noncomedogenic cosmetics. Oil from hair products and suntan lotions can also exacerbate acne. Female patients should be informed that acne usually worsens during the week before menses. Mechanical trauma can make acne worse. Therefore, patients should be encouraged to avoid picking at lesions, because doing so may cause more inflammation.

Russell JJ. Topical therapy for acne. *Am Fam Physician.* 2000;61:357–366.

46. Absence seizures are associated with which of the following features?
A) Subnormal intelligence
B) Three per second spike-and-wave electroencephalogram (EEG) pattern
C) Staring episodes that last 30 to 45 minutes
D) March-like progression of tonic–clonic activity
E) No genetic transmission

Answer and Discussion

The answer is B. Absence seizures (formerly called *petit mal seizures*) are characterized by brief, 10- to 30-second staring episodes, followed by a resumption of normal activity. Attacks may occur up to 100 times daily and can be precipitated by hyperventilation. The seizures usually affect children, and there is a genetic predisposition. Affected children usually have normal intelligence, and most cases resolve before 20 years of age. EEG findings show a characteristic 3/second bilateral spike-and-wave pattern. Treatment usually involves the use of valproic acid and/or ethosuximide and clonazepam.

Beers MH, Porter RS, eds. *The Merck manual of diagnosis and therapy,* Merck Research Laboratories, 18th ed. Whitehouse Station, NJ: Merck & Co.; 2006:1825, 1833.

47. Idiopathic aseptic necrosis of the femoral head is also known as
A) slipped capital femoral epiphyses
B) Osgood-Schlatter disease
C) Legg-Calvé-Perthes disease
D) Morton's neuroma
E) transient synovitis of the hip

Answer and Discussion

The answer is C. Idiopathic aseptic necrosis of the femoral head is also known as *Legg-Calvé-Perthes disease*. The disease is usually unilateral and is most common in boys 2 to 12 years of age. Symptoms include hip, groin, or thigh pain and difficulty ambulating, which is usually gradual in onset and progressive. Physical examination may show an abnormal gait (painless limp) and atrophy of the thigh muscles. Lateral radiographs (frog view) are required and show areas of lucency and fragmentation of the femoral head, which may progress to sclerosis and destruction. Radiographs are often normal early in the disease process; however, bone scans may show decreased uptake in the area of the femoral head. Treatment involves expectant observation both clinically and radiographically, abduction casts to contain the femoral head within the acetabulum, and surgery in select cases. It should be remembered that children who present with knee pain may have hip pathology.

Behrman RE, Kliegman RM, Jenson HB. *Nelson Textbook of Pediatrics,* 17th ed. Philadelphia: WB Saunders; 2004: 2276–2278.

48. Which of the following is associated with infectious mononucleosis?
A) submental lymphadenopathy
B) strawberry tongue
C) cobble-stoned appearance of posterior pharynx
D) palatal petechiae
E) negative heterophile antibody test

Answer and Discussion

The answer is D. Infectious mononucleosis is relatively common in patients 10 to 30 years of age who present with sore throat and fatigue, palatal petechiae, posterior cervical or auricular adenopathy, marked adenopathy, or inguinal adenopathy. An atypical lymphocytosis of at least 20% or atypical lymphocytosis of at least 10% plus lymphocytosis of at least 50% strongly supports the diagnosis, as does a positive heterophile antibody test. False-negative results of heterophile antibody tests are relatively common early in the course of infection. Symptomatic treatment, the mainstay of care, includes adequate hydration, analgesics, antipyretics, and adequate rest. Bed rest should not be strictly enforced, and the patient's energy level should guide activity. Corticosteroids, acyclovir, and antihistamines are not recommended for routine treatment of infectious mononucleosis, although corticosteroids may benefit patients with respiratory compromise or severe pharyngeal edema. Patients with infectious mononucleosis should be withdrawn from contact or collision sports for at least 4 weeks after the onset of symptoms. Fatigue, myalgias, and need for sleep may persist for several months after the acute infection has resolved.

Ebell MH. Epstein-Barr virus infectious mononucleosis. *Am Fam Physician.* 2004;70:1279–1287, 1289–1290.

49. Which of the following is routinely given at birth to prevent hemorrhagic disease of the newborn?
A) Erythromycin
B) Vitamin C
C) Vitamin K
D) Factor X
E) von Willebrand's factor

Answer and Discussion

The answer is C. Following birth, there is a modest decrease in the vitamin K (phytonadione)—dependent factors II, VII, IX, and X—that gradually return to normal in 7 to 10 days. The cause of this decrease is inadequate free vitamin K available from the mother and the newborn's inability to synthesize vitamin K because of a lack of intestinal flora. Therefore, 1 mg of vitamin K is administered intramuscularly at birth to prevent hemorrhagic disease of the newborn in term infants. Larger doses predispose to the development of hyperbilirubinemia and kernicterus. Breast milk is a poor source of vitamin K. As a result, hemorrhagic complications occur more frequently in breast-fed infants. Mothers taking medications that interfere with vitamin K function (i.e., phenobarbital and phenytoin) may have infants at increased risk for early onset bleeding.

Behrman RE, Kliegman RM, Jenson HB. *Nelson Textbook of Pediatrics,* 17th ed. Philadelphia: WB Saunders; 2004: 606–607.

50. Which of the following statements about Down syndrome is true?
A) Younger mothers are at increased risk for having a child affected with Down syndrome.
B) There is an increased risk of leukemia in children affected with Down syndrome.
C) Most children affected have normal intelligence quotients (IQs).
D) The condition is not passed on to children of affected mothers.
E) Those affected usually have a normal life expectancy.

Answer and Discussion

The answer is B. Down syndrome is a condition characterized by an extra chromosome 21. The incidence is reported to be 1 in 700 to 800 births, but it varies depending on maternal age. Older mothers (especially those older than 35) are at increased risk. The disease may result from trisomy 21, translocation, or mosaicism.

Signs and symptoms include a flattened, hypoplastic midface with a depressed nasal bridge, hypotonicity, retarded physical and mental development with decreased IQ, microcephaly with a flattened occiput, slanted eyes with epicanthal folds, Brushfield spots (gray to white spots around the periphery of the iris), Simian crease (single palmar crease), short fingers, and abnormal feet with a wide gap between the first and second toe. Other associated conditions include congenital heart disease (e.g., ventricular septal defects) and gastrointestinal anomalies (e.g., tracheoesophageal fistula, pyloric stenosis, duodenal atresia, and imperforate anus). The life expectancy of a child affected with Down syndrome is reduced by the presence of heart disease and an increased risk of acute leukemia. Some affected women are fertile; however, they have a 50% chance that their fetus will also have Down syndrome. Many of these affected fetuses abort spontaneously. All men with Down syndrome are infertile.

Beers MH, Porter RS, eds. *The Merck manual of diagnosis and therapy,* Merck Research Laboratories, 18th ed. Whitehouse Station, NJ: Merck & Co.; 2006:2449–2450.

Signs and symptoms of Down's syndrome include a flattened, hypoplastic midface with a depressed nasal bridge, hypotonicity, retarded physical and mental development with decreased IQ, microcephaly with a flattened occiput, slanted eyes with epicanthal folds, Brushfield spots (gray to white spots around the periphery of the iris), Simian crease (single palmar crease), short fingers, and abnormal feet with a wide gap between the first and second toe.

51. The most common cause of a limp in a 5-year-old boy is
A) stress fracture
B) transient synovitis of the hip
C) Legg-Calvé-Perthes disease
D) slipped capital femoral epiphyses
E) septic joint

Answer and Discussion

The answer is B. Transient synovitis of the hip is the most common cause of hip pain and limping in U.S. children. The condition usually follows an upper respiratory illness and resolves spontaneously within a few days. Children 3 to 10 years of age, particularly boys, are the most commonly affected. Physical examination shows a limp and limited motion of the hip, especially with internal rotation. The hip is usually kept flexed, abducted, and externally rotated. Radiographs are usually negative but may show soft tissue swelling associated with the hip joint. A complete blood count and the erythrocyte sedimentation rate are usually normal. Treatment involves rest and anti-inflammatory drugs. Symptoms usually resolve in 7 to 10 days. Traction of the hip in slight flexion may also be used. Follow-up radiographs (at 1 and 3 months from time of presentation or perhaps sooner if the child's limp persists) are recommended because of the risk for development of avascular necrosis of the femoral head. If septic arthritis is suspected, aspiration of the hip may be necessary.

Behrman RE, Kliegman RM, Jenson HB. *Nelson Textbook of Pediatrics,* 17th ed. Philadelphia: WB Saunders; 2004:606–607.

52. Which of the following statements concerning circumcision is true?

A) It is medically indicated for all males.
B) Premature infants should not be circumcised.
C) Infant males with posthitis should not be circumcised.
D) Hypospadias is not a contraindication for circumcision.
E) Circumcision can be performed in the office until 4 months of age.

Answer and Discussion

The answer is B. Controversy surrounds the necessity of circumcision. UTIs are 10 to 15 times more common in uncircumcised infants. Many recommend circumcision in infants who are predisposed to UTI, such as those with congenital hydronephrosis and vesicoureteral reflux. Other indications for circumcision include recurrent balanitis (inflammation of the glans), posthitis (inflammation of the foreskin), or paraphimosis (retraction of the prepuce behind the glans that may interfere with blood flow). Routine circumcision is often more a social issue than a medical indication. Because phimosis (tightness of the foreskin so that it cannot be retracted over the glans penis) cannot usually be detected before puberty, it is not an indication for circumcision. Contraindications for circumcision include prematurity, genital anomalies (including hypospadias or ambiguous genitalia), and bleeding disorders. Circumcision should be performed at least 12 to 24 hours after birth and within 6 weeks of birth, preferably before discharge from the hospital. If delay occurs beyond 6 weeks, circumcision should be postponed until after 1 year of age with general anesthesia. Most recommend using a dorsal penile nerve block with 1% lidocaine without epinephrine for local anesthesia. EMLA cream can also be applied.

Behrman RE, Kliegman RM, Jenson HB. *Nelson Textbook of Pediatrics,* 17th ed. Philadelphia: WB Saunders; 2004: 606–607.

53. Which of the following statements is true regarding infectious mononucleosis?

A) Guillain-Barré syndrome is an associated complication.
B) The disease can result in positive rheumatoid factor formation.
C) Heterophil agglutination tests are usually positive at the onset of the disease.
D) Rupture of the aorta can be associated with the disease.
E) Glaucoma is often seen with prolonged cases.

Answer and Discussion

The answer is A. Infectious mononucleosis is caused by the Epstein-Barr virus. It usually affects individuals between 10 and 35 years of age. Symptoms include fever, sore throat, anorexia, generalized fatigue, lymphadenopathy (especially affecting the posterior cervical chain), splenomegaly, and a maculopapular rash. Hepatitis with hepatomegaly is often seen with occasional jaundice. Laboratory findings include leukocytosis with many atypical lymphocytes (i.e., larger with vacuolated cytoplasm) and a positive monospot test (with heterophil agglutination) that becomes positive before the fourth week after the onset of the illness. The results of these tests are usually negative in infants and children younger than 4 years. False-positive rapid plasmin reagin and Venereal Disease Research Laboratory tests may occur, as well as abnormal liver function tests. Treatment involves supportive therapy with saline gargles, anti-inflammatories, and antipyretic medication. In severely ill patients with severe pharyngitis, corticosteroids can be used to help decrease inflammation. Complications include the development of Guillain-Barré syndrome, myocarditis, and encephalitis. Spleen rupture may also occur with trauma; therefore, contact sports should be avoided until the splenomegaly has resolved.

Ebell MH. Epstein-Barr virus infectious mononucleosis. *Am Fam Physician.* 2004;70:1279–1287, 1289–1290.

54. Which of the following is true regarding medications used in the treatment of acne?

A) A low estrogen-containing oral contraceptive can be helpful in the treatment of acne.
B) Doxycycline, tetracycline and minocycline are contraindicated before the age of 18.
C) Lipid values must be monitored when using isotretinoin.
D) Oral contraceptives are adequate to prevent pregnancy when administering isotretinoin.

Answer and Discussion

The answer is C. Topical retinoids, benzoyl peroxide, sulfacetamide, and azelaic acid are recommended in patients with mild or moderate comedones. Topical erythromycin or clindamycin can be used in addition in patients with mild to moderate inflammatory acne or mixed acne. A 6-month course of oral erythromycin, doxycycline, tetracycline, or minocycline can be prescribed in patients with moderate to severe inflammatory acne. A low-androgen containing oral contraceptive pill is also effective in women with moderate to severe acne. Isotretinoin is reserved for use in the treatment of the most severe or refractory cases of inflammatory cystic type acne. Because of its poor side effect profile and teratogenicity, isotretinoin (Accutane) must by prescribed by a physician who is registered with the System to Manage Accutane-Related Teratogenicity (SMART) program. Serious side effects of isotretinoin include hepatitis, hypertriglyceridemia, intracranial hypertension, arthralgia, myalgias, night blindness, and hyperostosis. Serum liver function tests and triglyceride levels must be monitored monthly in patients receiving isotretinoin. Isotretinoin is teratogenic and can result in severe fetal abnormalities involving several systems. As a result two forms of contraception must be used during isotretinoin therapy and for 1 month after treatment has been discontinued. To ensure that female patients are not pregnant when treatment is initiated, two negative urine pregnancy tests are required before isotretinoin is prescribed. Pregnancy status is rechecked at monthly visits. The link between isotretinoin and depression is controversial.

Feldman S, Careccia RE, Barham KL, et al. The diagnosis and treatment of acne. *Am Fam Physician.* 2004;69:2123–2130, 2135–2136.

55. A 2 year old presents with an erythematous rash on the face (slapped-cheek appearance) that has spread to involve the trunk; the extremities are spared. She also has a low-grade fever and malaise. Which of the following is the most likely diagnosis?
A) Measles
B) Congenital syphilis
C) Erythema infectiosum
D) Meningococcemia
E) Rubeola

Answer and Discussion

The answer is C. Erythema infectiosum is referred to as *fifth disease*, because it represents the fifth major viral childhood illness (which also includes measles, mumps, rubella, and rubeola). The disease is caused by parvovirus B19 and is characterized by mild constitutional symptoms, such as low-grade fever, malaise, and joint pain (particularly in adult women). Also, there is a classic indurated, erythematous maculopapular facial rash that may progress to the trunk and extremities (but spares the palms and soles). The rash is often pronounced on extensor surfaces. The rash is often referred to as a "slapped-cheek" appearance and can be exacerbated with exposure to sunlight, heat, emotional stress, or fever. The illness usually lasts 5 to 10 days, and only symptomatic treatment is necessary. Occasionally complications include arthropathies, myocarditis and a transient aplastic crisis. Fifth disease may occasionally cause fetal death secondary to fetal hydrops; therefore, pregnant women should avoid contact with affected patients. Children are not infectious once the rash develops because the rash and arthropathy (when present) are immune-mediated, postinfectious reactions. Therefore isolation from school and/or daycare is not necessary.

Behrman RE, Kliegman RM, Jenson HB. *Nelson Textbook of Pediatrics,* 17th ed. Philadelphia: WB Saunders; 2004: 1048–1050.

56. The treatment of choice for iron poisoning is
A) pralidoxime chloride
B) deferoxamine
C) penicillamine
D) edetate calcium disodium
E) plasmapheresis

Answer and Discussion

The answer is B. There are five stages described for iron intoxication:

- Stage 1. Hemorrhagic gastroenteritis, which occurs 30 to 60 minutes after the ingestion. Lasting for 4 to 6 hours, this may result in hematemesis, abdominal pain, irritability, explosive diarrhea, shock, coma, and metabolic acidosis.
- Stage 2. After these findings there is usually a symptom-free period that lasts up to 24 hours.
- Stage 3. The next 48 hours after ingestion is usually a period of delayed shock with iron levels >500 mg/dL. Cerebral dysfunction, fever, seizures, and coma may occur.
- Stage 4. Two to five days after ingestion liver damage starts to appear and may lead to hepatic failure. Other manifestations include coagulopathies and hypoglycemia.
- Stage 5. Gastrointestinal scarring, bowel obstruction, and pyloric stenosis may develop 2 to 5 weeks after the initial ingestion.

In addition to the previously mentioned symptoms, vomiting, hyperglycemia, leukocytosis, and an abdominal radiograph that shows the iron particles are usually related to a serum iron level > 300 mg/dL. Severe cases may cause seizures, coma, pulmonary edema, and vascular collapse. Treatment involves inducing vomiting, as well as gastric lavage, followed by use of the chelating agent deferoxamine. Charcoal does not bind iron. In severe cases, hemodialysis and exchange transfusion may be necessary.

Beers MH, Porter RS, eds. *The Merck manual of diagnosis and therapy,* Merck Research Laboratories, 18th ed. Whitehouse Station, NJ: Merck & Co.; 2006:2667–2668.

57. A 1-year-old infant is brought into the office by a concerned mother. The child has an erythematous diaper rash with small satellite lesions that have not improved with application of petroleum jelly. The most appropriate treatment is
A) zinc oxide
B) clotrimazole (Lotrimin) ointment
C) Neosporin ointment
D) mupirocin (Bactroban) ointment
E) hydrocortisone cream

Answer and Discussion

The answer is B. Diaper dermatitis secondary to *Candida albicans* is an intensely red and scorched-appearing rash that involves the perineal area. The rash may be well demarcated and possess vesicles that weep, pustules, papules, and the characteristic satellite lesions. Treatment consists of antifungal ointment (i.e., clotrimazole or nystatin) and, possibly, short-term use of hydrocortisone cream for severe dermatitis. Soothing cream (zinc oxide) should be applied with each diaper change. Also, keeping the area dry can help deter the development of yeast dermatitis.

Behrman RE, Kliegman RM, Jenson HB. *Nelson Textbook of Pediatrics,* 17th ed. Philadelphia: WB Saunders; 2004: 2234–2235.

58. Which of the following medications is recommended in the treatment of mild to moderate croup?
A) Acyclovir
B) Dexamethasone
C) Theophylline
D) Atropine
E) No medications have been found to be useful.

Answer and Discussion

The answer is B. Viral croup is the main cause of airway obstruction in children 6 months to 6 years of age. For children with mild croup, symptomatic care and mist therapy may be all that is necessary. Epinephrine has been used in the past to treat more severe cases of croup, but recent studies have found that glucocorticoid use is associated with shorter hospital stays, improvement in croup scores, and less use of epinephrine. Studies have shown that treatment with oral dexamethasone is as effective as intramuscular dexamethasone or nebulized budesonide. While more studies are needed to establish guidelines, oral dexamethasone can be used to treat mild to moderate croup with close follow-up and instructions for further care, if needed.

Knutson D, Aring A. Viral croup. *Am Fam Physician.* 2004; 69:535–540, 541–542.

59. Which of the following medications would not be a suitable alternative for second-line treatment of otitis media in a 6 year old?
A) Azithromycin
B) Cefaclor
C) Cefixime
D) Ciprofloxacin
E) Erythromycin

Answer and Discussion

The answer is D. Ciprofloxacin is generally not indicated for patients under age 18 because of the risk of damage to cartilage development. Although amoxicillin is considered the drug of choice the other options can be used as second line agents.

Behrman RE, Kliegman RM, Jenson HB. *Nelson Textbook of Pediatrics,* 17th ed. Philadelphia: WB Saunders; 2004:1788.

60. Immunizations (excluding hepatitis B) for premature infants should be
A) delayed because of the infant's immaturity
B) administered at same designated times as normal infants based on their age
C) withheld for 1 year
D) given earlier to help prevent diseases to which they are more susceptible
E) given in reduced amounts based on the child's weight

Answer and Discussion

The answer is B. Premature infants are predisposed to certain problems, including poor sucking and diminished gag and cough reflexes, which can lead to an increased risk of aspiration and difficulty feeding. Other problems include pulmonary immaturity, decreased ability to maintain body temperature, impaired renal excretion, limited iron stores with a predisposition to develop anemia, metabolic disturbances, and decreased ability to fight infection. Immunizations should take place at the same designated times as for term infants with no adjustments made for premature age. One exception to this recommendation is that hepatitis B vaccination should be delayed for 1 month if mothers are negative for hepatitis B surface antigen.

Behrman RE, Kliegman RM, Jenson HB. *Nelson Textbook of Pediatrics,* 17th ed. Philadelphia: WB Saunders; 2004:1182.

Premature infants are predisposed to certain problems, including poor sucking and diminished gag and cough reflexes, which can lead to an increased risk of aspiration and difficulty feeding.

61. Which of the following conditions is associated with children of teenage mothers?
A) Cognitive delays in IQ
B) Schizophrenia
C) Major depression
D) Manic–depressive disorder
E) Suicide

Answer and Discussion

The answer is A. The children of teenage mothers have been shown to have cognitive delays on IQ and vocabulary tests. They may also show problems of emotion, including rebelliousness, aggressiveness, uncontrollable anger, and impulsiveness. They are at greater risk for low birth weight and they have an increased risk of experiencing an accident within the home and of being hospitalized before the age of 5 years. There appears to be no link with major affective disorders.

Behrman RE, Kliegman RM, Jenson HB. *Nelson Textbook of Pediatrics,* 17th ed. Philadelphia: WB Saunders; 2004:673.

62. A 3-year-old boy presents with a bilateral conjunctivitis, cracking of his lips, cervical lymphadenopathy and swelling of his hands. The most likely diagnosis is
A) Kawasaki disease
B) infectious mononucleosis
C) scarlet fever
D) Rocky Mountain fever
E) Lyme disease

Answer and Discussion

The answer is A. Kawasaki disease was previously referred to as mucocutaneous lymph node syndrome. The cause of Kawasaki disease is unclear, and unfortunately a specific diagnostic test for its detection does not exist. The majority of affected patients are younger than age 5 years, and males are more frequently affected. Diagnosis is based on the following criteria and include fever for more than 5 days and at least four of the following features: (1) bilateral, painless, nonexudative conjunctivitis, (2) lip cracking and fissuring, strawberry tongue, inflammation of the oral mucosa, (3) cervical lymphadenopathy ($\geq$1.5 cm in diameter and usually unilateral), (4) exanthema, and (5) redness and swelling of the hands and feet with subsequent desquamation. Adverse cardiovascular effects are the most serious component of Kawasaki disease. Cardiovascular complications include myocarditis, pericarditis, valvular heart disease (usually mitral or aortic regurgitation), and coronary arteritis. Coronary artery lesions range from mild transient dilation of a coronary artery to large aneurysm formation. Those at greatest risk of aneurysm formation are males, children under the age of 6 months, and those not treated with intravenous immunoglobulin (IVIG). The gold standard for diagnosing coronary artery aneurysms is angiography, however two-dimensional echocardiography is highly sensitive and is the current standard screening test in children with Kawasaki disease. Fortunately, most coronary artery aneurysms resolve within 5 years of diagnosis. Giant aneurysms ($>$8 mm) are much less likely to resolve, and about half become stenotic. Of additional concern, acute thrombosis of an aneurysm can occur, resulting in a myocardial infarction, and can be fatal. The treatment of Kawasaki disease consists of therapy with IVIG and high-dose aspirin. This therapy is effective in decreasing the incidence of coronary artery dilation and aneurysm formation. Currently, corticosteroids are not felt to be effective in Kawasaki disease.

During the acute and subacute phases of the illness, patients should be monitored closely by serial electrocardiography, chest radiograph, and echocardiography. Selective coronary angiography is recommended in patients with evidence of myocardial ischemia.

American Heart Association: Diagnostic guidelines for Kawasaki disease. *Circulation* 2001;103(2):335.

Hay WW Jr, Levin MJ, Sondheimer JM, et al., eds. *Current pediatric diagnosis & treatment,* 18th ed. New York: McGraw-Hill; 2007:582–583.

63. A 2-year-old child is seen in the emergency room and diagnosed with multiple contusions in various stages of healing and a spiral-type fracture of the left radius secondary to falling down the stairs at home. The most appropriate initial treatment is
A) splinting of the fracture with orthopedic referral
B) hospitalization
C) social service consult
D) immediate reduction of the fracture and safety counseling for the child's parents
E) open reduction and internal fixation and follow-up in 3 days

Answer and Discussion

The answer is B. Child abuse is a difficult problem that must be identified as quickly as possible. Most children who die of child abuse are younger than 5 years. Most child abuse takes place in the home and is instituted by persons known to and trusted by the child. Although widely publicized, abuse in daycare and foster-care settings accounts for only a minority of confirmed cases of child abuse. Child abuse is 15 times more likely to occur in families in which spousal abuse occurs. Children are three times more likely to be abused by their fathers than by their mothers. Once a health care worker has any suspicion of child abuse, he or she is legally required to report the case for investigation. Protection of the child is the most important goal. The child should be hospitalized in a safe environment while further investigation by social workers is performed. Children younger than 3 years are the most commonly abused. Clinical findings include multiple fractures (especially spiral-type fractures), multiple bruises in different stages of healing, intestinal trauma injuries, burns, poor nutrition, poor development, and bizarre accidents reported by parents. More than 50% of fractures in children younger than 1 year are secondary to abuse. Before discharge from the hospital, the child's home environment must be determined to be safe by the appropriate protection agency. Further counseling for the child and family should be initiated after discharge. Unfortunately, therapy for child-abusing adults fails in approximately 33% of cases. As adults, children who were abused have a higher incidence of depression and drug abuse.

Behrman RE, Kliegman RM, Jenson HB. *Nelson Textbook of Pediatrics,* 17th ed. Philadelphia: WB Saunders; 2004: 121–131.

64. Which of the following animal bites requires rabies postexposure prophylaxis?
A) Fox
B) Squirrel
C) Hamster
D) Gerbil
E) Rat

Answer and Discussion

The answer is A. Rabies in humans is rare in the United States, but the CDC estimates that as many as 39,000 persons receive postexposure prophylaxis annually. The risk of infection must be carefully evaluated by the clinician in the management of potential human rabies exposures. Bats, skunks, raccoons, foxes, and most other carnivores should receive post exposure prophylaxis. Bites of squirrels, hamsters, guinea pigs, gerbils, chipmunks, rats, mice, other small rodents, rabbits, and hares almost never require antirabies postexposure prophylaxis. The CDC considers administration of postexposure prophylaxis to be a medical urgency, not a medical emergency, although ACIP emphasizes that decisions about using prophylaxis should not be put off.

From the Centers for Disease Control and Prevention. Human rabies prevention—United States, 1999; Recommendations of the Advisory Committee on Immunization Practices (ACIP). *MMWR Morb Mortal Wkly Rep.* 1999;48(RR-1):6.

Behrman RE, Kliegman RM, Jenson HB. *Nelson Textbook of Pediatrics,* 17th ed. Philadelphia: WB Saunders; 2004:1104.

65. Which of the following is a clinical finding of coarctation of the aorta?
A) Bounding femoral pulses
B) Blood pressure higher in the legs than in the arms in infants older than 1 year of age
C) Rib notching on chest radiograph
D) Diastolic murmur heard at the apex, radiating to the axilla
E) Dilation of the thoracic aorta near the ligamentum arteriosus

Answer and Discussion

The answer is C. Coarctation of the aorta is one of the more common congenital heart defects. Boys are more commonly affected than girls. The condition occurs when there is discrete narrowing of the thoracic aorta near the ligamentum arteriosus, leading to proximal hypertension and left ventricular overload. Other findings include a ventricular septal defect, patent ductus arteriosus, and bicuspid aortic valve. In most cases, those affected are asymptomatic during infancy. However, congestive heart failure can occur and may require immediate surgical intervention. Signs associated with coarctation of the aorta include diminished or absent femoral pulses, blood pressure higher in the arms than in the legs in infants older than 1 year, 2/6 to 3/6 systolic ejection murmur heard over the apex and upper left sternal border, rib notching on chest radiograph (which is a result of enlargement of the intercostal arteries), and left ventricular hypertrophy. Diagnosis is based on physical findings and echocardiography or with CT or MRI angiography. Treatment depends on the severity of coarctation and the heart's ability to maintain perfusion. In severe cases, prostaglandin E_1 may be used to keep a patent ductus arteriosus dilated until surgery or balloon angioplasty can be performed. In more stable patients, β-blockers and afterload-reducing agents can be used to postpone definitive treatment until the child is 3 to 5 years of age, when the treatment can be performed electively. Those patients who do well initially without evidence of congestive heart failure and requiring no surgery usually do quite well regarding further complications in childhood and adolescence. Those affected are at risk for hypertension and cardiac dysfunction as well as subacute infective endocarditis.

Beers MH, Porter RS, eds. *The Merck manual of diagnosis and therapy,* Merck Research Laboratories, 18th ed. Whitehouse Station, NJ: Merck & Co.; 2006:2667–2668.

66. Which of the following statements about cystic fibrosis is true?
A) It is an autosomal-dominant transmitted disease.
B) The condition is associated with pancreatic insufficiency.
C) It is commonly diagnosed with a pulmonary function test.
D) Those affected do not live beyond 20 years of age.
E) Fertility is not affected in those with cystic fibrosis.

Answer and Discussion

The answer is B. Cystic fibrosis is the most common fatal genetic disease in the United States. It is transmitted as an autosomal-recessive trait. The incidence in the United States is reported to be approximately 1:3,500 in whites and 1:17,000 in African Americans. Those who are heterozygous are unaffected. The disorder involves exocrine glands and affects predominantly the gastrointestinal and respiratory systems. Complications include meconium ileus present at birth, chronic cough and wheezing with copious mucous production, pancreatic insufficiency with possible development of insulin-dependent diabetes (up to 8%), retarded growth, infertility, and chronic obstructive pulmonary disease. The diagnosis is made by the pilocarpine iontophoresis sweat test. Levels of sodium and chloride >60 mEq/L are usually diagnostic. Survival beyond 30 years of age is occurring more frequently. Death usually results from pulmonary complications such as infections with *S. aureus, Pseudomonas aeruginosa*, and *H. influenzae*.

Behrman RE, Kliegman RM, Jenson HB. *Nelson Textbook of Pediatrics*, 17th ed. Philadelphia: WB Saunders; 2004: 1437–1450.

67. Of the following antibiotics, which one would be acceptable to use when treating penicillin-resistant *S. pneumoniae* otitis media?
A) Azithromycin
B) Clarithromycin
C) Cefuroxime
D) Cefaclor
E) Cephalexin

Answer and Discussion

The answer is C. Only five antibiotics—high-dose amoxicillin (80 mg/kg/day), amoxicillin–clavulanate (Augmentin), cefuroxime (Ceftin), cefprozil (Cefzil), and ceftriaxone (Rocephin)—have demonstrated a modest degree (60% to 80%) of clinical efficacy in the treatment of acute otitis media caused by penicillin-resistant *S. pneumoniae*.

Pichichero ME. Acute otitis media: Part II. Treatment in an era of increasing antibiotic resistance. *Am Fam Physician*. 2000;61:2410–2416.

Block SL, Harrison CJ, Hedrick JA, et al. Penicillin-resistant *Streptococcus pneumoniae* in acute otitis media: risk factors, susceptibility patterns and antimicrobial management. *Pediatr Infect Dis J*. 1995;14:751–759.

68. A 3-year-old boy presents to your office with a history of seven ear infections over the last year. Appropriate management of this child consists of
A) tonsillectomy and adenoidectomy
B) single-dose prophylactic antibiotics given at night
C) tympanostomy tube placement
D) long-term use of antihistamine-decongestant preparations
E) continued observation

Answer and Discussion

The answer is B. Chronic otitis media usually results from acute otitis media and eustachian tube dysfunction. Despite short courses of antibiotics, affected children have recurrent infections that appear to be more prevalent in the winter months. Persistent chronic otitis media may lead to hearing deficits and subsequent language delays. Prophylaxis should be attempted if the child experiences more than four infections in 1 year or three or more infections within 6 months. Treatment for this difficult problem consists of prophylactic antibiotics given in a single dose at bedtime. Medications for chronic suppression therapy include amoxicillin, sulfisoxazole, or trimethoprim-sulfamethoxazole. If a sulfonamide is used, the child should have a complete blood cell count periodically, and parents or guardians should be instructed to discontinue the medication immediately if a rash or mouth sore develops. Steroid use has not been advocated, and myringotomy tube placement should be reserved for children in whom prophylactic therapy fails.

Semchenko A, Baroody F, Culpepper L. Management of acute sinusitis and acute otitis media. *Am Fam Physician*. Monograph No. 1, 2001:16–17.

69. Which of the following statements about breast-feeding is true?
A) The infant should feed on each side for 8 to 15 minutes every 2 to 3 hours after birth.
B) Colostrum is excreted 7 to 10 days after delivery and contains important antibodies, high calories, and other nutrients.
C) The mother should weigh infants before and after feeding to quantify the amount consumed.
D) Breast-feeding usually provides adequate nutrition for 2 to 4 months—supplementation should begin at that point.
E) Breast-feeding should be based on timed intervals rather than on demand.

Answer and Discussion

The answer is A. Breast-feeding is encouraged for all mothers. Currently, as many as 50% of mothers (especially those in higher socioeconomic groups) are breast-feeding. In most cases, the infant should feed at each breast for 8 to 15 minutes every 2 to 3 hours after birth and can be started immediately after delivery. *Colostrum*, a yellowish fluid excreted from the breast immediately after delivery, contains important antibodies, high calories, and high proteins, as well as other nutrients and helps stimulate the passage of meconium. Some studies have shown that delaying breast-feeding, trying to quantify amounts of feeding with prefeed and postfeed weights, and providing infant formula decrease the percentage of women who breast-feed by discouraging the practice. Breast-feeding is usually adequate nutrition for 6 to 9 months. If mothers develop sore nipples, they should be counseled with regard to proper positioning of the baby's mouth on the breast. The production of a lubricant from Montgomery's glands occurs and helps protect the breast from excessive drying. Typically, breast-fed infants require more frequent feedings than bottle-fed infants. Breast-feeding should occur based on demand rather than by the clock. Breast engorgement can be avoided with more frequent feedings or manual expression of excessive milk production with breast pumps. New mothers should initiate breast-feeding as soon as possible after giving birth. When mothers initiate breast-feeding within one-half hour of birth, the baby's suckling reflex is strongest, and the baby is more alert. Early breast-feeding is associated with fewer nighttime feeding problems and better mother-infant communication. Babies who are put to breast earlier have been shown to have higher core temperatures and less temperature instability.

Moreland J, Coombs J. Promoting and supporting breast feeding. *Am Fam Physician.* 2000;61:2093–2100, 2103–2104.

70. The most common bacterial pathogen associated with lung infections in adolescents is
A) adenovirus
B) *Streptococcus pneumoniae*
C) *H. influenzae*
D) *Mycoplasma pneumoniae*
E) *Chlamydia*

Answer and Discussion

The answer is D. *Mycoplasma* is the most common pathogen responsible for lung infections in patients between 5 and 35 years of age. It may involve close contacts, school children, military recruits, and family members and is spread via respiratory droplets. Symptoms include malaise, sore throat, coryza, myalgias, and an increasing productive cough of mucopurulent or blood-streaked sputum. A maculopapular rash occurs in 10% to 20%. Unlike Spneumococcal pneumonia, the course is less severe. Bullous myringitis has also been associated with *Mycoplasma* infections. Chest radiographs of those affected with *Mycoplasma* pneumonia show patchy infiltrates in the lower lobes and, rarely, lobar consolidation. The white blood cell count may be normal or mildly elevated. Diagnosis can be made with acute and convalescent titers but is unnecessary. The drug of choice for treatment is a macrolide antibiotic. Alternative medications include fluoroquinolones and tetracyclines. Because the *Mycoplasma* organism does not have a cell wall, the β-lactam antibiotics are ineffective.

Beers MH, Porter RS, eds. *The Merck manual of diagnosis and therapy,* Merck Research Laboratories, 18th ed. Whitehouse Station, NJ: Merck & Co.; 2006:1487.

> *Mycoplasma* is the most common pathogen responsible for lung infections in patients between 5 and 35 years of age.

71. The major complication of slipped capital femoral epiphysis is
A) avascular necrosis of the hip
B) osteochonditis dissecans
C) leg length discrepancy
D) transient synovitis of the hip
E) in-toeing

Answer and Discussion

The answer is A. Slipped capital femoral epiphysis typically occurs during the adolescent growth spurt and is most frequent in obese children. In many cases both hips are affected. Most cases of slipped capital femoral epiphyses are stable and have a good prognosis if diagnosed early in their course. Unstable slipped capital femoral epiphysis has a worse prognosis because of the high risk of avascular necrosis. Early radiographic clues are the metaphyseal blanch sign and Klein's line. Once diagnosed, treatment in most cases includes surgical pinning.

Loder RT. Slipped capital femoral epiphysis. *Am Fam Physician.* 1998;57:2135.

Behrman RE, Kliegman RM, Jenson HB. *Nelson Textbook of Pediatrics,* 17th ed. Philadelphia: WB Saunders; 2004: 2278–2279.

72. In December, a 4-month-old infant is brought to the emergency room. The parents report the child has had a runny nose, fever, cough, and audible wheezing. The child is attending a daycare center, and other children have had similar symptoms. On examination, the child has some rales, wheezing, and intercostal retractions with grunting. The most likely infecting organism is
A) *S. pneumoniae*
B) *H. influenzae*
C) adenovirus
D) respiratory syncytial virus (RSV)
E) coxsackievirus

Answer and Discussion

The answer is D. Respiratory syncytial virus (RSV) is a pneumovirus that usually affects children between 1 and 6 months of age, with a peak incidence at 2 to 3 months of age. The commonly encountered virus gives rise to bronchiolitis and pneumonia. The virus occurs during the winter months and is characterized by rhinorrhea, fever, cough, and wheezing; in more severe cases, tachypnea, dyspnea, and hypoxia are present. The virus is spread by close contacts via fomites and respiratory secretions and tends to occur in outbreaks in places such as daycare centers. Physical examination shows nasal flaring, rales, and wheezing as well as intercostal retractions with grunting in infants. Laboratory evaluation usually shows a normal leukocyte count with elevated granulocytes. Chest radiographs may show hyperexpansion, areas of atelectasis, and/or bronchopneumonia. The virus may be quickly detected by immunofluorescence microscopy of nasal swabs or enzyme-linked immunoassay antigen detection tests. Treatment of upper respiratory infections is usually symptomatic. Lower respiratory infections may be treated with supplemental oxygen and hydration. Bronchodilators and corticosteroids are not generally helpful. Aerosolized ribavirin (an antiviral agent) is no longer recommended except in severely immunocompromised patients. Respiratory support may be necessary in severe cases.

Beers MH, Porter RS, eds. *The Merck manual of diagnosis and therapy,* Merck Research Laboratories, 18th ed. Whitehouse Station, NJ: Merck & Co.; 2006:1600.

73. Of the following, which is the first sign of sexual development in girls?
A) The presence of axillary hair
B) The development of pubic hair
C) Menstruation
D) Development of breast buds
E) Closure of the epiphyseal growth plate

Answer and Discussion

The answer is D. The development of breast buds (subareolar tissue) is usually the first sign of puberty (8 to 13 years of age). This is followed closely by the development of pubic hair (6 to 12 months later) and then axillary hair. The growth spurt often begins even before the development of breast buds. Menarche usually occurs 2.0 to 2.5 years after the development of the breast buds. Growth in height occurs predominantly before menarche and then slows thereafter. As the young girl's body changes, the percentage of body fat increases and redistributes, giving rise to adult contours. *Precocious puberty* is defined as the presence of breast development or pubic hair before 8 years of age. *Pubertal delay* is defined as absence of breast development before the age of 13 years or the lack of menstruation 5 years after breast growth.

Behrman RE, Kliegman RM, Jenson HB. *Nelson Textbook of Pediatrics,* 17th ed. Philadelphia: WB Saunders; 2004:53–55, 1863.

74. Which of the following patient group-treatment scenarios is appropriate for the treatment/exposure of bacterial meningitis?
A) Neonates—ampicillin and cefotaxime
B) 1 month to 10 years of age—ampicillin and gentamicin
C) 10 to 18 years old—cefuroxime and erythromycin
D) Adults—ampicillin and metronidazole
E) Isoniazid for individuals exposed to meningococcal meningitis

Answer and Discussion

The answer is A. The treatment of bacterial meningitis depends on the age of the patient. In neonates, the common infecting organisms include group B or D streptococci, *Listeria*, and gram-negative organisms such as *E. coli*. Recommended treatment includes ampicillin and cefotaxime until susceptibilities are known. In infants and children 1 month to 10 years of age, the common infecting organisms include pneumococci and meningococci. Combination therapy is recommended and includes ampicillin, vancomycin, and cefotaxime or ceftriaxone. Various combinations should be confirmed based on local sensitivities and most recent recommendations. For patients allergic to penicillin, vancomycin and rifampin may be considered. Family members, nursery school children, and other close contacts of those affected by meningococcal or *H. influenzae* meningitis should also receive rifampin as a prophylactic measure.

In addition to intravenous antibiotics, dexamethasone may decrease the incidence of permanent neurologic and audiologic complications and should be administered.

Beers MH, Porter RS, eds. *The Merck manual of diagnosis and therapy,* Merck Research Laboratories, 18th ed. Whitehouse Station, NJ: Merck & Co.; 2006:1860–1862.

75. Conductive hearing loss noted in children may be caused by
A) meningitis
B) medications
C) chronic eustachian tube dysfunction
D) intracranial hemorrhage
E) chronic exposure to loud noises

Answer and Discussion

The answer is C. Signs of hearing loss may include delayed speech development, behavioral problems, and impaired comprehension. Hearing loss can be categorized as conductive or sensorineural. Conductive hearing loss is usually caused by otitis media with effusion. Other causes include foreign bodies in the ear, allergies, or chronic eustachian tube dysfunction. Sensorineural hearing loss can be caused by meningitis and other congenital infections, intracranial hemorrhage, chronic noise exposure, congenital defects, medications that are ototoxic, and trauma. Although hearing screening has been mandated in 34 states for all children absolute indications for audiologic evaluation include premature birth (birth weight <2,500 g or birth weight >2,500 g with complications including asphyxia, seizures, intracranial hemorrhage, hyperbilirubinemia, persistent fetal circulation, and assisted ventilation), intrauterine infection, bacterial meningitis, anomalies of the first or second branchial arch, anomalies of the neural crest or ectoderm, family history of hereditary or unexplained deafness, parental concern, and delayed speech or language development or other disabilities (including mental retardation, autism, cerebral palsy, and blindness). Infants are tested using either otoacoustic emissions (OAE) or auditory brain stem–evoked responses (ABR). The auditory brain stem–evoked response uses external scalp electrodes to detect waveforms that occur in predictable patterns after an auditory stimulus. The prompt recognition of hearing problems in children can help prevent delays in language development.

Behrman RE, Kliegman RM, Jenson HB. *Nelson Textbook of Pediatrics,* 17th ed. Philadelphia: WB Saunders; 2004:2131.

76. In males, the first sign of puberty is
A) development of pubic hair
B) testicular enlargement
C) spermarche
D) enlargement of the penis
E) skeletal growth spurt

Answer and Discussion

The answer is B. At the onset of puberty males have testicular enlargement followed by the appearance of pubic hair, enlargement of the penis and spermarche. Skeletal and muscle growth are late events in male puberty. The age at which pubertal milestones are attained varies among the population studied and is influenced by activity level and nutritional status.

Behrman RE, Kliegman RM, Jenson HB. *Nelson Textbook of Pediatrics,* 17th ed. Philadelphia: WB Saunders; 2004:53–55, 1863.

Blondell RD, Foster MB, Dave KC. Disorders of puberty. *Am Fam Physician.* 1999;60:209–224.

77. Which of the following conditions is associated with giving whole milk to infants younger than 1 year?
A) Iron deficiency anemia
B) Inflammatory bowel disease
C) Mental retardation
D) Hirschsprung's disease
E) None of the above

Answer and Discussion

The answer is A. This condition has a variety of causes, including inadequate iron stores at birth because of prematurity, fetal-maternal blood loss, iron-deficient mother, or lack of iron ingestion by the child that fails to keep up with expanding blood volume as the child grows (especially between 9 and 18 months of age); in older adolescent patients, it may be caused by menstrual blood loss. Whole milk given to infants younger than 1 year may also cause chronic irritation of the colon, resulting in blood loss and development of iron deficiency anemia. The U.S. Preventative Services Task Force recommends that high-risk infants be screened for iron deficiency anemia between 6 and 12 months of age. Screening for iron deficiency anemia is not recommended in the general infant population because of low overall prevalence. The Centers for Disease Control and Prevention has developed specific criteria for anemia: hemoglobin levels <11.0 g/dL (110 g/L) for children between 6 months and 5 years of age. In 1993, it was estimated that the prevalence of iron deficiency anemia among children younger than 5 years was <3%, and most cases were mild; however, among high-risk groups, the prevalence may be up to 30%. Increased prevalence of iron deficiency anemia occurs among African Americans, Native Americans, Alaska Natives, persons of low socioeconomic status, preterm and low-birth-weight infants, immigrants from developing countries, and infants whose primary nutritional source is unfortified cow's milk.

Strategies to prevent iron deficiency anemia among infants are recommended. Family physicians should discuss issues of infant nutrition with expectant and new parents and encourage the consumption of iron-fortified formulas and cereals or encourage breast-feeding supplemented with iron-fortified cereals between the ages of 4 and 6 months.

Mahoney MC. Screening for iron deficiency anemia among children and adolescents. *Am Fam Physician.* 2000;62:671.

78. A 14-year-old boy presents with tenderness associated with the right breast. There are no other findings. Testicular examination is unremarkable. Appropriate management of this patient includes

A) mammogram
B) ultrasound of the breast
C) genetic typing
D) biopsy
E) reassurance and continued observation

Answer and Discussion

The answer is E. Benign gynecomastia of adolescence is a very common finding among boys in middle to late puberty. The breast tissue is usually asymmetric and often tender to palpation. Provided the history and physical examination, including palpation of the testicles, are unremarkable, reassurance and periodic reevaluation are all that is necessary. Most cases resolve in 1 to 2 years. Familial gynecomastia is a common genetic disorder transmitted as an X-linked recessive trait or a sex-limited dominant trait causing limited breast development around the time of puberty. It requires no further evaluation in an otherwise normal boy unless there is evidence of hypogonadism. In rare cases those with severe gynecomastia may require cosmetic surgery. Pathologic gynecomastia occurs in cases of Klinefelter's syndrome and prolactin-secreting adenomas and with a wide variety of drug use including marijuana and phenothiazines.

Blondell RD, Foster MB, Dave KC. Disorders of puberty. *Am Fam Physician.* 1999;60:209–224.

Behrman RE, Kliegman RM, Jenson HB. *Nelson Textbook of Pediatrics,* 17th ed. Philadelphia: WB Saunders; 2004:1930.

79. Which of the following is the medication of choice for the treatment of pinworms (*Enterobius vermicularis*)?

A) Mebendazole (Vermox)
B) Permethrin (Elimite)
C) Metronidazole (Flagyl)
D) Oral vancomycin (Vancocin)
E) Tetracycline (Achromycin)

Answer and Discussion

The answer is A. Pinworms is a common pediatric infection caused by the parasite *Enterobius vermicularis.* The parasite is a small (1 cm) white worm that lives in the bowel (usually the cecum) and often migrates out of the anus at night to deposit eggs on the perianal skin, giving rise to severe and intense pruritus. Children ages 5 to 10 years are predominantly affected. Young children may not be able to sleep, and rectal and vulvar inflammation may be evident. In many cases, the entire family may be affected through a fecal-oral route. Diagnosis can be made by visualizing the worms or applying cellophane tape to the anal area in the morning before bathing and observing for ova with microscopy (cellophane tape test). Treatment involves the administration of mebendazole (Vermox) in one dose, followed by a repeat dose 2 weeks later. Albendazole or pyrantel pamoate may be substituted for mebendazole. In most cases, the entire household should be treated. Other treatment recommendations include laundering of all bedclothes and underwear.

Beers MH, Porter RS, eds. *The Merck manual of diagnosis and therapy,* Merck Research Laboratories, 18th ed. Whitehouse Station, NJ: Merck & Co.; 2006:1551–1552.

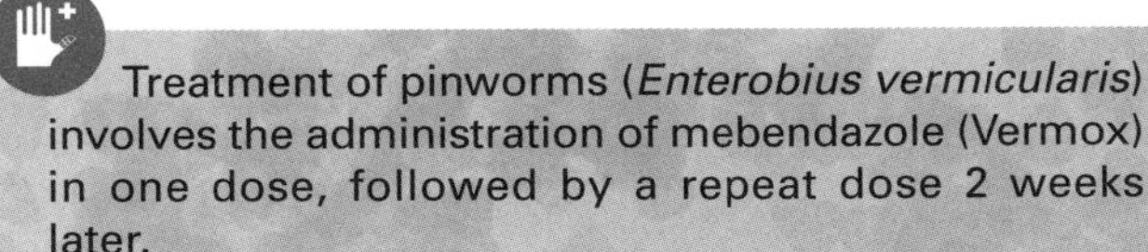

80. Which of the following drugs is concentrated in breast milk and should be avoided by women who are breast-feeding?

A) Heparin
B) Alcohol
C) Digoxin
D) Penicillin
E) Amitriptyline

Answer and Discussion

The answer is B. Medications that are classified as weak bases are usually concentrated in breast milk. Contraindicated drugs include anticancer drugs, therapeutic doses of radiopharmaceuticals, ergot and its derivatives (e.g., methysergide), lithium, chloramphenicol, atropine, thiouracil, iodides, and mercurials. These drugs should not be used in nursing mothers, or nursing should be stopped if any of these drugs is essential. Other drugs to be avoided in the absence of studies on their excretion in breast milk are those with long half-lives, those that are potent toxins to the bone marrow, and those given in high doses long-term. However, drugs that are so poorly absorbed orally that they are given (to the mother) parenterally pose no threat to the infant, who would receive the drug orally but not absorb it.

Nicotine and alcohol are concentrated in breast milk and should be avoided by mothers who are breast-feeding. Other drugs, including heparin, acetaminophen, insulin, diuretics, digoxin, β-blockers, penicillins, cephalosporins, most over-the-counter cold remedies, amitriptyline, codeine, and ibuprofen, do not show up in significant amounts in breast milk. Some oral contraceptives can depress lactation (particularly large-dose, estradiol-containing birth control pills), but in most cases are considered safe.

Beers MH, Porter RS, eds. *The Merck manual of diagnosis and therapy,* Merck Research Laboratories, 18th ed. Whitehouse Station, NJ: Merck & Co.; 2006:2227.

81. A 3 year old who attends day school is seen in the middle of June. The parent reports that the child has had profuse watery diarrhea. Laboratory tests of the stool sample show leukocytes, red blood cells, and small comma-shaped bacteria that have a corkscrew motion. The most likely diagnosis is

A) *Salmonella* infection
B) *Shigella* infection
C) *Rotavirus* infection
D) *Campylobacter* infection
E) *Escherichia coli* infection

Answer and Discussion

The answer is D. *Campylobacter* is an intestinal infection that can lead to profuse watery diarrhea. It is considered one of the most common causes of bacterial gastroenteritis. In many cases it affects young infants, particularly those in daycare centers; it is more common in the summer months. Associated foods include contaminated milk or water, poultry, and beef. Chickens are the classic source of *Campylobacter*; however, essentially all food sources can harbor the bacteria. In addition, pets can carry *Campylobacter*. Symptoms include loose, watery stools or bloody and mucus-containing stools. Fever, vomiting, malaise, and myalgia are common. Abdominal pain is usually periumbilical and cramping in nature. Children severely affected may show signs of dehydration. Laboratory tests of stool samples show leukocytes, red blood cells, and small comma-shaped bacteria that have a characteristic corkscrew motion. In most cases, antibiotics are unnecessary; however, because there is a carrier state, the use of antibiotics such as the quinolones (not used in children), erythromycin, doxycycline, and gentamicin can help to clear the stool of infecting organisms, particularly in an institutional setting. After treatment, repeat stool cultures should be performed to ensure eradication. Fecal shedding of the organisms can last up to 2 to 3 weeks in untreated patients. Severe cases or those immunosuppressed should be treated.

Behrman RE, Kliegman RM, Jenson HB. *Nelson Textbook of Pediatrics,* 17th ed. Philadelphia: WB Saunders; 2004:928.

82. In the United States, which of the following deficiencies is common in adolescents?

A) Iron
B) vitamin B_{12}
C) folate
D) thiamine
E) calcium

Answer and Discussion

The answer is E. In the United States, only a minority of adolescents receive the recommended daily allowance of calcium. As a result there is the possibility of a future epidemic of osteopenia or even osteoporosis in normal individuals who have calcium deficiency.

Greenspan FS, Gardner DG. *Basic and Clinical Endocrinology,* 7th ed. New York: McGraw-Hill; 2004.

83. A 6-month-old infant is brought in for a well-child visit. The growth chart shows the child's growth has slowed when compared to the growth curve expected for his age despite adequate caloric intake. The most appropriate action is

A) to increase feeding amounts
B) to reassure the family that this is a common finding and that no further workup is necessary
C) to order laboratory tests, including a complete blood cell count, electrolyte levels, serum glucose levels, and urinalysis
D) to consult social services
E) to start nutritional supplement

Answer and Discussion

The answer is C. Failure to thrive is a condition of infants. It is caused by a number of different factors. The condition is detected by following age-adjusted normals for height, weight, and head circumference. When the graph shows abnormalities (failure to meet the third percentile) or if there is a decrease in the expected rate of growth based on the child's previously defined growth curve, failure to thrive must be considered. Causes include birth defects (e.g., fetal infections, chromosomal abnormalities, inborn errors of metabolism), nutritional deficiencies with malabsorption, endocrine abnormalities, disturbances of bone development, disorders of oxygenation, malignancy, and neglect. Symptoms include poor weight gain, vomiting, diarrhea, muscle spasticity or hypotonia, developmental delay, apathy, withdrawn behavior, and poor hygiene. The diagnosis usually involves a detailed history and physical examination followed by an initial screening test, such as complete blood count, electrolyte levels, serum glucose levels, urinalysis, erythrocyte sedimentation rate, stool studies for ova, parasites, and blood. Other tests (e.g., thyroid function tests) may be indicated based on each case.

Beers MH, Porter RS, eds. *The Merck manual of diagnosis and therapy,* Merck Research Laboratories, 18th ed. Whitehouse Station, NJ: Merck & Co.; 2006:2395–2398.

84. Variation in a young patient's electrocardiogram pattern is noted with respiration. The rhythm remains sinus rhythm. The most appropriate action is

A) reassurance to patient and family
B) Holter monitoring
C) cardiology consultation
D) administration of β-blockers
E) synchronized cardioversion

Answer and Discussion

The answer is A. Sinus arrhythmia is usually noted in young, healthy patients and represents no concern for underlying pathology. The variation in heart rate is affected by normal respirations and is associated with the alternating increases and decreases in vagal and sympathetic tone. Patients report no symptoms, and no treatment is required.

Beers MH, Porter RS, eds. *The Merck manual of diagnosis and therapy,* Merck Research Laboratories, 18th ed. Whitehouse Station, NJ: Merck & Co.; 2006:676.

85. A 3-year-old boy is diagnosed with constitutional growth delay. The workup is unremarkable. The most appropriate management is

A) vitamin E supplementation
B) administration of prednisone
C) monitoring of thyroid function tests every 3 months
D) reassurance to parents
E) nutritional consult

Answer and Discussion

The answer is D. Constitutional growth delay is one variant of normal growth. Length and weight measurements of affected children are normal at birth, and growth is normal for the first 4 to 12 months of life. Growth then decelerates to near or below the third percentile for height and weight. By 2 to 3 years of age, growth resumes at a normal rate of 5 cm/year or more. The majority of these children are male and have a bone age that is appropriate for height age but are delayed relative to their chronologic age. Some of these children experience delayed puberty but eventually complete normal development without complications. Reassurance to the parent is the most appropriate management for children who are at Tanner stage 2 or 3, do not have underlying chronic disease, and have skeletal age-appropriate height as they grow older. The parents can be reassured that the child will go through a growth spurt in the near future, and no further testing is warranted. Although the child may end up being shorter than his or her peers, the child usually follows growth patterns of the parents. Only in extreme severe cases are medications such as anabolic and androgenic steroids considered.

Behrman RE, Kliegman RM, Jenson HB. *Nelson Textbook of Pediatrics,* 17th ed. Philadelphia: WB Saunders; 2004:1851.

86. A 3-year-old child presents with high fever, prostration, and purpuric rash. Appropriate management should be
A) administration of oral antibiotics with next-day follow-up
B) hospitalization, intravenous antibiotics, and close observation
C) to obtain throat culture and treat if positive for strep
D) symptomatic measures for likely viral infection
E) to check Lyme disease titers

Answer and Discussion

The answer is B. Meningococcemia is a severe infection that is caused by *Neisseria meningitidis*. The mode of transmission is through infected respiratory secretions. The onset is usually abrupt, and the course can be fulminant despite treatment. Symptoms include fever, chills, fatigue, and prostration. A distinctive petechial or purpuric rash develops. Fulminant disease can result in disseminated intravascular coagulopathy and septic shock. Children younger than 5 years are the most commonly affected. In many cases, meningitis results and can be fatal (5% of patients). Diagnosis can be made with an antigen detection test of the blood, cerebrospinal fluid, and urine. Cultures can also be used but typically require longer amounts of time. Treatment involves the use of high-dose intravenous penicillin G, ampicillin, central nervous system–penetrating cephalosporins, and chloramphenicol in an intensive care unit setting. Exposed household, day school, or school contacts should receive chemoprophylaxis with rifampin. Ceftriaxone and ciprofloxacin are also prophylactic substitutes for adults. Meningococcal vaccination should be given to individuals at risk (e.g., asplenic individuals, travelers in high-risk areas, college students living in dorms, military recruits, and patients with complement deficiencies). Newer recommendations may include universal administration.

Behrman RE, Kliegman RM, Jenson HB. *Nelson Textbook of Pediatrics,* 17th ed. Philadelphia: WB Saunders; 2004:896–899.

87. Which statement regarding metatarsus adductus is true?
A) metatarsus adductus is the rarest of foot disorders to affect children
B) intoeing rarely occurs as a result of metatarsus adductus
C) males are more commonly affected
D) surgery is rarely needed
E) stretching exercises are rarely effective

Answer and Discussion

The answer is D. Metatarsus adductus is the most common congenital foot deformity seen in children. Females are more commonly affected and the left side is more commonly affected. The most likely cause is positioning while in utero. Examination reveals adduction of the forefoot with a convex lateral border. The ankle has normal motion. The foot should be assessed for flexibility by holding the heel in neutral position and abducting the forefoot to at least a neutral position. If this cannot be done, then the deformity is rigid (i.e., metatarsus varus). The majority of cases of metatarsus adductus noted at birth resolve without treatment by 1 year of age. Flexible metatarsus adductus is managed by stretching exercises during the first 8 months of life. Parents are instructed to hold the infant's hindfoot in one hand, the forefoot in the other, and stretch the midfoot, opening the "C"-shaped curve and slightly overcorrecting it. Flexible deformities that persist beyond 8 months, and rigid deformities, may need a cast application. Improved results occur if treatment is started before 8 months of age. Casts should be changed biweekly with correction usually achieved after three or four casts. Residual adductus causes no long-term disability. Surgery is not typically recommended because of the risk of complications.

Sass P, Hassan G. Lower extremity abnormalities in children. *Am Fam Physician.* 2003;68:461–468.

88. Which of the following immunizations may result in a false negative PPD tuberculosis test?
A) Tetanus
B) Hepatitis B
C) Pneumococcal
D) Influenza
E) Measles, mumps, and rubella (MMR)

Answer and Discussion

The answer is E. Some persons (e.g., anergic patients, those with recent viral infections or those recently treated with live virus vaccines) may not react to the tuberculin skin test even though they are truly infected with *Mycobacterium tuberculosis*. Of those discussed, only the MMR is a live virus.

Kasper DL, Braunwald E, Fauci AS, et al., eds. *Harrison's principles of internal medicine,* 16th ed. New York: McGraw-Hill; 2005:964.

89. Which of the following is the treatment of choice for pertussis?
A) Penicillin G
B) Amphotericin B
C) Erythromycin
D) Ciprofloxacin
E) Metronidazole

Answer and Discussion

The answer is C. Pertussis is a highly contagious (gram-negative rod) bacterial disease caused by *Bordetella pertussis*. The disease is characterized by a short paroxysmal cough that ends with an inspiratory whoop. The incubation period is usually 7 to 21 days. Transmission occurs through a respiratory route. The disease is divided into three stages:

1. The *catarrhal stage* is characterized by sneezing, lacrimation, decreased appetite, fatigue, coryza, and a cough that usually becomes diurnal and lasts 10 to 14 days.

2. The *paroxysmal stage* is characterized by the whooping cough; vomiting as a result of the persistent cough may occur; this stage may last up to 4 weeks.
3. The *convalescent stage* involves a slow improvement of the cough and constitutional symptoms.

The entire illness may last up to 3 months. Diagnosis is made by obtaining a nasopharyngeal swab and performing an antibody test for detection of the gram-negative organism in the secretions. Treatment involves the use of erythromycin. Household or other close contacts should also be treated with oral erythromycin. Most patients may return to their regular activity 5 days after the administration of erythromycin. Routine childhood immunization is effective in the prevention of the disease, but not in all cases. Recently, *B. pertussis* has been increasingly responsible for chronic cough in adults. In adults and infants younger than 6 months, the classic whoop may not occur, but the diagnosis should be considered with a cough lasting more than 2 weeks. Parapertussis, caused by *Bordetella parapertussis*, is a similar illness and is clinically indistinguishable from pertussis, except it usually has a milder course and fewer complications.

Behrman RE, Kliegman RM, Jenson HB. *Nelson Textbook of Pediatrics*, 17th ed. Philadelphia; WB Saunders; 2004:908–912.

Parapertussis, caused by *Bordetella parapertussis*, is a similar illness and is clinically indistinguishable from pertussis, except it usually has a milder course and fewer complications.

90. A 4 year old presents with impetigo associated with the knee. No other areas are involved. The most appropriate treatment is
A) topical mupirocin
B) topical bacitracin
C) topical neomycin
D) topical polymyxin B
E) oral cefalexin

Answer and Discussion

The answer is A. Impetigo is a contagious superficial skin infection most commonly seen in children, with a peak incidence between the ages of 2 and 6 years. The condition is the most common skin infection affecting children. Causative agents include group A beta-hemolytic streptococci (GABHS) and *Staphylococcus aureus*. Complications such as cellulitis, lymphangitis, and septicemia are rare and result from spread of the infection. The infection is transmitted via direct contact with the lesion. Antibiotic administration is the mainstay of therapy. If the area of affected skin is limited, mupirocin is an effective topical therapy and has been shown to be more effective than the other topical antibiotics (i.e., neomycin, bacitracin, polymyxin B, and gentamicin). There is insufficient evidence to determine whether oral antibiotics are better than topical agents in patients with more extensive disease, although there are obvious practical reasons to choose oral agents if large amounts of skin are involved. Antibiotic categories to consider include penicillins, cephalosporins, and macrolides. Oral antibiotics have significantly more side effects, especially gastrointestinal effects, than topical agents.

Koning S, Verhagen AP, van Suijlekom-Smit LW, et al. Interventions for impetigo. *Cochrane Database Syst Rev.* 2004;(3):CD003261.

91. Which of the following is the most appropriate management of an asymptomatic umbilical hernia in a newborn?
A) Immediate surgical correction
B) Reassurance to parents that most hernias resolve in 6 to 8 weeks
C) Surgical correction if the hernia does not resolve before school age
D) Application of an elastic support to the mid-abdomen
E) None of the above

Answer and Discussion

The answer is C. Umbilical hernias are more commonly seen in premature, female, and African American infants. The condition results from imperfect closure or weakness of the umbilical ring. If noted before 6 months of age, most resolve spontaneously before 1 year of age. Although rare, incarceration of the bowel is the most dangerous condition associated with abdominal hernias. If the hernia does not close before school age, incarcerates the bowel, or becomes symptomatic, surgical correction should be considered. Reduction of the hernia with strapping devices is not useful.

Behrman RE, Kliegman RM, Jenson HB. *Nelson Textbook of Pediatrics*, 17th ed. Philadelphia: WB Saunders; 2004:609.

92. Early breast-feeding is associated with
A) improved growth in the first 2 months
B) lower risk of aspiration
C) less temperature instability
D) fewer apneic spells
E) higher rates of postpartum depression

Answer and Discussion

The answer is C. Mothers of newborn infants should initiate breast-feeding as soon as possible after giving birth. When mothers initiate breast-feeding within one-half hour of birth, the baby's suckling reflex is strongest, and the baby is more alert, which facilitates feeding. Early breast-feeding has been shown to be associated with fewer nighttime feeding problems and better mother-infant bonding. Additionally infants who are breast fed earlier have been shown to have higher core temperatures and less temperature instability.

Moreland J, Coombs J. Promoting and supporting breast-feeding. *Am Fam Physician.* 2000;61:2093–2100, 2103–2104.

93. A 5-year-old boy is brought in for a well-child visit. The child's parents are noted to be relatively short, and they have concerns because their child is shorter than most of the other children in his class. The child's skeletal maturation is consistent with his chronologic age. The most likely diagnosis is
A) parental neglect
B) hypothyroidism
C) genetic short stature
D) acromegaly
E) dwarfism

Answer and Discussion

The answer is C. Genetic short stature is a delay in growth and development that patterns the parents' growth and development. Typically, if the child has tall parents, the child will eventually be tall; if the parents are short, the child will eventually be short. Also, if the parents developed late in adolescence, then the child will mirror this development. Constitutional growth delay can be differentiated from genetic short stature by the level of skeletal maturation, which is consistent with chronologic age in the latter condition. There is no treatment necessary; however, the family may need reassurance that the child is normal and that no further treatment or evaluation is necessary.

Behrman RE, Kliegman RM, Jenson HB. *Nelson Textbook of Pediatrics,* 17th ed. Philadelphia: WB Saunders; 2004:54–57.

94. A 40-year-old woman who received killed measles vaccination in 1965 presents with high fever, headaches, abdominal pain, and a rash that began on her arms and spread to her trunk and face. Which of the following factors makes you suspicious that this is not typical measles?

A) Development of cough
B) Development of high fever
C) Presence of abdominal pain
D) Distribution of rash
E) Development of headaches

Answer and Discussion

The answer is D. A typical measles syndrome occurs in individuals who were immunized with the original killed virus vaccine, which was administered from 1963 to 1967. Some cases have been linked to the newer, live attenuated vaccine that was improperly stored. The disease is thought to result from a hypersensitive response in persons who have partial immunity. Symptoms are similar to regular measles and include high fever, headache, abdominal pain, cough, and a rash that begins on the extremities (unlike regular measles, in which the rash tends to form on the face first) 1 to 2 days after the onset of the initial symptoms. The rash may become purpuric or hemorrhagic. Koplik's spots are rarely seen in atypical measles.

Behrman RE, Kliegman RM, Jenson HB. *Nelson Textbook of Pediatrics,* 17th ed. Philadelphia: WB Saunders; 2004:1028.

95. Which of the following malignancies is most common in childhood?

A) Wilm's tumor
B) Retinoblastoma
C) Melanoma
D) Acute lymphoblastic leukemia (ALL)
E) Osteosarcoma

Answer and Discussion

The answer is D. Leukemia is the most common malignancy diagnosed in childhood. Acute lymphoblastic leukemia (ALL) is the most common type of leukemia in children. ALL typically occurs in children between 1 and 10 years of age, although it can occur at any age. This leukemia is more common in males and in Caucasians. Diagnosing acute lymphoblastic leukemia can be challenging. Frequently, the diagnosis is delayed because early symptoms are nonspecific and may resemble viral infections. Most children affected present with generalized malaise, loss of appetite and a low-grade fever. Additional symptoms include pallor, petechiae or ecchymoses, bone pain, and significant weight loss. The physical examination may not be revealing, but significant lymphadenopathy or hepatosplenomegaly should raise suspicion for leukemia. Hepatosplenomegaly is always an abnormal finding. A practical approach to the child with suspicious findings is to obtain a complete blood count (CBC) with a white blood cell differential and a reticulocyte count. The presence of blast cells on the peripheral smear is diagnostic of leukemia. However, many patients with leukemia only have blast cells in their bone marrow. The finding of anemia, especially if accompanied by reticulocytopenia or a high mean corpuscular volume, thrombocytopenia, leukopenia, or leukocytosis is likely associated with leukemia and deserves further evaluation. Illnesses that may mimic leukemia include infectious mononucleosis caused by Epstein-Barr virus or, less frequently, cytomegalovirus infection, collagen vascular disease, and aplastic anemia.

Young G, Toretsky JA, Cambell AB, et al. Recognition of childhood malignancies. *Am Fam Physician.* 2000;61:2144–2154.

96. Which of the following foods have been associated with the development of botulism in children younger than 1 year?

A) Corn syrup
B) Peanuts
C) Honey
D) Cereal
E) Animal crackers

Answer and Discussion

The answer is C. Botulism is caused by a toxin produced by the anaerobe *Clostridium botulinum*. Symptoms usually occur within 24 hours after ingestion of contaminated food (usually canned food). These symptoms include dry mouth, diplopia, dysarthria, dysphagia, decreased visual acuity, nausea, vomiting, abdominal cramps, and diarrhea. Neurologic disorders include weakness and eventual paralysis, which can lead to respiratory failure and death. Sensory function remains intact. Diagnosis is made by discovery of the botulinum toxin in the affected food or stool of affected patients. Treatment involves supportive therapy, including mechanical ventilation and the administration of a trivalent antitoxin. Mortality rates approach 25%. Prevention involves the use of pressure cookers, which provide temperatures higher than 100°C (212°F), for at least 10 minutes when canning vegetables; boiling food for at least 10 minutes before eating destroys any toxins present. Infant botulism is caused by the ingestion of botulinum spores, which produce the toxin *in vivo*. Unlike food-borne botulism, infant botulism is not caused by ingestion of a preformed toxin. Constipation is initially present in 90% of cases of infant botulism and is followed by neuromuscular paralysis beginning with the cranial nerves and proceeding to peripheral and respiratory musculature. Cranial nerve deficits typically include ptosis, extraocular muscle palsies, weak cry, poor suck, decreased gag reflex, pooling of oral secretions, and an expressionless face. Severity varies from mild lethargy and slowed feeding to severe hypotonia and respiratory insufficiency. Most infants affected are between the ages of 2 and 3 months. Finding *C. botulinum* toxin or organisms in the feces establishes the diagnosis. Honey has been shown to contain botulinum spores, and thus should be avoided in children younger than 1 year. Administration of the antitoxin may be considered (not in infants). Additionally antibiotics may be useful to treat secondary infections. Aminoglycosides should be avoided because they may potentiate the effects of the toxin. A clinical trial is being performed to determine the usefulness of human botulism immune globulin (derived from the plasma of persons immunized with *C. botulinum* toxoid) in the treatment of infant botulism.

Beers MH, Porter RS, eds. *The Merck manual of diagnosis and therapy,* Merck Research Laboratories, 18th ed. Whitehouse Station, NJ: Merck & Co.; 2006:1498–1499.

97. Which of the following is true regarding management of head lice?

A) Children should be kept out of school until no visible evidence of nits is noted.
B) Household members should only be treated if live lice or eggs are noted within 1 cm of the scalp.
C) Head lice programs have had a significant impact on lowering the incidence of head lice.
D) Cleaning of bedding has little impact on lice eradication.
E) The health of those exposed is more important than the confidentiality of the child affected.

Answer and Discussion

The answer is B. Practice guidelines published by the American Academy of Pediatrics (AAP) state that if a case of head lice is identified, all household members should be checked, and only those with live lice or eggs within 1 cm of the scalp should be treated. It is recommended to treat family members who share a bed with the person who is infected and to adequately clean hair care items and bed linens belonging to that person. A child with active head lice has likely had the infestation for a month or more by the time it is discovered and poses little risk to others. The child does not have a resulting hygiene or health problem and should stay in class but be discouraged from close, direct head contact with others. The child's parents should be notified immediately, and confidentiality should be maintained so the child is not embarrassed. A child should be allowed to return to school after proper treatment and should not miss school because of head lice. Head lice screening programs have not had a significant effect on the incidence of head lice in the school setting over time and are not cost effective.

Ressel GW. AAP releases clinical report on head lice. *Am Fam Physician.* 2003;67:1309.

98. Which of the following statements about osteoid osteoma is true?

A) It is a malignant tumor of long bones.
B) It is more common in girls.
C) It usually presents as a pathologic fracture.
D) Radiographs show radiolucent areas surrounded by sclerosis.
E) Treatment involves systemic chemotherapy.

Answer and Discussion

The answer is D. Osteoid osteoma is a benign tumor that usually involves the long bones of pediatric and adolescent patients. They are found more commonly in boys. Most cases present with pain, not fracture. Radiographs show a characteristic radiolucent area surrounded by sclerosis, which is usually associated with the ends of the tibia or femur. Technetium bone scans are helpful in determining the area involved. Treatment for severe refractory cases involves surgical resection, which is curative. Anti-inflammatories are often helpful for mild cases and can relieve the pain.

Adkins SB, Figler RA. Hip pain in athletes. *Am Fam Physician.* 2000;61:2109–2118.

99. Which of the following is *not* a suitable treatment for molluscum contagiosum?

A) Curettage
B) Cryotherapy
C) Trichloroacetic acid
D) Imiquimod (Aldara)
E) All are considered acceptable treatment.

Answer and Discussion

The answer is E. Molluscum contagiosum (MC) is a benign superficial eruption resulting from viral infections of the skin. Molluscum contagiosum eruptions are usually self-limited and without sequelae, although they can be more extensive especially in immunocompromised persons. In patients with HIV, MC infection frequently is not self-limited and can be much more extensive and even disfiguring. MC may serve as a cutaneous marker of severe immunodeficiency and sometimes is the first indication of HIV infection. Lesions usually spontaneously disappear but treatment by local destruction or immunologic modulation can shorten the disease course. Spontaneous disappearance of MC lesions with no residual scarring is common. This may occur after a period of inflammation and minor tenderness. Autoinoculation is associated with scratching of the lesions and transmission to others can occur. Lesion destruction may be mechanical (curettage, laser, or cryotherapy with liquid nitrogen or nitrous oxide cryogun), chemical [trichloroacetic acid, tretinoin (Retin-A)], or immunologic [imiquimod (Aldara)]. Advantages to imiquimod therapy include minimal side effects and convenience of application.

Stulberg DL, Hutchinson AG. Molluscum contagiosum and warts. *Am Fam Physician.* 2003;67:1233–1240, 1243–1244.

> Molluscum contagiosum lesion destruction may be mechanical (curettage, laser, or cryotherapy with liquid nitrogen or nitrous oxide cryogun), chemical (trichloroacetic acid, tretinoin [Retin-A]), or immunologic (imiquimod [Aldara]).

100. Which of the following statements about lead poisoning in children is true?

A) Symptoms include vomiting, irritability, weight loss, and abdominal pain.
B) Repeated ingestion of small amounts of lead is less dangerous than a single large ingestion.
C) All paints used in the home should be <25% lead.
D) It is treated with deferoxime.
E) Neurologic deficits are not routinely associated with lead poisoning.

Answer and Discussion

The answer is A. Lead poisoning is a particular concern for young children. Also known as *plumbism*, the condition is characterized by generalized weakness, vomiting, irritability, weight loss, changes in personality, ataxia, headache, and abdominal pain. Radiographic particles are often seen on abdominal films, and there is usually a visible lead line on the gums and involving bones at the metaphyseal zone. Further complications include delayed development with diminished IQ, decreased hearing, peripheral neuropathy, seizures, and coma in severe cases. The syndrome usually affects children younger than 5 years who have ingested lead. Some common sources of lead include leaded paint chips, solder, glazed pottery, and fumes from burning batteries. Repeated ingestion of small amounts of lead (>0.5 mg of lead absorbed per day) is more dangerous than one single large dose. All paints used in the home should be <1% lead. Drinking water is another important source of lead exposure if there are lead pipes or lead fixtures or fittings. The diagnosis of lead poisoning is made by laboratory determination of lead levels and is recommended for children at risk. Most experts recommend testing between 6 and 7 months unless it can be shown that the community in which the children live does not have a lead-poisoning problem. Levels >10 μg/dL should be further evaluated by public health officials to determine environmental exposure risk. The treatment of acute lead poisoning is achieved by the induction of vomiting and chelation therapy with the use of dimercaprol and edetate calcium disodium, followed by penicillamine once the patient can take oral medication. Close monitoring should be instituted to watch for renal failure and the development of seizures. Children should not be allowed to return to lead-contaminated environments until they are deemed safe by environmental agents.

Beers MH, Porter RS, eds. *The Merck manual of diagnosis and therapy,* Merck Research Laboratories, 18th ed. Whitehouse Station, NJ: Merck & Co.; 2006:2669–2670.

101. The first solid foods (iron-fortified cereal) should typically be administered to an infant at

A) 2 to 4 months
B) 4 to 6 months
C) 6 to 8 months
D) 8 to 12 months
E) only after 1 year

Answer and Discussion

The answer is B. Iron-fortified cereals should be the first solid food introduced to young infants at 4 to 6 months of age. These can be continued until approximately 18 months of age. When to start solid foods depends on the infant's needs and readiness, but infants do not need solids before 6 months of age. Neurologic development has progressed sufficiently for tongue and mouth movement to handle solids at approximately 4 months in full-term infants. Solid feedings given earlier than 4 months of age are extremely difficult to manage, because the infant's extrusion reflex causes the tongue to push solid food out of the mouth. Other foods, including fruit and vegetable baby food, may be started soon after the introduction of cereal. Typically one new food is added per week. Baby food meats can be added at 6 to 7 months; table food can be added at 8 to 12 months. Foods easily aspirated such as chunks of meat, popcorn, or nuts should be avoided. Whole milk can replace formula or breast milk at 12 months of age. And reduced fat milk is usually given at 2 years of age. To prevent food sensitivities, peanuts, eggs, and cow's milk should be avoided until the child is 1 year old. Honey should be avoided in children <1 year of age because of the risk of infant botulism.

Beers MH, Porter RS, eds. *The Merck manual of diagnosis and therapy,* Merck Research Laboratories, 18th ed. Whitehouse Station, NJ: Merck & Co.; 2006:2230.

102. A 4-year-old girl complains of vaginal itching, especially at night when she is going to bed. The most likely diagnosis is

A) ascariasis
B) cutaneous larva migrans
C) pinworms
D) pubic lice
E) molluscum contagiosum

Answer and Discussion

The answer is C. *Enterobius* (pinworms) is the most common parasite affecting children in the United States. Its prevalence approaches 100% in institutionalized children. Infestation usually results from hand to mouth transfer of ova from the perianal area to fomites (clothing, bedding, furniture, rugs, toys), from which the ova are picked up by the new host, transmitted to the mouth, and swallowed. Although less common, airborne ova may be inhaled and then swallowed. The pinworms reach maturity in the lower GI tract within 2 to 6 weeks. The female worm migrates to the perianal region (usually at night) to deposit ova. Movements of the female worm cause pruritus. The ova can survive on fomites as long as 3 weeks under normal conditions. Most persons who harbor pinworms have no symptoms or signs. Some will, however, experience the perianal itching and develop perianal excoriations from persistent scratching. Vaginitis in young females may be due to irritation from pinworms. Pinworm infestation can be diagnosed by finding the female worm, which is about 10 mm long (males average 3 mm), in the perianal region 1 or 2 hours after the child goes to bed at night or by microscopic identification of the ova. The ova are obtained in the early morning before the child arises by patting the perianal skinfolds with a strip of transparent adhesive tape. This procedure should be repeated on 5 successive mornings if necessary to rule out pinworm infestation. A single dose of mebendazole (regardless of age) is effective in eradicating pinworms (but not ova) in about 90% of cases. Pyrantel pamoate is also used and repeated after 2 weeks. Because multiple infestations within the household are the rule, treatment of the entire family is recommended. Extensive handwashing and housekeeping have little effect on the control or treatment of pinworm infestation.

Beers MH, Porter RS, eds. *The Merck manual of diagnosis and therapy,* Merck Research Laboratories, 18th ed. Whitehouse Station, NJ: Merck & Co.; 2006:1551–1552.

103. Retinopathy of prematurity is associated with

A) gestational diabetes
B) excessive oxygen administration
C) maternal hypothyroidism
D) maternal rubella infection
E) development of congenital cataracts

Answer and Discussion

The answer is B. Retinopathy of prematurity (ROP), or *retrolental fibroplasia,* is thought to be related to exposure of retinal vessels of premature infants to excessive oxygen concentrations; the condition rarely occurs otherwise. Other risk factors include respiratory distress, apnea, bradycardia, heart disease, infection, hypoxia, hypercarbia, acidosis, anemia and the need for transfusion. Most affected infants weigh <1,500 g, and the mechanism of injury is believed to be excessive oxygen exposure leading to the development of free radicals and neovascularization and eventual retinal detachment. Occasionally, if the neovascularization is mild, the abnormal vessels may spontaneously regress, preserving vision but usually leaving the infant with significant myopia. Prevention is aimed at carefully monitoring oxygen supplementation in minimal amounts to preserve brain tissue and, ultimately, prevention of premature birth. However, oxygen alone is neither sufficient nor necessary to produce ROP and no safe level of oxygen has been determined. Treatment involves the use of cryotherapy and laser photocoagulation, which may be beneficial in select cases. All infants who weigh <1,500 g should be evaluated by an ophthalmologist before discharge from the hospital and at least once at 6 months after birth.

Behrman RE, Kliegman RM, Jenson HB. *Nelson Textbook of Pediatrics,* 17th ed. Philadelphia: WB Saunders; 2004: 2113–2114.

104. The definition of delayed sexual maturation in boys includes
A) no testicular development by age 10 years
B) more than 5 years between the initial and completed growth of genitalia
C) lack of axillary hair growth by 13 years of age
D) lack of pubic hair growth 1 year after the growth spurt
E) no pubertal-related voice changes before age 15 years

Answer and Discussion

The answer is B. Delayed sexual maturation is defined as follows:

- *In boys*: no testicular development by age 14 years, no pubic hair by age 15 years, and more than 5 years between the initial and completed growth of the genitalia
- *In girls*: no breast development by age 13 years, no pubic hair before age 14 years, and no menstruation within 5 years of the development of breast buds, or if menstruation does not occur by age 16.

One of the major causes is *constitutional delay*, which is defined as an inherited delayed maturation affecting the child that is also often noted in the parents. In these cases, the prepubertal growth is normal, but the skeletal growth and adolescent growth spurt is delayed. Those affected develop sexually late but are considered completely normal. The condition is more common in males and can be treated with the use of testosterone supplementation. Girls with severe pubertal delay should be investigated for primary amenorrhea.

Beers MH, Porter RS, eds. *The Merck manual of diagnosis and therapy,* Merck Research Laboratories, 18th ed. Whitehouse Station, NJ: Merck & Co.; 2006:2370–2371.

105. Which of the following is a negative predictor for streptococcal pharyngitis?
A) Fever >38.3°C (100.9°F)
B) Exposure to a known *Streptococcus* pharyngitis contact
C) Pharyngeal or tonsillar exudates
D) Recent cough

Answer and Discussion

The answer is D. According to the Walsh Prediction Scale, the following are given equal weight in the diagnosis of strep pharyngitis:

- Fever >38.3°C (100.9°F)
- Exposure to a known streptococcus pharyngitis contact
- Pharyngeal or tonsillar exudates, enlarged or tender nodes

Recent cough actually was a negative predictor for strep pharyngitis. In patients with a low probability of streptococcal pharyngitis (score of −1), only follow-up is needed. Those in the intermediate group (score of zero or 1) could be tested further, treated, or followed, depending on physician preference. Patients with a high probability of disease (score of 2 or 3) should be treated empirically with an antibiotic.

McGinn TG, Deluca J, Ahlawat SK. Validation and modification of streptococcal pharyngitis clinical prediction rules. *Mayo Clin Proc.* 2003;78:289–293.

106. Which of the following statements about posterior urethral valves is true?
A) They affect only male children.
B) They cannot be detected by prenatal ultrasound.
C) Most cases resolve spontaneously.
D) They are secondary to abnormal valves found in the posterior calices of the kidney, giving rise to urinary diverticula.
E) They are not detected by a voiding cystourethrogram.

Answer and Discussion

The answer is A. Children with urinary tract infections do not always present with symptoms such as frequency, dysuria, or flank pain. Infants may present with fever and irritability or other subtle symptoms such as lethargy. Older children may also have nonspecific symptoms such as abdominal pain or unexplained fever. A urinalysis should be obtained in a child with unexplained fever or symptoms that suggest a urinary tract infection.

Posterior urethral valves are commonly the cause of urinary tract infections in young boys only. These valves are secondary to abnormal folds in the prostatic urethra that enlarge with voiding and cause obstruction of the urethral lumen. Symptoms include decreased urinary stream, overflow incontinence, and urinary tract infections with dysuria. Affected boys can be identified prenatally with maternal ultrasound, which shows bilateral hydronephrosis; a distended bladder; and, if obstruction is severe, oligohydramnios. Urinary tract infections noted in boys suspected of posterior urinary valves should undergo further evaluation, including voiding cystourethrogram, or perineal ultrasound, as soon as the diagnosis is suspected; this will help reduce the risk of kidney damage. Treatment involves surgical resection of the valves.

Behrman RE, Kliegman RM, Jenson HB. *Nelson Textbook of Pediatrics,* 17th ed. Philadelphia: WB Saunders; 2004: 1802–1803.

107. Of the following, the most appropriate treatment for cradle cap is
A) topical ketoconazole
B) aloe vera shampoo
C) topical moisturizers
D) vitamin E
E) topical hydrocortisone

Answer and Discussion

The answer is E. Newborns frequently develop seborrheic dermatitis, with a thick, yellow, crusted scalp lesion (cradle cap); fissuring and yellow scaling behind the ears; red facial papules; and an irritated diaper rash. In infants, a baby shampoo is used daily and 1% hydrocortisone cream is applied twice daily. Additionally the dermatitis usually responds to frequent zinc or tar shampoos.

Rudolph CD, Rudolph AM, Hostetter MK, et al. *Rudolph's Pediatrics,* 21st ed. New York: McGraw-Hill; 2003:1175.

108. A 4-year-old boy swallows a small button battery. The child undergoes a chest radiograph and abdominal series. The battery is located in the lower esophagus, above the lower esophageal ring. The most appropriate management is
A) observation
B) endoscopy to remove the battery
C) barium swallow study
D) ipecac administration
E) none of the above

Answer and Discussion

The answer is B. Children younger than 4 years are at particular risk for the ingestion of foreign bodies such as button batteries used in wristwatches and cameras. If a child ingests a battery, a radiograph of the child's chest and abdomen is indicated to locate the battery's position. If the battery is located distal to the lower esophageal ring, no further therapy is needed; however, if the battery is larger than 1.5 cm, a follow-up radiograph should be performed 48 hours later to make sure the battery has passed through the pylorus. If the battery is lodged in the esophagus, endoscopy should be performed to remove the foreign body. A battery lodged in the esophagus can lead to perforation if left for more than 4 hours.

Litovitz T, Schmitz BF. Ingestion of cylindrical and button batteries: an analysis of 2,382 cases. *Pediatrics*. 1992;89:747–757.

Beers MH, Porter RS, eds. *The Merck manual of diagnosis and therapy*, Merck Research Laboratories, 18th ed. Whitehouse Station, NJ: Merck & Co.; 2006:126–127.

109. A 12-year-old boy presents with pain over the tibial tubercle. His mother reports a recent growth spurt. The most likely diagnosis is

A) Legg-Calvé-Perthes disease
B) shin splints
C) Osgood-Schlatter disease
D) osteosarcoma
E) stress fracture

Answer and Discussion

The answer is C. Osgood-Schlatter disease is caused by inflammation of the tibial tubercle that usually occurs at the time of a child's growth spurt. It is aggravated by strenuous physical activity such as climbing or running. Boys are more affected than girls, the condition is usually unilateral, and most patients are between 10 and 15 years of age. Symptoms include pain, swelling, and tenderness over the tibial tubercle. The cause is repeated traction of the inferior patellar tendon on the developing epiphyseal insertion. Radiographs of the knee, although unnecessary for the diagnosis, usually show bone fragments at the site of the tibial tubercle. Treatment includes rest (especially from deep-knee bends), ice therapy, and anti-inflammatories. In severe cases, more aggressive therapy, including casting, cortisone injections, and surgery, to remove loose bodies may be necessary but is infrequent.

Rudolph CD, Rudolph AM, Hostetter MK, et al. *Rudolph's Pediatrics*, 21st ed. New York: McGraw-Hill; 2003:2432.

110. A 4-year-old boy is brought to your office by his mother. The child has evidence of a stomatitis and a vesicular rash that affects his hands and feet. The most likely cause is

A) coxsackievirus
B) adenovirus
C) syphilis
D) varicella
E) measles

Answer and Discussion

The answer is A. The coxsackievirus is responsible for several infections that usually affect the pediatric population. There are two types of the virus:

- *Coxsackievirus A*
  - A16 is responsible for hand, foot, and mouth disease, which is characterized by stomatitis and a vesicular rash that affects the hands and feet. It is usually mild, affects young children, and may occur in epidemics.
  - A2, A4, A5, A6, A7, and A10 are responsible for herpangina, which is a more severe febrile illness that sometimes leads to febrile seizures. Other symptoms include a severe sore throat; vesiculoulcerative lesions that affect the tonsils, soft palate, and posterior pharynx; headaches; myalgias; and vomiting.
- *Coxsackievirus B*
  - B1, B2, B3, B4, and B5 are responsible for pleurodynia with pain associated with the area of diaphragmatic attachment. Other symptoms include fever, headache, sore throat, malaise, and vomiting. Orchitis and pleurisy may also occur.

Coxsackievirus B infection is rare in persons older than 60 years and is more common in children and young adults. The infection is transmitted by hand-to-mouth contact and may become widespread in certain populations. This virus has been called "the great pretender" because of the variety of clinical syndromes it can produce. Many infections that are caused by the virus are subclinical. More serious conditions caused by coxsackievirus B include myocarditis, orchitis, myalgia, and pleurodynia. Pleurodynia may be severe and can occur in epidemics referred to as *Bornholm disease*, named after the original description of an early epidemic on the Danish island of Bornholm. Patients with pleurodynia are usually children or young adults who present with severe pleuritic pain, tachypnea, and systemic upset. The condition is usually self-limiting, but there can be serious, though rare, long-term sequelae. In most cases, the treatment of coxsackievirus is symptomatic, and most infections are self-limited. Antibiotics are usually unnecessary unless concomitant bacterial infection is suspected.

Walling AD. Family practice international—clinical information from the international family medicine literature. *Am Fam Physician*. 2000;61(12):3733.

In most cases, the treatment of coxsackievirus is symptomatic, and most infections are self-limited.

111. The most common cause of metabolic pancreatitis in children is

A) type I diabetes mellitus
B) primary hyperparathyroidism
C) primary hyperthyroidism
D) diabetes insipidus
E) Cushing's syndrome

Answer and Discussion

The answer is B. Hypercalcemia and hyperlipidemia are 2 recognized causes of pancreatitis, both in children and in adults. The hypercalcemia may be masked by the transient calcium-lowering effect of acute pancreatitis. Primary hyperparathyroidism related to adenoma or hyperplasia (sometimes secondary to multiple endocrine neoplasia, type IIa) is the most common cause of the hypercalcemia.

Uretsky G, Goldschmiedt M, James K. Childhood pancreatitis. *Am Fam Physician*. 1999;59:2507.

112. A 3-month-old boy is brought to your office by his parents. The child has an erythematous rash that spares the skin folds of the groin area. The most likely diagnosis is

A) diaper dermatitis
B) yeast dermatitis
C) heat rash
D) varicella
E) childhood eczema

Answer and Discussion

The answer is A. Diaper dermatitis, also known as *primary irritant dermatitis*, results from chronic exposure to urine and feces and its subsequent skin irritation. It is a shiny, erythematous rash that spares the skin folds in the groin area and usually affects infants after 3 months of age. In severe cases, the skin may ulcerate. Treatment involves adequate drying of the area with exposure to air. Frequent diaper changes may also speed recovery, as well as application of petroleum jelly and zinc oxide to the affected areas. If the condition lasts more than a few days, the diagnosis of candidiasis must be considered. Rubber or plastic pants inhibit moisture evaporation and should be avoided.

Rudolph CD, Rudolph AM, Hostetter MK, et al. *Rudolph's Pediatrics,* 21st ed. New York: McGraw-Hill; 2003:1176.

113. The anterior fontanel usually closes at

A) 3 months
B) 6 months
C) 12 months
D) 2 years
E) 5 years

Answer and Discussion

The answer is C. The diagnosis of an abnormal fontanel requires the physician to appreciate the wide variation of normal. At birth, an infant has six fontanels. The anterior fontanel is the largest and most important for clinical evaluation. The average size of the anterior fontanel is 2.1 cm, and the median time of closure is around 1 year of age. The most common causes of a large anterior fontanel or delayed fontanel closure are achondroplasia, hypothyroidism, Down syndrome, increased intracranial pressure, and rickets. A bulging anterior fontanel can be a result of increased intracranial pressure or intracranial and extracranial tumors, and a sunken fontanel usually is a sign of dehydration. A physical examination helps the physician determine which imaging modality, such as plain films, ultrasonography, computed tomographic scan, or magnetic resonance imaging, to use for diagnosis.

Kiesler J, Ricer R. The abnormal fontanel. *Am Fam Physician.* 2003;67:2547–2552.

114. An adequate level of fluoride supplementation in drinking water is equal to

A) 1,000 parts/million (ppm)
B) 500 ppm
C) 100 ppm
D) 10 ppm
E) 1 ppm

Answer and Discussion

The answer is E. Fluoride helps reduce the formation of dental caries. It is most effectively administered in drinking water. The need for supplementation depends on the amount of fluoride in the drinking water. Adequate levels are usually 1 ppm. Water with levels <0.6 ppm may require supplementation. Fluoride toothpaste is not a suitable alternative supplement. Supplementation should be initiated for infants given ready-to-feed formulas that do not contain fluoride and for infants who are breast-fed after 6 months of age. Excessive fluoride supplementation can cause fluorosis. The following recommendations are given by the American Academy of Pediatrics:

Supplemental Fluoride Dosage Schedule

Fluoride in Home Water (ppm)			
Age	<0.3	0.3–0.6	>0.6
Birth–6 mo	0[a]	0	0
6 mo–3 yr	0.25	0	0
3–6 yr	0.50	0.25	0
6–16 yr	1.0	0.50	0

[a]Milligrams of fluoride per day.

Behrman RE, Kliegman RM, Jenson HB. *Nelson Textbook of Pediatrics,* 17th ed. Philadelphia: WB Saunders; 2004:1212.

115. A 5-year-old boy is brought to the emergency room with inspiratory and expiratory stridor, high fever, and drooling. Initial treatment consists of

A) oxygen therapy
B) airway management by trained personnel
C) inhaled bronchodilators
D) lying the child in the supine position
E) administration of epinephrine

Answer and Discussion

The answer is B. Epiglottitis is a severe, life-threatening condition usually seen in children between 3 and 10 years of age. The condition was usually the result of a *Haemophilus* type B(Hib) infection. In recent years, the occurrence of epiglottitis has been reduced dramatically by the widespread use of the Hib vaccine. Other causes include bacterial infections by *Streptococcus* and *Staphylococcus* species. Manifestations include stridor with inspiration and expiration, high fever, dysphagia, drooling, and toxic appearance. Children may lean forward with their neck outstretched to minimize airway obstruction. Laboratory findings include an elevated white blood cell count and positive blood cultures. Arterial blood gases may show hypoxia. Lateral neck radiographs show a swollen epiglottis with obstruction of the airway (positive thumb sign). Treatment involves securing the child's airway, but this should be accomplished only by trained personnel. Before intubation, the child should not be moved nor placed in a supine position. Oxygen should also be avoided because of the risk of aggravating the child and possible complete obstruction of the airway. Intravenous antibiotics should be started immediately, and the child should be monitored in an intensive care setting.

Rudolph CD, Rudolph AM, Hostetter MK, et al. *Rudolph's Pediatrics,* 21st ed. New York: McGraw-Hill; 2003:1276.

116. The most appropriate treatment for school avoidance is

A) to return the child to school and then determine reasons for school avoidance
B) to allow the child to remain at home until reasons for avoidance are determined
C) to prescribe methylphenidate (Ritalin)

D) to begin inpatient psychotherapy
E) to change teachers or schools

Answer and Discussion

The answer is A. School avoidance/refusal is a problem encountered in many family physicians' offices. Children may manifest numerous complaints to their parents and teachers to avoid attending school. The beginning of the school year appears to increase significantly the incidence of headache. The first step in the treatment of a child refusing to go to school is to get him or her back into the classroom and, once that is accomplished, identify reasons why the child is avoiding school. Some common problems include difficulty with peer relationships; family discord at home; and poor school performance that may be caused by attention deficit disorder, dyslexia, and visual or hearing difficulties. Working closely with the child's family and teachers can be beneficial.

Behrman RE, Kliegman RM, Jenson HB. *Nelson Textbook of Pediatrics,* 17th ed. Philadelphia: WB Saunders; 2004:1212.

117. The normal heart rate for newborns is
A) 60 to100 beats/minute
B) 100 to 120 beats/minute
C) 120 to 160 beats/minute
D) 140 to 160 beats/minute

Answer and Discussion

The answer is C. The normal heart rate in newborns is 120 to 160 beats/minute.

Fuloria M, Kreiter S. The newborn examination: Part I. Emergencies and common abnormalities involving the skin, head, neck, chest, and respiratory and cardiovascular systems. *Am Fam Physician.* 2002;65:61–68.

118. Which of the following is a description of Prader-Willi syndrome?
A) Tall, large arm span, increased risk of aortic rupture
B) Obese, hypotonic, mental retardation, hypogonadism
C) Short, obese, frontal bossing, precocious puberty
D) Normal size, mental retardation, precocious puberty

Answer and Discussion

The answer is C. Prader-Willi syndrome is characterized by decreased fetal activity, obesity, hypotonia, mental retardation, and hypogonadotropic hypogonadism. The syndrome is caused by a defect on the proximal long arm of the paternal chromosome 15 or by a defect on the maternal chromosome 15. Associated features include failure to thrive due to hypotonia and feeding difficulties, which generally improve after 6 to 12 months of age. From about 12 to 18 months and beyond, uncontrollable appetite causes worsening weight gain as well as psychologic problems, as insatiable hunger with significant obesity becomes the most noticeable feature. Rapid weight gain continues but with ultimate short stature in adulthood. Behavioral features include emotional lability, poor gross motor skills, cognitive impairment, and insatiable hunger. Facial abnormalities include a narrow bitemporal dimension, almond-shaped eyes, and a mouth with thin upper lips and down-turned corners. Hypogonadotropic hypogonadism, cryptorchidism, and a hypoplastic penis and scrotum in males or hypoplastic labia in females are present. Skeletal abnormalities include scoliosis, kyphosis, and osteopenia. Limb abnormalities include small hands and feet.

Beers MH, Porter RS, eds. *The Merck manual of diagnosis and therapy,* Merck Research Laboratories, 18th ed. Whitehouse Station, NJ: Merck & Co.; 2006:2369.

119. A 6 month old is brought to your office in mid-January. The child's mother reports that the infant has had a low-grade fever, wheezing with coughing, and diminished appetite. The most likely diagnosis is
A) bronchiolitis secondary to RSV
B) pneumonia secondary to *S. pneumoniae*
C) aspiration pneumonia
D) asthma
E) bronchitis secondary to *H. influenzae*

Answer and Discussion

The answer is A. Bronchiolitis is a common disease of the lower respiratory tract of infants and results from inflammatory obstruction of the small airways. The condition affects young children (younger than 2 years), and the peak incidence is in infants 6 months of age. Bronchiolitis is caused in most cases (>50%) by respiratory syncytial virus (RSV). Other causes include parainfluenza virus and adenoviruses and *Mycoplasma*. It most commonly occurs in the winter months. Signs and symptoms include coughing, wheezing, fever, nasal flaring, tachypnea, delayed expiration, and chest wall retractions. The white blood cell count and differential are usually normal. Nasal swabs can be used for RSV cultures, and rapid antigen assays may be performed to aid in diagnosis. Chest radiographs are usually normal; however, hyperinflation and increased interstitial markings in the perihilar area may be noted. Treatment is accomplished with bronchodilators, humidified oxygen via a croup tent, and intravenous fluids. In severe cases, ribavirin aerosol, an antiviral agent, can be administered. Bronchiolitis is more likely to develop in infants who are exposed to cigarette smoke. RSV immune globulin given just before and during RSV season is effective in preventing severe RSV disease in at-risk infants with chronic lung disease.

Behrman RE, Kliegman RM, Jenson HB. *Nelson Textbook of Pediatrics,* 17th ed. Philadelphia: WB Saunders; 2004: 1076–1079.

120. Most children affected with rotavirus are
A) younger than 6 months
B) between 6 months and 2 years of age
C) older than 2 years
D) between 2 and 4 years of age
E) between 5 and 7 years of age

Answer and Discussion

The answer is B. Rotavirus is a viral intestinal infection commonly seen in children, predominantly during the winter months. Epidemics are common in daycare centers. Most of the children affected are between 6 months and 2 years of age, but any child can be affected. Symptoms include profuse, watery diarrhea with the absence of blood, mild fevers, mild abdominal cramping, and vomiting (which may precede the onset of diarrhea). Some children may have associated respiratory complaints. The diagnosis is usually made by the clinical presentation but can be confirmed with viral antigen detection kits. Stool tests for white blood cells are negative, supporting the diagnosis of a viral infection.

Treatment involves oral rehydration for mild cases and intravenous fluid replacement for moderate to severe dehydration. Lactose-containing foods should be avoided if they appear to exacerbate the symptoms. Breast-feeding should be continued during rehydration. The bananas, rice, cereal, applesauce, and toast diet has not been shown to be superior to a regular diet. Most cases resolve in 5 to 7 days. The rotavirus vaccine approved in 1998 was suspended from use in July of 1999 because of an association of intussusception.

Behrman RE, Kliegman RM, Jenson HB. *Nelson Textbook of Pediatrics*, 17th ed. Philadelphia: WB Saunders; 2004: 1081–1083.

Stool tests for white blood cells are negative with rotavirus, supporting the diagnosis of a viral infection.

121. Which of the following congenital heart defects is considered a cyanotic lesion?
A) Ventricular septal defect
B) Atrial septal defect
C) Patent ductus arteriosis
D) Coarctation of the aorta
E) Tetralogy of Fallot

Answer and Discussion

The answer is E. Congenital heart defects are classified into two broad categories: acyanotic and cyanotic lesions. The most common acyanotic lesions are ventricular septal defect, atrial septal defect, atrioventricular canal, pulmonary stenosis, patent ductus arteriosus, aortic stenosis, and coarctation of the aorta. Congestive heart failure is the primary risk in infants with acyanotic lesions.

- *Ventricular septal defect*: Ventricular septal defect is the most common CHD. It may occur in any location on the septal wall. The significance of a ventricular septal defect is related to the size of the defect and ranges from insignificant to severe. Spontaneous closure within the first 6 months of life occurs in 30% to 40% of defects and is more likely to occur in smaller defects than in larger defects. Congestive heart failure, which may begin to develop at 6 to 8 weeks of age, is managed with diuretics and digoxin (Lanoxin). Indications for surgical closure include impaired growth that is not responsive to medical management and development of pulmonary hypertension. Postoperative complications include conduction defects, such as transient right bundle branch block.
- *Atrial septal defect*: Atrial septal defects may occur as sinus venosus, secundum or primum type. The overall rate of spontaneous closure of the secundum type of atrial septal defect is approximately 85% in the first 4 years of life. Primum and sinus venosus types with defects >8 mm rarely close spontaneously, and surgical intervention is usually necessary. Most children with an atrial septal defect remain asymptomatic, but in those who develop congestive heart failure, medical management with diuretics and digoxin can be beneficial. Indications for surgical closure are persistence of the defect beyond 4 years of age, refractory congestive heart failure, and the presence of other associated defects, such as ventricular septal defect or valvular anomalies. Cardiac dysrhythmias and mitral valve prolapse may be late sequelae of treated or untreated atrial septal defect in children or adults. Pulmonary hypertension may develop in adults with an untreated atrial septal defect. Atrial flutter or fibrillation may also occur in adults with a history of atrial septal defect, regardless of the treatment.
- *Atrioventricular canal*: Atrioventricular canal is characterized by a combination of a primum type of atrial septal defect, a common atrioventricular valve, and an inlet type of ventricular septal defect. Most of the hemodynamic problems associated with this abnormality are caused by the ventricular septal defect, although mitral regurgitation or left-ventricle-to-right-atrium regurgitation, or both, may lead to pulmonary overload. The treatment of congestive heart failure in association with atrioventricular canal, the indications for surgical repair, and the postoperative complications are similar to those described for ventricular septal defect. Surgery should be performed before the onset of pulmonary vascular occlusive disease. Palliative pulmonary artery banding may be performed in infants who have refractory congestive heart failure and are too small for definitive repair.
- *Pulmonary stenosis*: Pulmonary stenosis may be valvular, subvalvular or supravalvular. The clinical manifestations of pulmonary stenosis may vary from an asymptomatic lesion to frank congestive heart failure. Newborns may respond to prostaglandin E_1 infusion. Balloon valvuloplasty, performed during cardiac catheterization, is the preferred method of treatment for the valvular type of pulmonary stenosis. If this treatment is not successful, surgery is necessary.
- *Patent ductus arteriosus*: Patent ductus arteriosus is a common problem in premature infants. Closure may be spontaneous; if medical closure is required, indomethacin is effective. In term infants, spontaneous closure is unlikely, and indomethacin is not effective. Congestive heart failure and recurrent pneumonia are likely complications if the flow through the ductus is substantial. Surgical ligation remains the preferred method of closure and should be performed as soon as possible. Cardiopulmonary bypass is not necessary. Nonsurgical techniques for correction of patent ductus arteriosus, such as catheter placement of an embolic device in term infants and indomethacin therapy in premature infants, are gaining in popularity. Patent ductus arteriosus is the only CHD that may be considered surgically "cured," with no long-term sequelae.
- *Aortic stenosis*: Aortic stenosis may be valvular, subvalvular or supravalvular. It may be asymptomatic or may cause symptoms of congestive heart failure. The pressure gradient across the stenosis increases with the child's growth, as the cardiac output increases. Surgical correction is the preferred treatment. Timing of the surgery is dependent on the child's cardiopulmonary status, the type of procedure planned (valvulotomy versus valve replacement), and the size of the valve if a graft is needed. Lifelong anticoagulation therapy is required if a prosthetic valve replacement is performed.
- *Coarctation of the Aorta*: Narrowing of the aorta may occur anywhere along its length, but the vast majority of cases occur just below the origin of the left subclavian artery. The classic clinical sign of coarctation of the aorta is a higher blood pressure in the arms than in the legs and pulses that are bounding in the arms but decreased in the legs. Surgical repair is usually performed between the ages of 2 and 4 years. Urgent surgical repair is performed in cases of circulatory shock, cardiomegaly, severe hypertension, or severe congestive heart failure.

The most common cyanotic lesions are tetralogy of Fallot and transposition of the great arteries. In infants with cyanotic lesions, hypoxia is more of a problem than congestive heart failure.

- *Tetralogy of Fallot*: Tetralogy of Fallot is the most common CHD seen after infancy, with surgical repair usually undertaken when the child reaches 3 years of age. It consists of a large ventricular septal defect, right outflow tract obstruction, right ventricular hypertrophy, and overriding of the aorta. The classic clinical presentation is characterized by hyperpnea, irritability, cyanosis, and decreased murmur intensity. Squatting decreases systemic venous return by trapping blood in the legs, breaking the overload-hypoxia cycle. If this maneuver is ineffective, pharmacologic treatment may be necessary. Medical management of tetralogy of Fallot includes education on ways to treat the symptoms, prevention of anemia, and prophylaxis for subacute bacterial endocarditis. Surgical palliation consists of placement of a shunt from the subclavian artery to the ipsilateral pulmonary artery. Several different types of shunt procedures are currently performed. Total repair includes placement of a ventricular septal defect patch and right ventricular outflow tract widening. Total repair is performed before the child is 4 years of age.
- *Transposition of the Great Arteries:* Complete transposition of the great arteries occurs in a small percentage of children with CHD. The aorta and pulmonary arteries are transposed, so that the two circulations are separate and parallel rather than in sequence. Infants with transposition of the great arteries are cyanotic at birth and often have congestive heart failure. Associated defects such as an atrial septal defect or patent ductus arteriosus, which permit the mixing of blood from the two sides of the vascular tree, are necessary for the infant's survival. Transposition of the great vessels requires that the ductus should be kept open by prostaglandin infusion until surgery can be performed. Metabolic abnormalities and severe hypoxia should be corrected before surgical repair is undertaken. The definitive surgical procedure of choice is the arterial switch operation, in which the aorta and the pulmonary artery are divided and reattached to their proper positions, resulting in a physiologic repair. It should be performed as soon as possible. Associated defects, such as ventricular septal defect, pulmonary stenosis, and patent ductus arteriosus, may necessitate a staged repair. Late complications of surgical repair include pulmonary or aortic stenosis, coronary artery obstruction, ventricular dysfunction, arrhythmias, and mitral regurgitation.

Suspicion of a congenital heart defect should be raised by the presence of feeding difficulties in association with tachypnea, sweating and subcostal recession, or severe growth impairment. More frequent follow-up is required if congestive heart failure is present.

Saenz RB, Beebe DK, Triplett LC. Caring for infants with congenital heart disease and their families. *Am Fam Physician.* 1999;59:1857.

Beers MH, Porter RS, eds. *The Merck manual of diagnosis and therapy,* Merck Research Laboratories, 18th ed. Whitehouse Station, NJ: Merck & Co.; 2006:2404–2421.

122. Which of the following is true regarding hepatitis B vaccination in healthy infants?

A) The first immunization should be given by 2 months of age, second immunization 1 to 2 months later, and third immunization given between 6 and 18 months.
B) Injections should be given in the buttock to increase immunogenicity.
C) Only infants at risk should receive hepatitis B vaccination.
D) Two doses will provide optimal results.
E) None of the above

Answer and Discussion

The answer is A. Hepatitis B immunizations currently available in the United States are recombinant vaccines (Recombivax, Engerix-B). Three intramuscular doses are required to induce optimal protective antibody responses. The vaccine should be administered in the anterolateral thigh muscle in infants and in the deltoid muscle in children, adolescents, and adults; injection in the buttocks or via the intradermal route may lead to diminished immunogenicity with lower seroconversion rates and serologic titers. Universal vaccination of infants is recommended. A three-dose schedule is required and should be initiated during the newborn period or by 2 months of age, a second dose given 1 to 2 months later, and a third dose given by 6 to 18 months of age. Most school districts now require hepatitis B immunization before admission to kindergarten or first grade. Susceptibility testing before vaccination is not routinely indicated, and postvaccination testing for immunity is not necessary after routine immunization.

Behrman RE, Kliegman RM, Jenson HB. *Nelson Textbook of Pediatrics,* 17th ed. Philadelphia: WB Saunders; 2004:1328.

123. A child is found to have higher blood pressures in the arms than in the legs and pulses are bounding in the arms but decreased in the legs. The most likely condition is

A) ventricular septal defect
B) tetralogy of Fallot
C) transposition of the great arteries
D) coarctation of the aorta
E) aortic stenosis

Answer and Discussion

The answer is D. Coarctation of the aorta involves narrowing of the aorta that may occur anywhere along its length, but the vast majority of cases occur just below the origin of the left subclavian artery. The classic clinical sign of coarctation of the aorta is a higher blood pressure in the arms than in the legs and pulses that are bounding in the arms but decreased in the legs. Surgical repair is usually performed between the ages of 2 and 4 years. Emergent surgical repair is performed in cases of circulatory shock, cardiomegaly, severe hypertension, or severe congestive heart failure.

Saenz RB, Beebe DK, Triplett LC. Caring for infants with congenital heart disease and their families. *Am Fam Physician.* 1999;59:1857.

124. A 4-year-old girl is brought to the emergency room. The mother reports that the child recently recovered from a viral upper respiratory tract infection, but over the past few days has developed nosebleeds and bleeding from the gums. She also has noticed bruising of the extremities. The most likely diagnosis is

A) meningococcemia
B) idiopathic thrombocytopenic purpura (ITP)
C) hemophilia A
D) ingestion of warfarin
E) vitamin K deficiency

Answer and Discussion

The answer is B. Ideopathic thrombocytopenic purpura (ITP) is a disorder that usually affects children between 2 and 6 years of age. Boys and girls are equally affected. The condition usually follows a febrile, viral illness (particularly varicella, Epstein-Barr, and cytomegalovirus) during the winter months. Petechiae, purpura, and bleeding from mucous membranes develop within 3 weeks after the infection. Laboratory results often show thrombocytopenia (platelet counts <20,000 mm^3), and bone marrow studies show an increase in megakaryocytes. Prothrombin time and partial thromboplastin time are normal, but bleeding times are increased. No treatment is necessary in mild cases. In more severe cases with platelet counts below 20,000 mm^3 or with active bleeding, corticosteroids, γ globulin, or other immunosuppressant agents that transiently elevate the platelet count can be used, but they do not alter the course of the illness. In severe cases, splenectomy or plasmapheresis may be necessary to achieve remission. Intracranial hemorrhage is the primary cause of death in severe cases. Most cases are mild and patients recover completely without complications.

There is a chronic form of ITP that usually affects patients between 20 and 50 years of age; women tend to be affected more than men. Treatment for this form is similar to acute ITP, and psychosocial issues involving the chronic state are similar to those of hemophilia.

Rudolph CD, Rudolph AM, Hostetter MK, et al. *Rudolph's Pediatrics*, 21st ed. New York: McGraw-Hill; 2003:1556–1557.

125. Which of the following congenital heart defects can be surgically cured with no permanent sequelae?

A) Coarctation of the aorta
B) Tetralogy of Fallot
C) Patent ductus arteriosis
D) Ventricular septal defect
E) Transposition of the great vessels

Answer and Discussion

The answer is C. Patent ductus arteriosus is the only congenital heart defect that may be considered surgically "cured," with no long-term sequelae.

Saenz RB, Beebe DK, Triplett LC. Caring for infants with congenital heart disease and their families. *Am Fam Physician*. 1999;59:1857.

126. A 2 year old is seen in your office. The parent reports that the child shows toeing in when walking. On examination, the child exhibits femoral anteversion. The most appropriate treatment is

A) reassurance to the parent that the condition usually corrects itself as the child grows older
B) referral to an orthopedist
C) referral to a physical therapist
D) bracing to correct internal rotation of the femurs
E) fitting for corrective shoes

Answer and Discussion

The answer is A. Femoral anteversion is a common orthopedic finding in young children. The condition results when femoral anteversion leads to excessive internal rotation of the femur. As a result, the child may exhibit "kissing knees," toeing-in, and the appearance of lack of coordination of the lower extremities. Maximal femoral anteversion occurs between 1 and 3 years of age. This abnormality usually corrects itself as the child becomes older. Significant abnormalities found after 8 years of age should be referred to an orthopedist. Activities that may help correct the condition include ballet, bicycling, and skating because of the rotation exercises involved. In most cases, bracing is not beneficial. Severe cases may require osteotomy for rotational correction.

Rudolph CD, Rudolph AM, Hostetter MK, et al. *Rudolph's Pediatrics*, 21st ed. New York: McGraw-Hill; 2003:2422–2424.

127. A 2 year old is brought into your office. The parent reports a purulent, malodorous, bloody discharge from the child's left nostril. The most likely diagnosis is

A) foreign body in the nose
B) acute sinusitis
C) Wegener's granulomatosis
D) cerebrospinal fluid leak
E) chronic tonsillitis

Answer and Discussion

The answer is A. Young children often lodge foreign bodies in their noses. Symptoms include unilateral purulent, malodorous, and often bloody nasal discharge. Other symptoms include nasal congestion and abnormal nasal sounds. Some children with clear nasal discharge or mild sinus congestion may harbor a foreign body. Foreign bodies should be removed anteriorly. An attempt at lavage should not be made because of the risk of pushing the foreign body further into the nasal cavity. Radiographs of the nasal area and sinuses may help localize the foreign body. There are several methods to remove nasal foreign bodies, including the use of an alligator forceps, ear curettes, and a Fogarty catheter (which is slipped behind the foreign body, inflated, and removed pulling the foreign body along with it); if the foreign body does not appear to have sharp edges, the practitioner can simply have the child blow the nose, forcing the foreign body out. If removal is unsuccessful, ear, nose, and throat referral and perhaps general anesthesia is in order. Inspection of the unaffected side and the ears should also be performed to ensure they are unaffected.

Beers MH, Porter RS, eds. *The Merck manual of diagnosis and therapy*, Merck Research Laboratories, 18th ed. Whitehouse Station, NJ: Merck & Co.; 2006:829.

128. Varicella-zoster immunoglobulin (VZIG) is recommended for which of the following groups?

A) All newborns
B) Newborns of mothers with onset of varicella 5 days before delivery
C) Hospitalized premature infants older than 28 weeks' gestation, regardless of the mother's history of chickenpox
D) Pregnant women just before delivery who have no history of varicella and were exposed at the time of conception
E) Newborns >4,500 g regardless of exposure history or mother's exposure history

Answer and Discussion

The answer is A. VZIG is indicated for the prevention of varicella and zoster infections in the following groups:

- Full-term infant born to mother who has chickenpox <1 week before delivery

- Every premature infant born to a mother with active chickenpox (even if present longer than 1 week)
- Newborns whose mothers had onset of varicella 5 days before delivery or within 2 days after delivery who are exposed to varicella
- Hospitalized premature infants (gestation of 28 weeks or more) whose mothers have no history of chickenpox
- Hospitalized premature infants (gestation of <28 weeks or ≤1,000 g) regardless of maternal history

VZIG is given by intramuscular injection. One vial (125 U) is given for each 10 kg of body weight, with a maximum dose of 625 U (five vials). For maximal effectiveness, VZIG should be given within 48 hours and preferably not more than 96 hours after exposure. Side effects are usually related to local discomfort at the injection site.

Current recommendations include routine vaccination of all infants with a single dose of live varicella virus vaccine (Varivax) at 12 to 18 months of age. Those older than 13 years with negative varicella titers require two doses given 4 to 8 weeks apart. The live virus is contraindicated in immunocompromised children. Varicella may occur in up to 6% of patients despite immunization; however, the illness is usually mild.

Gunn, VL, Nechyba C. *The Harriet Lane Handbook: A Manual for Pediatric House Officers*. St. Louis: Mosby; 2002:339–340.

129. The most common cause of lead exposure is
A) playing with toys made with lead
B) exposure to water from lead pipes
C) breathing lead particles from the atmosphere
D) ingesting food contaminated with lead
E) ingesting contaminated paint chips or house dust

Answer and Discussion

The answer is E. More than 4% of children in the United States have lead poisoning. Rates of lead poisoning are even higher in large cities and among people with low incomes. The most common cause of lead poisoning today is old paint with increased lead content. Lead has not been used in house paint since 1978. However, many older houses and apartment buildings (especially those built before 1960) have lead-based paint on their walls. Children can get lead poisoning by chewing on pieces of peeling paint or by swallowing house dust or soil that contains tiny chips of the leaded paint from these buildings (pica). Lead can also be in air, water, and food. Lead levels in the air have gone down greatly since lead was taken out of gasoline in the 1970s. Lead is still found in some old water pipes, although using lead solder to mend or put together water pipes is no longer allowed in the United States. Lead can also be found in food or juice stored in foreign-made cans or improperly fired ceramic containers.

Ellis MR, Kane KY. Lightening the lead load in children. *Am Fam Physician*. 2000;62:545–554, 559–560.

130. Which of the following statements about night terrors is true?
A) They affect adults more than children.
B) They are often remembered in vivid detail.
C) They occur during stage 3 or 4 of non–rapid eye movement (NREM) sleep.
D) They occur during REM sleep.
E) They are unaffected by benzodiazepines.

Answer and Discussion

The answer is C. Night terrors occur more frequently in children than in adults. Boys between 5 and 7 years are more commonly affected. Symptoms include sudden onset, fearful, screaming episodes that disrupt stages 3 and 4 NREM sleep cycle. They may accompany sleepwalking. They differ from nightmares in that nightmares occur during REM sleep and are frequently remembered in vivid detail, whereas night terrors are not remembered. A short course of diazepam (which suppresses stages 3 and 4 of sleep) or imipramine (Tofranil) is often helpful in patients with severe night terrors but is not helpful for patients who suffer from nightmares. An underlying emotional disorder should be investigated in children with persistent or prolonged night terrors.

Behrman RE, Kliegman RM, Jenson HB. *Nelson Textbook of Pediatrics*, 17th ed. Philadelphia: WB Saunders; 2004:18, 2010.

> **Symptoms of night terrors include sudden onset, fearful, screaming episodes that disrupt stages 3 and 4 NREM sleep cycle. Night terrors are not remembered.**

131. Which of the following statements is true regarding short stature in children?
A) Those with short stature and delayed bone age are considered to have constitutional short stature.
B) Those with genetic short stature rarely reach the height of their parents.
C) Those with constitutional short stature should undergo a comprehensive evaluation looking for secondary causes.
D) Chromosome studies should be performed on children suspected of genetic short stature.
E) Children with constitutional growth delay rarely reach normal adult height.

Answer and Discussion

The answer is A. Assessment of a child's growth rate is necessary when evaluating short stature. Most children in or below the fifth percentile for height have normal growth rates. In the absence of other clinical findings, no further assessment is needed; however, the child should be followed to ensure that the growth rate remains normal. Among children with short stature but normal growth rates, two specific groups can be identified based on bone age: those with (1) genetic short stature and (2) those with constitutional short stature. Children with short stature who have normal growth rates and normal bone age are considered to have genetic short stature. Their eventual adult stature will likely be similar to that of their parents. On the other hand, children with short stature and delayed bone age are considered to have constitutional short stature. Following a period of decreased growth rate in infancy, the growth rate in these children will return to normal for the remainder of their childhood. While these children may be considered short at some points during their childhood, they can be expected to eventually acquire normal adult height. In both groups, no further medical assessment or treatment is necessary. Children with short stature and decreased growth rates warrant a comprehensive evaluation for an underlying pathologic condition. The assessment should include a complete blood count, a urinalysis, a chemistry profile, and thyroid studies. Children should undergo a sweat chloride test if they have a history of recurrent pulmonary or gastrointestinal symptoms. Chromosome studies should be obtained if there are physical signs of Turner's syndrome. Growth hormone studies should not consist of a single random determination. Growth hormone stimulation methods are necessary. Consultation is warranted if the initial evaluation fails to reveal an etiology for the decreased stature.

Behrman RE, Kliegman RM, Jenson HB. *Nelson Textbook of Pediatrics,* 17th ed. Philadelphia: WB Saunders; 2004:61.

132. Measles (rubeola) is associated with which of the following conditions?

A) Small erythematous ulcerations on the tongue
B) Joint pain, rash, infertility
C) Unexplained brain deterioration with seizure formation, behavioral and intellectual deterioration, motor abnormalities, and possible death years after a measles attack
D) Petechial rash that develops on the trunk and spreads to involve the face and extremities
E) Disseminated intravascular coagulopathy

Answer and Discussion

The answer is C. Measles is a highly contagious disease that was common in children before the advent of immunization. Symptoms include the three Cs (cough, coryza, conjunctivitis), high fever, maculopapular rash, and pathognomonic Koplik's spots (small white spots that resemble flecks of sand surrounded by areas of erythema) on the buccal mucosa, usually opposite the first and second upper molar. The cause is a paramyxovirus that is spread by respiratory secretions. The disease is communicable 2 to 4 days before the onset of the characteristic rash, which usually develops on the face and spreads to involve the entire body approximately 2 weeks from the time of exposure. In 3 to 5 days, the patient usually improves and the fever and rash subside. Measles is usually self-limited and has a low mortality rate unless significant complications develop. Complications include pneumonia, bacterial superinfection, acute thrombocytopenic purpura, encephalitis, and subacute sclerosing panencephalitis (unexplained brain deterioration with seizure formation, motor abnormalities, and possible death years after the measles attack). Treatment for measles is directed toward the relief of symptoms and appropriate medication for any secondary infections. The use of immunoglobulin may also be indicated. Children should be immunized with the live attenuated MMR vaccination at 12 to 15 months and again at age 4 to 6 years. Measles vaccine is not recommended for pregnant women, immunocompromised patients, or HIV patients.

Behrman RE, Kliegman RM, Jenson HB. *Nelson Textbook of Pediatrics,* 17th ed. Philadelphia: WB Saunders; 2004: 1026–1031.

133. Diagnosis of mental retardation is

A) easily identified by clinicians
B) typically made by chromosomal analysis
C) dependent on a complete history, physical examination, and developmental assessment of the child
D) easily associated with an underlying etiology

Answer and Discussion

The answer is C. Mental retardation in young children is often missed by clinicians. The condition is present in 2% to 3% of the population, either as an isolated finding or as part of a syndrome or broader disorder. Causes of mental retardation are numerous and include genetic and environmental factors. In at least 30% to 50% of cases, physicians are unable to determine etiology despite thorough evaluation. Diagnosis is highly dependent on a comprehensive personal and family medical history, a complete physical examination and a careful developmental assessment of the child. These will guide appropriate evaluations and referrals to provide genetic counseling, resources for the family and early intervention programs for the child. The family physician is encouraged to continue regular follow-up visits with the child to facilitate a smooth transition to adolescence and young adulthood.

Daily DK, Ardinger HH, Holmes GE. Identification and evaluation of mental retardation. *Am Fam Physician.* 2000; 61:1059–1067, 1070.

134. Which of the following conditions is associated with congenital cataracts?

A) Maternal rubella infection
B) Maternal varicella infection
C) Congenital hypothyroidism
D) Acromegaly
E) Fetal hydrops

Answer and Discussion

The answer is A. A cataract is a proteinaceous opacity of the lens. Causes of congenital cataracts include ocular trauma, maternal rubella, diabetes mellitus, galactosemia, Marfan's syndrome, and Down syndrome. Monocular cataracts should be corrected as soon as possible (within the first 3 months of birth) so that vision can develop properly. Delayed intervention can lead to development of abnormal vision. Treatment of the amblyopia may be the most demanding and difficult step in the visual rehabilitation of infants and children with cataracts.

Behrman RE, Kliegman RM, Jenson HB. *Nelson Textbook of Pediatrics,* 17th ed. Philadelphia: WB Saunders; 2004: 2105–2106.

135. A child with Down syndrome is born, and you explain to the family

A) heart defects are very rare in Down syndrome children
B) some females are fertile; however, there is a 50% chance their children will have Down syndrome
C) fertility is not affected in males
D) IQ scores are rarely affected in Down syndrome children
E) the most common site for heart defects is associated with the atrial septum

Answer and Discussion

The answer is B. Newborns affected with Down syndrome are often placid, rarely cry, and demonstrate muscular hypotonia. Excess skin around the neck is common and can be detected by fetal ultrasound as edema of the neck. Physical and mental development are impaired; the mean intelligence quotient (IQ) is about 50. Microcephaly, a flattened occiput, and short stature are characteristic. The outer sides of the eyes are slanted upward, and epicanthal folds at the inner corner of the eye usually are present. Brushfield's spots (gray to white spots resembling grains of salt around the periphery of the iris) usually are visible and disappear during the first 12 months of life. The bridge of the nose is flattened, the mouth is often kept open because of a large protruding tongue that is furrowed and lacks the central fissure, and the ears are small and rounded. Hands are short and broad and often have a single palmar crease (simian crease); the fingers are short, with clinodactyly (incurving) of the fifth finger, which often has only two phalanges. The feet may have a wide gap between the first and second toes, and a plantar furrow often extends backward on the foot. Hands and feet show characteristic dermal prints (dermatoglyphics). Congenital heart disease, most commonly affecting the ventricular septum or the atrioventricular canal, occurs in about 40% of affected newborns. There is an increased incidence of almost all other congenital anomalies, particularly duodenal atresia. Many people with Down syndrome develop thyroid problems, which may be difficult to detect unless blood tests are done. Additionally, they are prone to developing hearing problems and problems with vision. Regular screening may be appropriate. At autopsy, all adult Down syndrome brains show the microscopic findings of Alzheimer's disease, and many persons also develop the associated clinical signs. Some affected women are fertile, and they have a 50% chance that their fetus will also have Down syndrome; however, many of these affected fetuses abort spontaneously. All men with Down syndrome are infertile.

Beers MH, Porter RS, eds. *The Merck manual of diagnosis and therapy,* Merck Research Laboratories, 18th ed. Whitehouse Station, NJ: Merck & Co.; 2006:2449–2450.

136. Which of the following findings is most commonly associated with fetal alcohol syndrome?

A) low birth weight
B) seizures
C) palmar erythema
D) peripheral neuropathy
E) cirrhosis

Answer and Discussion

The answer is A. Fetal alcohol syndrome is a constellation of symptoms in a newborn and is a result of maternal alcohol consumption. Physical findings include low birth weight, short palpebral fissures, midface hypoplasia, abnormal palmar creases, and cardiac abnormalities. Varying degrees of mental retardation may be present. Severe symptoms are usually the result of heavy ethanol consumption (i.e., 5 or more drinks daily); however, milder effects may be associated with consumption of smaller amounts. Because a safe level of alcohol consumption during pregnancy has not been established, pregnant women should be counseled to avoid all alcohol use during pregnancy.

Behrman RE, Kliegman RM, Jenson HB. *Nelson Textbook of Pediatrics,* 17th ed. Philadelphia: WB Saunders; 2004:612.

137. Klinefelter's syndrome is associated with

A) short stature and hirsutism
B) tall stature with disproportionately long arms and legs
C) increased development of homosexual behavior
D) low urinary excretion of FSH
E) universal cognitive defects

Answer and Discussion

The answer is B. Klinefelter's syndrome occurs in about 1/800 live male births. The extra X chromosome comes from the mother in 60% of cases. Affected persons tend to be tall, with disproportionately long arms and legs. They often have small, firm testes, and about one third develop gynecomastia. Puberty usually occurs at the normal age, but facial hair growth is often light. There is a predisposition for learning difficulties, and many have significant deficits. However, clinical variation is varied, and many 47, XXY males are normal in appearance and intellect and are found in the course of an infertility workup (probably all 47, XXY males are sterile) or in chromosomal surveys of normal populations. Boys from the latter group have been followed developmentally. There is no increased incidence of homosexuality. Testicular development varies from nonfunctional tubules to some production of spermatozoa, and urinary excretion of follicle-stimulating hormone is frequently increased. Some affected have 3, 4, and even 5 X chromosomes along with the Y. The more X chromosomes, the greater the severity of mental retardation.

Beers MH, Porter RS, eds. *The Merck manual of diagnosis and therapy,* Merck Research Laboratories, 18th ed. Whitehouse Station, NJ: Merck & Co.; 2006:2454.

138. A 5-year-old child has a chronic relapsing and pruritic superficial inflammation of the skin that affects the antecubital and popliteal fossas. The most likely diagnosis is

A) *Rhus* dermatitis
B) atopic dermatitis
C) hereditary angioedema
D) Cushing's disease
E) Lyme disease

Answer and Discussion

The answer is B. Atopic dermatitis is a condition characterized by chronic relapsing, superficial inflammation of the skin. The skin disorder is associated with severe pruritus and eczematous changes with erythematous papules or plaques that may show excoriations or lichenification. Many patients may show three different stages. The first stage is an infantile stage that begins at 2 to 3 months of age and lasts until 18 months of age. The eczematous rash affects the cheeks and scalp, may form oval-shaped patches on the trunk, and may eventually affect the extensor surfaces. The inflammation resolves in most cases. However, in 33% of patients, the rash progresses into stage 2, which is usually referred to as *childhood eczema*. The rash during this stage usually affects the flexor surfaces of the antecubital and popliteal fossas. Other areas of involvement include the neck, wrists, and, occasionally, the hands and feet. The third stage is adolescent eczema, which usually occurs around the age of 12 years. Only 33% of children with childhood eczema progress to adolescent eczema, which usually only involves the hands. Atopic dermatitis is less common after 30 years of age. The condition appears to be associated with asthma, hay fever, elevated IgE levels, and urticaria. There also appears to be a genetic predisposition to develop atopic dermatitis. Triggering factors include certain foods (e.g., cheese, wheat, nuts, legumes, egg whites) and inhaled irritants (e.g., pollens, perfumes, toxic fumes). Treatment involves the use of antihistamines, corticosteroid creams, emollients (Eucerin or Aquaphor), wet-to-dry dressing changes with Burow's solution, and antibiotics for secondary bacterial infections. Bathing should be kept to a minimum. A short course of oral steroids may be helpful for severe cases. The avoidance of triggering factors is also important. Extremes of temperature and humidity should be avoided.

Behrman RE, Kliegman RM, Jenson HB. *Nelson Textbook of Pediatrics,* 17th ed. Philadelphia: WB Saunders; 2004:774–778.

139. A child is born with excessive dorsal lymphedema of the hands and feet and with lymphedema or loose folds of skin over the posterior aspect of the neck. There is a low hairline on the back of the neck, ptosis, a broad chest with widely spaced nipples, multiple pigmented nevi, short 4th metacarpals and metatarsals, prominent finger pads, hypoplasia of the nails, and coarctation of the aorta. Based on the findings the most likely diagnosis is:

A) Klinefelter syndrome
B) Turner syndrome
C) Down syndrome
D) Marfan's syndrome
E) Prader-Willie syndrome

Answer and Discussion

The answer is B. Affected newborns with Turner syndrome may present with excessive dorsal lymphedema of the hands and feet and with lymphedema or loose folds of skin over the posterior aspect of the neck. However, many females with Turner syndrome are very mildly affected. Typically, short stature, webbing of the neck, low hairline on the back of the neck, ptosis, a broad chest with widely spaced nipples, multiple pigmented nevi, short fourth metacarpals and metatarsals, prominent finger pads, hypoplasia of the nails, coarctation of the aorta, bicuspid aortic valve, and increased carrying angle at the elbow occur. Renal anomalies and hemangiomas are common. Occasionally, telangiectasia occurs in the gastrointestinal tract, with resultant intestinal bleeding. Mental retardation is rare, but many have some diminution of certain perceptual ability and thus score poorly on performance tests and in mathematics, even though they score average or above in verbal IQ tests. Gonadal dysgenesis with failure to go through puberty, develop breast tissue, or begin menses occurs in the majority of affected persons. Replacement with female hormones will bring on puberty. The ovaries are replaced by bilateral streaks of fibrous stroma and are usually devoid of developing ova. However, 5% to 10% of affected girls do go through menarche spontaneously, and very rarely, affected women have been fertile and have had children.

Beers MH, Porter RS, eds. *The Merck manual of diagnosis and therapy,* Merck Research Laboratories, 18th ed. Whitehouse Station, NJ: Merck & Co.; 2006:2453–2454.

140. A 10-month-old girl is brought into the emergency room. The mother reports that the child pulls her legs up to her abdomen and cries for 5 to 10 minutes followed by episodes of relaxed silence. She also reports the child is passing blood and mucus in her stools. On examination, a tubular mass is felt in the upper right quadrant. The most likely diagnosis is

A) intussusception
B) volvulus
C) pyloric stenosis
D) viral gastroenteritis
E) ascariasis

Answer and Discussion

The answer is A. Intussusception is a cause of acute abdominal pain in young pediatric patients between 2 months and 6 years of age. The condition is rare before 3 months of age and decreases in frequency after 36 months. It is most commonly seen between the ages of 6 and 12 months. It is three times more common in males than in females. The cause is a telescoping of the bowel, which compromises blood flow. Symptoms include periumbilical, colicky, abdominal pain that occurs in periodic waves with some painless periods. Affected infants often pull their legs up to their abdomen to help relieve the discomfort and then rest comfortably after the waves of pain. Blood and mucus are passed in the stool (50% of patients), giving the stool a "currant jelly" appearance. There is usually a tender, sausage-like mass palpated in the right upper abdominal area. Vomiting is also usually present, especially in the early stages. Diagnosis and treatment may be achieved using a barium enema, which usually provides enough hydrostatic pressure to reduce the intussusception. In severe cases, laparotomy may be necessary to reduce the intussusception. A lead point may occur as a result of a polyp, duplication cyst, lymphoma, parasite, Meckel's diverticulum, hematoma associated with Henoch-Schönlein purpura, hypertrophied Peyer's patches, or ventriculoperitoneal shunt.

Hay WW Jr, Levin MJ, Sondheimer JM, et al., eds. *Current pediatric diagnosis & treatment,* 18th ed. New York: McGraw-Hill; 2007:616–617.

> With intussusception blood and mucus are passed in the stool (50% of patients), giving the stool a "currant jelly" appearance. Additionally there is usually a tender, sausage-like mass palpated in the right upper abdominal area.

141. Which of the following conditions is associated with atopic dermatitis?

A) Asthma
B) Vasomotor rhinitis
C) Elevated Ig A levels
D) Melanoma
E) Retinitis pigmentosa

Answer and Discussion

The answer is A. Atopic dermatitis is a chronic inflammatory condition of the skin that occurs in persons of all ages but is more common in children. The condition is characterized by intense pruritus and a course associated with exacerbations and remissions. Atopic dermatitis has been reported to affect as many as 10% of children. In the United States the symptoms of atopic dermatitis typically resolve by adolescence in 50% of affected children, but the condition can persist into adulthood. Poor prognostic features include a family history of the condition, early disseminated infantile disease, female gender, and coexisting allergic rhinitis and asthma. The diagnosis of atopic dermatitis is based on the findings of the history and physical examination. Exposure to possible exacerbating factors, such as aeroallergens, irritating chemicals, foods, and emotional stress, can cause exacerbations. There are no specific laboratory findings or histologic features that define atopic dermatitis, although elevated IgE levels are found in a majority of affected patients. In infants and young children with atopic dermatitis, pruritus commonly is present on the scalp, face (cheeks and chin), and extensor surfaces of the extremities. Over 50% of patients with atopic dermatitis have or develop asthma or allergic rhinitis. The majority of patients have a positive family history of atopy. Even if atopic dermatitis resolves with age, the predisposition for asthma and rhinitis persists.

Correale CE, Walker C, Murphy L, et al. Atopic dermatitis: a review of diagnosis and treatment. *Am Fam Physician.* 1999; 60:1191–1210.

Behrman RE, Kliegman RM, Jenson HB. *Nelson Textbook of Pediatrics,* 17th ed. Philadelphia: WB Saunders; 2004: 774–778.

142. Which of the following would concern a physician about a child's development?
A) Rolls over at 4 months
B) First words at 15 months
C) Walks at 12 months
D) Ties shoes at 5 years
E) Copies a circle at 3 years

Answer and Discussion

The answer is B. Some important developmental milestones for children include the following:

- *4 to 5 months:* Rolls over to supine position
- *6 months:* Sits without support
- *9 months:* Says "mama" and "dada" indiscriminately
- *9 months:* Creeps and crawls, pulls to stand, waves bye-bye
- *10 months:* Says "mama" and "dada" discriminately
- *12 months:* Walks alone
- *15 months:* Creeps up stairs, builds two-block towers, walks independently
- *18 months:* Points to four body parts
- *24 months:* Jumps, kicks ball, removes coat, verbalizes wants
- *3 years:* Copies circle; gives full name, age, and gender; throws ball overhand
- *4 years:* Hops on one foot, dresses with little assistance, shoes on the correct feet
- *5 years:* Ties shoes, prints first name, plays competitive games

Impairments in hearing can relate to delayed development. Therefore, the first step in the evaluation of a child with language delay is hearing assessment.

Behrman RE, Kliegman RM, Jenson HB. *Nelson Textbook of Pediatrics,* 17th ed. Philadelphia: WB Saunders; 2004:33–34.

143. The main reason the premature infants have difficulty maintaining body temperature is secondary to
A) large body surface to body mass index
B) inadequate hypothalamic function
C) poor sympathetic tone
D) excessive circulating norepinephrine
E) inability to produce neuromediated chills

Answer and Discussion

The answer is A. Premature infants have a large body surface area to body mass ratio; therefore, when exposed to temperatures below the neutral thermal environment they rapidly lose heat and have difficulty maintaining their body temperature.

Beers MH, Porter RS, eds. *The Merck manual of diagnosis and therapy,* Merck Research Laboratories, 18th ed. Whitehouse Station, NJ: Merck & Co.; 2006:2265.

144. Which of the following statements about measles immunizations is true?
A) Allergies to eggs or neomycin are not contraindications to the measles vaccine.
B) Those who received killed virus immunization between 1963 and 1967 should receive a live attenuated booster vaccination.
C) Infants receiving vaccination before 15 months of age do not need booster vaccinations.
D) The present immunization is a genetically derived recombinant vaccine.
E) Those born before 1956 should receive a measles booster vaccination.

Answer and Discussion

The answer is B. Measles immunization is accomplished with a live attenuated virus given at 12 to 15 months of age in the MMR vaccine and then as a booster with the preschool physical at 4 to 6 years of age. Those vaccinated with the killed virus (available in the United States from 1963 to 1967) should be given the live attenuated vaccine, because ineffectiveness is associated with the killed virus given during that period. Those born before 1956 are, in most cases, immune as a result of natural infection and therefore require no additional vaccination. Also, infants vaccinated before 12 months of age should receive two additional boosters. Prior anaphylactic reactions to eggs or neomycin are relative contraindications to the administration of the measles vaccine. A pediatric allergist or immunologist should be consulted before administration.

Abramson JS, Baker CJ, Baltimore RS. *Red Book Online* 2003: Report of the Committee on Infectious Diseases, American Academy of Pediatrics, accessed at http://aapredbook.aappublications.org on 6/19/06.

145. Premature infants are at increased risk for kernicterus. Which of the following statements is true regarding bilirubin in these children?
A) Decreased bowel motility increases the amount of excreted bilirubin in the stools.
B) Early feedings increase bowel motility and promote bilirubin excretion.
C) Feeding has little impact on the level of bilirubin excretion.
D) Enterohepatic circulation does not occur until the infant reaches 40 weeks.
E) Delayed clamping of the umbilical cord allows for better excretion of bilirubin.

Answer and Discussion

The answer is B. Premature infants develop hyperbilirubinemia more often than do full-term infants, and kernicterus may occur at serum bilirubin levels as low as 10 mg/dL (170 μmol/L) in underweight premature infants who are ill. The higher bilirubin levels in premature infants may be partially due to inadequately developed hepatic excretion mechanisms, including deficiencies in bilirubin's uptake from the serum, its hepatic conjugation to bilirubin diglucuronide, and its excretion into the biliary tree. Decreased bowel motility enables more bilirubin diglucuronide to be deconjugated within the intestinal lumen by enterohepatic circulation of bilirubin. On the other hand, early feedings increase bowel motility and reduce bilirubin reabsorption and can thereby significantly decrease the incidence and severity of physiologic jaundice. Uncommonly, delayed clamping of the umbilical cord can also increase the risk of significant hyperbilirubinemia by allowing the transfusion of a large RBC mass; RBC breakdown and bilirubin production are thus increased.

Beers MH, Porter RS, eds. *The Merck manual of diagnosis and therapy,* Merck Research Laboratories, 18th ed. Whitehouse Station, NJ: Merck & Co.; 2006:2267–2268.

146. Which of the following statements about insulin-dependent diabetes mellitus type I is true?
A) It usually develops in patients older than 30 years.
B) The disease is associated with insensitivity of the body's tissues to insulin.
C) Ninety percent of those affected present in nonketotic hyperosmolar coma.
D) There is a lack of insulin production as a result of destruction to the β cells in the islets of Langerhans.
E) Diabetic ketoacidosis is not associated with insulin-dependent diabetes mellitus type I.

Answer and Discussion

The answer is D. Insulin-dependent diabetes is the result of an insulin deficiency and appears to be a chronic autoimmune destruction of the β cells of Langerhans' islets. There is an increased risk among family members, and it is more common in individuals younger than 30 years. The most common symptoms are polyphagia, polyuria, polydipsia, increased thirst, weight loss despite increased appetite, fatigue, and blurred vision. One-third of patients have diabetic ketoacidosis at the time of presentation. Signs include severe dehydration, labored respirations (Kussmaul's respirations), altered mental status, abdominal pain, enuresis, and fruity breath. Laboratory results show hyperglycemia and glycosuria. Treatment involves the administration of exogenous insulin. Many patients (approximately 66%) experience a period of total or partial remission ("honeymoon period") within a few weeks or months after initiation of medication. The goals of treatment are replacing insulin, instituting diet and exercise regimens, and monitoring glucose levels.

Behrman RE, Kliegman RM, Jenson HB. *Nelson Textbook of Pediatrics,* 17th ed. Philadelphia: WB Saunders; 2004: 1947–1952, 1962–1963.

147. Which of the following is not associated with the development of acne?
A) Excessive sebum production
B) Diets high in fat
C) Hyperkeratinization with development of microcomedo
D) Accumulation of lipids and cellular debris
E) Bacterial colonization

Answer and Discussion

The answer is B. Acne is a disease associated with the pilosebaceous units in the skin. It is thought to be caused by four important factors.

1. Excessive sebum production secondary to sebaceous gland hyperplasia.
2. Subsequent hyperkeratinization of the hair follicle prevents normal shedding of the follicular keratinocytes, which then obstruct the follicle and form an inapparent microcomedo.
3. Lipids and cellular debris soon accumulate within the blocked follicle.
4. This microenvironment encourages colonization of *Propionibacterium acnes*, which provokes an immune response through the production of numerous inflammatory mediators. Inflammation is further enhanced by follicular rupture and subsequent leakage of lipids, bacteria, and fatty acids into the dermis.

Feldman S, Careccia RE, Barham KL, et al. Diagnosis and treatment of acne. *Am Fam Physician.* 2004;69:2123–2130, 2135–2136.

148. A 4-year-old boy is brought to the emergency room by his parents. They report that the child swallowed a penny. On examination, the child has no abdominal tenderness. Radiographs of the abdomen localize the coin in the duodenum. The appropriate management includes
A) laxative administration
B) esophagogastroduodenoscopy with removal of the coin
C) ipecac administration
D) charcoal administration
E) observation

Answer and Discussion

The answer is E. It is not uncommon for infants and small children who swallow coins to present to the family physician's office or emergency room. Most children are completely asymptomatic. A radiograph of the chest, neck, and abdominal area should help locate the radiopaque coin. If it is found below the diaphragm, the child only needs to be observed until the coin is passed. If the coin is lodged in the esophagus or if the child exhibits symptoms related to the ingested coin, an esophagogastroduodenoscopy may be necessary to remove the foreign body. In most cases, sharp objects should be retrieved by endoscopy (if possible) if they have not entered the small intestine. Follow-up radiographs of the abdomen can help locate and mark the progress of coins in the intestines. Hand-held metal detectors have also been used to locate the position of the coin. The use of ipecac, charcoal, or laxatives is not indicated.

Beers MH, Porter RS, eds. *The Merck manual of diagnosis and therapy,* Merck Research Laboratories, 18th ed. Whitehouse Station, NJ: Merck & Co.; 2006:126–127.

149. Which of the following statements is true regarding breast-feeding and nipple confusion?
A) The World Health Organization recommends avoiding the use of pacifiers or bottle-feeding to establish successful breast-feeding.
B) There is compelling evidence that pacifier use and bottle-feeding is detrimental to successful breast-feeding.
C) Early pacifier use is associated with increased breast-feeding at 1 month.
D) Supplementation with a cup or bottle increases the duration of breast-feeding.
E) Cup feeding was associated with a shorter duration of breast-feeding in comparison to bottle-feeding in mothers who had cesarean sections.

Answer and Discussion

The answer is A. The UNICEF/World Health Organization Baby Friendly Hospital Initiative recommends avoiding the use of pacifiers or bottle-feeding to ensure successful breast-feeding; however, the evidence supporting this recommendation is limited. Cup feeding has been advocated as a safe alternative to bottle-feeding in breastfed infants who require supplemental feedings to prevent "nipple confusion" or future problems with breastfeeding. Researchers conclude that early pacifier introduction is associated with fewer mothers exclusively breast-feeding at 1 month and decreased overall breast-feeding duration when compared with later pacifier introduction. Supplementation by cup or bottle led to a decrease in overall breast-feeding duration compared with infants receiving no supplementation. In mothers who had cesarean delivery, cup feeding was significantly associated with higher rates of exclusive breast-feeding and overall duration of breast-feeding compared with bottle-feeding.

Howard CR, Howard FM, Lanphear B. Randomized clinical trial of pacifier use and bottle-feeding or cupfeeding and their effect on breastfeeding. *Pediatrics.* 2003;111:511–518.

150. Which of the following statements about scoliosis is true?

A) The most common form is congenital.
B) The patient has a normal Adam's test.
C) Patients with abnormalities >5 degrees should be referred to an orthopedist.
D) Most curvature is to the right in the thoracic spine, causing the right shoulder to be higher than the left.
E) Syringomyelia is not associated with scoliosis.

Answer and Discussion

The answer is D. *Scoliosis* is defined as the presence of a lateral spinal curvature of 11 degrees or more. Its prevalence during adolescence is estimated to be between 2% and 3%. Curvatures >100 degrees can contribute to restrictive pulmonary disease; however, deviations of this magnitude are extremely rare. Scoliosis is classified as idiopathic (80% of cases), congenital (5%), neuromuscular (10%), or miscellaneous (5%). Severe scoliosis is more common in females. Idiopathic scoliosis is an inherited autosomal-dominant condition that occurs with variable penetrance. Most patients are asymptomatic; however, they may report backaches. The child should be examined with his or her back facing the examiner. The patient is asked to flex forward, and the scapula height is observed (known as the Adam's test). If scoliosis is present, asymmetry in scapular height is noted. In most cases, the right shoulder is higher than the left because of a convex curve of the spine to the right in the thoracic area and to the left in the lumbar area. Hip height and symmetry may also be affected. Radiographs should only be considered when a patient has a curve that might require treatment or could progress to a stage requiring treatment (usually 40 to 100 degrees). Radiographs should include posteroanterior and lateral views of the spine with the patient standing. Magnetic resonance imaging should be obtained in patients with an onset of scoliosis before 8 years of age, rapid curve progression of more than 1 degree/month, an unusual curve pattern such as left thoracic curve, neurologic deficit, or pain. Treatment depends on the degree of curvature. The primary goal of treating adolescent idiopathic scoliosis is preventing progression of the curve magnitude. Curves <10 to 15 degrees require no active treatment and can be monitored, unless the patient's bones are very immature and progression is likely. Moderate curves between 25 and 45 degrees in patients lacking skeletal maturity used to be treated with bracing, but this treatment has never been proven to prevent curve progression. Poor compliance with wearing a brace obviates any potential usefulness of the therapy. Much controversy surrounds brace indications, and trends since the mid-1980s have moved toward no bracing or bracing only the more significant curves (20 to 50 degrees). In more severe cases, braces (e.g., Milwaukee brace) or surgery may be indicated. Painful scoliosis may indicate underlying neurologic problems, such as syringomyelia or spinal cord lesion, and is less likely to be idiopathic.

Greiner KA. Adolescent idiopathic scoliosis: radiologic decision making. *Am Fam Physician.* 2002;65:1817–1822.

Mahoney MC. Screening for adolescent idiopathic scoliosis. *Am Fam Physician.* 2000;62:265.

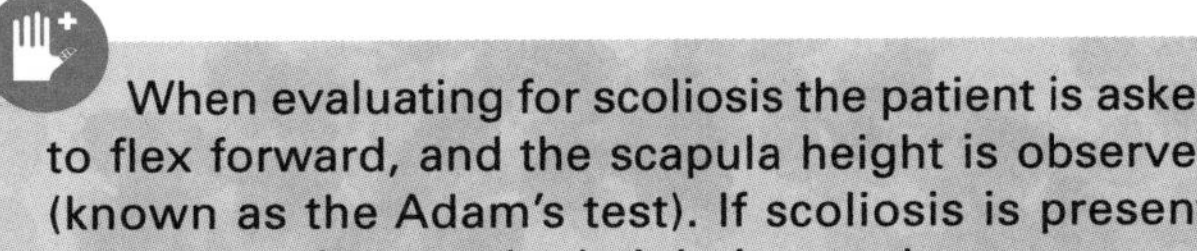

151. Which of the following organisms is most commonly associated with dental caries in children?

A) *Staphylococcus aureus*
B) *Bacteroides fragilis*
C) *Pasteurella multicida*
D) *Eikenella corrodens*
E) *Streptococcus mutans*

Answer and Discussion

The answer is E. The mutans streptococci (i.e., *Streptococcus mutans* and *Streptococcus sobrinus*) have been reported as the principal bacteria responsible for the initiation of dental caries in humans.

Douglass JM, AB Douglass. A guide to infant oral health. *Am Fam Physician.* 2004;70:2113–2120, 2121–2122.

152. A 3 year old is brought into the emergency room by her parents. The child has had a high fever, sore throat, and now has stridor. The child is sitting on a stretcher leaning forward with her neck extended. The most likely diagnosis is

A) strep throat
B) herpangina
C) meningitis
D) epiglottitis
E) herpes stomatitis

Answer and Discussion

The answer is D. Epiglottitis is a rapidly progressive and potentially fatal infection that causes swelling of the epiglottis and may lead to compromise of the child's airway. In the past it was most commonly caused by *H. influenzae.* The highest incidence occurs in children between 2 and 5 years of age. In recent years, the occurrence of epiglottitis has been reduced dramatically by the widespread use of the Hib vaccine. Symptoms include a sore throat, high fever, hoarseness, and dysphagia with drooling and stridor. Children affected usually lean forward and hyperextend the neck to open the compromised airway. Bacteremia is common. Because of the rapid course of the infection, the child should be immediately hospitalized and the airway secured. Inspection of the pharynx can precipitate a complete obstruction of the airway and should not be performed unless there are qualified personnel present who can simultaneously intubate the child during the inspection procedure if necessary. Lateral and anteroposterior soft tissue radiographs should be taken and can confirm the diagnosis. The characteristic "thumb sign" is noted on the lateral radiograph. In addition to securing an airway, parenteral antibiotics should be administered and the child monitored closely in an intensive care setting.

Rudolph CD, Rudolph AM, Hostetter MK, et al. *Rudolph's Pediatrics,* 21st ed. New York: McGraw-Hill; 2003:1276.

153. The most likely suspected cause for positional head deformities in children is
A) supine positioning
B) premature birth
C) genetic influences
D) child abuse
E) poorly developed sternocleidomastoid muscle

Answer and Discussion

The answer is A. In 1993, the American Society of Craniofacial Surgeons documented an increase in the incidence of posterior cranial deformities (occipital plagiocephaly) in infants who had no predisposing risk factors. The relationship of this increased incidence to the "Back to Sleep" campaign was proposed in 1996 and was supported by evidence of a rapid increase in positional head deformity without any significant change in the rate of synostotic plagiocephaly.

Behrman RE, Kliegman RM, Jenson HB. *Nelson Textbook of Pediatrics,* 17th ed. Philadelphia: WB Saunders; 2004:1992.

Argenta LC, David LR. Observations and thoughts on the changing constellation of cranial deformities. *J Craniofac Surg.* 1998;9:491–492.

154. Which of the following statements about Duchenne's muscular dystrophy is true?
A) Girls are affected more commonly than boys.
B) Early symptoms include mental retardation.
C) Distal muscles are affected before proximal muscles, and pseudohypertrophy of muscles can occur.
D) Creatinine kinase levels are low or undetectable.
E) Cardiomyopathy may result.

Answer and Discussion

The answer is E. Duchenne's muscular dystrophy is a genetically linked disorder (usually X-linked recessive) that usually affects boys between 2 and 5 years of age. The condition is caused by a mutation at the Xp21 locus, which results in the absence of dystrophin, a protein found inside the muscle cell membrane. It affects 1 in 3,600 live male births. Becker muscular dystrophy is the same fundamental disease with a genetic defect at the same locus but a milder clinical disease.

Many affected individuals have no family history of the disorder. Early manifestations include rapid fatigue on ambulation or running, clumsiness, waddling gait, and a distinctive pattern of climbing up on the legs from a sitting to standing position known as *Gowers' maneuver*. The proximal muscles are usually affected before the distal muscles; pseudohypertrophy of the gastrocnemius (seen in 90% of patients), triceps, and vastus lateralis may occur. Cardiomyopathy and mental retardation may occur in advanced cases, although intellectual impairment occurs in all patients. Diagnosis is usually accomplished by muscle biopsy, which shows degeneration of muscle fibers and proliferation in connective tissue. Electromyelography studies often distinguish between neuropathic and myopathic processes. Laboratory tests show a significantly elevated creatinine kinase level. Dystrophin analysis of muscle samples is also very helpful in the diagnosis; dystrophin is extremely low (<3%) or undetectable in patients with Duchenne's dystrophy. Mutation analysis of DNA isolated from peripheral blood leukocytes identifies deletions or duplications in the dystrophin gene in approximately 65% of patients and point mutations in approximately 25% of patients. Treatment involves physical therapy and braces. The prognosis is usually poor, with most patients dying of pneumonia before the age of 20 years.

Behrman RE, Kliegman RM, Jenson HB. *Nelson Textbook of Pediatrics,* 17th ed. Philadelphia: WB Saunders; 2004: 2060–2064.

155. Infant botulism is associated with
A) contaminated formula
B) ingestion of honey
C) baby food contamination
D) infant cereal

Answer and Discussion

The answer is B. Although the worldwide incidence of infant botulism is rare, the majority of cases are diagnosed in the United States. An infant can acquire botulism by ingesting Clostridium botulinum spores, which are found in soil or honey products. According to testing, up to 25% of honey products have been found to contain spores. A history of honey consumption is seen in 15% of the botulism cases reported to the CDC. As a result, honey should not be given to infants younger than 1 year.

Cox N, Hinkle R. Infant botulism. *Am Fam Physician.* 2002;65:1388–1392.

156. A 4-year-old girl is seen in the emergency room and is suspected of having meningitis. A positive Brudzinski's sign is noted. Which of the following describes a positive Brudzinski's sign?
A) The child dorsiflexes her feet when her head is flexed forward.
B) The child shows resistance when her legs are extended from a flexed position.
C) The child involuntarily flexes the hips with flexion of the neck.
D) The child involuntarily blinks with gentle tapping of the forehead.
E) The child shows extension-type posturing when her arms are flexed.

Answer and Discussion

The answer is C. Symptoms of bacterial meningitis include high-pitched cry, fever, anorexia, irritability, obtundation, lethargy, nausea, vomiting, neck stiffness, and a full fontanel (in infants).

In neonates, clinical clues to the presence of meningitis include temperature instability (hypothermia or hyperthermia), listlessness, high-pitched crying, fretfulness, lethargy, refusal to eat, a weak sucking response, irritability, vomiting, diarrhea, and respiratory distress. Because neonates usually do not have meningismus, a change in the child's affect or state of alertness is one of the most important signs. A bulging fontanel may occur late in the course of the disease in one-third of neonates. About 30% of neonates have seizures. Meningeal signs and fever are not always present in infants; however, meningeal signs are more reliable in older children and include the following:

- *Brudzinski's sign*: flexion of neck with the patient supine causes involuntary flexion at the hips
- *Kernig's sign*: attempts to extend the knees from a flexed position are met with resistance

The most common causes of bacterial meningitis include the following:

- *Neisseria meningitis* (meningococcal meningitis): usually seen in the first year of life
- *H. influenzae*: the Hib vaccination has dramatically reduced the incidence
- *Streptococcal pneumoniae*: the most common form of adult meningitis; immunization can help prevent this in children and adults
- *Group B or D streptococci and gram-negative organisms*: most common in neonates

Among U.S. children, there has been a substantial decrease in deaths and hospitalization from *H. influenzae* meningitis but not *S. pneumoniae* or *N. meningitidis* meningitis in the years after Hib conjugate vaccine licensure. This observation suggests that the declines in *H. influenzae* meningitis are due primarily to the use of Hib conjugate vaccines. The most common sequelae after meningitis include hearing loss and seizure disorders.

Beers MH, Porter RS, eds. *The Merck manual of diagnosis and therapy,* Merck Research Laboratories, 18th ed. Whitehouse Station, NJ: Merck & Co.; 2006:1860–1862.

157. Which of the following statements regarding colic is true?
A) Infants affected with colic are usually <10% on height and weight growth curves.
B) Symptoms are usually more severe at night.
C) The onset of colic occurs at birth.
D) Symptoms of colic last for approximately 1 year.
E) Colic has lasting negative effects on maternal mental health.

Answer and Discussion

The answer is B. Infant colic is characterized by excessive and inconsolable crying, hypertonicity, and wakefulness, mainly in the evening. An estimated 5% to 28% of infants have colic during the first few months of life. The widely cited "rule of threes" defines a colicky infant as one who is healthy and well-fed but cries for a total of at least 3 hours/day, more than 3 days in any 1 week. Onset is usually between the second and sixth weeks of life, and remission of symptoms generally occurs by 3 months of age. Although colic is thought to be a self-limited condition, it can be overwhelming to parents over a substantial number of weeks. One concern, moreover, is the potential lasting impact of colic on maternal mental health. Studies have shown that colic usually is a self-limited condition that does not result in long-lasting negative effects on maternal mental health.

Clifford TJ, Campbell MK, Speechley KN. Sequelae of infant colic. Evidence of transient infant distress and absence of lasting effects on maternal mental health. *Arch Pediatr Adolesc Med.* 2002;156:1183–1188.

158. A 7-year-old girl is seen in the emergency room. Her mother reports that she pulled the child up from the ground after the child fell. The child holds her left arm in a pronated position and refuses to use it. The most appropriate management is
A) radiographs to rule out fracture
B) firm stabilization of a flexed elbow and gentle pronation of the distal wrist
C) ice, anti-inflammatory medication, and rest
D) shoulder sling use for 2 weeks followed by physical therapy
E) orthopedic referral

Answer and Discussion

The answer is B. Nursemaid's elbow results when subluxation of the radial head occurs. The mechanism of injury occurs when a child's arm that is fully extended at the elbow is pulled. The injury usually affects children between 2 and 7 years of age. This injury occurs predominantly in toddlers, with a peak incidence between 2 and 3 years of age. Episodes in children younger than 6 months of age have been noted in the literature.

When examined, the child usually holds the forearm pronated and refuses to use it. Symptoms include pain and lack of movement of the affected extremity. Radiographs are unnecessary in most cases. Diagnosis is made by the history and usually involves a child that has been pulled abruptly from the ground with the elbow fully extended. To treat this, the physician places a finger on the head of the radius, and then firmly but gently supinates and flexes the distal arm until a pop is felt over the head of the radius. The child should then be observed for normal movement of the extremity. Parents should be counseled concerning the mechanism of injury to prevent recurrence. Usually there is sufficient development of the radial head to prevent subluxation of the annular ligament by age 4.

Behrman RE, Kliegman RM, Jenson HB. *Nelson Textbook of Pediatrics,* 17th ed. Philadelphia: WB Saunders; 2004: 2290–2291.

159. An 8 year old with a 5-year history of cystic fibrosis comes in to your office with increasing respiratory symptoms consisted with infection. Which of the following organisms is most likely involved?
A) *Streptococcus pneumoniae*
B) *Haemophilus influenzae*
C) *Mycoplasma pneumoniae*
D) *Pseudomonas aeruginosa*
E) *Moraxella catarrhalis*

Answer and Discussion

The answer is D. Early in the course of cystic fibrosis, *Staphylococcus aureus* is the pathogen most often isolated from the respiratory tract, but as the disease progresses, *Pseudomonas aeruginosa* is most frequently isolated. A mucoid variant of *Pseudomonas* is uniquely associated with CF.

Beers MH, Porter RS, eds. *The Merck manual of diagnosis and therapy,* Merck Research Laboratories, 18th ed. Whitehouse Station, NJ: Merck & Co.; 2006:2308–2313.

Early in the course of cystic fibrosis, *Staphylococcus aureus* is the pathogen most often isolated from the respiratory tract, but as the disease progresses, *Pseudomonas aeruginosa* is most frequently isolated.

160. Which of the following conditions may represent a contraindication for immunization?
A) Increase in body temperature to 38.5°C (101°F) after previous immunization
B) Allergy to neomycin
C) Recent mild upper respiratory infection in an otherwise healthy child
D) Current antibiotic use
E) Family history of seizure disorder

Answer and Discussion

The answer is B. The following conditions are in most cases contraindications to immunization practices:

- Previous severe reaction to the vaccine (anaphylaxis or persistent temperature >40.5°C [105°F])
- Allergy to eggs for influenza, yellow fever, and MMR vaccines
- Allergy to neomycin for MMR vaccine
- Immunocompromised patients or contacts for live attenuated vaccines such as MMR and varicella
- Chronic steroid therapy at moderate or high doses

Some health-care providers inappropriately consider certain circumstances to be contraindications to immunization. For example,

- Reaction to a previous DPaT dose that involved only soreness, redness, or swelling at the site of the injection or a temperature <105°F (40.5°C)
- Mild acute illness with low-grade fever in an otherwise healthy child
- Current antibiotic use
- Prematurity (however, hepatitis B immunization in most cases should be delayed)
- History of nonspecific allergies
- Allergies to duck meat or feathers
- Family history of convulsion in persons considered for pertussis or measles vaccination

Abramson JS, Baker CJ, Baltimore RS. *Red Book Online* 2003: Report of the Committee on Infectious Diseases, American Academy of Pediatrics. Accessed at http://aapredbook.aappublications.org on 6/21/06.

161. A 15-year-old presents with a painful area associated with the lower right leg. She is a volleyball player for her high school team. The pain is described as a dull, aching pain that has been present for the last several months. Recently it has become worse and is especially present at night. The most likely diagnosis is

A) osteosarcoma
B) shin splints
C) "growing pains"
D) Osgood-Schlatter's disease
E) stress fracture

Answer and Discussion

The answer is A. Patients with osteosarcoma typically present with dull, aching pain of several months' duration that may suddenly become more severe. The increase in pain severity may correlate with tumor penetration of cortical bone and irritation of the periosteum, or with pathologic fracture. Night pain is common and may awaken the patient from sleep. Chronic indolent night pain should not be dismissed as "growing pains," especially when it is unilateral. Patients frequently have a history of a minor injury, sprain, or muscle pull incurred while participating in a sport. The physical examination may reveal localized tenderness, restricted range of motion of the adjacent joint, a limp or muscle atrophy, and may confirm the presence of a mass, swelling, or deformity. Children frequently have referred pain; therefore, it is essential to perform a comprehensive examination of the joint above and below the area of complaint, as well as spinal and reflex examinations.

Wittig JC, Bickels J, Priebat D, et al. Osteosarcoma: a multidisciplinary approach to diagnosis and treatment. *Am Fam Physician.* 2002;65:1123–1132, 1135–1136.

162. A 2-year-old girl is brought in by her mother. The child has evidence of high fever for the past 9 days, conjunctivitis (without exudate), erythematous pharynx, and swollen lips that have fissured and cracked. The child is also noted to have a generalized erythematous, maculopapular rash associated with the hands and feet and early desquamation of the superficial layer of skin. The most likely diagnosis is

A) Lyme disease
B) scarlet fever
C) Kawasaki disease
D) Henoch-Schönlein purpura
E) herpangina

Answer and Discussion

The answer is C. Kawasaki disease, or *mucocutaneous lymph node syndrome*, is a disease of young children and is associated with an idiopathic vasculitis of the small- and medium-size blood vessels. The condition is characterized by prolonged high fever (>39°C [102°F]) that is often not relieved with antipyretics and the following:

- Conjunctival injection without exudate
- Erythematous mouth and pharynx with the development of strawberry tongue and red swollen lips, which may progress to fissuring and cracking by day 6 of disease
- Generalized maculopapular rash
- Induration of the hands and feet with erythema associated with the feet and hands, with desquamation during the second and third week of disease
- Unilateral cervical lymphadenopathy

For the diagnosis to be made, patients must have a fever for 5 days or more plus at least four of the aforementioned criteria. The rash appears within 3 days of the onset of fever and can vary in character. Frequently, the rash is scarlatiniform on the trunk and erythematous on the palms and soles with subsequent distal desquamation. Mucous membrane involvement is common and includes hyperemic bulbar conjunctiva; injected oropharynx; dry, cracked lips; and a strawberry tongue. Other symptoms include sterile pyuria, arthritis or arthralgias, aseptic meningitis, carditis with congestive heart failure, hydrops of the gallbladder, pericardial effusion, and arrhythmias. The physical examination may reveal nonsuppurative cervical lymphadenopathy (>1.5 cm in diameter). Coronary artery abnormalities develop in 20% to 25% of patients with Kawasaki disease. Cardiovascular complications are the major cause of short-term and long-term morbidity and mortality. Laboratory findings include leukocytosis with a bandemia, anemia, thrombocytosis, and an elevated erythrocyte sedimentation rate. Most affected individuals are younger than 5 years, with peak occurrence between 1 and 2 years of age. The condition is rare in children younger than 6 months and older than 12 years. Treatment involves supportive care and the use of aspirin and intravenous γ globulin. Steroid use is contraindicated and may increase the risk for coronary aneurysms. Antibiotics are unnecessary. Close follow-up with electrocardiography, chest radiographs, and echocardiography is necessary. Some patients may require coronary angiography to rule out aneurysm formation.

McKinnon HD, Howard T. Evaluating the febrile patient with a rash. *Am Fam Physician.* 2000;62:804–816.

163. An appropriate first step in the management of gastroesophageal reflux is

A) H_2-receptor antagonist
B) prokinetic agent

C) proton pump inhibitor
D) thickening feedings with dry rice cereal added to formula

Answer and Discussion

The answer is D. A common condition in infants is gastroesophageal reflux (GER), which causes parental anxiety resulting in numerous visits to the physician. The term GER implies a physiologic process in a healthy infant with no underlying systemic abnormalities. GER is a common condition involving regurgitation, or "spitting up," which is the passive return of gastric contents retrograde into the esophagus. The prevalence of GER peaks between 1 and 4 months of age, and usually resolves by 6 to 12 months of age. There is no gender predilection or definite peak age of onset beyond infancy. A more severe form is gastroesophageal reflux disease (GERD). GERD is a pathologic process in infants manifested by poor weight gain, signs of esophagitis, persistent respiratory symptoms, and changes in neurobehavior. After the first year of life, GERD is more resistant to complete resolution. Risk factors for GERD include: a history of esophageal atresia with repair; neurologic impairment and delay; hiatal hernia; bronchopulmonary dysplasia; asthma; and chronic cough. GERD is also associated with pulmonary aspiration, chronic bronchitis, and bronchiectasis. Conservative treatment for mild symptoms of GER involves thickened feedings and positional changes in infants, and dietary modification in children. Healthy infants who regurgitate without signs of GERD may be managed by thickening feedings with dry rice cereal added to formula. Thickened feeding reduces regurgitation and fussiness, and increases daily caloric intake. Smaller, more frequent feedings are recommended in older infants and children. The medications used for GERD include H_2-receptor antagonists, prokinetic agents, and proton pump inhibitors such as omeprazole (Prilosec) or lansoprazole (Prevacid) for patients with persistent esophagitis. Lansoprazole is also available in a liquid alkaline form for use in the childhood population.

Tsou VM, Bishop PR. Gastroesophageal reflux in children. *Otolaryngol Clin North Am.* 1998;31:419–434.

Jung AD. Gastroesophageal reflux in infants and children. *Am Fam Physician.* 2001;64:1853–1860.

164. The primary bacteria associated with the development of dental caries is
A) *Streptococcus mutans*
B) *Staphylococcus aureus*
C) *Streptococcus pneumoniae*
D) *Enterobacter* species
E) *Streptococcus viridans*

Answer and Discussion

The answer is A. Dental caries occur when the tooth's surface is susceptible to injury, bacteria are present, and there is a food source from which the bacteria can live and reproduce. The primary bacteria is *S. mutans*, which can manufacture lactic acid, damaging the tooth's protective covering. Excessive and repeated consumption of dietary carbohydrates places the patient at risk for the development of dental caries. Symptoms may include sensitivity to hot and cold fluids or foods, persistent pain, or visible caries formation. Diagnosis is usually made by probing the dental pits with a sharp dental instrument and detecting softened enamel. Radiographs may also show radiolucent areas. Treatment involves removal of the damaged enamel and replacement with restorative material. Prophylaxis involves proper brushing and flossing technique two times per day, combined with the use of fluoride and regular dental checkups to remove plaque buildup.

Douglass JM, AB Douglass. A guide to infant oral health. *Am Fam Physician.* 2004;70:2113–2120, 2121–2122.

165. A 1 week old is diagnosed with breast milk jaundice. You should instruct the mother to
A) maintain breast pumping and switch the child to formula and monitor bilirubin levels
B) stop breast-feeding and start phototherapy
C) continue breast-feeding and start phototherapy
D) schedule an exchange transfusion
E) avoid any future breast-feeding and switch to formula-feeding

Answer and Discussion

The answer is A. Breast milk jaundice usually peaks in the 6th to 14th days of life. This late-onset jaundice may develop in up to one-third of healthy breastfed infants. Total serum bilirubin levels vary from 12 to 20 mg/dL (340 μmol/L) and are not considered pathologic. The underlying cause of breast milk jaundice is not entirely known. Substances in maternal milk, such as β-glucuronidases, and nonesterified fatty acids may inhibit normal bilirubin metabolism. The bilirubin level usually decreases continually after the infant is 2 weeks old, but it may remain persistently elevated for 1 to 3 months. If the diagnosis of breast milk jaundice is in doubt or the total serum bilirubin level becomes markedly elevated, breastfeeding may be temporarily interrupted, although the mother should continue to express breast milk to maintain production. With formula substitution, the total serum bilirubin level should decline rapidly over 48 hours [at a rate of 3 mg/dL (51 μmol/L)/day], confirming the diagnosis. Breast-feeding may then be resumed.

Dennery PA, Seidman DS, Stevenson DK. Neonatal hyperbilirubinemia. *N Engl J Med.* 2001;344:581–590.

Gartner LM, Herschel M. Jaundice and breastfeeding. *Pediatr Clin North Am.* 2001;48:389–399.

166. A 15-year-old female dancer presents with pain, swelling, and a "give away" sensation in her knee. The patient reports that going up and down stairs aggravates the pain. Physical examination shows an increased Q angle. The most likely diagnosis is
A) anterior cruciate ligament rupture
B) Osgood-Schlatter disease
C) patellofemoral syndrome
D) tibial plateau fracture
E) iliotibial band syndrome

Answer and Discussion

The answer is C. Patellofemoral syndrome is a common overuse injury associated with the anterior knee. It commonly affects young women. In most cases, the syndrome is associated with poor conditioning and the initiation of a new activity, particularly running, but also other activities including dancing, gymnastics, and figure skating. Symptoms include pain, swelling, and a "give way" sensation associated with the knee. Ascending or descending hills or stairs and repeated squatting or weight bearing on a semi-flexed knee tend to aggravate symptoms. The contributing factor is weakness of the quadriceps muscles and particularly the vastus medialis. The condition is also associated with an increased Q angle (the angle formed from a line down the femur and a line formed by the patellar tendon) and a high-riding patella (patella alta). Radiographs (sunrise view) of the knees may show patellofemoral malalignment but are not necessary for the diagnosis. Treatment involves rest, ice, nonsteroidal anti-inflammatory agents, and quadriceps-strengthening exercises. Elastic neoprene knee sleeves worn during activities can help keep the patella in proper alignment and help prevent symptoms.

Behrman RE, Kliegman RM, Jenson HB. *Nelson Textbook of Pediatrics*, 17th ed. Philadelphia: WB Saunders; 2004:2311.

167. Of the following, the drug of choice for a pertussis infection is
A) penicillin
B) tetracycline
C) ciprofloxacin
D) chloramphenicol
E) erythromycin

Answer and Discussion

The answer is E. Pertussis is a potentially serious illness in children younger than 2 years. Mortality is about 1% to 2% in children younger than 1 year of age (highest in the first month of life). Most deaths are caused by bronchopneumonia and cerebral complications. Pertussis is troublesome but rarely serious in older children and adults, except in the elderly. Patients should be quarantined, particularly from susceptible infants, for at least 1 month from disease onset or until symptoms have subsided. Hospitalization is recommended for seriously ill infants to assess progression of disease and prevent and treat complications. Antibiotics given in the catarrhal stage may ameliorate the disease. After paroxysms are established, antibiotics usually have no discernible effect but are recommended to limit spread. The drug of choice is a macrolide antibiotic (e.g., erythromycin or azithromycin). Antibiotics should also be used for any bacterial complications such as bronchopneumonia and otitis media.

Beers MH, Porter RS, eds. *The Merck manual of diagnosis and therapy*, Merck Research Laboratories, 18th ed. Whitehouse Station, NJ: Merck & Co.; 2006:1465–1466.

168. Which of the following statements about isotretinoin (Accutane) is true?
A) It is recommended in the treatment of mild to moderate acne.
B) It has potential detrimental effects on the kidney.
C) It has beneficial effects on cholesterol levels.
D) Documentation of a negative pregnancy test is mandatory before its use in women.
E) A common side effect is tinnitus.

Answer and Discussion

The answer is D. Isotretinoin (Accutane) is used for moderate to severe nodulocystic acne unresponsive to conventional therapy. Therapy usually lasts 16 to 20 weeks followed by an 8-week drug vacation before the administration of the next course. It is absolutely contraindicated in pregnancy, and 2 to 3 contraceptive methods should be instituted before its administration. In addition, female patients should have a documented negative pregnancy test before isotretinoin (Accutane) administration. Side effects include xerosis, cheilitis, epistaxis, myalgias, and arthralgias. The effects of the drug may also alter the liver function test, blood counts, blood glucose, uric acid, and cholesterol and triglyceride levels, all of which may require frequent monitoring. There has been an association with pseudotumor cerebri development in patients who use isotretinoin. The administration is required to be monitored by certified provider.

Behrman RE, Kliegman RM, Jenson HB. *Nelson Textbook of Pediatrics*, 17th ed. Philadelphia: WB Saunders; 2004:2311.

The effects of isotretinoin (Accutane) may also alter the liver function test, blood counts, blood glucose, uric acid, and cholesterol and triglyceride levels, all of which may require frequent monitoring.

169. Which of the following anti-seizure medications is associated with weight loss?
A) Felbamate (Felbatol)
B) Gabapentin (Neurontin)
C) Lamotrigine (Lamictal)
D) Topiramate (Topamax)
E) Levetiracetam (Keppra)

Answer and Discussion

The answer is D. Several new medications for the treatment of epilepsy have become available in the recent past. The new drugs include: felbamate (Felbatol), gabapentin (Neurontin), lamotrigine (Lamictal), topiramate (Topamax), tiagabine (Gabitril), levetiracetam (Keppra), and zonisamide (Zonegran). Comparisons among these new drugs are difficult to make. In general, they are similar to each other in terms of efficacy. Therefore, the choice of a specific agent is often based on other factors, including side effect profile. All anti-epilepsy drugs are central nervous system depressants and are associated with sedation, dizziness, ataxia, cognitive and visual disturbances, and gastrointestinal symptoms. These side effects are predictable, benign, and dose- or rate-dependent. In most instances, the new anti-epileptic drugs are better tolerated than the older medications. However, significant differences exist among the drugs with regard to side effects, potential toxicity, and pharmacokinetics. Felbamate has a broad spectrum of activity in both partial and generalized seizures, but rare reports of fatal aplastic anemia and hepatic failure limit its use to patients for whom no other treatment alternative exists. Gabapentin is characterized by excellent tolerability. It is not protein bound, has no appreciable hepatic metabolism, and is excreted by the kidneys. Thus, gabapentin is appropriate for use in patients who require relatively quick titration, who have multiple drug intolerances, or who are taking multiple drugs with the potential for interaction, including the elderly. Lamotrigine has a broad spectrum of activity against multiple seizure types. Sedation is notably rare in monotherapy, and it even has an "alerting" response in some patients. One idiosyncratic side effect of lamotrigine, which is similar to effects of older antiepileptic drugs, is a rash. Infrequently the rash can be serious and may progress to Stevens-Johnson syndrome, which can be life-threatening. Rashes are more common in children when lamotrigine is taken in association with valproate sodium (Depakote) and with rapid dose adjustment. Topiramate also has a broad spectrum of activity. Weight loss has been noted, which can be a desirable side effect. The development of nephrolithiasis, which is rare, and paresthesias, which is common, likely reflects carbonic anhydrase inhibition. Tiagabine has no significant systemic or serious idiosyncratic adverse side effects, but it does have a relatively narrow spectrum of activity and must be adjusted slowly. One limitation of lamotrigine, topiramate, and tiagabine is that they need to be initiated at a low dosage and slowly increased in dosage over several weeks. Levetiracetam is unique among the new antiepileptic drugs because it is effective starting with the initial dose. It also has a mechanism of action that appears to be different from that of other antiepileptic drugs and, like gabapentin, its tolerability and pharmacokinetics are very acceptable. Levetiracetam is not metabolized by the liver (more than 60% is renally excreted unchanged), and <10% is protein bound. As a result, drug interactions are minimal.

Benbadis SR, Tatum WO IV. Advances in the treatment of epilepsy. *Am Fam Physician.* 2001;64:91–98, 105–106.

170. Which of the following statements about enuresis in children is true?

A) Primary enuresis is defined as the onset of bedwetting after a 6-month period of dryness.
B) Bed-wetting usually occurs in stage 1 of NREM sleep.
C) Most outgrow the condition before 12 years of age.
D) There is no approved treatment for enuresis.
E) Diagnosis should consist of cystoscopy to rule out structural causes.

Answer and Discussion

The answer is C. Nocturnal enuresis beyond 5 years of age in girls and 6 years of age in boys is a relatively common problem. *Primary enuresis* is defined as a patient who has never had an extended period of dryness since birth. *Secondary enuresis* is the onset of bed-wetting after 6 months of dryness. The condition is more common in young boys and firstborn children, and there is usually a positive family history. Bed-wetting usually occurs during the first REM sleep cycle, when sleep is relatively light. It may also occur in other stages, except for stage 1. The family and patient should be reassured that this is a common problem and is not associated with any underlying disorder. Diagnostic tests are usually limited to urinalysis to rule out infection. The bladder is usually a normal structural size but is functionally small. The physician should keep in mind that primary nocturnal enuresis is a diagnosis of exclusion, and all other causes of bed-wetting must be ruled out. Causes of secondary enuresis include neurogenic bladder and associated spinal cord abnormalities, urinary tract infections, and the presence of posterior urethral valves in boys or an ectopic ureter in girls. Posterior urethral valves cause significant voiding symptoms such as straining to void and diminished urinary stream. An ectopic ureter causes constant wetting. Treatment consists of observation. In older children, imipramine (Tofranil), oxybutynin (Ditropan), or nasal desmopressin (DDAVP) can be used. Other forms of treatment for older children include bell-and-pad conditioning. Most patients outgrow the condition before 12 years of age. Daytime enuresis may indicate underlying pathology or voiding dysfunction and requires further evaluation.

Thiedke CC. Nocturnal enuresis. *Am Fam Physician.* 2003;67:1499–1506, 1509–1510.

171. The majority of cases of occult bacteremia are caused by

A) *Streptococcus pneumoniae*
B) *Neisseria meningitides*
C) *Staphylococcus aureus*
D) *Haemophilus influenzae* type b (Hib)
E) *Salmonella*

Answer and Discussion

The answer is A. Occult bacteremia is caused by *Streptococcus pneumoniae* in 65% to 75% of cases, and the remainder by other bacteria, including *Neisseria meningitidis, Salmonella* spp., and *Staphylococcus aureus*. The incidence of bacteremia due to *Haemophilus influenzae* type b (Hib) has decreased substantially where Hib conjugate vaccine is part of routine childhood immunization. Occult bacteremia is detected in about 4% to 17% of febrile infants between 1 and 24 months of age. The majority of cases occur in infants between 6 and 24 months of age. Children who look well enough to be managed as outpatients but who later are found to be bacteremic usually are younger than 24 months of age. Incidence does not vary with sex or race.

Beers MH, Porter RS, eds. *The Merck manual of diagnosis and therapy,* Merck Research Laboratories, 18th ed. Whitehouse Station, NJ: Merck & Co.; 2006:1392–1393.

172. Substances that are contraindicated during breast-feeding include all of the following *except*

A) alcohol
B) tetracycline
C) penicillin
D) ciprofloxacin
E) bromocriptine

Answer and Discussion

The answer is C. Certain medications are contraindicated during breast-feeding, including quinolone antibiotics, tetracycline, chloramphenicol, bromocriptine, cyclosporine, cyclophosphamide, doxorubicin, methotrexate, lithium, and ergotamine. Other drugs that have relative contraindications include metronidazole, sulfonamides, salicylates, phenobarbital, other psychotropic medication, and antihistamines. Caffeine in large amounts should also be avoided. In addition, recreational drugs (e.g., alcohol, cocaine, marijuana) should be avoided.

Beers MH, Porter RS, eds. *The Merck manual of diagnosis and therapy,* Merck Research Laboratories, 18th ed. Whitehouse Station, NJ: Merck & Co.; 2006:2297.

173. Which of the following is not usually associated with autism?

A) Normal intelligence quotients (IQs)
B) Echolalia
C) Repetitive movements
D) Self-injury behaviors
E) Seizures

Answer and Discussion

The answer is A. The impairments noted in autistic persons are varied and result in good skills in some areas and poor skills in others. Echolalia, the involuntary repetition of a word or a sentence just spoken by another person, is a common feature of language impairment that, when present, may cause language skills to appear better than they really are. There may also be deficiencies in symbolic thinking, stereotypic behaviors (e.g., repetitive nonproductive movements of hands and fingers, rocking, meaningless vocalizations), self-stimulation, self-injury behaviors, and seizures. Mental retardation is not a diagnostic criterion, but it is frequently present in the moderate to severe range.

Prater CD, Zylstra RG. Autism: a medical primer. *Am Fam Physician.* 2002;66:1667–1674, 1680.

174. Which of the following statements about otitis media is true?

A) The most common organisms causing otitis media in newborns are *Streptococcus pneumoniae, Haemophilus influenzae* and *Moraxella catarrhalis.*
B) Ten percent of otitis media cases with *H. influenzae* as the causative organism are resistant to amoxicillin.
C) Close to 100% of otitis media cases with *M. catarrhalis* as the causative organism are resistant to amoxicillin.
D) The treatment of otitis media should include the use of antibiotics and an antihistamine/decongestant preparation.
E) Analgesic pain medication is rarely needed in the treatment of otitis media.

Answer and Discussion

The answer is C. Otitis media is one of the most frequent reasons parents bring their children to the physician. The condition occurs more frequently in the winter months and affects bottle-fed infants (especially those put to bed with bottles) more frequently than other infants; it also affects boys more often than girls, as well as premature infants or those enrolled in daycare more often than other infants. Infants with cleft palate or Down syndrome are also at increased risk. The most common etiologic agents for otitis media are as follows:

- *Streptococcus pneumoniae*
- *Moraxella (Branhamella) catarrhalis*
- *Non-typeable H. influenzae*

Newborns are more likely to be affected with *E. coli* and *S. aureus*. Children older than 5 years are less frequently affected by *Klebsiella pneumoniae* and *Bacteroides* rarely cause otitis media. Viruses, including RSV, rhinovirus, and adenovirus, can also cause otitis media and are often complicated with secondary bacterial organisms.

The major factor that contributes to otitis media is eustachian tube dysfunction and anatomic immaturity, which allows fluid and bacteria to reflux into the middle ear. Symptoms of otitis media include pain, fever, and occasionally purulent drainage if the tympanic membrane has ruptured. Younger children may be fussy, irritable, and show decreased appetite or sleep disturbances. Pulling at the ears may also be a sign of otitis media. Physical examination usually shows a bulging erythematous tympanic membrane with a loss of tympanic landmarks and lack of mobility with pneumatoscopy. Treatment involves the use of analgesics and first-line antibiotics, including amoxicillin, trimethoprim–sulfamethoxazole, and erythromycin. Amoxicillin remains the antibiotic of first choice, although a higher dosage (80 mg/kg/day) may be indicated to ensure eradication of resistant *S. pneumoniae*. Oral cefuroxime or amoxicillin-clavulanate and intramuscular ceftriaxone are suggested second-line choices for treatment failure.

Thirty percent to 60% of *S. pneumoniae* and close to 100% of *M. catarrhalis* strains are β-lactamase producers and are resistant to amoxicillin. Resistance may vary according to locality. If β-lactamase–producing infections are suspected, amoxicillin–clavulanate, erythromycin, trimethoprim–sulfamethoxazole, or cephalosporins are recommended. The use of antihistamines and decongestants has little or no benefit in the treatment of otitis media.

Pichichero ME. Acute otitis media: Part II. Treatment in an era of increasing antibiotic resistance. *Am Fam Physician* 2000; 61:2410–2416.

175. According to the American Academy of Pediatrics, at what age should a child begin formal swimming lessons?

A) After 1 year of age
B) After 2 years of age
C) After 3 years of age
D) After 4 years of age
E) After 5 years of age

Answer and Discussion

The answer is D. Children who are near water are at higher risk of drowning. The American Academy of Pediatrics (AAP) has updated its policy about swimming programs for infants and toddlers. While some aquatic programs may include water safety instructions for parents and children, these programs are clearly not designed to teach children how to swim. In fact, swimming skills are not the same as water safety skills, and parents should be clear about what is developmentally possible in different age groups. Rudimentary swimming movements (e.g., the dog paddle) are possible in a 1-year-old child, but traditional swimming strokes do not occur until a child is about 5 years of age. Children who have not yet reached their fourth birthday will not have the neuromuscular capability to adequately learn swimming skills. Taking swimming lessons at an earlier age does not mean that the child will master water skills earlier or be more proficient than children who take such lessons later. Training programs have been shown to improve water survival skills, but safety training has not been shown to decrease the risk of drowning. In fact, programs that emphasize making the child stop fearing water may, in fact, encourage children to enter the water without supervision. Therefore, the AAP recommends that children do not begin formal swimming lessons until after they are 4 years of age. Parents should not be encouraged to believe that a child's participation in an aquatic program will decrease the risk of drowning, and they should remain within arm's reach or able to touch the swimmer at all times (also known as *touch supervision*).

American Academy of Pediatrics Committee on Sports Medicine and Fitness and Committee on Injury and Poison Prevention. Swimming programs for infants and toddlers. *Pediatrics.* 2000;105:868–870.

176. The most common cause of septic joint in an immigrant 3-year-old boy with no prior immunizations is

A) *Neisseria gonorrhea*
B) *Pasteurella multocida*
C) *Mycoplasma pneumoniae*
D) *Streptococcus pneumoniae*
E) *Haemophilus influenzae*

Answer and Discussion

The answer is E. Bacterial infections are usually responsible for septic joints. In children (between 2 and 5 years of age), the most common pathogen associated with osteomyelitis is *Staphylococcus aureus*; other causes include *Staphylococcus*, *Streptococcus*, and gram-negative bacteria. In sexually active teenagers and young adults *Neisseria gonorrhea* is a common cause. Additionally, *Staphylococcus*, *group A streptococcus*, and *Streptococcus pneumoniae* are causes. Other agents include viruses, mycobacteria, or fungi. *H. influenzae* type B was most common before universal vaccination and may affect unimmunized immigrants. Salmonella and *S. aureus* are the two most common causes of osteomyelitis in children with sickle cell anemia. Patients with rheumatoid arthritis are at particular risk for septic joints. In adults, the most common joint affected is the knee, whereas, in children, the hip and knee are the most commonly affected. Typically, the child with a septic joint will have pain with any range of motion of the joint, whereas patients with trauma or toxic synovitis will allow some range of motion of the joint. Laboratory tests show an elevated white blood cell count and elevated sedimentation rate. Culture and Gram's stain of the joint fluid should be performed. Blood cultures are positive in 30% to 40%. Treatment involves surgical débridement as soon as possible if a bacterial source is suspected.

Behrman RE, Kliegman RM, Jenson HB. *Nelson Textbook of Pediatrics,* 17th ed. Philadelphia: WB Saunders; 2004:2298.

In sexually active teenagers and young adults *Neiserria gonorrhea* is a common cause of septic joints.

177. Which of the following sounds is associated with a positive Ortolani sign when assessing for developmental dysplasia of the hip (DDH)?
A) "Click"
B) "Clunk"
C) "Pop"
D) "Grinding"

Answer and Discussion

The answer is B. The American Academy of Pediatrics (AAP) has issued a clinical practice guideline about early detection of developmental dysplasia of the hip (DDH). It is important to remember that no physical examination finding is pathognomonic for DDH. The neonate should have a normal range of motion of abduction to 75 degrees and adduction to 30 degrees. A physical assessment should include evaluation for asymmetry as well as assessing Ortolani and Barlow signs. The Ortolani maneuver is performed with the infant supine and the hip flexed to 90 degrees. The leg is held in neutral rotation with the physician's index and middle finger along the greater trochanter and the thumb along the inner thigh. The hip is abducted as the leg is lifted anteriorly. A "clunk" (not a high-pitched click) indicates a positive Ortolani sign and occurs as the dislocated femoral head is reduced into the acetabulum. A positive Barlow sign occurs when there is a palpable "clunk" (or movement) of the femoral head being dislocated. Again, the infant has the hip flexed to 90 degrees; the leg is adducted while posterior pressure on the knee is applied to detect an unstable hip dislocating. High-pitched clicks are common with extension and flexion and are insignificant. With the infant prone, the physician should check for limb length discrepancy or asymmetric gluteal or thigh folds. In an older infant (about 3 months of age), limited abduction of the hip is a reliable sign of DDH. Again, asymmetry should be sought. Physical examination screening for DDH should occur at 2 to 4 days and at each well-child visit (1, 2, 4, 6, 9, and 12 months) until the child is 1 year old or is reliably able to walk.

Committee on Quality Improvement, Subcommittee on Developmental Dysplasia of the Hip. Clinical practice guideline: early detection of developmental dysplasia of the hip. *Pediatrics.* 2000;105:896–905.

178. Erythema infectiosum (fifth disease) is caused by
A) parvovirus
B) adenovirus
C) rhinovirus
D) paramyxovirus
E) herpes virus

Answer and Discussion

The answer is A. Parvovirus B19 is the causative agent responsible for erythema infectiosum, or fifth disease. The incubation period is 6 to 14 days. Outbreaks frequently occur at day schools, elementary schools, or junior high schools, and they frequently occur in the spring. Symptoms include a distinctive facial rash that has a "slapped-cheek" appearance, fever, arthralgias, and fatigue. Within 2 days, the facial rash gives rise to a generalized lace-like macular rash that involves the trunk. It has become increasingly clear over the past several years that parvovirus B19 causes arthritis and arthralgias in adults and children. Although parvovirus infections in adults are most commonly asymptomatic, an estimated 50% to 60% of women with symptomatic disease manifest arthropathy. Men appear to be affected much less frequently. Blood cell counts during the illness show leukopenia, lymphopenia, and thrombocytopenia with decreased reticulocytes. Because parvovirus B19 infects erythroid progenitor cells in the bone marrow and causes temporary cessation of red blood cell production, patients who have underlying hematologic abnormalities (and thus depend on a high rate of erythropoiesis) are prone to cessation of red blood cell production if they become infected. This can result in a transient aplastic crisis, which may occur in persons with chronic hemolytic anemia and conditions of bone marrow stress. Thus, patients with sickle cell anemia, thalassemia, acute hemorrhage, and iron deficiency anemia are at risk. The diagnosis of erythema infectiosum is made clinically, and laboratory studies are not needed under normal circumstances. Serologic tests are usually relied on for the diagnosis of parvovirus B19 infection in patients with transient aplastic crisis or arthropathy; a positive parvovirus B19–specific IgM antibody or a significant rise in parvovirus B19–specific IgG titer is indicative of an acute or recent infection. Exposure during pregnancy can lead to fetal hydrops, spontaneous abortion, and fetal death. Supportive care during an attack of fifth disease is usually adequate, and the illness is self-limited. The risk of respiratory transmission is decreased significantly when the rash starts to fade. Children with erythema infectiosum are not infectious and can attend school and daycare.

Young NS, Brown KE. Parvovirus B19. *N Engl J Med.* 2004;350:586–597.

179. When administering varicella vaccine, it is important to note that simultaneous administration of what other vaccine can diminish the effectiveness of the varicella vaccine?
A) Measles, mumps, rubella (MMR) vaccine
B) Hepatitis B vaccine
C) *Haemophilus influenzae* vaccine
D) Pneumococcal vaccine
E) Influenza vaccine

Answer and Discussion

The answer is A. Varicella is a highly contagious illness manifested by fever and a 3- to 5-day rash. Experts recommend live attenuated varicella zoster vaccine for healthy susceptible children (12 months and older), adolescents, and adults because of its high efficacy rate. Widespread use of the varicella vaccine has substantially decreased the rates of chickenpox and vaccine-related complications. Vaccinated persons develop milder symptoms with fewer skin lesions, which are more likely to be macular than vesicular. Residual scarring also is less common. However, atypical cases are making the diagnosis of varicella more difficult. Recent varicella exposure is the most useful clinical diagnostic hint because demonstration of viral antigen in skin scrapings or vesicular fluid is rarely available to the physician. It also is important to exclude similarly presenting conditions and to note that breakthrough varicella infection can be communicated to susceptible persons. Vaccination may be less effective in children younger than 15 months. However, because children 12 to 15 months of age are at risk and may not return at a later age for vaccination, the present recommendation remains to vaccinate at 12 months of age. Studies have found that children given a varicella vaccine within 30 days or less of receiving an MMR vaccine are at an increased risk of developing breakthrough varicella infection. Therefore, guidelines suggest separating the MMR and varicella zoster vaccines by 28 days if not given simultaneously.

Vãzquez M. Varicella infections and varicella vaccine in the 21st century. *Pediatr Infect Dis J.* 2004;23:871–872.

180. Transposition of the great vessels is associated with which of the following?
A) An aorta that arises from the left atrium
B) Cyanosis at birth with an intact ventricular septum
C) A pulmonary vein that empties into the right ventricle
D) A pulmonary artery that arises from the right ventricle
E) A superior vena cava that empties directly into the pulmonary circulation

Answer and Discussion

The answer is B. Transposition of the great vessels is a cause of cyanotic heart disease. Male term infants are more commonly affected than are females, as are infants of diabetic mothers. The condition is associated with an aorta that arises from the right ventricle and a pulmonary artery that arises from the left ventricle. There are basically two types:

- Transposition with an intact septum
- Transposition with a ventricular septal defect

Because the systemic blood must mix with the pulmonary circulation, an intact ventricular septum leads to immediate cyanosis and death if not treated. In many cases, the ductus arteriosus remains open for several days, and cyanosis does not develop until it has fully closed. In most cases, congestive heart failure develops and can lead to death. Retardation of growth and development is common. Many (but not all) children will have an associated systolic murmur, and some show significant cyanosis at the time of birth. Chest radiographs may be normal but can show mild cardiomegaly with an egg-shaped heart with a narrow superior mediastinum and increased pulmonary vascular markings ("egg on a string"). Cardiac catheterization is used for the diagnosis, and surgery is performed to return the normal anatomic circulation or to place an intra-atrial shunt to redirect blood flow to the appropriate circulation.

Behrman RE, Kliegman RM, Jenson HB. *Nelson Textbook of Pediatrics*, 17th ed. Philadelphia: WB Saunders; 2004: 1535–1538.

181. The most common organism isolated in periorbital cellulitis in vaccinated children in the absence of trauma is
A) *Haemophilus influenzae*
B) *Streptococcus pneumoniae*
C) *Moraxella catarrhalis*
D) *Staphylococcus aureus*
E) *Pseudomonas aeruginosa*

Answer and Discussion

The answer is B. Periorbital and orbital cellulitis may be caused by trauma (e.g., a wound, an insect bite), an associated infection (e.g., sinusitis), or seeding from bacteremia. Before widespread immunization, *Haemophilus influenzae* type b was the most common cause secondary to bacteremia (about 80% of cases) and remains so in nonimmunized populations. *Streptococcus pneumoniae* accounted for most of the remaining 20%. *S. pneumoniae* is the most likely agent in *Haemophilus influenzae* type b-vaccinated patients when sinusitis is present. The most common pathogens associated with external foci (trauma) are *Staphylococcus aureus* and *Streptococcus pyogenes,* but these are seldom isolated from the blood. In general, a bacterial pathogen is isolated from the blood in <33% of patients with periorbital cellulitis.

Beers MH, Porter RS, eds. *The Merck manual of diagnosis and therapy,* Merck Research Laboratories, 18th ed. Whitehouse Station, NJ: Merck & Co.; 2006:926–927.

182. A 4-year-old boy is noted to have impaired language development, compulsive repetitive behavior, impaired intelligence, and a preoccupation with inanimate objects. The most likely diagnosis is
A) conductive hearing loss
B) attention-deficit disorder
C) autism
D) manic–depressive disorder
E) dyslexia

Answer and Discussion

The answer is C. *Autism* is a condition that is associated with abnormal social relationships, impaired language development and understanding, compulsive repetitive behavior with a resistance to change, and impaired intelligence; most affected individuals are in the mentally retarded range. The condition affects boys more frequently than girls and, in most cases, manifests itself before 1 year of age. Symptoms include a lack of attachment; preoccupation with inanimate objects; avoidance of eye contact; resistance to change; outbursts of temper; repetitive, often self-destructive acts; delayed speech development or total muteness; and seizures in severely impaired children. Neurologic examination fails to show focal findings. CT scans of the head may show enlargement of the ventricles, and EEG studies are usually unremarkable. Most children are brought to their doctors because of poor speech development. Treatment involves psychotherapy; however, results have been limited with regard to improving the child's deficiencies and behavior. Most children require special schooling. Mainstream treatment consists of early, intensive education for parents, focusing on behavior and communication disorders. A highly structured environment with intensive individual instruction should be encouraged. Laboratory, metabolic, or genetic tests and diagnostic imaging provide little useful information, although an EEG is indicated in children in whom epilepsy is suspected. No specific pharmacologic therapies are available, but many patients do not require medication. When needed, medication is generally used for a particular manifestation or constellation of symptoms. Families may benefit from ongoing counseling and support, and specific instructions for dealing with tantrums and destructive behavior. Parents should be cautioned about costly and often questionable dietary, medical, and other unconventional therapies.

Prater CD, Zylstra RG. Autism: a medical primer. *Am Fam Physician.* 2002;66:1667–1674, 1680.

183. An 18-year-old woman presents with swelling, warmth, and spreading redness at the upper part of her ear, where she recently underwent an ear piercing. Appropriate antibiotic coverage includes

A) cephalexin
B) ciprofloxacin
C) azithromycin
D) penicillin
E) tetracycline

Answer and Discussion

The answer is B. The popularity of body piercing at sites other than the earlobe has grown since the mid-1990s. The tongue, lips, nose, eyebrows, nipples, navel, and genitals are frequent areas used for piercing. Complications include local and systemic infections, poor cosmetic results, and foreign body rejection. Swelling and damage to the dentition are common problems after tongue piercing. Minor infections, allergic contact dermatitis, keloid formation, and traumatic tearing may occur after piercing of the earlobe. "High" ear piercing through the ear cartilage is associated with more serious infections and disfigurement. Fluoroquinolone antibiotics are advised for treatment of auricular perichondritis because of their antipseudomonal activity. Navel, nipple, and genital piercings often have prolonged healing times.

Meltzer DI. Complications of body piercing. *Am Fam Physician.* 2005;72:2029–2034, 2035–2036.

184. Which of the following is NOT a contraindication for diphtheria-pertussis-tetanus (DPT) immunization?

A) Fever of 105°F (40.4°C) or higher within 48 hours after previous DPT dose
B) Current mild viral infection
C) Continuous crying for more than 3 hours after previous DPT dose
D) Convulsions within 3 days of a previous DPT dose
E) Progressive neurologic disorder that is not diagnosed

Answer and Discussion

The answer is B. Several conditions are a contraindication to the DTaP immunization:

- Fever of 105°F (40.4°C) or higher within 48 hours after previous dose
- Previous anaphylaxis to the vaccine
- Moderate to severe current illness; febrile illness
- Encephalopathy within 7 days after a previous DTaP dose
- Progressive neurologic disorder that is not diagnosed
- Continuous crying for more than 3 hours within 48 hours after a previous DTaP dose
- Convulsions occurring within 3 days after a previous DTaP dose

Abate M, Bates D, Berga SL, Ladenson PW. *PDR monthly prescribing guide.* Montvale NJ: Thompson PDR. 2006;5:290.

185. Which of the following medications has been shown to shorten hospital stays in children with croup?

A) Epinephrine
B) Dexamethasone
C) Albuterol
D) Antiviral medication
E) Ipratropium bromide

Answer and Discussion

The answer is B. Viral croup is the most common form of airway obstruction in children 6 months to 6 years of age. For children with mild croup, symptomatic care and mist therapy may be all that is necessary. Epinephrine has been used in the past to treat more severe cases of croup, but recent meta-analyses have found that glucocorticoid use is associated with shorter hospital stays, improvement in croup scores, and less use of epinephrine. Studies have shown that treatment with oral dexamethasone is as effective as intramuscular dexamethasone or nebulized budesonide. While more studies are needed to establish guidelines, oral dexamethasone can be used to treat mild to moderate croup with close follow-up and instructions for further care, if needed.

Knutson D, Aring A. Viral croup. *Am Fam Physician.* 2004;69:535–540, 541–542.

> Glucocorticoid use in children with croup is associated with shorter hospital stays, improvement in croup scores, and less use of epinephrine.

186. A 3-month-old girl is brought into your office. The parent reports that she has been having excessive nonpurulent tearing from the left eye for the past 4 weeks. The most likely diagnosis is

A) congenital cataracts
B) *Chlamydia trachomatis* infection
C) dacryostenosis
D) glaucoma
E) viral conjunctivitis

Answer and Discussion

The answer is C. Congenital stenosis of the nasolacrimal duct is associated with excessive tearing of usually one eye. The condition is rather common and usually affects children between 2 and 12 weeks of age. In most cases, the condition resolves by 6 months of age. Parents should be instructed to massage the duct 2 to 3 times daily. If no relief occurs by 12 months of age, the duct may need to be probed with the aid of anesthesia. Topical antibiotics should be administered if purulent discharge or conjunctivitis develops.

Behrman RE, Kliegman RM, Jenson HB. *Nelson Textbook of Pediatrics*, 17th ed. Philadelphia: WB Saunders; 2004:2099.

187. Which of the following (otherwise healthy) age groups is considered a priority group when administering influenza vaccine?

A) Birth to 6 months
B) 6 months to 23 months
C) 2 years to 5 years
D) Children under 7
E) Children in elementary school

Answer and Discussion

The answer is B. Given the uncertainties in doses and distribution, the AAFP and the CDC recommend that the following priority groups receive trivalent inactivated influenza vaccine (TIV):

- Persons age ≥65 years with comorbid conditions
- Residents of long-term care facilities
- Persons ages 2 to 64 years with comorbid conditions
- Persons ages ≥ 65 years without cormorbid conditions
- Children ages 6 to 23 months
- Pregnant women
- Health-care personnel who provide direct patient care
- Household contacts and out-of-home caregivers of children ages <6 months

CDC Update: Influenza vaccine supply and recommendations for prioritization during the 2005–2006 influenza season. *MMWR.* 2005;54(34):850.

188. Which of the following statements about transient cortical blindness is true?
A) It usually lasts 3 to 5 days.
B) It can be associated with head trauma.
C) It is associated with cerebral edema seen on computed tomography (CT) scans.
D) It is associated with permanent slowing seen on EEG.
E) It is commonly associated with other neurologic findings.

Answer and Discussion

The answer is B. Transient cortical blindness is blindness without other focal neurologic signs that resolves in 24 hours; it is usually caused by mild head trauma. Head CT scans are unremarkable, and there is no evidence of skull fractures. EEG results initially show some slowing, which resolves spontaneously as the blindness dissipates.

Behrman RE, Kliegman RM, Jenson HB. *Nelson Textbook of Pediatrics,* 17th ed. Philadelphia: WB Saunders; 2004: 2087–2089.

189. Which of the following medications is *not* approved for the treatment of influenza A in a 15-year-old adolescent?
A) Amantadine (Symmetrel)
B) Rimantadine (Flumadine)
C) Zanamivir (Relenza)
D) Oseltamivir (Tamiflu)

Answer and Discussion

The answer is B. Four influenza antiviral agents are available in the United States: amantadine (Symmetrel), rimantadine (Flumadine), zanamivir (Relenza), and oseltamivir (Tamiflu). Amantadine and rimantadine are chemically related antiviral drugs known as adamantanes with activity against influenza A viruses, but not influenza B viruses. Amantadine was approved in 1966 for chemoprophylaxis of influenza type A virus infections among adults and children 1 year old or older. Rimantadine was approved in 1993 for treatment and chemoprophylaxis of influenza A inflection among adults and prophylaxis among children. Although rimantadine is approved only for chemoprophylaxis of influenza A infection among children, rimantadine treatment for influenza A among children can be beneficial. Zanamivir and oseltamivir are chemically related antiviral drugs known as neuraminidase inhibitors that have activity against both influenza A and B viruses. Both zanamivir and oseltamivir were approved in 1999 for treating uncomplicated influenza infections. Zanamivir is approved for treating persons 7 years or older, and oseltamivir is approved for treatment of persons 1 year or older. In 2000, oseltamivir was approved for chemoprophylaxis of influenza among persons 13 years or older.

CDC. Prevention and control of influenza. Recommendations of the Advisory committee on Immunization Practices (ACIP). *MMWR.* 2005;54(No. RR-8):1–40.

190. A painless, cystic structure in the scrotum that transilluminates but is not associated with the presence of sperm is most likely a
A) spermatocele
B) hydrocele
C) varicocele
D) epididymis
E) testicular tumor (Leydig cell)

Answer and Discussion

The answer is B. Hydrocele is a common condition in which a collection of fluid forms between the tunica vaginalis and the tunica albuginea surrounding the testicle. It usually is noted as a painless, enlarging, cystic structure that transilluminates. It is usually an idiopathic congenital finding but can be associated with injury, infection, and, rarely, tumor. Most cases require no further treatment unless the patient is symptomatic or a hernia occurs; surgical consultation is then recommended. Ultrasound examination is usually not necessary, unless there is a question about the diagnosis or the mass does not transilluminate; in these cases, other conditions such as testicular tumors should be ruled out. In some cases, a communicating hydrocele may start out small in the early morning and enlarge throughout the day, or it may enlarge with Valsalva-type maneuvers (e.g., coughing, crying, changing position). Most hydroceles seen in newborns resolve during the first year, and parents need only to be reassured about the condition.

Behrman RE, Kliegman RM, Jenson HB. *Nelson Textbook of Pediatrics,* 17th ed. Philadelphia: WB Saunders; 2004:1820.

191. Which of the following statements regarding inhalant abuse is true?
A) Approximately 5% of children in middle school and high school have experimented with inhaled substances.
B) No associated fetal abnormalities have been associated with inhalant abuse during pregnancy.
C) Drug testing can help aid in the diagnosis of inhalant abuse.
D) Inhalant abuse can become addictive.
E) Reversal of inhalant effects can be achieved with the administration of naloxone (Narcan).

Answer and Discussion

The answer is D. Inhalant abuse is a prevalent and common form of substance abuse in teenagers. Study results consistently show that nearly 20% of children in middle school and high school have experimented with inhaled substances. The method of delivery is inhalation of a solvent from its container, a soaked rag, or a bag. Solvents include almost any household cleaning agent or propellant, paint thinner, glue, or lighter fluid. Inhalant abuse typically can cause a euphoric feeling and can become addictive. Acute effects include sudden sniffing death syndrome, asphyxia, and serious injuries (e.g., falls, burns, frostbite). Chronic inhalant abuse can damage cardiac, renal, hepatic, and neurologic systems. Inhalant abuse during pregnancy can cause fetal abnormalities. Diagnosis of inhalant abuse is difficult and relies almost entirely on a thorough history and a high index of suspicion. No specific laboratory tests confirm solvent inhalation. Treatment is generally supportive, because there are no reversal agents for inhalant intoxication. Education of young persons and their parents is essential to decrease experimentation with inhalants.

Anderson CE, Loomis GA. Recognition and prevention of inhalant abuse. *Am Fam Physician.* 2003;68:869–874, 876.

192. Tick paralysis is associated with all of the following *except*
A) the bite of the *Dermacentor* or *Amblyomma* species of tick
B) muscle weakness, anorexia, lack of coordination, ascending flaccid paralysis
C) a bacteria harbored by the tick that serves as its vector
D) a neurotoxin produced by the tick's salivary gland
E) rapid recovery once the tick is removed

Answer and Discussion

The answer is C. Ticks are capable of carrying many diseases. The *Dermacentor* and *Amblyomma* species of ticks found in North America have been linked to a condition called *tick paralysis*. Children, especially those with long hair that can hide ticks, are usually those affected. Manifestations include muscle weakness, anorexia, lack of coordination, lethargy, nystagmus, and an ascending flaccid paralysis. Sensory examinations and lumbar punctures are normal. In severe cases, respiratory and bulbar paralysis can occur. The paralysis is thought to be caused by inoculation of a neurotoxin that is found in the tick's salivary gland; it is not thought to represent a disease carried by the tick. Therefore, antibiotics are not indicated for affected patients; removal of the tick usually starts the recovery. Treatment of tick paralysis is symptomatic. In severe cases, mechanical ventilation may be necessary if respiratory paralysis occurs. Mortality rates can be as high as 10% for those with severe cases that go untreated. Removal of the tick usually results in improvement within a few hours and total recovery in a few days.

Behrman RE, Kliegman RM, Jenson HB. *Nelson Textbook of Pediatrics,* 17th ed. Philadelphia: WB Saunders; 2004: 2074–2075.

193. Which of the following is true regarding *Neisseria meningitides*?
A) Serogroup B that accounts for the highest incidence of disease in young infants is prevented with administration of the vaccine.
B) Young adults affected with *Neisseria* meningitis typically have better outcomes than other age groups.
C) Eleven- to twelve-year-old adolescents should be vaccinated against *Neisseria meningitides*.
D) Antibiotic prophylaxis is only recommended for household contacts.
E) Even high-risk adults should not receive *Neisseria meningitides* vaccination because of potential side effects.

Answer and Discussion

The answer is C. *Neisseria meningitidis* has an average annual incidence of one case per 100,000 in the United States. The disease can cause rapid death or result in severe neurologic and vascular damage despite antibiotic therapy. Antibiotic chemoprophylaxis with rifampin, ciprofloxacin, or ceftriaxone is recommended for household and other close contacts. The majority of cases of meningococcal disease are sporadic, but outbreaks can occur, and vaccination of the affected population often is required. Serogroup B accounts for the highest incidence of disease in young infants but is not included in any vaccine licensed in the United States. Adolescents and young adults 15 to 24 years of age have a higher incidence of disease and a higher fatality rate than other populations. Because 70% to 80% of these infections in the United States are caused by meningococcal serogroups C, Y, and W-135, which are contained in the tetravalent meningococcal vaccines, they can be prevented. The U.S. Food and Drug Administration recently approved a meningococcal conjugate vaccine containing serogroups A, C, Y, and W-135. The Advisory Committee on Immunization Practices recommends that this vaccine be given to 11- and 12-year-old adolescents, to adolescents entering high school, and to college freshmen living in dormitories. The vaccine also may be given to persons 11 to 55 years of age who belong to certain high-risk groups.

Kimmel SR. Prevention of meningococcal disease. *Am Fam Physician.* 2005;72:2049–2056.

194. Syringomyelia may expand during adolescent years. Typically, the first neurologic deficit is with
A) coordination
B) motor function
C) pain and temperature sensation
D) lower-extremity reflexes
E) mentation

Answer and Discussion

The answer is C. A syringomyelia is a fluid accumulation that involves the spinal canal and is usually associated with the cervical area; however, it may extend to involve the entire spinal cord. The lesion may expand during adolescent years and can give rise to symptoms, including loss of sensation involving the distal extremities, upper shoulders, and back; spasticity; asymmetric or absent reflexes; and weakness with muscle wasting. Pain and temperature sensation are usually lost first. A rapidly progressing scoliosis may be the initial manifestation of syryngomyelia. The congenital abnormality is associated with an Arnold-Chiari malformation, with cerebellar tissue extending into the spinal canal. Diagnosis involves the use of CT scans, magnetic resonance imaging (the test of choice), and myelography. Treatment involves surgery to remove the pocket of fluid.

Behrman RE, Kliegman RM, Jenson HB. *Nelson Textbook of Pediatrics,* 17th ed. Philadelphia: WB Saunders; 2004:2051.

195. Which of the following conditions is associated with meconium ileus?
A) Pyloric stenosis
B) Malrotation
C) Cystic fibrosis
D) Duodenal atresia
E) Hirshsprung's disease

Answer and Discussion

The answer is C. Meconium ileus is almost always an early sign of cystic fibrosis. The thick meconium in meconium ileus is easily differentiated from the rubbery meconium plug of meconium plug syndrome. In meconium ileus the meconium adheres to the bowel mucosa and causes obstruction at the level of the terminal ileum. Distal to the obstruction, the colon is narrow in diameter and contains dry meconium pellets. The relatively empty colon of small caliber is termed a *microcolon*. Loops of distended small bowel can sometimes be palpated through the abdominal wall.

Beers MH, Porter RS, eds. *The Merck manual of diagnosis and therapy*, Merck Research Laboratories, 18th ed. Whitehouse Station, NJ: Merck & Co.; 2006:2309.

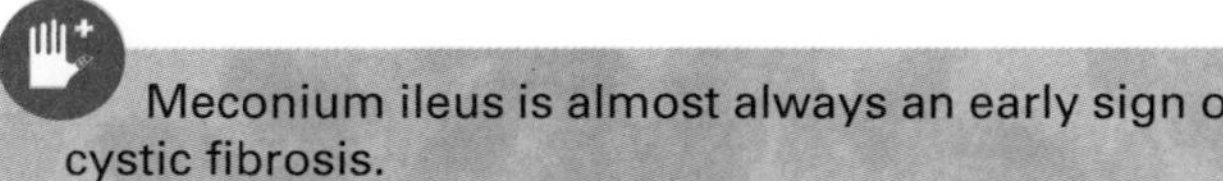
Meconium ileus is almost always an early sign of cystic fibrosis.

196. Which of the following statements about immunoglobulin A (IgA) deficiency is true?
A) It is the most common immunodeficiency.
B) It is associated with influenza vaccination administration.
C) Symptoms include night blindness, skin necrosis, and joint pain.
D) Treatment involves (scheduled) monthly antibiotic administration.
E) Most individuals affected die before age 20 years.

Answer and Discussion

The answer is A. IgA deficiency is the most common immunodeficiency and results in a lack of IgA in secretions. It is the mildest form of immunodeficiency and affects 1 in 600 individuals. The condition has been associated with phenytoin administration, congenital intrauterine infections, and abnormalities of chromosome 18. Most affected individuals are asymptomatic. However, some affected individuals may have decreased immune status resulting in frequent respiratory infections, allergies, recurrent diarrhea, and various autoimmune disorders (e.g., lupus erythematosus, rheumatoid arthritis). In most cases, treatment is unnecessary. However, patients with recurrent respiratory infections may use antibiotics frequently. In some cases, the patient may experience spontaneous remission. Some patients may have antibody development to IgA, which can lead to anaphylactic reactions during blood transfusion.

Behrman RE, Kliegman RM, Jenson HB. *Nelson Textbook of Pediatrics*, 17th ed. Philadelphia: WB Saunders; 2004:691.

197. When do symptoms of pyloric stenosis usually become noticeable?
A) After the first few feedings
B) Within the first week
C) At 4 to 6 weeks after birth
D) At 3 to 4 months of age
E) Pyloric stenosis does not typically cause symptoms

Answer and Discussion

The answer is C. Pyloric stenosis may cause almost complete gastric outlet obstruction. Hypertrophy is rare at birth but develops over the initial 4 to 6 weeks of life, when signs of upper intestinal obstruction usually first appear. Males are affected more than females (4:1). Forceful projectile vomiting of feedings without bile usually begins late in the first month of life. Delayed diagnosis may lead to repeated vomiting, dehydration, failure to gain weight, and hypochloremic metabolic alkalosis (from losses of hydrochloric acid). Diagnosis is suspected by palpation of a discrete, 2- to 3-cm, firm, movable pyloric "olive-like mass" deep in the right side of the epigastrum and confirmed by identification of the hypertrophied pyloric muscle by abdominal ultrasonography. If the diagnosis is uncertain, a barium swallow will show delayed gastric emptying and the typical "string sign" of a markedly narrowed, elongated pyloric lumen. The treatment of choice is a longitudinal pyloromyotomy, which leaves the mucosa intact and separates the incised muscle fibers. Postoperatively, the infant usually tolerates feedings within a few days.

Beers MH, Porter RS, eds. *The Merck manual of diagnosis and therapy*, Merck Research Laboratories, 18th ed. Whitehouse Station, NJ: Merck & Co.; 2006:2284.

198. The most important recommendation a family physician can make regarding reducing the risk of death while riding a bicycle is
A) always wear shoes while riding
B) look both ways before crossing an intersection
C) use proper hand signals
D) make sure the bike is properly fitted
E) wear a helmet while riding

Answer and Discussion

The answer is E. The peak incidence of bicycle-related injuries and fatalities is in the 9- to 15-year age group with a male-to-female ratio of 2 to 3:1. Important risk factors for bicycle-related injuries include not wearing a helmet, crashes involving motor vehicles, an unsafe riding environment, and male gender. In adolescents and young adults, alcohol and substance abuse can be associated with bicycle injury. Most injuries occur in boys and are associated with riding at high speed; most serious injuries and fatalities result from collisions with motor vehicles. Although superficial soft tissue injuries and musculoskeletal trauma are the most common injuries, head injuries are responsible for most fatalities and long-term disabilities. Overuse injuries may contribute to a variety of musculoskeletal complaints, compression neuropathies, perineal complaints, and genital complaints. Physicians treating such patients should consider medical factors, as well as suggest adjusting various components of the bicycle, such as the seat height and handlebars. Encouraging bicycle riders to wear helmets is key to preventing injuries; protective clothing and equipment and general safety advice also may offer some protection.

Thompson MJ, Rivara FP. Bicycle related injuries. *Am Fam Physician*. 2001;63:2007–2014, 2017–2018.

199. Which of the following is true regarding lice infestations?
A) They are obligate human parasites.
B) They frequently jump onto new hosts.
C) Person-to-person contact is not necessary for transmission.
D) Head and pubic lice may cause systemic disease.
E) The incidence of head lice is decreasing.

Answer and Discussion

The answer is A. The three lice species that infest humans are *Pediculus humanus capitis* (the head louse), *Phthirus pubis* (the crab or pubic louse), and *Pediculus humanus corpus* (the body louse). All three species are obligate human parasites. Contrary to popular belief, these insects do not hop, jump, or fly. Instead, they are transmitted by person-to-person contact. Despite the introduction of new treatments, the frequency of lice infestation may be increasing. One explanation may be the development of resistance to current treatments. Fortunately, head and pubic lice do not transmit systemic disease. Hence, treatment is directed at relieving symptoms and preventing reinfestation and transmission.

Flinders DC, De Schweinitz P. Pediculosis and scabies. *Am Fam Physician.* 2004;69:341–348, 349–350.

200. Which of the following is the antibiotic of choice for treating infected dog bites?
A) Amoxicillin
B) Cephalexin
C) Azithromycin
D) Penicillin
E) Amoxicillin–clavulanate

Answer and Discussion

The answer is E. Almost one-half of all dog bites involve an animal owned by the victim's family or neighbors. A large percentage of dog bite victims are children. Although some breeds of dogs have been identified as being more aggressive than other breeds, any dog may attack when threatened. All dog bites carry a risk of infection, but immediate copious irrigation can significantly decrease that risk. Only 15% to 20% of dog bite wounds become infected. Crush injuries, puncture wounds, and hand wounds are more likely to become infected than scratches or tears. Most infected dog bite wounds yield polymicrobial organisms. *P. multocida* and *S. aureus* are the most common aerobic organisms. Amoxicillin–clavulanate potassium (Augmentin) is the antibiotic of choice for an infected dog bite. For patients who are allergic to penicillin, doxycycline (Vibramycin) is an acceptable alternative, except for children younger than 8 years and pregnant women. Erythromycin can also be used, but the risk of treatment failure is greater because of antimicrobial resistance. Assessment for the risk of tetanus and rabies virus infection should be made. The dog bite injury should be documented with photographs and diagrams when appropriate. Patients who have been bitten by a dog should be instructed to elevate and immobilize the involved area. Most bite wounds should be reexamined in 24 to 48 hours, especially bites to the hands. Family physicians should educate parents and children on ways to prevent dog bites.

Presutti RJ. Prevention and treatment of dog bites. *Am Fam Physician.* 2001;63:1567–1572, 1573–1574.

201. A 7 year old with a history of mild asthma presents to your office complaining of wheezing and shortness of breath that have developed over the last 24 hours. She has not used any medication. Which of the following medications would be initially indicated?
A) Albuterol
B) Salmeterol
C) Cromolyn sodium
D) Inhaled corticosteroids
E) Theophylline

Answer and Discussion

The answer is A. The prevalence of asthma in children has increased 160% since 1980, and the disease currently affects nearly 5 million children in the United States. Asthma triggers include allergens from dust mites or mold spores, animal dander, cockroaches, pollen, indoor and outdoor pollutants, irritants (e.g., tobacco smoke, smoke from wood-burning stoves or fireplaces, perfumes, cleaning agents), pharmacologic triggers (e.g., aspirin or other nonsteroidal anti-inflammatory drugs, β-blockers, sulfites), physical triggers (e.g., exercise, hyperventilation, cold air), and physiologic factors [e.g., stress, gastroesophageal reflux, respiratory infection (viral, bacterial), rhinitis]. The National Asthma Education and Prevention Program provides guidelines for improved asthma care. The four components of asthma management include regular assessment and monitoring, control of factors that contribute to or aggravate symptoms, pharmacologic therapy, and education of children and their caregivers. The guidelines recommend a stepwise approach to pharmacologic treatment, starting with aggressive therapy to achieve control and followed by a "step down" to the minimal therapy that maintains control. Quick relief of symptoms can be achieved preferentially by the use of short-acting β_2 agonists. Medications for long-term control should be considered for use in children with persistent symptoms. Inhaled corticosteroids are the most potent long-term anti-inflammatory medications. Other options include long-acting β_2 agonists (usually reserved for patients when other treatments have failed), cromolyn sodium and nedocromil, antileukotriene agents, and theophylline. All have advantages and disadvantages in individual situations. Poor compliance is a major problem in pediatric asthma management, and several factors play a role in this. These include the route of administration (oral therapy is preferred to inhaled medication), frequency of dosing (once- or twice-daily regimens are preferred), medication effects (a slow onset of action and long duration on discontinuance have poor adherence rates), and the risk or concern of side effects. The goals of pharmacologic therapy are to minimize daytime and nocturnal symptoms, the number of asthma episodes, and the use of short-acting β agonists to improve peak exploratory flow to 80% or more of personal best and to allow the child to maintain normal activities without producing adverse medication side effects.

Kemp JP, Kemp JA. Management of asthma in children. *Am Fam Physician.* 2001;63:1341–1348, 1353–1354.

202. Which of the following statements is true regarding sexual abuse in children?
A) Less than 10% of girls at age 18 years have been sexually abused.
B) Sexual acting out is a normal child activity and represents little concern.
C) Secondary enuresis can be a symptom of sexual abuse.
D) Physicians should make a careful decision if there is enough evidence to report parents suspected of sexual abuse.
E) A person who reports sexual abuse may be held liable if no abuse is found.

Answer and Discussion

The answer is C. It is estimated that by the age of 18 years, 12% to 25% of girls and 8% to 10% of boys have been victims of sexual abuse. With this high prevalence, it is likely that primary care physicians will encounter child victims of abuse in their practice. Suspicion of sexual abuse should be raised when children exhibit behavioral changes or have anogenital or other medical problems. Behavioral changes include sexual acting out, aggression, problems in school, regression (e.g., return to thumb sucking, use of a security blanket), sleep disturbances, depression, and eating disturbances. Sexual acting-out behavior is the most specific indicator of possible sexual abuse. Medical problems include anogenital trauma, bleeding, irritation or discharge, dysuria, frequent urinary tract infections, encopresis, enuresis (especially after continence has been achieved), pregnancy, diagnosis of a STD, and oral trauma. Children may present with somatic complaints such as recurrent abdominal pain or frequent headaches resulting from the psychologic stress. Physicians are mandated to report suspected cases of child sexual abuse to the local child protective services agency. When sexual abuse is suspected or when a child discloses a sexual abuse event, a report should be made. In most states, the person who reports the suspected abuse case will not be held liable if the report is made in "good faith."

Lahoti SL, McClain N, Girardet R, et al. Evaluating a child for sexual abuse. *Am Fam Physician.* 2001;63:883–892.

203. Which of the following statements regarding colic in infants is true?
A) Newborns are usually noted to be colicky before discharge from the hospital.
B) Inadequate parenting is a common cause of colic.
C) Treatment consists of swaddling the infant firmly in a blanket.
D) Infants rarely respond to being held, rocked, or being patted.
E) Colic rarely occurs at predictable times of day.

Answer and Discussion

The answer is C. The term *infant colic* is referred to as a symptom constellation that consists of paroxysms of crying, apparent abdominal pain, and irritability. Colic can begin shortly after a baby comes home from the hospital but more often begins some weeks later and may persist until age 3 or 4 months. Typically, the colicky infant eats and gains weight well. He or she may seem excessively hungry and often sucks vigorously on almost anything available. However, bouts of crying may represent significant stress to the family and parents. Colic often occurs at a predictable time of day or night, but a few infants cry almost incessantly. Excessive crying causes aerophagia, which results in flatulence and abdominal distention. The diagnosis of colic is a diagnosis of exclusion. Identifiable conditions must be ruled out by physical examination, blood count, urinalysis, or other studies as needed. In most cases no testing is necessary. Parents should be reassured that the baby's irritability is not due to poor parenting. The infant may respond to being held, rocked, or patted gently. An infant with a strong sucking urge who fusses soon after a feeding may need to suck more. A pacifier also may quiet the infant. A very active, restless infant may respond to being swaddled firmly with a small blanket. A milk-substitute formula may be tried briefly to ascertain whether milk intolerance exists. Parents should be assured that the colicky infant is healthy, that this behavior will cease in a few weeks, and that too much crying is not harmful.

Beers MH, Porter RS, eds. *The Merck manual of diagnosis and therapy,* Merck Research Laboratories, 18th ed. Whitehouse Station, NJ: Merck & Co.; 2006:2236.

204. An 18 month old is brought into your emergency room after being involved in a motor vehicle accident. The child's blood pressure is low and he is tachycardic and lethargic. His capillary refill is delayed and his mucous membranes are dry. Appropriate management consists of
A) oral rehydration
B) intravenous lactated Ringer's, 20 mL/kg given over 30 to 60 minutes
C) intravenous 0.45 normal saline, 20 mL/kg given over 30 to 60 minutes
D) intravenous D5 with normal saline, 20 mL/kg given over 30 to 60 minutes
E) intravenous D5 W, 20 mL/kg given over 30 to 60 minutes

Answer and Discussion

The answer is B. Emergent resuscitation of infants and children typically involves fluid replacement. Fluid deficits can result from a host of conditions including infection, trauma, or dehydration. A short-term weight loss >1% body weight/day is presumed to represent a fluid deficit. The rate at which the deficit is replaced depends on the severity of dehydration and the rate of fluid loss. In general, when signs of circulatory compromise exist, 20 mL/kg of lactated Ringer's solution or 0.9% sodium chloride solution is rapidly infused intravenously to restore adequate perfusion. If circulation does not improve satisfactorily, more fluid is infused. Children in severe hypovolemic shock may require and tolerate fluid boluses totaling 60 to 80 mL/kg within the first 1 to 2 hours of presentation. The need for additional fluid should alert the physician to anticipate complications of acute shock. The remainder of the deficit can be replaced over 8 to 48 hours, depending on clinical need.

Behrman RE, Kliegman RM, Jenson HB. *Nelson Textbook of Pediatrics,* 17th ed. Philadelphia: WB Saunders; 2004:299.

205. Pseudostrabismus is best diagnosed using a
A) Snellen's eye chart
B) funduscopic examination
C) cover/uncover test
D) corneal light reflex test
E) slit-lamp examination

Answer and Discussion

The answer is D. Visual acuity improves as children become older. All children older than 8 years should be able to achieve 20/20 visual acuity using eyeglass correction. Younger children should be referred to an ophthalmologist if there is a difference between the right and left eyes of two or more lines on a Snellen's chart visual evaluation. Strabismus is the most common cause of amblyopia (decreased visual acuity). All infants should have consistent, synchronized eye movement by 5 to 6 months of age. Strabismus most often results from an altered reflex arc in the central nervous system. It can also result from cranial nerve palsies, neuromuscular disorders, or structural abnormalities. Amblyopia is not necessarily related to the degree of strabismus. Small deviations can result in significant vision loss. Strabismus is categorized as medial deviation (esotropia), lateral deviation (exotropia), or vertical deviation (hypertropia). Vertical deviation is the least common type. Deviations that are always manifested are called *tropias,* whereas those that are only elicited by provocative testing are called *phorias.* Intermittent strabismus occurs when there is inconsistent alignment. Usually, the angle between the normal eye and the strabismic eye stays constant through all directions of eye movement and is not influenced by the eye used for fixation. This is termed *concomitant strabismus.* When the eye divergence worsens in some gaze directions, the strabismus is nonconcomitant. This is characteristic of restrictive or paralytic etiologies. In the majority of cases, strabismus develops between 18 months and 6 years of age. Pseudostrabismus is an apparent esotropia that occurs when a child has a wide nasal bridge and prominent epicanthal folds. The corneal light reflex is symmetric with pseudostrabismus. No treatment is needed. Amblyopia is treated by forcing the use of the suppressed eye with a patch over the preferred eye. A schedule whereby the patch is removed for 1 to 2 waking hours each day reduces the risk of a deprivation amblyopia in the good eye. Once the visual goal is achieved, part-time patching is needed to prevent relapse and is often continued for many months to years. The shorter the time that amblyopia is present and the later the age at which it began, the better the prognosis.

Broderick P. Pediatric vision screening for the family physician. *Am Fam Physician.* 1998;58:691.

Behrman RE, Kliegman RM, Jenson HB. *Nelson Textbook of Pediatrics,* 17th ed. Philadelphia: WB Saunders; 2004: 1975–1976, 2084–2085.

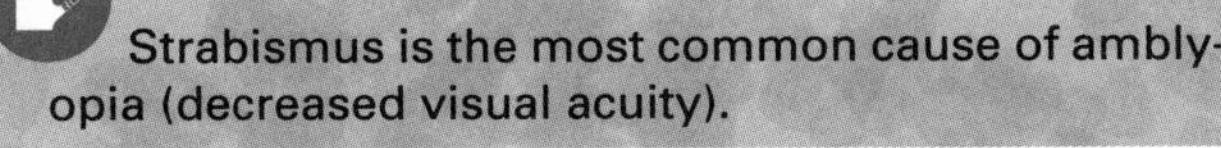

Strabismus is the most common cause of amblyopia (decreased visual acuity).

206. Which of the following is recommended in pediatric adolescent screening?

A) Lipid profiles for all teenagers before age 18 years.
B) Blood chemistries to include electrolytes and complete blood cell count determination.
C) Routine screening for sexually transmitted diseases (STDs) in sexually active teens.
D) Tuberculosis screening for all teens.
E) Urinalysis for all girls over the age of 18 years.

Answer and Discussion

The answer is C. Goals for Adolescent Pediatric Screening (GAPS) consists of 24 recommendations that encompass health care delivery, health guidance, screening, and immunizations. The objective of GAPS is to improve health-care delivery to adolescents using primary and secondary interventions to prevent and reduce adolescent morbidity and mortality. Following are the 24 recommendations made:

1. From ages 11 to 21 years, all adolescents should have an annual routine health visit.
2. Preventive service should be age and developmentally appropriate and should be sensitive to individual and sociocultural differences.
3. Physicians should establish office policies regarding confidential care for adolescents.
4. Parents or other adult caregivers of adolescents should receive health guidance at least once during early adolescence, once during middle adolescence, and, preferably, once during late adolescence.
5. All adolescents should receive general health guidance annually.
6. All adolescents should receive guidance annually to promote the reduction of injuries.
7. All adolescents should receive guidance annually about dietary habits.
8. All adolescents should receive guidance annually about the benefits of exercise and should be encouraged to engage in safe exercise on a regular basis.
9. All adolescents should receive guidance annually regarding responsible sexual behaviors, including abstinence. Latex condoms to prevent STDs (including HIV infection) and appropriate methods of birth control should be made available with instructions on ways to use them effectively.
10. All adolescents should receive guidance annually to promote avoidance of tobacco, alcohol and other abusable substances, and anabolic steroids.
11. All adolescents should be screened annually for hypertension according to the protocol developed by the National Heart, Lung, and Blood Institute's Task Force on Blood Pressure Control in Children.
12. Selected adolescents should be screened to determine their risk of developing hyperlipidemia and adult coronary heart disease, following the protocol developed by the Expert Panel on Blood Cholesterol Levels in Children and Adolescents.
13. All adolescents should be screened annually for eating disorders and obesity.
14. All adolescents should be asked annually about their use of tobacco products, including cigarettes and smokeless tobacco.
15. All adolescents should be asked annually about their use of alcohol and other abusable substances, and about their use of over-the-counter or prescription drugs, including anabolic steroids, for nonmedical purposes.
16. All adolescents should be asked annually about involvement in sexual behaviors that may result in unintended pregnancy and STDs, including HIV infection.
17. Sexually active adolescents should be screened for STDs.
18. Adolescents at risk for HIV infection should be offered confidential HIV screening. (Newer guidelines recommend longer screening intervals.)
19. Female adolescents who are sexually active and women 18 years or older should be screened annually for cervical cancer by use of a Papanicolaou test.
20. All adolescents should be asked annually about behaviors or emotions that indicate recurrent or severe depression or risk of suicide.
21. All adolescents should be asked annually about a history of emotional, physical, or sexual abuse.
22. All adolescents should be asked annually about learning or school problems.
23. Adolescents should receive a tuberculin skin test if they have HIV, have been exposed to active tuberculosis, have lived in a homeless shelter, have been incarcerated, have lived in or come from an area with a high prevalence of tuberculosis, or currently work in a health care setting.
24. All adolescents should receive prophylactic immunizations according to the guidelines established by the federally convened Advisory Committee on Immunization Practices.

Elster AB, Kuzsets NJ, eds. AMA guidelines for adolescent preventive services (GAPS). Recommendations and rationale. *Arch Pediatr Adolesc Med.* 1997 Sept;151(a):958–959.

Behrman RE, Kliegman RM, Jenson HB. *Nelson Textbook of Pediatrics,* 17th ed. Philadelphia: WB Saunders; 2004:643–646.

207. The major difference between stuttering and developmental dysfluency is

A) stuttering involves repetition of word parts and prolongation of sounds
B) stuttering involves repetition of whole words and phrases
C) stutterers tend to speak more slowly than those with developmental dysfluency
D) those affected with developmental dysfluency are more easily frustrated
E) those with developmental dysfluency may display inappropriate articulating postures

Answer and Discussion

The answer is A. The etiology of stuttering is controversial. Today, the prevailing theory is that stutterers have subtle neurophysical dysfunctions that disrupt the precise timing required to produce speech. Stutterers also have difficulty coordinating airflow, articulation, and resonance. In addition, small asynchronies have also been found in the fluent speech of stutterers. Stuttering is a common disorder that usually resolves by adulthood. Boys are more frequently affected, and there appears to be an increased genetic risk. Generally, there is cause for concern if a patient's speech has five or more breaks per 100 words. Almost 80% of children who stutter recover fluency by the age of 16 years. Mild stuttering is self-limited, but more severe stuttering requires speech therapy, which is the mainstay of treatment. Delayed auditory feedback and computer-assisted training are currently used to help slow down speech and control other speech mechanisms. Pharmacologic therapy is seldom used, although haloperidol has been somewhat effective. Differentiating between normal developmental dysfluency and stuttering is important. In general, developmental dysfluency involves the repetition of whole words and phrases, whereas stuttering involves the repetition of word parts and the prolongation of sounds. In addition, stutterers frequently speak at a faster tempo, display silent pauses, have inappropriate articulating postures, become more dysfluent in response to stress, and are more easily frustrated.

Lawrence M, Barclay DM. Stuttering: a brief review. *Am Fam Physician.* 1998;57:2175.

Behrman RE, Kliegman RM, Jenson HB. *Nelson Textbook of Pediatrics,* 17th ed. Philadelphia: WB Saunders; 2004:102.

208. Which of the following is an acceptable criterion for discharging a premature infant from the neonatal unit?
A) Body temperature is maintained in an open crib.
B) The child is maintaining its birth weight.
C) The child is gaining weight of 5 g/day.
D) The child can tolerate tube feeds.
E) The child can react to external stimuli.

Answer and Discussion

The answer is A. Because of the increased survival rate and because many neonatal intensive care units now allow early discharge, family physicians are increasingly likely to provide care to small, premature infants after discharge from the hospital. Most neonatal units have no minimum weight requirement for discharge (although most are at least 1,800 to 2,100 g). Medical guidelines for discharge are as follows:

- Body temperature is maintained while the infant is in an open crib, usually at 34 weeks of gestational age or at 2,000 g (4 lb, 6 oz) of weight
- The infant feeds by mouth well enough to have a weight gain of 10 to 30 g/day
- The infant is not receiving medications that require hospital management
- No recent major changes in medications or oxygen administration have occurred
- No recent episodes of apnea or bradycardia

During the first 2 years of life, growth is plotted using age corrected for prematurity. Growth charts for the "average" premature infant have been designed for this purpose. After the infant reaches 2 years of age, a standard growth chart for chronologic age may be used. The infant's development during the first 2 years should be plotted from the infant's estimated due date rather than the infant's birth date. The Denver Prescreening Developmental Questionnaire, the Denver Developmental Screening Test, and the Gesell Screening Inventory are all accepted tests. Using a standardized developmental test is more important than the choice of test. The timing of immunizations in the physician's office should be based on the infant's chronologic age, not the gestational age. The only exception is hepatitis B vaccination. The American Academy of Pediatrics Committee on Infectious Diseases has issued a statement indicating that it may be advisable to delay administration of hepatitis B vaccine until the infant weighs 2,000 g (4 lbs, 6 oz). The full dose of all immunizations should be given. As with term infants, premature infants should be given the acellular pertussis vaccine when it is available. Influenza vaccine should be given to infants older than 6 months with chronic medical problems, especially lung disease. With all premature infants, consideration should also be given to administering influenza vaccine before the influenza season to parents and other frequent visitors in the home. Administration of the pneumococcal vaccine at 2 years of age may be beneficial in infants with chronic problems such as lung disease; more recently, the heptavalent vaccine (Prevnar) has been given.

Behrman RE, Kliegman RM, Jenson HB. *Nelson Textbook of Pediatrics,* 17th ed. Philadelphia: WB Saunders; 2004: 557–558.

Chapter 3

Obstetrics and Gynecology

Questions

Each of the following questions or incomplete statements below is followed by suggested answers or completions. Select the ONE BEST ANSWER in each case.

1. Which of the following statements is true regarding herpes simplex virus (HSV) infections in newborns?
A) Most children have no symptoms related to their infection.
B) Most infants affected present with vesicular skin lesions.
C) Even in cases that are limited to the skin significant morbidity and mortality occur.
D) Disseminated disease can result in learning disabilities.
E) Diagnosis is easily made at the time of birth.

Answer and Discussion

The answer is D. The diagnosis of neonatal HSV can be difficult initially. Signs and symptoms are nonspecific and include irritability, lethargy, fever, or failure to feed at about 1 week of age. Infants often do not have skin lesions (<50% of infants with encephalitis or disseminated disease). Unfortunately, by the time diagnosis is made, many infants have severe disease and have developed complications. When diagnosis is delayed, mortality is high despite antiviral therapy. There is virtually no mortality among infants with disease limited to the skin, eyes, and mouth, but mortality increases to 15% among infants with encephalitis and 57% among infants with disseminated disease, even with antiviral therapy. Long-term morbidity is common in infants who survive with encephalitis or disseminated disease, and may include seizures, psychomotor retardation, spasticity, blindness, or learning disabilities.

Rudnick CM, Hoekzema GS. Neonatal herpes simplex virus infections. *Am Fam Physician*. 2002;65:1138–1142, 1143.

2. A 21-year-old woman who is 12 weeks' pregnant with her first child presents to your office. A urinalysis shows evidence of bacteriuria. She is completely asymptomatic. Appropriate management at this time includes
A) no treatment; repeat urinalysis at her next visit
B) continue observation and reassure the patient that antibiotic administration is not necessary; she should notify you if she develops symptoms
C) no antibiotic treatment; ask the patient to drink more fluids and cranberry juice daily
D) discontinue urinalysis at OB visits because of the high rate of false positives
E) treat the patient with a 7-day course of amoxicillin

Answer and Discussion

The answer is E. Asymptomatic bacteriuria, defined as more than 100,000 colonies of a single bacterial species per milliliter of urine, cultured from midstream sample, is present in 2% to 7% of pregnant women. The most commonly associated bacteria is *Escherichia coli*. Pregnancy does not increase the incidence of asymptomatic bacteriuria; however, pyelonephritis develops in a significant number of pregnant women with untreated asymptomatic bacteriuria. Asymptomatic bacteriuria in women is associated with a higher preterm delivery rate than women without bacteriuria. Treatment of group B *Streptococcus* (GBS) bacteriuria has also been shown to decrease the rate of preterm delivery. Additionally, GBS bacteriuria has been associated with heavy GBS genitourinary colonization. The Centers for Disease Control and Prevention (CDC) recommends that pregnant women with GBS bacteriuria be treated at the time of diagnosis and during labor. Intrapartum antibiotic prophylaxis is used to prevent early GBS infection in newborns. In most cases, women who do not have asymptomatic bacteriuria at the initial prenatal visit will not develop bacteriuria later in the pregnancy. Accordingly, routine screening for asymptomatic bacteriuria should be performed at the initial prenatal visit. Treatment options include a 3- to 7-day course of (1) oral amoxicillin, (2) nitrofurantoin (Macrobid), or (3) cephalexin (Keflex). After therapy is completed, a urine culture should be repeated to ensure eradication of infection. This repeat culture also identifies patients with persistent or recurrent bacteriuria. For patients who have persistent or recurrent bacteriuria, consideration should be given to administering suppressive doses of antibiotics.

Cram LF, Zapata MI, Toy EC, et al. Genitourinary infections and their association with preterm labor. *Am Fam Physician*. 2002;65:241–248.

Asymptomatic bacteriuria in women is associated with a higher preterm delivery rate than women without bacteriuria.

3. *Preterm labor* is defined as regular contractions with cervical change before
A) 40 weeks' gestation
B) 39 weeks' gestation
C) 38 weeks' gestation
D) 37 weeks' gestation
E) 36 weeks' gestation

Answer and Discussion

The answer is D. According to the American College of Obstetricians and Gynecologists (ACOG), *preterm labor* is defined as regular contractions associated with cervical change before 37 weeks' gestation.

American College of Obstetricians and Gynecologists. Assessment of risk factors for preterm birth. ACOG Practice Bulletin; no. 31, *Obstet Gynecol.* 2001;98:709–716.

4. Which of the following bacterial infections is *not* generally associated with preterm labor?
A) *Ureaplasma urealyticum*
B) *Mycoplasma hominis*
C) *Gardnerella vaginalis*
D) *Bacteroides* species
E) All are associated with preterm labor.

Answer and Discussion

The answer is E. Several bacterial infections have been associated with preterm labor, including *Ureaplasma urealyticum*, *Mycoplasma hominis*, *Gardnerella vaginalis*, and *Peptostreptococcus* and *Bacteroides* species. These organisms are usually of low virulence, and it is unclear whether they are etiologic or associated with an acute inflammatory response of another etiology.

American College of Obstetricians and Gynecologists. Assessment of risk factors for preterm birth. ACOG Practice Bulletin; no. 31, *Obstet Gynecol.* 2001;98:709–716.

5. Which of the following tests has been shown to be a good predictor of preterm labor in the general obstetrical population and results in fewer preterm deliveries?
A) Home Uterine Activity Monitoring (HUAM)
B) Measurement of salivary estriol
C) Screening for bacterial vaginosis
D) Fetal fibronectin screening
E) None of the above

Answer and Discussion

The answer is E. The following have been mentioned for detection of preterm labor; however, none have been shown to be beneficial:

- *Home Uterine Activity Monitoring (HUAM).* HUAM has been suggested as a method for predicting preterm birth in high-risk women. It combines telemetric recordings of uterine contractions using a tocodynamometer and daily telephone calls from a physician to offer support and advice. Because of study limitations, varying results, and flawed study designs, there is uncertainty about the usefulness of HUAM. The U.S. Preventive Services Task Force (USPSTF) and the U.S. Food and Drug Administration (FDA) concluded that the device was not effective. Data are insufficient to support HUAM in preventing preterm birth, and it is not recommended.
- *Salivary estriol.* Observational studies have shown that maternal levels of serum estradiol and salivary estriol increase before the onset of spontaneous term and preterm labor. A test using salivary estriol levels was designed to predict preterm delivery, but maternal estriol levels peak at night and may be suppressed by betamethasone administration. The test carries a high percentage of false-positive results and can add significantly to the cost of prenatal care if used in the low-risk population. Trials with salivary estriol testing have failed to establish its usefulness for anything more than investigational purposes.
- *Bacterial vaginosis.* The presence of bacterial vaginosis has been associated with preterm delivery independent of other known risk factors. Bacterial vaginosis is a common alteration of the normal vaginal flora and has been found in 10% to 25% of patients in general gynecology and obstetric patients, with 50% being asymptomatic. Trials of screening and treatment for bacterial vaginosis in pregnant women to reduce the incidence of preterm birth have been conducted in mixed populations with varying results. Some trials have shown an association with the presence of bacterial vaginosis and preterm delivery, but most results have failed to show if treatment for this condition can prevent preterm birth. There is insufficient data to support screening and treating women at low and high risk.
- *Fetal fibronectin screening.* Numerous trials have shown an association with the presence of the fetal fibronectin protein and preterm birth and a decrease in the risk of preterm birth when the test result for this protein is negative. Although a negative test result appears to be useful in ruling out preterm delivery within 2 weeks, the clinical implications of a positive result have not been evaluated fully because no intervention has been shown to decrease the risk of preterm delivery. The test has limited usefulness in low-risk women. For high-risk women, the following criteria should be met: intact amniotic membranes; minimal cervical dilatation; testing should be performed no earlier than 24 weeks, 0 days of gestation, and no later than 34 weeks, 6 days of gestation; and results must be available in time to allow for decision making, ideally within 24 hours.
- *Cervical ultrasonography.* Transvaginal cervical ultrasonography is a reliable and reproducible way to assess the length of the cervix. Results of a prospective trial showed that the relative risk of preterm delivery increased as the cervical length decreased. Despite the usefulness of measuring cervical length as a predictor of preterm delivery, it is not recommended because of lack of effective treatments.

ACOG has made the following recommendation: screening for risk of preterm labor by means other than historic risk factors is not beneficial in the general obstetric population.

American College of Obstetricians and Gynecologists. Assessment of risk factors for preterm birth. ACOG Practice Bulletin; no. 31, *Obstet Gynecol.* 2001;98:709–716.

6. Which of the following sports is contraindicated in pregnancy?
A) Walking
B) Stationary bicycle
C) Low-impact aerobics
D) Snow skiing
E) Swimming

Answer and Discussion

The answer is D. Concerns have been raised about the safety of some forms of exercise during pregnancy. Because of the body changes associated with pregnancy as well as the hemodynamic response to exercise, some precautions should be observed. The physician should identify any contraindications to exercise and encourage patients to avoid overly vigorous activity, especially in the third trimester, when most pregnant women have a decreased tolerance for weight-bearing exercise. Adequate hydration and appropriate ventilation are important in preventing the possible teratogenic effects of overheating. Pregnant women should avoid exercise that involves the risk of abdominal trauma, falls, or excessive joint stress, as in contact sports and vigorous racquet sports. In the absence of any obstetric or medical complications, most women can maintain a regular exercise regimen during pregnancy. Some studies have found a greater sense of well-being, shorter labor, and fewer obstetric interventions in physically well-conditioned women as compared with other women.

DeCherney AH, Nathan L. *Current Obstetric and Gynecologic Diagnosis and Treatment*, 9th ed. New York: Lange/McGraw-Hill; 2003:211.

7. During pregnancy, it is important to counsel pregnant patients to add an additional _____ calories to their dietary intake for normal activity.
A) 150
B) 300
C) 500
D) 1000
E) 1500

Answer and Discussion

The answer is B. An increase of 300 calories per day is required in pregnancy. Caloric demands with exercise are even higher, although no studies have focused on exact requirements. The competing energy demands of the exercising mother and the growing fetus raise the theoretic concern that excessive exercise might adversely affect fetal development.

Rakel RE. *Textbook of Family Practice*, 6th ed. Philadelphia: WB Saunders; 2002:520–521.

8. Which of the following is *not* a contraindication to exercise during pregnancy?
A) Pregnancy induced hypertension (PIH)
B) Incompetent cervix
C) Preterm labor during a prior pregnancy
D) Placenta previa
E) All are contraindications

Answer and Discussion

The answer is E. Although supportive data is limited, there appears to be no reason why women who are in good health should not be permitted to engage in exercise while pregnant. However, women with medical or obstetric complications should be encouraged to avoid vigorous physical activity. Given the current lack of data, a conservative approach is warranted when doubt exists. Contraindications to exercise during pregnancy include PIH, preterm rupture of membranes, preterm labor during the prior or current pregnancy, incompetent cervix or cerclage placement, persistent second- or third-trimester bleeding, placenta previa, and intrauterine growth retardation.

DeCherney AH, Nathan L. *Current Obstetric and Gynecologic Diagnosis and Treatment*, 9th ed. New York: Lange/McGraw-Hill; 2003:211.

9. Maternal temperature elevations above _____ can be detrimental to the fetus in the first trimester of pregnancy.
A) 98.6°F
B) 100.0°F
C) 101.0°F
D) 102.0°F
E) Maternal temperature has no detrimental effects on the fetus.

Answer and Discussion

The answer is D. Some data suggest a teratogenic potential when maternal temperatures rise above 39.2°C (102.6°F), especially in the first trimester.

Clapp JF III. Exercise in pregnancy: a brief clinical review. *Fetal Med Rev.* 1990;2:89–101.

10. Which of the following medications is generally avoided during pregnancy?
A) Acetaminophen
B) Chlorpheniramine
C) Pseudoephedrine
D) Diphenhydramine
E) Aspirin

Answer and Discussion

The answer is E. High-dose aspirin has been theoretically associated with increased perinatal mortality, neonatal hemorrhage, decreased birth weight, prolonged gestation and labor, and possible birth defects, and in general should be avoided in pregnancy. Low-dose aspirin in combination with heparin has been used successfully in the treatment of antiphospholipid syndrome in pregnancy.

Cunningham FG, Gant NF, Leveno KJ, et al. *Williams Obstetrics*, 21st ed. New York: McGraw-Hill; 2001:1027.

High-dose aspirin has been associated theoretically with increased perinatal mortality, neonatal hemorrhage, decreased birth weight, prolonged gestation and labor, and possible birth defects, and in general should be avoided in pregnancy.

11. During labor, the fetal heart tracing shows repeated late decelerations. You suspect
A) uteroplacental insufficiency
B) abnormal presentation
C) head engagement
D) rapid descent of the fetus
E) normal progression of labor

Answer and Discussion

The answer is A. Repetitive late decelerations of the fetal heart rate may signal uteroplacental insufficiency.

Cunningham FG, Gant NF, Leveno KJ, et al. *Williams Obstetrics*, 21st ed. New York: McGraw-Hill; 2001:340.

12. Repetitive variable decelerations noted on fetal heart tracings suggest
A) umbilical cord compression
B) placenta previa
C) uterine rupture
D) polyhydramnios
E) normal progression of labor

Answer and Discussion

The answer is A. Repetitive variable decelerations suggest umbilical cord compression, especially in the presence of oligohydramnios or amniotomy.

Cunningham FG, Gant NF, Leveno KJ, et al. *Williams Obstetrics*, 21st ed. New York: McGraw-Hill; 2001:341.

13. A 26-year-old woman is having difficulty delivering her first child. You suspect shoulder dystocia and ask the mother to stop pushing and notify your staff. The next appropriate step is
A) place the mother in the left lateral position
B) perform McRoberts' maneuver
C) apply fundal pressure
D) the Rubin maneuver (reverse Woods screw)
E) perform a cesarean section

Answer and Discussion

The answer is B. The recommended sequence for reducing shoulder dystocia begins with calling for help and asking the mother to stop her pushing efforts. The first step is the McRoberts' maneuver, in which assistants hyperflex the mother's hips against her abdomen, thereby rotating the symphysis pubis anteriorly and decreasing the forces needed to deliver the fetal shoulders. A recent retrospective study found this maneuver to be the safest and most successful technique for relieving shoulder dystocia. An assistant can add gentle posterolateral suprapubic pressure while the physician continues moderate posterior traction on the fetal head. Fundal pressure should be avoided, because it tends to increase the impaction.

DeCherney AH, Nathan L. *Current Obstetric and Gynecologic Diagnosis and Treatment*, 9th ed. New York: Lange/McGraw-Hill; 2003:382, 473.

14. The drug of choice for controlling eclamptic seizures is
A) hydralazine
B) phenobarbital
C) phenytoin
D) diazepam
E) magnesium sulfate

Answer and Discussion

The answer is E. In the United States, magnesium sulfate is considered the drug of choice for controlling eclamptic seizures. Fewer intubations are required in the neonates of eclamptic women who are treated with magnesium sulfate. In addition, fewer newborns require placement in neonatal intensive care units. In the treatment of eclampsia and preeclampsia, magnesium sulfate is often given according to established protocols. If serum magnesium levels exceed 10 mEq/L (5 mmol/L), respiratory depression can occur. This problem may be counteracted by the rapid intravenous infusion of 10% calcium gluconate. Magnesium sulfate should be used with caution in patients with impaired renal or cardiac status. It should not be used in patients with myasthenia gravis.

DeCherney AH, Nathan L. *Current Obstetric and Gynecologic Diagnosis and Treatment*, 9th ed. New York: Lange/McGraw-Hill; 2003:347.

15. The diagnosis of preeclampsia consists of all of the following *except*
A) elevated blood pressure
B) proteinuria
C) seizures
D) all are components of preeclampsia

Answer and Discussion

The answer is C. The classic preeclamptic triad includes elevated blood pressure, proteinuria, and edema. More recently, edema has been removed as part of the criteria. Seizures are the distinguishing component of eclampsia.

Cunningham FG, Gant NF, Leveno KJ, et al. *Williams Obstetrics*, 21st ed. New York:McGraw-Hill; 2001:595–609.

16. The most common cause of postpartum bleeding is
A) retained placenta
B) vaginal laceration
C) uterine atony
D) coagulopathy
E) HELP syndrome

Answer and Discussion

The answer is C. Hemorrhage after placental delivery should prompt vigorous fundal massage while the patient is rapidly given oxytocin in their intravenous fluid. If the fundus does not become firm, uterine atony is the presumed (and most common) diagnosis. While fundal massage continues, the patient may be given methylergonovine (Methergine) intramuscularly, with the dose repeated at 2- to 4-hour intervals if necessary. Methylergonovine may cause cramping, headache, and dizziness. The use of this drug is contraindicated in patients with hypertension. Carboprost (Hemabate), 15-methyl prostaglandin F_{2a}, may be administered intramuscularly or intramyometrially every 15 to 90 minutes, up to a maximum dosage. As many as 68% of patients respond to a single carboprost injection, with 86% responding by the second dose. Because oxygen desaturation has been reported with the use of carboprost, patients should be monitored by pulse oximetry.

Cunningham FG, Gant NF, Leveno KJ, et al. *Williams Obstetrics*, 21st ed. New York: McGraw-Hill; 2001:637.

17. An 18-year-old woman pregnant with her first child is in the second stage of labor. She complains of abdominal pain between uterine contractions. You suspect
A) posterior presentation
B) breech presentation
C) abruption placenta
D) vasa previa
E) uterine atony

Answer and Discussion

The answer is C. The patient in labor who develops abdominal pain between uterine contractions or a tender uterus must be presumed to have abruptio placentae. Ultrasound examination has a high false-negative rate in diagnosing abruption and as a result this complication is diagnosed clinically. In one prospective study, 78% of patients with abruptio placentae presented with vaginal bleeding, 66% with uterine or back pain, 60% with fetal distress, and only 17% with uterine contractions or hypertonus. The management of abruptio placentae is primarily supportive and entails both aggressive hydration and monitoring of maternal and fetal well-being. Coagulation studies should be performed, and fibrinogen and D-dimers or fibrin-degradation products should be measured to screen for disseminated intravascular coagulation (DIC). Packed red blood cells should be typed and held. If the fetus appears viable but compromised, urgent cesarean delivery should be considered.

DeCherney AH, Nathan L. *Current Obstetric and Gynecologic Diagnosis and Treatment*, 9th ed. New York: Lange/McGraw-Hill; 2003:357–362.

18. A 25-year-old presents to your office complaining of abnormal vaginal bleeding. Your first consideration in the differential diagnosis is
A) infection
B) trauma
C) foreign body
D) pregnancy
E) coagulopathy

Answer and Discussion

The answer is D. Pregnancy is the first consideration in women of childbearing age who present with abnormal uterine bleeding.

Shwayder JM. Pathophysiology of abnormal uterine bleeding. *Obstet Gynecol Clin North Am.* 2000;27:219–234.

Oriel KA, Schrager S. Abnormal uterine bleeding. *Am Fam Physician.* 1999;60:1371–1380.

19. Patients undergoing cesarean section should
A) always receive a preoperative antibiotic
B) not receive antibiotics because of the risk of resistant organisms
C) receive antibiotics only if the surgery is prolonged (>1.5 hours)
D) not receive antibiotics if they are considered low risk
E) receive antibiotics only if infection is suspected

Answer and Discussion

The answer is A. According to ACOG, all high-risk patients undergoing cesarean delivery should receive prophylaxis with narrow-spectrum antibiotics such as cephalosporin. Several well-designed studies have documented the efficacy of prophylactic antibiotics in reducing the rates of postpartum endometritis and wound infection in patients who have undergone a cesarean delivery and are at high risk for infection. High-risk patients include those who have had cesarean deliveries after membrane rupture or labor and patients who undergo emergency procedures for which preoperative cleansing may have been inadequate. Other patients who may be at increased risk for postoperative infection include patients whose surgeries last for more than one hour and those who experience high blood loss. Risks of febrile morbidity, urinary tract infection, and wound infection also are reduced by antibiotic prophylaxis. Whether patients at lower risk for infection benefit from antibiotic therapy is less clear. No differences in rates of wound infection, endometritis, urinary tract infection, pneumonia, or febrile morbidity were noted in a randomized controlled study of 480 women undergoing cesarean delivery. In a prospective study of 82 women, the incidence of febrile morbidity and endometritis was reduced by antibiotic prophylaxis. Although the evidence is inconclusive, prophylactic antibiotics are recommended in low-risk patients undergoing cesarean delivery.

American College of Obstetricians and Gynecologists. Prophylactic antibiotics in labor and delivery. ACOG Practice Bulletin; no. 47, *Obstet Gynecol.* 2003;102:875–882.

20. In discussing the risk of placing an epidural during labor, you explain to your patient that
A) The ACOG recommends that epidural anesthesia in nulliparous women is not recommended until cervical dilation has reached 4 to 5 cm regardless of maternal request, because
B) early epidural anesthesia increases the risk of cesarean section
C) early epidural anesthesia may increase the rate of vacuum extraction
D) early epidural anesthesia has no effect on the rate of mid- to low forceps delivery
E) epidural anesthesia is of little help with pain management in early labor

Answer and Discussion

The answer is C. Epidural analgesia during labor is an effective pain reliever that has become more commonly used. Despite wide acceptance of this use, the timing of epidural placement remains controversial, with conflicting reports on the risk for subsequent cesarean deliveries and the length of the latent phase of labor. Because of these concerns, ACOG recommended using other forms of analgesia in nulliparous women until they reach dilatation of 4 to 5 cm. However, some institutions did not follow these guidelines for all women in labor, so ACOG released a follow-up report recommending that maternal request is a sufficient indication for epidural analgesia during labor and that it should not be denied on the basis of cervical dilatation. To develop better information about epidural analgesia, Vahratian and colleagues compared the effect of early epidural analgesia with that of early intravenous analgesia on labor progression. The proportion of cesarean deliveries remained the same (18%) in both groups. In the epidural group, the use of outlet forceps or vacuum extraction increased from 10% to 14%, and the use of mid- to low forceps or vacuum extraction decreased from 14% to 10%. The authors conclude that it is unnecessary to withhold epidural analgesia before 4 cm of cervical dilatation is achieved. In their study, the only difference in labor progression between epidural and intravenous analgesia was at 4 to 5 cm and not in the early phase of labor.

Vahratian A, Zhang J, Hasling J. The effect of early epidural versus early intravenous analgesia use on labor progression: a natural experiment. *Am J Obstet Gynecol.* 2004;191:259–265.

> Maternal request is a sufficient indication for epidural analgesia during labor. It should not be denied on the basis of cervical dilatation.

21. When using a vacuum extractor, the procedure should be abandoned after
A) 5 minutes
B) 10 minutes
C) 5 attempts
D) 3 attempts

Answer and Discussion

The answer is D. Vacuum extraction should not be attempted if the head is not engaged. The procedure should be abandoned if delivery is not achieved or the labor does not progress. Under ordinary circumstances, the procedure should be abandoned after three attempts. The procedure should also be stopped if there is any evidence of fetal scalp trauma.

Cunningham FG, Gant NF, Leveno KJ, et al. *Williams Obstetrics*, 21st ed. New York: McGraw-Hill; 2001:506.

22. Proper placement of the vacuum extractor is
A) placed as far anteriorly as possible
B) over the sagittal suture extending to the posterior fontanel
C) covering the posterior fontanel
D) over the sagittal suture and 3 cm in front of the posterior fontanel
E) anywhere on the exposed cranium

Answer and Discussion

The answer is D. When the vacuum extractor is placed on the fetal scalp, the center of the cup should be over the sagittal suture and about 3 cm (1.2 in.) in front of the posterior fontanel. As a general guide, the cup is generally placed as far posteriorly as possible. This cup placement maintains flexion of the fetal head and avoids traction over the anterior fontanel. In positioning the cup, the physician should be careful to avoid trapping maternal soft tissue (e.g., labia) between the cup and the fetal head.

Cunningham FG, Gant NF, Leveno KJ, et al. *Williams Obstetrics*, 21st ed. New York: McGraw-Hill; 2001:504.

23. Pregnant patients with established HIV infection
A) should avoid all antiviral medications because of their teratogenic potential
B) should receive only zidovidine at the time of delivery
C) should be treated the same as adults with HIV who are not pregnant
D) should avoid zidovidine because of its limited effectiveness
E) receive only zidovidine if their CD4+ counts are unacceptably low

Answer and Discussion

The answer is C. Recommendations from the Centers for Disease Control and Prevention (CDC) regarding optimal antiretroviral therapy are to treat pregnant women infected with HIV the same as adults infected with HIV who are not pregnant, using clinical, virologic, and immunologic status to guide treatment decisions. One difference for pregnant women is to include zidovudine in every treatment regimen, given the extensive data demonstrating its benefits. A follow-up study trial showed that zidovudine was beneficial independent of its effect on viral load and regardless of the CD4+ lymphocyte count and viral load at the initiation of therapy.

Cunningham FG, Gant NF, Leveno KJ, et al. *Williams Obstetrics*, 21st ed. New York: McGraw-Hill; 2001:1502.

24. When repairing perineal lacerations, it has been shown that
A) skin sutures may increase the incidence of perineal pain
B) skin sutures are required for adequate skin approximation
C) interrupted transcutaneous sutures are superior to running subcuticular sutures
D) sutures should begin at the anterior point of the skin laceration
E) repair with skin sutures leads to better outcomes

Answer and Discussion

The answer is A. When the perineal muscles are repaired anatomically, the overlying skin is usually well approximated, and skin sutures generally are not required. Skin sutures have been shown to increase the incidence of perineal pain at 3 months after delivery. If the skin requires suturing, running subcuticular sutures have been shown to be superior to interrupted transcutaneous sutures. The 4-0 polyglactin 910 sutures should start at the posterior apex of the skin laceration and should be placed approximately 3 mm from the edge of the skin.

Kettle C, Johanson RB. Continuous versus interrupted sutures for perineal repair. *Cochrane Database Syst Rev.* 2003;(1):CD000947.

25. Laser conization and LEEP procedures have been associated with
A) premature rupture of membranes (PROM)
B) increased peripartum mortality
C) increased cesarean rates
D) higher rates of endometritis during pregnancy
E) no adverse effects during pregnancy

Answer and Discussion

The answer is A. A recent study concludes that there is an increased risk of PROM and preterm labor, but not overall preterm deliveries, following laser conization or LEEP. Although PROM leads to preterm deliveries, these were higher in the untreated group after adjustments compared with the treated group. The authors attribute this incongruity to the higher rate of iatrogenic preterm deliveries in the untreated group. The authors of the study suggest careful adherence to CIN management guidelines, avoidance of unnecessary excisions, and appropriate counseling of previously treated women when they become pregnant.

Sadler L, Saftlas A, Wang W. Treatment for cervical intraepithelial neoplasia and risk of preterm delivery. *JAMA.* 2004;291:2100–2106.

26. A 39-year-old mother presents to your office for preconception counseling. She has one child affected with neural tube defect. Appropriate counseling concerning folic acid supplementation should include ____ daily
A) 100 mcg
B) 400 mcg
C) 1 mg
D) 4 mg
E) none needed based on her current age

Answer and Discussion

The answer is D. Taking folic acid supplementation before conception reduces the incidence of neural tube defects, including spina bifida and anencephaly. The average woman receives about 100 mcg of folic acid per day, mostly from fortified breads and grains. Supplementation should begin at least 1 month before conception and continue through the first 3 months of pregnancy; women should take a daily vitamin supplement containing at least 400 mcg of folic acid. Higher dosages are indicated for special-risk groups. A dosage of 1 mg per day is recommended for women with diabetes mellitus or epilepsy. Mothers who have given birth to children with neural tube defects should take 4 mg of folic acid per day for subsequent pregnancies.

Botto LD, Moore CA, Khoury MJ, et al. Neural-tube defects. *N Engl J Med.* 1999;341:1509–1519.

Werler MM, Louik C, Mitchell AA. Achieving a public health recommendation for preventing neural tube defects with folic acid. *Am J Public Health.* 1999;89:1637–1640.

Iqbal MM. Prevention of neural tube defects by periconceptional use of folic acid. *Pediatr Rev.* 2000;21:58–66.

27. A 36-year-old woman has a history of a prior deep venous thrombosis (DVT). She is pregnant for the first time. In view of her prior history of DVT, you should recommend
A) warfarin (Coumadin)
B) heparin
C) aspirin
D) clopidogrel (Plavix)
E) no prophylaxis is necessary

Answer and Discussion

The answer is B. Women who have a personal or family history of venous thromboembolism should be offered testing for coagulopathy before pregnancy. Women with a prior history of DVT have a 7% to 12% risk of recurrence during pregnancy. Heparin (in regular or low-molecular-weight form) is indicated for prophylaxis and should be started as early in pregnancy as possible. Women receiving warfarin (Coumadin) as maintenance therapy for DVT should be switched to heparin before conception, because warfarin is teratogenic.

American College of Obstetricians and Gynecologists. Thromboembolism in pregnancy. ACOG Practice Bulletin; no. 19. *Obstet Gynecol.* 2000;96:1–10.

28. When advising mothers concerning anti-seizure medications during pregnancy, which of the following statements is true?
A) Multiple medications are preferred to maintain lower levels of medication.
B) Anti-seizure medications should be discontinued at the time pregnancy is determined.
C) Seizure activity in mothers has no impact on fetal outcomes.
D) Most anti-seizure medications are considered safe (category B).
E) Single agents are preferred over multiple medications.

Answer and Discussion

The answer is E. Children of mothers with epilepsy have a 4% to 8% risk of congenital anomalies, which may be caused by anticonvulsant medication or may be related to an increased genetic risk. These children also have an increased risk of developing epilepsy. Preconception counseling should include optimizing seizure control, prescribing folic acid supplements of 1 to 4 mg per day, and offering referral to a genetic counselor. When possible, use of multiple anticonvulsants should be discouraged. It is advisable to aim to use the best single agent for the seizure type at the lowest protective level. There is no single drug of choice. The older agents are classified as FDA pregnancy risk category D and the newer agents are poorly studied. If the patient has been seizure-free for 2 years or longer, drug discontinuation with a long taper period (3 months) may be successful.

Malone FD, D'Alton ME. Drugs in pregnancy: anticonvulsants. *Semin Perinatol.* 1997;21:114–123.

Brundage SC. Preconception health care. *Am Fam Physician.* 2002;65:2507–2514, 2521–2522.

29. Which of the following statements is true regarding smoking during pregnancy?
A) Smoking increases the risk of attention-deficit disorder in the child.
B) Nicotine patches are a safe alternative during pregnancy.
C) Bupropion (Zyban) should be avoided during pregnancy.
D) Regardless of when she stops smoking, infants born to mothers with a smoking history are more at risk for neonatal complications.
E) When compared to total abstinence, reducing the number of cigarettes smoked has no effect on fetal outcomes.

Answer and Discussion

The answer is A. Smoking increases the risk of miscarriage, low birth weight, perinatal mortality, and attention-deficit disorder in the child. If the mother smokes less than 1 pack of cigarettes per day, the risk of a low-birth-weight infant increases by 50%; with more than 1 pack per day, the risk increases by 130%. If the mother quits smoking by 16 weeks of pregnancy, the risk to the fetus is similar to that of a nonsmoker. Behavioral techniques, support groups, and family assistance may be beneficial. Nicotine patches or gum may be helpful before conception, but most authorities recommend avoiding them during pregnancy. Bupropion (Zyban) may be used during pregnancy. If the patient cannot stop smoking, the physician should help her establish a goal to decrease her number of cigarettes to fewer than 10 per day, because many of the adverse effects are dose related.

Brundage SC. Preconception health care. *Am Fam Physician.* 2002;65:2507–2514, 2521–2522.

30. The use of benzodiazepines during pregnancy has been associated with
A) polydactily
B) cleft lip
C) spina bifida
D) growth retardation
E) developmental delay

Answer and Discussion

The answer is B. Maternal use of benzodiazepines during pregnancy has been associated with anomalies such as cleft lip and palate, as well as a withdrawal syndrome in the newborn.

Brundage SC. Preconception health care. *Am Fam Physician.* 2002;65:2507–2514, 2521–2522.

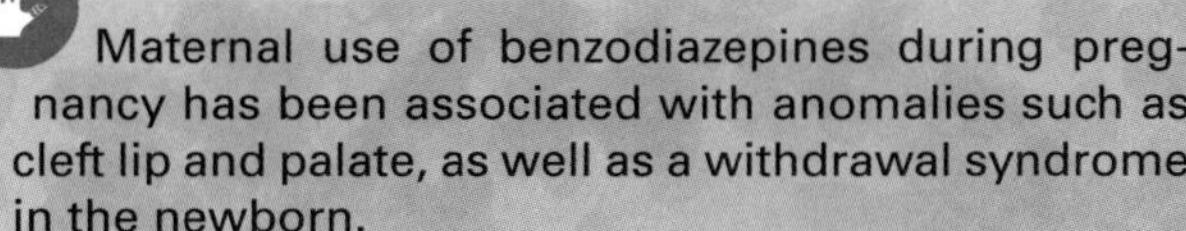

Maternal use of benzodiazepines during pregnancy has been associated with anomalies such as cleft lip and palate, as well as a withdrawal syndrome in the newborn.

31. Which of the following is not associated with maternal obesity during pregnancy?
A) hydrocephalus
B) maternal hypertension
C) preeclampsia
D) maternal diabetes
E) macrosomic infant

Answer and Discussion

The answer is A. Obesity and being underweight increase pregnancy risks. Obesity increases the risks of maternal hypertension, preeclampsia, diabetes, and delivering a macrosomic infant. Women who are obese should diet prior to conception and then alter their consumption to a maintenance diet of 1,800 calories per day while trying to conceive.

Brundage SC. Preconception health care *Am Fam Physician.* 2002;65:2507–2514, 2521–2522.

32. A 26-year-old primagravida presents to your office. She is pregnant with a twin gestation and is in her third trimester. She complains of pruritic, vesicular skin lesions that have developed on her abdomen. Her face, palms and soles are spared. You suspect

A) varicella
B) scabies
C) pruritic urticarial papules and papules of pregnancy (PUPPP)
D) herpes zoster
E) hyperbilirubinemia

Answer and Discussion

The answer is C. Pruritic urticarial papules and plaques of pregnancy (PUPPP), also known as *polymorphic eruption of pregnancy,* is the most common dermatologic complaint of pregnancy, occurring in up to 1 in 160 pregnancies, with an increased incidence in multiple gestations. It usually occurs in primigravidas in the third trimester and recurrence in subsequent pregnancies is unusual. The rash may first appear postpartum. PUPPP typically has a marked pruritic component, the onset of which coincides with the skin lesions. The rash typically begins over the abdomen, commonly involving the striae gravidarum, and may spread to the breasts, upper thighs, and arms. The face, palms, soles, and mucosal surfaces usually are spared. The lesions typically consist of polymorphous, erythematous, nonfollicular papules, plaques, and sometimes vesicles. The lesions can be painful. The rash usually resolves near term or in the early postpartum period. Topical moisturizers and moderately potent steroids in combination with oral antihistamines can provide symptomatic relief.

Kroumpouzos G, Cohen LM. Dermatoses of pregnancy. *J Am Acad Dermatol.* 2001;45:1–19.

33. Which of the following statements is true regarding pruritus gravidarum?

A) The condition is associated with a lacy, erythematous rash that affects the entire body.
B) The rash is limited to the soles of the feet and palms of the hand.
C) The onset is typically in the third trimester.
D) Emollients and antihistamines offer no relief.
E) The condition has no obvious dermatosis.

Answer and Discussion

The answer is E. Pruritus gravidarum is a poorly defined condition of pregnancy associated with itching without an obvious dermatosis. The term pruritus gravidarum is classically associated with pruritus in the first trimester. Its etiology and incidence are unknown. The symptoms of pruritus gravidarum usually can be relieved by emollients and antihistamines.

Kroumpouzos G, Cohen LM. Dermatoses of pregnancy. *J Am Acad Dermatol.* 2001;45:1–19.

34. A 26-year-old woman who is 30 weeks' pregnant is involved in a motor vehicle accident. She has suspected neck trauma and is in need of transport. You suggest placing her

A) in the left lateral decubitus position
B) in the Trendelenberg position
C) prone position on a backboard
D) supine on a backboard with her right hip elevated
E) supine on a backboard

Answer and Discussion

The answer is D. After 20 weeks of gestation, the enlarged uterus may compress the great vessels when a pregnant woman is in a supine position. This compression can cause a decrease of up to 30 mm Hg in maternal systolic blood pressure, a 30% decrease in stroke volume, and a consequent decrease in uterine blood flow. Manual deflection of the uterus laterally or placement of the patient in the lateral decubitus position avoids uterine compression. Because of suspected neck trauma in this patient, placing her supine on a backboard with her right hip elevated 4 to 6 in with towels is the safest treatment.

Grossman NB. Blunt trauma in pregnancy. *Am Fam Physician.* 2004;70:1303–1310, 1313.

35. Which of the following statements about the evaluation of infertility is true?

A) The woman should be evaluated before the man with a postcoital test.
B) A hysterosalpingogram should be performed as the first step in an infertility workup.
C) The first step is evaluation of the male factor with a sperm analysis.
D) Hormone level determination is the first test that should be ordered for the woman before the workup for the man.
E) An endometrial biopsy on the woman is the first test to consider in the workup of infertility.

Answer and Discussion

The answer is C. Infertility affects as many as 10% to 15% of couples in the United States and appears to be increasing in incidence. The definition of infertility is the lack of conception after 1 year of unprotected intercourse. As many as 40% of infertility cases are the result of the male factor (i.e., inadequate sperm production, abnormal sperm motility, or abnormally formed sperm). Other factors involve the female factor and include previous pelvic infections with fallopian tube damage, anovulation, low progesterone levels, hypothyroidism, hyperprolactinemia, or the presence of antisperm antibodies. In the evaluation of infertility, the man is usually evaluated first with a sperm analysis, because the female evaluation may be more extensive. If the sperm is found to be adequate, the woman can be evaluated with a postcoital test, hormone level determination, endometrial sampling, and hysterosalpingogram, which determine patency of the fallopian tubes. Measurement of basal body temperature may show a 0.5°F to 1.0°F increase in temperature supporting ovulation. Further evaluation may require endocrine testing or CT scanning of the head to rule out pituitary tumors or testing to rule out polycystic ovary disease.

Beers MH, Porter RS, eds. *The Merck manual of diagnosis and therapy*, Merck Research Laboratories, 18th ed. Whitehouse Station, NJ: Merck & Co.; 2006:2138–2143.

36. Which of the following conditions is characterized by infarction of the pituitary gland during labor and delivery?
A) Asherman's syndrome
B) Stein-Leventhal syndrome
C) Sheehan's syndrome
D) Cushing's disease
E) Nelson's syndrome

Answer and Discussion

The answer is C. Sheehan's syndrome is a complication of childbirth that results from shock and excessive peripartum bleeding. During pregnancy the pituitary gland usually enlarges and is vulnerable to infarction if excessive bleeding compromises blood flow. Necrosis of the pituitary can occur with varying loss of pituitary function. Symptoms of Sheehan's syndrome include lack of postpartum milk production as a result of low prolactin levels, breast atrophy, loss of pubic or axillary hair, amenorrhea, depressed mental status, low blood pressure, loss of libido, and lack of sweating. Laboratory findings include evidence of hypothyroidism, adrenal insufficiency, and decreased gonadotropin hormone secretion. Treatment involves the replacement of inadequate hormones, including thyroxine, glucocorticoids, and sex hormones.

Cunningham FG, Gant NF, Leveno KJ, et al. *Williams Obstetrics*, 21st ed. New York: McGraw-Hill; 2001:638.

37. Which of the following factors is associated with preterm labor?
A) Long cervix (>30 mm by vaginal ultrasound)
B) Positive fibronectin assay
C) Braxton-Hicks contractions
D) Nipple stimulation
E) Orgasm

Answer and Discussion

The answer is B. Preterm labor is defined as labor pains occurring regularly at frequent intervals (generally more than 4 per hour, accompanied by cervical dilation between 20 and 37 weeks' gestation. Causes include infections, uterine abnormalities, cervical incompetency, premature rupture of membranes, multiple gestations, and other abnormalities (e.g., polyhydramnios, fetal abnormalities). A long cervix (>30 mm by transvaginal ultrasound) and a negative fibronectin assay both have an excellent negative predictive value for preterm labor. Treatment involves the correction of underlying factors (e.g., treatment of infection), bed rest, and the use of tocolytics, such as ritodrine, nifedipine, terbutaline, and magnesium sulfate.

Rakel RE. *Textbook of Family Practice*, 6th ed. Philadelphia: WB Saunders; 2002:534.

38. Which of the following statements is true regarding seatbelt use in pregnancy?
A) The use of seatbelts can increase the risk of fetal injury.
B) The lap belt should be placed under the gravid uterus and over the thighs with the shoulder harness placed between the breast and over the uterus.
C) The air bag should be disabled.
D) Seat belt-restrained women who are in motor vehicle crashes have the same fetal mortality rate as women who are not in motor vehicle crashes.
E) The shoulder harness should not be used during pregnancy.

Answer and Discussion

The answer is D. Proper seat belt use is the most significant preventative measure in decreasing maternal and fetal injury and mortality after motor vehicle crashes. Seat belt-restrained women who are in motor vehicle crashes have the identical fetal mortality rate as women who are not in motor vehicle crashes, but unrestrained women who are in crashes are more than twice as likely to lose their fetuses. Prenatal care should include three-point seat belt instruction. The lap belt should be placed under the gravid abdomen, snugly over the thighs, with the shoulder harness off to the side of the uterus, between the breasts and over the midline of the clavicle. Seat belts placed directly over the uterus can cause fetal injury. Airbags should not be disabled during pregnancy.

Grossman NB. Blunt trauma in pregnancy. *Am Fam Physician.* 2004;70:1303–1310, 1313.

39. An ultrasound evaluation at 12 weeks' gestation detects nuchal translucency in the fetus. Based on the ultrasound report, you suspect
A) Down syndrome
B) brachial cleft cyst
C) spina bifida
D) anencephaly
E) normal development

Answer and Discussion

The answer is A. There is no evidence that directly links improved fetal outcomes with routine ultrasound screening. However, there is sufficient evidence that early ultrasonography (i.e., before 14 weeks' gestation) accurately determines gestational age, decreases the need for labor induction after 41 weeks' gestation, and detects multiple pregnancies. Ultrasonography at 10 to 14 weeks' gestation can measure nuchal translucency as a screening test for Down syndrome. Pregnant women should be offered an ultrasound evaluation to search for structural anomalies between 18 and 20 weeks' gestation. Diagnostic ultrasound exposure has not been proved to harm the mother or fetus.

Kirkham C, Harris S, Grzybowski S. Evidence-based prenatal care: Part I. General prenatal care and counseling issues. *Am Fam Physician.* 2005;71:1307–1316, 1321–1322.

Ultrasonography at 10 to 14 weeks' gestation can measure nuchal translucency as a screening test for Down syndrome.

40. The addition of progesterone to estrogen replacement therapy (ERT) prevents the development of
A) adenomyosis
B) fibroid tumors
C) cervical cancers
D) ovarian cancer
E) endometrial hyperplasia

Answer and Discussion

The answer is E. Estrogen use without progesterone can lead to endometrial hyperplasia, a precursor to endometrial cancer. Thus, in postmenopausal women with an intact uterus, estrogen (0.625 mg/day) should be given along with low-dose progesterone (2.5 mg/day) in a continuous combined method; the more traditional cyclical pattern is 0.625 mg/day estrogen with 5 or 10 mg/day progesterone given on days 19 through 25. Transdermal estrogen is also available, but is less beneficial with regard to lipid metabolism. The addition of progesterone for at least 10 days per month reliably prevents the development of endometrial hyperplasia. Abnormal vaginal bleeding should be further evaluated with an endometrial biopsy and ultrasound of the uterus. If the endometrial thickness is less than or equal to 5 mm, the risk of endometrial hyperplasia or cancer is low. Significant controversy surrounds the use of estrogen replacement secondary to results from the Women's Health Initiative Survey. Many favor avoiding the use in postmenopausal women except in specific cases.

Beers MH, Porter RS, eds. *The Merck manual of diagnosis and therapy*, Merck Research Laboratories, 18th ed. Whitehouse Station, NJ: Merck & Co.; 2006:2121.

41. What percentage of babies born to human immunodeficiency virus (HIV)–positive mothers is HIV positive?

A) 0% to 1%
B) 20% to 30%
C) 50% to 75%
D) 90% to 100%
E) 100%

Answer and Discussion

The answer is B. Prenatal screening for HIV should be offered to all pregnant women. Approximately 20% to 30% of babies who are born to mothers with HIV are HIV positive. Cesarean section is controversial, but generally recommended if the HIV-1 ribonucleic acid load is greater than 1,000 copies per milliliter. After delivery, if the infant screening test is negative, breast-feeding should be discouraged. HIV has been isolated from mothers' breast milk, and the potential for transmission exists. Azidothymidine administered during the second and third trimesters and then given to infants during the first 6 weeks of life decreases the risk of HIV transmission. A protease inhibitor (i.e., indinavir, ritonavir, or saquinavir) should also be offered to pregnant women, although recommendations are constantly changing with regard to treatment.

Cunningham FG, Gant NF, Leveno KJ, et al. *Williams Obstetrics*, 21st ed. New York: McGraw-Hill; 2001:1501–1503.

42. The most appropriate management for fetal demise includes

A) observation for up to 4 weeks until the mother goes into labor
B) immediate cesarean section
C) administration of oxytocin (Pitocin) after the application of prostaglandin gel and laminaria tents to the cervix
D) administration of terbutaline after application of prostaglandin gel to the cervix
E) heparin plus antibiotic prophylaxis and observation for up to 4 weeks

Answer and Discussion

The answer is C. The risk of DIC is increased if a dead fetus has been retained in utero for more than 3 to 4 weeks. Therefore, it is practical to provide expectant management for patients with in utero fetal demise for up to 2 weeks. However, because many mothers experience significant psychological stress from carrying a dead fetus, aggressive measures—including the administration of oxytocin and laminaria tents to provide cervical dilation, as well as prostaglandin E_2—can be taken to facilitate cervical ripening and eventual delivery and should be performed as soon as a firm diagnosis is made.

Beers MH, Porter RS, eds. *The Merck manual of diagnosis and therapy*, Merck Research Laboratories, 18th ed. Whitehouse Station, NJ: Merck & Co.; 2006:2101–2202.

43. A standard dose of Rh immune globulin (300 μg) prevents sensitization from fetomaternal hemorrhage of up to

A) 30 ml of whole blood
B) 60 ml of whole blood
C) 100 ml of whole blood
D) 500 ml of whole blood
E) any amount of whole blood

Answer and Discussion

The answer is A. Rh immune globulin (RhIg) must be administered to an Rh-negative mother immediately after abortion or delivery (live or stillborn) unless the infant is Rh_0(D) and D^u negative, the mother's serum already contains anti-Rh_0(D), or the mother refuses. The standard dose of intramuscular RhIg (300 μg) prevents sensitization from fetomaternal hemorrhage of up to 30 mL whole blood. It is necessary to identify women with fetomaternal hemorrhage to calculate the doses needed to prevent sensitization via a screening rosette test, which, if positive, is followed by a quantitative test (e.g., Kleihauer-Betke).

Beers MH, Porter RS, eds. *The Merck manual of diagnosis and therapy*, Merck Research Laboratories, 18th ed. Whitehouse Station, NJ: Merck & Co.; 2006:2195.

44. Which of the following statements regarding varicella during pregnancy is true?

A) If a pregnant woman has no history of varicella and tests negative for antibodies, she should be immunized as soon as possible.
B) Varicella vaccination should be avoided in breastfeeding women.
C) Susceptible pregnant women who are exposed to varicella are candidates for varicella zoster immune globulin.
D) Pregnancy should be delayed 6 months after varicella vaccination.
E) A single dose of varicella vaccine is safe during pregnancy and can be administered to help protect the fetus.

Answer and Discussion

The answer is C. If varicella testing is performed in the preconception period, women can be offered two doses of varicella vaccine at least 1 month apart. Pregnancy should be delayed 1 month after vaccination. Varicella vaccine is contraindicated in pregnant women. Women found to be nonimmune during pregnancy should be counseled to avoid exposure to chickenpox and to report exposure immediately. Susceptible pregnant women who are exposed to varicella are candidates for varicella zoster immune globulin. Nonimmune women should be offered postpartum varicella vaccination. The vaccine is considered safe in breastfeeding women.

Kirkham C, Harris S, Grzybowski S. Evidence-based prenatal care: Part II. Third-trimester care and prevention of infectious diseases. *Am Fam Physician*. 2005;71:1555–1560, 1561–1562.

45. Rh_0 (D) immune globulin (RhoGAM) is indicated when

A) the mother has type AB blood
B) the father is Rh negative

C) the mother is Rh positive
D) none of the above

Answer and Discussion

The answer is D. If the antibody test is negative, Rh-negative mothers should be given RhoGAM (an immune globulin preparation) at 28 weeks' gestation to prevent erythroblastosis fetalis. If the father is also Rh negative, the administration is unnecessary; however, extramarital pregnancies should be considered. If the antibody test is positive, the mother should be referred to a specialist. A dose of RhoGAM should also be given at the time of delivery. This dose can be determined by the Kleihauer-Betke (FetalDex) test, which measures the amount of fetal erythrocytes in the maternal blood. If the newborn is Rh negative, there is no need for RhoGAM administration. RhoGAM should also be given to Rh-negative women after elective or spontaneous abortion, placental abruption, ectopic pregnancy, or amniocentesis. Typically, the standard RhoGAM dose is 300 μg, which protects up to 10 mL of Rh-positive fetal red cells.

DeCherney AH, Nathan L. *Current Obstetric and Gynecologic Diagnosis and Treatment*, 9th ed. New York: Lange/McGraw-Hill; 2003:296–299.

46. When there is first-trimester bleeding, fetal viability can be determined by which of the following tests?
A) Qualitative β–human chorionic gonadotropin (hCG) determination
B) Serial quantitative β-hCG determinations
C) α-Fetoprotein testing
D) Kleihauer-Betke test
E) Biophysical profile

Answer and Discussion

The answer is B. Approximately 25% of pregnant women experience vaginal spotting or heavier bleeding during the first trimester of pregnancy, and 25% to 50% of these pregnant women experience spontaneous abortion. Genetic anomalies are the most common cause of spontaneous abortion in the first trimester. When first-trimester bleeding is present, viability of the fetus can be determined with a quantitative β-hCG determination, which is repeated 3 to 5 days later. The β-hCG level should double every 48 hours when a viable pregnancy is present. Other causes for first-trimester bleeding, such as infection, should be ruled out. A fetus should be seen with vaginal ultrasound by the 33rd to 35th day after the last menstrual period, or when the β-hCG level has reached 1,500 mIU/mL. If the β-hCG level exceeds 1,500 to 2,000 mIU/mL and no intrauterine pregnancy is found with vaginal ultrasound, an ectopic pregnancy should be suspected, especially if an adnexal mass is palpated on physical examination or the expecting mother experiences lower abdominal pain. Progesterone levels of <5 ng/dL indicate a nonviable pregnancy.

Cunningham FG, Gant NF, Leveno KJ, et al. *Williams Obstetrics*, 21st ed. New York: McGraw-Hill; 2001:884–893.

47. Which of the following is an acceptable form of exercise during pregnancy?
A) Horseback riding
B) Skiing
C) Volleyball
D) Tennis
E) Aerobics (high impact)

Answer and Discussion

The answer is D. ACOG makes specific recommendations concerning exercise during pregnancy that include the following:

- Regular exercise (at least three times per week) is preferable.
- Extreme heat or humidity should be avoided.
- Ballistic or jerking-type movements should be avoided.
- Extreme flexion or extension of joints should be avoided.
- The warm-up should last for at least 5 minutes' minimum duration; the patient should also perform cooling-off exercises after the workout.
- Heart rate at peak activity should be measured.
- The patient should be aware of symptoms of orthostatic hypotension and make sure that she does not become dehydrated.
- The patient should drink plenty of fluids to avoid dehydration.
- The patient should begin with a light exercise program and advance the program slowly.
- The amount of exercise should be maintained at approximately the same level as before pregnancy.

In addition, the mother's core temperature should not exceed 38°C. Women who are at more than 4 months' gestation should avoid exercise in the supine position. They should also avoid repeated Valsalva maneuvers, and caloric intake should be adjusted to support maternal and fetal needs.

Racket sports, swimming, bicycling, and light weightlifting are acceptable as long as proper breathing techniques are used and the mother avoids Valsalva maneuvers. Horseback riding, volleyball, skiing, and high-impact aerobics are not recommended. Contraindications to exercise include cervical incompetence, uterine bleeding, previous premature labor, uncontrolled hypertension, or diabetes and significant anemia.

American College of Obstetrics and Gynecology. Exercise during pregnancy and the postpartum period. ACOG Technical Bulletin No. 189. *Int J Gynaecol Obstet.* 1994;45:65–70.

Cunningham FG, Gant NF, Leveno KJ, et al. *Williams Obstetrics*, 21st ed. New York: McGraw-Hill; 2001:238–239.

48. A 29-year-old woman is now in her 14th week of pregnancy and developed an initial outbreak of genital herpes. You explain to her
A) genital herpes that is acquired during pregnancy does not seem to increase rates of neonatal illness or congenital HSV infection as long as HSV seroconversion has completed by the time labor begins.
B) the fetus has a higher risk of congenital infection even if seroconversion has completed and in the absence of lesions at the time of delivery.
C) termination of the pregnancy should be considered.
D) the risk of fetal malformations is higher for her child.
E) antiviral medications such as acyclovir (Zovirax) cannot be used in pregnancy if she develops recurrent attacks.

Answer and Discussion

The answer is A. Genital herpes that is acquired during pregnancy does not seem to increase rates of neonatal illness or congenital HSV infection as long as HSV seroconversion has completed by the time labor begins. Women with recurrent HSV infection should be counseled about the use of acyclovir (Zovirax) at term to decrease the rate of cesarean delivery, the role of cesarean delivery in decreasing vertical transmission, and avoiding postpartum transmission to the infant through direct contact.

Kirkham C, Harris S, Grzybowski S. Evidence-based prenatal care: Part II. Third-trimester care and prevention of infectious diseases. *Am Fam Physician.* 2005;71:1555–1560, 1561–1562.

Genital herpes that is acquired during pregnancy does not seem to increase rates of neonatal illness or congenital herpes simplex virus (HSV) infection as long as HSV seroconversion has completed by the time labor begins.

49. Which of the following is *not* a risk factor for group B β-streptococcal infection?
A) Twin gestation
B) Less than 37 weeks' gestation
C) Prolonged rupture of membranes
D) Maternal fever
E) All are risk factors

Answer and Discussion

The answer is A. Group B β-streptococcal (GBS) infection is responsible for a significant amount of neonatal morbidity and mortality. Up to 30% of women are colonized by GBS. Risk factors for neonatal infection include: less than 37 weeks' gestation, prolonged rupture of membranes (>18 hours), and maternal fever. Multiple organizations recommend that all women be offered GBS screening by vaginorectal culture at 35 to 37 weeks' gestation and that colonized women be treated with intravenous antibiotics [e.g., high-dosage penicillin or clindamycin (Cleocin)] at the time of labor or rupture of membranes. GBS bacteriuria indicates heavy maternal colonization. Women with GBS bacteriuria or a previous infant with GBS infection should be offered intrapartum antibiotics routinely and therefore do not require vaginorectal culture.

American College of Obstetricians and Gynecologists. Prevention of early-onset group B streptococcal disease in newborns. ACOG committee opinion; no. 279. *Obstet Gynecol.* 2002; 100:1405–1412.

50. Patients who have difficulty with infertility may have antisperm antibodies. Which of the following medications may help lower antisperm antibodies?
A) Medroxyprogesterone (Depo-Provera)
B) Oral contraceptive pills
C) Gonadotropin-releasing hormone (GnRH) agonist
D) Corticosteroids
E) None of the above

Answer and Discussion

The answer is D. Immunologic infertility can occur in women as a result of the development of local and circulating antisperm antibodies. In men, there may also be circulating antibodies that prevent conception. Men with previous vasectomies have an increased risk of antisperm antibodies. Immunologic tests are now available for the detection of these antibodies. In some cases, spontaneous remission of antibodies has occurred. In cases in which they persist, steroids may be useful in lowering the levels of antibodies, thus allowing pregnancy.

Haas G, Cines D, Schreiber A. Immunologic infertility: identification of patients with antisperm antibodies. *N Engl J Med.* 1980;303:722–726.

Beers MH, Porter RS, eds. *The Merck manual of diagnosis and therapy*, Merck Research Laboratories, 18th ed. Whitehouse Station, NJ: Merck & Co.; 2006:2138.

51. A 26-year-old woman presents to your office with questions regarding an intrauterine device (IUD) for birth control. Which of the following statements is true?
A) The first IUD that was developed is still available and has now been determined to be safe to use.
B) Failure rates can be as high as 15%.
C) Newer IUDs pose less risk for pelvic inflammatory disease (PID).
D) Placement of an IUD may affect future fertility.
E) Copper IUDs have been associated with an increased risk for cervical cancer.

Answer and Discussion

The answer is C. An IUD is a contraceptive method that involves placing a foreign body through the cervical os and into the uterus. Interest in the IUD started in the 1960s, and its use in this country increased over the next decade. A 1974 study, however, linked the Dalkon Shield to maternal death and found it to have a disproportionately higher rate of infection than any other IUD. The cause of infection was the multifilament string (or tail), which was a modification of the monofilament tails used by other IUDs. This multifilament tail provided a pathway for bacteria, enabling them to bypass the immunologic barrier provided by the endocervix. This design flaw caused a fivefold increase in PID and an increase in septic abortion. After the Dalkon Shield was removed from the market, the use of IUDs declined in the United States. Currently, the ParaGard copper T308A is a type of IUD that can be left in place for 8 to 10 years. The levonorgestrel-secreting IUD is effective for 5 years. The mechanism of action is through the prevention of implantation. Failure rates are <5%. Contraindications for the use of IUDs include cervical or uterine infections and pregnancy. Relative contraindications include a history of PID, ectopic pregnancy, multiple sexual partners, menorrhagia, or diabetes. If a pelvic infection is suspected, an IUD should be removed. The risk of ectopic pregnancy is slightly increased for those who use IUDs compared with those using oral contraceptives. A pregnancy test should be performed in patients who present with abdominal pain and an IUD in place. More recent IUDs have an improved design, and reevaluation has shown them to be a safe, efficacious, and cost-effective form of birth control. Careful patient selection and preinsertion counseling are crucial to success with the device. Recent studies conclude that the IUD poses little or no increased risk of PID or infertility when used by appropriately selected patients. Multiple studies have shown no increased risk for cervical or uterine malignancies in IUD users. Several reviews have indicated that women who use copper IUDs actually have a decreased risk of cervical malignancies with increasing duration of use, suggesting that copper ions may protect against cervical malignancies.

Canavan TP. Appropriate use of the intrauterine device. *Am Fam Physician.* 1998;58:2083.

Beers MH, Porter RS, eds. *The Merck manual of diagnosis and therapy*, Merck Research Laboratories, 18th ed. Whitehouse Station, NJ: Merck & Co.; 2006:2135–2136.

52. An 18-year-old woman has noted darkened areas of skin on her face following the initiation of oral contraceptives. The most likely diagnosis is
A) melasma
B) lupus pernio
C) malignant melanoma
D) sebaceous hyperplasia
E) adrenal hyperplasia

Answer and Discussion

The answer is A. Melasma occurs in some women taking oral contraceptives. The condition is characterized by areas of darkened pigmentation that may affect the face. The condition is also seen in pregnancy. The condition is more common in African Americans and Latinas. Sun exposure can worsen the condition. Usually, the areas fade when pregnancy is complete or oral contraceptives are discontinued. Oral contraceptives do not increase the risk of malignant melanoma.

Beers MH, Porter RS, eds. *The Merck manual of diagnosis and therapy*, Merck Research Laboratories, 18th ed. Whitehouse Station, NJ: Merck & Co.; 2006:2135–2136.

53. Which of the following is the drug of choice for the prevention of group B β–streptococcal infection in the peripartum period?
A) Intramuscular ceftriaxone
B) Oral ciprofloxacin
C) Intravenous penicillin G
D) Intravenous vancomycin
E) Oral amoxicillin

Answer and Discussion

The answer is C. Intravenous penicillin G is the preferred antibiotic for the prevention of group B β–streptococcal infection in newborns, with ampicillin as an alternative. Penicillin G should be administered at least 4 hours before delivery for maximum effectiveness. Cefazolin is recommended in women allergic to penicillin who are at low risk of anaphylaxis. Clindamycin and erythromycin are options for women at high risk for anaphylaxis, and vancomycin should be used in women allergic to penicillin and whose cultures indicate resistance to clindamycin and erythromycin or when susceptibility is unknown.

Schrag S, Gorwitz R, Fultz-Butts K, et al. Prevention of perinatal group B streptococcal disease. Revised guidelines from CDC. *MMWR Recomm Rep.* 2002;51(RR-11):1–22.

54. The diagnostic test of choice for the detection of ectopic pregnancy is
A) quantitative β-subunit human chorionic gonadotropin (β-hCG) levels
B) computed tomography (CT) of pelvis
C) magnetic resonance imaging (MRI) of the pelvis
D) ultrasound of the pelvis
E) hysteroscopy

Answer and Discussion

The answer is D. Ectopic pregnancy is the most common cause of pregnancy-related death in the first trimester and a common diagnostic and management challenge. Because of its relatively high incidence, ectopic pregnancy represents a risk of mortality from ectopic rupture. When diagnosed early, ectopic pregnancy may be treated medically rather than surgically. Therefore, ectopic pregnancy should be considered and quickly ruled out in all women of reproductive age who present with abdominal pain or vaginal bleeding. Ultrasonography remains the diagnostic test of choice, but it is less specific in patients with low β-subunit human chorionic gonadotropin (β-hCG) levels and may not be available 24 hours a day in some hospitals and clinics.

Buckley RG, et al. History and physical examination to estimate the risk of ectopic pregnancy: validation of a clinical prediction model. *Ann Emerg Med.* 1999;34:589–594.

55. Which of the following statements about molar pregnancy is true?
A) Malignant transformation is monitored by serial α-fetoprotein levels.
B) Further pregnancies should be discouraged after a molar pregnancy.
C) It is usually associated with hyperemesis gravidarum.
D) Risk for recurrent molar pregnancy is not increased in women who have had previous molar pregnancies.
E) The majority of molar pregnancies result in malignant transformation.

Answer and Discussion

The answer is C. A molar pregnancy (hydatidiform mole) occurs when the placenta undergoes trophoblastic transformation and results in a neoplasm of the placenta. The abnormal placenta is usually swollen, edematous, and vesicular, resembling a cluster of grapes. The condition usually affects women younger than 20 and older than 40 years of age, and those with a prior history of hydatidiform mole are at increased risk. Hydatidiform moles are usually associated with hyperemesis gravidarum and preeclampsia that occur before the third trimester. Other associated conditions include vaginal bleeding; signs and symptoms of hyperthyroidism; trophoblastic embolization that may cause cough, tachypnea, and cyanosis; enlarged uterus associated with gestation; and theca lutein cysts resulting in ovarian enlargement. In 80% of patients, the molar pregnancy resolves spontaneously without complications; however, in 20%, there is a malignant transformation of the tissue. Therefore, serum hCG determination (which is usually significantly elevated) should be monitored every 2 weeks after evacuation of the uterus until the value drops to nonpregnant values and then every 1 to 2 months for 1 year. Repeated pelvic examinations should be performed on a monthly basis after a molar pregnancy for the first year. In addition, a chest x-ray should be performed at the time of evacuation and 4 to 8 weeks after evacuation to check for metastasis. The lungs are the most common sites for metastasis. Patients should avoid pregnancy for at least 1 year after the development of a molar pregnancy. Those who have had prior molar pregnancies have an increased risk for recurrent molar pregnancies, and those who have recurrent molar pregnancies are at an increased risk for malignant transformation. Malignant transformation is usually treated with methotrexate.

Cunningham FG, Gant NF, Leveno KJ, et al. *Williams Obstetrics*, 21st ed. New York: McGraw-Hill; 2001:836–844.

Hydatidiform moles are usually associated with hyperemesis gravidarum and preeclampsia that occur before the third trimester.

56. A 44-year-old woman presents with irregular vaginal bleeding. Appropriate initial management includes
A) endometrial biopsy
B) trial of oral contraceptives
C) medroxyprogesterone injection
D) surgical referral

Answer and Discussion

The answer is A. Women who are reproductively mature, are older than 40, and experience irregular vaginal bleeding should be evaluated with endometrial biopsy to rule out endometrial hyperplasia or carcinoma. In addition, other tests to rule out thyroid dysfunction and bleeding disorders should be considered. Adolescents with abnormal vaginal bleeding can be regulated with oral contraceptive medications once pregnancy and infection have been ruled out. Vaginal bleeding before the age of 9 and after the age of 52 in the absence of hormone replacement is cause for concern and requires investigation.

Beers MH, Porter RS, eds. *The Merck manual of diagnosis and therapy*, Merck Research Laboratories, 18th ed. Whitehouse Station, NJ: Merck & Co.; 2006:2066–2069.

57. In the management of a pregnant patient, medications are classified based on their risk to the fetus. Category A medications
A) should never be given during pregnancy
B) are considered safe during pregnancy
C) should only be given in life-threatening situations
D) have unknown risk for the fetus
E) are associated with teratogenicity in animals

Answer and Discussion

The answer is B. The following medication classifications are used to determine the risk of their use during pregnancy:

- *Category A*: Controlled studies in women fail to demonstrate risk to the fetus in the first trimester; considered safe with no harmful effects on the fetus.
- *Category B*: Animal studies do not indicate a risk; however, there are no human studies. Considered relatively safe during pregnancy.
- *Category C*: Unknown fetal risk with no human studies to support or disprove safety.
- *Category D*: Some risk has been proved for the fetus; these drugs should be used only in life-threatening situations.
- *Category X*: Proven harm to the fetus; should not be used in pregnancy.

Cunningham FG, Gant NF, Leveno KJ, et al. *Williams Obstetrics*, 21st ed. New York: McGraw-Hill; 2001:1009.

58. Which of the following medications has been shown to be comparable to laparoscopic salpingostomy in the treatment of small ectopic pregnancy that has not ruptured?
A) Bromocriptine
B) Methotrexate
C) Thalidomide
D) Misoprostol
E) Oxytocin

Answer and Discussion

The answer is B. In recent years, intramuscular methotrexate has been advocated as an alternative to salpingostomy for management of ectopic pregnancy. In addition, there is also interest in using serum human chorionic gonadotropin (hCG) or progesterone levels to monitor resolution of ectopic pregnancy after intervention. Based on study results a single dose of intramuscular methotrexate is comparable to laparoscopic salpingostomy for the treatment of a small, unruptured ectopic pregnancy. The fact that serum progesterone levels resolved faster than serum hCG levels suggests that serum progesterone may be a better marker for monitoring resolution of ectopic pregnancy.

Saraj AJ, Wilcox JG, Najmabadi S. Resolution of hormonal markers of ectopic gestation: a randomized trial comparing single-dose intramuscular methotrexate with salpingostomy. *Obstet Gynecol.* 1998:92: 989–994.

Cunningham FG, Gant NF, Leveno KJ, et al. *Williams Obstetrics*, 21st ed. New York: McGraw-Hill; 2001:904.

59. Which of the following medications is used for cervical ripening and labor induction?
A) Terbutaline
B) Methotrexate
C) Thalidomide
D) Misoprostol
E) Bromocriptine

Answer and Discussion

The answer is D. Misoprostol (Cytotec) has been extensively investigated in the past few years for use in cervical ripening and labor induction. Marketed as a gastric cytoprotective agent, the drug is also an effective, safe, and inexpensive agent for cervical ripening and labor induction, although it is not FDA-labeled for that purpose.

Wing DA, Paul RH. Misoprostol for cervical ripening and labor induction: the clinician's perspective and guide to success. *Contemp Ob/Gyn.* 1999;44:46–61.

60. Which of the following statements about uterine adenomyosis is true?
A) The condition is associated with the invasion of myometrial tissue into the peritoneal cavity.
B) The condition commonly causes intense pelvic pain, dysuria, and dyspareunia.
C) Those affected with uterine adenomyosis have an increased risk of endometrial cancer.
D) The condition is considered benign and usually causes no associated symptoms.
E) The condition results from uterine atony after delivery.

Answer and Discussion

The answer is D. Uterine adenomyosis is defined as the invasion of endometrial tissue into the myometrium. This common disorder is benign and usually causes no symptoms. Those who do have symptoms complain of menorrhagia, irregular vaginal bleeding, pelvic pain, and bladder or rectal discomfort. Pelvic examination may reveal an enlarged uterus that feels softer in consistency; there may be associated fibroid tumors. Hysterectomy may be indicated for those beyond their childbearing years if symptoms are severe. Oral contraceptives and GnRH agonists are not very effective in treatment. Uterine adenomyosis is more likely to cause secondary dysmenorrhea than fibroids, endometrial polyps, cervical papillomas, or polycystic ovary disease.

DeCherney AH, Nathan L. *Current Obstetric and Gynecologic Diagnosis and Treatment*, 9th ed. New York: Lange/McGraw-Hill; 2003:669–670.

61. A 17-year-old girl is seen in the emergency room. She reports high fever, nausea, vomiting, myalgias, and lethargy. On examination, she is found to have hypotension and a generalized erythematous rash and desquamation of the hands and feet. Laboratory tests show an increased white blood cell count, increased blood urea nitrogen, and increased serum creatinine with decreased urine output. The most likely diagnosis is
A) gonorrhea
B) Lyme disease
C) toxic shock syndrome
D) tertiary syphilis
E) PID

Answer and Discussion

The answer is C. Toxic shock syndrome is a condition that is characterized by high fever, nausea and vomiting, myalgias, mental status changes, and an erythematous, sandpaper-like skin rash with the development of severe hypotension and vascular collapse. Desquamation of the hands and feet is also common. First recognized in 1978, the condition tends to affect young menstruating women and is associated with the use of vaginal tampons. The syndrome is a result of staphylococcal or streptococcal infection that produces an exotoxin. Occasionally, the syndrome is associated with postoperative infections, diaphragm use, contraceptive sponges, septic abortions, insect bites, and other infections that involve staphylococcal and streptococcal organisms. Complications include multisystem failure, adult respiratory distress syndrome (ARDS), and even death in severe cases. Laboratory studies often reveal an elevated white blood cell count, increased blood urea nitrogen and serum creatinine with decreased urine output, and thrombocytopenia followed by thrombocytosis. Mortality may be as high as 5% to 15%. Recurrence is common if the woman continues to use tampons within the first 4 months after an infection. Treatment with a β-lactamase–resistant penicillin or cephalosporin is recommended, as is supportive treatment to replace fluid loss and electrolytes. Steroids may be indicated for severe cases. Patients with toxic shock syndrome should be encouraged not to use high-absorbency tampons or diaphragms. Oral contraceptives may help to reduce the number of recurrent cases.

Taylor RB, David AK, Fields SA, et al. *Family Medicine: Principles and Practice*, 6th ed. New York: Springer; 2003:915–916.

62. A 35-year-old woman presents to your office complaining of a copious white vaginal discharge. Microscopic examination shows evidence of pseudohyphae. The most appropriate treatment is
A) penicillin G
B) doxycycline
C) terconazole (Terazol) vaginal cream
D) metronidazole (Flagyl)
E) topical acyclovir

Answer and Discussion

The answer is C. Yeast vaginitis (monilial vaginitis) is caused by *Candida albicans*. Predisposing factors include the recent use of wide-spectrum antibiotics, the use of oral contraceptives, pregnancy, menstruation, diabetes mellitus, constrictive undergarments, the use of immunosuppressive drugs (e.g., steroids), or immunodeficient states [e.g., acquired immunodeficiency syndrome (AIDS)]. As part of their vaginal flora, 20% of women harbor *C. albicans* and are asymptomatic. Symptoms include intense vulvar irritation, pruritus, and vaginal discomfort. Erythema that affects the vulvar area, vaginal lining, and cervix is usually present. A copious, white, cottage cheese–like vaginal discharge also generally occurs. Diagnosis is made by microscopic examination of vaginal secretions following the application of potassium hydroxide to a glass slide. Characteristic budding yeast-like cells are noted with projections of pseudohyphae. Vaginal pH is less than 4.5. Treatment consists of local antifungal vaginal cream [miconazole (Monistat), terconazole (Terazol) and others] applied nightly for 3 to 7 days; the newer oral antifungals usually produce satisfactory results.

Beers MH, Porter RS, eds. *The Merck manual of diagnosis and therapy*, Merck Research Laboratories, 18th ed. Whitehouse Station, NJ: Merck & Co.; 2006:2086.

63. Which of the following is true of oxytocin administration?
A) The drug must be given through a controlled infusion device.
B) Oxytocin be administered as a continuous infusion or in "pulsed" doses.
C) The medication can have an antidiuretic effect with high doses.
D) Hyperstimulation can result from oxytocin administration.
E) All of the above.

Answer and Discussion

The answer is E. Oxytocin is mixed for use by placing 10 U in 1 L of isotonic intravenous solution to achieve a concentration of 10 mU/mL. Because severe hypotension can occur, especially during rapid intravenous administration, and because the drug is infused into the main intravenous line, a controlled infusion device *must* be used to determine its rate. It can be administered as a continuous infusion or in "pulsed" doses. Oxytocin's effect is noted within 3 to 5 minutes, and a steady state is achieved within 15 to 30 minutes. Studies show a wide range of effective dosages and change intervals, and no regimen has been shown to be clearly superior. Oxytocin has many advantages. The medication is potent and easy to titrate, has a short half-life (1 to 5 minutes), and is generally well tolerated. Dose-related adverse effects can occur. Because oxytocin is close to vasopressin in structure, it has an antidiuretic effect when given in high dosages (40 mU/min); thus, water intoxication is a possibility in prolonged inductions. Uterine hyperstimulation and uterine rupture can also occur. When the resting uterine tone remains >20 mm Hg, uteroplacental insufficiency and fetal hypoxia can result. This outcome emphasizes the importance of continuous fetal monitoring while administering oxytocin.

Harman JH Jr, Kim A. Current trends in cervical ripening and labor induction. *Am Fam Physician*. 1999;60:477–484.

64. Which of the following medications has been used with success in gestational diabetes?
A) Glipizide (Glucotrol)
B) Glyburide (Micronase, Diabeta)
C) Glimepiride (Amaryl)
D) Rosiglitazone (Avandia)
E) Repaglinide (Prandin)

Answer and Discussion

The answer is B. Gestational diabetes mellitus (GDM) is carbohydrate intolerance that occurs during pregnancy. Those affected are at risk of developing diabetes and related conditions later in life and face a range of complications during pregnancy, including hypertension, preeclampsia, and cesarean delivery. Macrosomia is more common in infants exposed to GDM, as are the risks of operative delivery, shoulder dystocia, birth trauma, and obesity during childhood. Although the U.S. Preventive Services Task Force concluded that there was insufficient evidence to recommend universal screening for GDM, >90% of obstetric physicians report screening all patients. Screening based on risk factors such as obesity, family or personal history of diabetes, or previous adverse pregnancy outcome misses approximately one half of mothers with GDM. The most commonly used test is the 50-g 1-hour glucose challenge. The accepted optimal limits vary, but at the recommended level of 130 mg/dL (7.2 mmol/L), the screening test has an estimated sensitivity of 79% and a specificity of 87%. The diagnostic test specific to pregnancy and with the most supporting data is the 100-g 3-hour oral glucose tolerance test. Women with GDM are often treated initially with diets designed to achieve normal glycemic levels and avoid ketoacidosis. However, an acceptable diet has not been determined, and calorie restriction may increase the chance of ketosis. Several trials have demonstrated reduced fetal macrosomia if the mother is treated with insulin. Although insulin treatment is common in GDM, only 9% to 40% of treated mothers benefit. Treatment aims to achieve glucose levels of 130 mg/dL 1 hour postprandially. Oral hypoglycemic agents, with the exception of glyburide, are contraindicated in pregnancy. In one study, glyburide provided outcomes comparable to those achieved with insulin in patients with GDM who had failed to achieve adequate glycemic control with diet alone. When glycemic control is satisfactory and no complications occur, mothers with GDM routinely do not require early or operative delivery. Nevertheless, the high incidence of macrosomia and other complications often results in cesarean or other operative delivery.

American College of Obstetricians and Gynecologists. *Gestational diabetes*. ACOG Practice Bulletin no. 30. *Obstet Gynecol.* 2001;98:525–538.

Macrosomia is more common in infants exposed to gestational diabetes mellitus (GDM), as are the risks of operative delivery, shoulder dystocia, birth trauma, and obesity during childhood.

65. The diagnosis of endometriosis is generally made by
A) detection of increased estrogen levels
B) endometrial biopsy
C) pelvic ultrasound
D) laparoscopy
E) computed tomography (CT) of the pelvis

Answer and Discussion

The answer is D. Endometriosis is the presence of endometrial tissue outside the uterus. Locations include the ovaries, fallopian tubes, uterosacral ligaments, peritoneal cul-de-sac, and uterovesical peritoneum. Rare locations include the nasal mucosa and lungs. Theories for the development of endometriosis are abundant, and include the migration of endometrial tissue through the fallopian tubes and into the peritoneal cavity or transformation of existing epithelium into endometrial-type tissue. Symptoms include dysmenorrhea, dyspareunia, infertility, dysuria, irregular vaginal bleeding, and pelvic pain. As many as 33% of affected individuals have no symptoms. Risk factors include nulliparity and a positive family history. Most patients have normal examination results; however, some have a tender retroverted uterus or adnexal masses that are tender with palpation. Diagnosis is usually accomplished with laparoscopy. Treatment involves the use of analgesics, progesterone, and oral contraceptives to regulate cycles for mild disease. More advanced disease can be treated with danazol (Danocrine), an anabolic steroid that has androgen activity. Side effects of danazol therapy include weight gain, fluid retention, fatigue, acne, chloasma, irregular vaginal bleeding, cholestatic jaundice with prolonged use, and hepatic dysfunction in patients who receive high doses. GnRH agonists are also used for treatment. Severe cases may require surgery.

Winkel CA. Evaluation and management of women with endometriosis. *Obstet Gynecol.* 2003;102:397–408.

66. Symptoms that present the greatest concern in pregnant women include
A) visual disturbances
B) nausea
C) heartburn
D) abnormal cravings
E) mild edema

Answer and Discussion

The answer is A. Symptoms noted in early pregnancy that present concern to the physician include vaginal bleeding or fluid vaginal discharge, severe headaches, visual disturbances, chronic vomiting, fever or chills, dysuria, swelling of the face or hands, and pelvic pain. Abnormal cravings, nausea, mild lower extremity edema, and heartburn are common complaints of pregnancy.

Cunningham FG, Gant NF, Leveno KJ, et al. *Williams Obstetrics*, 21st ed. New York: McGraw-Hill; 2001:238–244.

67. Which of the following statements about primary dysmenorrhea is true?
A) The condition usually worsens with the use of oral contraceptives.
B) It is thought to be associated with excessive prostaglandin activity.
C) The onset of symptoms typically begins after 30 years of age.
D) Endometriosis is a common cause.
E) The condition is related to adenomyosis.

Answer and Discussion

The answer is B. *Primary dysmenorrhea* is defined as menstrual-related pain that occurs during menstruation with the absence of pelvic pathology. The onset is usually before 20 years of age, and it affects women during the first day or two after the onset of menstruation. The cause is thought to be secondary to excessive prostaglandin activity, which leads to uterine contractions and ischemia, giving rise to pelvic discomfort. Other symptoms include headache, nausea, and occasionally vomiting, constipation, diarrhea, and urinary frequency. Premenstrual symptoms, including water retention, irritability, nervousness, and depression, may also persist during the early period of menstruation. Treatment usually involves reassurance, nonsteroidal anti-inflammatory agents (NSAIDs), and heating pads to the lower abdomen. A trial of oral contraceptives may be beneficial. In women who do not desire hormonal contraception, there is some evidence of benefit with the use of the Japanese herbal remedy toki-shakuyaku-san; thiamine, vitamin E, and fish oil supplements; a low-fat vegetarian diet; and acupressure.

In secondary dysmenorrhea, patients report the same symptoms as those of primary dysmenorrhea, except that there is evidence of pelvic pathology (i.e., endometriosis, fibroids, chronic PID, IUD use, cervical stenosis, or adenomyosis). The age of onset is usually older than 20 years, and the course can be progressive. The treatment is correction of the underlying cause.

French L. Dysmenorrhea. *Am Fam Physician.* 2005;71:285–291, 292.

68. A 33-year-old woman who delivered last week presents to your office with questions about her gestational diabetes that developed during the first trimester. You explain
A) her risk of developing type 2 diabetes in the future is no different than anyone else
B) she should be checked yearly for diabetes
C) no further monitoring is necessary unless she develops symptoms of diabetes
D) she should be tested for diabetes 6 months after delivery via fasting blood glucose measurements on two occasions or a 2-hour oral 75-g glucose tolerance test

Answer and Discussion

The answer is B. Women with gestational diabetes are at high risk for developing type 2 diabetes in the future and should be tested for diabetes 6 weeks after delivery via fasting blood glucose measurements on two occasions or a 2-hour oral 75-g glucose tolerance test. Normal values for a 2-hour glucose tolerance test are less than 140 mg/dL. Values between 140 and 200 mg/dL (11.1 mmol/L) represent impaired glucose tolerance, and greater than 200 mg/dL are diagnostic of diabetes. Screening for diabetes should be repeated annually thereafter, especially in patients who had elevated fasting blood glucose levels during pregnancy.

Kim C, Newton KM, Knopp RH. Gestational diabetes and the incidence of type 2 diabetes: a systematic review. *Diabetes Care.* 2002;25:1862–1868.

69. Which of the following medications is contraindicated for the management of hypertension in pregnancy?
A) Methyldopa
B) Hydralazine
C) Labetalol
D) Nitroprusside
E) Losartan

Answer and Discussion

The answer is E. Most hypertensive women of childbearing age have stage I or II hypertension (systolic blood pressure of 140 to 179 mm Hg or diastolic blood pressure of 90 to 109 mm Hg) without target organ damage. Therefore, the risk for acute cardiovascular consequences during pregnancy is very low. Improved maternal or neonatal outcomes with antihypertensive therapy have not been documented in this group. Accordingly, the Working Group advises that antihypertensive medication might be safely withheld in such patients, provided that blood pressure remains less than 150 to 160 mm Hg systolic and 100 to 110 diastolic while the patient is off medications. Continuing previous antihypertensive medication is another option, although angiotensin-converting enzyme (ACE) inhibitors and angiotensin-receptor blockers should not be used during pregnancy. Because methyldopa (Aldomet) has the longest track record of safety in pregnancy, it is preferred by many clinicians. Hydralazine, nifedipene, labetalol, and nitroprusside (for severe cases) are also used.

Report of the National High Blood Pressure Education Program Working Group on High Blood Pressure in Pregnancy. *Am J Obstet Gynecol;* 2000;183(1):S1–S22.

70. Which of the following is most commonly associated with nongonococcal urethritis?
A) Gonorrhea
B) *Ureaplasma*
C) *Chlamydia*
D) *Trichomonas*
E) Syphilis

Answer and Discussion

The answer is C. Nongonococcal urethritis is commonly caused by chlamydia infections (approximately 50% of cases). Chlamydia is currently the most common sexually transmitted disease in the United States. Other causes include *Trichomonas*, *Ureaplasma urealyticum*, genital herpes, *Mycoplasma genitalium*, and *Candida*. Symptoms include clear vaginal or penile discharge, dysuria, pruritus, and occasionally meatal erythema. Women are often completely asymptomatic. Symptoms, when they are present, include vaginal discharge, dysuria, frequency, pelvic pain, and dyspareunia. The incubation period is between 7 and 28 days. Diagnosis of chlamydia infections is often difficult because it is an obligate intracellular parasite; diagnosis is usually accomplished by tissue cultures but can also be made with fluorescent antibody tests using smears of genital secretions. Chlamydia can result in infertility in women, and complications for men include epididymitis. Treatment of chlamydia is accomplished with oral doxycycline, 100 mg, taken twice a day for 7 days. Other alternatives include tetracycline, erythromycin, azithromycin, and ofloxacin.

Beers MH, Porter RS, eds. *The Merck manual of diagnosis and therapy*, Merck Research Laboratories, 18th ed. Whitehouse Station, NJ: Merck & Co.; 2006:1651–1652.

71. Dysfunctional uterine bleeding is most common
A) during pregnancy
B) after sexual intercourse
C) at the time of menopause
D) with the development of PID
E) in premenarchal women

Answer and Discussion

The answer is C. *Dysfunctional uterine bleeding* is defined as abnormal uterine bleeding in the absence of inflammation, pregnancy, or tumors. The condition is most commonly associated with anovulation. It usually occurs just after menarche or around the time of menopause. Treatment depends on the age of the patient, the desire for fertility and contraception, and the duration and severity of bleeding. If the patient is young and healthy and the bleeding is not profuse, she can be treated medically with high-dose oral estrogens every 6 hours, which usually stops the bleeding within the first 24 hours. After the cessation of bleeding, the patient should continue with daily estrogen for the rest of the month, followed by the administration of progesterone during the final 10 days of the month. After the addition of the progesterone, withdrawal bleeding should occur within a few days, and the patient can then begin oral contraceptive pills to regulate her menstrual cycles. If bleeding continues, further evaluation with an endometrial biopsy or dilation and curettage may be necessary. Older women in the perimenopausal state may initially need endometrial biopsy and possible dilation and curettage to rule out endometrial hyperplasia or endometrial cancer.

Taylor RB, David AK, Fields SA, et al. *Family Medicine: Principles and Practice*, 6th ed. New York: Springer; 2003:878, 879–880.

72. Which of the following statements about exercise-induced amenorrhea is true?
A) The condition is rarely reversible with weight gain.
B) It usually affects women who weigh >115 lb or those who have gained >10% to 15% in muscle mass.
C) Osteoporosis can be associated.
D) It is usually associated with prolactinomas.
E) Hormone therapy is contraindicated in those affected.

Answer and Discussion

The answer is C. Exercise-induced amenorrhea is a condition that is noted in competitive female athletes. The cause appears to be associated with the athlete's weight and weight loss. Menstrual irregularities or amenorrhea are most likely to develop in women who weigh <115 lb or those who have lost >10 lb (10% to 15% of normal weight) while training. The basis of amenorrhea is unknown but may be associated with hypothalamic dysfunction. In most cases, weight gain reverses the condition; however, many women are unwilling to gain the additional weight. The female athlete triad is defined as the combination of disordered eating, amenorrhea, and osteoporosis. This disorder often goes unrecognized. The consequences of lost bone mineral density can be devastating for the female athlete. Premature osteoporotic fractures can occur, and lost bone mineral density may never be regained. Early recognition of the female athlete triad can be accomplished by the family physician through risk factor assessment and screening questions. Instituting an appropriate diet and moderating the frequency of exercise may result in the natural return of menses. Hormone therapy should be considered early to prevent the loss of bone density.

Hobart JA, Smucker DR. The female athlete triad. *Am Fam Physician.* 2000;61:3357–3364, 3367.

73. Painless and profuse vaginal bleeding in the third trimester is most likely
A) placenta acreda
B) placenta previa
C) vaso previa
D) bloody show
E) cervical ripening

Answer and Discussion

The answer is B. Painless hemorrhage is the hallmark sign of placenta previa. Although spotting may occur during the first and second trimesters of pregnancy, the first episode of hemorrhage usually begins at some point after the 28th week and is characteristically described as being sudden, painless, and profuse. With the onset, clothing or bedding is saturated by an impressive amount of bright red, clotted blood, but the blood loss usually is not extensive, seldom produces shock, and is almost never fatal. In about 10% of cases there is some initial pain because of coexisting placental abruption, and spontaneous labor may be expected over the next few days in 25% of patients. In rare cases, bleeding is less dramatic or does not begin until after spontaneous rupture of the membranes or the onset of labor. Occasionally, nulliparous patients can reach term without bleeding, possibly because the placenta has been protected by an intact cervix.

DeCherney AH, Nathan L. *Current Obstetric and Gynecologic Diagnosis and Treatment*, 9th ed. New York: Lange/McGraw-Hill; 2003:362–365.

74. The normal amount of blood loss for a vaginal delivery is
A) 250 mL
B) 500 mL
C) 1000 mL
D) 1500 mL
E) 2000 mL

Answer and Discussion

The answer is B. The normal pregnant patient typically loses 500 mL of blood at the time of vaginal delivery and 1,000 mL during a cesarean delivery. Appreciably more blood can be lost without clinical evidence of a volume deficit as a result of the 40% expansion in blood volume that occurs by the 30th week of pregnancy.

Benedetti TJ. Chapter 17: Obstetric hemorrhage. In: Gabbe SG, Niebyl JR, Simpson JL, eds. *Obstetrics: normal and problem pregnancies.* 4th ed. New York: Churchill Livingstone; 2003:503.

75. Which of the following statements about epidural anesthesia is true?
A) It provides anesthesia only for lumbar and sacral nerve roots.
B) It should only be used for multigravida women.
C) It can be used in hemophiliacs.
D) It can be associated with hypotension.
E) Placement of the catheter should be at the L2–L3 level.

Answer and Discussion

The answer is D. Epidural anesthesia is used as a regional block during childbirth. The procedure is performed by inserting a needle in the L3–L4 interspace and threading a catheter into the epidural space. The catheter is then aspirated to check for the presence of cerebrospinal fluid. If this occurs, the catheter must be repositioned. A test dose is then administered to reconfirm position. When position is confirmed, a full dose of anesthetic is administered through the catheter. Analgesia is usually established with fentanyl plus a small dose of bupivacaine. Fentanyl works better for the visceral pain that is associated with labor, whereas bupivacaine is more effective for somatic pain. The dose may need to be repeated to maintain anesthesia during delivery. In most cases, a full dose provides anesthesia of nerve roots T10–S5. Risks that are involved with epidural anesthesia include drug reaction, hypotension, and rare neurologic complications. If the dura is penetrated, a spinal headache eventually develops in many patients. Contraindications to epidural anesthesia include adverse affects to anesthesia, bleeding tendency, infection of the lumbar area, or underlying neurologic defects. Some studies have reported that epidural anesthesia may prolong labor, leading to an increased cesarean delivery rate.

Cunningham FG, Gant NF, Leveno KJ, et al. *Williams Obstetrics*, 21st ed. New York: McGraw-Hill; 2001:373–379.

Some studies have reported that epidural anesthesia may prolong labor, leading to an increased cesarean delivery rate.

76. Which of the following statements regarding anencephaly is true?
A) Intracerebral shunts can be used effectively in preventing central nervous system complications.
B) The condition should be suspected with elevations in α-fetoprotein levels.
C) Children who are affected may need additional tutoring during school.
D) Nicotinic acid may help prevent anencephaly when given antepartum.
E) Urinary tract infections are common in those affected.

Answer and Discussion

The answer is B. The condition of anencephaly occurs when the cerebral hemispheres are absent. In some cases there may be some cystic neural remnants. In many instances the spinal cord and brainstem are affected. Diagnosis is suspected with elevated α-fetoprotein levels obtained at 16 to 18 weeks' gestation and confirmed with ultrasound examination. Unfortunately, the condition is incompatible with life, and these infants are usually stillborn or die within a few hours or days after birth. The use of prenatal vitamins that contain at least 0.4 mg folic acid can help to prevent neural tube defects such as anencephaly.

Beers MH, Porter RS, eds. *The Merck manual of diagnosis and therapy*, Merck Research Laboratories, 18th ed. Whitehouse Station, NJ: Merck & Co.; 2006:2442.

77. Which of the following medications is *not* used in the treatment of preterm labor?
A) Ritodrine
B) Magnesium sulfate
C) Terbutaline
D) Propanolol
E) Nifedipene

Answer and Discussion

The answer is D. *Tocolysis* is the process of stopping preterm labor contractions with medication. Medications that are used for tocolysis include β-sympathomimetics, magnesium sulfate, prostaglandin synthetase inhibitors (indomethacin), and calcium-channel blockers (nifedipine). Of these, ritodrine (Yutopar), a β-sympathomimetic, although still used, is not used as frequently for labor tocolysis, and terbutaline is now often utilized because of its ease of administration. Tocolysis is usually not successful if the cervix has dilated to >4 cm and should be reserved for pregnancies between 20 and 36 weeks' gestation. Contraindications to tocolysis include fetal distress, fetal anomalies, significant risk to the mother, abruptio placentae, or placenta previa with heavy bleeding.

DeCherney AH, Nathan L. *Current Obstetric and Gynecologic Diagnosis and Treatment*, 9th ed. New York: Lange/McGraw-Hill; 2003:290.

78. Which of the following is *not* considered as part of the Amsel criteria for diagnosing bacterial vaginosis?
A) Milky, homogeneous, adherent discharge
B) Vaginal pH greater than 4.5
C) Positive whiff test
D) Presence of clue cells on light microscopy
E) Vaginal itching

Answer and Discussion

The answer is E. The Amsel criteria are considered to be the standard diagnostic approach to bacterial vaginosis and continue to be used for the diagnosis. The criteria include the following: milky, homogeneous, adherent discharge; vaginal pH >4.5; positive whiff test (the discharge typically has a fishy smell); and presence of clue cells in the vaginal fluid on light microscopy. If three of the four criteria are met, there is a 90% likelihood of bacterial vaginosis.

Sobel JD. Vaginitis. *N Engl J Med.* 1997;337:1896–1903.

79. A 24-year-old woman is noted to have the presence of *Trichmonas* found on a routine Pap smear that is performed at the student health center. Although the center diagnoses a number of cases each year, she is entirely asymptomatic. Appropriate management should be to
A) reassure patient that no treatment is necessary
B) repeat cultures after the next menstrual cycle and treat if the organism is present
C) treat only if the patient is pregnant
D) treat regardless of symptoms
E) treat only if symptoms are present

Answer and Discussion

The answer is D. Unlike women with asymptomatic *Gardnerella vaginalis* or *Candida* colonization, women with asymptomatic *Trichomonas vaginalis* infection should be treated. *Trichomonas vaginalis* is highly transmissible and is associated with other sexually transmitted diseases (STDs). Asymptomatic infection may also increase the risk of acquiring HIV. When trichomoniasis is found during routine Pap testing, management should be based on the pretest probability of infection in the patient, which is determined by the prevalence of *T. vaginalis* infection in the community; information on prevalence usually can be obtained from the local health department.

Wiese W, Patel SR, Patel SC, et al. A meta-analysis of the Papanicolaou smear and wet mount for the diagnosis of vaginal trichomoniasis. *Am J Med.* 2000;108:301–308.

80. Which of the following statements about neural tube defects is true?
A) Laboratory testing is not useful in the diagnosis of neural tube defects.
B) Elevated α-fetoprotein levels should be further evaluated by obstetric ultrasound.
C) Nicotinic acid has been shown to help prevent neural tube defects.
D) α-fetoprotein testing should be done at 24 to 28 weeks' gestation.
E) Elevated α-fetoprotein levels are not associated with normal pregnancies.

Answer and Discussion

The answer is B. Neural tube defects (e.g., spina bifida, meningomyelocele, anencephaly) can be screened for by performing a serum α-fetoprotein blood test, which is done at 16 to 18 weeks' gestation. Evaluation is based on maternal weight and length of gestation. The accuracy of the test approaches 95%. Causes for elevations of maternal α-fetoprotein include inaccurate gestation dates, multiple gestations, abdominal wall defects in the fetus, congenital nephrotic syndrome, fetal demise, and neural tube defects. In addition, normal pregnancies may be associated with elevations in α-fetoprotein levels. Low levels of α-fetoprotein are associated with inaccurate gestation dates, chromosome trisomy such as Down syndrome, molar pregnancy, and fetal demise. In addition, normal pregnancies may exhibit low α-fetoprotein levels. In most cases, an obstetric ultrasound should be performed if the α-fetoprotein level is abnormal. Recent studies have shown that the administration of folic acid before pregnancy may help to prevent neural tube defects. The current recommendations are that women who plan to conceive should consume at least 0.4 mg folate/day (which is usually contained in a prenatal vitamin). Preconception counseling should include a discussion of folic acid supplementation.

Cunningham FG, Gant NF, Leveno KJ, et al. *Williams Obstetrics*, 21st ed. New York: McGraw-Hill; 2001:980–982.

81. A 28-year-old woman who recently delivered a child presents with pelvic pain, fever, vaginal discharge, and nausea with vomiting. Examination shows a positive Chandelier sign. The most likely diagnosis is
A) ectopic pregnancy
B) pyelonephritis
C) PID
D) bacterial vaginosis
E) yeast vaginitis

Answer and Discussion

The answer is C. Pelvic inflammatory disease (PID) is a condition that includes infection of the fallopian tubes, cervix, endometrium, or ovaries. It is usually seen in women younger than 30 years of age who are sexually active or who have recently experienced childbirth. Causative agents include chlamydia, gonorrhea, gram-negative and gram-positive bacteria, *Mycoplasma,* and viral infections. Many cases involve polymicrobial infections. Symptoms include pelvic pain, fever, vaginal discharge, dyspareunia, nausea, and vomiting. Physical examination reveals adnexal, uterine, and cervical motion tenderness (positive Chandelier sign). Laboratory findings include an elevated white blood cell count and elevated erythrocyte sedimentation rate. The differential diagnosis includes multiple conditions, including appendicitis, ectopic pregnancy, urinary tract infection, and peritonitis. Complications of PID include chronic PID, infertility, and ectopic pregnancy. Treatment consists of ceftriaxone (Rocephin) and doxycycline. Outpatient therapy with oral antibiotics can be used in the majority of patients with PID. Follow-up care must be available within 72 hours to evaluate the response to treatment. Hospitalization of patients with PID is recommended only in certain instances. The use of condoms lowers the risk of PID. The use of IUDs and multiple sex partners increases the risk.

Miller KE, Graves JC. Update on the prevention and treatment of sexually transmitted disease. *Am Fam Physician.* 2000;61:379–386.

82. A 27-year-old asymptomatic pregnant woman is found to have hyperthyroidism. Which of the following medications is the drug of choice for treatment?
A) Propylthiouracil
B) Radioactive iodine
C) Methimazole
D) Propranolol
E) Levothyroxine

Answer and Discussion

The answer is A. Hyperthyroidism during pregnancy is usually associated with Graves' disease. Other causes include toxic nodular goiter, choriocarcinoma, hydatidiform mole, ovarian teratoma, and iatrogenic thyrotoxicosis. Symptoms may include weight loss, tachycardia, exophthalmos, pretibial myxedema, generalized weakness, and tremor. Laboratory findings include an elevated triiodothyronine, thyroxine, and low sensitive thyroid-stimulating hormone. Treatment depends on the situation. Antithyroid medications readily cross the placenta and inhibit fetal thyroid function. Propylthiouracil and methimazole cross the placenta but are used in the treatment of hyperthyroidism during pregnancy. Propylthiouracil does not cross the placenta as easily as methimazole and is the drug of choice. Radioactive iodine ablation of the thyroid is contraindicated during pregnancy. Close monitoring of thyroid hormones is required when administering antithyroid medications during pregnancy. Side effects of the medications include rash, urticaria, arthralgias, and agranulocytosis, which may predispose to maternal infection. Surgery is reserved for severe refractive cases. Untreated hyperthyroidism during pregnancy can lead to premature delivery, neonatal thyrotoxicosis, and spontaneous abortion.

DeCherney AH, Nathan L. *Current Obstetric and Gynecologic Diagnosis and Treatment*, 9th ed. New York: Lange/McGraw-Hill; 2003:441–442.

83. Which of the following is a characteristic of atrophic vaginitis?
A) Vaginal pH of 5 to 7
B) Milky discharge
C) Increased vaginal rugae
D) Endometrial cells noted on wet-mount microscopic examination
E) Increased glycogen levels

Answer and Discussion

The answer is A. The decline in estrogen levels during perimenopause and after menopause can cause vaginal atrophy and resulting atrophic vaginitis. One important physiologic change is thinning of the vaginal epithelium; another is loss of glycogen, which leads to changes in the vaginal pH and flora. Many women with these vaginal changes are minimally symptomatic and require only explanation and reassurance. In women with more severe changes, vaginal irritation, dyspareunia, and fragility may become problems. Atrophy is diagnosed by the presence of a thin, clear or bloody discharge, a vaginal pH of 5 to 7, loss of vaginal rugae, and the finding of parabasal epithelial cells on microscopic examination of a wet-mount preparation.

Owen MK, Clenney TL. Management of vaginitis. *Am Fam Physician.* 2004;70:2125–2132, 2139–2140.

84. A 45-year-old woman is noted to have four yeast infections in 1 year. Appropriate management of this patient should be
A) continued observation and treatment only if symptomatic
B) further evaluation for hypothyroidism
C) blood test to look for the presence of diabetes
D) prophylactic therapy with weekly metronidazole
E) examination for endometrial structural abnormalities

Answer and Discussion

The answer is C. Recurrent vulvovaginal candidiasis is defined as four or more yeast infections in 1 year. The possibility of uncontrolled diabetes mellitus or immunodeficiency should be considered in women with recurrent vulvovaginal candidiasis. When it has been determined that no reversible causes are present (e.g., antibiotic therapy, uncontrolled diabetes, oral contraceptive pill use) and initial therapy has been completed, maintenance therapy may be appropriate. Selected long-term regimens include the use of clotrimazole and fluconazole. The role of boric acid and lactobacillus therapy remains in question.

Sobel JD. Recurrent vulvovaginal candidiasis (RVVC). *Int J STD AIDS.* 2001;12(suppl 2):9.

The possibility of uncontrolled diabetes mellitus or immunodeficiency should be considered in women with recurrent vulvovaginal candidiasis.

85. Which of the following statements about dysfunctional uterine bleeding is true?
A) The condition is most common during the middle of a woman's reproductive years.
B) It typically occurs during pregnancy.
C) Most cases are seen with anovulatory cycles.
D) Gynecologic malignancies are related to dysfunctional uterine bleeding.
E) Inflammation is a commonly associated condition.

Answer and Discussion

The answer is C. *Dysfunctional uterine bleeding* is defined as abnormal uterine bleeding in the absence of inflammation, pregnancy, or tumors. It is the most common form of abnormal uterine bleeding and is seen most commonly at the extremes of the reproductive cycle (menarche and menopause). Most cases are seen with anovulatory cycles. Causes include exogenous estrogen use, polycystic ovary syndrome, hyperthyroidism, and hypothyroidism.

Beers MH, Porter RS, eds. *The Merck manual of diagnosis and therapy*, Merck Research Laboratories, 18th ed. Whitehouse Station, NJ: Merck & Co.; 2006:2077–2078.

86. An 18-year-old woman presents to your office complaining of pelvic pain, dysuria, and a purulent yellowish-green vaginal discharge. A Gram's stain of cervical secretions shows gram-negative diplococci. The most appropriate medication is
A) ceftriaxone + doxycycline
B) penicillin G + azithromycin
C) cefuroxime + tetracycline
D) cefoxitin + doxycycline
E) metronidazole + doxycycline

Answer and Discussion

The answer is A. Gonorrhea is caused by a gram-negative diplococcus, *Neisseria gonorrhoeae*. Symptoms include purulent, yellowish-green vaginal, rectal, or penile discharge; urethritis; and genital irritation and discomfort. Other symptoms include scrotal pain, abdominal or pelvic pain, and pharyngeal discomfort. Some patients, especially women, are completely asymptomatic. Disseminated gonococcal infection can give rise to polyarthralgias, tenosynovitis, and a hemorrhagic papular or pustular skin rash that affects the genitalia, hands, feet, and other areas of the body. The disease is spread by sexual contact. Incubation is 2 to 14 days for men and 7 to 21 days for women. Diagnosis is accomplished with Gram's stains that show leukocytes with intracellular gram-negative diplococci and more accurately with cultures made on Thayer-Martin chocolate agar media. Treatment is ceftriaxone, 125 mg, given intramuscularly. Alternatives include cefixime, azithromycin, ciprofloxacin, norfloxacin, or ofloxacin given orally and spectinomycin, cefoxitin with probenecid, ceftizoxime, cefotaxime, or cefotetan given intramuscularly. Repeat cultures should be performed to ensure eradication, and sexual partners should also be treated. Because chlamydia may also coexist, most patients are treated with a course of doxycycline or azithromycin as well. Other sexually transmitted diseases (e.g., syphilis, HIV, hepatitis) may also coexist and need appropriate diagnosis and treatment.

Taylor RB, David AK, Fields SA, et al. *Family Medicine: Principles and Practice*, 6th ed. New York: Springer; 2003:349–350.

87. Which of the following fetal heart rate tracings is a warning sign of uteroplacental insufficiency?
A) Early accelerations
B) Late accelerations
C) Early decelerations
D) Late decelerations
E) Variable decelerations

Answer and Discussion

The answer is D. Late decelerations on fetal heart tracings are defined as repetitive decelerations in fetal heart rate (usually <15–20 bpm from the baseline) that occur late in the contraction phase during labor. Usually, there are no associated accelerations. Late decelerations indicate uteroplacental insufficiency and fetal hypoxia. In most cases, this is a worrisome sign and a potentially dangerous situation. Other worrisome features include fetal tachycardia and loss of fetal heart rate variability. Treatment involves actions to improve fetal oxygenation and includes positioning the mother on her side, administering oxygen, discontinuing oxytocin, administering fluids to help relieve maternal hypotension, performing a vaginal examination to rule out a prolapsed cord, fetal scalp monitoring, and immediate delivery (possibly via cesarean section) if late decelerations persist.

Cunningham FG, Gant NF, Leveno KJ, et al. *Williams Obstetrics*, 21st ed. New York: McGraw-Hill; 2001:341.

88. You perform a Pap smear on a 48-year-old woman and the results reveal the presence of benign appearing endometrial cells. She reports no vaginal bleeding or any other associated symptoms. Appropriate management consists of
A) endometrial biopsy
B) ultrasound examination of the uterus
C) dilation and curettage
D) colposcopy
E) no further evaluation

Answer and Discussion

The answer is E. Endometrial cancer is a relatively common gynecologic malignancy in the United States. Despite recent advances, approximately 6,000 deaths result from endometrial cancer each year. Several studies have suggested a correlation between endometrial cells (both normal and abnormal) on Papanicolaou smears and endometrial cancer, mainly in postmenopausal women. Kerpsack and associates conducted a study to evaluate a possible correlation between the presence of endometrial cells on a Pap smear and significant endometrial pathology. The study concludes that asymptomatic patients who have benign endometrial cells on a Pap smear but no abnormal vaginal bleeding do not require further evaluation. However, even if the endometrial cells are described as benign, a patient with abnormal vaginal bleeding should receive further evaluation with dilatation and curettage.

Kerpsack JT, Finan MA, Kline RC. Correlation between endometrial cells on Papanicolaou smear and endometrial carcinoma. *South Med J.* 1998;91:749–752.

89. A 56-year-old woman presents for her well-woman exam. She has been seen yearly for the last 10 years and is otherwise healthy. She has not had an abnormal Pap smear and is in a monogamous relationship with her husband of 30 years. She inquires about her Pap smear. An appropriate response is

A) A yearly Pap smear is necessary in her age group because of the risk of cervical cancer.
B) Pap smears are no longer required for women in her age group.
C) An appropriate interval for repeat Pap smear screening is 5 years.
D) An appropriate interval for Pap smear screening is 3 years.
E) She would need a repeat Pap smear only if she had another sexual partner.

Answer and Discussion

The answer is D. Annual cervical cancer screening in women with three previously normal Pap smears provides a negligible benefit, and the screening interval may be extended safely to every 3 years in this low-risk group.

Sawaya GF, et al. Risk of cervical cancer associated with extending the interval between cervical-cancer screenings. *N Engl J Med.* 2003;349:1501–1509.

90. Live virus vaccines, such as measles, mumps, and rubella, should be administered to pregnant women

A) at the first prenatal visit following conception
B) at least 3 months before conception
C) during the third trimester
D) at 18 to 20 weeks' gestation

Answer and Discussion

The answer is B. Immunizations with live attenuated vaccines, such as measles, mumps, rubella, varicella, and the oral vaccine for polio, are contraindicated in pregnancy and 3 months before conception. Immunizations with inactivated virus, such as influenza, *Pneumococcus,* tetanus, rabies, and the injectable poliovirus, as well as the hepatitis B recombinant vaccine, are safe to administer.

Cunningham FG, Gant NF, Leveno KJ, et al. *Williams Obstetrics*, 21st ed. New York: McGraw-Hill; 2001:241.

91. Women immunized for rubella should be counseled to avoid pregnancy for

A) 1 month
B) 3 months
C) 6 months
D) 1 year
E) Rubella immunization presents no dangers before or during pregnancy.

Answer and Discussion

The answer is B. Rubella ("German measles") is a highly contagious childhood disease that can affect pregnant mothers. As many as 15% of mothers do not have antibodies to the rubella virus. Symptoms include fever, cough, and conjunctivitis. Other symptoms include headaches, malaise, myalgias, arthralgias, and postauricular and suboccipital lymphadenopathy. An erythematous morbilliform rash usually develops on the face and spreads inferiorly. Generally, the symptoms of rubella are less severe than those of rubeola, and there is usually no prodrome seen with rubella (unlike with rubeola). Spontaneous abortion occurs two to four times more frequently in pregnancies that are complicated by rubella. Transmission to the fetus occurs by direct infection. If the woman is affected during the first trimester, the risk of birth defects is higher than if she is affected during the last two trimesters. Effects of the virus on the fetus (congenital rubella syndrome) include cataracts, glaucoma, blindness, cardiac abnormalities, deafness, mental retardation, cerebral palsy, growth retardation, hemolytic anemia, and cleft palate. In cases of maternal rubella, therapeutic abortion can be considered if infection occurs in the first two trimesters. All women should receive routine rubella testing during pregnancy. If negative the patient should be vaccinated during the immediate postpartum period. Women who are immunized with the live attenuated virus should not become pregnant for 3 months following immunization. The use of immune globulin for pregnant women who are exposed to rubella is not recommended.

Cunningham FG, Gant NF, Leveno KJ, et al. *Williams Obstetrics*, 21st ed. New York: McGraw-Hill; 2001:1467.

92. An 18-year-old woman presents to your office complaining of irregular periods. On examination, she is found to be obese, has evidence of excessive facial hair, and reports that her mother had similar problems. Laboratory studies show normal estrogen levels, increased luteinizing hormone, low follicle-stimulating hormone, elevated testosterone level, and elevated urinary 17-ketosteroids. The most likely diagnosis is

A) pregnancy
B) Cushing's disease
C) polycystic ovary syndrome
D) adrenal adenoma
E) acromegaly

Answer and Discussion

The answer is C. Polycystic ovary syndrome (Stein-Leventhal syndrome) is an inherited condition characterized by cystic ovaries, hirsutism, amenorrhea, and obesity. It is the most common cause of anovulation and hirsutism. Some patients present with primary amenorrhea, some have abnormal irregular periods, and some have normal periods. Laboratory studies show normal or increased levels of estrogen, increased luteinizing hormone, normal or decreased follicle-stimulating hormone, normal or increased testosterone, and increased urinary 17-ketosteroids. Pelvic ultrasound can also aid in the diagnosis by demonstrating bilateral enlargement of the ovaries. Administration of progesterone usually results in withdrawal bleeding for patients with amenorrhea. Glucose intolerance with increased insulin levels may also be present. Therapy includes the use of oral contraceptives to suppress hirsutism and small doses of glucocorticoid (dexamethasone) at bedtime to suppress the adrenal gland. Bromocriptine has shown some benefit for the menstrual irregularities and hirsutism. Antiandrogens can be combined with oral contraceptive pills for the treatment of hirsutism. If used alone, antiandrogens may produce irregular uterine bleeding. The most commonly used antiandrogens are spironolactone (Aldactone), flutamide (Eulexin), and cyproterone (Cyprostat). These agents should not be used in pregnant women. Spironolactone, in a dosage of 25 to 100 mg administered twice a day, is the most commonly used antiandrogen because of its safety, availability, and low cost. Flutamide is usually given in a dosage of 250 mg twice a day, and cyproterone is given in a dosage of 25 to 50 mg/day for 10 days each month.

GnRH analogs such as luprolide (Lupron) should be reserved for use in women who do not respond to combination hormonal therapy or cannot tolerate oral contraceptive pills. The GnRH analogs should be used cautiously, with particular attention given to long-term consequences (e.g., hot flushes, bone demineralization, atrophic vaginitis) that can occur secondary to hypoestrogenemia induced by these agents. Surgery (wedge resection of the ovary) has also been shown to restore ovulatory periods and fertility.

Hunter MH, Sterrett JJ. Polycystic ovary syndrome: it's not just infertility. *Am Fam Physician*. 2000;62:1079–1088, 1090.

93. A 48-year-old otherwise healthy woman has undergone a hysterectomy secondary to abnormal vaginal bleeding. Pathology results confirm no evidence of malignancy. She asks you how often she should have a Pap smear. The appropriate response is

A) yearly Pap smears for an additional 3 years are recommended
B) Pap smears should be reinstituted if she develops atrophic vaginitis
C) Pap smears should be repeated every 3 years
D) Pap smears should be performed every 5 years
E) no further Pap smears are necessary

Answer and Discussion

The answer is E. Multiple studies have concluded that vaginal cuff smear testing is not necessary in women who have undergone hysterectomy for benign conditions.

Videlefsky A, Grossl N, Denniston M. Routine vaginal cuff smear testing in post-hysterectomy patients with benign uterine conditions: when is it indicated? *J Am Board Fam Pract*. 2001;13:233–238.

94. A Pap smear result shows atypical cells of undetermined significance (ACS-US). HPV typing is negative for high-risk HPV. Appropriate management at this time includes

A) repeat Pap smear at one year
B) repeat Pap smear at 6 months
C) colposcopy
D) LEEP procedure
E) cervical cryotherapy

Answer and Discussion

The answer is A. Women with ACS-US who test negative for high-risk HPV types can have repeat cytology at 12 months. Colposcopy is recommended for women who test positive for oncogenic HPV types. If initial colposcopy does not identify a lesion, repeating the cytology at 6 and 12 months is acceptable. If the woman is HPV-positive and repeat cytology still reveals ASC-US or greater, repeat colposcopy is recommended. It is also acceptable to perform repeat HPV DNA testing at 12 months and refer the patient for colposcopy if oncogenic HPV types persist.

Wright TC Jr, Cox JT, Massad LS, et al. 2001 Consensus guidelines for the management of women with cervical cytological abnormalities. *JAMA*. 2002;287:2120–2129.

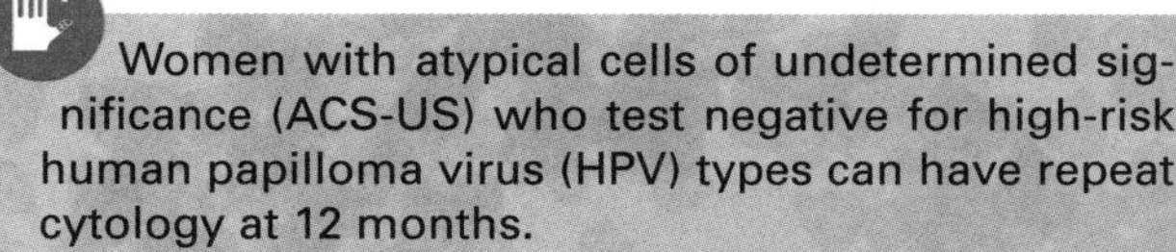

95. Which of the following is the most common cause of postpartum hemorrhage?

A) Uterine atony
B) Uterine rupture
C) Lacerations of the cervix
D) Retained placenta
E) Primagravida birth

Answer and Discussion

The answer is A. Postpartum hemorrhage is conventionally defined as the loss of >500 mL of blood after delivery. It occurs in approximately 4% of deliveries. The following are the most common causes of postpartum hemorrhage:

- Uterine atony: lack of contraction of the uterus after delivery; the most common cause
- Lacerations of the vagina, cervix, or perineum especially after a difficult or forceps delivery
- Hematomas: usually seen in association with lacerations
- Uterine rupture: seen in patients with fibroids, hyperstimulation of the uterus with oxytocin (Pitocin), or prolonged labor
- Retained placenta: seen in cases in which delayed hemorrhage occurs
- Uterine inversion
- Coagulation disorders
- Low placental implantation

Resuscitation with normal saline usually requires three times the volume of the estimated blood loss. It is best not to use glucose-containing fluids.

Cunningham FG, Gant NF, Leveno KJ, et al. *Williams Obstetrics*, 21st ed. New York: McGraw-Hill; 2001:635–652.

96. The most common cause of galactorrhea is

A) psychotropic medication
B) hypothyroidism
C) prolactinoma
D) nipple stimulation
E) sexual intercourse

Answer and Discussion

The answer is C. Galactorrhea is defined as the presence of lactation in the absence of pregnancy. It can occur in men and in women. The most common cause is a prolactinoma in the pituitary gland. Other causes include psychotropic medications, opioids, antihypertensive drugs (α-methyldopa), hypogonadism, nipple stimulation, bronchogenic carcinomas, herpes zoster, hypothyroidism, and trauma. Many women who are affected may also have amenorrhea. Diagnosis involves determination of prolactin levels and CT scanning or MRI scans of the sella turcica to exclude pituitary adenomas. Visual field defects may also be present if tumors impinge on the optic chiasm. Other testing may be necessary to exclude other precipitating causes, such as medication-induced hyperprolactinemia. Patients who are affected with small microadenomas can be treated with bromocriptine;

however, those with macroadenomas are usually treated with surgery or radiation.

Beers MH, Porter RS, eds. *The Merck manual of diagnosis and therapy*, Merck Research Laboratories, 18th ed. Whitehouse Station, NJ: Merck & Co.; 2006:1187–1189.

97. The definition of *dyspareunia* is
A) painful intercourse
B) abnormal hip alignment
C) disturbed pelvic sensation
D) altered menstrual cycles
E) difficult labor

Answer and Discussion

The answer is A. Dyspareunia is painful intercourse, and the causes can be organic or psychogenic. Organic causes include inflammatory diseases of the vulva or vagina; infections, including fungal, bacterial, and viral (herpes, condyloma); tight-fitting clothes; a contracted vaginal orifice (caused by scarring from previous episiotomy or trauma); atrophic vaginitis; lack of lubrication; foreign bodies; an intact or constricted hymen; or a reaction to chemicals that are involved in contraception, deodorant sprays, and douches. Other pelvic disorders, including pelvic infections, masses, or endometriosis, can lead to dyspareunia. Psychogenic causes may include fear, anxiety, disinterest, or previous abuse or rape. Treatment involves adequate lubrication, correction of organic causes, and psychotherapy and education for psychogenic causes.

Beers MH, Porter RS, eds. *The Merck manual of diagnosis and therapy*, Merck Research Laboratories, 18th ed. Whitehouse Station, NJ: Merck & Co.; 2006:2100–2101, 2104.

98. A Pap smear result comes back atypical cells of undetermined significance and the report cannot exclude high-grade intraepithelial lesion (ASC-H). Appropriate management at this time includes
A) repeat Pap smear at 1 year
B) repeat Pap smear at 6 months
C) colposcopy
D) LEEP procedure
E) cervical cryotherapy

Answer and Discussion

The answer is C. Although ASC-H is less common than ASC-US, the risk of underlying grade 2 or 3 CIN is higher and colposcopy is recommended. If CIN is identified by biopsy, management is based on the grade of the lesion. If no lesion is found on colposcopy, a review of the colposcopic, cytologic, and histologic findings is recommended. If the diagnosis remains the same after the review, repeat cytology at 6 and 12 months or HPV DNA testing at 12 months is acceptable. If the diagnosis changes, physicians should follow accepted management guidelines.

Wright TC Jr, Cox JT, Massad LS, et al. 2001 Consensus guidelines for the management of women with cervical cytological abnormalities. *JAMA.* 2002;287:2120–2129.

99. A 40-year-old woman's Pap smear result comes back atypical glandular cells–not otherwise specified (AGC-NOS). Appropriate management at this time includes
A) repeat Pap smear at 1 year
B) repeat Pap smear at 6 months
C) colposcopy
D) colposcopy and endometrial sampling
E) HPV testing and colposcopy only if high risk HPV identified

Answer and Discussion

The answer is D. The category of atypical glandular cells (AGC) is divided into "not otherwise specified" (AGC-NOS) and "favor neoplasia" or adenocarcinoma-in-situ (AIS). Although AGC is an uncommon cytologic diagnosis, up to 54% of women with AGC have an underlying SIL, 8% have AIS, and up to 9% may have an invasive squamous or adenocarcinoma. Cervical cytology has low sensitivity for detection of glandular lesions, and it is unknown if HPV DNA testing has a role in management of AGC. Therefore, colposcopy with endocervical sampling is recommended in women with all categories of AGC. Endometrial sampling at the time of colposcopy is recommended in women older than 35 years and in younger women with unexplained vaginal bleeding.

Wright TC Jr, Cox JT, Massad LS, et al. 2001 Consensus guidelines for the management of women with cervical cytological abnormalities. *J Lower Genital Tract Dis.* 2002;6:127–143.

100. When testing fetal well-being, which of the following factors is *not* measured with a biophysical profile?
A) Fetal tone
B) Amniotic fluid
C) Fetal heart rate
D) Fetal size
E) Body movements

Answer and Discussion

The answer is D. Biophysical profile testing is a more extensive method of testing fetal well-being than nonstress testing. Indications include the following:

- Maternal hypertension
- Maternal diabetes
- Postterm pregnancies
- Multiple gestations
- Oligohydramnios
- Intrauterine growth deficiencies
- Placental abnormalities
- Decreased fetal movement
- Previous abnormal pregnancies

The test involves the testing of five different aspects of fetal well-being with real-time ultrasound, including the following:

- Fetal breathing
- Body movements
- Fetal tone
- Amniotic fluid volume
- Fetal heart rate monitoring (nonstress test)

Each aspect is given either a score of 0 for abnormal findings or 2 for normal findings. A score of 4 or less is a poor prognostic indicator, whereas a score of 8 or 10 is reassuring for fetal well-being. A score of 6 is suspicious for chronic asphyxia.

Cunningham FG, Gant NF, Leveno KJ, et al. *Williams Obstetrics*, 21st ed. New York: McGraw-Hill; 2001:1104–1105.

101. The most sensitive method to diagnose endometrial cancer is with
A) Papanicolaou (Pap) smear
B) ultrasound

C) CT of the pelvis
D) endometrial biopsy
E) fractionated endometrial curettage

Answer and Discussion

The answer is E. Adenocarcinoma of the endometrium usually occurs in postmenopausal women between 50 and 60 years of age. It usually arises from the columnar cells of the endometrial lining. Associated conditions that constitute risk factors include adenomatous hyperplasia; unopposed estrogen use; delayed menopause; infertility (nulliparity); Stein-Leventhal syndrome; previous breast, colon, or ovarian cancer; diabetes; chronic tamoxifen use; hypertension; and obesity. The hallmark symptom is unexplained irregular vaginal bleeding, particularly in postmenopausal women. The diagnosis can be made with Pap smears in 40% of patients; however, because of the relatively high rate of false-negative results, diagnosis is better made with endometrial biopsy, ultrasound, or the gold standard fractionated endometrial curettage. Treatment involves surgical excision with total abdominal hysterectomy and bilateral oophorectomy followed by lymph node sampling. Chemotherapy using cytotoxic drugs as well as progesterone and radiation is also used in the treatment of endometrial cancer. Prognosis depends on the stage and differentiation of the cancer. Well-differentiated, well-localized tumors have a 5-year survival rate of close to 95%, whereas poorly differentiated tumors with metastasis have less than a 20% 5-year survival rate.

Kasper DL, Braunwald E, Fauci AS, et al., eds. *Harrison's principles of internal medicine*, 16th ed. New York: McGraw-Hill; 2005:556.

102. Which of the following is recommended for postpartum breast engorgement?
A) Firm binding of breast with a comfortable wrap
B) Cabbage leaves
C) Bromocriptine
D) Initiation of oral contraceptives
E) Topical vitamin E

Answer and Discussion

The answer is A. The best way to prevent postpartum breast engorgement is to bind the breasts firmly with a comfortable wrap. Other suggestions include cold packs, analgesics, and the avoidance of direct warm water during showering. The use of bromocriptine (a dopamine agonist) to stop lactation is associated with rebound lactation after discontinuation of the medication, hypotension, hypertension, seizures, and stroke; it is no longer approved by the U.S. Food and Drug Administration for this use. Other medications, such as estrogen and testosterone combinations, are not recommended because of their increased risk for thromboembolism and hair growth, respectively. In most cases, breast engorgement resolves within 72 hours.

Cunningham FG, Gant NF, Leveno KJ, et al. *Williams Obstetrics*, 21st ed. New York: McGraw-Hill; 2001:412.

103. A 38-year-old woman has a Pap smear result of atypical glandular cells (AGC)–favor neoplasia. She undergoes colposcopy and no invasive disease is found. Appropriate management at this time includes
A) repeat Pap smear at 1 year
B) repeat Pap smear at 6 months
C) repeat colposcopy at 6 months
D) LEEP procedure
E) cold-knife conization procedure

Answer and Discussion

The answer is E. The category of atypical glandular cells (AGC) is divided into "not otherwise specified" (AGC-NOS) and "favor neoplasia" or adenocarcinoma-in-situ (AIS). Women with AGC-favor neoplasia or AIS who are not found to have invasive disease on initial colposcopic evaluation should undergo a diagnostic excisional procedure, preferably cold-knife conization to avoid thermal artifact from the loop electrosurgical excision procedure, which may preclude a diagnosis.

Geier CS, Wilson M, Creasman W. Clinical evaluation of atypical glandular cells of undetermined significance. *Am J Obstet Gynecol.* 2001;184:64–69.

104. Which of the following medications is associated with an increased risk of endometrial carcinoma?
A) Bromocriptine (Parlodel)
B) Oral contraceptives
C) Progesterone
D) Alendronate (Fosamax)
E) Tamoxifen (Nolvadex)

Answer and Discussion

The answer is E. Risk factors for endometrial cancer include anovulatory cycles, obesity, nulliparity, age greater than 35 years, unopposed estrogen use, and tamoxifen therapy.

Ries LA, Eisner MP, Kosary CL, et al., eds. *SEER cancer statistics review, 1975–2000.* Bethesda, MD: National Cancer Institute, 2003. Accessed December, 12, 2004, at http://seer.cancer.gov/csr/1975_2000.

Risk factors for endometrial cancer include anovulatory cycles, obesity, nulliparity, age greater than 35 years, unopposed estrogen use, and tamoxifen therapy.

105. Which of the following is an absolute contraindication of tocolysis?
A) Chorioamnionitis
B) 4-cm cervical dilation
C) Biophysical profile score of 8
D) Oligohydramnios
E) Hyperthyroidism

Answer and Discussion

The answer is A. The arresting of labor has certain contraindications that must be ruled out before tocolytics are given. Absolute contraindications include the following:

- Severe abruptio placentae
- Infection (chorioamnionitis)
- Severe bleeding
- Severe pregnancy-induced hypertension
- Fetal anomalies that are incompatible with life
- Fetal death
- Severe growth retardation
- Fetal distress

Relative contraindications include the following:

- Hyperthyroidism
- Uncontrolled diabetes
- Maternal heart disease
- Hypertension
- Mild abruptio placentae
- Stable placenta previa
- Fetal distress
- Mild growth retardation
- Cervical dilation greater than 5 to 6 cm

Corticosteroids are recommended to help prevent RDS if there is premature rupture of membranes before 34 weeks' gestation. Delay of labor for >1 week after rupture of membranes is usually not recommended unless the fetus is very small (<1,250 g).

DeCherney AH, Nathan L. *Current Obstetric and Gynecologic Diagnosis and Treatment*, 9th ed. New York: Lange/McGraw-Hill; 2003:288.

106. When testing fetal well-being, which of the following statements about the nonstress test is true?

A) Two or more fetal heart accelerations (at least 15 beats above baseline) that last for 15 seconds in a 20-minute period are reassuring.
B) Late decelerations are usually noted with fetal movements.
C) An abnormal nonstress test should be followed by a contraction stress test.
D) The presence of oligohydramnios is accurately predicted with the results of a nonstress test.
E) Nonstress tests should be routinely performed beginning at 38 weeks until delivery.

Answer and Discussion

The answer is A. Nonstress tests are used for antenatal well-being studies. Nonstress testing includes the use of a fetal heart monitor and contraction monitor. Testing is usually reserved for difficult problem pregnancies (e.g., intrauterine growth retardation, gestational diabetes, pregnancy-induced hypertension, multiple gestations, previous difficulties in childbirth) or postdate pregnancy. A reassuring nonstress test shows two or more fetal movements with a fetal heart rate acceleration of at least 15 beats/sec above the baseline that last for at least 15 seconds during a 20-minute period. If this criterion is not met, a biophysical profile should be performed. Late or variable decelerations are concerning findings. Oligohydramnios is a risk for cord compression but is not well predicted by nonstress testing. Simplistically, the nonstress test is primarily a test of fetal well-being, whereas the contraction stress test is a test of uteroplacental function.

Cunningham FG, Gant NF, Leveno KJ, et al. *Williams Obstetrics*, 21st ed. New York: McGraw-Hill; 2001:1100–1102.

107. RhoGAM should be given to Rh-negative mothers at

A) first prenatal visit and at delivery
B) 12 and 36 weeks' gestation
C) 16 weeks' gestation and delivery
D) 28 weeks' gestation and delivery
E) 28 and 36 weeks' gestation

Answer and Discussion

The answer is D. The condition of erythroblastosis fetalis is the result of blood incompatibility between the mother and fetus. It results when an Rh-negative woman is impregnated by an Rh-positive man. Red blood cells (RBCs) cross the placenta into the mother's bloodstream and evoke the production of her antibodies to the child's RBCs. The antibodies can cross the placenta and result in severe anemia that may cause death to the fetus. To compensate, the fetal bone marrow releases immature RBCs and erythroblasts (thus, the name *erythroblastosis fetalis*). The condition rarely affects the first pregnancy, and the risk for sensitization increases with each pregnancy. As a result of the antibody destruction of RBCs, there is an increased production of bilirubin that can result in kernicterus, which is characterized by poor feeding, apnea, poor fetal tone, mental retardation, seizures, and death. In the United States, approximately 15% of marriages involve Rh-positive fathers and Rh-negative mothers, but the potential may be underestimated because of the number of children who are born out of wedlock with unknown fathers. Of this 15%, only 1 in 27 are affected with erythroblastosis fetalis. Prevention of the disease is accomplished by administering RhoGAM, an anti-Rh antibody, to the mother. RhoGAM attacks and destroys the fetal blood cells when they cross the placenta, before they can involve the production of antibodies. RhoGAM is administered at 28 weeks' gestation and then at the time of delivery. It should also be given if abortion or ectopic pregnancy occurs or in any case in which there is fetal–maternal transfer of blood. All mothers should be screened for Rh status at their initial prenatal visit.

Beers MH, Porter RS, eds. *The Merck manual of diagnosis and therapy*, Merck Research Laboratories, 18th ed. Whitehouse Station, NJ: Merck & Co.; 2006:2194–2195.

108. A 17-year-old woman presents to your office complaining of dysfunctional uterine bleeding. Appropriate management consists of

A) endometrial sampling
B) ultrasound examination of the uterus
C) endometrial sampling and ultrasound evaluation
D) dilation and curettage
E) use of oral contraceptives and observation

Answer and Discussion

The answer is E. Endometrial cancer is rare in 15- to 18-year-old women. Therefore, most adolescents with dysfunctional uterine bleeding can be treated safely with hormone therapy and observation, without diagnostic testing.

Elford KJ, Spence JE. The forgotten female: pediatric and adolescent gynecological concerns and their reproductive consequences. *J Pediatr Adolesc Gynecol.* 2002;15:65–77.

109. In treating atrophic vaginitis, which of the following statements is true?

A) In women with an intact uterus, progestin treatment is not needed for short-term local estrogen treatment.
B) Current breast cancer is not a contraindication for topical estrogens.
C) Topical estrogen can be used in women with a history of endometrial cancer.
D) Topical estrogen can be used during breast feeding.
E) Postmenopausal bleeding during use of topical estrogen can be observed.

Answer and Discussion

The answer is A. Vaginal estrogen therapy is indicated for short-term (6 months or less) treatment of symptoms related to vaginal atrophy in postmenopausal women. In women with an intact uterus, progestin treatment is not needed for short-term local estrogen treatment. However, data are limited about the use of local estrogen therapy for longer than 6 months. Patients should not be prescribed vaginal estrogens if they have undiagnosed vaginal bleeding, current breast cancer, history of endometrial cancer, or a thromboembolic disorder, or are pregnant or breastfeeding. Local estrogen therapy should be used with caution in patients with impaired liver function. Postmenopausal bleeding in women using local estrogen therapy should be evaluated as in any other postmenopausal patient. Manufacturers of topical estrogens available in the United States recommend limiting treatment to 3 to 6 months. However, many physicians prescribe vaginal estrogens for periods much longer than 3 to 6 months, but data on long-term safety are lacking. Further trials that provide data on long-term safety of local estrogen therapy are needed.

Willhite LA, O'Connell MB. Urogenital atrophy: prevention and treatment. *Pharmacotherapy*. 2001;21:464–480.

110. Fibroid tumors can be associated with which of the following conditions?
A) Amenorrhea
B) Renal lithiasis
C) Postpartum hemorrhage
D) Increased risk of ovarian carcinoma
E) Increased risk for endometrial hyperplasia

Answer and Discussion

The answer is C. Fibroid tumors are irregular enlargements of the uterus. They are the most common benign tumors of the female genital tract, with as many as 20% of 40-year-old women affected. The tumors are composed of smooth muscle and connective tissue. In most cases, the condition is asymptomatic; however, it can cause dysmenorrhea with heavy menstrual blood loss leading to anemia and irregular periods. Occasionally, the fibroids degenerate, giving rise to intense pelvic pain and the development of pelvic infections. In some cases, infertility can occur when a fibroma blocks the fallopian tube. Other complications include difficult pregnancies with dystocia and excessive postpartum hemorrhage and urinary frequency or difficulty in defecating when the tumors press on the bladder or colon. Diagnosis is usually made with ultrasound, CT scan, MRI, or hysteroscopy. Treatment involves GnRH analogs (leuprolide), which may decrease the size of the fibroid; however, regrowth often occurs after the medication is discontinued. For severe cases, surgery, including myomectomy or hysterectomy, may be indicated. Treatment with estrogen can produce growth of the tumors and worsening of symptoms.

DeCherney AH, Nathan L. *Current Obstetric and Gynecologic Diagnosis and Treatment*, 9th ed. New York: Lange/McGraw-Hill; 2003:693–699.

111. The most appropriate medication for the treatment of pyelonephritis in pregnancy is
A) ampicillin + gentamicin
B) trimethoprim–sulfamethoxazole
C) tetracycline
D) nitrofurantoin
E) ciprofloxacin

Answer and Discussion

The answer is A. Pyelonephritis is one of the most common serious complications in pregnancy. It occurs in approximately 2% of pregnancies and more frequently in the third trimester. Symptoms include fever, chills, dysuria, flank pain, nausea, vomiting, and malaise. Treatment of choice is ampicillin or cefazolin, with the possible addition of an aminoglycoside (gentamicin) for severe cases. Sulfonamides are contraindicated in the third trimester of pregnancy because of the risk of kernicterus in newborns. Quinolone antibiotics (e.g., ciprofloxacin) interfere with cartilage development and should be avoided. Tetracyclines are contraindicated because they can cause yellowish discoloration in the child's teeth. Nitrofurantoin is used frequently in pregnancy but can induce hemolysis in patients who are deficient in glucose-6-phosphate dehydrogenase (G6PD; affects approximately 2% of African Americans). Treatment of pyelonephritis is necessary because of the increased risk of premature labor. All pregnant patients with pyelonephritis should be hospitalized, and periodic fetal monitoring should be instituted. Follow-up cultures are indicated to ensure eradication.

DeCherney AH, Nathan L. *Current Obstetric and Gynecologic Diagnosis and Treatment*, 9th ed. New York: Lange/McGraw-Hill; 2003:422–423.

112. Which of the following tests is indicated at the time of the first prenatal visit in a healthy mother?
A) α-Fetoprotein testing
B) Quantitative β-HCG
C) Antibody test (indirect Coomb's test)
D) Glucose tolerance test
E) Sensitive thyroid-stimulating hormone

Answer and Discussion

The answer is C. Prenatal testing is usually performed at the initial prenatal visit. Tests include Pap smear, complete blood count, urinalysis with culture, ABO blood type, Rh status, antibody test (indirect Coombs' test), rubella antibody titer, VDRL, and hepatitis B surface antigen. Other tests may include cervical cultures for chlamydia and gonorrhea, tuberculosis skin test, sickle cell prep, cytomegalovirus titers, and toxoplasmosis, and HIV testing should be offered to all patients. α-fetoprotein testing is usually done at 15 to 18 weeks' gestation, glucola test at 24 to 28 weeks' gestation, hematocrit determination at 28 to 32 weeks' gestation, and Rh antibody screening if indicated at 36 weeks' gestation. Patients at high risk for sexually transmitted diseases may need repeated cultures later in pregnancy. Routine ultrasound examination is controversial, but is generally performed in most pregnancies.

Cunningham FG, Gant NF, Leveno KJ, et al. *Williams Obstetrics*, 21st ed. New York: McGraw-Hill; 2001:86–87.

113. Which of the following would support the diagnosis of menopause in a woman taking no medications?
A) Vaginal pH >4.5
B) FSH level <10 mIU/mL
C) Endometrial cells noted on Pap smear
D) TSH >5.6
E) Progesterone >10 ng/dL

Answer and Discussion

The answer is A. A vaginal pH >4.5 indicates menopause in women who are without vaginitis and are not receiving estrogen therapy. Studies have shown that vaginal pH is similar to FSH levels in establishing the diagnosis of low estrogen levels or menopause, and that a vaginal pH of 4.5 or less can be used to monitor adequate response to estrogen replacement therapy. Bacterial vaginosis can also cause a vaginal pH to be >4.5.

Roy S, Caillouette JC, Roy T. Vaginal pH is similar to follicle-stimulating hormone for menopause diagnosis. *Am J Obstet Gynecol*. 2004;190:1272–1277.

114. Which of the following is an absolute contraindication for the use of oral contraceptives in women over the age of 35?

A) Family history of stroke
B) Hypertension without vascular disease
C) Mild hyperlipidemia
D) Diabetes with neuropathy
E) Smoker (<10 cigarettes/day)

Answer and Discussion

The answer is D. Risks associated with combination oral contraceptive pills (OCPs) may limit their use in women older than 35 years of age. Most concerns are based on early studies of oral contraceptive formulations with a high ethinyl estradiol content, rather than more recent studies of lower dose formulations. Although use of OCPs increases the risk of venous thromboembolism, the degree of risk appears to be the same in women taking formulations that contain 20 to 35 mcg of estrogen. The absolute risk of venous thromboembolism is very low (1 case per 10,000 OCP users per year). Oral contraceptive pills also contain progestins, including desogestrel and gestodene. These two progestins have been associated with an increased risk of venous thromboembolism. The risk of myocardial infarction may be increased in women using OCPs, especially if smoking (>10 cigarettes per day) or other cardiovascular risk factors are present. The association between OCP use and ischemic stroke is not clear, although increased risk has been demonstrated in OCP users who have migraines. There is no documentation of an increased risk of breast cancer in women who use OCPs. One study has found a slightly increased risk of gallstones, although the risk was lower in women older than 35 years of age than in younger women. The potential benefits of OCP use in women older than 35 years of age include effective birth control, reduced risk of ovarian and endometrial cancers, possible reduced risk of colon cancer, improvement of perimenopausal symptoms, improvement of acne, and increased bone mineral density (although improved fracture rates have not yet been demonstrated). Before use of OCPs is initiated, a thorough medical history should be obtained and blood pressure should be measured. If a patient has risk factors for cardiovascular disease or a family history of dyslipidemia, a routine fasting lipid panel is recommended. Mild lipid abnormalities do not contraindicate use of OCPs, but lipid levels should be monitored. Because OCPs can increase blood pressure, they should be prescribed with caution in patients with mild hypertension and patients who smoke. Absolute contraindications include:

- Pregnancy
- Postpartum less than 6 weeks and breastfeeding
- Age more than 35 years and heavy smoker (>15 cigarettes per day)
- Systolic blood pressure >160 mm Hg, diastolic blood pressure greater than 99 mm Hg
- Hypertension with vascular disease
- Diabetes with neuropathy, retinopathy, nephropathy, or vascular disease
- History of deep venous thrombosis or pulmonary embolism
- Major surgery with prolonged immobilization
- History of ischemic heart disease
- History of stroke
- Complicated valvular disease (with atrial fibrillation, pulmonary hypertension, bacterial endocarditis)
- Severe headaches with focal neurologic symptoms
- Current breast cancer
- Active viral hepatitis, severe cirrhosis, benign or malignant liver tumors

The best OCP in women over 35 is the one with the lowest effective estrogen dose. Side effects are most common during the first 3 months. The most frequent adverse effects are abnormal menstrual bleeding, nausea, weight gain, mood changes, breast tenderness, and headache. Follow-up should include annual blood pressure measurements, lipid profiles in patients with a baseline abnormality, and a review of symptoms that could signify an important adverse effect. Breakthrough bleeding is common and usually resolves spontaneously after a few months. The incidence of breakthrough bleeding appears to be higher with formulations containing lower estrogen doses.

Seibert C, Barbouche E, Fagan J. Prescribing oral contraceptives for women older than 35 years of age. *Ann Intern Med*. 2003;138:54–64.

> The potential benefits of oral contraceptive pill (OCP) use in women older than 35 years of age include effective birth control, reduced risk of ovarian and endometrial cancers, possible reduced risk of colon cancer, improvement of perimenopausal symptoms, improvement of acne, and increased bone mineral density (although improved fracture rates have not yet been demonstrated).

115. Which of the following is associated with preeclampsia?

A) Blood pressure elevations of 30 mm Hg systolic or 15 mm Hg diastolic over baseline
B) Trace proteinuria
C) Mild edema
D) Seizures
E) Scotomata

Answer and Discussion

The answer is A. Preeclampsia is defined as follows:

- Hypertension (>90 mm Hg diastolic and >140 mm Hg systolic after 20 weeks on two separate occasions taken 6 hours apart; also blood pressure elevations of 30 mm Hg systolic or 15 mm Hg diastolic over baseline)
- Proteinuria (>300 mg/24 hours or 1+ on urine dipstick)
- Other laboratory abnormalities: increased uric acid, thrombocytopenia, and elevated liver function test

Note: Edema has been removed from the criteria

Risk factors include age younger than 20 or older than 40 years, primigravid state, previous preeclampsia, twin pregnancy, diabetes mellitus, hydatidiform mole, fetal hydrops, or chronic hypertension. *Eclampsia* is defined as the above criteria plus the development of seizures that cannot be attributed to other causes. Warning signs for the development of eclampsia may include severe headache, scotomas, blurred vision, and vomiting. HELLP syndrome (*h*emolysis, *e*levated *l*iver function tests, and *l*ow *p*latelets) may also occur.

DeCherney AH, Nathan L. *Current Obstetric and Gynecologic Diagnosis and Treatment*, 9th ed. New York: Lange/McGraw-Hill; 2003:338–349.

116. Gestational diabetic screening during pregnancy should take place
A) at the first prenatal visit
B) at 12 to 16 weeks' gestation
C) at 24 to 28 weeks' gestation
D) at 30 to 34 weeks' gestation
E) randomly throughout pregnancy

Answer and Discussion

The answer is C. Diabetes during pregnancy is associated with a number of abnormalities that affect the fetus, including increased risk of spontaneous abortion, congenital anomalies (e.g., neural tube defects, cardiac defects, skeletal abnormalities, malformations of the intestinal and urinary tract), and fetal macrosomia. White's criteria are used to classify gestational diabetes:

- *A1*: gestational diabetes not requiring insulin
- *A2*: gestational diabetes requiring insulin
- *B*: onset in a patient older than 20 years of age or lasting less than 10 years
- *C*: onset at 10 to 20 years of age or duration of 10 to 20 years
- *D*: onset in patients younger than 10 years of age or duration of more than 20 years
- *F*: nephropathy
- *R*: proliferative retinopathy or vitreous hemorrhage
- *H*: atherosclerotic heart disease that is clinically evident
- *T*: renal transplant

Risk factors for gestational diabetes include maternal age older than 35 years, obesity, positive family history of diabetes, and prior history of gestational diabetes. All pregnant women should be screened for diabetes between weeks 24 and 28 of gestation with the glucola (1-hour 50-g oral glucose) screening test. If values are >140 mg/dL, a 3-hour glucose tolerance test should be performed. In patients with White's classification A2 to D, periodic monitoring with contraction stress testing is recommended. Although most women experience a resolution of diabetes immediately postpartum, they are at increased risk of developing type II diabetes mellitus later in life.

Cunningham FG, Gant NF, Leveno KJ, et al. *Williams Obstetrics*, 21st ed. New York: McGraw-Hill; 2001:1361.

117. Which of the following test results is associated with pregnancy?
A) Increased white blood cell count
B) Decreased alkaline phosphatase
C) Increased hemoglobin
D) Decreased lactic dehydrogenase
E) Decreased fibrinogen level

Answer and Discussion

The answer is A. Many laboratory values are affected during pregnancy:

- Hemoglobin/hematocrit: decreased
- White blood cell count: increased
- Fibrinogen level: increased
- Erythrocyte sedimentation rate: increased
- Albumin level: decreased
- Fasting blood glucose: decreased
- Lactic dehydrogenase: increased
- Creatinine phosphokinase: increased
- Alkaline phosphatase: increased
- Calcium (total): decreased
- Cortisol: increased
- Prolactin: increased
- Thyroxine total: increased

Mild glycosuria and proteinuria are also common during pregnancy. Excessive amounts should prompt for further evaluation to rule out gestational diabetes and preeclampsia.

Cunningham FG, Gant NF, Leveno KJ, et al. *Williams Obstetrics*, 21st ed. New York: McGraw-Hill; 2001:143–163.

118. Studies have shown that the use of depot medroxyprogesterone acetate (DMPA) contraception is associated with
A) accelerated bone loss
B) increased migraines
C) increased endometrial cancer
D) increased pregnancy risk
E) increased teratogenicity in future pregnancies

Answer and Discussion

The answer is A. Depot medroxyprogesterone acetate (DMPA) use for 12 months or more is associated with a loss of bone mineral density, whereas oral contraceptive use is associated with gains in bone strength. This effect is likely related to low serum levels of ethinyl estradiol and the finding calls for further studies.

Berenson AB, Radecki CM, Grady JJ. A prospective, controlled study of the effects of hormonal contraception on bone mineral density. *Obstet Gynecol.* 2001;98:576–582.

119. Which of the following tests would support the diagnosis of polycystic ovary syndrome (PCOS)?
A) Low dehydroepiandrosterone sulfate (DHEAS) levels
B) Low androstenedione levels
C) Low free testosterone levels
D) LH to FSH ratio of 3:1
E) Fasting glucose to insulin level >4.5

Answer and Discussion

The answer is D. Although there is no agreement as to which laboratory tests should be used to diagnose polycystic ovary syndrome (PCOS), most experts agree that the evaluation should screen for hyperandrogenemia as well as for abnormalities that have serious consequences. Often, the presentation is readily apparent from the history and physical findings. Elevated bioavailable (free) testosterone levels may support the diagnosis, especially in a nonhirsute woman with other signs and symptoms of PCOS. Hyperandrogenemia also might be established by elevated serum levels of dehydroepiandrosterone sulfate (DHEAS) and androstenedione. Both free testosterone and sex hormone-binding globulin may be useful in monitoring the efficacy of androgen suppression therapy. Total testosterone levels greater than 20 ng/dL (0.7 nmol/L) or DHEAS levels greater than 700 ng/mL (1.9 μmol/L) are suggestive of androgen-secreting tumors; these patients should be referred for further gynecologic investigation. Morning 17a-hydroxyprogesterone (17-OHP) determination is important to exclude nonclassic adrenal hyperplasia secondary to 21-hydroxylase deficiency. When elevated 17-OHP is discovered, the next step should be a short adrenocorticotropic hormone stimulation test to further delineate the enzymatic defect. The ratio of LH to FSH is greater than 3:1 in about 30% of women with PCOS and may be diagnostically helpful in nonhirsute women with mild ovulatory dysfunction. Because nearly 30% of women with PCOS have impaired glucose tolerance, determinations of glucose tolerance and insulin resistance are of major importance. One approach is to perform standard oral glucose tolerance testing with insulin levels. Peak levels of insulin >100 μU/mL (718 pmol/L) are suggestive of insulin resistance. A more efficient assessment may be to use the ratio of fasting levels of glucose to insulin. When <4.5, this ratio has a significant correlation with insulin resistance and has been studied for use as a screening test in obese patients with PCOS. Assessments of total, HDL, and LDL cholesterol levels as well as triglyceride levels may assist in planning and follow-up of recommended dietary modifications to reduce obesity and cardiovascular risk. Finally, endometrial biopsy is helpful to rule out endometrial hyperplasia in patients with prolonged amenorrhea (more than 5 months).

Legro RS, Finegood D, Dunaif A. A fasting glucose to insulin ratio is a useful measure of insulin sensitivity in women with polycystic ovary syndrome. *J Clin Endocrinol Metab*. 1998;83:2694–2698.

Richardson M. Current perspectives in polycystic ovary syndrome. *Am Fam Physician*. 2003;68:697–704.

120. Which of the following is the most common endocrinopathy among women of reproductive age?
A) Diabetes mellitus
B) Hypothyroidism
C) Cushing's syndrome
D) Addison's disease
E) Polycystic ovary syndrome (PCOS)

Answer and Discussion

The answer is E. PCOS is the most common endocrinopathy among women of reproductive age and is estimated to affect up to 10% of the U.S. population.

Hull MG. Epidemiology of infertility and polycystic ovarian disease: endocrinological and demographic studies. *Gynecol Endocrinol*. 1987;1:235–245.

121. Which of the following medications is used in polycystic ovary syndrome to restore menstrual cyclicity and induce ovulation?
A) Bromocriptine (Parlodel)
B) Misoprostol (Cytotec)
C) Rosiglitazone (Avandia)
D) Metformin (Glucophage)
E) Bupropion (Wellbutrin)

Answer and Discussion

The answer is D. Metformin (Glucophage), a biguanide and insulin-sensitizing agent, has been used to restore menstrual cyclicity and induce ovulation in PCOS without the use of additional fertility drugs. Use of this agent is associated with reductions in serum levels of bioavailable androgen, LH, and atherogenic lipids. Metformin is presently classified as a category "B" risk in pregnancy, which indicates that there are no apparent fetal defects associated with its use in the late trimester of pregnancy, based on animal studies. Because the human effects of first-trimester use are unknown, discontinuation of therapy at the onset of pregnancy confirmation has been standard. However, a recent prospective study of women with PCOS who continued metformin therapy through the first trimester of pregnancy showed no evidence of fetal harm, calling into question this recommendation. Metformin therapy is associated with a slight risk of lactic acidosis and is not used in patients with impaired liver or renal function.

Velazquez EM, Mendoza S, Hamer T, et al. Metformin therapy in polycystic ovary syndrome reduces hyperinsulinemia, insulin resistance, hyperandrogenemia, and systolic blood pressure, while facilitating normal menses and pregnancy. *Metabolism*. 1994;43:647–654.

Richardson M. Current perspectives in polycystic ovary syndrome. *Am Fam Physician*. 2003;68:697–704.

122. Which of the following statements concerning oral contraceptive use is true?
A) Oral contraceptives may decrease the risk of cervical cancer.
B) Oral contraceptives increase the risk of cholelithiasis.
C) Women who use oral contraceptives have a higher incidence of ectopic pregnancy.
D) The use of oral contraceptives is associated with a higher incidence of PID.
E) Women who use oral contraceptives have a higher incidence of endometrial carcinoma.

Answer and Discussion

The answer is B. The use of oral contraceptives for birth control is widely accepted and prescribed. Properly used, the pill approaches 100% effectiveness in preventing pregnancy. Its mechanism of action involves the prevention of ovulation by the regulation of hormones [suppression of follicle-stimulating hormone (FSH) and luteinizing hormone (LH)] during the menstrual cycle, induction of atrophic changes to the endometrium that are not conducive to implantation, and the alteration of cervical mucus. Basically, there are two types: combination pills that include estrogen and progestin components and pills that contain only progestin. Pills that contain only progestin are best suited for women older than 35 years, smokers, or those who cannot tolerate estrogen. Additionally, oral contraceptives are divided into monophasic (fixed combination of estrogen and progestin component) and multiphasic (varying amount of progestin during each of the 3 weeks of medication with a fixed amount of estrogen). Overall, the multiphasic oral contraceptives are highly effective and may provide a lower dose of estrogen and progestin. Absolute contraindications to oral contraceptives include pregnancy, active liver disease, uncontrolled hypertension, significant hyperlipidemia, diabetes with vascular changes, previous deep venous thrombosis, coronary artery disease, stroke, or estrogen-related cancers. Relative contraindications include migraine headaches, hypertension, smoking, diabetes, major surgery within 1 month, sickle cell disease, gallbladder disease, immobilization of the lower extremities, undiagnosed vaginal bleeding, and age older than 40 years with cardiovascular risk factors. Complications associated with oral contraceptive use include increased blood pressure, midcycle bleeding between periods, headaches, weight gain, hirsutism, acne, increased risk of cholelithiasis, melasma, increased risk for myocardial infarction in smokers older than 35 years, and, rarely, benign hepatic lipomas. Women who use oral contraceptives are at decreased risk for ovarian cancer, endometrial cancer, PID, and ectopic pregnancy. No consistent association has been found between breast cancer and oral contraceptive use, except for the possibility of a slightly elevated risk in users of oral contraceptives for more than 3 years before 25 years of age. Women who are taking antiepileptic medication have an increased risk for oral contraceptive failure because of the enzyme-inducing action of the antiseizure medication. Antibiotic use may also decrease the effectiveness of oral contraceptives.

DeCherney AH, Nathan L. *Current Obstetric and Gynecologic Diagnosis and Treatment*, 9th ed. New York: Lange/McGraw-Hill; 2003:634–638.

123. Pap smears should be performed
A) typically 3 to 5 years before a woman becomes sexually active
B) every 5 years for sexually active women
C) every 2 to 3 years for women who are at low risk for cervical cancer and have had negative Pap smears in the past
D) until 50 years of age, when they can be discontinued
E) yearly, regardless of age, in sexually active women

Answer and Discussion

The answer is C. Pap smears are used to detect abnormal cervical cells. The possibility of false-negative results may occur between 10% and 30% of the time. Most experts agree that Pap smears should be performed on a yearly basis once a woman becomes sexually active. Those at low risk for cervical cancer may elect for screening every 2 to 3 years if they have had previous normal Pap smears. If a patient is older than 65 years and has had previous normal Pap smears, some recommendations state the smears can be discontinued.

Beers MH, Porter RS, eds. *The Merck manual of diagnosis and therapy*, Merck Research Laboratories, 18th ed. Whitehouse Station, NJ: Merck & Co.; 2006:2125.

Those at low risk for cervical cancer may elect for screening every 2 to 3 years if they have had previous normal Pap smears.

124. Which of the following statements about the use of a cervical cap is true?
A) Cervical caps are more effective when used in multiparous women.
B) Use of the cervical cap increases the risk of vaginal and urinary tract infections.
C) Failure rates with cervical caps are significantly lower than with diaphragms.
D) The cervical cap can be left in place for no more than 12 hours.
E) Cervical cap use is higher in the United States than in Europe.

Answer and Discussion

The answer is B. The cervical cap is a birth control method. The cap is similar to the diaphragm but is smaller in size and only covers the cervix and the cervical os. It comes in four different sizes and needs to be fitted by a physician before its use. The cervical cap is more effective in nulliparous than in multiparous women. It can be left in place for up to 72 hours. Failure rates are improved with the use of spermicidal gel and are similar to those of the diaphragm (approximately 8% to 15%). Use of the cervical cap increases the risk of vaginal and urinary tract infections. Patients should have a negative Pap smear before the use of the cervical cap, and a repeat Pap smear should be taken after 3 months of use. Use during menstruation should be discouraged because of the theoretical risk of the development of endometriosis. Reasons for discontinuing the cervical cap include patient or partner discomfort, difficulty with proper insertion, and unplanned pregnancy. The cervical cap is used more widely in Europe than in the United States and because of the difficulty in fitting the cap and routine insertion required it is unlikely to play an important role in contraception in the United States.

DeCherney AH, Nathan L. *Current Obstetric and Gynecologic Diagnosis and Treatment*, 9th ed. New York: Lange/McGraw-Hill; 2003:633.

125. Which of the following statements is true regarding the placement of an Intrauterine device (IUD)?
A) IUDs should only be inserted during menses.
B) Multiparous women have a higher risk of expulsion.
C) Routine prophylactic antibiotics are recommended before the procedure.
D) Antibiotic prophylaxis in patients at risk for endocarditis is necessary before IUD insertion or removal.
E) An IUD should not be inserted if the depth of the uterus is <6 cm.

Answer and Discussion

The answer is E. IUDs may be inserted anytime during the menstrual cycle. Documentation of a negative pregnancy test is recommended. Insertion may be performed during menstruation to provide additional reassurance that the woman is not pregnant. If insertion is planned during the luteal phase, another nonhormonal contraceptive should be used until completion of the next menses. A pregnancy test at this time cannot always rule out early pregnancy. An IUD should not be inserted in a woman with an STD. The American College of Obstetricians and Gynecologists recommends a pelvic examination before insertion to screen for Chlamydia and gonorrhea. Routine prophylactic antibiotic administration is not necessary. According to the American Heart Association, antibiotic prophylaxis in patients at risk for endocarditis is not necessary before IUD insertion or removal. IUDs are for parous women who are in a stable, mutually monogamous relationship, with no history of PID. Although not contraindicated in this group, nulliparous women tend to have higher expulsion and failure rates, and also offer more challenging insertion because they have a smaller uterine cavity. An adequate uterine depth is between 6 and 9 cm and should be documented in the patient's record. An IUD should not be inserted if the depth of the uterus is less than 6 cm.

Johnson BA. Insertion and removal of intrauterine devices. *Am Fam Physician*. 2005;71:95–102.

Grimes DA, Schulz KF. Antibiotic prophylaxis for intrauterine contraceptive device insertion. *Cochrane Database Syst Rev*. 2001;(1):CD001327. [Update in: *Cochrane Database Syst Rev*. 2001;(2):CD001327.]

Dajani AS, Taubert KA, Wilson W, et al. Prevention of bacterial endocarditis. Recommendations by the American Heart Association. *Circulation*. 1997;96:358–666.

126. The progestin-releasing IUD can be used for
A) 3 years
B) 5 years
C) 10 years
D) 15 years
E) indefinitely, as long as it's kept in proper placement

Answer and Discussion

The answer is B. The progestin-releasing IUD can be used for 5 years. The copper-releasing IUD can be used for 10 years before replacement.

Johnson BA. Insertion and removal of intrauterine devices. *Am Fam Physician.* 2005;71:95–102.

127. Which of the following oral contraceptives is approved by the FDA for the treatment of acne vulgaris in women and adolescent females?
A) Ethinyl estradiol–norelgestromin (OrthoEvra patch)
B) Ethinyl estradiol–levonorgestrel (Preven)
C) Norethindrone (Micronor)
D) Ethinyl estradiol–drospirenone (Yasmin)
E) Ethinyl estradiol–norgestimate (Ortho Tri-Cyclen)

Answer and Discussion

The answer is E. Oral contraceptives may be a useful adjunctive therapy for all types of acne in women and adolescent girls. Sebum production is controlled by androgens, and oral contraceptives are known to decrease androgen levels by increasing sex hormone binding globulin levels, thus reducing the availability of biologically active free testosterone. The third-generation progestin norgestimate has lower intrinsic androgenicity than other currently available progestins and is effective in treating moderate inflammatory acne. Ortho Tri-Cyclen is a triphasic combination of norgestimate and ethinyl estradiol that has been labeled by the U.S. Food and Drug Administration (FDA) for the treatment of acne vulgaris in women and adolescent girls. Other contraceptive agents that contain norgestimate (Ortho-Cyclen) or desogestrel (Desogen) are also reasonable choices. Two to 4 months of therapy may be required before improvement is noted, and relapses are common if medication is stopped.

Johnson BA, Nunley JR. Use of systemic agents in the treatment of acne vulgaris. *Am Fam Physician.* 2000;62:1823–1830, 1835–1836.

128. When considering treatment for osteoporosis which of the following is true?
A) Impaired eyesight is not a factor to consider in the decision to start medication.
B) Less than 30% of White women have an osteoporotic fracture at some point in their lifetime.
C) Bone mineral density testing is recommended in all women ages 65 and older, regardless of additional risk factors.
D) Bone mineral density testing should be performed only in postmenopausal women under age 65 who have two or more additional risk factors for osteoporosis (in addition to menopause).
E) Weight-bearing exercise should be avoided in postmenopausal women.

Answer and Discussion

The answer is C. The National Osteoporosis Foundation (NOF) has issued recommendations for the prevention, risk factor assessment, diagnosis and treatment of osteoporosis, including specific guidelines on the use of bone mineral density tests.

- All women should be counseled about the risk factors for osteoporosis. Risk factors for osteoporotic fracture include personal history of fracture as an adult, history of fracture in a first-degree relative, white race, advanced age, female sex, dementia, poor health/frailty, cigarette smoking, low body weight [<127 lb (58 kg)], estrogen deficiency, lifelong low calcium intake, alcoholism, impaired eyesight despite adequate correction, recurrent falls, and inadequate physical activity. According to the NOF, osteoporosis is a "silent" risk factor for fracture; one out of two White women will have an osteoporotic fracture at some point in her lifetime.
- The NOF recommends that all postmenopausal women with a fracture be evaluated for osteoporosis using bone mineral density testing to determine if the woman has osteoporosis and to determine disease severity. According to the NOF, measurements of bone mineral density at any skeletal site can predict the risk of fracture, but a measurement of the hip is the best predictor of hip fractures, and hip measurement can predict fractures at other sites as well. The measurement of bone density can also be used to monitor changes in bone density associated with medical conditions or therapy.
- The NOF recommends bone mineral density testing in all postmenopausal women under age 65 who have one or more additional risk factors for osteoporosis (in addition to menopause).
- Bone mineral density testing is also recommended in all women ages 65 and older, regardless of additional risk factors.
- All adults should be advised to consume an adequate intake of dietary calcium (at least 1,200 mg/day, including supplements if necessary) and vitamin D (400 to 800 IU/day for persons at risk of deficiency).
- All patients should be counseled to avoid smoking and to limit alcohol intake to moderate levels. All patients should be encouraged to participate in regular weight-bearing and muscle-strengthening exercise to reduce the risk of falls and fractures.
- Physicians should consider osteoporosis treatment for all postmenopausal women who present with vertebral fractures or hip fractures. The NOF emphasizes that these sites are the most common sites for osteoporotic fractures.
- Bone mineral tests provide physicians with a T score expressed in standard deviation; the more negative the number, the greater the risk of fracture. Each standard deviation represents a 10% to 12% bone loss, and a T score of −2.5 indicates osteoporosis. The NOF recommends therapy to reduce fracture risk in women with a bone mineral density T score below −2.0 in the absence of risk factors, and in women with a T score below −1.5 if other risk factors are present.

The National Osteoporosis Foundation (NOF) guidelines accessed at http://www.nof.org/osteoporosis/sgr_release.htm on 12/18/2005. Accessed 6/1/06.

129. Which of the following factors makes appendicitis during pregnancy difficult to diagnose?
A) Location of the appendix
B) Presence of fever
C) Rectal tenderness
D) Rebound tenderness
E) Presence of pyuria

Answer and Discussion

The answer is A. Appendicitis during pregnancy may be difficult to diagnose. The white blood cell count is mildly elevated during a normal pregnancy, making it difficult to distinguish the leukocytosis seen with infection. In addition, as pregnancy progresses, the position of the appendix migrates superiorly (usually above the iliac crest in patients at more than 5 months' gestation). Therefore, there is a greater risk for perforation in those with appendicitis as pregnancy progresses. In addition, there is a greater risk of perinatal mortality when the appendix is perforated. In early pregnancies, the appendix is usually removed through a midline vertical incision; however, with more advanced pregnancies, an incision is generally made over the point of maximal tenderness. The complications involved with appendectomy include premature labor and infection. The differential diagnosis of abdominal pain during pregnancy is extensive and includes gastroenteritis, inflammatory bowel disease, cholecystitis, intestinal obstruction, pancreatitis, pyelonephritis, nephrolithiasis, spontaneous abortion, round ligament pain, ectopic pregnancy, uterine contractions, placental abruption, and pelvic infections.

Cunningham FG, Gant NF, Leveno KJ, et al. *Williams Obstetrics*, 21st ed. New York: McGraw-Hill; 2001:1281–1282.

130. The treatment of choice for bacterial vaginosis is
A) metronidazole
B) doxycycline
C) ceftriaxone
D) nystatin vaginal tablets
E) vinegar douche

Answer and Discussion

The answer is A. Bacterial vaginosis is a condition that is caused by proliferation of a number of organisms, including *Gardnerella vaginalis, Mobiluncus* species, *Mycoplasma hominis*, and *Peptostreptococcus* species. The condition accounts for as many as 50% of all cases of vaginitis and is characterized by a gray, often frothy, foul-smelling vaginal discharge. When 10% to 20% potassium hydroxide is applied, the discharge gives off a characteristic amine-like fishy odor. Patients often report vaginal irritation and a foul-smelling discharge. Microscopic examination of the discharge shows "clue cells" (epithelial cells that are covered with coccobacilli on the cell walls). The vaginal secretion pH is >4.5. Treatment of choice is metronidazole. Topical 2% clindamycin cream can also be used. Cultures are not helpful because *Gardnerella* may be a normal inhabitant of the vagina. Studies indicate that treating the male sexual partner of a woman with bacterial vaginosis is not beneficial and that even women who are not sexually active can have the infection. Additional risk factors for bacterial vaginosis include the use of IUDs, douching, and pregnancy. Evidence suggests that bacterial vaginosis is a risk factor for premature rupture of membranes and preterm labor. Treating the infection in pregnancy decreases this risk. In pregnant women with bacterial vaginosis, treatment should be administered after the first trimester to lower the risk of premature rupture of membranes. Additional possible adverse outcomes include an increased frequency of abnormal Pap smears, PID, and endometritis. Vaginal cuff cellulitis, PID, and endometritis can occur if invasive gynecologic procedures or surgeries are performed when a patient has bacterial vaginosis.

Egan ME, Lipsky MS. Diagnosis of vaginitis. *Am Fam Physician*. 2000;62:1095–1104.

131. Which of the following statements about sexual intercourse and uncomplicated pregnancy is true?
A) Intercourse should be avoided until 36 weeks' gestation because of the risk of premature labor.
B) Intercourse should be avoided 2 weeks before the estimated date of confinement because of the risk of infection.
C) Intercourse is safe during pregnancy; however, orgasm should be avoided because of the risk of preterm labor.
D) Intercourse is not considered dangerous during normal pregnancy.
E) Intercourse should be avoided during pregnancy because of the risk for placental abruption.

Answer and Discussion

The answer is D. Sexual intercourse during pregnancy is generally considered safe as long as the mother has not had complications during pregnancy that would put the infant at risk (e.g., preterm labor, abnormal vaginal bleeding, premature rupture of membranes). Orgasm with uterine contractions does not induce labor; however, milk ejection may occur and is a normal response. In many cases, the woman has an increased desire for intercourse during pregnancy; however, other women may have a decrease in desire. Both responses are considered normal. Abstention from sexual intercourse was formerly recommended during the final months of pregnancy; however, it is no longer considered a risk in normal pregnancies.

Cunningham FG, Gant NF, Leveno KJ, et al. *Williams Obstetrics*, 21st ed. New York: McGraw-Hill; 2001:240.

132. The vaginal ring contraceptive can be left in place for
A) 3 days
B) 1 week
C) 3 weeks
D) 3 months
E) 1 year

Answer and Discussion

The answer is C. After three weeks, the contraceptive vaginal ring is removed for 1 week, and a new ring is inserted. Withdrawal bleeding occurs during the ring-free week.

Herndon EJ, Zieman M. New contraceptive options. *Am Fam Physician*. 2004;69:853–860.

133. How long can the vaginal ring be out of the vagina before an additional form of contraception is necessary?
A) 30 minutes
B) 1 hour
C) 3 hours
D) 24 hours
E) 1 week

Answer and Discussion

The answer is C. If the ring is removed from the vagina for more than 3 hours, additional back-up contraception should be used until the ring has been back in place for 7 days.

Bjarnadottir RI, Tuppurainen M, Killick SR. Comparison of cycle control with a combined contraceptive vaginal ring and oral levonorgestrel/ethinyl estradiol. *Am J Obstet Gynecol*. 2002;186:389–395.

If a vaginal ring is removed from the vagina for more than 3 hours, additional back-up contraception should be used until the ring has been back in place for 7 days.

134. A hypertensive woman uses enalapril for her blood pressure management. She has excellent control. Which of the following oral contraceptives when used with enalapril can lead to hyperkalemia?
A) ethinyl estradiol–norelgestromin (OrthoEvra patch)
B) ethinyl estradiol–levonorgestrel (Preven)
C) norethindrone (Micronor)
D) ethinyl estradiol–drospirenone (Yasmin)
E) ethinyl estradiol–norgestimate (Ortho Tri-Cyclen)

Answer and Discussion

The answer is D. A combination OCP that contains the new progestogen drospirenone (Yasmin) has been available for the last several years. Drospirenone has antimineralocorticoid activity and has been shown to decrease the water retention, negative affect, and appetite changes that commonly are associated with menstrual cycle changes. Serum potassium levels should be monitored when using this OCP in conjunction with other medicines that also raise potassium levels, because of the risk of developing hyperkalemia.

Herndon EJ, Zieman M. New contraceptive options. *Am Fam Physician*. 2004;69:853–860.

135. The oral contraceptive levonorgestrel–ethinyl estradiol (Seasonale) is different from other oral contraceptives as a result of
A) a lower dose of ethinyl estradiol
B) once-a-month dosing
C) increased effectiveness
D) the duration of hormone therapy between periods
E) the addition of levonorgestrel

Answer and Discussion

The answer is D. The U.S. Food and Drug Administration (FDA) recently approved the use of levonorgestrel ethinyl estradiol (Seasonale) in an extended OCP regimen consisting of 84 days of active pills and 7 days of nonhormonal pills.

Herndon EJ, Zieman M. New contraceptive options. *Am Fam Physician*. 2004;69:853–860.

136. A 15-year-old girl presents to the office complaining that she has not had a period in 3 months. The young girl emphatically states that she is not pregnant, and her mother assures you she is not pregnant. The most appropriate initial test would be
A) urine pregnancy test
B) thyroid function test
C) serum prolactin level
D) progesterone challenge test
E) serum cortisol level

Answer and Discussion

The answer is A. Abnormal menses are normal in the immediate pubertal period. Lack of menses for 3 to 4 months presents no concern if there is no possibility that the girl is pregnant. However, the history given by young, sexually active girls often cannot be trusted. The first step in the evaluation of amenorrhea is to determine if the patient is pregnant. Other tests for the workup of amenorrhea include a serum prolactin level and sensitive thyroid-stimulating hormone. If these tests are normal and the pregnancy test is negative, a progesterone challenge test can be performed. In this test, medroxyprogesterone acetate is given for 7 to 10 days, and withdrawal bleeding is usually induced after administration. If withdrawal bleeding occurs (positive test), the diagnosis of anovulation can be made. If no withdrawal bleeding occurs (negative test), the differential diagnosis includes polycystic ovary syndrome or an adrenal enzyme deficiency that leads to an excess of progesterone. If amenorrhea continues on a regular basis and the patient is diagnosed with anovulation, a daily dose of medroxyprogesterone can be prescribed for the first 10 days of alternative months. Pathologic amenorrhea is divided into primary amenorrhea (absence of menses before the age of 16) and secondary amenorrhea (absence of menses for 3 months or more in patients who have had previous periods).

Taylor RB, David AK, Fields SA, et al. *Family Medicine: Principles and Practice*, 6th ed. New York: Springer; 2003:874–878.

137. Which of the following statements about postpartum depression is true?
A) Postpartum depression usually occurs 9 to 12 months after delivery.
B) Social support has little impact on the development of postpartum depression.
C) Those with obstetric complications are at increased risk.
D) Those affected are at increased risk for postpartum depression with subsequent pregnancies.
E) Patients who have postpartum depression have no higher risk of developing depression in later years when compared to the general population.

Answer and Discussion

The answer is D. Mild postpartum depression (also referred to as the "baby blues") is usually seen within the first few days after delivery. The incidence ranges up to 25%, and those with poor social support are more commonly affected. There appears to be no relationship with obstetric complications. Symptoms vary but are usually mild and self-limited. In most cases, reassurance that these feelings are common is all that is needed. In more severe cases, in which the mother's symptoms last for extended periods or if the mother shows a lack of interest in the newborn, has suicidal or homicidal thoughts or gestures, or shows psychotic behavior, further therapy (including medication and psychotherapy) may be needed. Women who are affected with severe postpartum depression are at risk for development of further depressive episodes and recurrent postpartum depression with subsequent pregnancies.

Taylor RB, David AK, Fields SA, et al. *Family Medicine: Principles and Practice*, 6th ed. New York: Springer; 2003:139.

138. Prenatal vitamins are important during pregnancy because they help to reduce the incidence of neural tube defects. Which of the following is responsible for this protective effect?
A) Calcium
B) Iron
C) Folic acid
D) Vitamin C
E) Vitamin B_{12}

Answer and Discussion

The answer is C. Prenatal vitamins are recommended for pregnant women when dietary intake does not satisfy nutritional needs (multiple gestations, drug abusers, vegetarians, epileptics, and women with hemoglobinopathies) and in those who are planning pregnancy. The supplementation of iron during pregnancy is needed to prevent severe anemia and is usually accomplished by the use of prenatal vitamins. The following are the recommended requirements for pregnant women:

- Calcium, 1,200 to 1,500 mg/day
- Iron, 30 mg/day
- Folic acid, at least 0.4 mg/day

The use of prenatal vitamins before pregnancy can supply adequate folic acid, which has been shown to help prevent neural tube defects. Excessive use of vitamin A supplements should be avoided because of a small number of case reports that suggest a link to birth defects. Furthermore, if the infant is breast-fed, the use of prenatal vitamins for the mother is usually encouraged.

Cunningham FG, Gant NF, Leveno KJ, et al. *Williams Obstetrics*, 21st ed. New York: McGraw-Hill; 2001:234–238.

139. Which of the following statements is true regarding bacterial vaginosis during pregnancy?
A) All studies have shown an increased risk of premature labor in women affected with bacterial vaginosis.
B) Symptomatic women should be treated.
C) Routine screening is recommended for all pregnant patients.
D) Vaginal pH <4.5 is supportive of bacterial vaginosis.
E) Treatment should be avoided until after pregnancy.

Answer and Discussion

The answer is B. Routine screening of all pregnant women for bacterial vaginosis (BV) is not recommended. Well-designed studies of BV screening in women with a history of preterm delivery found inconsistent results. Physicians may consider screening women at increased risk of preterm labor with Gram stain or Amsel criteria (i.e., three of the following signs: homogeneous white or gray noninflammatory vaginal discharge, presence of clue cells, vaginal secretion pH of 4.5 or greater, and amine odor of vaginal discharge before or after addition of 10% potassium hydroxide [KOH]). Symptomatic women should be treated.

U.S. Preventive Services Task Force. Screening for bacterial vaginosis in pregnancy: recommendations and rationale. *Am J Prev Med.* 2001;20(3 suppl):59–61.

Guise JM, Mahon SM, Aickin M, et al. Screening for bacterial vaginosis in pregnancy. *Am J Prev Med.* 2001;20(3 suppl):62–72.

140. A 65-year-old woman presents to your office concerned about uterine prolapse. During her examination, you note the cervix is visible outside of the vaginal introitus. The uterus is not visible. Based on your findings, you classify her as having ____________.
A) first-degree prolapse
B) second-degree prolapse
C) third-degree prolapse
D) no prolapse

Answer and Discussion

The answer is B. Uterine prolapse is classified by degree. In first-degree uterine prolapse, the cervix is visible when the perineum is depressed. In second-degree prolapse, the cervix is visible outside of the vaginal introitus while the uterine fundus remains inside. In third-degree prolapse, or *procidentia,* the entire uterus is outside of the vaginal introitus. Uterine prolapse is associated with urinary incontinence, vaginitis, cystitis, and, possibly, uterine malignancy.

Viera AJ, Larkins-Pettigrew M. Practical use of the pessary. *Am Fam Physician.* 2000;61:2719–2726, 2729.

141. The most common cause of first-trimester spontaneous abortion is
A) incompetent cervix
B) chromosomal abnormalities
C) increased maternal age
D) inadequate levels of progesterone during the luteal phase
E) lupus anticoagulant

Answer and Discussion

The answer is B. It is estimated that spontaneous abortions during the first trimester affect 20% of all pregnancies. Because many cases go unreported, the true incidence may be much higher (50% to 75%). The most common cause is chromosomal abnormalities (usually autosomal trisomies), which are incompatible with life. Other factors that may contribute to spontaneous abortion include maternal smoking, increased maternal age, maternal illness, incompetent cervix, lupus anticoagulant, and inadequate levels of progesterone during the luteal phase of the menstrual cycle. Patients usually report vaginal bleeding and uterine cramps. Expulsion of fetal material generally occurs spontaneously, but in some cases dilation and curettage is needed. Misoprostol provides a safe and effective means of initial treatment for spontaneous abortion with retained products of conception. Although gastrointestinal side effects are common with medical management, they are seldom severe. The addition of misoprostol to routine management of spontaneous abortion can significantly reduce the need for surgical intervention and ultimately reduce the overall rate of complications. Patients should receive emotional support and reassurance. Vaginal bleeding develops in 25% of pregnant women during the first half of pregnancy, and 50% of those patients eventually abort.

Chung TK, Lee DT, Cheung LP, et al. Spontaneous abortion: a randomized, controlled trial comparing surgical evacuation with conservative management using misoprostol. *Fertil Steril.* 1999;71:1054–1059.

Cunningham FG, Gant NF, Leveno KJ, et al. *Williams Obstetrics*, 21st ed. New York: McGraw-Hill; 2001:874–875.

142. The presence of sterile pyuria in a sexually active individual is most commonly associated with
A) gonorrhea
B) syphilis
C) chlamydia
D) herpes genitalis
E) human papillomavirus virus

The answer is C. Chlamydia is a sexually transmitted disease that is caused by *Chlamydia trachomatis*. Approximately 50% of nongonococcal urethritis and most cases of cervicitis are caused by chlamydia. Men usually report discomfort associated with the urethra, dysuria, or a clear to mucopurulent discharge that occurs 1 to 3 weeks after exposure. Most women are asymptomatic, although they may report dysuria, pelvic discomfort with dyspareunia, and vaginal discharge that may have a clear to yellow mucopurulent appearance. The cervix may bleed easily and is usually swollen and covered with a yellowish-green discharge. Diagnosis is made with immunologic studies performed on urine, secretions, or culture. The presence of sterile pyuria in a sexually active individual should raise the suspicion of chlamydia. The presence of gonorrhea must be ruled out and patients should be treated for gonorrhea if chlamydia is found, and vice versa. Because chlamydial infection is often asymptomatic and the sequelae can be serious, routine screening for disease during annual examinations is recommended in young sexually active women. Single-dose therapy with azithromycin is as effective as a 7-day course of doxycycline (Vibramycin). Doxycycline is less expensive, but azithromycin may be cost beneficial because it provides single-dose, directly observed therapy. Erythromycin and ofloxacin (Floxin) also can be used to treat *C. trachomatis*. Erythromycin is less efficacious than azithromycin and doxycycline, and its adverse gastrointestinal effects may decrease patient compliance. Ofloxacin is as effective as the recommended regimens but offers no dosing or cost advantages. Doxycycline and ofloxacin are contraindicated in pregnant women.

Beers MH, Porter RS, eds. *The Merck manual of diagnosis and therapy*, Merck Research Laboratories, 18th ed. Whitehouse Station, NJ: Merck & Co.; 2006:1651–1652.

143. Treatment for vaginismus includes which of the following?
A) Desensitization therapy with continued regular intercourse until it becomes comfortable.
B) Treatment with muscle relaxants.
C) Kegel exercises.
D) Dilation with vaginal probes.
E) Transcutaneous electrical nerve stimulation treatment.

Answer and Discussion

The answer is D. Vaginismus is a condition that is characterized by involuntary spasm of the lower vaginal muscles, resulting in an unconscious effort to prevent penile penetration. Causes include psychiatric factors, local trauma, infection, or mechanical factors, including vaginal stenosis or dryness. Women report extreme discomfort with attempts at penetration. Treatment involves correction of reversible causes, sexual counseling, and gradual and repeated attempts at vaginal dilation with vaginal or (shorter) rectal probes. Treatment can be continued by the patient at home in a private environment after the appropriate technique is learned. Intercourse can be attempted once the patient is able to tolerate larger dilators without discomfort. Communication with the patient's partner often is helpful in overcoming the patient's fears.

Beers MH, Porter RS, eds. *The Merck manual of diagnosis and therapy*, Merck Research Laboratories, 18th ed. Whitehouse Station, NJ: Merck & Co.; 2006:2100–2104.

144. Which of the following is *not* useful in treating premenstrual syndrome?
A) Vitamin B_6
B) Vitamin E
C) Calcium supplementation
D) Folate

Answer and Discussion

The answer is D. A meta-analysis of randomized, placebo-controlled trials was conducted to ascertain the effectiveness of vitamin B_6 in PMS management. The researchers concluded that vitamin B_6, in dosages of up to 100 mg/day, is likely to benefit patients with premenstrual symptoms and premenstrual depression. In another study, the reviewers concluded that calcium supplementation in a dosage of 1,200 to 1,600 mg/day is a treatment option in women with PMS. Calcium supplementation (using Tums E-X) was found to reduce core premenstrual symptoms by 48%. Vitamin E, an antioxidant, seems to reduce the affective and physical symptoms of PMS. Tryptophan, a substrate for serotonin, may also benefit some patients.

Steinberg S, Annable L, Young SN, et al. A placebo-controlled clinical trial of l-tryptophan in premenstrual dysphoria. *Biol Psychiatry*. 1999;45:313–320.

Wyatt KM, Dimmock PW, Jones PW, et al. Efficacy of vitamin B-6 in the treatment of premenstrual syndrome. *BMJ*. 1999;318:1375–1381.

Ward MW, Holimon TD. Calcium treatment for premenstrual syndrome. *Ann Pharmacother*. 1999;33:1356–1358.

145. Which of the following statements is true regarding post-coital emergency contraception?
A) Birth defects often occur if the method is unsuccessful.
B) Emergency contraception is 95% effective.
C) Emergency contraception is most effective if administered within 72 hours.
D) Plan B has more side effects than Preven.
E) The dose of Plan B should be split to avoid side effects.

Answer and Discussion

The answer is C. Women have the option to use emergency contraception to prevent pregnancy after known or suspected failure of birth control or after unprotected intercourse. Emergency contraception has been an off-label use of oral contraceptive pills since the 1960s. Products including the Yuzpe regimen (Preven) and levonorgestrel (Plan B) were marketed in the United States after 1998, but had been available in Europe for years before that. The Plan B option consists of two tablets, each containing 0.75 mg of levonorgestrel. (This amount differs from the 0.075 mg dose of norgestrel in certain progestin-only pills.) There is a general consensus that the levonorgestrel emergency contraception should be given in preference to the Yuzpe regimen where available because it is more effective and has fewer side effects. In addition, a World Health Organization (WHO) multicenter randomized trial shows that the levonorgestrel dose does not have to be split, but can be taken as a single 1.5-mg dose. One dose simplifies the use of levonorgestrel without causing an increase in side effects. A third approved method of emergency contraception is the insertion of an intrauterine device. Emergency contraception is about 75% to 85% effective. It is most effective when initiated within 72 hours after unprotected intercourse. The mechanism of action may vary, depending on the day of the menstrual cycle on which treatment is started. Despite the large number of women who have received emergency contraception, there have been no reports of major adverse outcomes. If a woman becomes pregnant after using emergency contraception, she may be reassured about the lack of negative effects emergency contraception has on fetal development.

Weismiller DG. Emergency contraception. *Am Fam Physician*. 2004;70:707–714, 717–718.

Emergency contraception is about 75% to 85% effective. It is most effective when initiated within 72 hours after unprotected intercourse.

146. Oligohydramnios is associated with an increased risk of
A) placenta previa
B) cord prolapse
C) Down syndrome
D) prolonged labor
E) endometritis

Answer and Discussion

The answer is B. *Oligohydramnios* is defined as an amount of amniotic fluid that is less than what is expected for gestational age. In cases in which there is a lack of amniotic fluid, fetal movement is restricted and there is an increased risk of cord prolapse with fetal injury and demise. Other associated conditions include abnormal facies, limb contractures, and pulmonary hypoplasia. The cause of oligohydramnios is related to either a fluid loss with premature rupture of membranes or lack of amniotic fluid production with renal disturbances, including renal agenesis, dysplasia, or obstruction. The condition is more common in postterm pregnancies. Oligohydramnios seen early in pregnancy is a poor prognostic sign. The amount of amniotic fluid is usually quantified with ultrasound determination, including fluid pocket measurements. If the largest area of fluid accumulation is <1 cm $\times$ 1 cm, it is considered diagnostic for oligohydramnios. Fluid pockets of <2 cm $\times$ 2 cm are considered borderline. If the mother is suspected of having oligohydramnios, close monitoring by an obstetrician is usually recommended. Treatment of oligohydramnios as a result of spontaneous rupture of membranes can be achieved with amnioinfusion of warmed saline solution. If cord prolapse does occur, emergency cesarean section is necessary.

Cunningham FG, Gant NF, Leveno KJ, et al. *Williams Obstetrics*, 21st ed. New York: McGraw-Hill; 2001:821–824.

147. Which of the following statements about acute pyelonephritis during pregnancy is true?
A) It is associated with an increased risk of premature labor.
B) The medication of choice is a sulfonamide antibiotic.
C) Prophylaxis should never be instituted during pregnancy.
D) Most cases can be treated on an outpatient basis.
E) The drug of choice is intravenous ciprofloxacin.

Answer and Discussion

The answer is A. An important complication that is seen in pregnancy is pyelonephritis. The most common infecting agents are *E. coli* and *Klebsiella pneumoniae*. In most cases, hospitalization is necessary. The drug of choice is ampicillin, usually combined with the aminoglycoside gentamicin. Sulfonamides should not be used during pregnancy because of the increased risk of kernicterus, and trimethoprim has been associated with teratogenicity. Tetracyclines should be avoided because their use is associated with discoloration of the infant's teeth and with bone abnormalities. Nitrofurantoin is often used but has been associated with hemolysis in women who are deficient in glucose-6-phosphate dehydrogenase (2% of African-American women) and therefore should be avoided. Extended-spectrum penicillins and third-generation cephalosporins are suitable alternatives. Prophylaxis should be considered for patients who have had more than two infections during pregnancy. Infections that involve the urinary tract are usually associated with an increased risk for premature labor.

Cunningham FG, Gant NF, Leveno KJ, et al. *Williams Obstetrics*, 21st ed. New York: McGraw-Hill; 2001:1256–1257.

148. Rubella infection during pregnancy
A) rarely affects the fetus
B) has its most devastating effects during the third trimester
C) is associated with cataracts, cardiac defects, and cleft palate
D) is associated with neural tube defects
E) can be prevented with immunization during the pregnancy

Answer and Discussion

The answer is C. Rubella infection ("German measles") during pregnancy can have devastating effects on the fetus. They are most severe for those fetuses that are affected during the first trimester. Clinical findings of congenital rubella include cataracts, blindness, and cardiac abnormalities (including patent ductus arteriosus, pulmonary valve stenosis, and ventricular septal defect). Other findings include pigmented birthmarks, hemolytic anemia, cleft palate, deafness, mental retardation, cerebral palsy, and fetal death. Treatment is aimed at prevention by immunizing all prospective mothers. The vaccine should be given at least 3 months before conception because of the live attenuated vaccine.

Cunningham FG, Gant NF, Leveno KJ, et al. *Williams Obstetrics*, 21st ed. New York: McGraw-Hill; 2001:1465.

149. The most frequently reported symptom in women with vulvar cancer is
A) bleeding
B) dyspareunia
C) vaginal dryness
D) itching
E) vaginal discharge

Answer and Discussion

The answer is A. The most frequently reported symptom of vulvar cancer is vaginal bleeding. Other common presenting symptoms include vulvar itching, discharge, dysuria, and pain. The most common presenting sign of vulvar cancer is a vulvar lump or mass. Rarely, patients present with a large, fungating mass.

Beers MH, Porter RS, eds. *The Merck manual of diagnosis and therapy*, Merck Research Laboratories, 18th ed. Whitehouse Station, NJ: Merck & Co.; 2006:2129.

150. A 70-year-old woman has been treated for 6 months with topical estrogen for chronic lichen sclerosus. Despite treatment she continues to have vaginal pruritus. Appropriate treatment at this point includes
A) addition of moisturizing cream
B) oral estrogen replacement therapy
C) cryotherapy of the area affected
D) administration of topical antifungal cream
E) punch biopsy and tissue examination

Answer and Discussion

The answer is E. Lichen sclerosus is a type of vulvar non-neoplastic epithelial disorder (VNED) that is thought to be a predisposing factor in the development of HPV-negative vulvar cancer. According to the "itch-scratch-lichen sclerosus hypothesis," lichen sclerosus, by causing a severe pruritus, sets up an itch-scratch cycle that over a period of time causes the development of squamous cell hyperplasia. Further progression of the condition results in atypical formation, followed by VIN and eventual invasive squamous cell cancer. This hypothesis suggests that treatment of lichen sclerosus with topical steroids would prevent vulvar cancer in these patients, and some research may support this recommendation. Aggressive evaluation and treatment of VNEDs could have a dramatic impact on the incidence of vulvar cancer in this subgroup of patients.

Scurry J. Does lichen sclerosus play a central role in the pathogenesis of human papillomavirus negative vulvar squamous cell carcinoma? The itch-scratch lichen sclerosus hypothesis. *Int J Gynecol Cancer*. 1999;9:89–97.

151. A major risk factor for shoulder dystocia includes which of the following?
A) Young maternal age
B) Gestational diabetes
C) Precipitous delivery
D) Preterm delivery
E) Thin body habitus

Answer and Discussion

The answer is B. Shoulder dystocia occurs in 1 of 300 deliveries. Risk factors include diabetes, postterm pregnancy, obesity, previous shoulder dystocia, prolonged second stage of labor, advanced maternal age, and multiparity. Warning signs for shoulder dystocia include a prolonged second stage of labor and retraction of the fetal head tightly against the vaginal introitus after delivery of the head. Complications include a fractured clavicle or humerus, brachial plexus injuries, anoxic brain injuries, and even death of the fetus. Treatment consists of moderate suprapubic pressure, McRobert's maneuver (i.e., flexing the patient's thighs at the hips back to the woman's abdomen and applying firm pressure to the suprapubic area), which may help dislodge the fetus' anterior shoulder that is lodged behind the pubic bone. A large episiotomy should be performed before the procedure. If McRobert's maneuver is unsuccessful, Wood's maneuver can be used, in which the infant's shoulders are rotated 180 degrees to dislodge the blocked shoulder by pulling on the posterior presenting arm. This maneuver is associated with a higher incidence of injury to the arm and clavicle.

Further efforts include an attempt to fracture the clavicle to facilitate delivery or pushing the infant's head back into the vagina and performing emergent cesarean section. In all cases in which dystocia is suspected, a newborn resuscitation team should be alerted. Risk of shoulder dystocia is related to the size of the fetus:

- Less than 3,000 g = 0%
- 3,001 to 3,500 g = 0.3%
- 3,501 to 4,000 g = 1.0%
- 4,001 to 4,500 g = 5.4%
- Greater than 4,500 g = 19%
- All weights = 0.9%

Cunningham FG, Gant NF, Leveno KJ, et al. *Williams Obstetrics*, 21st ed. New York: McGraw-Hill; 2001:450–464.

152. Which of the following tumor markers can be used to follow the effectiveness of ovarian cancer treatment?
A) α-fetoprotein
B) Carcinoembryonic antigen
C) CA 125
D) β-hCG
E) None of the above

Answer and Discussion

The answer is C. Ovarian carcinoma usually affects women in their 50s. It is the fifth most common cancer that affects women, and approximately 25,000 new cases are diagnosed yearly in the United States. Because of the difficulty in diagnosis, most cases have metastasized outside the pelvis at the time of diagnosis; therefore, prognosis is usually poor. Risk factors include a positive family history, *BRCA1* gene mutation on chromosome 17, White race, high-fat diet, asbestos or talc exposure, and nulliparity or low parity. The use of oral contraceptives may be protective. Any ovarian mass >5 cm deserves careful follow-up. Postmenopausal women usually have atrophic ovaries that are not palpable; thus, any palpable ovary in a postmenopausal woman deserves further investigation. The types of tumors are divided histologically into those that arise from the ovarian epithelium:

- Serous cystadenocarcinomas (most common)
- Clear cell carcinomas
- Mucinous cystadenocarcinomas
- Endometrioid tumors
- Celioblastomas (Brenner tumors)
- Tumors not classified

In addition, tumors arise from germ cells and stroma, such as

- Sertoli-Leydig cell tumors
- Malignant teratomas
- Dysgerminomas
- Granulosa–theca cell tumors

Patients may report lower abdominal fullness or discomfort, gastrointestinal complaints, abnormal vaginal bleeding, or pelvic pain. Diagnosis is usually aided with ultrasound or CT examination. Treatment of ovarian carcinoma depends on the staging and cell type but involves surgical excision and in some cases chemotherapy or radiation. Metastasis is usually to lung or bone. The blood test CA 125 can be used to follow patients for recurrence of tumor after surgery or the response to chemotherapy but is not a suitable screening test. Benign masses that affect the ovary include functional cysts, which usually resolve within 2 months, and benign cystic teratoma (dermoid tumor), which may contain hair follicles or tooth formations. Another condition that may be seen with ovarian masses is Meigs' syndrome, which is associated with ascites, right hydrothorax, and benign fibroma or thecoma.

Kasper DL, Braunwald E, Fauci AS, et al., eds. *Harrison's principles of internal medicine,* 16th ed. New York: McGraw-Hill; 2005:553.

153. The most common side effect of the "morning after" pill is
A) nausea and vomiting
B) breast tenderness
C) insomnia
D) pelvic pain
E) headache

Answer and Discussion

The answer is A. Emergency postcoital contraception, a method used to prevent pregnancy after unprotected sexual intercourse, is a highly effective but underused birth control option. Two hormone regimens, ethinyl estradiol (100 μg) with levonorgestrel (0.5 mg) or high-dose levonorgestrel (0.75 mg), given within 72 hours of intercourse and repeated 12 hours later, are available for this purpose. The two new dedicated products, Preven and Plan B, are now available. Plan B is available for purchase in pharmacies via physician prescription, having previously been distributed only in Title 10 clinics, Planned Parenthood clinics, state and county health departments, and university campus health centers. Preven has been available through pharmacies, but still is not readily available in many locations. Both dedicated products should become more accessible in all locations according to physician demand. The high-dose contraceptives cause shedding of the endometrium and prevent implantation of the fertilized ovum. Side effects include nausea and vomiting that may require antiemetics and disruption of the woman's normal menstrual cycle.

Wertheimer RE. Emergency postcoital contraception. *Am Fam Physician*. 2000;62:2287–2292.

154. Which of the following is true regarding symptoms of ovarian cancer?
A) Most women are asymptomatic.
B) Symptoms are less severe than in benign processes.
C) Symptoms are less frequent than in benign processes.
D) Symptoms are of greater duration than in benign processes.
E) Symptoms often involve a combination of gastrointestinal and genitourinary symptoms.

Answer and Discussion

The answer is E. No effective screening test exists for ovarian cancer. The symptoms most commonly reported in patients with ovarian cancer include bloating, increased abdominal size, abdominal or pelvic pain, and urinary tract symptoms, although these also are common in women with benign masses. Symptoms tend to be more severe, more frequent, and of shorter duration in women with malignant masses than in women with benign masses. Women with ovarian cancer also are more likely to present with a combination of symptoms.

Goff BA, Mandel LS, Melancon CH. Frequency of symptoms of ovarian cancer in women presenting to primary care clinics. *JAMA*. 2004;291: 2705–2712.

> The symptoms most commonly reported in patients with ovarian cancer include bloating, increased abdominal size, abdominal or pelvic pain, and urinary tract symptoms, although these also are common in women with benign masses.

155. A 61-year-old woman is found to have a new 2.5 cm unilocular ovarian cyst (confirmed by ultrasound) during her routine well woman examination. Her CA 125 level is normal. Appropriate management at this time includes
A) serial ultrasounds and CA 125 levels
B) laparoscopic surgical removal
C) hysteroscopic evaluation and biopsy
D) cone radiation ablation
E) no further monitoring is necessary

Answer and Discussion

The answer is A. In postmenopausal women, most ovarian cysts <50 mm in diameter are benign and can be managed safely by regular monitoring of cyst size and serum CA 125 level.

Nardo LG, Kroon ND, Reginald PW. Persistent unilocular ovarian cysts in a general population of postmenopausal women: is there a place for expectant management? *Obstet Gynecol.* 2003;102:589–593.

156. Which of the following statements about striae distensae (stretch marks) is true?
A) They usually respond to topical corticosteroids.
B) They rarely fade after pregnancy.
C) They may be related to excessive corticosteroids that are produced during pregnancy.
D) The condition is secondary to excessive weight gain (>40 lb) during pregnancy.
E) None of the above.

Answer and Discussion

The answer is C. Striae distensae, also known as stretch marks, are abnormal skin findings that are noted with varying degree during pregnancy. They affect up to 50% of pregnant women. Typically, they are initially erythematous, pink or purple, and slightly raised to form ridges. They can occur in different areas but are usually found associated with the abdomen, breast, or hips. The cause of stretch marks was once believed to be excessive stretching of the skin; however, more recently it has been thought that they are secondary to excessive corticosteroids produced endogenously during pregnancy, combined with the body changes that occur with pregnancy. Excessive weight gain is not the reason for striae development. Unfortunately, there is no effective treatment for stretch marks. They usually fade after pregnancy and are barely noticeable.

DeCherney AH, Nathan L. *Current Obstetric and Gynecologic Diagnosis and Treatment*, 9th ed., New York: Lange/McGraw-Hill; 2003:434.

157. At what month during pregnancy does the mother's appendix move upward to a level above the iliac crest?
A) Third month
B) Sixth month
C) Ninth month
D) The appendix does not change location.
E) When the fetal head engages in the pelvis.

Answer and Discussion

The answer is B. Because of the normal changes during pregnancy, such as leukocytosis, nausea, vomiting, anorexia, and abdominal discomfort, the diagnosis of appendicitis may be difficult. The condition occurs with equal frequency during each trimester of pregnancy. As the sixth month approaches, the appendix moves upward, above the iliac crest. The risk for perforation is particularly increased in the third trimester. With perforation, the perinatal risk is increased. Complications of appendectomy include premature labor and wound infection. The differential diagnosis includes placental abruption, round ligament pain, acute pyelonephritis, renal colic, and cholecystitis.

Cunningham FG, Gant NF, Leveno KJ, et al. *Williams Obstetrics*, 21st ed. New York: McGraw-Hill; 2001:1281–1282.

158. An increase in blood pressure that is seen with oral contraceptive use is
A) rarely a problem in patients with underlying hypertension
B) more common in women with a positive family history for hypertension

C) not associated with increased age of the patient
D) related to a permanent increase in blood pressure despite discontinuation of the drug
E) most commonly associated with underlying renal disease

Answer and Discussion

The answer is B. A slight increase in blood pressure (systolic, 5 to 6 mm Hg; diastolic, 1 to 2 mm Hg) is expected in some women who take oral contraceptives. In fact, hypertension is five to six times more likely to develop in women who use oral contraceptives than in those who do not use them. Women who are older or who have a positive family history for hypertension and those using oral contraceptives for longer durations are at increased risk. It is thought that hypertension is related to the progestin component, although estrogens may induce the synthesis of the renin substrate angiotensinogen, which increases the formation of angiotensin and leads to increases in blood pressure. Blood pressure increases may occur within weeks; however, it may not be noted for months or even years after starting medication. Switching to an oral contraceptive with lower progestin may alleviate the problem. Discontinuation of oral contraceptives in most patients allows the blood pressure to decrease to normal levels. Patients should be seen for a blood pressure check within 3 months after the initiation of the contraceptive. If significant increases occur, oral contraception medication should be discontinued. Underlying preexisting hypertension is a relative contraindication for oral contraceptive use.

Cunningham FG, Gant NF, Leveno KJ, et al. *Williams Obstetrics*, 21st ed. New York: McGraw-Hill; 2001:1529.

159. Which of the following is an independent risk factor for the development of vulvar cancer?
A) Diabetes
B) Hypertension
C) Obesity
D) Syphilis
E) Human papillomavirus virus

Answer and Discussion

The answer is E. Vulvar intraepithelial neoplasia (VIN) is clearly a premalignant finding and is associated with HPV infection, particularly subtypes 16 and 18. Hypertension, diabetes mellitus, and obesity have been found to coexist in up to 25% of patients, although they are not considered independent risk factors. In the past, syphilis and other granulomatous diseases have been associated with vulvar cancer.

Canavan TP, Cohen D. Vulvar cancer. *Am Fam Physician.* 2002;66:1269–1274, 1276.

160. In addition to a loss of menses and disordered eating, what other component of the female athlete triad causes significant problems for women?
A) Loss of libido
B) Sleep disturbances
C) Osteoporosis
D) Poor mentation
E) Thyroid dysfunction

Answer and Discussion

The answer is C. The female athlete triad is defined as the combination of disordered eating, amenorrhea, and osteoporosis. This disorder often goes undiagnosed. The consequences of lost bone mineral density can be debilitating for the female athlete. Premature osteoporotic fractures can occur, and lost bone mineral density may never be regained. Early recognition of the female athlete triad is important. Instituting an appropriate diet and moderation of exercise may result in the natural return of menses. Hormone replacement therapy should be considered early to prevent the loss of bone density. A collaborative effort among coaches, athletic trainers, parents, athletes, and physicians is optimal for the recognition and prevention of the triad. Increased education of parents, coaches, and athletes in the health risks of the female athlete triad can prevent a potentially life-threatening illness.

Hobart JA, Smucker DR. The female athlete triad. *Am Fam Physician.* 2000;61:3357–3364, 3367.

161. Which of the following statements regarding estrogen replacement therapy (ERT) is true?
A) The addition of progesterone slightly raises the risk for endometrial carcinoma.
B) ERT lowers the risk for ovarian carcinoma.
C) All forms of estrogen delivery are equally effective in lowering cholesterol.
D) Patients with a prior history of thrombosis should avoid ERT.
E) Studies show that there is no increased risk for breast cancer with ERT.

Answer and Discussion

The answer is D. The use of estrogen in postmenopausal women is controversial. Benefits include the prevention of osteoporosis and symptoms associated with estrogen deficiency (i.e., hot flashes, vaginal atrophy, vulvar irritation, mood swings, and dysuria). Recent studies have shown increases in the risk for breast cancer after years of estrogen use. Relative contraindications for ERT include undiagnosed abnormal genital bleeding, known or suspected pregnancy, a previous diagnosis of breast cancer, liver disease, and thromboembolic disease. If the patient has an intact uterus, estrogen should be given along with progesterone, which decreases the risk of endometrial hyperplasia. Different methods of administration have been developed:

- *Transdermal patches*: Some of the lipid-lowering benefits are eliminated with this route of administration.
- *Cyclical combined low-dose therapy (0.625 mg/day estrogen and 10 mg progesterone given the first 10 to 14 days or last 10 to 14 days of the month)*: This regimen usually results in the development of mild menstruation after progesterone withdrawal.
- *Continuous combined low-dose therapy (0.625 mg/day estrogen and 2.5 mg/day progesterone)*: This may result in irregular vaginal bleeding for up to 6 months after administration.

Taylor RB, David AK, Fields SA, et al. *Family Medicine: Principles and Practice*, 6th ed. New York: Springer; 2003:882–886.

162. Female children of women who are exposed to diethylstilbestrol during their pregnancy are at increased risk for which of the following?
A) Early menopause
B) Clear cell carcinoma of the vagina
C) Ovarian carcinoma
D) Severe limb defects in their offspring
E) Mental retardation

Answer and Discussion

The answer is B. Diethylstilbestrol was widely used from the 1940s to the early 1970s to help prevent spontaneous abortion in diabetic pregnant women. Approximately 2 to 3 million fetuses were exposed to the medication. Unfortunately, later studies showed that girls who were born to mothers who took the medication while they were pregnant were at increased risk of developing clear cell carcinoma of the vagina as well as cervical and vaginal intraepithelial neoplasia. These patients are also at risk for vaginal adenosis (most common anomaly associated with exposure), septated vagina, cervical collar, hypoplasia of the cervix, and uterine abnormalities. In addition to lower genital tract anomalies, upper genital tract anomalies occur in 50% of patients. The most common is a T-shaped uterus and small uterine cavity. Daughters of women who took this drug may have difficulty in conceiving, higher rates of ectopic pregnancy, spontaneous abortion, and premature births as well as a slightly increased risk for breast cancer. All exposed women are encouraged to undergo thorough vaginal examinations, including colposcopy, starting at menarche or age 14, whichever comes first. Male children of women who took the medication may show testicular or epididymal abnormalities and low sperm counts.

Beers MH, Porter RS, eds. *The Merck manual of diagnosis and therapy*, Merck Research Laboratories, 18th ed. Whitehouse Station, NJ: Merck & Co.; 2006:1147.

163. Which of the following is a contraindication for vaginal birth after cesarean section (VBAC)?
A) Deliveries that require oxytocin administration
B) Two previous cesarean sections
C) Previous transverse incision in the lower segment of the uterus
D) Multiple gestation

Answer and Discussion

The answer is D. VBAC has advantages that include increased maternal satisfaction and acceptance, lower morbidity and mortality, and less expense than repeat cesarean section, although these are controversial. Women who have had a previous cesarean section with a classic vertical incision should undergo repeat cesarean section for delivery because of the risk of uterine rupture. Other contraindications to VBAC may include multiple gestation, macrosomia (>4,000 g), abnormal presentation, and inadequate facilities for close monitoring. Those who have had previous cesarean section with a low transverse incision should be allowed a trial of labor and are quite successful (approximately 60% to 80%) in vaginal deliveries with subsequent births. Even if the woman has had multiple previous cesarean sections, there is not a definite contraindication for a vaginal delivery if low transverse incisions are used with previous cesarean sections. Women with previous cesarean sections (low transverse incision) can also receive oxytocin during labor, but the contractions and the fetus should be closely monitored.

DeCherney AH, Nathan L. *Current Obstetric and Gynecologic Diagnosis and Treatment*, 9th ed. New York: Lange/McGraw-Hill; 2003:529.

> Women who have had a previous cesarean section with a classic vertical incision should undergo repeat cesarean section for delivery because of the risk of uterine rupture.

164. Which of the following is associated with oral contraceptive use?
A) Increased risk of endometrial cancer
B) Increased risk of ovarian cancer
C) Decreased risk of cervical cancer
D) Decreased risk of liver cancer
E) Fewer ectopic pregnancies

Answer and Discussion

The answer is E. The neoplastic effects of oral contraceptives have been extensively studied, and recent meta-analyses indicate that there is a reduction in the risk of endometrial and ovarian cancer, a possible small increase in the risk for breast and cervical cancer, and an increased risk of liver cancer. Benefits include reduction in menstrual-related symptoms, fewer ectopic pregnancies, a possible increase in bone density, and possible protection against pelvic inflammatory disease.

Burkman R, Schlesselmann JJ, Zieman M. Safety concerns and health benefits associated with oral contraception. *Am J Obstet Gynecol*. 2004;190(4 Suppl. S):S5–S22.

165. Which of the following is the most common cause of hair loss in women?
A) Androgenetic alopecia
B) alopecia areata
C) Telogen effluvium
D) Cicatricial alopecia
E) Traumatic alopecia

Answer and Discussion

The answer is A. Alopecia can be divided into disorders in which the hair follicle is normal but the cycling of hair growth is abnormal, and disorders in which the hair follicle is damaged. Androgenetic alopecia is the most common cause of hair loss in women. Other disorders include alopecia areata, telogen effluvium, cicatricial alopecia, and traumatic alopecias.

Thiedke CC. Alopecia in women. *Am Fam Physician*. 2003;67:1007–1014, 1017–1018.

166. Which of the following has been shown to help prevent neural tube defects in newborns?
A) Magnesium
B) Calcium
C) Folic acid
D) Vitamin B_{12}
E) Vitamin C

Answer and Discussion

The answer is C. The use of folic acid in the prenatal period can help to prevent neural tube defects, such as spina bifida and anencephaly. The use of prenatal vitamins that contain at least 0.4 mg/day folic acid are given before conception and are recommended during the entire pregnancy. Other sources of folic acid include leafy green vegetables, broccoli, mushrooms, and liver.

DeCherney AH, Nathan L. *Current Obstetric and Gynecologic Diagnosis and Treatment*, 9th ed. New York: Lange/McGraw-Hill; 2003:207.

167. Which of the following statements about diaphragm contraception is true?
A) The diaphragm should be left in place for no more than 4 hours after intercourse.
B) The diaphragm should not be used with contraceptive jelly because of the risk of slippage.
C) The diaphragm is associated with an increase in vaginal and urinary infections.
D) The diaphragm can be prescribed based on patient's height and weight.
E) Diaphragm use is associated with an increased risk of cervical cancer.

Answer and Discussion

The answer is C. The diaphragm is a contraceptive device. It is a round, dome-shaped piece of rubber that has a spring incorporated on the outer edge. The device is placed in the vagina and positioned so that it covers the cervix. The diaphragm should be placed in the vagina before intercourse and left in place for 8 hours after intercourse. Contraceptive foam or jelly should always be used with the diaphragm to improve its effectiveness. When used properly, pregnancy rates are approximately 3% but can be as high as 15% with improper use. The diaphragm is associated with an increased risk of vaginal and urinary infections. Patients who desire to use a diaphragm should have it fitted by a physician, and they should demonstrate proper diaphragm positioning to the physician before leaving the office to ensure proper use.

DeCherney AH, Nathan L. *Current Obstetric and Gynecologic Diagnosis and Treatment*, 9th ed. New York: Lange/McGraw-Hill; 2003:633.

168. Pregnancy-induced hypertension is associated with
A) systolic blood pressure >140 mm Hg and diastolic blood pressure >90 mm Hg
B) proteinuria
C) edema
D) microscopic hematuria
E) seizures

Answer and Discussion

The answer is A. Pregnancy-induced hypertension is defined as systolic blood pressure that is greater than 140 mm Hg or diastolic blood pressure >90 mm Hg or a rise >30 mm Hg over baseline systolic or a rise of 15 mm Hg over baseline diastolic blood pressure. Unlike preeclampsia, no proteinuria or edema is noted. Risk factors for pregnancy-induced hypertension include primigravida state, multiple gestation, family history of the condition, polyhydramnios, hydatidiform mole, or underlying vascular disease. Laboratory tests often reveal elevated uric acid levels with decreased chloride levels. In most cases, treatment is initiated with diastolic pressures >100 mm Hg. Initial treatment consists of bed rest and sodium restriction. The drug of choice used in the treatment of pregnancy-induced hypertension is α-methyldopa. Patients with this condition should be followed closely to watch for signs of preeclampsia. Other medications that are used in the acute treatment of hypertension during pregnancy include labetalol and hydralazine.

DeCherney AH, Nathan L. *Current Obstetric and Gynecologic Diagnosis and Treatment*, 9th ed. New York: Lange/McGraw-Hill; 2003:338–346.

169. Which of the following is *not* an option for treating an abnormal Pap smear with results showing squamous cells of undetermined significance (ASCUS) with LSIL (low-grade squamous intraepithelial lesion)?
A) Immediate colposcopy
B) Repeat Pap smear and referral for colposcopy if high-grade squamous intraepithelial lesions (HSILs) are present
C) Screening for human papillomavirus (HPV) DNA and referral for colposcopy if HPV is detected
D) Cryotherapy

Answer and Discussion

The answer is D. Significant controversy surrounds the optimal management of abnormal squamous cells of undetermined significance (ASCUS) reported on Papanicolaou (Pap) screening for cervical cancer. The recommendations of the ASCUS LSIL (low-grade squamous intraepithelial lesion) Triage Study (ALTS) have been controversial. Currently, for minimally abnormal Pap smears (ASCUS LSIL) there are basically three management options:

1. The option of immediate colposcopy is considered appropriate.
2. Repeat Pap screening is also retained as a recommended option, but the indications for referral to colposcopy are more stringent, requiring high-grade squamous intraepithelial lesions (HSIL) on follow-up screening to avoid colposcopy in women with minimal lesions.
3. The new option introduces screening for human papillomavirus (HPV) DNA and referral for colposcopy if HPV is detected. The overall goal is to detect the maximum proportion of cancer cases with the minimum number of colposcopies.

Solomon D, Schiffman M, Tarone R. ASCUS LSIL triage study (ALTS) conclusions reaffirmed: response to a November 2001 commentary. *Obstet Gynecol*. 2002;99:671–674.

170. An 18-year-old man is diagnosed with Chlamydia after complaining of penile discharge. The patient has not been compliant with your recommendations in the past. Appropriate therapy for this infection is
A) azithromycin
B) doxycycline
C) erythromycin
D) ofloxacin
E) none of the above

Answer and Discussion

The answer is A. Chlamydia genital infections are common among adolescents and young adults who are sexually active. *C. trachomatis* infection can be associated with pelvic inflammatory disease (PID), ectopic pregnancy and infertility. Chlamydial infection is often asymptomatic but the complications can be serious. As a result, routine screening for disease during annual examinations is recommended. Single-dose therapy with azithromycin is as effective as a 1-week course of doxycycline (Vibramycin). Doxycycline is cheaper, but azithromycin may be cost-beneficial because it provides single-dose, directly observed therapy. When compliance is an issue it is clearly superior. Erythromycin and ofloxacin (Floxin) also may be used to treat *C. trachomatis*. Erythromycin is less efficacious than azithromycin and doxycycline, and its adverse gastrointestinal effects may decrease patient compliance. Ofloxacin is as effective as the recommended regimens but offers no dosing or cost advantages. Doxycycline and ofloxacin are contraindicated in pregnant women. In addition, the safety and efficacy of azithromycin in pregnant women has not been established; therefore, a 7-day course of either erythromycin or amoxicillin is recommended in this group. Because neither regimen is considered highly effective, cultures should be repeated in 3 weeks.

Woodward C, Fisher MA. Drug treatment of common STDs: Part I. Herpes, syphilis, urethritis, chlamydia, and gonorrhea. *Am Fam Physician*. 1999;60:1387–1394.

171. Which of the following statements about premenstrual syndrome (PMS) is true?
A) Women with fibroids are more commonly affected.
B) Symptoms begin 3 to 7 days after menstruation.
C) Diuretics have no beneficial role in treatment.
D) Fluoxetine (Prozac) can be used in treatment.
E) Niacin has been shown to help reduce symptoms.

Answer and Discussion

The answer is D. Premenstrual syndrome (PMS) is characterized by cyclical nervousness, irritability, emotional mood swings, depression, headaches, water retention with edema, abdominal bloating, and breast tenderness. The syndrome usually begins 7 to 10 days before the onset of menses and disappears once menstruation begins. A key feature is a symptom-free period after the completion of menstruation during the follicular stage of the menstrual cycle. The symptoms are attributed to hormone changes involving estrogen and progesterone. The type, duration, and severity of symptoms vary among individuals but in some women can be very debilitating. As many as 40% of women experience PMS. Diagnosis can be obtained by charting symptoms and comparing them with the patient's menstrual cycle. Treatment involves restriction of salt, caffeine, and fats; vitamin B_6 supplementation; use of diuretics during periods of water retention; use of prostaglandin inhibitors; and use of oral contraceptives. For more severe cases, tranquilizers, fluoxetine (Prozac), progesterone vaginal suppositories, danazol, and bromocriptine have been used. More recently, calcium and magnesium supplementation have been advocated in the treatment of PMS.

DeCherney AH, Nathan L. *Current Obstetric and Gynecologic Diagnosis and Treatment*, 9th ed. New York: Lange/McGraw-Hill; 2003:623–626.

172. Which of the following is the most important risk factor in the transmission of HIV from an infected mother to her newborn?
A) Preterm delivery (<34 weeks' gestation)
B) Low birth weight
C) Low maternal CD4 count
D) Prolonged rupture of membranes (>4 hours)
E) Intravenous drug use during pregnancy

Answer and Discussion

The answer is D. HIV infection types 1 and 2 are diagnosed by the enzyme-linked immunosorbent assay (ELISA) test initially. If the ELISA is positive, the ELISA test should be repeated first, and then, if still positive, the results should be confirmed with the Western blot test. Antibodies to HIV generally appear in the circulation 2 to 12 weeks after infection. Detection in the newborn is more difficult when the mother is infected with HIV, because the child will be positive for the ELISA and the Western blot as a result of maternal transmission of the antibody transplacentally. Because of this, the HIV DNA (deoxyribonucleic acid) PCR (polymerase chain reaction) testing is the preferred test in developed countries. Almost 40% of infected newborns have positive tests in the first 2 days of life, with more than 90% testing positive by 2 weeks of age. Reported rates of transmission from mother to child have varied; most large studies in the United States and Europe have documented transmission rates in untreated women of between 12% and 30%. Rates are reported to be higher in Africa and Haiti. Perinatal treatment of HIV-infected mothers with antiretroviral drugs has dramatically decreased these rates to <8%. Several risk factors increase the rate of vertical transmission:

- Preterm delivery (<34 weeks' gestation)
- Low birth weight
- Low maternal antenatal CD4 count (<29%)
- Intravenous drug use during pregnancy
- Prolonged rupture of membranes (>4 hours), which is the most important variable that increases risk

Cesarean section combined with prenatal, intrapartum, and neonatal zidovudine therapy decreases the transmission rate by 87%. HIV can be transmitted via breast milk and colostrum. Homosexuals who practice the insertive role in intercourse are eight times more likely to get hepatitis B than HIV. Practicing the receptive role in intercourse increases the risk of HIV transmission. If a patient has either virus, he or she is at risk for contracting the other. Needle-stick injuries result in the transmission of HIV in approximately 0.3% of cases.

Kasper DL, Braunwald E, Fauci AS, et al., eds. *Harrison's principles of internal medicine,* 16th ed. New York: McGraw-Hill; 2005:1079.

173. Which laboratory test would best support lung maturity in a fetus whose mother has shown signs of premature labor?
A) Lecithin–sphingomyelin (L/S) ratio of 1.75
B) L/S ratio of 1.5
C) Absence of phosphatidylinositol
D) Absence of phosphatidylglycerol (PG)
E) L/S ratio of 1.8 with a positive PG level

Answer and Discussion

The answer is E. Premature birth can result in severe lung-related problems secondary to inadequate lung development. A number of different medications have been advocated to improve lung maturation. Currently, the use of antenatal corticosteroids reduces mortality and the incidence of RDS and intraventricular hemorrhage in new preterm infants. They are typically administered between 24 and 34 weeks. The benefits usually peak at 24 hours and continue for 7 days. Treatment consists of betamethasone given in two intramuscular doses 12 hours apart. Antenatal steroids should be administered unless immediate delivery is anticipated. Thyroid-releasing hormone (TRH) has been advocated but not proven to be beneficial for lung maturation in fetuses younger than 28 weeks' gestation. Because thyroid hormone does not pass across the placenta, TRH is used. TRH crosses the placenta and increases fetal thyroxine levels that are thought to improve lung maturation. Surfactant is also used for lung maturation, and studies support its beneficial use. Tests for lung maturity include the L/S ratio, phosphatidylinositol, and PG levels. The levels are measured by obtaining amniotic fluid via amniocentesis. RDS is rare if the L/S ratio is >2 and PG is present. If the L/S ratio is <2 but PG is present, RDS develops in <5% of infants. Meconium lowers the L/S ratio, and blood tends to normalize the value to 1.4. Other tests for lung maturation include the foam stability index and the lamellar body number density. Both are relatively fast tests and may be more accurate and useful than the L/S ratio.

Beers MH, Porter RS, eds. *The Merck manual of diagnosis and therapy*, Merck Research Laboratories, 18th ed. Whitehouse Station, NJ: Merck & Co.; 2006:2303–2304.

Respiratory distress syndrome (RDS) is rare if the lecithin-sphingomyelin ratio (L/S ratio) is greater than 2 and phosphatidylglycerol (PG) is present.

174. A 22-year-old man is diagnosed with primary syphilis. He has no allergies and is otherwise healthy. The drug of choice is
A) oral penicillin
B) oral azithromycin
C) intramuscular ceftriaxone
D) parenteral penicillin G
E) oral ciprofloxacin

Answer and Discussion

The answer is D. Syphilis is a systemic disease caused by the sexual transmission of *Treponema pallidum*. It can occur as primary, secondary, or tertiary disease. Primary disease presents with one or more painless ulcers or chancres at the inoculation site. Secondary disease manifestations include rash and adenopathy. Cardiac, neurologic, ophthalmic, auditory, or gummatous lesions characterize tertiary infections. Latent disease may be detected by serologic testing, without the presence of signs and symptoms. Early latent disease is defined as disease acquired within the preceding year. All other cases of latent syphilis are considered late latent disease or disease of unknown duration. The recommended treatment regimens have not changed since the 1993 CDC Guidelines. Parenteral penicillin G is still the preferred drug for treating all stages of syphilis, including disease in pregnant women.

Woodward C, Fisher MA. Drug treatment of common STDs: Part I. Herpes, syphilis, urethritis, chlamydia, and gonorrhea. *Am Fam Physician*. 1999;60:1387–1394.

175. Which of the following is *not* an acceptable treatment for uncomplicated gonococcal infections of the cervix?
A) Doxycycline
B) Cefixime
C) Ceftriaxone
D) Ciprofloxacin
E) Ofloxacin

Answer and Discussion

The answer is A. Four single-dose regimens are now available for treatment of uncomplicated gonococcal infections of the cervix, urethra, and rectum. They include cefixime (Suprax), ceftriaxone, ciprofloxacin, and ofloxacin.

Woodward C, Fisher MA. Drug treatment of common STDs: Part I. Herpes, syphilis, urethritis, chlamydia, and gonorrhea. *Am Fam Physician*. 1999; 60:1387–1394.

176. Which of the following is considered the drug of choice to treat preterm labor?
A) Magnesium sulfate
B) Terbutaline
C) Ritodrine
D) Indomethacin
E) Nifedipine

Answer and Discussion

The answer is A. The drug of choice for preterm labor is magnesium sulfate given intravenously. Magnesium sulfate works by competing with calcium for entry into muscle cells. This results in myometrial relaxation. The levels of the medication need to be monitored to maintain optimal therapeutic levels. Adjustments need to be made in patients with renal disease and abnormal creatinine clearance. Once the preterm labor has been arrested, the patient can be switched to oral magnesium sulfate. A minor side effect of magnesium sulfate is warmth or flushing with the first administration. Respiratory depression can occur with levels of 12 to 15 mg/dL, and cardiac effects may occur with higher levels. With magnesium sulfate administration the fetus (if delivered) may show signs of decreased muscle tone and drowsiness, resulting in lower Apgar scores. These effects are often prolonged in premature infants because of decreased renal clearance.

DeCherney AH, Nathan L. *Current Obstetric and Gynecologic Diagnosis and Treatment*, 9th ed. New York: Lange/McGraw-Hill; 2003:290–291.

177. Which of the following fetal presentations should always be delivered via cesarean section?
A) Complete breech
B) Footling breech
C) Frank breech
D) Vertex presentation

Answer and Discussion

The answer is B. Three types of vaginal breech delivery are performed:

- *Spontaneous breech delivery*: The fetus is delivered spontaneously without manipulation by the physician other than support of the fetus.
- *Partial (or assisted) breech extraction*: The fetus is delivered spontaneously until the umbilicus is at the introitus, at which point the fetus is extracted.
- *Total breech extraction*: The physician extracts the entire body of the fetus.

Incomplete or footling breech presentations should be delivered via cesarean section because the risk of cord prolapse is greater and entrapment of the fetus by the cervix is greater.

The risk of birth trauma is greater with breech deliveries, particularly brachial plexus injuries, if the fetus weighs >3,600 g. In many communities the standard of care is cesarean section for breech presentation; however, this is controversial. Premature infants are generally delivered by cesarean section because of the disparity between head and body size.

DeCherney AH, Nathan L. *Current Obstetric and Gynecologic Diagnosis and Treatment*, 9th ed. New York: Lange/McGraw-Hill; 2003:369–376.

178. Which of the following is a contraindication for external cephalic version?
A) 36 weeks' gestation
B) Maternal age of 35
C) Polyhydramnios

D) Maternal diabetes
E) Obesity

Answer and Discussion

The answer is A. External cephalic version can be attempted on fetuses that are detected before the onset of labor and after 37 weeks' gestation. A tocolytic medication is delivered, and abdominal manipulation is performed under ultrasound guidance. Version before 37 weeks is not recommended because of the risk that the fetus may revert to a breech presentation before delivery and the risk of delivery of a premature infant. The success rate is approximately 75%. The procedure should be performed in the hospital so that cesarean section can be done if complications arise. The most common complications are placental abruption and cord compression. Contraindications for external cephalic version include uteroplacental insufficiency, hypertension, intrauterine growth retardation, oligohydramnios, or history of prior uterine surgery.

DeCherney AH, Nathan L. *Current Obstetric and Gynecologic Diagnosis and Treatment*, 9th ed. New York: Lange/McGraw-Hill; 2003:378–379.

179. Which of the following is not an acceptable test for the detection of chlamydia and gonorrhea?
A) Polymerase chain reaction (PCR) on urine samples in women.
B) Transcription-mediated amplification on urine samples in men.
C) Strand displacement amplification on urine samples in women.
D) Polymerase chain reaction (PCR) on urine samples in men.
E) Transcription-mediated amplification on urine samples in women.

Answer and Discussion

The answer is A. Until recently, testing patients for chlamydia and gonorrhea involved collecting samples from the cervix or urethra and sending them for cultures. The discomfort and embarrassment associated with sampling these sites may deter some high-risk patients from seeking testing for these infections. An alternative to cervical or urethral cultures is nucleic acid amplification tests (NAATs) that can be performed on urine samples. Three types of NAAT are commercially available: polymerase chain reaction (PCR), transcription-mediated amplification, and strand displacement amplification. With the exception of PCR for detection of gonorrhea in women, urine samples perform as well as samples collected from other sites.

Cook RL, Hutchison SL, Ostergaard L. Systematic review: noninvasive testing for *Chlamydia trachomatis* and *Neisseria gonorrhoeae*. *Ann Intern Med.* 2005;142:914–925.

180. Which of the following is used infrequently in the treatment of pubic lice because of concerns of neurotoxicity, resistence, and slow killing time?
A) Malathion
B) Permethrin
C) Pyrethrum
D) Lindane

Answer and Discussion

The answer is D. Pubic lice are readily transmitted sexually. There is some evidence that occasionally they may be transmitted through contaminated clothing or towels, although this is controversial. The presence of pubic lice should prompt an evaluation for other common sexually transmitted diseases, such as chlamydial infection and gonorrhea. Treatment is the same as for head lice. Sexual contacts also should be treated if infested. Recent evidence-based reviews found that malathion, permethrin, and pyrethrum insecticides were equally effective in treating head lice infestations. A 1% lindane shampoo is also used to treat resistant lice infestations. However, lindane shampoo is used infrequently now because of concerns about neurotoxicity, resistance, and slow killing time.

Flinders DC, De Schweinitz P. Pediculosis and scabies. *Am Fam Physician.* 2004;69:341–348, 349–350.

181. Which of the following ultrasound parameters is best used for estimating gestational age during the first trimester?
A) Crown–rump length
B) Biparietal diameter
C) Femur length
D) Head–foot length
E) Estimated weight

Answer and Discussion

The answer is A. The practice of performing routine ultrasound examinations to confirm accurate dates is controversial. Many advocate no testing, whereas others believe that an ultrasound at 14 to 20 weeks helps to confirm dates and looks for fetal abnormalities or perhaps twins. The ultrasound can be used to measure crown–rump length, biparietal diameter, and femur length, all of which can be used to confirm dates. The crown–rump length is more accurate during the first trimester, whereas the biparietal diameter and femur length are used more during the second trimester. The ultrasound is best used in the first trimester for estimating age of the fetus. As pregnancy progresses estimation of age is more difficult to assess using ultrasound examination.

DeCherney AH, Nathan L. *Current Obstetric and Gynecologic Diagnosis and Treatment*, 9th ed. New York: Lange/McGraw-Hill; 2003:266.

182. The maximum acceptable cumulative dose of ionizing radiation during pregnancy is
A) 100 rads
B) 50 rads
C) 10 rads
D) 5 rads
E) 1 rad

Answer and Discussion

The answer is D. The accepted cumulative dose of ionizing radiation during pregnancy is 5 rads, and no single diagnostic study exceeds this maximum. The amount of exposure to the fetus from a two-view chest x-ray of the mother is only 0.00007 rads. The most sensitive time period for central nervous system teratogenesis is between 10 and 17 weeks of gestation. The fetal malformations that are most commonly caused by high-dose radiation are central nervous system changes, especially microcephaly and mental retardation. Nonurgent radiologic testing should be avoided during this time. Rare consequences of prenatal radiation exposure also include a slight increase in the incidence of childhood leukemia and, possibly, a very small change in the frequency of genetic mutations. Such exposure is not an indication for pregnancy termination. Appropriate counseling of patients before radiologic studies are performed is critical. Physicians should carefully weigh the risks and benefits of any radiographic study and include the mother in the decision-making process whenever possible.

Toppenberg KS, Hill DA, Miller DP. Safety of radiographic imaging during pregnancy. *Am Fam Physician.* 1999;59: 1813–1818.

183. Which of the following statements regarding ectopic pregnancy is correct?

A) The number of ectopic pregnancies has decreased significantly over the last few decades.
B) Symptoms are rarely present.
C) Diagnosis should be suspected if there is no gestational sac and the β-hCG level is >1,500 mIU/mL (1,500 IU/L).
D) Methotrexate is best for large ectopic pregnancies that have ruptured the fallopian tube.
E) Symptoms are usually delayed for 10 to 12 weeks.

Answer and Discussion

The answer is C. The number of ectopic pregnancies has increased dramatically in the past few decades. Ectopic pregnancy is more often detected in women older than 35 years of age and in non-White ethnic groups. The hallmark symptoms of ectopic pregnancy are abdominal pain with spotting, usually occurring 6 to 8 weeks after the last normal menstrual period. This remains the most common presentation of tubal pregnancy in symptomatic patients. Other presentations depend on the location of the ectopic pregnancy. Less commonly, ectopic pregnancy presents with pain that radiates to the shoulder, vaginal bleeding, syncope, and/or hypovolemic shock. The condition should be suspected if a transvaginal ultrasound shows no intrauterine gestational sac when the β-hCG level is >1,500 mIU/mL (1,500 IU/L). If the β-hCG level plateaus or fails to double in 48 hours and the ultrasound examination fails to identify an intrauterine gestational sac, uterine curettage may determine the presence or absence of chorionic villi. Although past treatment consisted of an open laparotomy and salpingectomy, current laparoscopic techniques for unruptured ectopic pregnancy emphasize tubal preservation. Other treatment options include the use of methotrexate therapy for small, unruptured ectopic pregnancies in hemodynamically stable patients. Expectant management may have a role when β-hCG levels are low and declining.

Tenore JL. Ectopic pregnancy. *Am Fam Physician.* 2000; 61: 1080–1088.

The hallmark symptoms of ectopic pregnancy are abdominal pain with spotting, usually occurring 6 to 8 weeks after the last normal menstrual period.

184. In premenopausal women the best time to perform a clinical breast examination (CBE) is

A) 1 week prior to menses
B) 1 week after menses
C) during menses
D) at the time of ovulation
E) 1 day prior to menses

Answer and Discussion

The answer is B. A CBE includes an assessment of both breasts and the chest, axillae, and regional lymphatics. In premenopausal women, the CBE is best done the week following menses, when breast tissue is least engorged. With the patient in an upright position, the physician visually inspects the breasts, noting asymmetry, nipple discharge, obvious masses, and skin changes, such as dimpling, inflammation, rashes, and unilateral nipple retraction or inversion.

Klein S. Evaluation of palpable breast masses. *Am Fam Physician.* 2005;71:1731–1738.

Barton MB, Harris R, Fletcher SW. The rational clinical examination. Does this patient have breast cancer? The screening clinical breast examination: should it be done? How? *JAMA.* 1999;282:1270–1280.

185. Which of the following statements regarding breast conservation therapy is true?

A) The risk of recurrent cancer is higher.
B) The fear of recurrence is higher in these women.
C) Women have more depression with breast conservative therapy.
D) Women have more anxiety with breast conservative therapy.
E) Women have fewer episodes of insomnia with breast conservative therapy.

Answer and Discussion

The answer is E. The patient's desires should always be considered when deciding breast cancer treatment. For most patients, mastectomy does not influence the likelihood of survival, but may have an impact on quality of life. Women whose breasts are preserved have fewer episodes of depression, anxiety, and insomnia. A recent study of patients with early-stage breast cancer found women who undergo breast conservation therapy have improved body image, higher satisfaction with treatment, and no more fear of recurrence compared with women treated with mastectomy.

McArdle JM, Hughson AV, McArdle CS. Reduced psychological morbidity after breast conservation. *Br J Surg.* 1990;77: 1221–1223.

Curran D, van Dongen JP, Aaronson NK, et al. Quality of life of early-stage breast cancer patients treated with radical mastectomy or breast-conserving procedures: results of EORTC Trial 10801. *Eur J Cancer.* 1998;34:307–314.

186. The most common cause of neonatal sepsis in the United States is

A) *Staphylococcus aureus*
B) *Streptococcus pneumoniae*
C) Group B *Streptococcus*
D) *Escherichia coli*
E) *Haemophilus influenzae*

Answer and Discussion

The answer is C. Group B *Streptococcus* is considered part of the normal flora of humans. The majority of the bacteria exist in the gastrointestinal tract; however, the bacteria may also be found in the vagina, cervix, throat skin, urethra, and urine of healthy individuals. The organism affects as many as 40% of pregnant or sexually active women. The diagnosis is made by culture or rapid assays that are now available. Transmission to the fetus at the time of birth ranges from 35% to 70%, with the highest rates associated with heavy vaginal colonization. Risk factors for transmission include preterm labor or delivery, premature rupture of membranes, low birth weight, prolonged rupture of membranes (>12–18 hours), intrapartum fever, and a history of delivering an infected infant. Group B *Streptococcus* is the most common cause of neonatal sepsis in the United States. It is the second-most common cause of bacteriuria in pregnancy. Affected children may experience respiratory distress, pneumonia, and meningitis (30%). Septicemia, shock, and death may occur despite the use of antibiotics. Treating carriers in labor reduces the rate of transmission to the infant. All women should be tested at 35 to 37 weeks. Empiric treatment in during labor and subsequent delivery is recommended. Treatment usually consists of ampicillin, penicillin, and clindamycin for those with penicillin allergies.

Cunningham FG, Gant NF, Leveno KJ, et al. *Williams Obstetrics*, 21st ed. New York: McGraw-Hill; 2001:1472–1473.

187. Which of the following statements regarding vasectomy is true?

A) Vasectomy requires surgical intervention and has many risks that prevent it from being a cost-effective birth control method.
B) Patients should be monitored in a controlled setting for 2 days following a vasectomy.
C) Sperm analysis should be performed twice to confirm azoospermia before the discontinuation of alternative birth control methods.
D) After vasectomy the patient should be counseled not to lift heavy objects for 4 weeks.
E) Intercourse should be avoided for 4 to 6 weeks after vasectomy.

Answer and Discussion

The answer is C. Vasectomy is among the most dependable and cost-effective methods of contraception. Family physicians perform approximately 15% of the estimated 500,000 vasectomies that are done each year in the United States. Vasectomy can be performed using various techniques, although each requires isolation and division of the vas and operative management of the vasal ends. Removal of at least 15 mm vas is recommended. Division of the vas without removal of a segment is effective if the technique is combined with other methods for treating the vasal ends, such as thermal luminal fulguration and proximal fascial interposition. Ligation of the ends without the aid of surgical clips may result in necrosis and sloughing of the ends, which may cause early failure. Leaving the testicular end of the vas open has been shown to be effective and to result in a lower incidence of epididymal congestion and sperm granuloma. The no-scalpel technique offers shorter operating time, less pain and swelling, and faster recovery. Appropriate postoperative recommendations include intermittent ice applications to the scrotum for 8 hours, bed rest and scrotal support for 48 hours, and avoidance of heavy exertion for 1 week. Acetaminophen usually produces sufficient analgesia, although occasionally narcotic analgesics are necessary. Sexual activity should be avoided for 1 week. Another method of contraception should be used until semen analysis has confirmed azoospermia on two separate occasions. The possible link with vasectomy and coronary artery disease has not been proven to exist by large studies.

Clenney TL, Higgins JC. Vasectomy techniques. *Am Fam Physician*. 1999;60:137–152.

188. Which of the following tests is most useful in diagnosing cystic breast masses?

A) Mammograms
B) Ultrasound
C) Fine-needle biopsy
D) Magnetic resonance imaging (MRI)
E) Computed tomography (CT)

Answer and Discussion

The answer is B. Approximately 180,000 new cases of breast cancer are diagnosed annually, accounting for about 48,000 deaths/year in the United States. Although somewhat controversial, annual mammograms and clinical breast examinations are recommended for women older than 40 years. Women older than 20 years should be encouraged to do monthly breast self-examinations, and women between 20 and 39 years of age should have a clinical breast examination every 3 years. Screening guidelines are modified for women with risk factors. Risk factors include increasing age and female sex. Family history is highly significant in a first-degree relative (e.g., mother, sister, daughter), especially if the cancer has been diagnosed premenopausally. Women who have premenopausal first-degree relatives with breast cancer have a three- to fourfold increased risk of developing breast cancer than women who do not. Important to note is that most women with breast cancer have no identifiable risk factors. Approximately 8% of all cases of breast cancer are hereditary. About one-half of these cases are attributed to mutations in two breast cancer susceptibility genes, *BRCA1* and *BRCA2*. Hereditary breast cancer commonly occurs in premenopausal women and is more frequently bilateral than is nonhereditary breast cancer. Several family members are affected over three generations or more and can include women from the paternal side of the family. Screening tests are available that detect *BRCA* mutations. Abnormal breast examinations and mammograms should be further evaluated. Ultrasonographic studies are most useful to evaluate cystic breast masses. For solid masses, diagnostic biopsy techniques include fine-needle aspiration, core biopsy, and excisional biopsy.

Apantaku LM. Breast cancer diagnosis and screening. *Am Fam Physician*. 2000;62:596–602, 605–606.

189. A 43-year-old woman is diagnosed with stage II breast cancer. One year later she is asymptomatic. Appropriate follow up consists of

A) at least yearly mammograms
B) bone scan to rule out metastatic disease
C) CT of the head to rule out metastatic disease
D) liver function test every 6 months to rule out metastatic disease
E) serial calcium levels to monitor for metatstatic disease

Answer and Discussion

The answer is A. A baseline mammogram should be obtained approximately 6 months after tumor excision and the completion of all treatments. Mammography should then be done at least annually. Other imaging studies may be necessary in symptomatic patients. Patients with bone pain should be screened by bone scan for bone associated metastasis. Detailed laboratory follow-up is expensive and has not been shown to improve survival. Randomized control trials have not shown survival benefit from the routine use of bone scan and computed tomographic scan for asymptomatic patients with stage I or stage II breast cancer.

Cady B, Bland K, Copeland E. Choice of operations for early breast cancer: an expanding role for breast conservation instead of mastectomy. In: Bland KI, Copeland EM, eds. *The breast: comprehensive management of benign and malignant diseases.* 2nd ed. Philadelphia: WB Saunders; 1998:1130–1152.

190. Which of the following HPV subtypes is most associated with the development of cervical cancer?

A) Types 43 and 54
B) Types 7 and 9
C) Types 16 and 18
D) Types 24 and 28
E) Types 33 and 40

Answer and Discussion

The answer is C. A preponderance of evidence suggests a causal link between HPV infection and cervical neoplasia. This link is strongest for certain HPV types, particularly types 16 and 18.

Beers MH, Porter RS, eds. *The Merck manual of diagnosis and therapy*, Merck Research Laboratories, 18th ed. Whitehouse Station, NJ: Merck & Co.; 2006:1652.

A preponderance of evidence suggests a causal link between HPV infection types 16 and 18 and cervical neoplasia.

Chapter 4

Psychiatry

Questions

Each of the following questions or incomplete statements is followed by suggested answers or completions. Select the ONE BEST ANSWER in each case.

1. Cognitive therapy involves

A) repetition of negative thoughts that eventually dissipate
B) changing a thought that involves a situation that leads to a change of mood, behavior, or reaction
C) repeated acts of fearful situations that allow adaptation
D) negative reinforcement of harmful activities
E) none of the above

Answer and Discussion

The answer is B. Cognitive therapy is a psychological treatment method that helps patients correct false self-beliefs that contribute to certain moods and behaviors. The basic principle behind cognitive therapy is that a thought precedes a mood, and that both are interrelated with a person's environment, physical reaction, and subsequent behavior. Therefore, changing a thought that arises in a given situation changes mood, behavior, and physical reaction. Although it is unclear who benefits most from cognitive therapy, motivated patients who have an internal center of control and the capacity for introspection likely would benefit most.

Ramana R, Paykel ES, Cooper Z, et al. Remission and relapse in major depression: a two-year prospective follow-up study. *Psychol Med.* 1995;25:1161–1170.

The basic principle behind cognitive therapy is that a thought precedes a mood, and that both are interrelated with a person's environment, physical reaction, and subsequent behavior.

2. The most common side effect of high dose St. John's Wort is

A) transient photosensitivity
B) hoarseness
C) myalgias
D) hypertension
E) tremor

Answer and Discussion

The answer is A. Transient photosensitivity is generally the most common side effect of St. John's Wort and occurs more commonly at higher dosages. Other side effects include gastrointestinal upset, increased anxiety, minor palpitations, fatigue, restlessness, dry mouth, headache, and increased depression.

Brockmoller J, Reum T, Bauer S, et al. Hypericin and pseudohypericin: pharmacokinetics and effects on photosensitivity in humans. *Pharmacopsychiatry.* 1997;30(suppl 2):94–101.

3. Which of the following medications can be affected by the concurrent use of St. John's Wort?

A) Amoxicillin
B) Gabapentin
C) Oral contraceptives
D) Glipizide
E) Hydrochlorothiazide

Answer and Discussion

The answer is C. Due to the induction of CYP 3A4, concurrent use of St. John's Wort may reduce the effectiveness of oral contraceptives. Women using oral contraceptives should be counseled regarding possible breakthrough bleeding and might consider a barrier method of contraception when taking St. John's Wort.

Hall SD, Wang Z, Huang SM, et al. The interaction between St. John's Wort and an oral contraceptive. *Clin Pharmacol Ther.* 2003;74:525–535.

4. Which of the following is the definition of *adjustment disorder with depressed mood?*

A) Tearfulness related to the death of a loved one 1 year ago.
B) Development of emotional or behavioral symptoms in response to an identifiable stressor that occurs within 3 months of the stressor.
C) Thoughts of death and morbid preoccupation with worthlessness with no prior triggering event.
D) Lifetime obsession with morbid thoughts.
E) Transient, normal depressive responses or mood changes to stress.

Answer and Discussion

The answer is B. *Adjustment disorder with depressed mood* is defined as development of emotional or behavioral symptoms in response to an identifiable stressor that occurs within 3 months of the stressor. Symptoms include depressed mood, tearfulness, and hopelessness, and occur in excess of what would usually be expected from exposure to the stressor and cause significant impairment in social and occupational/academic functioning. Once the stressor (or its consequences) has terminated, the symptoms resolve within 6 months. Acute episodes last for less than 6 months, and chronic episodes last 6 months or more.

Son SE, Kirchner JT. Depression in children and adolescents. *Am Fam Physician.* 2000;62:2297–2308, 2311–2312.

5. Which of the following medications would be the best selection to treat chronic neuropathic pain in a frail elderly man with a history of cardiac conduction abnormalities?
A) Fluoxitene (Prozac)
B) Amitryptiline (Elavil)
C) Gabapentin (Neurontin)
D) Phenytoin (Dilantin)
E) Cyclobenzaprine (Flexaril)

Answer and Discussion

The answer is C. An antiepileptic drug [e.g., gabapentin (Neurontin)] is preferred if the patient cannot tolerate the side effects of tricyclic antidepressants, has cardiac contraindications to the use of tricyclic antidepressants (e.g., conduction abnormalities, recent cardiac event), or is a "frail elder." Of the second-generation antiepileptic drugs, gabapentin (Neurontin) has the best documented efficacy in the treatment of neuropathic pain.

Son SE, Kirchner JT. Depression in children and adolescents. *Am Fam Physician.* 2000;62:2297–2308, 2311–2312.

6. Which of the following medications is limited by potentially life-threatening rashes?
A) Phenytoin (Dilantin)
B) Lamotrigine (Lamictal)
C) Carbamazepine (Tegretol)
D) Gabapentin (Neurontin)
E) Tramadol (Ultram)

Answer and Discussion

The answer is B. Lamotrigine (Lamictal) has been proved to be modestly effective in patients with trigeminal neuralgia, neuropathy associated with human immunodeficiency virus (HIV) infection, and poststroke pain. The drug is ineffective in patients with unspecified refractory neuropathic pain. The use of lamotrigine is limited by potentially life-threatening rashes.

Son SE, Kirchner JT. Depression in children and adolescents. *Am Fam Physician.* 2000;62:2297–2308, 2311–2312.

7. Which of the following means is the most common for suicide completion?
A) Firearms
B) Prescription medication overdose
C) Illicit drug overdose
D) Carbon monoxide poisoning
E) Hanging

Answer and Discussion

The answer is A. Access to means to attempt suicide is an important precipitating cause. This is true even after controlling for other risk factors such as depression or substance use. Firearms are the most common means for suicide completion. Other means include medications, illicit drugs, toxic chemicals, carbon monoxide, hanging, and cutting. Almost anything can be used as a means to attempt suicide, but access to the most lethal means often is preventable.

Brent DA, Perper JA, Allman CJ. Alcohol, firearms, and suicide among youth. Temporal trends in Allegheny County, Pennsylvania, 1960 to 1983. *JAMA.* 1987;257:3369.

Brent DA, Perper JA, Allman CJ, et al. The presence and accessibility of firearms in the homes of adolescent suicides. A case-control study. *JAMA.* 1991;266:2989.

Kennebeck S, Bonin L. Epidemiology and risk factors for suicidal behavior in children and adolescents. Up to Date, version 14.1. Accessed 3/6/06.

8. Which of the following statements is true regarding the use of haloperidol?
A) The drug has been approved for intravenous use.
B) Haloperidol is considered safe in those with a known seizure disorder.
C) The drug can cause prolongation of the QT interval.
D) ECG monitoring is not necessary when the drug is given intravenously.
E) None of the above.

Answer and Discussion

The answer is C. Haloperidol has not been approved for intravenous use, although it is commonly used by this route and is generally thought to be safe. The drug may cause prolongation of the QT interval; as a result, electrocardiographic monitoring is necessary. Haloperidol should be avoided if possible in patients with a known seizure disorder.

Fife A, Schreiber J. Psychiatric emergencies: agitation or aggression. Up to Date, version 14.1. Accessed 3/6/06.

9. Domestic violence
A) is higher in gay and lesbian relationships
B) affects males and females equally
C) rarely affects the elderly
D) increases during pregnancy
E) is rarely associated with a spouse

Answer and Discussion

The answer is D. Studies show that women are much more likely than men to be the victims of chronic physical abuse. Domestic violence in gay and lesbian relationships appears to be as common as in heterosexual relationships. Domestic violence is also a significant problem among the elderly. Elder abuse is associated with an increase in reports of chronic pain, depression, number of health conditions, and an increased mortality. The abuser is most commonly a relative (usually the spouse). Domestic violence often begins or, if already present, increases during pregnancy and the postpartum period.

Hillard PJ. Physical abuse in pregnancy. *Obstet Gynecol.* 1985;66:185.

Sillman JS. Diagnosing, screening and counseling for domestic violence. Up to Date, version 14.1. Accessed 3/6/06.

Studies show that women are much more likely than men to be the victims of chronic physical abuse. Domestic violence in gay and lesbian relationships appears to be as common as in heterosexual relationships.

10. When considering light therapy for seasonal affective disorder (SAD), which of the following is *not* a factor that predicts a positive result?
A) Hypersomnia
B) High number of vegetative symptoms
C) Increased intake of sweet foods in the afternoon
D) History of reactivity to ambient light
E) Positive family history of SAD

Answer and Discussion

The answer is E. Light therapy involves exposure to minimum 2,500 lux of visible light. 10,000 lux for 30 minutes/day has been shown to be effective. Factors that have predicted a positive response to light therapy include hypersomnia, high rate of vegetative symptoms, an increased intake of sweet foods in the afternoon, and a history of reactivity to ambient light. A positive family history does not necessarily increase a positive response to light therapy.

Oren DA, Jacobsen FM, Wehr TA, et al. Predictors of response to phototherapy in seasonal affective disorder. *Compr Psychiatry.* 1992; 33:111.

Saeed SA, Bruce TJ. Seasonal affective disorder. Up to Date, version 14.1. Accessed 3/8/06.

11. Which of the following statements regarding lesbians and health care is true?
A) Approximately 1% of the women in the United States identify themselves as lesbian.
B) Lesbians tend to overutilize health care.
C) Lesbians typically present later for health care than heterosexual women.
D) Lesbian women are usually of higher socioeconomic status than gay men.
E) Lesbian awareness rarely affects their health care.

Answer and Discussion

The answer is C. Approximately 4% to 10% of women in the United States identify themselves as lesbians. Lesbians, like other marginalized groups of women, underutilize clinical care services and present later for health care than heterosexual women. Some reasons for these deficiencies are health-care providers who lack awareness of the health issues of lesbians, who discriminate against them, and who create negative experiences. In addition, women are often of lower socioeconomic status than gay men, without spousal or family benefits such as health insurance. Lesbians also use health-care services that focus on contraception and reproduction less frequently; these services are entry points to the health-care system for many women.

Denenberg R. Report on lesbian health. *Womens Health Issues.* 1995;5:81.

O'Hanlan KA. Lesbian health and homophobia: Perspectives for the treating obstetrician/ gynecologist. *Curr Probl Obstet Gynecol Fertil.* 1995;18:99.

Carroll NM. Gynecologic and obstetric care for lesbians. Up to Date, version 14.1. Accessed 3/8/06.

12. Risk factors for smoking include all of the following *except*
A) exposure to secondhand smoke
B) presence of a smoker in the family
C) poor academic performance
D) single parent at home
E) lack of concern over weight and body image, particularly in women

Answer and Discussion

The answer is E. Risk factors for smoking include exposure to secondhand smoke, presence of a smoker in the household, comorbid psychiatric disorders, strained relationship with parent and/or single parent at home, low level of expressed self-esteem and self-worth, poor academic performance, increased adolescent perception of parental approval of smoking, affiliation with smoking peers, and availability of cigarettes. An additional risk factor for boys is high levels of aggression and rebelliousness; among girls, preoccupation with weight and body image is a separate risk factor.

Hurt RD, Sachs DPL, Glover ED, et al. A Comparison of sustained-release bupropion and placebo for smoking cessation. *N Engl J Med.* 1997;337:1195.

Rennard RI, Daughton DM. Overview of smoking cessation. Up to Date, version 14.1. Accessed 3/8/06.

13. Smoking is associated with an increased risk of all of the following *except*
A) infertility
B) spontaneous abortion
C) ectopic pregnancy
D) premature menopause
E) multiple births

Answer and Discussion

The answer is E. Smoking is associated with infertility, spontaneous abortion, ectopic pregnancy, and premature menopause.

Smoking and infertility. *Fertil Steril.* 2004;81:1181.

Rennard RI, Daughton DM. Overview of smoking cessation. Up to Date, version 14.1. Accessed 3/8/06.

14. Which of the following has been shown to be beneficial in smoking cessation?
A) Fluoxetine
B) Venlafaxine
C) Bupropion
D) Sertraline
E) Doxepin

Answer and Discussion

The answer is C. Bupropion (also marketed as Wellbutrin) has been available for use as an antidepressant in the United States since 1989, and is thought to act by enhancing central nervous system noradrenergic and dopaminergic function. A sustained-release formulation of the drug (Zyban) is licensed as an aid to smoking cessation.

Rennard RI, Daughton DM. Overview of smoking cessation. Up to Date, version 14.1. Accessed 3/8/06.

15. Urges or impulses for repetitive intentional behavior performed in a stereotyped manner in an attempt to relieve anxiety is termed
A) adaptation
B) congruence

C) compulsion
D) obsession
E) transference

Answer and Discussion

The answer is C. *Obsessions* are persistent thoughts, ideas, and images that invade into conscious awareness, are recognized as a product of one's mind, and are perceived as senseless and intrusive. In many cases these obsessions have a theme that an insignificant oversight will result in tremendous catastrophe. Other common themes are contamination, a need for ordering things, aggressive impulses, and sexual imagery. *Compulsions* are urges or impulses for repetitive intentional behavior performed in a stereotyped manner (e.g., touching, counting, arranging) in an attempt to alleviate the anxiety that most frequently results from the obsessions. Often these behaviors are believed to help defend the patient and others from potential harm.

Ciechanowski P, Katon W. Overview of obsessive-compulsive disorder. Up to Date, version 14.1. Accessed 3/8/06.

16. Which of the following medications is used in the classic treatment of bipolar disorder?
A) Lithium
B) Sertraline
C) Amitriptyline
D) Phenytoin
E) Alprazolam

Answer and Discussion

The answer is A. Bipolar disorder is most commonly diagnosed in persons between 18 and 24 years of age. The clinical presentations of this disorder are diverse and include mania, hypomania, and psychosis. Frequently associated conditions include substance abuse and anxiety disorders. Patients with acute mania must be evaluated urgently. Treatment involves the use of mood stabilizers such as lithium, valproic acid, and carbamazepine.

Grisswold KS, Pessar LF. Management of bipolar disorder. *Am Fam Physician.* 2000;62:1343–1353, 1357–1358.

17. A 21 year old presents with complaints of an inflated self-esteem, decreased need for sleep, and distractibility. The most likely diagnosis is
A) depression
B) hypothymia
C) borderline personality
D) mania
E) antisocial personality

Answer and Discussion

The answer is D. The diagnosis of mania consists of at least three of the following:

1. Inflated self-esteem or grandiosity
2. Decreased need for sleep (e.g., feels rested after only 3 hours of sleep)
3. More talkative than usual, or pressure to keep talking
4. Flight of ideas, or subjective experience that thoughts are racing
5. Distractibility (i.e., attention too easily drawn to unimportant or irrelevant external stimuli)
6. Increase in goal-directed activity (either socially, at work or school, or sexually) or psychomotor agitation
7. Excessive involvement in pleasurable activities that have a high potential for painful consequences (e.g., engaging in unrestrained buying sprees, sexual indiscretions, foolish business investments)

American Psychiatric Association. *Diagnostic and statistical manual of mental disorders,* 4th ed. Washington, DC: American Psychiatric Association; 2000:327, 332.

18. Which of the following is the greatest risk factor for suicide?
A) Unemployment
B) Single status
C) Low income status
D) Resident of urban area
E) History of admission to a psychiatric hospital

Answer and Discussion

The answer is E. Suicide rates were higher in residents of urban areas compared with nonurban residents. The risk of suicide was also increased with unemployment, single status, low income, and receipt of pension or social security benefit. The strongest risk factor concerned admission to a psychiatric hospital. Almost one half of the persons who committed suicide had a history of admission to psychiatric facilities. Regardless of diagnosis, the greatest risk was during hospital admission and in the first week following discharge.

Mortensen PB, Agerboo E, Erikson T. Psychiatric illness and risk factors for suicide in Denmark. *Lancet.* 2000;355:9–12.

> The risk of suicide is increased with unemployment, single status, low income, and receipt of pension or social security benefit. The strongest risk factor is admission to a psychiatric hospital.

19. In a dying patient, which of the following is used to detect depression?
A) Pervasive hopelessness
B) Weight loss
C) Crying
D) Dependency
E) Concern over being a burden

Answer and Discussion

The answer is A. A person who is grieving maintains a sense of hope. Hope may change from the hope for a cure to the hope for prolonging life to the hope to live comfortably and without pain for the duration of life, but it is not lost in persons who are dying. Pervasive hopelessness, however, is a hallmark of depression.

Periyakoil VS, Hallenbeck J. Identifying and managing preparatory grief and depression at the end of life. *Am Fam Physician.* 2002;65:883–890, 897–898.

20. Which of the following electrolyte abnormalities is associated with bulimic patients?
A) Metabolic acidosis
B) Respiratory acidosis
C) Metabolic alkalosis
D) Respiratory alkalosis
E) Normal electrolytes

Answer and Discussion

The answer is C. Symptoms and signs of bulimia include reflux esophagitis, abdominal cramping, diarrhea, and rectal bleeding. Electrolyte abnormalities and metabolic alkalosis signal extreme purging habits in a bulimic patient. Patients with anorexia generally have laboratory test results within normal limits until the very late stage of the condition.

Mehler PS. Diagnosis and care of patients with anorexia nervosa in the primary care setting. *Ann Intern Med.* 2001; 134:1048–1059.

21. A 42-year-old man is seen in your office. He has recently seen a psychiatrist and is being treated for severe depression. The patient cannot recall the medication that he is taking, but he remembers that the psychiatrist told him not to eat cheeses or aged meats. Which of the following agents is this patient most likely taking?
A) Tricyclic antidepressant
B) Selective serotonin release inhibitor
C) Monoamine oxidase (MAO) inhibitor
D) Neuroleptic
E) Anxiolytic

Answer and Discussion

The answer is C. Antidepressant medications fall into three basic categories:

- Tricyclic antidepressants: These include amitriptyline, imipramine, nortriptyline, and desipramine. Tricyclic antidepressants have been commonly used in the treatment of depression since the mid-1980s. These medications may require 2 to 6 weeks before full therapeutic effect is noted. Many have anticholinergic side effects. Amitriptyline has the most anticholinergic properties, including dry mouth, blurred vision, constipation, ileus, urinary retention, and even delirium. In most cases, these side effects improve with time. Drug selection should depend on the symptoms and the side effect profile of the medication.
- *Selective serotonin reuptake inhibitors (SSRIs)*: These include fluoxetine, paroxetine, citalopram, escitalopram, and sertraline. SSRIs are popular mainly because of their reduced side effect profile and once-a-day dosing. These medications are very effective in the treatment of depression and are associated with a lower incidence of side effects compared with tricyclic antidepressants. The risk of death from overdose is very low with these medications. They are activating and should be given during the day.
- *Serotonin modulators:* The medications block primarily the 5-HT2 receptor and inhibit reuptake of 5-HT and norepinephrine. The group includes nefazodone, trazadone, and mirtazapine.
- *Serotonin-norepinephrine reuptake inhibitors:* This group includes venlafaxine and duloxetine. They have dual 5-HT and norepinephrine mechanism of action.
- *Dopamine-norepinephrine reuptake inhibitors:* The only drug in this class is bupropion.
- *MAO inhibitors*: These include phenelzine and tranylcypromine. MAO inhibitors are not used as frequently for the treatment of depression because of the potential for severe side effects. Interactions with sympathomimetic medications or tyramine-containing foods (e.g., cheeses, wines, beers, aged meats and fruits, beans, liver, yeast extracts) can lead to a hypertensive crisis. Orthostatic hypotension, nausea, insomnia, and sexual dysfunction are also common.

Beers MH, Porter RS, eds. *The Merck manual of diagnosis and therapy,* Merck Research Laboratories, 18th ed. Whitehouse Station, NJ: Merck & Co.; 2006:1708–1709.

22. Which of the following is considered tertiary prevention?
A) Pneumococcal (Pneumovax) immunization
B) Purified protein derivative determination in a patient who is affected with tuberculosis
C) Smoking cessation counseling in a patient who is known to have chronic obstructive pulmonary disease
D) Administration of erythromycin eye drops to neonates
E) Hepatitis A vaccination for travelers

Answer and Discussion

The answer is C. The following are three types of prevention:

1. *Primary prevention*: These types of treatments prevent the development of disease. Examples include tetanus, influenza, or pneumovax vaccination and intraocular administration of erythromycin to prevent neonatal chlamydia or gonorrhea.
2. *Secondary prevention*: These are steps taken in the early course of illness and help identify those who are affected. Examples include purified protein derivative determination in patients affected with tuberculosis or Venereal Disease Research Laboratory (VDRL) determination in those with syphilis.
3. *Tertiary prevention*: These are steps that are taken after the development of a condition to help rehabilitate the patient. Examples include counseling a patient with emphysema or chronic bronchitis to stop smoking.

Rakel RE. *Textbook of Family Practice*, 4th ed. Philadelphia: WB Saunders; 1990:209, 210, 217.

23. A 30-year-old woman presents with fatigue, difficulty with concentration, weight loss, and insomnia. She is an avid equestrian, but recently has not been interested in riding. The most likely diagnosis is
A) somatoform disorder
B) depression
C) anorexia nervosa
D) bulimia
E) cyclothymia

Answer and Discussion

The answer is B. Common symptoms that are associated with clinical depression include depressed mood, diminished interest or pleasure, significant appetite or weight change, sleep disturbances, agitation, fatigue, feelings of worthlessness or guilt, difficulty with concentration, or suicidal thoughts. Symptoms must be present for at least 2 weeks before the diagnosis is made. In addition, symptoms must be present almost daily and must represent a change from the patient's previous level of functioning. Other contributing causes must be ruled out. Either a depressed mood or a loss of pleasure in most activities must be present for the diagnosis.

American Psychiatric Association. *Diagnostic and Statistical Manual of Mental Disorders,* 4th ed. Washington, DC: American Psychiatric Association; 2000:78.

24. In young women with an eating disorder, at what point would you expect her menstrual periods to resume?
A) 75% of ideal body weight
B) 80% of ideal body weight

C) 90% of ideal body weight
D) 100% of body weight
E) It is unusual for menstrual cycles to resume with any weight gain.

Answer and Discussion

The answer is C. Menstruation usually resumes in women affected with anorexia when the patient approaches 90% of ideal body weight.

Mehler PS. Diagnosis and care of patients with anorexia nervosa in the primary care setting. *Ann Intern Med.* 2001; 134:1048–1059.

25. Which of the following behaviors is associated with bulimia?
A) Self-mutilation
B) Anxiety
C) Substance abuse
D) Unprotected sexual activity
E) All of the above

Answer and Discussion

The answer is E. Young women with bulimia characteristically have low self-esteem, are depressed and/or anxious, and have poor impulse control. They typically engage in other risky behaviors, such as substance abuse, unprotected sexual activity, self-mutilation, and suicide attempts.

Kaplan A, Seidenfeld ME, Rickert VI. Impact of anorexia, bulimia and obesity on the gynecologic health of adolescents. *Am Fam Physician.* 2001;64:445–450.

26. Which of the following statements regarding obsessive-compulsive disorder (OCD) is true?
A) Obsessions are repetitive behaviors.
B) Most affected patients have obsessions as well as compulsions.
C) Compulsions are thoughts or ideas that recur.
D) Anxiety is a central feature.
E) Patients are usually unaware of their actions and thoughts and are resistant to them.

Answer and Discussion

The answer is D. OCD is characterized by recurrent actions or ideas that interfere with normal daily activities. The patient is usually aware of the actions and thoughts and feels a strong inner resistance toward them. *Obsessions* are defined as thoughts or ideas that recur, and the patient tries to repress them. Common obsessions include fear of dirt, germs, or contamination; disgust with bodily waste or secretions; fear of harming a family member or friend; concern with order, symmetry (balance), and exactness; worry that a task has been done poorly, even when the person knows this is not true; fear of thinking evil or sinful thoughts; constantly thinking about certain sounds, images, words, or numbers; or a constant need for reassurance. Compulsions are repetitive behaviors that are performed in response to the obsessions. Common compulsions include cleaning and grooming rituals, such as excessive hand-washing, showering, and tooth-brushing; checking rituals involving drawers, door locks, and appliances to be sure they are shut, locked, or turned off; repeating rituals, such as going in and out of a door, sitting down and getting up from a chair, and touching certain objects several times; putting items in a certain order or arrangement; counting over and over to a certain number; saving newspapers, mail, or containers when they are no longer needed; or seeking reassurance and approval. Obsessions and compulsions can have an aggressive or sexual attachment. Fewer than 10% of patients have both obsessions and compulsions; however, individuals may exhibit multiple obsessions or multiple compulsions. Anxiety is a central feature of this disorder, but it is generated by internal thoughts as opposed to external circumstances. The neurosis affects men and women equally and usually is found in those of a higher socioeconomic class with above-average intelligence. The condition usually becomes apparent in childhood. Until recently, OCD has been a difficult illness to treat. However, we now have better medicines. Clomipramine (Anafranil) helps many people with OCD and usually decreases symptoms to mild levels. Si3de effects from this drug, such as dry mouth, constipation and drowsiness, and sometimes an inability to achieve orgasm, are common. Fluoxetine, sertraline, paroxetine, and fluvoxamine (Luvox) can also help some patients with OCD.

American Academy of Family Physicians. Information from your family doctor—Obsessive-compulsive disorder: what it is and how to treat it. *Am Fam Physician.* 2000;61(5):1537.

27. High fever, tachycardia, tachypnea, diaphoresis, hypertension, and seizures develop in a psychiatric patient who is receiving haloperidol. The most likely diagnosis is
A) malignant hyperthermia
B) rhabdomyolysis
C) neuroleptic malignant syndrome
D) sepsis
E) serotonin syndrome

Answer and Discussion

The answer is C. Neuroleptic malignant syndrome is an uncommon idiosyncratic condition that is associated with the use of dopamine antagonist (i.e., antipsychotic medications). Usually associated with the more potent medications, such as haloperidol and piperazine phenothiazines, the symptoms include high fever (102°F to 104°F), tachycardia, tachypnea, diaphoresis, autonomic dysfunction, mental status changes, hypertension and hypotension, tremors, seizures, muscle rigidity, and leukocytosis. Significant elevations of serum creatinine kinase may signal rhabdomyolysis. Other complications include respiratory failure, myocardial infarction, and renal and hepatic failure. Disseminated intravascular coagulopathy may also occur. The treatment involves stopping the antipsychotic, supportive care, and the use of intravenous dantrolene. Bromocriptine, amantadine, and benzodiazepines can also be used. Mortality approaches 30%.

Beers MH, Porter RS, eds. *The Merck manual of diagnosis and therapy,* Merck Research Laboratories, 18th ed. Whitehouse Station, NJ: Merck & Co.; 2006:1671.

28. *Panic disorder* is defined as recurrent attacks that may involve which of the following symptoms?
A) Flight of ideas
B) Hallucinations
C) Feelings of envy
D) Impulsivity
E) Choking

Answer and Discussion

The answer is E. As much as 33% of the population may have a panic episode during the year, but far fewer are affected with panic disorder. According to the *Diagnostic and Statistical Manual of Mental Disorders*, 4th ed. (*DSM-IV-TR*), the diagnosis of *panic attack* is a discrete period of intense fear or discomfort in which four (or more) of the following symptoms develop abruptly and reach a peak within 10 minutes:

1. Shortness of breath
2. Dizziness, fainting
3. Palpitations or tachycardia
4. Shaking
5. Diaphoresis
6. Choking
7. Nausea or abdominal discomfort
8. Depersonalization
9. Paresthesia
10. Flushing or chills
11. Chest discomfort
12. Fear of dying
13. Fear of insanity or doing something uncontrolled

Panic disorder is divided into panic disorder with or without agoraphobia. Criteria consist of

1. Recurrent unexpected panic attacks.
2. At least one of the attacks has been followed by 1 month (or more) of the following:
   - Persistent concern about additional attacks.
   - Worry about the implications of the attack or its consequences.
   - Significant change in behavior related to the attacks.
3. Panic attacks are not due to the direct physiologic effects of a substance (drug abuse, medication).
4. Panic attacks are not better accounted for by another mental disorder.

Treatment involves counseling, antidepressants (paroxetine), buspirone, and benzodiazepines (alprazolam).

Saddock BJ, Saddock VA. *Kaplan and Saddock's Concise Textbook of Psychiatry*, 2nd ed. Philadelphia: Lippincott Williams & Wilkins; 2004:216–217.

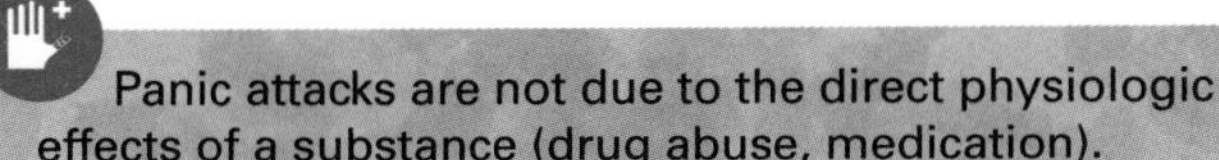

29. Which of the following medications is best indicated in a patient with Parkinson's disease who experiences psychosis?
A) Haloperidol (Haldol)
B) Olanzapine (Zyprexa)
C) Quetiapine (Seroquel)
D) Risperidone (Risperdal)
E) Thioridazine (Mellaril)

Answer and Discussion

The answer is C. Quetiapine (Seroquel) has shown promise in the treatment of psychosis in elderly patients with Alzheimer's disease and Parkinson's disease. It improves psychosis in patients with Parkinson's disease without exacerbating movement disorders. This feature has led some experts to recommend it as the first-line agent for treatment of psychosis in patients with Parkinson's disease. Haloperidol (Haldol) and thioridazine (Mellaril) can cause drug-induced parkinsonism, akathisia, acute dystonia, and tardive dyskinesia. Risperidone (Risperdal) exacerbates movement disorders in patients with Parkinson's disease. In patients with Parkinson's disease, olanzapine (Zyprexa) was found to increase motor symptoms.

Dewey RB Jr, O'Suilleabhain PE. Treatment of drug-induced psychosis with quetiapine and clozapine in Parkinson's disease. *Neurology.* 2000;55:1753–1754.

30. Which of the following is a potential side effect of quetiapine (Seroquel)?
A) Agranulocytosis
B) Cataract formation
C) Hepatotoxicity
D) QT interval prolongation
E) Thrombocytopenia

Answer and Discussion

The answer is B. Quetiapine should be initiated at a dosage of 12.5 mg at bedtime and titrated every 3 to 5 days until the desired effect is achieved or side effects emerge. Common side effects include sedation, headache, and orthostatic hypotension. Cataract formation was noticed in pre-marketing studies, but a causal relationship has not been found. Screening for cataract formation is recommended at the initiation of therapy and at 6-month intervals thereafter.

Mosby's GenRx: a comprehensive reference for generic and brand prescription drugs, 11th ed. St. Louis: Mosby; 2001.

31. Which of the following statements about fluoxetine (Prozac) is true?
A) Side effects often include dry mouth, urinary retention, and blurred vision.
B) The treatment of panic disorder typically requires higher doses than the recommended starting dose for depression.
C) The mechanism of action involves the reuptake of dopamine at the postsynaptic junction.
D) The drug has significant anticholinergic activity.
E) Treatment of bulimia typically requires higher doses than the recommended starting dose for depression.

Answer and Discussion

The answer is E. Fluoxetine (Prozac) is used for the treatment of depression, OCD, and bulimia nervosa. Other uses include the treatment of dysthymic disorder, panic disorder, social phobia, premenstrual syndrome, and bipolar disorder depression. The medication is an SSRI and has advantages when compared with the older tricyclic antidepressants. SSRIs have very little anticholinergic activity (which can cause blurred vision, urinary retention, and dry mouth); thus, they are better tolerated. The starting dose of fluoxetine is usually 10 to 20 mg/day, which is then titered up to 80 mg/day to achieve a clinical response. The full therapeutic response may take up to 4 weeks. Treatment of bulimia and OCD requires a dose of 60 mg/day. The treatment of panic disorder often requires smaller initial doses. Initial doses of 20 mg often precipitate panic attacks and lead to a high discontinuation rate. Side effects include headaches, anxiety, nervousness, excessive sweating, insomnia, anorexia, weight loss, nausea, diarrhea, and rash. Depressed patients should be monitored closely for suicidal thoughts or gestures, especially once their depression starts to improve. In most cases, medication for depression is complemented with counseling and is more effective than medication alone.

Saddock BJ, Saddock VA. *Kaplan and Saddock's Concise Textbook of Psychiatry*, 2nd ed. Philadelphia: Lippincott Williams & Wilkins; 2004:482.

32. The treatment of choice for seasonal affective disorder (SAD) is
A) tricyclic antidepressants
B) electroconvulsive shock treatment
C) psychotherapy
D) intense white light therapy
E) MAO inhibitors

Answer and Discussion

The answer is D. SAD is a pattern of major depressive episodes that occur and remit with changes in seasons. Two patterns have been identified. The most often recognized is the fall-onset type, also known as *winter depression*, in which major depressive episodes begin in the late fall to early winter months and remit during the summer months. Atypical signs and symptoms of depression predominate in cases of winter depression and include the following:

- Increased rather than decreased sleep
- Increased rather than decreased appetite and food intake with carbohydrate craving
- Marked increase in weight
- Irritability
- Interpersonal difficulties (especially rejection sensitivity)
- Leaden paralysis (a heavy, leaden feeling in the arms or legs)

A spring-onset pattern (summer depression) also has been described in which the severe depressive episode begins in late spring to early summer and is characterized by typical vegetative symptoms of depression, such as decreased sleep, weight loss, and poor appetite. Patients with winter depression usually reside in the more northern regions, and symptoms tend to develop when the days become shorter and nighttime is more prolonged. Treatment with intense white light has proved to be successful in controlling symptoms. Light therapy is initiated with a 10,000-lux light box directed toward the patient at a downward slant. The patient's eyes should remain open throughout the treatment session, although staring directly into the light source is unnecessary and is not advised. The patient should start with a single 10- to 15-minute session per day, gradually increasing the session's duration to 30 to 45 minutes. Sessions should be increased to twice a day if symptoms worsen. Ninety minutes a day is the conventional daily maximum duration of therapy, although there is no reason to limit the duration of sessions if side effects are not severe.

Kasper DL, Braunwald E, Fauci AS, et al., eds. *Harrison's principles of internal medicine,* 16th ed. New York: McGraw-Hill; 2005:1560, 2554.

33. Which of the following is a characteristic of antisocial personality disorder?
A) Those who are affected suppress their conflicts
B) Symptoms include severe agoraphobia
C) Schizophrenia may coexist
D) Many patients have a record of stealing, fighting, rape, or arson
E) Adolescents under the age of 18 are commonly affected

Answer and Discussion

The answer is D. Patients with antisocial personality disorder must be older than 18 years of age and act out their conflicts or go against the rules of social normalcy. They are often impulsive, reckless, and immoral. They often had previous problems concerning truancy, cruelty to animals and other individuals, and initiation of fights and use of weapons with fighting. They usually have a record of stealing, possible rape, arson, and falsifying the truth since childhood. The definition also requires that a pattern of irresponsible behavior must be present since the age of 15, with school suspension, employment problems, poor parenting, lack of monogamy (no monogamous relationship lasting more than 1 year), and failed financial obligations in the absence of schizophrenia or manic episodes. In most cases, those affected lack regard for other people's rights.

American Psychiatric Association. *Diagnostic and Statistical Manual of Mental Disorders*, 4th ed. Washington, DC: American Psychiatric Association; 2000:327, 332.

34. Which of the following is not classified as a selective serotonin reuptake inhibitor (SSRI)?
A) Sertraline (Zoloft)
B) Mirtazapine (Remeron)
C) Escitalopram (Lexapro)
D) Paroxetine (Paxil)
E) Fluoxetine (Prozac)

Answer and Discussion

The answer is B. Mirtazapine (Remeron) is a tetracyclic antidepressant unrelated to tricyclic antidepressants and SSRIs. It is unique in its action among the currently available antidepressants. It is referred to as a *serotonin modulator.* Mirtazapine is a presynaptic α_2-adrenergic receptor antagonist plus a potent antagonist of postsynaptic 5-HT_2 and 5-HT_3 receptors. The net outcome of these effects is stimulation of the release of norepinephrine and serotonin. The drug has antidepressant and anxiolytic effects but does not cause sexual dysfunction. It can cause sedation and weight gain.

Beers MH, Porter RS, eds. *The Merck manual of diagnosis and therapy,* Merck Research Laboratories, 18th ed. Whitehouse Station, NJ: Merck & Co.; 2006:1709.

35. Which of the following is most likely to cause withdrawal symptoms with abrupt discontinuation?
A) Fluoxetine (Prozac)
B) Sertraline (Zoloft)
C) Paroxetine (Paxil)
D) Citalopram (Celexa)
E) none of the SSRIs cause withdrawal symptoms

Answer and Discussion

The answer is C. Studies have shown that when comparing fluoxetine, sertraline, paroxetine, and citalopram, withdrawal from paroxetine was shown to cause more severe symptoms that may occur more quickly, even after the second missed dose. Because of its long half-life, fluoxetine may have the least severe symptoms. Methods to prevent antidepressant discontinuation syndrome include tapering the drug and educating the patient to avoid sudden cessation of the medication. Reintroduction of the medication will usually reverse severe symptoms within 24 hours.

Haddad PM. Antidepressant discontinuation syndromes. *Drug Saf.* 2001;24:183–197.

Michelson D, Fava M, Amsterdam J, et al. Interruption of selective serotonin reuptake inhibitor treatment: double-blind, placebo-controlled trial. *Br J Psychiatry.* 2000;176: 363–368.

Studies have shown that when comparing fluoxetine, sertraline, paroxetine, and citalopram, withdrawal from paroxetine was shown to cause more severe symptoms that may occur more quickly, even after the second missed dose.

36. A 20-year-old college student presents to her dentist. Her vital signs are normal, and her weight is 120 lb. On examination, extensive upper dental erosion is noted. The most likely diagnosis is
A) obsessive-compulsive disorder
B) anorexia nervosa
C) hypothyroidism
D) bulimia nervosa
E) Crohn's disease

Answer and Discussion

The answer is D. Bulimia nervosa is an eating disorder that usually affects young, white, middle- and upper-class women (typically college women). The disorder is characterized by episodes of secret binge eating followed by self-induced vomiting. Other manifestations include excessive exercise and the misuse of diuretics, laxatives, or enemas. Although the etiology of this disorder is unknown, genetic and neurochemical factors have been implicated. Bulimia nervosa is ten times more common in females than in males and affects up to 3% of young women. The condition usually becomes symptomatic between the ages of 13 and 20 years, and it has a chronic, sometimes episodic course. Unlike anorexia nervosa, those affected with bulimia are within 15% of their desirable weight. Menstrual cycles are rarely affected; in anorexia, menstrual cycles are commonly absent or extremely irregular. Most affected individuals have feelings of guilt and depression. Severe cases may result in

- Gastric dilation
- Dental erosions, particularly the upper dentition (the lower dentition is protected by the tongue during vomiting)
- Salivary gland enlargement
- Esophagitis
- Electrolyte abnormalities
- Aspiration
- Pancreatitis

Treatment involves psychotherapy with behavior modification and the use of antidepressants (tricyclic antidepressants and SSRIs, especially fluoxetine). Many patients relapse and require long-term therapy.

Yager J, ed. Treatment of bulimia nervosa and binge eating disorder [Monograph]. University of South Florida College of Medicine. 2003.

37. Which of the following factors is associated with dysthymic disorder?
A) Substance abuse
B) Sleep disturbances
C) Mania
D) Myasthenia gravis
E) Flight of ideas

Answer and Discussion

The answer is B. Dysthymia is a condition characterized by depressed mood for at least 2 years with at least two of the following factors:

- Appetite changes
- Sleep disturbances
- Fatigue
- Low self-esteem
- Poor concentration
- Feelings of hopelessness

The symptoms must not have an organic cause and must never be interrupted for more than 2 months. Major depression has many of the same symptoms, but they are more severe. Cyclothymia is dysthymia followed by episodes of mild mania. The diagnosis of dysthymia requires that the patient has no history of substance abuse, mania, hypomania, major depression, or psychotic disorders.

American Psychiatric Association. *Diagnostic and Statistical Manual of Mental Disorders*, 4th ed. Washington, DC: American Psychiatric Association; 2000:327, 332.

38. Children who exhibit symptoms of school avoidance with nausea, vomiting, and abdominal pain may benefit from
A) antidepressant medication
B) methylphenidate
C) psychotherapy
D) benzodiazepines
E) mood stabilizers

Answer and Discussion

The answer is C. It is a normal developmental response for children to cry when their parents leave the room beginning at approximately 8 months of age and continuing up to 2 years of age. The response varies with each child. Many first-time parents overreact and fear that the child is emotionally harmed by the separation. Reassuring the parents that this is a normal response is appropriate for treatment. Occasionally, a child exhibits symptoms of nausea, vomiting, and abdominal pain, which signal an abnormal response. Separation anxiety disorder affects children under the age of 18 years and consists of developmentally inappropriate and excessive anxiety concerning separation from home or a major attachment figure that lasts for at least 4 weeks. Periods of exacerbations and remissions are typical. These children (in many cases, school-aged children with school avoidance) often have no siblings and come from an extremely close family. Boys and girls are equally affected. Psychotherapy may be necessary for these children. Medication is not recommended.

American Psychiatric Association. *Diagnostic and Statistical Manual of Mental Disorders*, 4th ed. Washington, DC: American Psychiatric Association; 2000:327, 332.

39. Which of the following medications is least likely to cause sexual side effects?
A) Fluoxetine (Prozac)
B) Sertraline (Zoloft)
C) Venlafaxine (Effexor)
D) Citalopram (Celexa)
E) Bupropion (Wellbutrin)

Answer and Discussion

The answer is E. Sexual side effects, usually delayed ejaculation or anorgasmia, may occur in both men and women who are taking SSRIs and venlafaxine (Effexor). Treatment consists of several options: reducing the dosage, switching to another agent, or adding another agent to overcome the sexual side effects. Sexual dysfunction typically resolves within 1 to 3 days after discontinuation of the antidepressant and returns on reintroduction. Recovery after withdrawal from fluoxetine (Prozac) may occur within 1 to 3 weeks. Studies suggest that the addition of bupropion (Wellbutrin) may decrease sexual side effects.

Ables AZ, Baughman AO III. Antidepressants: update on new agents and indications. *Am Fam Physician.* 2003;67:547–554.

40. After discontinuing fluoxetine, how long should a clinician wait before prescribing a monoamine oxidase inhibitor (MAOI)?
A) 1 day
B) 3 days
C) 1 week
D) 5 weeks
E) No delay is necessary.

Answer and Discussion

The answer is D. Because of its long half-life, patients should allow at least 5 weeks between discontinuation of fluoxetine (Prozac) and commencement of monoamine oxidase inhibitor (MAOI) therapy.

Hines Burnham T, et al., eds. *Drug facts and comparisons,* 55th ed. St. Louis: Facts and Comparisons; 2001:345.

41. Which of the following statements is associated with adjustment disorder?
A) The patient has an expected reaction to a known stressor.
B) The condition is usually chronic, lasting for several years or more.
C) Depression and anxiety are commonly associated.
D) Medication is usually indicated for treatment.
E) Support groups are rarely of any benefit.

Answer and Discussion

The answer is C. An *adjustment disorder* is defined as an excessive maladaptive reaction to an identifiable psychosocial stressor (e.g., death of a loved one, loss of a job, marital discord, divorce) that has occurred within the previous 3 months. The reaction may affect social relationships or the ability to function effectively at work or school. The disturbance cannot last for more than 6 months, and other mental disorders must be ruled out. In most cases, depression and anxiety are major manifestations. The best treatment is psychosocial support to help enhance the patient's ability to cope and adapt to stressful conditions. In most cases, medication is not necessary; rather, psychotherapy (individual, family, behavioral, and self-help groups) is used in treatment.

Saddock BJ, Saddock VA. *Kaplan and Saddock's Concise Textbook of Psychiatry*, 2nd ed. Philadelphia: Lippincott Williams & Wilkins; 2004:333–334.

42. Which of the following statements about somatization disorder is true?
A) Men are more commonly affected than women.
B) Patients exhibit multiple physical complaints that usually have an identifiable physiologic basis.
C) The condition usually develops after age 50.
D) Symptoms rarely affect the patient's interpersonal relationships.
E) Treatment involves frequent office visits and reassurance to the patient.

Answer and Discussion

The answer is E. Somatization disorder is a condition characterized by multiple physical symptoms that have no identifiable physiologic basis or are in excess of any physical findings made. The symptoms are usually defined in vague or exaggerated terms. The condition generally develops in the teen years and always before 30 years of age. Women are more commonly affected than men, and there is usually a positive family history. The symptoms generally interrupt one's job and interpersonal relationships. Suicide can occur in those affected. Currently, eight symptoms are required, which must meet a specific pattern: four different sites of pain, two different gastrointestinal symptoms, one sexual or reproductive system other than pain, and one pseudoneurologic symptom. The subjective severity of the symptoms must be sufficient to lead the patient to consult a physician, take medicine, or make lifestyle changes. It appears that there is no effective treatment; however, reassurance with frequent office visits and sensitivity to the patient's needs is usually beneficial. Costly tests and repeated subspecialty consultations are discouraged unless there are questions with the diagnosis.

Saddock BJ, Saddock VA. *Kaplan and Saddock's Concise Textbook of Psychiatry*, 2nd ed. Philadelphia: Lippincott Williams & Wilkins; 2004:216–217.

43. Which of the following statements about the use of buspirone (Buspar) is true?
A) The drug is used in the treatment of acute anxiety.
B) The drug may cause displacement of tightly bound drugs, such as phenytoin and warfarin, leading to toxicity.
C) Side effects include dizziness, fatigue, nervousness, and headache.
D) The medication is commonly associated with abuse.
E) The drug can be used in combination with MAO inhibitors to treat resistant depression.

Answer and Discussion

The answer is C. Buspirone (Buspar) is an antianxiety medication that is used for chronic anxiety. It is not associated with abuse, drowsiness, or functional limitations. Buspirone is not useful in the treatment of acute anxiety, because it often takes several days to weeks (depending on the patient) to produce its therapeutic effect. The drug's mechanism of action involves serotonin, norepinephrine, and dopamine receptors, and it indirectly affects GABA receptors. The medication does not affect other tightly bound drugs, such as warfarin, propranolol, or phenytoin, but may affect less tightly bound drugs, such as digoxin. Patients receiving MAO inhibitors should not use buspirone because of the risk of elevated blood pressure and hypertensive crisis. Side effects reported with the use of buspirone include dizziness, fatigue, nervousness, headache, decreased concentration, palpitations, nausea, and abdominal complaints.

Saddock BJ, Saddock VA. *Kaplan and Saddock's Concise Textbook of Psychiatry*, 2nd ed. Philadelphia: Lippincott Williams & Wilkins; 2004:442–443.

44. Which of the following is rated the greatest problem in children 8 to 15 years of age by children of that age?
A) Racism
B) Pressure to have sex
C) Pressure to drink alcohol
D) Pressure to do drugs
E) Bullying

Answer and Discussion

The answer is E. Childhood bullying has been viewed as an inevitable part of growing up. However, recent survey data show that American children 8 to 15 years of age rate bullying as a greater problem than racism or pressure to have sex or use alcohol and other drugs.

Kaiser Family Foundation. Children Now. Talking with kids about tough issues. Accessed online March 12, 2006, at: http://www.childrennow.org/nickelodeon/new-booklet.pdf.

Lyznicki JM, McCaffree MA, Robinowitz CB. Childhood bullying: implications for physicians. *Am Fam Physician.* 2004;70:1723–1728, 1729–1730.

45. A 42-year-old woman presents to your office. Her life appears chaotic and she transfers many of her dysfunctional feelings and conflicts to you her physician. She is at times paranoid, depressed, and angry. She has a history of multiple unstable interpersonal relationships. The most likely diagnosis is
A) borderline personality disorder
B) antisocial behavior
C) narcissistic disorder
D) histrionic disorder
E) none of the above

Answer and Discussion

The answer is A. Treating borderline personality disorder can be difficult and challenging. Because of their instability in the multiple areas of interpersonal relationships, self image, affects, and impulsivity, these affected patients can present with a wide range of symptoms, including depression, anger, paranoia, extreme dependency, self mutilation, and alternating idealization and devaluation of the physician. Their lives tend to be chaotic. They transfer many of their dysfunctional feelings and conflicts to the treating physician and the medical encounter. A detached professional stance and clear limit setting in terms of availability, appointment frequency, appropriate behavior, and medication use are necessary to manage these patients successfully. It is important to monitor one's own feelings, and to refrain from responding inappropriately to verbal attacks and manipulation. The development of a formal behavioral treatment plan and insistence on participation in psychiatric care may be required to establish an effective working relationship.

Ward RK. Assessment and management of personality disorders. *Am Fam Physician.* 2004;70:1505–1512.

When treating borderline personality disorder a detached professional stance and clear limit setting in terms of availability, appointment frequency, appropriate behavior, and medication use are necessary to manage these patients successfully.

46. A 17-year-old girl is brought to your office by her parents. She has been having hallucinations over the past year and recently experienced a psychotic episode that lasted for 2 weeks. She has been out of school for 3 years and has not been able to hold a job. Her mother reports that the girl often remains in her room. The most likely diagnosis is
A) agoraphobia
B) panic attacks
C) schizophrenia
D) school avoidance
E) major depression

Answer and Discussion

The answer is C. Schizophrenia is one of the most common psychiatric disorders and usually has a strong family history. Typically, patients are in the late teens or early 20s when the condition is identified. The definition describes a condition in which there is chronic impairment of functioning that involves disturbances of thinking, feeling, and behavior. Specific criteria involve the following:

- Episodes of psychosis, including delusions, hallucinations, incoherent behavior, and a decrease in social functioning.
- Signs must be present for at least 6 months, with one psychotic episode that lasts at least 1 week.
- Other features include social isolation, difficulties with social functioning or job requirements, peculiar behavior, impaired hygiene, abnormal thought processes, inappropriate affect, and lack of energy or interest.

Treatment involves the use of antipsychotics and psychotherapy. The prognosis in patients with schizophrenia is worsened the longer the duration of psychosis before institution of effective antipsychotic therapy and the greater the number of psychotic relapses. Use of traditional antipsychotic medications has been limited by their side effects and failure to achieve long-term control of symptoms in some cases. New "atypical" antipsychotic drugs (clozapine, risperidone, and olanzapine) are used for the treatment of resistant cases of schizophrenia and improvement in patient tolerance and compliance. These medications have been more successful than traditional antipsychotic drugs in treating the negative symptoms of schizophrenia, such as social withdrawal and apathy. The atypical antipsychotic drugs produce fewer extrapyramidal side effects and no tardive dyskinesia or dystonia. However, they are associated with neuroleptic malignant syndrome, and clozapine can produce fatal agranulocytosis. Use of these medications in selected patients who do not benefit from, or cannot tolerate, traditional agents is an important step in improving the lives of individuals with schizophrenia. Despite advancement in medication, relapses are common, and some patients require institutionalization.

Beers MH, Porter RS, eds. *The Merck manual of diagnosis and therapy,* Merck Research Laboratories, 18th ed. Whitehouse Station, NJ: Merck & Co.; 2006:1722–1728.

47. A 7-year-old boy is brought to your office. The parents report that the child has had problems in school for the last 6 months. His teacher reports lack of concentration and excessive fidgeting. The child typically interrupts others and often loses objects. The most appropriate treatment is
A) reassurance
B) stimulant medication
C) antidepressant medication

D) short-acting benzodiazepines
E) strict discipline

Answer and Discussion

The answer is B. Attention deficit disorder, also known as *hyperactivity*, is a condition characterized by a short attention span or distractibility that persists for longer than 6 months. Other symptoms include fidgeting or squirming in one's seat, restlessness, inability to remain seated when required to do so, difficulty in awaiting one's turn, blurting out answers to questions before they are completed, difficulty in completing cognitive tasks (not related to oppositional behavior or lack of comprehension), and excessive talking. Affected children often interrupt others, frequently lose objects, do not listen to instructions, and engage in dangerous activities without consideration of the consequences. Boys are more commonly affected, and the onset typically occurs before 7 years of age. The clinical history is usually all that is needed to determine the diagnosis, although psychological and educational testing may help to support the diagnosis. Treatment is accomplished with stimulants, such as methylphenidate and dextroamphetamine, which have a paradoxical calming effect on young patients. Atomoxetine (Staterra) is a selective norepinephrine reuptake inhibitor that is approved for use in children over age 6. Most children show improvement with medication; drug holidays (at least 2 weeks/year) are important during chronic therapy to see if further medication is necessary. Behavior modification for the child and family counseling may also be helpful.

Ferri FF. *Ferri's Clinical Advisor, Instant Diagnosis and Treatment.* Philadelphia: Elsevier/Mosby; 2006:107–108.

48. Which of the following statements about suicide is true?
A) Males make more suicide attempts.
B) Women are more successful.
C) Anxiety is the most common contributing factor.
D) Most suicides occur during December.
E) Married people have the lowest risk for suicide.

Answer and Discussion

The answer is E. Suicide is an ever-increasing problem in the United States. Men tend to be more successful at suicide attempts, whereas women make more attempts. Underlying depression is the most common contributing factor. Persons in the 40- to 50-year age range are at particular risk, as are those with chronic diseases (e.g., acquired immunodeficiency syndrome, cancer, and respiratory illnesses, and patients who require hemodialysis). Groups that are particularly affected include those who feel overwhelmed with their personal problems, those who attempt to control others with their actions, those with severe depression who are overwhelmed by a stressful situation or accusation, and those with underlying psychotic illness. Other risk factors include drug abuse, family history of suicide, previous suicide attempts, lack of social support system, and recent loss of a loved one, particularly in older patients. The number of suicides increases slightly in the spring and summer; however, contrary to popular belief, suicides do not increase in December and holiday periods. Married people have the lowest suicide rates.

Saddock BJ, Saddock VA. *Kaplan and Saddock's Concise Textbook of Psychiatry*, 2nd ed. Philadelphia: Lippincott Williams & Wilkins; 2004:389–395.

49. A 31-year-old woman you are treating is emotional and seductive in her behavior. She is very focused on her appearance to others and wants to be the center of attention. You note she has a difficult time making decisions. The most likely diagnosis is
A) borderline personality disorder
B) antisocial behavior
C) narcissistic disorder
D) histrionic disorder
E) none of the above

Answer and Discussion

The answer is D. Histrionic patients are not satisfied if they are not the center of attention. They tend to be emotional and seductive, and use their appearance to attract the attention of others. As a result, the implications of illness and aging may have a profound impact on their psychologic functioning. When faced with these patients the physician should maintain an awareness of the patients' interpersonal style, and be empathetic to their issues, while at the same time avoiding inappropriate emotional or seductive behaviors. Additionally, these patients have difficulties in dealing with facts, details, and decision making. As a result, they may require extra assistance in processing medical information.

Ward RK. Assessment and management of personality disorders. *Am Fam Physician.* 2004;70:1505–1512.

50. Before the diagnosis of post-traumatic stress disorder (PTSD) is made, symptoms should be present for at least
A) 1 year
B) 6 months
C) 3 months
D) 1 month
E) 1 week

Answer and Discussion

The answer is D. PTSD can occur after any major traumatic event. Symptoms include disturbing thoughts and nightmares about the traumatic event, avoidance behavior, numbing of general responsiveness, increased irritability, and hypervigilance. To fulfill the DSM-IV criteria for PTSD, an individual must have been exposed to a traumatic event; have at least one re-experiencing, three avoidance, and two hyperarousal phenomena; have had the symptoms for at least 1 month; and the symptoms must cause clinically important distress or reduced day-to-day functioning. Acute stress disorder occurs within the first month after a major traumatic event and requires the presence of symptoms for at least 2 days. It is similar to PTSD, but dissociative symptoms are required to make the diagnosis. Treatments for PTSD may have similar effects, regardless of the traumatic event that precipitated PTSD. However, caution should be applied when generalizing among types of trauma.

Bisson J. Post-traumatic stress disorder. *Clin Evid Concise.* 2005;13:306–309.

51. Which of the following agents is the most appropriate treatment for a patient with bipolar disorder?
A) Haloperidol (Haldol)
B) Chlorpromazine (Thorazine)
C) Diazepam (Valium)
D) Lithium (Eskalith)
E) Fluoxetine (Prozac)

Answer and Discussion

The answer is D. Bipolar disorder is characterized by episodes of mania (e.g., flight of ideas, excessive spending, aggressive and grandiose behavior, little sleep, activities that are later regretted) followed by major depressive attacks (e.g., anhedonia, inability to concentrate, withdrawal from activities, chronic fatigue, loss of sexual drive, insomnia, anorexia with weight loss). Bipolar I disorder is typically diagnosed when patients are in their early 20s. Manic symptoms can rapidly escalate over a period of days and frequently follow psychosocial stressors. Some patients initially seek treatment for depression. Others may appear irritable, disorganized, or psychotic. Differentiating true mania from mania that results from secondary causes can be challenging. Initially, during the manic phase, these behaviors may attract other people; however, in the long term, they lead to significant interpersonal difficulties and conflicts. The episodes, which begin abruptly and are often precipitated by life stresses, may last for up to several months; manic episodes are typically shorter in duration. Bipolar II disorder typically is brought to medical attention when the patient is depressed. A careful history usually illuminates the diagnosis. Some depressed patients exhibit hypomania when given antidepressants. This variation is sometimes referred to as bipolar III disorder. Spring and summer months tend to be peak times for the development of symptoms. The condition may occur at any age but is most common in the second or third decade of life. The treatment for bipolar disorder is accomplished with lithium (Eskalith). It is important to remember that lithium levels need to be followed, and abnormalities associated with the kidneys and thyroid can be induced with medication. Valproic acid (Depakene) can also be used to treat the manic symptoms. If the patient is psychotic, a neuroleptic medication is also given. Long-acting benzodiazepines can be used for treating agitation. However, in patients with a substance abuse history, benzodiazepines should be used with caution because of the addictive potential of these agents. When the patient with bipolar disorder becomes depressed, an SSRI or bupropion is recommended. The use of tricyclic antidepressants should be avoided because of the possibility of inducing rapid cycling of symptoms.

Griswold KS, Pessar LF. Management of bipolar disorder. *Am Fam Physician*. 2000;62:1343–1353, 1357–1358.

52. Tardive dyskinesia is associated with
A) use of lithium
B) chronic blockade of dopaminergic receptors
C) use of serotonin reuptake inhibitors
D) short-term use of phenothiazine neuroleptics
E) anti-Parkinson's medications

Answer and Discussion

The answer is B. Tardive dyskinesia is a condition characterized by repetitive, involuntary, and purposeless choreiform movements of the extremities and buccal, oral, and lingual structures. Although often considered an extrapyramidal symptom, tardive dyskinesia is a separate, mechanistically distinct phenomenon. The condition is thought to be secondary to chronic blockage of dopamine receptors in the brain. It is usually associated with side effects of long-term use of phenothiazine neuroleptics and anticholinergic medication. Older patients and those with previous brain injury have a higher incidence of tardive dyskinesia. In most cases, the symptoms do not resolve when the medication is discontinued. Treatment with lithium, tricyclic antidepressants, and baclofen has shown some limited benefit.

Gurvich T, Cunningham JA. Appropriate use of psychotropic drugs in nursing homes. *Am Fam Physician*. 2000;61:1437–1446.

53. Laboratory findings seen in anorexia nervosa include
A) hyperkalemia
B) leukocytosis
C) prolonged QT interval on electrocardiogram
D) metabolic acidosis
E) elevated sedimentation rate

Answer and Discussion

The answer is C. Anorexia nervosa is a psychiatric problem that centers on a disturbed sense of body image and extreme fear of obesity. Among women, the lifetime prevalence of anorexia nervosa is 0.5% to 3.7%. Symptoms include self-induced vomiting and extreme exercise routines in the setting of extreme thinness. Women account for 95% of those affected. Onset is usually during adolescence but can occur earlier. Severe cases can be fatal. Most patients are described as being compulsive, intelligent, and meticulous; they are usually high achievers. Physical findings include cachexia (>15% less than ideal weight), amenorrhea, loss of sexual desire, low body temperature, cold intolerance, bradycardia, dental erosions, hypotension, hypothermia, edema, and hirsutism. Depression may also be present. Laboratory findings include electrolyte disorders (e.g., hypokalemia), metabolic alkalosis, increased blood urea nitrogen secondary to dehydration, thrombocytopenia, leukopenia, low or normal erythrocyte sedimentation rate, and prolonged QT interval on electrocardiogram. Short-term treatment involves active intervention to restore weight (which may require hospitalization), correction of electrolytes, and preservation of vital functions; long-term treatment involves psychiatric counseling to restore a healthy body image and to treat possible underlying depression. The goals of treatment for anorexia nervosa are to restore patients to a healthy weight, treat the physical complications, enhance the patient's motivation to cooperate with treatment, and provide education about healthy nutrition and eating habits. Other goals of treatment include correcting maladaptive thoughts, attitudes, and feelings related to the eating disorder; treating associated psychiatric conditions; enlisting family support; and attempting to prevent relapse. Medication should be considered in the treatment of anorexia but should not be the sole or primary treatment.

American Psychiatric Association. Practice guideline for the treatment of patients with eating disorders (revision). *Am J Psychiatry*. 2000;157[Suppl]:1–39.

54. An 80-year-old man is hospitalized secondary to pneumonia. On day 2 of his hospitalization, the nurse calls and tells you he is confused and calling out from his room. He has made multiple attempts to leave his room. You suspect delirium. He has no history of drug or alcohol abuse. Appropriate medication would include
A) diazepam (Valium)
B) lorazepam (Ativan)
C) haloperidol (Haldol)
D) mirtazapine (Remeron)
E) fluoxetine (Prozac)

Answer and Discussion

The answer is C. The management of delirium involves identifying and correcting the underlying medical problem, and symptomatically managing any behavioral or psychiatric symptoms. Low doses of antipsychotic drugs can help to control agitation. The use of benzodiazepines should be avoided except in cases of alcohol or sedative-hypnotic withdrawal. Environmental interventions, including frequent reorientation of patients by nursing staff and education of patients and families, should be instituted in all cases.

Gleason OC. Delirium. *Am Fam Physician.* 2003;67:1027–1034.

The management of delirium involves identifying and correcting the underlying medical problem, and symptomatically managing any behavioral or psychiatric symptoms.

55. When patients participated in weekly alcoholics anonymous meetings after discharge from a treatment program, the 1-year abstinence rate is

A) 1% to 5 %
B) 10% to 20%
C) 25% to 30%
D) 56% to 60%
E) 80% to 90%

Answer and Discussion

The answer is E. The abstinence-based method is commonly used to treat alcohol/drug addiction (95% of programs reviewed). This method utilizes cognitive behavior techniques and referral to 12-step recovery programs, such as Alcoholics Anonymous (AA) and Narcotics Anonymous (NA). One-year abstinence rates of 80% to 90% were accomplished when patients participated in weekly continuing care and/or AA meetings after discharge from the treatment program. Also, 1-year abstinence rates were associated with reduced rates of medical and psychiatric utilization.

Miller NS. *Treatment of the Addictions: Applications of Outcome Research for Clinical Management.* New York: Haworth; 1995.

56. Which of the following is considered the "date rape" drug?

A) 3,4-Methylenedioxymethamphetamine (MDMA)
B) Flunitrazepam (Rohypnol)
C) Ketamine (Ketalar)
D) Cocaine
E) Cannabis

Answer and Discussion

The answer is B. The most widely used club drugs are 3,4-methylenedioxymethamphetamine (MDMA), also known as ecstasy; gamma-hydroxybutyrate (GHB); flunitrazepam (Rohypnol); and ketamine (Ketalar). These drugs are popular because they are inexpensive and are conveniently dispensed as small pills, powders, or liquids. Club drugs usually are taken orally and may be taken in combination with each other, with alcohol, or with other drugs. Adverse effects of MDMA ingestion result from sympathetic overload and include tachycardia, mydriasis, diaphoresis, tremor, hypertension, arrhythmias, parkinsonism, esophoria (tendency for eyes to turn inward), and urinary retention. However, the most dangerous potential outcome of MDMA ingestion is hyperthermia and the associated "serotonin syndrome." Serotonin syndrome is manifested by grossly elevated core body temperature, rigidity, myoclonus, and autonomic instability; it can result in end-organ damage, rhabdomyolysis and acute renal failure, hepatic failure, adult respiratory distress syndrome, and coagulopathy. GHB produces euphoria, progressing with higher doses to dizziness, hypersalivation, hypotonia, and amnesia. Overdose may result in Cheyne-Stokes respiration, seizures, coma, and death. Coma may be interrupted by agitation, with flailing activity described similar to a drowning swimmer fighting for air. Bradycardia and hypothermia are present in about one third of patients admitted to a hospital for using GHB and appear to be correlated with the level of consciousness. Chronic use of GHB may produce dependence and a withdrawal syndrome that includes anxiety, insomnia, tremor, and in severe cases, treatment-resistant psychoses. In the United States, imported Rohypnol came to prominence in the 1990s as an inexpensive recreational sedative and the "date rape" drug. Effects of rohypnol occur about 30 minutes after ingestion, peak at 2 hours, and may last up to 8 to 12 hours. The effects are much greater with the concurrent ingestion of alcohol or other sedating drugs. Some users experience hypotension, dizziness, confusion, visual disturbances, urinary retention, or aggressive behavior. Ketamine is difficult to develop; therefore, most of the illegal supply is obtained from human and veterinary anesthesia products. Ketamine is distributed in a liquid form that can be ingested or injected. In clubs, it usually is smoked in a powder mixture of marijuana or tobacco, or is taken intranasally. A typical method uses a nasal inhaler, called a "bullet" or "bumper"; an inhalation is called a "bump." Ketamine often is taken in "trail mixes" of methamphetamine, cocaine, sildenafil citrate (Viagra), or heroin. Effects of ketamine ingestion appear rapidly and last about 30 to 45 minutes, with sensations of floating outside the body, visual hallucinations, and a dream-like state. Along with these "desired" effects, users also commonly experience confusion, anterograde amnesia, and delirium. They also may experience tachycardia, palpitations, hypertension, and respiratory depression with apnea. "Flashbacks" or visual disturbances can be experienced days or weeks after ingestion. Some chronic users become addicted and exhibit severe withdrawal symptoms that require detoxification.

Gahlinger PM. Club Drugs: MDMA, Gamma-hydroxybutyrate (GHB), Rohypnol, and Ketamine. *Am Fam Physician.* 2004;69: 2619–2626, 2627.

57. Galactorrhea is associated with which of the following medications?

A) Benzodiazepines
B) Tricyclic antidepressants
C) MAO inhibitors
D) Antipsychotic medication
E) Dopamine agonist

Answer and Discussion

The answer is D. Antipsychotic (neuroleptic) medications are dopamine receptor antagonist and include the following:

- Phenothiazines—chlorpromazine (Thorazine), thioridazine (Mellaril), mesoridazine (Serentil), perphenazine (Trilafon), trifluoperazine (Stelazine), and fluphenazine (Prolixin)
- Thioxanthenes—thiothixene (Navane)
- Butyrophenones—haloperidol (Haldol)
- Dihydroindolones—molindone (Moban)
- Dibenzoxazepine—loxapine (Loxitane)

Side effects of these medications are extensive and include anticholinergic effects such as dry mouth, blurred vision, urinary retention, delayed gastric emptying, acute glaucoma in patients with narrow anterior chamber angles, orthostatic hypotension, sexual dysfunction, cardiac arrhythmias, and endocrine abnormalities (hyperglycemia and hyperprolactinemia with galactorrhea). Extrapyramidal symptoms include akathisias (the desire to be in constant motion), acute dystonias (bizarre muscle spasms of the head, neck, and tongue), drug-induced parkinsonism (pill-rolling tremor, rigidity, and bradykinesia), and tardive dyskinesia (abnormal repetitive movements of the face, tongue, trunk, or limbs). The medications are indicated in the treatment of schizophrenia, psychoses, and mania. The risk for tardive dyskinesia increases with age and the length of administration of the medication. Neuroleptic malignant syndrome is a severe life-threatening side effect of antipsychotics that requires prompt recognition and treatment. Newer atypical antipsychotics have fewer side effects and are dopamine-serotonin antagonists.

Saddock BJ, Saddock VA. *Kaplan and Saddock's Concise Textbook of Psychiatry*, 2nd ed. Philadelphia: Lippincott Williams & Wilkins; 2004:454–455.

58. Good parenting is associated with which of the following?
A) Bargaining
B) Redirecting
C) Dependence
D) Variability
E) Inconsistency

Answer and Discussion

The answer is B. The use of positive reinforcement can be a powerful determinate of a child's behavior. Parents need to be instructed that positive reinforcers, such as candy, toys, and increased attention, given to children who disobey only serve to encourage poor behavior. However, failure to reward good behavior discourages further obedience. Therefore, parents should attempt to use positive reinforcers when they are pleased with their child's behavior. Parents must also remain consistent in their parenting practices. Children require reliable standards and expectations that are clearly demonstrated by their parents. Parents must be in agreement with regard to discipline. It is important to foster a sense of independence and responsibility in children. The goal of discipline is to teach children self-control. One good method for infants and toddlers is called *redirecting*. When one redirects a child, one replaces an unwanted (bad) behavior with an acceptable (good) behavior. For example, if throwing a ball inside the house is not allowed, a parent can take the child outside to throw the ball. For older children, it is important that they see the consequences of their actions and take responsibility for them.

American Academy of Family Physicians. Information from your family doctor—Tips for better parenting. *Am Fam Physician.* 1999;59(6):1591.

59. A recognized symptom of depression includes which of the following?
A) Sense of entitlement
B) Changes in weight
C) Hallucination
D) Flight of ideas
E) Depersonalization

Answer and Discussion

The answer is B. Depression is one of the most common problems seen by family physicians. Women are more affected than men, and the most common age range is 20 to 50 years. *DSM-IV* requires that at least five of the following symptoms are present for at least 2 weeks. The patient must show anhedonia or dysphoria and

- Depressed or irritable mood, or both (most of the day)
- Diminished interest or pleasure, or both, in most activity
- Significant change in weight or appetite, or both, with no effort
- Insomnia; hypersomnia
- Psychomotor retardation or agitation
- Fatigue; decreased activity
- Feelings of worthlessness or inappropriate guilt
- Poor concentration; indecisiveness
- Recurrent thoughts of death or suicide, or both

The patient must have no evidence of previous psychiatric diagnosis, no organic contributing cause, and no recent emotional loss. Many patients have a family history of depression and substance abuse. Evaluation should be performed to rule out causative factors such as anemia, infections, hypothyroidism, medication-related side effects, and alcohol or illegal drug abuse. Psychotherapy and antidepressant medication are the mainstays of treatment. Electroconvulsive therapy is reserved for severe cases. Hospitalization is indicated if a patient is suicidal.

American Psychiatric Association. *Diagnostic and Statistical Manual of Mental Disorders*, 4th ed. Washington, DC: American Psychiatric Association; 2000:327, 332.

60. Which of the following statements is true regarding inhalant abuse?
A) Twenty percent of children in middle school and high school have experimented with inhalants.
B) Inhalant use is not addictive.
C) A comprehensive drug screen can help identify the inhalant used.
D) Reversing agents can assist with recovery from an inhalant toxicity.
E) Hepatic damage is not associated with inhalant abuse because of the lack of enterohepatic circulation of the substance.

Answer and Discussion

The answer is A. Inhalant abuse is prevalent in adolescents. Studies show that nearly 20% of children in middle school and high school have experimented with inhalants. The method of delivery is inhalation of a solvent from its container, a soaked rag, or a bag. Solvents include household cleaning agents or propellants, paint thinners, glue, and lighter fluid. Inhalant abuse typically can cause a euphoric feeling and can become addictive. Acute effects include sudden sniffing death syndrome, asphyxia, and serious injuries (e.g., falls, burns, frostbite). Chronic inhalant abuse can cause cardiac, renal, hepatic, and neurologic damage. Inhalant abuse during pregnancy can lead to fetal abnormalities. Diagnosis of inhalant abuse is difficult and relies almost entirely on a thorough history and a high index of suspicion. No specific laboratory tests confirm solvent inhalation. Treatment is generally supportive, because there are no reversal agents for inhalant intoxication.

Anderson CE, Loomis GA. Recognition and prevention of inhalant abuse. *Am Fam Physician.* 2003;68:869–874, 876.

61. Which of the following is true regarding attention-deficit/hyperactivity disorder (ADHD)?
A) The condition is more common in females.
B) Combining psychosocial therapy with medication has proven to be superior to medication alone.
C) ADHD is best diagnosed using the DSM-IV diagnostic criteria and the Conners' Parent and Teacher Rating Scales.
D) Symptoms tend to increase over time.
E) Other psychiatric co-morbidities are rare.

Answer and Discussion

The answer is C. ADHD presents as inappropriate hyperactivity, impulsivity, and inattention in reference to the patient's age. ADHD cannot be easily diagnosed by a specific test or biologic marker, and it is unclear if the disorder is a truly pathologic condition or just one end of the behavioral spectrum. ADHD is more frequently diagnosed in children with behavioral difficulties and academic underachievement. Based on study results the pooled prevalence of ADHD is between 6.8% and 10.3%, with boys having a threefold higher rate. Psychiatric comorbidities, including oppositional-defiant disorder, conduct disorder, depressive disorder, and anxiety disorders are common. The Conners' ADHD Index and symptom scales from the *Diagnostic and Statistical Manual of Mental Disorders,* 4th ed. (DSM-IV), which are ADHD-specific checklists, have a high sensitivity for identification of children with the disorder. Reviews of the pharmacologic management of ADHD with methylphenidate hydrochloride, dextroamphetamine sulfate, and pemoline show these drugs to be effective. Nonpharmacologic treatments that have some beneficial effect on behavior and academic performance are behavioral modification and intensive contingency management therapy. Combining drug therapy with psychosocial therapy shows no clear advantage when compared to drug therapy alone. However, the addition of behavioral therapies to medication may have some benefit, including reduction of anxiety and improvement in social skills. ADHD is best diagnosed using the DSM-IV diagnostic criteria and the Conners' Parent and Teacher Rating Scales. Other psychiatric comorbidities are common and should be identified and properly managed. The symptoms of ADHD tend to decrease over the long-term but may continue into adolescence and adulthood. The most common treatment is stimulant medication.

Guevara JP. Attention deficit hyperactivity disorder. *West J Med.* 2001;175:189–192.

Hunt RD, Paquin A, Payton K. An update on assessment and treatment of complex attention-deficit hyperactivity disorder. *Pediatr Ann.* 2001 30;3:162–172.

62. Chronic alcohol abuse is associated with which of the following?
A) Hyperuricemia
B) Alanine aminotransferase–aspartate aminotransferase ratio of 2:1
C) Decreased mean corpuscular volume
D) Decreased γ-glutamyl transferase
E) Decreased triglycerides

Answer and Discussion

The answer is A. Alcohol abuse is usually described as an impairment of social or occupational functioning because of alcohol use. Symptoms include chronic anxiety or tension, insomnia, depression, headaches, legal and marital problems, gastrointestinal discomfort, frequent falls, and minor injuries. Complications include gastritis, peptic ulcer disease, cirrhosis, sexual dysfunction, nutritional deficiencies, neuropathy, and pancreatitis. Laboratory findings may include mild elevations of liver function tests. The aspartate aminotransferase–alanine aminotransferase ratio is often 2:1. A macrocytosis with an elevated mean corpuscular volume is usually the result of folate deficiency. Hypertriglyceridemia, hyperuricemia, and elevations in γ-glutamyl transferase are also seen. Treatment is aimed at abstinence of alcohol, and participation in rehabilitation programs such as Alcoholics Anonymous should be encouraged. Close monitoring, including hospitalization, may be necessary if withdrawal symptoms are anticipated.

Ferri FF. *Ferri's Clinical Advisor, Instant Diagnosis and Treatment.* Philadelphia: Elsevier/Mosby; 2006:36–38.

63. A patient whose spouse recently died presents to your office complaining of anxiety, insomnia, depressed mood, and anorexia. She reports that she continues to work and remains active playing bridge. The most appropriate treatment is
A) antidepressant medications
B) major tranquilizers
C) frequent office visits to receive biofeedback
D) inpatient psychiatric counseling
E) short-acting sedative to help with sleep

Answer and Discussion

The answer is E. Grief or bereavement reaction occurs in response to significant loss or separation. Situations such as the death of a loved one, marital separation, loss of a girlfriend or boyfriend, or a move to a different and unfamiliar location can give rise to the condition. The reaction is a normal process that usually improves with time. Symptoms include anxiety, insomnia, depressed mood, anorexia, and mood swings. Treatment involves frequent, short office visits to allow patients to express their grief. The use of major tranquilizers and antidepressants is unnecessary and may interfere with the normal grieving process. However, nighttime sedatives can be used for patients with insomnia. It is common for relapses to occur after the resolution of the grieving process, especially during the holidays or special events. Patient reassurance is usually all that is needed. In severe cases, in which there is significant functional impairment or psychomotor retardation, antidepressants may become necessary.

Beers MH, Porter RS, eds. *The Merck manual of diagnosis and therapy,* Merck Research Laboratories, 18th ed. Whitehouse Station, NJ: Merck & Co.; 2006:2768.

> The use of major tranquilizers and antidepressants during a significant loss is unnecessary and may interfere with the normal grieving process.

64. A 28-year-old man is noted to have impairment in social situations and job-related problems because of a pervasive pattern of grandiosity, lack of empathy, and extreme sensitivity to criticism. Coworkers report he frequently takes advantage of others for self-promotion. The most likely diagnosis is
A) borderline personality disorder
B) bipolar disorder
C) narcissistic personality disorder

D) paranoid personality disorder
E) antisocial personality disorder

Answer and Discussion

The answer is C. Patients who are affected with narcissistic personality disorder fulfill the following DSM-IV criteria and exhibit impairment in social or job situations with a pervasive pattern of grandiosity, lack of empathy, and extreme sensitivity to the evaluation and judgment of others. They must exhibit at least five of the following behaviors:

1. Reacts with rage, shame, or humiliation to criticism by others
2. Takes advantage of others for self-promotion
3. Requires constant attention and admiration of others
4. Lacks empathy toward others
5. Obsessed with feelings of envy
6. Possesses a sense of entitlement
7. Possesses a sense of self-importance
8. Remains preoccupied with fantasies of unlimited success
9. Believes own problems are unique and only understood by other special people

Patients with narcissistic personality disorder often experience depression and severe bouts of envy toward others. Occasionally, those who are affected become delusional in their thoughts. The treatment is psychoanalytic therapy that emphasizes acceptance of failures and the development of appreciation toward others. Success is limited but can be achieved. The course of this disease is chronic; however, narcissistic symptoms tend to diminish after the age of 40, when pessimism usually develops.

Saddock BJ, Saddock VA. *Kaplan and Saddock's Concise Textbook of Psychiatry*, 2nd ed. Philadelphia: Lippincott Williams & Wilkins; 2004:347.

65. Traditionally, what is the cutoff for a normal score on the Mini-Mental Status Examination in a college graduate?
A) 18
B) 20
C) 24
D) 27
E) 30

Answer and Discussion

The answer is C. A total maximal score on the MMSE is 30 points. Generally, a score of <24 points is suggestive of dementia or delirium. Using a cutoff of 24 points, the MMSE had a sensitivity of 87% and a specificity of 82% in a large population–based sample. However, the test is not sensitive for mild dementia, and scores may be influenced by age and education, as well as language, motor, and visual impairments. In one study, for example, the median MMSE score was 29 for individuals with at least 9 years of schooling, 26 for those with 5 to 8 years of schooling, and 22 for those with 4 years of schooling or less. The use of higher cutoff scores on the MMSE improves sensitivity but lowers specificity. The MMSE also has utility in assessing competency in decision making. Studies suggest that high scores (≥23) and low scores (<19) can be highly predictive in discriminating competency from incompetency. Intermediate scores warrant more detailed competency evaluation.

Crum RM, Anthony JC, Bassett SS, et al. Population-based norms for the Mini-Mental State Examination by age and educational level. *JAMA*. 1993;269:2386.

66. Which of the following statements is true regarding Tourette's syndrome?
A) Only 1% of the population is affected.
B) Tourette's syndrome is a familial disorder.
C) Patients with tic disorders rarely have other associated psychological conditions.
D) Tricyclic antidepressants are the treatment of choice.
E) The long-term prognosis for treatment is poor.

Answer and Discussion

The answer is B. Tic disorders and Tourette's syndrome are conditions that are rather common in the general population. Up to 20% of children have at least a transient tic disorder at some point. Once thought to be rare, Tourette's syndrome is now known to be a more common disorder that represents the most complex and severe manifestation of the spectrum of tic disorders. Tourette's syndrome is a chronic familial disorder with a fluctuating course; the long-term outcome is generally favorable. Although the exact underlying pathology has yet to be determined, evidence indicates a disorder localized to the frontal-subcortical neural pathways. Tourette's syndrome is associated with attention-deficit/hyperactivity disorder, obsessive-compulsive disorder, behavior problems, and learning disabilities. These associated conditions can make the management of Tourette's syndrome more difficult. Use of antipsychotic medications (resperidone, pimozide, olanzapine, and haloperidol) and clonidine can be effective but may be associated with significant side effects.

Bagheri MM, Kerbeshian J, Burd L. Recognition and management of Tourette's syndrome and tic disorders. *Am Fam Physician*. 1999;59:2263–2274.

67. Obligatory running is associated with
A) OCD
B) manic-depressive disorder
C) panic disorder
D) antisocial personality disorder
E) borderline personality disorder

Answer and Discussion

The answer is A. In some individuals who run on a regular basis, an obsession with running develops. The obsession can lead to a significant disruption in a person's life. Extreme inflexibility, adherence to running schedules, and extreme commitment to running can lead to pathologic behavior. If the patient cannot run, depression, fatigue, insomnia, irritability, and anxiety may occur. As in the alcoholic, interpersonal relationships can also be affected. The disorder has elements of a neurotic obsessive disorder. Psychotherapy may be necessary if symptoms are severe.

Dishman RK. Medical psychology in exercise and sport. *Med Clin North Am*. 1985;69:123–143.

Mellion MB, ed. *Office management of sports injuries and athletic problems*. Philadelphia: Hanley & Belfus; 1988:136–137.

68. Which of the following would be the drug of first choice for the treatment of mild Tourette's syndrome?
A) Carbamazepine
B) Phenobarbital
C) Primidone
D) Phenytoin
E) Lorazepam

Answer and Discussion

The answer is E. Tourette's syndrome is a genetically transmitted disorder that begins in childhood as a simple tic, progressing to multiple tics as the patient ages. Tics may begin as grunts or barks and progress to involuntary compulsive utterances called *coprolalia*. These outbursts may become severe and significantly disable the patient from a physical or social standpoint. Tics tend to be more complex than myoclonus but less flowing than choreic movements, from which they must be differentiated. The patient may voluntarily suppress them for seconds or minutes. Simple tics may respond to benzodiazepines. For simple and complex tics, clonidine is effective in some patients. Long-term use of clonidine does not cause tardive dyskinesia; its limiting adverse effect is hypotension. Intermediate-acting benzodiazepines (e.g., lorazepam) may be useful as adjuvant treatment. For more severe cases, antipsychotics, such as haloperidol, olanzapine, resperidone or pimozide, may be required. Side effects of dysphoria, parkinsonism, akathisia, and tardive dyskinesia may limit their use. Antipsychotics should be started cautiously, and patients should be told about potential adverse outcomes.

Beers MH, Porter RS, eds. *The Merck manual of diagnosis and therapy,* Merck Research Laboratories, 18th ed. Whitehouse Station, NJ: Merck & Co.; 2006:2379.

69. Which of the following statements about conversion disorder is true?
A) An underlying conflict or need does not have to be present.
B) Symptoms often have a physiologic or pathophysiologic explanation.
C) Men are more commonly affected.
D) Treatment usually involves pharmacotherapy.
E) Those who are affected subject themselves to unnecessary medical testing.

Answer and Discussion

The answer is E. Conversion disorder, also known as *hysterical neurosis*, occurs because of an underlying psychological conflict or need. The symptoms are not voluntarily controlled, and there is no physiologic or pathophysiologic explanation for the symptoms. Reported symptoms include paresis, paralysis, seizures, blindness, abdominal pain, and vomiting. Most patients present with symptoms in adolescence, but the disorder may occur at any age. Women are more commonly affected than men. Episodes may occur over time but may be limited to a single episode. Stress often precipitates the episode. In most cases, the episode is short, and most symptoms resolve quickly. The diagnosis may be difficult initially because the patient believes that the symptoms stem from a physical disorder. Also, physicians are taught almost exclusively to consider (and exclude) physical disorders as the cause of physical symptoms. Commonly, the diagnosis is considered only after extensive physical examinations and laboratory tests fail to reveal a disorder that can fully account for the symptom and its effects. Although ruling out a possible underlying physical disorder is crucial, early consideration of conversion may avoid tests that increase the costs and risks to the patient and that may unduly delay diagnosis. The best clue is that conversion symptoms rarely conform fully to known anatomic and physiologic mechanisms. Most patients, because of their complaints, subject themselves to unnecessary medical tests. Treatment usually involves psychotherapy. Medication is generally not warranted.

Beers MH, Porter RS, eds. *The Merck manual of diagnosis and therapy,* Merck Research Laboratories, 18th ed. Whitehouse Station, NJ: Merck & Co.; 2006:1737–1738.

70. Which of the following medications should be monitored in the blood of newborns when treating the mother for postpartum depression?
A) Fluoxetine (Prozac)
B) Sertraline (Zoloft)
C) Bupropion (Wellbutrin)
D) Paroxetine (Paxil)
E) Mirtazapine (Remeron)

Answer and Discussion

The answer is A. Because of the long elimination half-life of fluoxetine (Prozac), if a woman who was taking this drug during pregnancy wishes to breast feed while continuing fluoxetine treatment, she should have the infant's blood tested after about 6 weeks of breast-feeding to rule out drug accumulation. In infants exposed to any antidepressant through breast milk, plasma concentrations of the drug should be determined if they are exhibiting persistent unexplained irritability.

Epperson CN. Postpartum major depression: detection and treatment. *Am Fam Physician.* 1999;59:2247–2259.

71. Which of the following should be used initially in conjunction with benzodiazepines in the treatment of serotonin syndrome?
A) Diphenhydramine
B) Prednisone
C) Cyproheptadine
D) Dantrolene
C) Nitroprusside

Answer and Discussion

The answer is C. The initial pharmacologic treatment of serotonin syndrome is with benzodiazepines and cyproheptadine (an antihistamine with serotonin antagonist properties). Other medications may include dantrolene and methysergide. If muscular rigidity and hyperthermia do not respond to these interventions, neuromuscular paralysis with endotracheal intubation is appropriate.

Boyer EW, Shannon M. The serotonin syndrome. *N Engl J Med.* 2005;352:1112.

72. Which of the following statements is true regarding lithium administration?
A) Hepatotoxicity can develop after 4 weeks of therapy.
B) The drug may affect thyroid function.
C) Renal function can be improved with the use of lithium.
D) Peripheral neuropathy is a possible side effect.
E) Drug levels remain constant and rarely need monitoring.

Answer and Discussion

The answer is B. Lithium is used in the treatment of bipolar disorder. In most cases, it takes 1 week before the effects are noted. Side effects of the medication include tremor, polydipsia, polyuria, gastrointestinal irritation, and diarrhea. Hypothyroidism and renal toxicity are other complications of lithium administration. Toxicity is characterized by lethargy, seizures, nephropathy, and coma. Blood levels should be monitored carefully and adjusted as necessary. In addition, serum creatinine and thyroid function tests should be evaluated periodically. Drugs that decrease renal clearance, such as nonsteroidal anti-inflammatory agents, should be used cautiously in patients receiving lithium.

Saddock BJ, Saddock VA. *Kaplan and Saddock's Concise Textbook of Psychiatry*, 2nd ed. Philadelphia: Lippincott Williams & Wilkins; 2004:458–460.

73. A 30-year-old woman makes frequent visits to your office with vague somatic complaints that have no medical justification. In addition, she has frequent mood swings and unstable interpersonal relationships. In the past, she has had problems with alcohol. She is very interested in your personal life and thinks you are a "wonderful doctor." The most likely diagnosis is
A) borderline personality disorder
B) bipolar disorder
C) schizophrenia
D) dysthymic disorder
E) narcissistic personality disorder

Answer and Discussion

The answer is A. Borderline personalities are often encountered in the family physician's office. Characteristics of this disorder include impulsiveness, unstable and intense interpersonal relationships, substance abuse, and self-destructive behavior with accident proneness. Those who are affected lack self-control, lack self-fulfillment, and have identity problems. Their behaviors include aggressive and suicidal actions with frequent mood swings. In many cases, they present with vague, unexplainable somatic complaints; do not follow therapeutic recommendations; and are very frustrating to their physicians. Most affected persons present during adolescence. Treatment involves adequate communication, supportive limit-setting, frequent office visits, and occasionally medication. Acute crisis may require hospitalization. Patients with this disorder have high comorbidity with other psychiatric disorders and high rates of suicidal ideation, and they cause particular treatment difficulties, including hostility toward caregivers and low rates of treatment compliance. The central feature of patients with borderline personality disorder is a morbid fear of abandonment, with consequential pathologic responses to perceived rejection. Such patients may demand inappropriate amounts of time or support from a primary care physician, and they may become hostile and demanding or suicidal if these needs are not met. The family practitioner should be alert to the following "red flags": a history of doctor shopping; a history of legal suits against physicians or other professionals; a history of suicide attempts; a history of several brief marriages or intimate relationships; an immediate idealization of you as a "wonderful doctor," especially if the patient compares you with disappointing caregivers of the past; and excessive interest in your personal life, eventually leading to invitations to socialize with you. Behavior of this type implies boundary violations, and its purpose is to cement a relationship with the physician, allaying the patient's ever-present fear of abandonment.

Beers MH, Porter RS, eds. *The Merck manual of diagnosis and therapy*, Merck Research Laboratories, 18th ed. Whitehouse Station, NJ: Merck & Co.; 2006:1719.

74. Which of the following drugs has been shown to be beneficial in the treatment of premenstrual dysphoric disorder?
A) Haloperidol
B) Progesterone
C) Fluoxetine
D) Furosemide
E) Lithium

Answer and Discussion

The answer is C. Premenstrual dysphoric disorder is associated with mood-related symptoms leading to functional impairment that distinguish it from premenstrual syndrome. Patients must have a symptom-free postmenopausal week, and they typically experience the symptom of being overwhelmed or out of control during the most affected time. The symptoms must be present during the luteal phase of the menstrual cycle (from ovulation to the onset of menses), and there must not be an underlying psychiatric disorder. The most common symptom reported is depressed mood, followed by anxiety or tension, mood swings, and anger or irritability. At least one of these must be present to make the diagnosis. The time of greatest well-being is just before ovulation. The average age of presentation is 36. Many report that their symptoms began when they were in their 20s and worsened over time. Those who are affected are at higher risk for development of a major depressive disorder. Fluoxetine (Sarafem, Prozac) was found to be beneficial in treating symptoms, as was sertraline (Zoloft).

Saddock BJ, Saddock VA. *Kaplan and Saddock's Concise Textbook of Psychiatry*, 2nd ed. Philadelphia: Lippincott Williams & Wilkins; 2004:207–208.

Premenstrual dysphoric disorder is associated with mood-related symptoms leading to functional impairment that distinguish it from premenstrual syndrome.

75. Which of the following is most commonly associated with tricyclic antidepressant toxicity?
A) Third-degree AV block
B) Prolongation of the PR interval
C) Prolongation of the QT interval
D) Widened QRS interval
E) T-wave elevation

Answer and Discussion

The answer is C. The tricyclic antidepressants are used less frequently as first-line agents with the development of the SSRIs and other newer antidepressants. This is mainly due to the less benign side-effect profile of the cyclic antidepressants. These drugs interact with a wide variety of brain-receptor types that result in their antidepressant efficacy and side-effect profiles. Most serious is the toxicity of the cyclic antidepressants in overdose. In comparison to the SSRIs, the cyclic antidepressants can be fatal in doses as little as five times the therapeutic dose. The toxicity is usually due to prolongation of the QT interval, leading to arrhythmias.

Ray WA, Meredith S, Thapa PB, et al. Cyclic antidepressants and the risk of sudden cardiac death. *Clin Pharmacol Ther.* 2004;75:234.

76. Which of the following has the least amount of sexual side effects?
A) Fluoxetine (Prozac)
B) Sertraline (Zoloft)
C) Bupropion (Wellbutrin)

D) Paroxetine (Paxil)
E) Citalopram (Celexa)

Answer and Discussion

The answer is C. Bupropion appears to have no or only a limited effect on sexual function.

Zajecka J. Strategies for the treatment of antidepressant-related sexual dysfunction. *J Clin Psychiatry.* 2001;62 (Suppl) 3:35.

77. A 41 year old presents with feelings of being "choked up." The symptoms are rather constant and are not made worse with swallowing. He denies that food is stuck in the throat, and he has had no recent weight change. Eating and drinking help to relieve symptoms. The most likely diagnosis is
A) globus hystericus
B) panic attacks
C) Barrett's esophagus
D) reflux esophagitis
E) Zenker's diverticulum

Answer and Discussion

The answer is A. *Globus hystericus* is defined as the subjective sensation of a lump or mass in the throat. No specific cause or mechanism has been determined, although there is some evidence to suggest that increased cricopharyngeal (upper esophageal sphincter) pressures or abnormal hypopharyngeal motility exist during the time of symptoms. The sensation may result from gastroesophageal reflux or from frequent swallowing and drying of the throat associated with anxiety or other emotional states. Although not related to a specific psychiatric disorder, globus may be a symptom of certain mood states. Suppression of sadness is most often implicated. Symptoms resemble the normal sensation of being "choked up." With globus, symptoms do not become worse during swallowing, food does not stick in the throat, and eating or drinking often provides relief. No pain or weight loss occurs. Chronic symptoms may be experienced during grief reactions and may be relieved by crying. The diagnosis is based on the history and physical examination and is a diagnosis of exclusion. The treatment involves treating the underlying psychological condition.

Beers MH, Porter RS, eds. *The Merck manual of diagnosis and therapy,* Merck Research Laboratories, 18th ed. Whitehouse Station, NJ: Merck & Co.; 2006:69–70.

78. A 7 year old is brought to your office by his parents at the request of his teachers. The child appears to have understanding of spoken language but has a reading disorder that involves single word decoding. The parents report that the father has similar problems that were detected during his schooling. The most likely diagnosis is
A) attention deficit disorder
B) autism
C) dyslexia
D) congenital hearing loss
E) mental retardation

Answer and Discussion

The answer is C. The inability to learn derivational rules of printed language is often considered part of dyslexia. Affected children may have difficulty in determining root words or word stems and determining which letters in words follow others and form specific sound-symbol associations, such as vowel patterns, affixes, syllables, and word endings. The cause of dyslexia is unknown, but a strong genetic link has been established. Cerebrovascular accidents, prematurity, and intrauterine complications have been linked to dyslexia. Most experts agree that dyslexia is left hemisphere–related and is associated with deficiencies or dysfunctions in the areas of the brain that are responsible for language association (Wernicke's area) and sound and speech production (Broca's area) and in the interconnection of these areas. Most dyslexics are not identified until kindergarten or first grade, when symbolic learning is taught. However, dyslexia in preschool children may manifest itself as delayed language production, speech articulation problems, and difficulties in remembering the names of letters, numbers, and colors, particularly in children with a family history of reading or learning problems. Many dyslexics confuse letters and words with similar configurations or have difficulty in visually selecting or identifying letter patterns and clusters (sound-symbol association) in words. Reversals or visual confusions tend to be seen frequently during the early school years. Most reading and writing reversals occur because dyslexics forget or confuse the names of letters and words that have similar structures; subsequently, *d* becomes *b, m* becomes *w, h* becomes *n, was* becomes *saw,* and *on* becomes *no,* for example. Students with a history of delayed language acquisition use or who are not accelerating in word learning by the middle or end of first grade, or who are not reading at the level expected for their verbal or intellectual abilities at any grade level, should be evaluated. Many dyslexics develop functional reading skills with direct instruction, although dyslexia is a lifelong problem, and many dyslexics never reach full literacy. Compensatory approaches, such as taped texts, readers, and scribes, are used to assist the dyslexic with higher-order learning.

Beers MH, Porter RS, eds. *The Merck manual of diagnosis and therapy,* Merck Research Laboratories, 18th ed. Whitehouse Station, NJ: Merck & Co.; 2006:2490–2491.

79. Medication for the treatment of premature ejaculation includes
A) finasteride (Proscar)
B) tamsulosin (Flomax)
C) sildenafil (Viagra)
D) sertraline (Zoloft)
E) progesterone (Provera)

Answer and Discussion

The answer is D. *Premature ejaculation* is best defined as persistent or recurrent ejaculation with minimal stimulation before, on, or shortly after penetration and before the sexual partner wishes it. Premature ejaculation is thought to be the most common form of male sexual dysfunction, with an estimated prevalence of up to 40%. Treatment of ejaculatory dysfunction centers on relationship counseling, behavioral therapy, and pharmacologic interventions. Behavioral therapy has been considered the gold standard of treatment. Techniques include the Semen's pause maneuver, the Masters and Johnson pause-squeeze technique, and the Kaplan stop-start method. These techniques are directed at the induction of male sexual arousal to the point of ejaculation followed by relaxation before orgasm is allowed to occur. The methods can be self-applied, although with suboptimal outcomes; hence, involvement of the sexual partner is essential. Because of the limitations of behavioral therapy, pharmacologic interventions are often used to treat premature ejaculation. Anorgasmia and delayed ejaculatory response are well-known side effects of tricyclic antidepressants (clomipramine) and SSRIs. Recent studies have shown that these drugs modify the ejaculatory response in men with premature ejaculation. Results appear better with clomipramine, but sertraline was better tolerated and had a better safety profile.

Epperly TD, Moore KE. Health issues in men (Part I). Common genitourinary disorders. *Am Fam Physician*. 2000;61:3657–3664.

80. When initiating antidepressants in children, the risk of suicide is maximum during

A) the first hours of medication administration
B) during the first few weeks
C) during the first few months
D) usually a year or more after starting therapy
E) the risk of suicide is not increased

Answer and Discussion

The answer is B. The FDA advisory panel concluded there is a small, but real, increased risk of suicidal thoughts or behavior in children taking antidepressants compared to placebo. The risk appears to be greatest in the first few weeks after initiation of therapy.

Hammad TA. Review and evaluation of clinical data. Center for Drug Evaluation and Research, FDA. August 16, 2004. Available at www.fda.gov/ohrms/dockets/ac/04/briefing/2004-4065b1.htm. Accessed on March 17, 2006.

Jick H, Kaye JA, Jick SS. Antidepressants and the risk of suicidal behaviors. *JAMA*. 2004; 292:338.

81. Which of the following has the best side-effect profile?

A) Amitriptyline
B) Nortriptyline
C) Desipramine
D) Clomipramine
E) Fluoxetine

Answer and Discussion

The answer is E. The tricyclic antidepressants are used less frequently as first-line agents with the development of the SSRIs and other newer antidepressants. This is mainly due to the less benign side-effect profile of the cyclic antidepressants.

Ray WA, Meredith S, Thapa PB, et al. Cyclic antidepressants and the risk of sudden cardiac death. *Clin Pharmacol Ther.* 2004;75:234.

82. Which of the following factors may contribute to an increased risk of domestic violence?

A) More than three children in the home
B) Power differential in the relationship
C) Women with depression
D) Prior divorce
E) One spouse undergoing schooling

Answer and Discussion

The answer is B. Studies have not identified any consistent psychiatric diagnoses among abusers, but abusive men share some common characteristics such as rigid sex role stereotypes, low self-esteem, depression, a high need for power and control, a tendency to minimize and deny their problems or the extent of their violence, a tendency to blame others for their behavior, violence in the family of origin (particularly witnessing parental violence), and drug and alcohol abuse (which are not causative but are often associated). Some but not all batterers meet the criteria in the DSM-IV for personality disorders or depression. Men who have alcoholism combined with a major depressive disorder or antisocial personality disorder are more likely to commit domestic violence than are men with either of these conditions alone. Most researchers believe that abusive behavior is the result of multiple factors, including individual characteristics, a family history of violence, and the culturally rooted belief that violence is an acceptable means of solving problems and that violence toward women is acceptable or tolerated. Factors that specifically relate to partner abuse include the following:

- A power differential in the relationship in which one partner is financially or emotionally dependent on the other.
- A temporary or permanent disability (including pregnancy).
- A force orientation—a belief on the part of the perpetrator that violence is an acceptable solution to conflicts and problems.
- A personal or family history of abuse.

Signs that often indicate a need to further assess the risk of abuse include excessive work loss, sleep disturbances, substance abuse, anxiety, sexual dysfunction, depression, frequent injuries, or being "accident prone." It is imperative to discuss events noted in these records with the patient and to assess any discrepancy between an injury and its reported causative mechanism, because injuries that are related to battering are often attributed to falling on the stairs or some other household accident. In such cases, the patient should be asked to describe the accident in more detail, or the physician should ask about precipitating factors (e.g., "Were you pushed?"). Ancillary tests should be obtained as indicated for the specific injury or infection. The physician should be especially alert for pregnancy complications and sexually transmitted infections, including human immunodeficiency virus infection.

U.S. Preventive Services Task Force. Screening for family and intimate partner violence: recommendation statement. *Ann Intern Med.* 2004;140:382–386.

83. Which of the following statements regarding the use of psychotropic agents in a nursing home setting is true?

A) Phenobarbital does not require monitoring.
B) Sedative-hypnotics should be used to sedate patients who are at risk for falls.
C) Periodic dose reductions should be performed.
D) The physician is ultimately responsible for drug monitoring.
E) Tranquilizers, regardless of their effectiveness in patients before admission to the nursing home, should not be used.

Answer and Discussion

The answer is C. All psychotropic drugs (antidepressants, anxiolytics, sedative-hypnotics, and antipsychotics) are subject to the "unnecessary drug" regulation of the Omnibus Budget Reconciliation Act (OBRA). According to the federal government guidelines, "nursing home residents must be free of unnecessary drugs," which are defined as those that are duplicative, excessive in dose or duration, or used in the presence of adverse effects or without adequate monitoring or indication. Medical, environmental, and psychosocial causes of behavioral problems must be ruled out, and nonpharmacologic management must be attempted before psychotropic drugs are prescribed to nursing home residents. Because treatment with psychotropic medications is indicated only to maintain or improve functional status, diagnoses and specific target symptoms or behaviors must be documented, and the effectiveness of drug therapy must be monitored. Specific dosage limits must be observed, and periodic dosage reductions or drug discontinuations must be undertaken. Side effects (of antipsychotics in particular) must be monitored. Barbiturates and certain other older tranquilizers may not be prescribed unless they were being used successfully before a patient was admitted to a long-term care facility. Phenobarbital can be used only to control seizures. OBRA restricts the use of antipsychotic drugs only in patients with dementia. None of the OBRA dosage restrictions or monitoring requirements apply in patients with psychotic disorders (e.g., schizophrenia). Each nursing home is surveyed annually. Because facilities that do not meet the federal government's requirements may be denied Medicare reimbursement, physicians who prescribe medications for nursing home residents must document the medical necessity of noncompliance with regulations (e.g., drug prescriptions in excess of OBRA-mandated dosages). In most cases, a local consultant pharmacist reviews all charts monthly and assists with compliance. According to the OBRA strategy, the long-term care facility, rather than the prescribing physician, is accountable for monitoring drug use. Regardless of where final responsibility lies, physicians need to be aware of the federal government's interpretive guidelines for the fulfillment of OBRA requirements.

Gurvich T, Cunningham JA. Appropriate use of psychotropic drugs in nursing homes. *Am Fam Physician.* 2000;61: 1437–1446.

84. Which of the following antidepressant medications has the lowest risk of drug interactions?
A) Fluoxetine (Prozac)
B) Paroxetine (Paxil)
C) Sertraline (Zoloft)
D) Citalopram (Celexa)
E) Amitriptyline (Elavil)

Answer and Discussion

The answer is D. Most SSRIs are associated with significant drug interactions. Fluoxetine, paroxetine, and, to a lesser extent, sertraline inhibit the metabolism of warfarin (Coumadin), cisapride (Propulsid), benzodiazepines, quinidine, tricyclic antidepressants, theophylline, and some statins. In patients who are at risk for these interactions, citalopram, an SSRI that is now available in the United States, may offer an advantage. Studies have shown that compared with other SSRIs, citalopram has less of an inhibitory effect on the cytochrome P-450 system. It is as effective as fluoxetine and sertraline in the treatment of depression.

Gurvich T, Cunningham JA. Appropriate use of psychotropic drugs in nursing homes. *Am Fam Physician.* 2000;61:1437–1446.

> Compared with other SSRIs, citalopram has less of an inhibitory effect on the cytochrome P-450 system.

85. A 47-year-old man complains of a depressed mood over the last 3 years. He complains of low energy and low self-esteem. The condition has not prevented him from working nor has it seemed to interfere with his family life. You explain to him he has the diagnosis of
A) major depression
B) dysthymia
C) dissociation disorder
D) attention deficit disorder
E) introvert personality disorder

Answer and Discussion

The answer is B. Dysthymia is a more chronic, low-intensity mood disorder. By definition, symptoms must be present for more than 2 years consecutively. It is characterized by anhedonia, low self-esteem, and low energy. It may have a more psychologic than biologic explanation and tends to respond to medication and psychotherapy equally. Long-term psychotherapy is frequently able to establish a permanent change in dysthymic individuals. There are often unrealistic and neurotic expectations stemming from adolescence in this disorder.

American Psychiatric Association. *Diagnostic and Statistical Manual of Mental Disorders*, 4th ed. Washington, DC: American Psychiatric Association; 2000:327, 332.

86. Selective serotonin reuptake inhibitors (SSRIs) are
A) associated with GI bleeding in patients taking NSAIDs
B) contraindicated in diabetics
C) not associated with withdrawal symptoms
D) cardiotoxic in doses that approach therapeutic range
E) contraindicated in patients with a history of suicidal attempts

Answer and Discussion

The answer is A. Studies have suggested that SSRIs are associated with an increased risk of upper gastrointestinal (UGI) bleeding, particularly in patients taking NSAIDs.

de Abajo FJ, Garcia Rodriguez LA, Montero D. Association between selective serotonin reuptake inhibitors and upper gastrointestinal bleeding: Population-based case-control study. *BMJ.* 1999;319:1106.

87. Bupropion (Wellbutrin) is structurally related to
A) anxiolytics
B) stimulants
C) barbiturates
D) alcohol
E) antibiotics

Answer and Discussion

The answer is B. Bupropion (Wellbutrin, Zyban) is used for the treatment of depression and also in treatment for tobacco abuse. Because bupropion is structurally related to stimulants, bedtime administration should be avoided. The most common adverse reactions include tremor, headaches, rash, and urticaria. Other adverse effects include insomnia and dry mouth. Bupropion in dosages >400 mg/day is associated with seizures.

Gurvich T, Cunningham JA. Appropriate use of psychotropic drugs in nursing homes. *Am Fam Physician.* 2000;61: 1437–1446.

88. Children whose parents divorce are at increased risk for
A) lower academic achievement
B) more conduct problems

C) poorer self-concept
D) more maladjustment problems
E) all of the above

Answer and Discussion

The answer is E. Marital conflict and divorce are prevalent in our society. Women who divorce during middle age face age-specific stresses, including loss of long-held social position, the possibility of overdependence on young adult children, a shrinking remarriage pool, socially denigrated body changes, and unfair labor market conditions. In assisting women who are going through divorce, family physicians need to focus initially on the patient's grief and mourning and then emphasize behavior modification and improved coping skills, which can be accomplished with the aid of a therapist. As a group, children (especially boys) of parents who are going through a high-conflict divorce are two to four times more likely to have clinical emotional and behavioral disturbances compared with national norms. Court-ordered joint physical custody and a frequent visitation arrangement in high-conflict divorce tend to be associated with poorer outcomes in children, especially girls. Thus, a child's ultimate adjustment to divorce depends on several factors, including the following:

- The level of interparental conflict that precedes and follows divorce. The number of stressful life events that accompany and follow divorce
- The custodial parent's psychological adjustment and parenting skills
- The amount and quality of contact with the noncustodial parent
- The degree of economic hardship to which children are exposed

After a divorce, children may experience sadness and depression, aggressive behavior, frequent illnesses, abdominal pain, headaches, difficulty in school, eating problems, and sleeping disturbances. Children who experience parental divorce, compared with children in intact two-parent families, exhibit more conduct problems, more symptoms of psychologic maladjustment, lower academic achievement, more social difficulties, and poorer self-concept. Similarly, adults who experienced parental divorce as children, compared with adults raised in continuously intact two-parent families, score lower on a variety of indicators of psychologic, interpersonal, and socioeconomic well-being. However, the overall differences between offspring from divorced and intact families are small, with considerable diversity existing in children's reactions to divorce.

Meurer JR, Meurer LN, Holloway RL. Clinical problems and counseling for single-parent families. *Am Fam Physician.* 1996;54(3):864.

89. Teen pregnancy is most closely associated with
A) higher birth weight infants
B) improved Apgar scores
C) higher risk of gestational diabetes
D) higher risk of preeclampsia
E) higher risk of deep venous thrombosis

Answer and Discussion

The answer is D. Each year, approximately 1 million adolescents become pregnant in the United States, and nearly half of them give birth and become parents. Risk factors that are predictive of early sexual activity and subsequent pregnancy include poverty, poor academic ability and achievement, and a lack of educational goals. Pregnant adolescents are at greater risk than older mothers for nutritional deficiencies, anemia, preeclampsia, and cephalopelvic disproportion, due partly to inadequate prenatal care. In addition, pregnancy increases the teenager's risk of dropping out of school, leading to fewer career opportunities, chronic unemployment, and societal dependence. Infants who are born to adolescents are at high risk for premature birth, low birth weight, and infant death. They experience more illnesses, have more cognitive delays, and perform less well in school than children with more mature parents. The children of adolescent parents are at risk themselves for early sexual activity and teenage pregnancy, thereby perpetuating the cycle.

Kasper DL, Braunwald E, Fauci AS, et al., eds. *Harrison's principles of internal medicine,* 16th ed. New York: McGraw-Hill; 2005:281.

90. Which of the following is the primary treatment of schizophrenia?
A) Cognitive therapy
B) Behavioral therapy
C) Interpersonal therapy
D) Psychodynamic psychotherapy
E) Pharmacotherapy

Answer and Discussion

The answer is E. Pharmacotherapy is the primary treatment for schizophrenia and other psychotic disorders.

Kopelowicz A, Liberman RP. Psychosocial treatments for schizophrenia. In: Nathan PE, Gorman JM, eds. *A guide to treatments that work.* New York: Oxford University Press; 1998:190.

91. Which of the following foods is safe to eat if the patient is taking a monoamine oxidase inhibitor (MAOI)?
A) Fermented cheese
B) Soy sauce
C) Bananas
D) Smoked sausage
E) Wheat bread

Answer and Discussion

The answer is E. MAO inhibitors are often avoided because of their potential to precipitate enhanced sympathetic activity and severe hypertension with the concomitant ingestion of tyramine containing foods (e.g., fermented cheeses; imported beer; Chianti, champagne, some other wines; soy sauce; avocados; bananas; overripe or spoiled food; and any fermented, smoked, or aged fish or meat).

Paulson RH, Katon W, Ciechenowski P. Treatment of depression in adults. Up to Date, version 14.1. Accessed 3/17/06.

92. Which of the following drugs used in the treatment of attention deficit disorder hyperactivity disorder has been associated with hepatotoxicity?
A) Methylphenidate (Ritalin)
B) Dextroamphetamine (Dexedrine)
C) Pemoline (Cylert)
D) Clonidine (Catapres)
E) Desipramine (Norpramin)

Answer and Discussion

The answer is C. Attention deficit hyperactivity disorder is the most common pediatric psychiatric disorder, involving 1 of every 20 children. It is often a disabling condition and is frequently accompanied by high levels of frustration and comorbidity. Diagnosis of attention deficit hyperactivity disorder requires a detailed history from the family and use of rating scales to collect observations from two or more settings. Effective treatment, including behavior management, appropriate educational placement, and stimulant medication, improves academic performance and behavior in most patients. Children in whom initial management fails or for whom the diagnosis is unclear or complicated should be referred to appropriate mental health professionals. Medications that are used for treatment include methylphenidate, dextroamphetamine, and pemoline. Although these medicines have a stimulating effect in most, they have a calming effect in children and adults with attention deficit hyperactivity disorder. Other medications include atomoxetine, clonidine, desipramine, imipramine, and bupropion. Side effects include headaches, gastrointestinal symptoms, anorexia and weight loss, insomnia, and palpitations. Pemoline has been associated with hepatotoxicity and is no longer used. Dosing of medications should be 30 to 45 minutes before meals (breakfast and lunch). Lunchtime doses can be given at school for some children. An alternative is the use of longer-acting preparations. The long-acting form of these medications should not be crushed, broken, or chewed before swallowing. The long-acting forms are dosed (usually) once a day, before breakfast.

Guevara J, Paquin A, Payton K. Attention deficit hyperactivity disorder. *West J Med.* 2001;175:189–192.

Hunt RD, et al. An update on assessment and treatment of complex attention-deficit hyperactivity disorder. *Pediatr Ann.* 2001;30(3):162–172.

93. Which of the following side effects is associated with the use of St. John's Wort?

A) Photosensitivity
B) Peripheral neuropathy
C) Hepatotoxicity
D) Renal toxicity
E) Rhabdomyolysis

Answer and Discussion

The answer is A. St. John's Wort *(Hypericum perforatum)* is an herbal medicine that is used for the treatment of depression. Several studies have shown beneficial responses with use of the medication, although criticism of the research exists. St. John's Wort should not be combined with the use of SSRIs. In addition there is concern about the side effect of photosensitivity with prolonged use. Other side effects include delayed hypersensitivity, gastrointestinal tract upset, dizziness, dry mouth, sedation, restlessness, and constipation. No effect on cardiac conduction has been found. Contraindications include pregnancy, lactation, exposure to strong sunlight, and pheochromocytoma. The drug should not be used with MAO inhibitors. A recent review concluded that *Hypericum* is at least as safe and possibly safer than conventional antidepressant medications.

Beers MH, Porter RS, eds. *The Merck manual of diagnosis and therapy,* Merck Research Laboratories, 18th ed. Whitehouse Station, NJ: Merck & Co.; 2006:2732–2733.

94. Kava is included in an herbal remedy that is used in the treatment of

A) depression
B) impotence
C) anxiety
D) memory loss
E) attention deficit disorder

Answer and Discussion

The answer is C. The term *kava* refers to a Pacific Island plant *(Piper methysticum)* and the beverage that is prepared from it. The drug may be beneficial in the management of anxiety and tension of nonpsychotic origin and does not adversely affect cognitive function, mental acuity, or coordination. Long-term use of high doses has been associated with scaling of the skin on the extremities. Kava may potentiate the action of other centrally mediated agents and interact with alcohol.

Beers MH, Porter RS, eds. *The Merck manual of diagnosis and therapy,* Merck Research Laboratories, 18th ed. Whitehouse Station, NJ: Merck & Co.; 2006:2732.

> Kava may be beneficial in the management of anxiety and tension of nonpsychotic origin and does not adversely affect cognitive function, mental acuity, or coordination.

95. Which of the following conditions is commonly seen in patients with mental retardation?

A) Hyperthyroidism
B) Hyperparathyroidism
C) Diabetes mellitus
D) Osteoporosis
E) Pernicious anemia

Answer and Discussion

The answer is D. Osteoporosis is a common condition seen in patients with mental retardation, particularly among non-weight-bearing patients. It has been estimated that as many as 50% of adults with mental retardation have osteoporosis or osteopenia. Conditions associated with an increased risk of osteoporosis include cerebral palsy, Down syndrome, use of antiepileptics, special diets (e.g., ketogenic diet for seizure control), and hypogonadism. Aggressive evaluation of traumatic injuries with radiographic studies may be justified even when there are few physical findings. Furthermore, osteoporosis and use of antiepileptics may predispose patients to degenerative disk disease with spinal cord compromise, leading to functional decline.

Prater CD, Zylstra RG. Medical care of adults with mental retardation. *Am Fam Physician.* 2006;73:2175–2183, 2184.

96. Which of the following medications is more likely to have a paradoxical reaction in patients affected with mental retardation?

A) Haloperidol
B) Lorazepam
C) Phenobarbitol
D) Phenytoin
E) Buspirone

Answer and Discussion

The answer is B. In patients affected with mental retardation, many of the most challenging behaviors are caused by the same neuropsychiatric disorders that affect the general population and most respond to the same treatments. One notable exception is benzodiazepine therapy, which can precipitate paradoxical reactions of increased irritability and aggression in 10% to 15% of patients with mental retardation.

Kalachnik JE, Hanzel TE, Sevenich R, et al. Benzodiazepine behavioral side effects: review and implications for individuals with mental retardation. *Am J Ment Retard.* 2002;107:376–410.

97. Valerian is an herbal remedy that is used for the treatment of
A) sleep disorders
B) mania
C) depression
D) menstrual disorders
E) bulimia

Answer and Discussion

The answer is A. Valerian is derived from the perennial herb *Valerian officinalis*. The herb is used in the treatment of anxiety and sleep disorders. It interacts with the inhibitory neurotransmitter GABA. Valerian may potentiate the effects of other central nervous system depressants. The incidence of adverse side effects with its use appears to be low; however, more research is needed.

Beers MH, Porter RS, eds. *The Merck manual of diagnosis and therapy,* Merck Research Laboratories, 18th ed. Whitehouse Station, NJ: Merck & Co.; 2006:2733.

98. Patients with which of the following conditions should use ginkgo biloba with caution?
A) Peptic ulcer disease
B) Peripheral neuropathy
C) Cardiac conduction defects
D) Renal insufficiency
E) Prior deep venous thrombosis

Answer and Discussion

The answer is A. An extract of the dried leaves of the *Ginkgo biloba* tree is used in Europe to alleviate symptoms that are associated with a range of cognitive problems and has been approved in Germany for the treatment of dementia. Ginkgo is thought to have antioxidant properties, although its exact mechanism of action is unclear. Le Bars and colleagues conducted a randomized, double-blind, placebo-controlled trial to test the efficacy of ginkgo in the management of patients with Alzheimer's disease and multi-infarct dementia. Adverse events were not significantly different between the treatment and placebo groups and were considered to be mild to moderate in intensity. The authors conclude that treatment with extract of *Ginkgo biloba* is safe for up to 1 year in patients with dementia and can improve cognitive performance and functioning. The improvement was significant enough to be identified by the patient's caregiver. The most common adverse affect is headache. Caution should be exercised when using ginkgo combined with anticoagulant treatment including aspirin when there is risk of bleeding as in peptic ulcer disease and subdural hematoma. Safety in pregnancy and in lactation has not been determined.

Le Bars PL, Katz MM, Berman N, et al. A placebo-controlled, double-blind, randomized trial of an extract of ginkgo biloba for dementia. *JAMA.* 1997;278:1327–1332.

99. Yohimbine has been associated with which of the following?
A) Colon polyps
B) Priapism
C) Cataract formation
D) Skin pigmentation
E) Hypertensive complications

Answer and Discussion

The answer is E. Yohimbine is an indole alkaloid that is obtained from the bark of a West African tree *(Pausinystalia yohimba)*. The product is an α-adrenergic receptor antagonist that is marketed for the treatment of impotence. Results of studies have shown consistent ability of the drug to enhance erectile functioning. Yohimbine increases sympathetically mediated plasma norepinephrine, which in turn produces a pressor response. Therefore, yohimbine should be administered with caution to patients with high blood pressure or those who are undergoing concomitant treatment with tricyclic antidepressants or other drugs that interfere with neuronal uptake or metabolism of norepinephrine. The drug may induce panic attacks in patients with anxiety disorders.

Saddock BJ, Saddock VA. *Kaplan and Saddock's Comprehensive Textbook of Psychiatry*, 7th ed. Philadelphia: Lippincott Williams & Wilkins. 2000:2014.

100. *Cognitive therapy* is defined as:
A) repeated exposure to one's fears to overcome associated anxiety
B) a treatment that helps patients reverse false self-beliefs that lead to certain moods and behaviors
C) a confrontation with the patient that exposes certain inadequacies in social interaction
D) an exhaustive review of past events that outlines previous failures
E) an introspective review of past behaviors that highlights poor judgment

Answer and Discussion

The answer is B. Cognitive therapy is defined as a treatment process that helps patients reverse false self-beliefs that lead to certain moods and behaviors. The basic principle behind cognitive therapy is that a thought comes before a mood, and that both are associated with a person's environment, physical reaction, and subsequent behavior. As a result, changing a thought that arises in a given situation changes mood, behavior, and physical reaction. Motivated patients who have an internal locus of control and the capacity for introspection likely would benefit most. During cognitive therapy, the therapist assists the patient with several steps. First, the patient accepts that some of his or her perceptions and interpretations of reality may be false (because of past experience or hereditary or biological reasons) and that these interpretations lead to negative thoughts. Next, the patient learns to recognize the negative (surface or "automatic") thoughts and discovers alternative thoughts that reflect reality more closely. The patient then decides internally whether the evidence supports the negative thought or the alternative thought. Ideally, the patient will recognize distorted thinking and "reframe" the situation. As cognitive therapy progresses, it focuses more on reframing deeply held or "core" beliefs about self and the world. In cognitive behavior therapy (CBT) for depression, behavioral principles are used to overcome a patient's reluctance at the beginning of therapy and to reinforce positive activities. An important part of CBT for depression is having the patient participate in pleasurable activities, especially with others, that usually give positive reinforcement. Other CBT techniques include assigning projects and tasks and acting out difficult behavioral situations.

Rupke SJ, Blecke D, Renfrow M. Cognitive therapy for depression. *Am Fam Physician.* 2006;73:83–86, 93.

101. Which of the following medications is preferred in the treatment of alcohol withdrawal syndrome?
A) Haloperidol
B) Lorazepam
C) Phenytoin
D) Phenobarbitol
E) Carbamazepine

Answer and Discussion

The answer is B. Pharmacologic treatment of alcohol withdrawal syndrome involves the use of medications that are cross-tolerant with alcohol. Benzodiazepines have been shown to be safe and effective, particularly for preventing or treating seizures and delirium, and are the preferred agents for treating the symptoms of alcohol withdrawal syndrome.

Bayard M, McIntyre J, Hill KR, et al. Alcohol withdrawal syndrome. *Am Fam Physician.* 2004;69:1443–1450.

102. Which of the following medications is least likely to cause problems with libido?
A) Risperidone (Risperdal)
B) Cimetidine (Tagamet)
C) Bupropion (Wellbutrin)
D) Fluoxetine (Prozac)
E) Citalopram (Celexa)

Answer and Discussion

The answer is C. The loss of libido is a common problem that is addressed by family physicians. Many individuals have coexisting depression that is being treated. Patients whose depression improves with treatment but who continue to experience a lowered libido should be asked about their use of other medications. Several antipsychotic agents, including haloperidol, thioridazine, and risperidone, can decrease libido. Cimetidine, in contrast to ranitidine, has been found to lower libido and cause erectile dysfunction. Perimenopausal women who take oral contraceptives and postmenopausal women who are given estrogen replacement therapy may experience an improvement of depressive symptoms but a lowering of libido as a result of estrogen-induced deficiency of free testosterone. Testosterone testing and supplementation should be considered in women who experience a decline in libido after starting estrogen therapy. Testosterone testing should also be considered in men who have a gradual loss of libido and no improvement despite adequate treatment for depression. Psychologic and interpersonal factors commonly affect depression and sexual desire. These factors include stressful life events (loss of job or family trauma), life milestones (children leaving home), and ongoing relationship problems. Alcohol and narcotics are known to decrease libido, arousal, and orgasm. Consistent evidence shows that, with the exception of bupropion (Wellbutrin), mirtazipine (Remeron), and trazodone (Desyrel), antidepressant medications may cause a decline in libido or sexual functioning despite improvement of depression. Up to one-half of patients surveyed before and after starting therapy with the SSRIs fluoxetine, paroxetine, fluvoxamine, citalopram, and sertraline reported a decline in libido with medication use.

Phillips RL, Slaughter JR. Depression and sexual desire. *Am Fam Physician.* 2000;62:782–786.

103. Adenosylmethionine (SAMe) is thought to affect levels of the neurotransmitter
A) acetylcholine
B) gamma-aminobutyric acid (GABA)
C) serotonin
D) norepinephrine

Answer and Discussion

The answer is C. SAMe is an alternative medication that is used for the treatment of depression. The rationale for the use of SAMe in depression stems from its role in the metabolism of serotonin, dopamine, and melatonin. Oral and intravenous SAMe supplementation has been shown to increase SAMe levels significantly in cerebrospinal fluid, indicating SAMe's crossover through the blood-brain barrier. This has been associated with increased levels of serotonin metabolites in cerebrospinal fluid. Depressed patients may have low serotonin levels associated with low levels of SAMe. Because no studies have yet validated the long-term safety or efficacy of SAMe, further large long-term studies should be conducted before it receives widespread recommendation.

Morelli V, Zoorob RJ. Alternative therapies (Pt I). Depression, diabetes, obesity. *Am Fam Physician.* 2000;62:1051–1060.

104. Puerperal psychosis typically develops
A) during the first month after delivery
B) 3 to 4 months after delivery
C) 6 to 12 months after delivery
D) after the child has reached the age of 1 year

Answer and Discussion

The answer is A. When trying to determine if the presence of a symptom is a sign of depression or a normal postpartum reaction, the physician should consider the circumstances. Loss of energy and diminished concentration are frequently the result of sleep deprivation. However, for a postpartum woman to have no energy or to have such difficulty in concentrating that she frequently loses her train of thought or has considerable difficulty in making decisions is not normal. Determining how much time has elapsed since delivery helps the physician to distinguish PMD from subclinical mood fluctuations, which occur with such frequency during the first 2 weeks after delivery that they are considered part of the normal postpartum experience. Many women experience the "baby blues," which are characterized by mild depressive symptoms, tearfulness (often for no discernible reason), anxiety, irritability, mood lability, increased sensitivity, and fatigue. The blues peak 4 to 5 days after delivery, may last hours to days, and resolve by the tenth postnatal day. Women who experience them have an increased risk for PMD later in the postpartum period, especially if the blues symptoms were severe. Subclinical mood swings in either direction (high vs. low) after delivery are an indication for more intensive follow-up later in the postpartum period.

Finally, PMD must be distinguished from puerperal psychosis. Most puerperal psychoses have their onset within the first month of delivery and are related to mania. An inability to sleep for several nights, agitation, expansive or irritable mood, and avoidance of the infant are early warning signs that herald the onset of puerperal psychosis. Because the woman is at risk of harming herself or her baby (or both), postpartum psychosis is a medical emergency. Most patients with puerperal psychosis are treated in a hospital with neuroleptic agents and mood stabilizers. Before a definitive diagnosis of PMD is made, depression caused by a medical condition such as thyroid dysfunction or anemia must be ruled out.

Epperson CN. Postpartum major depression: detection and treatment. *Am Fam Physician.* 1999;59:2247–2254, 2259–2260.

Many women experience the "baby blues," characterized by mild depressive symptoms, tearfulness (often for no discernible reason), anxiety, irritability, mood lability, increased sensitivity, and fatigue.

105. Alcohol affects which of the following neurotransmitters?
A) Gamma-aminobutyric acid (GABA)
B) Dopamine
C) Norepinephrine
D) Acetylcholine
E) None of the above

Answer and Discussion

The answer is A. Alcohol enhances the effect of GABA on GABA-A neuroreceptors, resulting in decreased overall brain excitability. Chronic exposure to alcohol results in a compensatory decrease of GABA-A neuroreceptor response to GABA, evidenced by increasing tolerance of the effects of alcohol.

Bayard M, McIntyre J, Hill KR, et al. Alcohol withdrawal syndrome. *Am Fam Physician.* 2004;69:1443–1450.

106. A 56-year-old business executive with a history of alcoholism and associated liver disease presents to your office and would like to stop drinking. In order to prevent alcohol withdrawal, you select which of the following medications?
A) Lorazepam
B) Clonazepam
C) Diazepam
D) Flurazepam
E) Buspirone

Answer and Discussion

The answer is A. An evidence-based guideline from the American Society of Addiction Medicine recommends benzodiazepines as a first-line agent for the treatment of alcohol withdrawal. The guideline notes that although agents with a longer duration of action may provide fewer breakthrough symptoms, those with a shorter duration of action, such as lorazepam (Ativan), may be preferred when there is concern about prolonged sedation (e.g., in patients with significant comorbidities or liver disease).

Ntais C, Pakos E, Kyzas P. Benzodiazepines for alcohol withdrawal. *Cochrane Database Syst Rev.* 2005;(3):CD005063.

107. Which of the following statements regarding mass psychogenic illness is true?
A) Outbreaks are usually slow to develop.
B) Causes are usually readily identifiable.
C) Children and adolescents are rarely affected.
D) Incidents precede an environmental trigger.
E) Media coverage can escalate the outbreak.

Answer and Discussion

The answer is E. *Mass psychogenic illness* has been defined as a constellation of symptoms that are suggestive of organic illness with no identifiable cause and little clinical or laboratory evidence of disease that occurs among persons who share beliefs regarding their symptoms. Outbreaks often involve acute onset and rapid spread of symptoms with minimal physical or abnormal laboratory findings (except those that are associated with hyperventilation). Person-to-person spread within minutes has been called pathognomonic of this illness, although it is not always present. Symptoms include headache, dizziness, light-headedness, abdominal cramps, nausea, cough, irritated eyes, dyspnea, chest tightness or pain, inability to concentrate, vomiting, and nervousness. Symptoms may suggest an environmental cause, but no such cause can be identified, and other putatively exposed persons do not become ill. Rash has been described in several outbreaks of psychogenic illness. Outbreaks affect women disproportionately more often than men, and frequently involve adolescents or children. Incidents often follow an environmental trigger such as an odor, and many outbreaks are preceded by illness in an index case that generates a substantial emergency response. Illness can spread through exposure to audiovisual cues and by *"line-of-sight" transmission*. The latter term refers to the apparent spread of symptoms among persons who see others become ill. Symptoms can recur in the setting of the initial outbreak. Media coverage frequently escalates such outbreaks.

Jones TJ. Mass psychogenic illness: role of the individual physician. *Am Fam Physician.* 2000;62:2649–2653, 2655–2656.

108. Which of the following is not associated with anorexia nervosa in adolescent females?
A) Bradycardia
B) Low blood pressure
C) Low bone density
D) Low estradiol levels
E) Precocious puberty

Answer and Discussion

The answer is E. Adolescent girls with anorexia nervosa have an increased risk for hematologic, metabolic (low estradiol levels), hemodynamic, and skeletal abnormalities (low bone density), including bradycardia, low blood pressure, and pubertal delay, compared with healthy girls.

Misra M, Aggarwal A, Miller KK. Effects of anorexia nervosa on clinical, hematologic, biochemical, and bone density parameters in community-dwelling adolescent girls. *Pediatrics.* 2004;114:1574–1583.

109. When distinguishing delirium from preexisting psychiatric disorders, which of the following is characteristic of delirium?
A) Slow onset with a variable course
B) Slowing on EEG recordings
C) Auditory hallucinations

D) Memory impairment
E) Feelings of hopelessness

Answer and Discussion

The answer is B. Specific signs and symptoms can assist physicians in distinguishing between delirium and a preexisting psychiatric disorder. Visual hallucinations are an indicator of an underlying metabolic disturbance or adverse effect of medication or substance abuse. Although visual hallucinations can occur in patients with primary psychiatric illnesses such as schizophrenia, they are much less common than auditory hallucinations. In primary psychiatric disorders, visual hallucinations are associated with other, more characteristic signs and symptoms of the disorders. Visual hallucinations that occur in patients with delirium can be formed (e.g., people, animals) or unformed (e.g., spots, flashes of light). Electroencephalography (EEG) can be useful in differentiating delirium from other conditions. In patients with delirium, the EEG displays a diffuse slowing of the background rhythm. An exception is patients with delirium tremens, where the EEG shows fast activity. EEGs are also useful in detecting ictal and postictal seizure activity, as well as nonconvulsive status epilepticus, all of which can present as delirium. Abnormal EEG readings would not be expected in patients with psychotic disorders or depression. However, slowing may occur in patients with dementia. Additionally, the acute onset and fluctuating nature of delirium are hallmark features in distinguishing it from primary psychiatric disorders. Patients are often unable to provide an adequate history. It is important to interview family members and caregivers to determine the time of onset of symptoms and other pertinent medical and psychiatric information, including a review of medications and a history of substance abuse. It is also important to know how patients are currently different from their normal cognitive state. Psychiatric symptoms that arise in persons 50 years and older without a prior psychiatric history or the development of new symptoms in patients with preexisting psychiatric illness should undergo a thorough medical work-up.

Gleason OC. Delirium. *Am Fam Physician.* 2003;67:1027–1034.

> Although visual hallucinations can occur in patients with primary psychiatric illnesses such as schizophrenia, they are much less common than auditory hallucinations.

Chapter 5

Surgery

Questions

Each of the following questions or incomplete statements is followed by suggested answers or completions. Select the ONE BEST ANSWER in each case.

1. A 21 year old is brought to your clinic in status epilepticus. What drug should be administered initially?
A) Lorazepam
B) Phenytoin
C) Phenobarbital
D) Pentobarbital
E) Fosphenytoin

Answer and Discussion

The answer is A. Lorazepam should be administered intravenously and approximately 1 minute allowed to assess its effect. Diazepam or midazolam may be substituted if lorazepam is not available. If seizures continue at this point, additional doses of lorazepam should be infused and a second intravenous catheter placed in order to begin a concomitant phenytoin (or fosphenytoin) loading infusion. Even if seizures terminate after the initial lorazepam dose, therapy with phenytoin or fosphenytoin is generally indicated to prevent the recurrence of seizures.

MM Stecker. Status epilepticus in adults. Up to Date, version 14.1. Accessed 3/18/2006.

2. A 42-year-old carpenter presents with wrist pain and grip weakness. On exam he is found to have pain over the radial aspect of the wrist that is aggravated by flexing the thumb and applying ulner flexion. The most likely diagnosis is
A) carpal tunnel syndrome
B) scaphoid fracture
C) de Quervain's tenosynovitis
D) boxer's fracture
E) hamate fracture

Answer and Discussion

The answer is C. The combination of wrist pain and grip weakness is characteristic of de Quervain's tenosynovitis. The pain is generally located on the radial aspect of the wrist and reproduced with direct palpation of the involved tendons. Pain is aggravated by passively stretching the thumb tendons over the radial styloid in thumb flexion (the Finkelstein maneuver).

Sheon RP, Anderson BC. de Quervain's tenosynovitis. Up to Date, version 14.1. Accessed 3/18/2006.

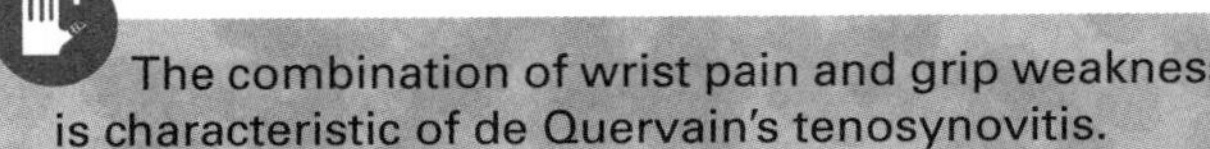
The combination of wrist pain and grip weakness is characteristic of de Quervain's tenosynovitis.

3. Which of the following statements is true regarding corneal injuries?
A) Patients should have the affected eye patched for 24 hours.
B) Topical antibiotics are recommended to prevent superinfection.
C) Foreign bodies should not be removed because of potential further injury to the cornea.
D) Topical anesthetics should be given to treat the discomfort.
E) None of the above.

Answer and Discussion

The answer is B. Controlled studies have not found patching to improve the rate of healing or comfort in patients with traumatic or foreign body abrasions. Patients should be treated with topical antibiotics to prevent superinfection. If a corneal foreign body is detected, an attempt can be made to remove it by irrigation. Topical anesthetics should never be administered or prescribed for pain relief because they delay corneal epithelial healing.

Jacobs DS. Corneal abrasions and corneal foreign bodies. Up to Date, version 14.1. Accessed 3/18/2006.

4. Which finger is most likely to be affected with disruption of the flexor digitorum profundus tendon (also known as a *jersey finger*)?
A) Thumb
B) Index finger
C) Third finger
D) Ring finger
E) Fifth finger ("pinky")

Answer and Discussion

The answer is D. Disruption of the flexor digitorum profundus tendon, also known as jersey finger, commonly occurs when an athlete's finger catches on another player's clothing, usually while playing a tackling sport such as football or rugby. The injury causes forced extension of the DIP joint during active flexion. The ring finger is the weakest finger and accounts for 75% of jersey finger cases.

Leggit JC, Meko CJ. Acute finger injuries: Part I. Tendons and ligaments. *Am Fam Physician.* 2006;73:810–816, 823.

5. Injury to the extensor tendon at the DIP joint is also known as
A) boutonnière deformity
B) jersey finger
C) mallet finger
D) swan necking
E) "jammed" finger

Answer and Discussion

The answer is C. Injury to the extensor tendon at the DIP joint is also known as mallet finger. The condition is the most common closed tendon injury of the finger. Mallet finger usually is caused by an object (e.g., a ball) striking the finger, creating a forced flexion of an extended DIP. The extensor tendon may be strained, partially torn, or completely ruptured or separated by a distal phalanx avulsion fracture. Those affected with mallet finger complain of pain at the dorsal DIP joint; inability to actively extend the joint; and, often, with a characteristic flexion deformity. It is critical to isolate the DIP joint during the evaluation to ensure extension is from the extensor tendon and not the central slip. The absence of full passive extension may indicate bony or soft tissue entrapment requiring surgical intervention.

Marx JA, Hockberger RS, Walls RM, et al., eds. *Rosen's emergency medicine: concepts and clinical practice,* 6th ed. Philadelphia: Elsevier/Mosby; 2006:604–608, 2002.

6. Which of the following would indicate the patient must be monitored in an intensive care unit setting following an overdose?
A) PaCO2 >45 mmHg
B) Seizures
C) QRS duration ≥ 0.12 seconds
D) Second- or third-degree atrioventricular block
E) All of the above

Answer and Discussion

The answer is E. The presence of any of eight clinical criteria predict a complicated hospital course that could be best managed in an ICU:

- PaCO2 >45 mmHg
- A need for emergency intubation
- The presence of postingestion seizures
- Unresponsiveness to verbal stimuli
- A non-sinus cardiac rhythm
- Second- or third-degree atrioventricular block
- Systolic blood pressure <80 mmHg
- QRS duration ≥ 0.12 seconds

Brett AS, Rothschild N, Gray R, et al. Predicting the clinical course in intentional drug overdose: Implications for use of the intensive care unit. *Arch Intern Med.* 1987;147:133.

7. Where are most Morton's neuromas found?
A) In the tarsal tunnel
B) At the first metatarsal phalangeal joint
C) The second and third interdigital space
D) At the attachment of the plantar fascia
E) At the head of the fifth metatarsal

Answer and Discussion

The answer is C. The interdigital spaces of the foot are common sites for painful neuromas, a condition termed *Morton's neuroma.* The second and third common digital branches of the medial plantar nerve are the most frequent sites for development of interdigital neuromas. Morton's neuromas develop as a result of chronic trauma and repetitive stress, as occurs in persons wearing tight-fitting or high-heeled shoes. Pain and paresthesias are usually mild at onset and are located in the interdigital space of the affected nerve. In some cases, the interdigital space between the affected toes may be widened as a result of an associated ganglion or synovial cyst. Pain is noted in the affected interdigital space when the metatarsal heads of the foot are squeezed together. Injection with 1% lidocaine (Xylocaine) can assist in confirming the diagnosis.

Wu KK. Morton's interdigital neuroma: a clinical review of its etiology, treatment, and results. *J Foot Ankle Surg.* 1996;35: 112–119.

8. Which of the following tests is the most sensitive and specific for the detection of renal stones?
A) KUB plain film
B) Ultrasound
C) Intravenous pyelography
D) Noncontrast helical CT

Answer and Discussion

The answer is D. Compared with abdominal ultrasonography and KUB radiography, intravenous pyelography has greater sensitivity (64% to 87%) and specificity (92% to 94%) for the detection of renal calculi. Noncontrast helical CT is being used increasingly in the initial assessment of renal colic. This imaging modality is fast and accurate, and it readily identifies all stone types in all locations. Its sensitivity (95% to 100%) and specificity (94% to 96%) suggest that it may definitively exclude stones in patients with abdominal pain.

Chen MY, Zagoria RJ. Can noncontrast helical computed tomography replace intravenous urography for evaluation of patients with acute urinary tract colic? *J Emerg Med.* 1999;17:299–303.

Vieweg J, Teh C, Freed K, et al. Unenhanced helical computerized tomography for the evaluation of patients with acute flank pain. *J Urol.* 1998;160:679–684.

9. Which of the following statements regarding cholecystectomy is *false*?
A) Between 5% and 26% of patients undergoing elective laparoscopic cholecystectomy require conversion to an open procedure.
B) A common reason for conversion to an open procedure is failure to identify the anatomy.
C) Laparoscopic cholecystectomy is safer than an open procedure.
D) Laparoscopic cholecystectomy has a lower rate of common bile duct injury.
E) Common bile duct injuries are extremely difficult to repair.

Answer and Discussion

The answer is D. Between 5% and 26% of patients undergoing elective laparoscopic cholecystectomy require conversion to an open procedure. A common reason for conversion is the inability to clearly identify the biliary anatomy. In a recent meta-analysis, researchers compared the outcomes of laparoscopic cholecystectomy for more than 78,000 patients in 98 studies with the outcomes of open cholecystectomy for more than 12,000 patients in 28 studies. The researchers found a decreased mortality rate in patients undergoing laparoscopic cholecystectomy compared with those undergoing open cholecystectomy (8.6 to 16 deaths/10,000 patients versus 66 to 74 deaths/10,000 patients, respectively), but also noted a higher rate of common bile duct injury (36 to 47 injuries/10,000 patients versus 19 to 29 injuries/10,000 patients, respectively). Common bile duct injuries associated with cholecystectomy can be extremely difficult to repair, and management at a tertiary care center with surgeons experienced in biliary injuries should be strongly considered.

Shea JA, Healey MJ, Berlin JA, et al. Mortality and complications associated with laparoscopic cholecystectomy. A meta-analysis. *Ann Surg.* 1996;224:609–620.

10. Which of the following medications is associated with a reduction of cardiac-related mortality in perioperative patients with known or suspected coronary heart disease?
A) Lisinopril
B) Metoprolol
C) Aspirin
D) Simvastatin
E) Warfarin

Answer and Discussion

The answer is B. Use of perioperative beta blockers reduces cardiac-related mortality in patients with known or suspected coronary heart disease.

Mangano DT, Layug EL, Wallace A, et al. Effect of atenolol on mortality and cardiovascular morbidity after noncardiac surgery. Multicenter Study of Perioperative Ischemia Research Group. *N Engl J Med.* 1996;335:1713–1720.

Poldermans D, Boersma E, Bax JJ, et al. The effect of bisoprolol on perioperative mortality and myocardial infarction in high-risk patients undergoing vascular surgery. Dutch Echocardiographic Cardiac Risk Evaluation Applying Stress Echocardiography Study Group. *N Engl J Med.* 1999;341:1789–1794.

11. When vancomycin is used as a preoperative prophylactic antibiotic, it should be administered within ______ minutes of the start of surgery.
A) 15
B) 30
C) 60
D) 120
E) At the time of incision

Answer and Discussion

The answer is D. Ideally, a preoperative dose of antibiotic should provide a sufficient antibiotic serum level throughout the surgery to combat organisms most likely to cause a site infection. It is recommended that the first dose be timed to occur within 60 minutes before the surgical incision is made. If a fluoroquinolone or vancomycin is chosen for prophylaxis, the first dose should be administered within 120 minutes of the start of surgery. If the surgery involves the use of a tourniquet (e.g., hip or knee arthroplasty), the antibiotic infusion should be completed before inflation of the tourniquet. For most surgeries, it is recommended that use of prophylactic antibiotics end within 24 hours after surgery.

Bratzler DW, Houck PM. Antimicrobial prophylaxis for surgery: an advisory statement from the National Surgical Infection Prevention Project. *Clin Infect Dis.* 2004;38:1706–1715.

Ideally, a preoperative dose of antibiotic should provide a sufficient antibiotic serum level throughout the surgery to combat organisms most likely to cause a site infection.

12. Which of the following is *not* an absolute contraindication for breast conservative therapy?
A) Estrogen/progesterone receptor positive tumor
B) Two tumors are located in different quadrants
C) Diffuse micocalcifications that appear malignant
D) Prior breast radiation
E) Positive surgical margins

Answer and Discussion

The answer is A. When there are two or more primary tumors located in different quadrants of the breast or there are associated diffuse microcalcifications that appear malignant, breast-conserving therapy is not considered appropriate. Additionally, a woman with previous breast irradiation is also not a candidate for breast conservation treatment. Breast irradiation cannot be given during pregnancy, but it may be possible to perform breast-conserving surgery in the third trimester and administer irradiation after delivery. Positive surgical margins are also an absolute contraindication.

Winchester DP, Cox JD. Standards for breast-conservation treatment. *CA Cancer J Clin.* 1992;42:134–162.

Apantaku LM. Breast-conserving surgery for breast cancer. *Am Fam Physician.* 2002;66:2271–2278, 2281.

13. Which of the following antibiotics given alone is adequate for prophylaxis when performing an appendectomy?
A) Cephalexin
B) Ceftriaxone
C) Cefotaxime
D) Metronidazole
E) Ampicillin

Answer and Discussion

The answer is B. Ceftriaxone and cefotaxime provide effective prophylaxis for abdominal surgeries, but cefotaxime does not provide adequate coverage for appendectomy without the addition of metronidazole. Overall, ceftriaxone is more effective, particularly against *Staphylococcus aureus*, and has a longer half-life and no active metabolites. Despite being more expensive, this agent is a more versatile choice for antibiotic prophylaxis in abdominal surgery.

Woodfield JC, Van Rij AM, Pettigrew RA. A comparison of the prophylactic efficacy of ceftriaxone and cefotaxime in abdominal surgery. *Am J Surg.* 2002;185:45–459.

14. Which of the following may have an antiplatelet activity and should be stopped before surgery?
A) Ephedra
B) Ginseng

C) Valerian
D) St. John's wort
E) Kava

Answer and Discussion

The answer is B. Ginseng is touted to protect the body against stress. Pharmacologically, ginseng lowers blood glucose levels (even in patients without diabetes mellitus) and, therefore, may cause intraoperative complications, especially in patients who fasted before surgery. Ginseng may also have a platelet inhibitory effect, and this effect may be irreversible. It should be discontinued at least 7 days before surgery.

Ang-Lee MK, Moss T, Yuan CS. Herbal medicines and perioperative care. *JAMA*. 2001;286:208–216.

15. After hip surgery, DVT prophylaxis should be maintained for at least
A) 24 hours
B) 3 days
C) 1 week
D) 1 month
E) indefinitely

Answer and Discussion

The answer is C. In patients not receiving DVT prophylaxis who are having elective hip or knee replacement or hip fracture surgery, the risk of postoperative DVT is at least 40%, and the risk of pulmonary embolus can be as high as 30%. Low-molecular-weight heparin is considered safe and effective following surgery for hip replacement. It has been shown in a recent study to be superior to low-dose subcutaneous heparin, and its use resulted in significantly fewer hemorrhagic complications. Studies comparing low-molecular-weight heparin with low-dose warfarin (Coumadin) therapy [maintaining an International Normalized Ratio (INR) between 2.0 and 3.0] showed that low-molecular-weight heparin is slightly more effective, although the difference is small. As a result the decision to use low-molecular-weight heparin or warfarin should be based on convenience and cost. Low-molecular-weight heparin is given subcutaneously twice daily, and laboratory monitoring is not required. Treatment with either warfarin or low-molecular-weight heparin should be continued for a minimum of 7 days postoperatively.

Imperiale TF, Speroff T. A meta-analysis of methods to prevent venous thromboembolism following total hip replacement. *JAMA*. 1994;271:1780–1785.

16. A general surgeon contacts you regarding preoperative clearance for an otherwise healthy 42 year old scheduled for an appendectomy. The patient has no history of excessive bleeding, no family history of bleeding disorders, and is on no medications. He inquires about the need for coagulation studies, which have not been performed. A correct response is
A) a PT/PTT must be performed before surgery
B) a bleeding time is sufficient for assessing the risk of bleeding
C) a prior normal PT/PTT test performed within the last year is sufficient to clear this patient for surgery
D) no further testing is necessary to clear this patient for surgery
E) none of the above

Answer and Discussion

The answer is D. Coagulation times are not routinely indicated in patients undergoing surgery. Studies have shown that the yield is very low and that abnormal results are expected or do not significantly affect management. Coagulation studies would be indicated if the patient is receiving anticoagulant therapy, has a family or personal history that suggests a bleeding disorder, or has evidence of liver disease.

King MS. Preoperative evaluation. *Am Fam Physician*. 2000;62:387–396.

17. A 56-year-old female is found to have biliary colic. You explain to her that the risk of developing acute cholecystitis is
A) 10%
B) 25%
C) 50%
D) 75%
E) 90%

Answer and Discussion

The answer is A. Acute cholecystitis develops in up to 10% of patients with symptomatic gallstones and is caused by the complete obstruction of the cystic duct.

Friedman GD. Natural history of asymptomatic and symptomatic gallstones. *Am J Surg*. 1993;165:399–404.

Bellows CF, Berger DH, Crass RA. Management of gallstones. *Am Fam Physician*. 2005;72:637–642.

18. You receive a call from the newborn nursery and are told that there is a breast-fed newborn who is vomiting bile-stained emesis. The most appropriate management is
A) decrease feeding frequency
B) switch to formula feedings
C) administration of rectal promethazine (Phenergan)
D) barium enema
E) nasogastric feedings

Answer and Discussion

The answer is D. *Intestinal malrotation* is a condition that results during development of the fetus. As the bowel develops outside the abdomen, it returns to the body cavity with a counterclockwise rotation. When malrotation occurs, the bowel returns in a clockwise rotation, and intestinal obstruction can result. Presenting symptoms include vomiting of bile-stained material, abdominal distention, and dehydration soon after birth. Diagnosis is usually accomplished by a barium enema revealing an abnormal cecal position. An upper gastrointestinal barium series of a patient with volvulus typically shows twisting of the bowel (i.e., the site of obstruction) at the level of Treitz's ligament. Treatment is usually surgical.

Beers MH, Berkow R, eds. *The Merck manual of diagnosis and therapy*, Merck Research Laboratories, 17th ed. Whitehouse Station, NJ: Merck & Co.; 1999:2215.

19. Which of the following statements about lumbar disc disease is true?
A) It usually involves the L5–S1 interspace.
B) It typically involves anterior herniation of the nucleus pulposus.
C) It usually requires surgical intervention.
D) Treatment involves strict bed rest for 1 to 2 weeks.
E) Forward flexion of the trunk often helps relieve symptoms.

Answer and Discussion

The answer is A. Lumbar disc disease usually results from posterior herniation of the nucleus pulposus that impinges on the spinal cord. The most common site is the L5–S1 interspace, which affects the first sacral nerve root. Patients typically recall a precipitating event such as lifting a heavy object. Symptoms include severe back pain that radiates to the legs and is aggravated by coughing, sneezing, or forward flexion of the trunk. The condition is the most common cause of sciatica. Examination may show decreased sensation in a dermatome pattern, weakness, decreased reflexes, and a positive straight leg–raising test. In severe cases, patients may experience bowel or bladder incontinence. Radiographs and laboratory tests are generally unnecessary, except in the few patients in whom a serious cause is suspected based on a comprehensive history and physical examination. Surgical evaluation is indicated in patients with worsening neurologic deficits or intractable pain that is resistant to conservative treatment. The current recommendation is 2 or 3 days of bed rest for patients with acute radiculopathy. The treatment plan should be reassessed in patients who do not return to normal activity within 4 to 6 weeks. Most mild cases can be treated with the limitation of aggravating activity, anti-inflammatory agents, and muscle relaxants.

Patel AT, Ogle AA. Diagnosis and management of acute low back pain. *Am Fam Physician.* 2000;61:1779–1786,1789–1790.

20. Which of the following is *not* an indication for referral for Mohs' micrographic surgery?
A) Lesion in close proximity to nose
B) Lesion size >2 cm
C) Lesion with indistinct margin
D) Recurrent lesions
E) Lesion is identified as an actinic keratosis

Answer and Discussion

The answer is E. Patients with nonmelanoma skin cancer measuring >2 cm, lesions with indistinct margins, recurrent lesions, and those close to important structures, including the eyes, nose, and mouth, should be considered for referral for complete excision via Mohs' micrographic surgery. The Mohs' surgeon can confirm the complete removal of the lesion by immediately reviewing the pathology during a staged excision, which, in these high-risk settings, can require removal of much more tissue than might have been clinically apparent initially. If a complicated repair is anticipated or a poor cosmetic result is expected, referral is appropriate.

Stulberg DC, Crandell B, Fawcett RS. Diagnosis and treatment of basal cell and squamous cell carcinomas. *Am Fam Physician.* 2004;70:1481–1488.

Patients with non-melanoma skin cancer measuring >2 cm; lesions with indistinct margins, recurrent lesions; and those close to important structures, including the eyes, nose, and mouth, should be considered for referral for complete excision via Mohs' micrographic surgery.

21. A newborn who develops aspiration pneumonia should be evaluated for
A) tracheoesophageal fistula
B) hypothyroidism
C) cystic fibrosis
D) human immunodeficiency virus
E) tetralogy of Fallot

Answer and Discussion

The answer is A. Tracheoesophageal fistula is a congenital defect seen in newborns. The incidence is 1 in 1,500 to 3,000 live births. Boys and girls are equally affected. The condition is commonly associated with esophageal atresia. Cases have been associated with Down syndrome and trisomy 18. Symptoms include excessive secretions with coughing and aspiration after feedings. Complications include the development of cyanosis and aspiration pneumonia. Diagnosis can be established by the inability to pass a red-rubber catheter or nasogastric tube into the stomach. Frontal and lateral radiographs confirm the level of obstruction. If gas is noted below the diaphragm, then an associated fistula is present. If not, the patient most likely is affected with esophageal atresia alone. Care must be taken to avoid aspiration of dye during diagnostic tests. Treatment involves withholding oral feedings and providing surgical correction. Prognosis is generally good; however, some patients may develop incompetence of the lower esophageal sphincter with chronic reflux symptoms.

Townsend CM, ed. *Sabiston textbook of surgery*, 16th ed. Philadelphia: WB Saunders; 2001:1467.

22. Extracorporeal shock wave therapy for renal stones
A) requires stones to be present in the renal pelvis
B) rarely requires repeated treatment regardless of stone size
C) is more effective for stones <2 cm in diameter
D) requires less energy for calcium oxalate and cystine stones
E) rarely achieves optimal results

Answer and Discussion

The answer is C. Lithotripsy has been used to fragment and remove kidney stones. The procedure involves placing the patient on a lithotripsy gantry so the calculus overlies a circular window in the table containing the water bath and is focused on the calculus. The procedure is more effective for stones <2 cm in diameter. Calcium oxalate and cystine stones are usually dense and require increased energy. Large stones may require repeated treatments. Previously, extracorporeal shock wave therapy was reserved primarily for renal calculi, but now it may be used for calculi within the kidney, ureter, or bladder with a 90% chance of rendering the patient stone free within 3 months.

Taylor R, David AK, Johnson TA Jr, et al., eds. *Family medicine: principles and practice*, 5th ed. New York: Springer-Verlag; 1998:878.

23. Topical lidocaine is used with ______________ to treat chronic anal fissures
A) nifedipine
B) cocaine
C) nitroglycerin
D) nystatin
E) mupirocin

Answer and Discussion

The answer is A. Topical nifedipine in addition to lidocaine gel is effective and well tolerated in the treatment of chronic anal fissures.

Perrotti P, Bove A, Antropoli C. Topical nifedipine with lidocaine ointment vs. active control for treatment of chronic anal fissure: results of a prospective, randomized, double-blind study. *Dis Colon Rectum.* 2002;45:1468–1475.

24. A 24-year-old woman presents to your office. She is quite concerned that she is bleeding internally, because her stools have been dark, tarry black. Further questioning reveals that she has been having episodes of diarrhea, which have resolved with the use of Pepto-Bismol. She denies abdominal pain, light-headedness, nausea, vomiting, or fevers. The most likely cause of her dark stools is
A) upper gastrointestinal bleeding source
B) lower gastrointestinal bleeding source
C) rectal outlet bleeding
D) bismuth ingestion
E) None of the above

Answer and Discussion

The answer is D. Melena is the passage of black tarry stools, which is secondary to gastrointestinal bleeding. In most cases, the source is located in the upper gastrointestinal tract; however, a source in the distal right colon or small intestine can also cause melena. Approximately 100 to 200 mL of blood loss is needed to cause melena. Other causes for black stools that are often confused with melena include iron, bismuth, licorice, and a variety of other food ingestions.

Beers MH, Berkow R, eds. *The Merck manual of diagnosis and therapy*, Merck Research Laboratories, 17th ed. Whitehouse Station, NJ: Merck & Co.; 1999:241.

25. Which of the following local anesthetics has the longest duration of action?
A) Procaine (Novocaine)
B) Bupivacaine (Marcaine)
C) Mepivacaine (Carbocaine)
D) Lidocaine (Xylocaine)
E) All are about the same

Answer and Discussion

The answer is B. The following local anesthetics have the following durations of action:

- Procaine (Novocaine): <30 minutes
- Bupivacaine (Marcaine): 180 to 360 minutes, the longest-acting anesthetic; good for nerve blocks
- Mepivacaine (Carbocaine): 45 to 75 minutes
- Lidocaine (Xylocaine): 60 to 180 minutes

The use of epinephrine should be avoided in areas such as the fingers, nose, penis, and toes or other distal appendages. The vasoconstrictive effect can lead to ischemic necrosis. The most common reason for inadequate anesthesia is not allowing enough time for the anesthetic to take effect. In most cases, the surgeon should wait at least 5 minutes after injection before starting a procedure.

Townsend CM, ed. *Sabiston textbook of surgery*, 16th ed. Philadelphia: WB Saunders; 2001:286.

26. Blunt objects in the esophagus (with the exception of button batteries) may be observed for ___________ before performing endoscopy for removal.
A) 4 hours
B) 24 hours
C) 3 days
D) 1 week
E) 10 days

Answer and Discussion

The answer is B. Most blunt objects (with the exception of button batteries) in the esophagus may be observed for up to 24 hours. If the object fails to pass into the stomach, it should be removed or possibly pushed into the stomach. Objects that have been lodged in the esophagus for >24 hours or for an unknown duration should be removed endoscopically. If the object has been lodged in the esophagus for >2 weeks, there is significant risk of erosion into surrounding structures, and surgical consultation should be obtained before attempting removal. Early intervention is indicated for patients who have swallowed button or disc batteries because of the potential for voltage burns and direct corrosive effects. Burns can occur as early as 4 hours after ingestion.

Eisen GM, Baron TH, Dominitz JA, et al. Guideline for the management of ingested foreign bodies. *Gastrointest Endosc.* 2002;55:802–806.

27. Which of the following statements regarding preoperative evaluations is correct?
A) A patient with a previous coronary bypass graph 2 years earlier should undergo cardiac stress testing before clearance, regardless of the presence of cardiac symptoms
B) Urine pregnancy testing should be considered for women of childbearing age
C) Coagulation studies should be included in your laboratory assessment of all surgical candidates
D) Patients who have had angioplasty within 6 months are not required to have further cardiology assessment
E) A baseline renal function study should be assessed for all surgical candidates

Answer and Discussion

The answer is B. Before elective surgery, a preoperative examination should be performed to review a patient's history. Preoperative laboratory studies once routinely included a complete blood count, extensive blood chemistry profile, urinalysis, prothrombin time, partial thromboplastin time, electrocardiogram (ECG), and chest radiographs. Current recommendations allow for fewer routine tests and for selective ordering of laboratory tests based on the specific indications in a given patient. In addition, the availability of previous laboratory testing can obviate the need for additional preoperative tests. A hemoglobin measurement is useful in detecting unsuspected anemia and providing a baseline level, which can be helpful information postoperatively, particularly for surgeries with potential bleeding complications. Renal and liver function studies are not routinely needed but may be indicated for patients who have a medical condition or medication use that would serve as indications for these tests. Preoperative glucose determination should be obtained in patients 45 years or older, as there are currently recommendations to screen everyone older than 45 years for diabetes mellitus and the presence of diabetes increases perioperative risks. A urine pregnancy test should be considered for women of childbearing age. Coagulation times are not routinely indicated, as studies have shown that the yield is very low and that abnormal results are expected or do not significantly affect management. Coagulation studies would be indicated if the patient is receiving anticoagulant therapy, has a family or personal history that suggests a bleeding disorder, or has evidence of liver disease. An ECG is also not routinely indicated in patients 40 years or younger, but it should be obtained in patients older than 40 years or in patients with cardiac indications based on the medical history. Chest radiographs should be obtained on the basis of findings from the medical history or physical examination. Assessing risk for cardiac patients is important. In general, patients in whom cardiac stress testing was normal within the previous 2 years or who have had coronary bypass surgery within the previous 5 years and are without symptoms require no further assessment. Clinically stable patients who have undergone angioplasty between 6 months and 5 years previously require no further assessment. However, patients who have had angioplasty within the previous 6 months may require cardiac reevaluation and/or consultation with a cardiologist before surgery. Patients at high risk for complications usually warrant cardiology consultation and possibly angiography. Cardiac stress testing should be performed in patients at intermediate risk and with poor functional capacity or who are undergoing high-risk procedures such as vascular surgery. For patients with minor clinical predictors, only patients who have poor functional capacity and are undergoing a high-risk procedure require stress testing. Patients with positive stress test results warrant cardiology consultation before proceeding with surgery. Assessment of left ventricular function is not routinely indicated for preoperative evaluation whether or not the patient has cardiac disease. The preoperative assessment guideline from the American College of Physicians notes that radionuclide or echocardiographic assessment of left ventricular function does not appear to improve the risk prediction provided by the clinical examination alone. In summary, recommendations do not call for preoperative cardiac testing in all patients. The need for further cardiac evaluation before surgery is determined by the clinical risk predictors identified from the patient's history, physical examination, ECG, and functional status, along with the risk associated with the operation itself. Pulmonary function testing may be helpful in diagnosing and assessing disease severity. Baseline chest radiographs may be helpful in at-risk patients. Preoperative guidelines do not define the degree of pulmonary function impairment that would prohibit surgery other than that for lung resection. With lung resection surgery, patients with a forced expiratory volume in 1 second of <2L require preoperative ventilation/perfusion studies to determine the predicted postoperative forced expiratory volume in 1 second. An estimated postoperative forced expiratory volume in 1 second of 800 mL or more is required before lung resection is performed. Patients who smoke cigarettes should be advised to quit smoking for 8 weeks before surgery. Asthma should be under control before surgery, if possible. Steroid therapy for asthma can be continued throughout the perioperative period without excess surgical morbidity. Patients with asthma or chronic obstructive pulmonary disease can be given pre- and postoperative bronchodilators to increase pulmonary function.

> King MS. Preoperative evaluation. *Am Fam Physician.* 2000;62:387–396.

28. A 65-year-old retired secretary presents with a painful bump that is associated with the medial first metatarsal joint. She reports that the bump has developed over the past 10 to 20 years. The most likely diagnosis is

A) hallux valgus
B) Morton's neuroma
C) chronic gout
D) metatarsalgia
E) bunionette

Answer and Discussion

The answer is A. Hallux valgus (bunions) is more common in women than in men. Symptoms include a painless or painful bump (exostosis) that forms on the medial aspect of the first metatarsal joint. Contributing physical factors include hyperelasticity syndromes, metatarsus varus, short first metatarsal joint, and pes valgus. Other factors include a family history of bunions and the prolonged use of narrow high-heeled shoes. Conservative treatment is usually all that is needed and includes wide shoes, the use of bunion pads, ice, rest, and anti-inflammatory agents for acute pain. Most cases referred for surgery have intermetatarsal angles greater than 10 degrees or fail to improve with conservative measures. Absolute contraindications for surgery include peripheral vascular disease and local tissue infections, whereas relative contraindications include narcissistic personality disorders, painless cosmetic bunions, and age 65 years or older. A bunionette is a bony prominence on the lateral aspect of the fifth metatarsal head.

> Taylor R, David AK, Johnson TA Jr, et al., eds. *Family medicine: principles and practice*, 5th ed. New York: Springer-Verlag; 1998:985.

29. When injecting a local anesthetic with epinephrine, which of the following locations should be avoided?

A) Lip
B) Distal finger
C) Forehead
D) Back
E) Scalp

Answer and Discussion

The answer is B. Epinephrine administration should be avoided near the terminal arterial branches in the digits, tip of the nose, ear lobes, or tip of the penis.

> Avina R. Primary care local and regional anesthesia in the management of trauma. *Clin Fam Pract.* 2000;2:533–550.

30. Which of the following is the standard treatment for subacute bacterial endocarditis (SBE) prophylaxis for minor procedures in low-risk adult patients?

A) Amoxicillin: 1 g given intravenously at the time of the procedure
B) Amoxicillin: 2 g given orally 1 hour before the procedure
C) Ampicillin: 2 g given intravenously plus gentamicin (1.5 mg/kg intravenously) 30 minutes before the procedure; dose repeated 8 hours after the procedure
D) Ampicillin: 500 mg given orally 1 hour before the procedure and 250 mg given 6 hours after the procedure
E) Amoxicillin 3 g orally 1 hour before the procedure and 1.5 g given 6 hours after

Answer and Discussion

The answer is B. Standard regimens for SBE prophylaxis involve the following:

- Minor or repetitive procedures in low-risk patients (dental procedures, oral, respiratory tract procedures, or esophageal procedures): amoxicillin, 2 g orally given 1 hour before procedure; the follow-up dose is no longer recommended; those unable to take oral medication are given ampicillin, 2 g intravenously or intramuscularly
- Gastrointestinal and genitourinary surgery and instrumentation or those at high risk for other procedures (prosthetic heart valves), excluding esophageal procedures: ampicillin, 2 g intravenously or intramuscularly plus gentamicin (1.5 mg/kg

intravenously or intramuscularly—not to exceed 120 mg) 30 minutes before procedure and ampicillin (1 g) intramuscularly or intravenously or amoxicillin (1 g) orally 6 hours later

If the patient is allergic to penicillin, then cephalexin, cefadroxil, azithromycin, clarithromycin, or clindamycin may be given orally (for low risk), and vancomycin may be substituted for ampicillin intravenously (for high risk).

Gilbert DN, Moellering RC, Sande MA. *The Sanford guide to antimicrobial therapy, 2000*. Hyde Park, VT: Antimicrobial Therapy, Inc. 2000:118–119.

When administering subacute bacterial endocarditis (SBE) prophylaxis, if the patient is allergic to penicillin, then cephalexin, cefadroxil, azithromycin, clarithromycin, or clindamycin may be given orally (for low-risk procedures), and vancomycin may be substituted for ampicillin intravenously (for high-risk procedures).

31. Diverticulosis is a condition associated with
A) increased risk of colon cancer
B) herniations of the bowel mucosa and submucosa through the muscular layers of the bowel wall
C) inflammatory bowel disease
D) a 90% risk of developing diverticulitis
E) predominantly the proximal colon

Answer and Discussion

The answer is B. Diverticulosis, an outpouching of the bowel wall, increases in frequency after 40 years of age. Acquired diverticular disease affects approximately 5% to 10% of the Western population older than 45 years and approximately 80% of persons older than 85 years. It is more common in the sigmoid and distal colon. Colonic diverticula are related primarily to two factors: increased intraluminal pressure and a weakening of the bowel wall. Patients with known diverticula have been found to have elevated resting colonic pressures. The Western diet, which tends to be low in dietary fiber and high in refined carbohydrates, is also believed to be a contributing factor. The condition occurs when there is herniation of bowel mucosa and submucosa through muscular layers of the colon. Inflammation of the small herniations, referred to as *diverticulitis,* occurs in approximately 10% to 20% of patients with diverticulosis and more commonly in men. Most patients with diverticulosis remain asymptomatic. Symptoms of diverticulitis include lower abdominal pain usually located on the left that may be steady or cramping and is sometimes relieved with a bowel movement, anorexia, nausea, vomiting, and constipation. Physical examination usually shows abdominal tenderness and guarding and, occasionally, a palpable abdominal or rectal mass with abscess formation. Occult blood is present in approximately 20% of patients. Fever and an increased white blood cell count may also be present. Previously, diverticular disease was diagnosed using a contrast barium enema. However, because of the possibility of an obstructing fecalith being dislodged by insufflation and causing bowel perforation, CT scanning is now the diagnostic procedure of choice. Treatment of diverticulitis can take place on an outpatient basis for a patient with a mild first attack who is able to tolerate oral hydration and an antibiotic. Treatment consists of a liquid diet and 7 to 10 days of therapy with broad-spectrum antimicrobials such as metronidazole and ciprofloxacin. Patients with severe illness, or those who cannot tolerate oral hydration or who have pain severe enough to require narcotic analgesia, should be hospitalized. Because feeding increases intracolonic pressure, patients should receive nothing by mouth and should be treated with intravenous triple therapy consisting of ampicillin, gentamicin, and metronidazole. Alternative monotherapy includes piperacillin or tazobactam. If narcotics are required for pain control, meperidine is recommended because morphine sulfate causes colonic spasm. If the pain, fever, and leukocytosis do not resolve within 3 days, further imaging studies are indicated. If an abscess is uncovered and is >5 cm in size, CT-guided drainage and adequate antibiotic coverage should be considered. Approximately 20% of patients with diverticulitis require surgery. Bowel resection is usually recommended for recurrent episodes of diverticulitis or if fistulas are present.

Ferzoco LB, Raptopoulos V, Silen W. Acute diverticulitis. *N Engl J Med.* 1998;338:1521–1526.

32. Of the following, which local anesthetic has the fastest onset of action?
A) Lidocaine
B) Mepivicaine
C) Bupivicaine
D) Procaine
E) Tetracaine

Answer and Discussion

The answer is A. Lidocaine has the fastest onset of action.

Salam GA. Regional anesthesia for office procedures: Part I. Head and neck surgeries. *Am Fam Physician.* 2004;69:585–590.

33. Which of the following sutures is *not* absorbable?
A) Catgut
B) Vicryl
C) Polypropylene
D) Dexon
E) Chromic catgut

Answer and Discussion

The answer is C. The goal of suturing is to approximate the skin and eliminate unnecessary dead space. Tension at the wound site should be minimized. To achieve maximal cosmetic result, a suture is chosen based on the clinical situation. Monofilament sutures have significantly lowered the incidence of infection compared with multifilament sutures that can harbor bacteria. Nonabsorbable sutures (i.e., nylon, silk, polypropylene, braided polyester, and polybutester) are usually used to close the superficial layer of skin; absorbable sutures (i.e., catgut, chromic catgut, Dexon, Maxon, and Vicryl) are used to close deep layers of skin. Silk is often used on oral lacerations because of its tolerability in the mouth.

Graber MA, Toth PP, Herting RL Jr. *University of Iowa: The Family Practice Handbook*, 3rd ed. St. Louis: Mosby; 1997:385.

34. Which of the following statements regarding cervical cancer screening is true?
A) The death rate from cervical cancer continues to increase despite Pap smear screening.
B) Immunosuppression has not been identified as a risk factor for cervical cancer.
C) Human papillomavirus (HPV) types 1 and 3 are most closely linked to cervical cancer.

D) Smoking has been linked to the development of cervical cancer.
E) Most cases of cervical cancer occur between the ages of 20 and 30 years.

Answer and Discussion

The answer is D. Cervical cancer before 20 years of age is rare. Most cases occur between the ages of 45 and 55 years. Since the mid-1970s, the death rate has decreased significantly as the result of Pap smear screening. Women who are at risk for developing cellular abnormalities include those who smoke and those with a history of sexually transmitted diseases, HPV infection, low socioeconomic status, two or more lifetime sexual partners, or immunosuppression. The latter factors cause frequent exposure to potential carcinogens, and their requisite presence supports the hypothesis that cervical cancer is a sexually transmitted disease. Smoking also contributes to the development of cervical cancer. Although nicotine is not considered a causative agent, smoking may predispose a woman to the development of cervical cancer by lowering her immune surveillance at the cellular level. Smokers also may engage in behaviors that increase their susceptibility to malignant change. A preponderance of evidence suggests a causal link between HPV infection and cervical neoplasia. This link is strongest for certain HPV types, particularly types 16 and 18. The American College of Obstetricians and Gynecologists, the American Academy of Family Physicians, and the U.S. Preventive Services Task Force recommend that all women receive screening Pap smears at the onset of sexual activity or at 18 years of age. Once three normal annual Pap smears are documented, the interval for continued surveillance with screening Pap smears may be lengthened at the discretion of the physician and the patient.

Canavan TP, Doshi NR. Cervical cancer. *Am Fam Physician.* 2000;61:1369–1376.

35. Of the following, which local anesthetic has the longest duration of action?
A) Lidocaine
B) Mepivicaine
C) Bupivicaine
D) Procaine
E) Tetracaine

Answer and Discussion

The answer is C. Bupivicaine has the longest duration of action (2 to 4 hours).

Salam GA. Regional anesthesia for office procedures: Part I. Head and neck surgeries. *Am Fam Physician.* 2004;69:585–590.

36. A 32-year-old woman is brought to the emergency room by ambulance. She was involved in a motor vehicle accident. Close observation shows that her chest expands with expiration and contracts with inspiration. The most likely diagnosis is
A) ruptured thoracic aorta
B) pneumothorax
C) ruptured esophagus
D) flail chest
E) cardiac contusion

Answer and Discussion

The answer is D. In cases of severe blunt trauma to the chest, multiple rib fractures may lead to flail chest. By definition, a flail chest occurs in the presence of two or more fractures in three or more consecutive ribs, causing instability of the chest wall; however, the condition can also occur after costochondral separation. The diagnosis is made by noting paradoxical chest wall motion in which the chest wall depresses with inspiration and expands with expiration. There may be coexisting intrathoracic or intraabdominal injuries. Patients report dyspnea, and respiratory failure occurs in severe cases. Treatment is accomplished in most cases by intubation and mechanical ventilation with peak-end expiratory pressure as long as pain control is adequate. Further evaluation of underlying cardiac and pulmonary injury should be initiated once the patient's respiratory status has stabilized.

Townsend CM, ed. *Sabiston textbook of surgery*, 16th ed. Philadelphia: WB Saunders; 2001:327.

37. Which of the following can be added to lidocaine to reduce the burning sensation when it is administered?
A) Sodium bicarbonate
B) Epinephrine
C) Normal saline
D) Lactated Ringer's solution
E) Aluminum hydroxide

Answer and Discussion

The answer is A. Sodium bicarbonate may be added to neutralize the acidic local anesthetic and to reduce the burning sensation associated with anesthetic administration.

Salam GA. Regional anesthesia for office procedures: Part I. Head and neck surgeries. *Am Fam Physician.* 2004;69:585–590.

38. Which of the following statements about total parenteral nutrition (TPN) is true?
A) Lipid emulsions can lead to fatty emboli and are not added to TPN solutions.
B) Electrolytes should be monitored closely until stable.
C) In most cases, TPN is administered through peripheral access.
D) Equivalent amounts of calories can be delivered via a central or peripheral access.
E) Because glucose is delivered in standard amounts at predetermined rates, there is little need to follow glucose on a regular basis.

Answer and Discussion

The answer is B. TPN is nutritional support given intravenously to patients who suffer from malnutrition. TPN supplies all of the patient's daily nutritional requirements. A peripheral vein may be used for short periods, but longer periods of use with concentrated solutions can readily lead to thrombosis. Therefore, central venous access is usually required. For shorter periods requiring TPN, peripheral access may be used; however, fewer calories can be given via this route. TPN requires water (30 to 40 mL/kg/day) and energy (30 to 60 kcal/kg/day) depending on energy expenditure and amino acids (1 to 3 g/kg/day) depending on the degree of catabolism. Lipid emulsions supplying essential fatty acids and triglycerides may be used in addition to a basic solution. Indications include malnourished patients scheduled for surgery, chemotherapy, or radiation. Patients with severe burns, anorexia, coma, Crohn's disease, ulcerative colitis, or pancreatitis may benefit from TPN. The following should be monitored daily: weight, plasma urea and glucose (several times daily until stable), complete blood cell count, blood gases, accurate fluid balance, 24-hour urine, and electrolytes. When the patient becomes stable, the frequency of these tests can be reduced considerably. Liver function tests should be performed, and plasma proteins; prothrombin time; plasma and urine osmolality; and calcium, magnesium, and phosphate (not during glucose infusion) should be measured twice weekly. Progress should be followed on a flowchart. Nutritional assessment and C3 complement should be repeated at 2-week intervals.

Beers MH, Berkow R, eds. *The Merck manual of diagnosis and therapy*, Merck Research Laboratories, 17th ed. Whitehouse Station, NJ: Merck & Co.; 1999:17–21.

39. Patients with gallbladder carcinoma
A) typically have a life expectancy of more than 5 years
B) may have a history of chronic cholecystitis
C) rarely develop jaundice
D) rarely have metastasis at the time of diagnosis
E) are typically of middle age (35 to 65 years of age)

Answer and Discussion

The answer is B. Cancer of the gallbladder is rare, affects predominantly the elderly, and is very difficult to detect clinically. In most cases, it is found during surgery and has metastasized at the time of diagnosis. Ninety percent are adenocarcinomas. Symptoms, when they are present, include right-upper quadrant pain that radiates to the back, jaundice, weight loss, and anorexia. A palpable gallbladder with obstructive jaundice usually signifies cancer of the gallbladder. Treatment is limited, and surgery is used only in certain situations to relieve biliary obstruction. The prognosis is poor; few patients survive longer than 6 months. Chronic calculus cholecystitis increases the risk for cancer of the gallbladder, and cholecystectomy is recommended. Elective cholecystectomy with no indication to prevent carcinoma of the gallbladder carries a significant surgical risk and is not recommended.

Townsend CM, ed. *Sabiston textbook of surgery*, 16th ed. Philadelphia: WB Saunders; 2001:331.

Chronic calculus cholecystitis increases the risk for cancer of the gallbladder, and cholecystectomy is recommended.

40. When diagnosing an acute appendicitis, which of the following tests has the highest accuracy rate?
A) Plain films of the abdomen
B) Barium enema
C) CT of the abdomen
D) HIDA scan
E) Abdominal ultrasound

Answer and Discussion

The answer is C. Acute appendicitis is the most common reason leading to emergent abdominal surgery. The overall diagnostic accuracy achieved by traditional history, physical examination, and laboratory tests has been approximately 80%. The accuracy of diagnosis varies and is more difficult in women of childbearing age, children, and elderly persons. If the diagnosis of acute appendicitis is clear from the history and physical examination, prompt surgical referral is warranted. In atypical presentations, ultrasonography and computed tomography (CT) may help lower the rate of false-negative appendicitis diagnoses, reduce morbidity from perforation, and lower medical expenses. Ultrasonography is safe and readily available, with accuracy rates between 71% and 97%, although it is highly operator dependent and difficult in patients with a large body habitus. Although there is controversy regarding the use of contrast media and which CT technique is best, the accuracy rate of CT scanning is between 93% and 98%. Disadvantages of CT include radiation exposure, cost, and possible complications from contrast media.

Old JL, Dusing RW, Yap W, et al. Imaging for suspected appendicitis. *Am Fam Physician.* 2005;71:71–78.

41. Pain over the anatomic "snuff box" may indicate
A) Colles' fracture
B) cuboid fracture
C) scaphoid fracture
D) hook of the hamate fracture
E) boxer's fracture

Answer and Discussion

The answer is C. Scaphoid fractures account for approximately 60% of carpal bone fractures and are often missed on the initial radiograph. Symptoms include pain over the anatomic "snuff box" (area between the extensor pollicis brevis and the extensor pollicis longus tendons) and pain with radial deviation of the wrist. Reduction is seldom necessary; however, the arm, wrist, and thumb should be immobilized with a thumb spica cast for at least 6 weeks. If pain persists for longer than 4 months, there is an increased risk of nonunion or avascular necrosis with development of arthritis. Surgery may be indicated for this condition. If clinically suspected, radiographs (including scaphoid views) should be performed initially. Plain wrist films usually do not detect these fractures. In some cases, a bone scan or tomograms may be necessary to confirm the diagnosis. Bony electrical stimulation has also been shown to be effective in the healing of scaphoid fractures. Displaced fractures require open reduction with screw fixation.

Townsend CM, ed. *Sabiston textbook of surgery*, 16th ed. Philadelphia: WB Saunders; 2001:1576–1577.

42. Relief of hip pain after hip replacement occurs
A) almost immediately
B) after 3 months
C) after 6 months
D) usually after 1 year
E) rarely; hip replacement mostly improves functionality

Answer and Discussion

The answer is A. Hip arthroplasty is usually reserved for elderly patients with severe degenerative or rheumatoid arthritis. Indications include intractable pain or severe limitation of motion that interferes with the patient's activity level. Those patients with rheumatoid arthritis have longer and more lasting improvement than those with osteoarthritis. Complications include bleeding, infection, and the major immediate complication of thromboembolism. Bone resorption is a major complication that may affect the life of the prosthesis. Long-term complications include loosening of the prosthesis, which may require further surgery. In most cases, relief is immediate after hip replacement, and 90% of hip replacements are never revised.

NIH Consensus Development Panel on Total Hip Replacement. NIH consensus conference: Total hip replacement. *JAMA.* 1995;273:1950–1956.

43. A *felon* is a/an
A) prominence of the distal fifth toe
B) form of a cleft lip
C) neuroma associated with the flexor tendon
D) asymmetric nevus
E) abscess of the distal fingertip

Answer and Discussion

The answer is E. A felon is an abscess of the distal pulp or phalanx pad of the fingertip.

Harrison BP, Hilliard MW. Emergency department evaluation and treatment of hand injuries. *Emerg Med Clin North Am.* 1999;17:793–822.

44. Which of the following conditions is an indication for SBE prophylaxis?
A) Previous pacemaker placement
B) Previous coronary artery bypass graft
C) Previous episode of bacterial endocarditis
D) Mitral valve prolapse without regurgitation
E) History of ventricular septal defect successfully repaired 10 years ago

Answer and Discussion

The answer is C. Indications for SBE prophylaxis include the following:

- Previous episode of endocarditis
- Mitral valve prolapse with regurgitation (or thickened or redundant valve)
- Prosthetic cardiac valves
- Congenital cardiac defects (except for those specified)
- Hypertrophic cardiomyopathy
- Previous valvular surgery
- Rheumatic valvular dysfunction
- Surgically constructed systemic pulmonic shunts or conduits
- Dental or surgical indications for SBE prophylaxis
- Dental or surgical procedures likely to cause mucosal bleeding
- Tonsillectomy/adenoidectomy
- Surgery involving the respiratory or gastrointestinal mucosa
- Rigid bronchoscopy
- Sclerotherapy of esophageal varices
- Esophageal dilation
- Gallbladder surgery
- Urinary tract surgery if infection is present
- Prostatic surgery
- Cystoscopy
- Ureteral dilation
- Incision and drainage of infected tissue
- Vaginal delivery in the presence of infection

SBE prophylaxis is not necessary for ventricular septal defects, patent ductus arteriosus, and isolated secundum atrial septal defects if they have been repaired for at least 6 months without complications, physiologic murmurs, previous rheumatic fever without valve dysfunction, history of coronary artery bypass surgery, coronary stent placement, transesophageal echocardiogram, previous pacemaker or defibrillator placement, or history of Kawasaki disease without valve dysfunction. Also, SBE prophylaxis is not necessary for dental procedures not likely to cause gingival bleeding (fillings above the gum line, adjustment of orthodontic equipment, etc.), injection of intraoral anesthetics, shedding of primary teeth, tympanostomy tube placement, skin biopsy, cesarean section, endotracheal intubation, flexible bronchoscopy with or without biopsy, cardiac catheterization, endoscopy with or without biopsy, routine urinary catheterization (no infection present), dilation and curettage, uncomplicated vaginal delivery, abortion, insertion and removal of intrauterine devices, sterilization procedures, or laparoscopy.

Gilbert DN, Moellering RC, Sande MA. *The Sanford Guide to Antimicrobial Therapy, 2000.* Hyde Park, VT: Antimicrobial Therapy, Inc.; 2000:118–119.

45. A pipe smoker is found to have a white elevated plaque on his buccal mucosa during a general medical examination. The area cannot be wiped away with sterile gauze. The most likely diagnosis is
A) squamous cell carcinoma
B) thrush
C) gingivitis
D) leukoplakia
E) periodontitis

Answer and Discussion

The answer is D. Leukoplakia is a precancerous lesion that appears as a white, elevated, plaque-like growth that usually has asymmetric borders and usually affects the oral mucosa. It cannot be wiped off. The lesions tend to occur on the lip, mouth, buccal mucosa, or vaginal mucosa. Those at risk are cigarette smokers, pipe smokers, smokeless tobacco users, and heavy alcohol users. Others at risk include those with chronic oral infections, chronic malocclusion, or chronic ultraviolet light exposure. If suspected, these lesions should be biopsied to rule out malignancy. Approximately 10% may show malignant transformation. *Candida* infections can resemble leukoplakia, but *Candida* can be removed using a cotton swab.

Taylor R, David AK, Johnson TA Jr, et al., eds. *Family medicine: principles and practice*, 5th ed. New York: Springer-Verlag; 1998:1043.

46. Which of the following statements is true regarding screening for abdominal aortic aneurysms?
A) Screening is not beneficial for any subgroups of the populations.
B) Both women and men over the age of 50 should be screened.
C) Only men older than 75 should be screened.
D) Only men ages 65 to 75 with prior history of smoking should be screened.
E) Abdominal CT scanning is recommended for screening.

Answer and Discussion

The answer is D. The U.S. Preventive Services Task Force (USPSTF) recommends a single screening for abdominal aortic aneurysm (AAA) by ultrasonography in men ages 65 to 75 years who have previously smoked (defined as 100 or more cigarettes in a person's lifetime). The USPSTF found adequate evidence from large population-based studies in the United Kingdom that screening for AAA and surgical repair of large AAAs lead to decreased AAA-specific mortality. Almost all deaths from ruptured AAAs occur in men older than 65 years; most AAA-related deaths occur in men younger than 80 years. For most men, 75 years may be considered an upper age limit for screening, because increased comorbidities in patients 75 years and older decrease the likelihood that they will benefit from screening. Because few AAA-related deaths occur in women, and those AAAs that do rupture occur after 80 years of age when there are competing causes of mortality, the potential benefit of screening for AAA among women is low. Physicians must individualize recommendations for men and women depending on a patient's risk and likelihood of benefit. One-time screening to detect an AAA using ultrasonography is sufficient. Death from AAA rupture after negative results on a single ultrasound scan at age 65 is rare.

U.S. Preventive Services Task Force. Screening for abdominal aortic aneurysm: recommendation statement. *Ann Intern Med.* 2005;142:198–202.

47. A 65-year-old man presents to your office complaining of abdominal pain. His vital signs are stable. Examination reveals a pulsatile mass in the mid-abdomen. The most appropriate test is

A) magnetic resonance imaging (MRI) of the abdomen
B) laboratory tests, including complete blood count, electrolytes, and erythrocyte sedimentation rate
C) ultrasound examination of the abdomen
D) upper gastrointestinal series
E) barium enema

Answer and Discussion

The answer is C. Abdominal aortic aneurysms result from a weakening in the wall of the aorta. Most cases occur inferior to the renal arteries and are asymptomatic; however, back pain or abdominal pain may precede rupture. Most aneurysms are the result of atherosclerotic disease that results in weakening of the vessel. Strong evidence suggests a genetic susceptibility to abdominal aortic aneurysms. Patients with these aneurysms have a 20% chance of having a first-degree relative with the same condition. Male siblings are at particular risk. Approximately 75% of abdominal aortic aneurysms are asymptomatic and are detected during routine physical examination or during an unrelated radiologic or surgical procedure. Symptoms of an abdominal aortic aneurysm may result from expansion or rupture of the aneurysm, pressure on adjacent structures, embolization, or thrombosis. The most commonly reported symptom is any type of abdominal, flank, or back pain. Pressure on adjacent viscera may result in compression of the bowel. Patients may present with early satiety and, occasionally, nausea and vomiting. Rarely, ureteral compression may result in a partial ureteral obstruction. Thrombus and atheromatous material, which line nearly all abdominal aortic aneurysms, may occasionally result in distal arterial embolization and, rarely, aneurysm thrombosis. The abrupt onset of severe, constant pain in the abdomen, flank, or back, unrelieved by positional changes, is characteristic of expansion or rupture of the aneurysm. Physical examination often reveals a pulsating abdominal mass. Obesity, uncooperativeness, ascites, tortuosity of the aorta, and excessive lumbar lordosis are conditions that may make diagnosis by palpation difficult. Examination of the abdominal aorta is facilitated by having the patient lie on the examination table with the knees slightly flexed. The aorta is palpated during exhalation. A pulsatile abdominal mass left of midline—between the xiphoid process and the umbilicus—is highly suggestive of an abdominal aortic aneurysm. Diagnosis is made with ultrasound or CT examination. B-mode ultrasound is the screening method of choice for asymptomatic abdominal aortic aneurysms. It is available in most hospitals, is relatively inexpensive (approximately $150/examination), does not require ionizing radiation, reveals details of the vessel wall and associated atherosclerotic plaques, and allows accurate measurement of the aneurysm in longitudinal and transverse dimensions. Typically, aneurysms >6 cm are treated surgically, whereas smaller aneurysms are observed for any changes. Endovascular repair is safer, results in shorter hospital stays and quicker recovery, and translates into significant cost savings when compared with conventional surgery. The operative mortality rate is usually <5%. The mortality rate of patients with aneurysms >6 cm is approximately 50% in 1 year; patients with aneurysms between 4 and 6 cm have a mortality rate of 25% in 1 year.

Santilli JD, Santilli SM. Diagnosis and treatment of abdominal aortic aneurysms. *Am Fam Physician.* 1997;56(4):1081.

48. Which of the following can impede the healing of decubitus ulcers?

A) Wet-to-dry dressing changes
B) Doughnut cushions
C) Frequent position changes
D) Air-fluidized mattresses
E) Débridement of nonviable tissue

Answer and Discussion

The answer is B. Decubitus ulcers occur when there is prolonged pressure of skin against an external object such as a bed or a wheelchair. It occurs most often in patients who are debilitated and have impaired sensory function. The sacrum, ischia, greater trochanters, external malleoli, and heels are at particular risk for tissue breakdown. There are four stages in the development of a decubitus ulcer:

- *Stage 1*—nonblanchable erythema of intact skin
- *Stage 2*—partial thickness dermal or epidermal loss causing a blister, shallow crater, or abrasion
- *Stage 3*—full thickness necrosis causing a deep crater down to fascia
- *Stage 4*—full thickness destruction of muscle, bone, or supporting structures

Intrinsic and extrinsic factors play a role in the development of pressure ulcers. Intrinsic factors include loss of pain and pressure sensations (which ordinarily prompt the patient to shift position and relieve the pressure) and minimal fat and muscle padding between bony weight-bearing prominences and skin. Disuse atrophy, malnutrition, anemia, and infection also contribute. In a paralyzed patient, loss of vasomotor control leads to lowered tone in the vascular bed and lowered circulatory rate. Spasticity, especially in patients with spinal cord injuries, can place a shearing force on the blood vessels to further compromise circulation. Extrinsic factors include pressure due to infrequent shifting of the patient's position; friction, irritation, and pulling of the skin from ill-adjusted supports or wrinkled bedding or clothing also contribute. In an immobilized patient, severe pressure can impair local circulation in less than 3 hours, causing local tissue anoxia that, if unrelieved, progresses to necrosis of the skin and subcutaneous tissues. Moisture (e.g., from perspiration or incontinence) leads to tissue maceration and predisposes to pressure sores. The treatment of decubitus ulcers includes wet-to-dry dressing changes and the use of air-fluidized beds, particularly for large ulcers. Ulcers that have not advanced beyond stage 3 may heal spontaneously if the pressure is removed and the area is small. New hydrophilic gels and hydrocolloid dressings speed healing. Stage 4 ulcers require débridement or more extensive surgery. When the ulcers are filled with pus or necrotic debris, dextranomer beads or newer hydrophilic polymers may hasten débridement without surgery. Conservative débridement of necrotic tissue with forceps and scissors should be instituted. Some ulcers may be débrided by cleansing them with hydrogen peroxide. Whirlpool baths may also assist débridement. The use of egg-crate mattresses, sheepskins, and doughnut cushions are not adequate to prevent ulcers; doughnut cushions can actually decrease the blood flow to the area of the body in the center of the cushion, thereby impeding the healing process. The use of antibiotics is unnecessary unless cellulitis, osteomyelitis, or sepsis is present. The use of topical antiseptics and antibiotics may also impede the healing process by damaging fibroblasts, which are needed for healing.

Beers MH, Berkow R, eds. *The Merck manual of diagnosis and therapy*, Merck Research Laboratories, 17th ed. Whitehouse Station, NJ: Merck & Co.; 1999:834–835.

49. Of the following measurements, which would be considered the threshold for surgical intervention in treating a man with an abdominal aortic aneurysm?

A) 4.0 cm
B) 5.0 cm
C) 6.0 cm
D) 7.0 cm
E) 8.0 cm

Answer and Discussion

The answer is B. There is some debate about aneurysms. A recent study recommends delaying surgical repair of abdominal aortic aneurysms 5.5 cm in diameter. The risk of aneurysm rupture is four times as high in women. Although there should be a lower threshold for surgical repair in women, the authors of the study did not think that a specific numeric cutoff could be recommended, based on the data.

Powell JT, Greenhalgh RM. Small abdominal aortic aneurysms. *N Engl J Med.* 2003;348:1895–1901.

In patients with abdominal aortic aneurysms with a diameter >6 cm, the risk of rupture is increased markedly, and surgical repair is indicated if the patient can tolerate the intervention.

50. A 51-year-old woman presents to the office with a 2-day history of right-upper quadrant, colicky abdominal pain, as well as nausea and vomiting. Examination shows significant pain with palpation in the right-upper quadrant. Laboratory findings include an elevated white blood cell count, alkaline phosphatase, and bilirubin level. The most likely diagnosis is

A) viral gastroenteritis
B) dissecting abdominal aneurysm
C) acute pancreatitis
D) acute cholecystitis
E) perforated duodenal ulcer

Answer and Discussion

The answer is D. Cholecystitis is an acute inflammation of the gallbladder wall. The condition usually results from an obstruction of the bile ducts as a result of biliary stones (most commonly cholesterol). Risk factors for cholesterol gallstone formation include age, obesity, rapid weight loss, pregnancy, female gender, use of exogenous estrogens, diabetes, certain gastrointestinal conditions, and certain medications. Symptoms include colicky right-upper quadrant abdominal pain that starts out mild and crescendos into more severe pain that may last several hours before resolving spontaneously. Patients may also report nausea and vomiting and low-grade fevers. Physical examination usually shows marked right-upper quadrant tenderness with a positive Murphy's sign (marked abdominal pain and inspiratory arrest with palpation of the right-upper quadrant). A palpable gallbladder is present in as many as 30% to 40% of patients. Jaundice is present in 15% of patients. Laboratory findings include an elevated white blood cell count, increased serum transaminases, alkaline phosphatase, bilirubin levels, and, in some cases, amylase levels. The diagnosis is usually made with ultrasound; however, cholescintigraphy (HIDA scan) is the most sensitive test to document obstruction in the biliary system. Oral cholecystograms are rarely used for diagnosing acute cholecystitis. CT scans are not superior to ultrasound and are more expensive. Up to one-half of stones in the common bile duct are not detected on ultrasonography. In the gallbladder, stones <2 mm in diameter may be missed or misdiagnosed as sludge. Endoscopic retrograde cholangiopancreatography is the test of choice to detect stones in the common bile duct. If infection is suspected, antibiotics—including ampicillin plus sulbactam (Unasyn), or a third-generation cephalosporin plus metronidazole—are indicated. Pain can be managed with ketorolac or meperidine. Morphine should be avoided, because it may cause spasm of the sphincter of Oddi and increase pain. Treatment usually involves surgical excision.

Ahmad M, Cheung RC, Keeffe EB, et al. Differential diagnosis of gallstone-induced complications. *South Med J.* 2000;93:261–264.

51. Which of the following cardiac arrhythmias is associated with lightning strikes?

A) Asystole
B) Ventricular fibrillation
C) Atrial fibrillation
D) Atrioventricular dissociation
E) Third-degree heart block

Answer and Discussion

The answer is A. More people are killed each year in the United States by lightning than by any other natural disaster. Lightning injuries are direct current injuries. They differ from alternating current injuries, because victims can suffer from a shock-wave phenomenon that may violently throw them and cause multiple trauma. Therefore, the cervical spine must be protected after a lightning strike. The major cardiac effect is asystole, whereas a high-voltage alternating current injury usually causes ventricular fibrillation. A flashover effect in which the main current travels peripherally over the victim's body may also occur. Leaf-like patterns of burned skin result. Wet clothing can cause excessive skin injury. Treatment should follow advanced cardiac life-support protocol and can be successful if initiated immediately after the injury. Other complications include vitreous hemorrhage, retinal detachment, and ruptured tympanic membranes. Lightning rarely, if ever, produces entry and exit wounds and seldom causes muscle damage or myoglobulinuria, because the duration of current is too short to break down the skin and tissues. Lightning flashes over the person, producing little internal damage other than electrical short-circuiting of systems (e.g., heart asystole, brain confusion, loss of consciousness, neuropsychologic sequelae). Some form of amnesia generally results. Neuropsychologic damage, pain syndromes, and sympathetic nervous system damage are the most common long-term sequelae. Cardiopulmonary arrest is the most common cause of death.

Beers MH, Berkow R, eds. *The Merck manual of diagnosis and therapy*, Merck Research Laboratories, 17th ed. Whitehouse Station, NJ: Merck & Co.; 1999:2442.

52. Which of the following factors would be favorable in deciding if a patient would benefit from a carotid endarterectomy?
A) Female sex
B) Patient is older than 75 years
C) Surgery to be performed 4 weeks after their ischemic event
D) Patient has diabetes
E) Bilateral carotid stenosis is present

Answer and Discussion

The answer is B. The European Carotid Surgery Trial and the North American Symptomatic Carotid Endarterectomy Trial included 95% of patients in trials of carotid endarterectomy surgery. The participants had experienced recent clinical events in the distribution of the carotid artery, and the symptomatic vessel was visualized by angiography. Participants were randomized to medical or surgical treatment, and follow-up was conducted by neurologists or by subspecialists in stroke. Follow-up data were obtained for 5,893 patients over an average of 66 months. Of the 3,157 patients treated with endarterectomy, 222 (7%) had operative deaths or strokes. The perioperative risk of death or stroke was increased in women, patients with diabetes, patients with occlusion of the other carotid artery, patients with ulcerated or irregular plaques, and patients who had hemispheric (rather than retinal) events preceding clinical events. Age, sex, and time since last symptomatic event greatly modified the outcome of surgery. When all variables were included in the analysis, the benefits from surgery were greatest in men, patients older than 75 years, and those who had surgery within 2 weeks of their last ischemic event.

Rothwell PM, Eliasziw M, Gutnikov SA. Endarterectomy for symptomatic carotid stenosis in relation to clinical subgroups and timing of surgery. *Lancet*. 2004;363:915–924.

53. A 25-year-old patient arrives in the emergency room after being involved in a high-speed motor vehicle accident. The patient is conscious, hypotensive, and complains of abdominal pain. The most appropriate management includes
A) flat and upright abdominal series
B) diagnostic peritoneal lavage
C) abdominal ultrasound
D) emergent abdominal computed tomography (CT) scan
E) exploratory laparotomy

Answer and Discussion

The answer is B. Patients who have experienced significant abdominal trauma, have abdominal pain, or are unstable and the diagnosis remains unclear should undergo diagnostic peritoneal lavage once they arrive in the emergency room. The procedure involves making a small incision between the umbilicus and pubis after local anesthesia is administered. A small 1-cm incision is then made in the peritoneal fascia, and a peritoneal dialysis catheter is placed. The catheter is directed to the posterior sacral area and 1,000 mL of normal saline is infused into the peritoneal cavity and allowed to return by gravity. A return of at least 10 mL of gross blood; a bloody lavage effluent; an RBC count greater than 100,000/mm^3; a white blood cell count greater than 500/mm^3; an amylase greater than 175 IU/dL; or the detection of bile, bacteria, or food fibers in the aspirated fluid is considered a positive response and requires immediate laparotomy to look for an internal bleeding site. Patients who are clinically stable may undergo CT or ultrasound to further evaluate the abdomen when blunt trauma has occurred. Diagnostic peritoneal lavage is highly sensitive for the presence of intraperitoneal blood; however, specificity is low.

Townsend CM, ed. *Sabiston textbook of surgery*, 16th ed. Philadelphia: WB Saunders; 2001:331.

54. A 33-year-old street person presents to the emergency room. While scavenging in garbage cans, the patient cut his left hand. He does not recall if he has ever had immunization for tetanus before. The most appropriate immunization is
A) adult diphtheria tetanus toxoid (dT)
B) diphtheria-pertussis-tetanus vaccine (DPT)
C) dT and tetanus immunoglobulin (TIG)
D) observation

Answer and Discussion

The answer is C. Tetanus immunization for adults is recommended every 10 years with an adult dT. If the patient has not received adequate immunization before injury and the wound is dirty and tetanus-prone, they should receive tetanus and diptheria toxiod and tetanus immune globulin.

	Inadequate or unknown immunization (<3 doses)	Adequate immunization (at least 3 doses and a booster within 10 years)
Wound		
Clean	Adult dT	—
Dirty	dT, TIG	dT[a]

[a]If immunization occurred >5 years ago.

Gilbert DN, Moellering RC, Sande MA. *The Sanford Guide to Antimicrobial Therapy, 2000*. Hyde Park, VT: Antimicrobial Therapy, Inc.; 2000:128.

55. Which of the following statements is true regarding hip fractures?
A) Most hip fractures do not require surgery for repair.
B) Avascular necrosis of the femoral head is a serious complication.
C) Nonunion or malunion does not occur with hip fractures.
D) Location of the fracture has no bearing on the outcome.
E) None of the above.

Answer and Discussion

The answer is B. The distinction between intracapsular and extracapsular hip fracture has prognostic value for the patient's outcome. Early detection of intracapsular fractures is especially important, because these fractures are prone to complications for two primary reasons. First, interuption of the blood supply to the femoral head frequently occurs and can lead to avascular necrosis. Second, the head fragment of the fracture is often a shell containing fragile cancellous bone that provides poor attachment for a fixation device, a situation that often increases the possibility of nonunion or malunion.

Caviglia HA, Osorro PQ, Comando D. Classification and diagnosis of intracapsular fractures of the proximal femur. *Clin Orthop.* 2002;(399):17–27.

56. Which of the following types of polyps is associated with the greatest risk of malignant transformation?
A) Hyperplastic polyp
B) Tubular adenoma
C) Villous adenoma
D) Mixed tubulovillous adenoma
E) All have equal risk.

Answer and Discussion

The answer is C. The development of colon polyps has been associated with a high-fat, low-fiber diet. They also occur more frequently in patients with a positive family history (two to four times more common than in the healthy population). Polyps are divided into differing histologic types, including the following:

1. Tubular adenoma: 5% chance of cancer development
2. Villous adenoma: 40% chance of cancer development
3. Mixed tubulovillous adenoma: 22% chance of cancer development

Although controversial, the U.S. Agency for Health Care Policy and Research has recommended screening for average-risk persons older than 50 years using one of the following techniques: fecal occult blood testing each year, flexible sigmoidoscopy every 5 years, fecal occult blood testing every year combined with flexible sigmoidoscopy every 5 years, double-contrast barium enema every 5 to 10 years, or colonoscopy every 10 years. Screening of persons with risk factors should begin at an earlier age, depending on the situation. The detection of adenomatous polyps should prompt thorough evaluation and removal using colonoscopy. The risk of synchronous polyps affecting the proximal colon is as high as 35%. For those with a positive family history of colon cancer, more frequent and earlier periodic colonoscopy should be considered.

Read TE, Kodner IJ. Colorectal cancer: risk factors and recommendations for early detection. *Am Fam Physician.* 1999;59:2975.

57. A 40-year-old woman is found to have chronic cholestasis. The most serious complication is the development of
A) intractable hiccups
B) primary biliary cirrhosis
C) cholelithiasis
D) hypercholesterolemia
E) chronic urticaria

Answer and Discussion

The answer is B. Primary biliary cirrhosis is a condition that is characterized by chronic cholestasis, which can damage the liver and ultimately result in the development of cirrhosis. The cause is unknown but may be associated with an underlying autoimmune disorder. The condition typically affects women between 35 and 70 years of age; the condition can occur in men. The disease usually involves four stages:

1. Bile duct inflammation
2. Periportal fibrosis
3. Progressive scarring
4. Cirrhosis

Symptoms include itching secondary to elevations of bilirubin, fatigue, and jaundice. Physical findings include hepatosplenomegaly, skin xanthomas (especially around the eyelids and involving the tendons), clubbing, and jaundice. Laboratory tests show elevated alkaline phosphatase, bilirubin, γ-glutamyl transferase, aspartate aminotransferase, and alanine aminotransferase. Serum cholesterol is also usually elevated. Diagnostic procedures include ultrasound, endoscopic retrograde cholangiopancreatography, and liver biopsy. Unfortunately, no specific treatment is available; however, those affected may be candidates for liver transplantation if they develop cirrhosis with hepatic failure. Cholestyramine may be beneficial for the pruritus. Those affected have a variable prognosis, depending on the severity of the disease. Those with slow progression may be minimally affected. Chronic urticaria may be associated with underlying urticarial vasculitis and is diagnosed by skin biopsy.

Beers MH, Berkow R, eds. *The Merck manual of diagnosis and therapy*, Merck Research Laboratories, 17th ed. Whitehouse Station, NJ: Merck & Co.; 1999:375.

58. A 54-year-old male with no prior history of DVT presents with unilateral swelling of the right lower extremity after a recent prolonged plane flight. The patient is found to have a below-the-knee DVT associated with the calf. He has no contraindication for anticoagulation therapy. What is the appropriate therapy?
A) Heparin therapy followed by oral anticoagulation for 6 to 12 weeks.
B) No anticoagulation and monitor for proximal for proximal extension with duplex ultrasound two times per week for 2 weeks.
C) No anticoagulation and monitor for proximal for proximal extension with duplex ultrasound once a week for 4 weeks.
D) No anticoagulation and application of compressive stockings.
E) No anticoagulation and elevation of the extremity and early mobilization.

Answer and Discussion

The answer is A. Patients with a first episode of calf DVT with a transient risk factor should receive heparin therapy followed by oral anticoagulation for 6 to 12 weeks. If anticoagulation is contraindicated, physicians should monitor for proximal thrombus extension with duplex ultrasound twice weekly for 2 weeks. The use of low-molecular-weight heparin (LMWH), outpatient therapy, compression stockings, elevation of the extremity, and early mobilization may be beneficial based on extrapolation from studies of proximal DVT.

Diagnosis and treatment of deep venous thrombosis and pulmonary embolism. Evidence Report/Technology Assessment No. 68. AHRQ Publication No. 03-E012. Rockville, MD: Agency for Healthcare Research and Quality, January 2003. Accessed online March 19, 2006, at: http://www.ahrq.gov/clinic/epcsums/dvtsum.htm.

Lagerstedt CI, Olsson CG, Fagher BO, et al. Need for long-term anticoagulant treatment in symptomatic calf-vein thrombosis. *Lancet.* 1985;2:515–518.

59. A 45-year-old woman complains of rectal discomfort and bleeding aggravated by bowel movements. The patient reports a long history of constipation. On examination, there is a small fissure at the lateral 9 o'clock position. Which of the following statements is true?

A) Rectal spasms increase blood flow and accelerate healing.
B) A cause other than trauma should be considered.
C) Bowel movements help relieve symptoms.
D) Exercise often leads to development of fissures.
E) Corticosteroid creams should be avoided because of the risk of bacterial overgrowth.

Answer and Discussion

The answer is B. Anal fissures are small tears in the mucosa of the anal canal. They often produce pain disproportionate to the size of the lesion. The cause is thought to be secondary to traumatic tearing of the mucosa with the passage of large, hard stools. Other causes include proctitis as a result of previous rectal surgery, hemorrhoids, or rectal cancer. Because of its location in the area of the rectal sphincter, spasms may keep the area from healing. Fissures are most commonly located anterior or posterior to the anus. When fissures are found laterally, syphilis, tuberculosis, occult abscesses, leukemic infiltrates, carcinoma, herpes, acquired immunodeficiency syndrome, or inflammatory bowel disease should be considered as causes. Symptoms include rectal pain and bleeding, which is aggravated with bowel movements. Treatment involves the use of stool softeners and laxatives, hydrocortisone creams, benzocaine ointments, and sitz baths, as well as increased oral fluids and adequate exercise. Another nonsurgical treatment for anal fissure is nitroglycerin ointment. Surgery may be indicated for severe cases that are refractive to these measures.

Pfenninger JL, Zainea GG. Common anorectal conditions: Part II. Lesions. *Am Fam Physician.* 2001;64:77–88.

60. How long should an isolated calf DVT be treated with anticoagulation?
A) 1 month
B) 3 months
C) 6 months
D) 9 months
E) 12 months

Answer and Discussion

The answer is B. In the Seventh Conference on Antithrombotic and Thrombolytic Therapy, the American College of Chest Physicians (ACCP) recommends treating symptomatic isolated calf DVT with anticoagulation for 3 months (INR 2 to 3).

Buller HR, Agnelli G, Hull RD, et al. Antithrombotic therapy for venous thromboembolic disease: the Seventh ACCP Conference on Antithrombotic and Thrombolytic Therapy [published correction appears in *Chest.* 2005;127:416]. *Chest.* 2004;126(3 suppl):S401–S428.

61. The best test for the diagnosis of acute obstructive cholecystitis is
A) ultrasound examination
B) radionuclide excretion test (HIDA scan)
C) CT examination
D) oral cholecystography
E) MRI

Answer and Discussion

The answer is B. Cholecystitis (inflammation of the gallbladder) usually results as a complication of cholelithiasis (gallstones) and obstruction of the biliary duct by gallstones. The condition is seen more commonly in women than in men. The incidence increases with age. Symptoms include rapid onset of intermittent cramping abdominal pain in the upper-right quadrant, which gradually becomes worse and lasts for several hours; fever, nausea, and vomiting may be present in some cases. Physical findings include right-upper quadrant pain, guarding, and a positive Murphy's sign (significant tenderness with palpation in the right-upper quadrant with inspiration). Chronic cholelithiasis follows a more indolent course with less severe symptoms that are shorter in duration and are recurrent. Diagnosis of acute and chronic cholelithiasis is commonly made with ultrasound examination; however, the best test for detection of acute obstructive cholelithiasis is the radionuclide excretion test (HIDA scan), particularly if the ultrasound is normal or nondiagnostic. Laboratory tests usually show elevations in white blood cell count, liver function tests, amylase, alkaline, phosphatase, and bilirubin during attacks of biliary colic. Patients with chronic cholecystitis rarely have abnormal laboratory studies. Laparoscopic cholecystectomy is the procedure of choice for uncomplicated acute and chronic cholecystitis. Stones can be composed of cholesterol (most common), pigment, and mixed stones. Oral cholecystography is no longer commonly used in the diagnosis of cholecystitis. Prophylactic cholecystectomy for asymptomatic cholelithiasis is generally not recommended.

Taylor R, David AK, Johnson TA Jr, et al., eds. *Family medicine: principles and practice*, 5th ed. New York: Springer-Verlag; 1998:805–806.

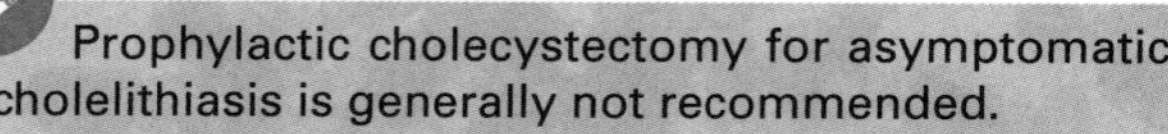

Prophylactic cholecystectomy for asymptomatic cholelithiasis is generally not recommended.

62. What is the annual risk of major hemorrhage when treating a DVT?
A) 2%
B) 25%
C) 50%
D) 75%
E) 98%

Answer and Discussion

The answer is A. Oral anticoagulation for DVT carries a steady 2% annual risk of major hemorrhage plus risk of minor hemorrhage.

Diagnosis and treatment of deep venous thrombosis and pulmonary embolism. Evidence Report/Technology Assessment No. 68. AHRQ Publication No. 03-E012. Rockville, MD: Agency for Healthcare Research and Quality, January 2003. Accessed online March 19, 2006, at: http://www.ahrq.gov/clinic/epcsums/dvtsum.html.

63. Which of the following statements about an abnormal breast lesion is true?
A) Cystic lesions are usually benign.
B) A risk factor for breast cancer is early menopause.
C) Mammograms can be used to determine whether the lesion is cystic or solid.
D) Baseline mammogram screening should begin at 50 years of age.
E) Mammograms have less than a 5% false-negative rate.

Answer and Discussion

The answer is A. The development of a breast mass requires a thorough evaluation to rule out a possible malignancy. Risk factors for breast cancer include increased age, early menarche, late menopause,

BRCA gene mutation, being nulliparous, having a first-degree relative with breast cancer, or having cancer in the contralateral breast. A palpable mass can be evaluated with fine-needle or excisional biopsy. It is important to remember that mammograms have a 10% to 15% false-negative rate; therefore, a palpable solid mass should, in most cases, be biopsied despite a negative mammogram. In addition, a solid lesion is more worrisome for malignancy than a cystic lesion, and ultrasound may be used to differentiate between the two. If the mass is cystic, it can be watched closely with serial ultrasounds or aspirated. The screening guidelines for the diagnosis of breast cancer are continually changing. Because of increased awareness of the signs and symptoms of breast cancer and the use of screening mammograms, breast cancers are increasingly being diagnosed at earlier stages. Annual mammograms and clinical breast examinations are recommended for women older than 40 years. Women older than 20 years should be encouraged to do monthly breast self-examinations, and women between 20 and 39 years of age should have a clinical breast examination every 3 years. These guidelines are modified for women with risk factors, particularly those with a strong family history of breast cancer.

Beers MH, Berkow R, eds. *The Merck manual of diagnosis and therapy*, Merck Research Laboratories, 17th ed. Whitehouse Station, NJ: Merck & Co.; 1999:1974–1976.

64. A 71-year-old hospitalized patient who previously underwent bowel resection and is now receiving TPN is noted to have a mild elevation in his liver function test. The most appropriate action is

A) observation
B) ultrasound examination of the liver, pancreas, and gallbladder
C) exploratory laparoscopy
D) discontinuation of parenteral nutrition
E) liver biopsy

Answer and Discussion

The answer is A. TPN is the intravenous administration of a patient's daily nutritional requirements. Generally, the concentrated solution is given through central vein access, although peripheral access can be used for short durations. Patients who may be candidates for TPN include burn victims, malnourished patients in the perioperative period, or patients who have severe trauma or are in a comatose state. Formulations include daily nutritional requirements, including vitamin supplementation. Patients should be monitored closely with laboratory tests, daily weights, and accurate intakes and outputs. Complications involve nutritional deficiencies and administration complications (e.g., infection of intravenous sites). Laboratory abnormalities may include elevated liver function tests, hepatosplenomegaly, thrombocytopenia, or hyperlipidemia. Peripheral TPN typically provides less calories than centrally administered TPN.

Beers MH, Berkow R, eds. *The Merck manual of diagnosis and therapy*, Merck Research Laboratories, 17th ed. Whitehouse Station, NJ: Merck & Co.; 1999:17–21.

65. Which of the following statements regarding dipstick urinalysis is *false*?

A) In women with classic UTI symptoms, in the absence of vaginal symptoms, empiric treatment may be considered without dipstick testing.
B) In low-risk patients with a low pretest probability of UTI, the dipstick adequately rules out infection when both leukocyte esterase and nitrites are negative.
C) Given the more serious consequences of a missed diagnosis of UTI in children, a backup urine culture is recommended.
D) Even in women with classic UTI symptoms, treatment over the telephone should not be performed.
E) Dipstick urinalysis are not sufficiently accurate to make a diagnosis.

Answer and Discussion

The answer is D. In women with classic UTI symptoms, particularly in the absence of vaginal symptoms, the probability of a UTI is so high that empiric treatment may be considered without dipstick testing. This might allow treatment by telephone, without necessitating a patient visit resulting in improved cost savings and patient convenience. In a patient with nonspecific complaints such as dysuria and vaginal discharge, a dipstick might be useful. In low-risk patients with a low pretest probability of UTI, the dipstick adequately rules out infection when both leukocyte esterase and nitrites are negative. This also has the benefit of cost containment because fewer urine cultures are needed in low-risk patients. Given the more serious consequences of a missed diagnosis of UTI in children, a backup urine culture is recommended.

Wright OR, Safranek S. FPIN's clinical inquiries: urine dipstick for diagnosing urinary tract infection. *Am Fam Physician*. 2006;73:129.

66. Which of the following statements is true regarding vasectomies?

A) Early failure rate is approximately 1 in 300.
B) Development of sperm antibodies occurs in <1%.
C) Sperm antibodies are related to the future development of coronary artery disease.
D) The incidence of testicular cancer increases after vasectomy.
E) Patients may resume unprotected intercourse after one sperm-free semen analysis.

Answer and Discussion

The answer is A. Vasectomies are performed to provide sterilization for men. Before the procedure, the possibility of complications should be discussed with the patient. The most important complication to discuss is the failure rate of vasectomy as a contraceptive method. Pregnancy occurs after a vasectomy in most cases because the couple had sexual intercourse before azoospermia was documented by two separate semen samples. Early failure occurs in approximately 1 out of 300 vasectomies. Late recanalization is thought to be rare after vasectomy. As many as 50% to 66% of patients develop sperm antibodies after vasectomy. Previous concern about the damage of coronary vessels by these antibodies has not been substantiated. Except for the development of epididymitis, orchitis, and sperm granulomas, those with vasectomies have no higher incidence of disease (including testicular cancer) than control groups. Patients who develop sperm granulomas are at increased risk for recannulation of the vas deferens and should have periodic sperm samples checked. After vasectomy, approximately 15 to 20 ejaculations are required to clear the sperm. The patient should not be considered sterile until two sperm-free specimens are obtained. Contraindications for vasectomy include bleeding disorders, current infection, coercion by family or friends, or anatomic abnormalities.

Clenney TL, Higgins JC. Vasectomy techniques. *Am Fam Physician*. 1999;60:137–152.

67. Which of the following deters healing of anal fissures?
A) Sitz baths
B) Internal sphincter spasms
C) Poor blood supply to the dentate line
D) External hemorrhoids
E) Rectal rugae

Answer and Discussion

The answer is B. Fissures of the anal canal are usually due to traumatic lacerations as a result of chronic constipation with perhaps an underlying infection of the lesion. Other associated conditions include chronic proctitis, rectal carcinoma, hemorrhoids, or previous rectal surgery. The lesion is often associated with the internal sphincter and can cause spasms that can deter healing. Symptoms include pain and bleeding during and after defecation. Physical examination usually shows evidence of a linear fissure located in the midline. Treatment involves the use of stool softeners, fiber supplements, sitz baths, and hydrocortisone- or benzocaine-containing cream, which may aid in decreasing any associated pain or inflammation and promote healing. Surgery is reserved for cases that fail to respond to medical therapy.

Pfenninger JL, Zainea GG. Common anorectal conditions: Part II. Lesions. *Am Fam Physician.* 2001;64:77–88.

68. A 16-year-old gymnast suffers a fall onto an outstretched hand. On exam she appears to have an unstable distal radioulnar joint. Which of the following injuries is most likely?
A) Greenstick fracture of the radius
B) de Quervain's tenosynovitis
C) Colles' fracture
D) Injury to the triangular fibrocartilage complex (TFCC)
E) Scaphoid fracture

Answer and Discussion

The answer is D. Ulnar wrist pain and weakness caused by a fall onto an outstretched hand may suggest injury to the TFCC, which is the primary stabilizer of the distal radioulnar joint. TFCC injury is common in gymnasts and in racquetball, tennis, and hockey players.

Rettig AC. Athletic injuries of the wrist and hand. Part I: traumatic injuries of the wrist. *Am J Sports Med.* 2003;31: 1038–1048.

69. Which of the following blood types is considered the universal donor?
A) AB positive
B) O positive
C) AB negative
D) O negative
E) B negative

Answer and Discussion

The answer is D. In trauma settings, the use of intravenous fluid is important to maintain adequate perfusion to vital tissues and organs. The use of blood for fluid replacement requires typing and proper storing, making it impractical to use in emergent settings in which time is extremely valuable. Because of this, a trauma patient should receive two large-bore (16-gauge or larger) intravenous lines and normal saline or lactated Ringer's solution until proper blood can be given in a controlled setting. For adults, 1,000 mL of crystalloid solution should be given as an initial bolus—children should receive 20 mL/kg. In some emergent situations, O-negative blood, the universal donor blood, can be given until appropriately typed blood arrives.

Ritchie WP, Steele G, Dean RH. *General Surgery.* Philadelphia: JB Lippincott Co.; 1995:923.

> In some emergent situations, O-negative blood (the universal donor blood) can be given until appropriately typed blood arrives.

70. The most common form of malignant melanoma is
A) lentigo maligna melanoma
B) superficial spreading melanoma
C) nodular melanoma
D) acrolentiginous melanoma

Answer and Discussion

The answer is B. Malignant melanoma is not as common as squamous cell carcinoma and basal cell carcinoma but is more serious and life threatening because of the potential for distant metastasis. It is the leading cause of death as a result of a skin disease, and the incidence is increasing. Studies have shown that the prevalence of melanoma increases with proximity to the equator. Persons with skin types that are sensitive to the effects of ultraviolet radiation—red or blond hair, freckles, and fair skin that burns easily and tans with difficulty—are at higher risk. Although cumulative sun exposure is linked to nonmelanoma skin cancer, intermittent intense sun exposure seems to be more related to melanoma risk. Other risk factors for melanoma include melanocytic precursor lesions (atypical moles), increased numbers of acquired nevi (>50), a family history of melanoma, a personal history of nonmelanoma skin cancer, giant congenital nevi (>20 cm), and immunosuppression. Melanomas are classified into the following:

- *Lentigo maligna melanoma.* This usually affects older patients in their 60s and 70s. These lesions usually show variegation of color including black, brown, reddish lesions and are rather large (measuring 2 to 6 cm).
- *Superficial spreading melanoma.* This is the most common type. These lesions are usually smaller (2 to 3 cm in diameter) and tend to affect patients in their 50s and 60s.
- *Nodular melanoma.* These patients are usually younger (average, 30 to 50 years of age). These lesions are usually smaller than the other two types and are slightly raised and uniform in color. Unfortunately, these lesions tend to spread deeply into the underlying tissue and have the worst prognosis.
- *Acrolentiginous melanoma.* This condition is rare and is associated with lesions affecting the palmar and plantar surface of the extremities as well as the subungual skin. It is similar to lentigo maligna melanoma.

Rare before puberty, malignant melanoma may tend to bleed or ulcerate. Early metastasis occurs through the lymph nodes; late metastasis occurs through a hematogenous route and may affect the skin, liver, or lungs. A properly performed biopsy is essential for the diagnosis. If melanoma is diagnosed, the histologic interpretation of the biopsy determines the prognosis and treatment plan. General recommendations include performing an excisional biopsy whenever possible. Accepted techniques for excisional biopsy include punch, saucerization, and elliptic excision. Shave biopsy is not recommended. A shave biopsy will not miss a diagnosis of melanoma, but may interfere with the staging process of determining the depth of invasion. Treatment involves a full-thickness wide excision of the lesion and node dissection for advanced tumors. Prognosis depends on the depth of invasion.

Edman RL, Wolfe JT. Prevention and early detection of malignant melanoma. *Am Fam Physician.* 2000;62:2277–2285.

71. When treating anaphylaxis, which of the following, in addition to intravenous fluid, is considered the mainstay of treatment?
A) Diphenhydramine
B) Prednisone
C) Propanolol
D) Epinephrine
E) Naproxen

Answer and Discussion

The answer is D. Anaphylaxis is a life-threatening reaction with respiratory, cardiovascular, cutaneous, or gastrointestinal manifestations that results from an exposure to a precipitating agent, usually a food, insect sting, medication, or physical factor. It causes approximately 1,500 deaths in the United States annually. The differential includes septic or other forms of shock, asthma, airway foreign body, panic attack, or other entities. Urinary and serum histamine levels and plasma tryptase levels drawn after onset of symptoms may help in the diagnosis. Prompt treatment of anaphylaxis is crucial, with subcutaneous or intramuscular epinephrine and intravenous fluids remaining the mainstay of management. Adjunctive measures include airway protection, antihistamines, steroids, and beta agonists. Patients taking β-blockers may require additional treatment. Patients should be observed for delayed or protracted anaphylaxis and instructed how to initiate urgent treatment for future episodes.

Tang AW. A practical guide to anaphylaxis. *Am Fam Physician.* 2003;68:1325–1332, 1339–1340.

72. The first step in the management of a lower gastrointestinal hemorrhage is to
A) obtain a CT scan of the abdomen
B) perform a bleeding scan
C) resuscitate the unstable patient
D) perform a colonoscopy
E) obtain a surgical consult

Answer and Discussion

The answer is C. Gastrointestinal bleeding suspected from a lower source may be secondary to diverticular disease, angiodysplasia, ulcerative colitis, ischemic colitis, neoplasm, or hemorrhoids. The immediate response to significant bleeding is to resuscitate the patient if they are unstable. Further evaluation includes bowel studies, including flexible sigmoidoscopy or colonoscopy. Radioisotope bleeding scans may be helpful in identifying the site of bleeding if the volume is >0.1 to 0.4 mL/minute. However, positive findings in this type of testing must be verified with an alternative test because of a relatively high number of false-positive results. Angiography may be useful in patients with active bleeding >0.5 mL/minute and can identify highly vascular nonbleeding lesions such as angiodysplasia and neoplasms.

Clinical Practice and Practice Economics committee, American Gastroenterological Association. AGA technical review on the evaluation and management of occult and obscure gastrointestinal bleeding. *Gastroenterology.* 2000;118:201–221.

73. Which of the following patients affected with chronic knee pain is best suited for joint replacement?
A) 45-year-old mailman
B) 52-year-old weekend golfer
C) 70-year-old retired banker
D) 20-year-old college athlete with hopes of a professional career
E) 42-year-old business executive

Answer and Discussion

The answer is C. Joint replacement is reserved for patients with intractable pain that does not respond to other medical regimens (i.e., nonsteroidal anti-inflammatory agents, gold or antimalarials, exercise and physical therapy, corticosteroids, and immunosuppressants). Surgery is usually reserved for patients older than 65 years who have severe arthritis. Osteoarthritis of the knee that is complicated by internal derangement may be treated with arthroscopic débridement or joint lavage. Osteotomy may be performed if significant malalignment of the knee or hip joints is present. Total joint arthroplasty usually has an excellent outcome and markedly improves quality of life. The life expectancy of the replaced joint varies, but is usually between 15 and 20 years.

Manek NJ, Lane NE. Osteoarthritis: current concepts in diagnosis and management. *Am Fam Physician.* 2000;61:1795–1804.

74. Which of the following is *false* regarding latex allergies?
A) Approximately 10% of health-care workers experience some form of allergic reaction to latex.
B) Latex is not found in catheters.
C) Persons allergic to latex also may be sensitive to fruits such as bananas, kiwis, pears, pineapples, grapes, and papayas.
D) Latex allergies became an important problem with the institution of universal precautions.
E) Many consumer products contain latex.

Answer and Discussion

The answer is B. Latex allergy has become a significant problem since the widespread adoption of universal precautions against infection. As many as 17% of health-care workers experience some form of allergic reaction to latex, although not all are anaphylaxis. Recognizing latex allergy is crucial, because physicians may inadvertently expose the patient to more latex during treatment. Latex is in gloves, catheters, and numerous other medical supplies, as well as consumer products. Persons allergic to latex also may be sensitive to fruits such as bananas, kiwis, pears, pineapples, grapes, and papayas.

Latex Hypersensitivity Committee of the American College of Allergy, Asthma, and Immunology. Latex allergy—an emerging healthcare problem. *Ann Allergy Asthma Immunol.* 1995;75:19–21.

Tang AW. A practical guide to anaphylaxis. *Am Fam Physician.* 2003;68:1325–1332, 1339–1340.

75. Risk factors for colon cancer include all of the following *except*
A) history of breast cancer
B) Asian descent
C) inflammatory bowel disease
D) Peutz-Jeghers syndrome
E) prior hyperplastic polyps

Answer and Discussion

The answer is E. Colorectal cancer is the leading cause of death due to cancer in the United States. Risk factors for colon cancer include the following:

- Personal or family history of colon cancer (two to four times risk when a first-degree relative is affected)
- Women with histories of breast or genital cancer
- Asian descent
- High-fat, low-fiber diet (although this is a controversial factor)
- Inflammatory bowel disease (greater risk with ulcerative colitis than with Crohn's disease)
- Gardner's syndrome
- Peutz-Jeghers syndrome
- Prior uterosigmoidostomy
- Advanced age (older than 50 years)
- History of colorectal polyps (adenomas)

The majority of cancers arise from preexisting adenomas and rarely do they form de novo. Warning signals for colorectal cancer include changes in bowel movements, abdominal pain, blood in the stool, fever, malaise, fatigue, or weight loss. A collaborative group of experts convened by the U.S. Agency for Health Care Policy and Research has recommended screening for average-risk persons older than 50 years using one of the following techniques:

- fecal occult blood testing each year
- flexible sigmoidoscopy every 5 years
- fecal occult blood testing every year combined with flexible sigmoidoscopy every 5 years
- double-contrast barium enema every 5 to 10 years or colonoscopy every 10 years

Screening of persons with risk factors should begin at an earlier age, depending on the family history of colorectal cancer or polyps. Medicare has recently agreed to provide reimburse-ment for screening colonoscopy. The U.S. Agency for Health Care Policy and Research panel recommended that persons who have first-degree relatives with colorectal cancer or adenomatous polyps undergo screening for colorectal neoplasia beginning at 40 years of age or 10 years before the age at which the diagnosis was made in the affected relative, whichever is earlier. Because patients whose first-degree relatives developed colorectal cancer before the age of 50 years may be at higher risk, complete colonic evaluation with colonoscopy should be strongly considered. Persons with a family history of familial adenomatous polyposis should undergo flexible sigmoidoscopy or colonoscopy at puberty. Lower endoscopy should be repeated every 1 to 2 years, because adenomatous polyps throughout the bowel generally precede cancer. Genetic testing should be considered, especially in large families with many at-risk members; in such situations, genotyping may be more cost-effective than repeated endoscopy. Expert panels convened by the U.S. Agency for Health Care Policy and Research and the Cancer Genetics Studies Consor-tium recommend that persons who are members of a family that fits the clinical criteria for hereditary non-polyposis colorectal cancer undergo colonoscopy at 20 to 25 years of age and every 1 to 3 years thereafter. In addition, these patients and their family members should be referred for genetic counseling. Patients with ulcerative colitis (or Crohn's disease) are commonly screened every 1 to 2 years by colonoscopy with multiple random biopsy samples to look for dysplasia. This screening is initiated 7 to 8 years after the diagnosis of pancolitis and 12 to 15 years after the diagnosis of left-sided colitis.

Read TE, Kodner IJ. Colorectal cancer: risk factors and recommendations for early detection. *Am Fam Physician.* 1999;59:2975.

76. A 56-year-old man presents to your office. He reports persistent, severe chest pain after repeated bouts of vomiting over the past 24 hours. The most appropriate management involves

A) chest x-ray
B) administration of H_2 antagonists
C) treadmill exercise testing
D) administration of proton pump inhibitor
E) observation with antiemetics

Answer and Discussion

The answer is A. Esophageal rupture, also known as *Boerhaave's syndrome*, is a rare, life-threatening condition that can lead to mediastinitis and pleural effusions. A delay in the diagnosis can lead to a poor prognosis. Symptoms include midsternal chest pain after a severe episode of vomiting. Associated conditions include peptic ulcer disease, alcoholism, and other neurologic disorders. The differential diagnosis includes myocardial infarction, pulmonary embolism, pancreatitis, peptic ulcer disease with rupture, or a dissecting aortic aneurysm. Chest radiographs and CT scans of the chest usually show pneumomediastinum, and a barium swallow showing communication between the esophagus and pleural space can be used to confirm the diagnosis. Treatment involves immediate surgery and drainage of any associated fluid collection.

Townsend CM, ed. *Sabiston textbook of surgery*, 16th ed. Philadelphia: WB Saunders; 2001:724–726.

77. Facial sutures should be removed at

A) 24 hours
B) 3 to 5 days
C) 7 to 10 days
D) 14 days
E) Only absorbable sutures should be used on the face.

Answer and Discussion

The answer is B. Postoperative care for lacerations does not include routine use of prophylactic antibiotics unless there is evidence of bacterial contamination or a risk factor is evident. Sutured or stapled lacerations should be covered with a protective, nonadherent dressing for at least 24 to 48 hours to avoid contamination. Patients should be instructed to observe the wound for the presence of warmth, redness, swelling, or drainage. Sutures or staples should be removed after approximately 7 days. Facial sutures should be removed within 3 to 5 days. Sutures in areas subject to high tension should be left in place for 10 to 14 days.

Hollander JE, Singer AJ. Laceration management. *Ann Emerg Med.* 1999;34:356–367.

78. The most appropriate treatment for cholesteatoma is

A) oral antibiotics
B) antibiotic otic drops
C) oral steroids
D) tympanostomy tube placement
E) surgical removal

Answer and Discussion

The answer is E. A cholesteatoma results from a chronic otitis media and perforation of the tympanic membrane. Prolonged dysfunction of the eustachian tube with the development of chronic negative pressure results in the formation of a squamous epithelial lined sac, which remains chronically infected. Cholesteatomas may be recognized during otoscopic examination by the white debris in the middle ear and the destruction of the ear canal bone adjacent to the perforation. Bone destruction due to an otherwise unsuspected cholesteatoma may be demonstrated on a CT scan. Aural polyps are usually associated with cholesteatomas. A cholesteatoma, particularly with an attic perforation, greatly increases the probability of a serious complication (e.g., purulent labyrinthitis, facial paralysis, intracranial suppuration). A cholesteatoma typically erodes the temporal bone and may destroy the small ossicle bones. With time, they can erode into the facial nerve or into the brain. Treatment involves surgical removal.

Beers MH, Berkow R, eds. *The Merck manual of diagnosis and therapy*, Merck Research Laboratories, 17th ed. Whitehouse Station, NJ: Merck & Co.; 1999:677.

A cholesteatoma typically erodes the temporal bone and may destroy the small ossicle bones.

79. A 27-year-old woman presents to the emergency room complaining of periumbilical pain, anorexia, and vomiting. Physical findings show a fever of 101.5° F, rebound tenderness, and extreme pain with rectal examination. The patient is also found to have positive psoas and obturator signs. The most likely diagnosis is

A) bowel infarction
B) acute appendicitis
C) acute cholecystitis
D) torsion of the ovary
E) ectopic pregnancy

Answer and Discussion

The answer is B. Appendicitis is the most common acute surgical condition of the abdomen. Approximately 7% of the population will have appendicitis in their lifetime, with the peak incidence occurring between the ages of 10 and 30 years. Despite technologic advances, the diagnosis of appendicitis is still based primarily on the patient's history and the physical examination. Prompt diagnosis and surgical referral may reduce the risk of perforation and prevent complications. The mortality rate in nonperforated appendicitis is less than 1%, but it may be as high as 5% or more in young and elderly patients in whom diagnosis may often be delayed, thus making perforation more likely. Appendicitis occurs when there is an obstruction in the appendiceal lumen. Although the symptoms are not always consistent, the typical presentation involves dull periumbilical pain that migrates to the right-lower abdomen. Anorexia, nausea, and vomiting usually accompany the onset of the abdominal pain. It is more common in adolescents; diagnosis in infants, the elderly, and obese and pregnant patients is often more difficult. Physical findings often include a low-grade fever, right-lower quadrant pain, rebound tenderness, and spasms of the overlying abdominal muscles with guarding. A positive psoas sign (i.e., pain with passive extension of the right hip) and obturator sign (i.e., pain with internal and external rotation of the flexed right hip) are strongly supportive of the diagnosis. Rectal examination may reveal localized tenderness. Laboratory results usually show a moderate leukocytosis (10,000 to 20,000 white blood cells/mm^3) with a left shift; however, this finding neither confirms nor excludes the diagnosis. Hematuria, proteinuria, and pyuria may be present. Visualization of the appendiceal lumen with a barium enema rules out the diagnosis. Ultrasound and CT examination may be helpful in determining the diagnosis in complicated cases. CT, specifically the technique of appendiceal CT, is more accurate than ultrasonography. Appendiceal CT consists of a focused, helical, appendiceal CT after a gastrografin saline enema (with or without oral contrast) and can be performed and interpreted within 1 hour. Intravenous contrast is unnecessary. The accuracy of CT is due in part to its ability to identify a normal appendix better than ultrasonography. An inflamed appendix is more than 6 mm in diameter, but the CT also demonstrates periappendiceal inflammatory changes. If appendiceal CT is not available, then a standard abdominal/pelvic CT with contrast remains highly useful and may be more accurate than ultrasonography. In most cases, diagnostic testing is unnecessary for the typical presentation of appendicitis. If the patient is suspected of having appendicitis, he or she should be given nothing by mouth, and surgical consultation should be pursued.

Hardin DM. Acute appendicitis: review and update. *Am Fam Physician.* 1999;60:2027–2034.

80. Application of tissue adhesives is useful in repairing lacerations; which of the following statements regarding adhesives is not true?

A) They are resistant to bacterial growth.
B) They have lower tensile strength when compared to sutures.
C) They are not useful on the hand.
D) Exposure to water has little effect on adhesives.
E) Adhesives are not recommended over high-tension areas.

Answer and Discussion

The answer is D. Tissue adhesives are used to close lacerations and have some advantages and disadvantages when compared to traditional suturing. Adhesives are resistant to bacterial growth and they have lower tensile strength when compared to sutures. They are not useful on the hand, and exposure to water is contraindicated. Adhesives are not recommended over high-tension areas.

Hollander JE, Singer AJ. Laceration management. *Ann Emerg Med.* 1999;34:356–367.

81. Diagnosis of corneal abrasions can best be accomplished in a family physician's office with

A) fluorescein dye examination
B) slit-lamp examination
C) hand-held ophthalmoscope
D) visual field testing
E) Schiøtz's tonometer

Answer and Discussion

The answer is A. Eye injuries are frequently encountered in the family physician's office. The following are some of the most common:

- *Corneal abrasions.* Corneal abrasions occur when there is localized loss of epithelium from the cornea typically caused by trauma. Symptoms include pain, foreign body sensation, tearing, and injection. A fluorescein dye examination is used to diagnose corneal abrasions. Treatment involves instilling a topical anesthetic before an examination is performed, followed by administering the fluorescein dye. A Wood's light is then used to examine all four quadrants of the globe. If an abrasion is detected, antibiotic drops are applied and the eye is covered for 24 hours (some recent evidence shows that patching may not always be necessary and may delay healing). The patient should be reexamined in 24 hours when the patch is removed. Visual acuity should be tested at the time of presentation and again the day after. Repeated patching with reexamination every 24 hours may be necessary until the abrasion heals. Antibiotic drops are usually continued for an additional 5 days.

- *Foreign bodies.* Inspection of the entire cornea is necessary to identify foreign bodies. The upper and lower eyelid should also be inspected. Foreign bodies should be removed by flushing with normal saline, cotton swab, eye spud, or 25-gauge needle. Fluorescein dye examination should be performed to rule out an abrasion. Rust rings should be examined for and removed as much as possible by an ophthalmologist; however, complete removal is unnecessary.
- *Blunt trauma.* Blunt trauma can cause orbital wall fractures. Signs and symptoms include diplopia, epistaxis, ecchymosis, crepitus, hypesthesia in the infraorbital nerve distribution, and restricted upward gaze secondary to inferior rectus entrapment. CT of the orbits is necessary for diagnosis. Surgical referral is indicated.
- *Subconjunctival hemorrhage.* This condition is present when there is a well-demarcated area of injection from the rupture of small subconjunctival vessels. Causes include trauma, coughing, vomiting, straining, or viral hemorrhagic conjunctivitis. Blood in the anterior chamber indicates a hyphema and requires immediate ophthalmologic referral.

Graber MA, Toth PP, Herting RL Jr. *University of Iowa: The Family Practice Handbook*, 3rd ed. St. Louis: Mosby; 1997:525.

82. Which of the following statements about epistaxis is true?
A) Unless there are previous symptoms of infection, the use of antibiotics while nasal packs are in place is unwarranted.
B) Nasal packs should be left in place for at least 72 hours.
C) In most cases, anterior bleeding originates from Kiesselbach's area.
D) The use of silver nitrate or electric cautery is contraindicated in the nose.
E) Patients with chronic obstructive pulmonary disease are not affected by nasal packing, because the majority are mouth breathers.

Answer and Discussion

The answer is C. Nosebleeds can be caused by a number of different mechanisms including trauma, nose picking, infection, foreign bodies, excessive drying of the nasal mucosa, and bleeding disorders. Most bleeding originates from a plexus of vessels in the anteroinferior septum called *Kiesselbach's plexus*. In most cases, pinching the nasal ala together for 10 to 15 minutes stops the bleeding. If nasal bleeding continues, identifying the source is the goal. Once the source is located, nasal packing or cauterization with silver nitrate or electric cautery may be necessary. If the nose is packed, antibiotics such as trimethoprim-sulfamethoxazole should be started while the packing is in place. Packs should not be left in place more than 48 hours. If bleeding continues, a posterior source is most likely the cause, and a posterior pack should be placed by an otolaryngologist. Hospitalization for observation is indicated with serial blood counts in posterior bleeds. For severe nosebleeds, a bleeding time and von Willebrand's factor should be checked to rule out bleeding disorders. Caution should be used when placing nasal packs in patients with chronic obstructive pulmonary disease, because the nasopulmonary reflex can produce a 15 mm Hg drop in PO_2.

Graber MA, Toth PP, Herting RL Jr. *University of Iowa: The Family Practice Handbook*, 3rd ed. St. Louis: Mosby; 1997:699–700.

83. A patient collapses in your office. A cardiac monitor is placed and the rhythm is determined to be ventricular fibrillation. Despite three defibrillation shocks, intravenous epinephrine, and a further attempt at defibrillation there is no change. The patient is unconscious. What is the most appropriate next step?
A) Another attempt at defibrillation
B) Administer lidocaine
C) Administer amiodarone
D) Administer procainamide
E) Administer magnesium sulfate

Answer and Discussion

The answer is C. Intravenous amiodarone appears to be more effective than lidocaine, as demonstrated in the ALIVE trial of 347 patients with persistent or recurrent VF despite three defibrillation shocks, intravenous epinephrine, and a further attempt at defibrillation.

Dorian P, Cass D, Schwartz B, et al. Amiodarone as compared with lidocaine for shock-resistant ventricular fibrillation. *N Engl J Med.* 2002;346:884.

84. A 60-year-old man presents with pain in the upper legs that is exacerbated with walking. Symptoms are relieved with sitting. Peripheral pulses are intact. The most likely diagnosis is
A) spinal stenosis
B) claudication
C) dissecting aortic aneurysm
D) incarcerated inguinal hernia
E) myasthenia gravis

Answer and Discussion

The answer is A. Spinal stenosis is a condition characterized by pain in the legs, calves, thighs, and buttocks that occurs with walking, running, or climbing stairs. Symptoms are often relieved by flexing at the spine or sitting. Conversely, lying prone or in any position that extends the lumbar spine exacerbates the symptoms, presumably because of ventral infolding of the ligamentum flavum in a canal already significantly narrowed by degenerative osseus changes. Middle-age patients and the elderly are most commonly affected. Typically, the earliest complaint is back pain, which is relatively nonspecific and may result in delayed diagnosis. Patients then often experience leg fatigue, pain, numbness, and weakness, sometimes several months to years after the back pain was first noticed. Patients may undergo minor trauma that can exacerbate symptoms, which may lead to a more rapid diagnosis. Once the leg pain begins, it is most commonly bilateral, involving the buttocks and thighs and spreading distally toward the feet, typically with the onset and progression of leg exercise. In some patients, the pain, paresthesias, and/or weakness are limited to the lower legs and feet, remaining present until movement ceases. The lower extremity symptoms are almost always described as burning, cramping, numbness, tingling, or dull fatigue in the thighs and legs. Disease onset is usually insidious; early symptoms may be mild and progress to become extremely disabling. Symptom severity does not always correlate with the degree of lumbar canal narrowing. Causes include osteoarthritis, spondylolisthesis with associated edema in the area of the cauda equina, and Paget's disease affecting the lower spine. Spinal stenosis may be difficult to distinguish from claudication; however, with spinal stenosis, there are usually neurologic deficits present and peripheral pulses are normal. MRI scanning, with its multiplanar-imaging capability, is currently the preferred modality for establishing a diagnosis and excluding other conditions. The MRI depicts soft tissues, including the cauda equina, spinal cord, ligaments, epidural fat, subarachnoid space, and intervertebral discs, with exquisite detail in most instances. Loss of epidural fat on T_1-weighted images, loss of cerebrospinal fluid signal around the dural sac on T_2-weighted images, and degenerative disc disease are common features of lumbar stenosis on MRI. Treatment for symptomatic lumbar stenosis is usually surgical decompression. Medical treatment alternatives such as bed rest, pain management, and physical therapy should be reserved for use in debilitated patients or patients whose surgical risk is prohibitive as a result of concomitant medical conditions.

Alvarez JA, Hardy RH Jr. Lumbar spine stenosis: a common cause of back and leg pain. *Am Fam Physician.* 1998;57:1825.

85. A 31-year-old man is brought to the emergency room after suffering severe injuries in a motorcycle accident. A dipstick urinalysis shows hemoglobin. However, the microscopic examination fails to show red blood cells (RBCs). The most likely diagnosis is

A) renal trauma
B) urethral rupture
C) laboratory error
D) myoglobinuria
E) underlying urinary tract infection

Answer and Discussion

The answer is D. Myoglobinuria is a condition that results when there is massive muscle destruction known as *rhabdomyolysis*. The condition occurs as a result of severe infection, toxic insult, inflammation, or metabolic or traumatic damage to the muscles. Laboratory findings include elevated creatinine kinase, lactate dehydrogenase, aspartate aminotransferase, alanine aminotransferase, and a positive urine test for blood with the absence of RBCs. Specific tests for the detection of myoglobinuria are done with immunoassay. Treatment involves correcting the underlying causative factor and administering fluids. Renal failure may require further treatment.

Beers MH, Berkow R, eds. *The Merck manual of diagnosis and therapy*, Merck Research Laboratories, 17th ed. Whitehouse Station, NJ: Merck & Co.; 1999:1808.

86. At what age do children develop anticipatory pain when faced with a potentially painful situation?

A) 3 months
B) 6 months
C) 12 months
D) 24 months
E) 36 months

Answer and Discussion

The answer is B. Children's perception of pain is influenced by age, cognitive level, and past experiences of painful experiences. Other factors affecting pain perception include the perceived cause and expected duration of the pain, extent of control over the situation, and parental response. The response to pain differs with the level of development and age of the child. Treatment approaches should account for these differences. Following are some characteristics:

- *Younger than 6 months:* Infants do not express anticipatory fear. Their level of anxiety reflects that of the parent. Typical responses are facial grimacing, thrashing of extremities, withdrawal from the painful stimulus, and crying a few seconds after the event.
- *6 to 18 months:* Infants begin to develop fear of painful experiences and withdraw when pain is anticipated (e.g., when they see a needle).
- *18 to 24 months:* Children express pain with words such as "hurt" or "boo boo."
- *3 years:* Children more reliably assess the pain they feel. They begin to localize pain and identify external causes. However, they depend on a visual injury or cause for adequate localization and are unable to understand a reason for pain. Control over certain aspects of a procedure (e.g., when and where it is performed) improves their tolerance.
- *5 to 7 years:* Children in this age group have improvements in understanding of pain, the ability to localize internal pain, and cooperation.

Comprehension continues to grow as the child becomes older. By adolescence, patients become more adept at qualifying and quantifying pain, and they develop cognitive coping strategies that help to diminish physical pain.

Joseph MH, Brill J, Zeltzer LK. Pediatric pain relief in trauma. *Pediatr Rev.* 1999;20:75.

87. Duodenal obstruction is associated with which of the following radiographic signs?

A) Bird's beak sign
B) Hampton's hump
C) Double bubble sign
D) Kerley B lines
E) Scalloping of the diaphragm

Answer and Discussion

The answer is C. Duodenal obstruction is a congenital abnormality that can be caused by several different abnormalities, including duodenal atresia, duodenal stenosis, and malrotation of the intestine. Infants with Down syndrome are at increased risk. Symptoms include projectile vomiting after the first few feedings. Polyhydramnios may also be present during pregnancy and is caused by a failure of absorption of amniotic fluid in the distal intestine. Diagnosis is usually made radiographically. Plain radiographs show the characteristic "double bubble" sign—one large bubble in the stomach with a smaller adjacent bubble that represents the duodenum. If atresia is present, no abdominal gas is seen in the distal bowel; however, if stenosis is present, a small amount of gas may be present. A barium swallow helps localize the site of obstruction. Treatment involves nasogastric suction to decompress the stomach and surgery to correct the obstruction.

Townsend CM, ed. *Sabiston textbook of surgery*, 16th ed. Philadelphia: WB Saunders; 2001:1469.

Duodenal obstruction is associated with a "double bubble" radiographic sign.

88. When repairing a facial laceration, it is important to test all aspects of the facial nerve. Which of the following tasks tests the zygomatic branch?

A) Contract the forehead and elevate the eyebrow
B) Open and shut the eyes

C) Smile
D) Frown
E) Contract the platysma muscle

Answer and Discussion

The answer is B. When repairing a facial laceration the facial nerve function should be tested in all five branches as follows:

- *Temporal:* Contract the forehead and elevate the eyebrow
- *Zygomatic:* Open and shut eyes
- *Buccal:* Smile
- *Mandibular:* Frown
- *Cervical:* Contract the platysma muscle

Trott AT. Wounds and Lacerations. St. Louis: Mosby-Year Book, 1991.

89. A 42-year-old woman following the American Cancer Society guidelines should have a mammogram
A) beginning at 50 years of age
B) every 2 years
C) every year
D) every 3 years
E) every 5 years

Answer and Discussion

The answer is C. Breast cancer is the most common cancer that affects women. Approximately 1 in 9 to 10 women will have breast cancer during her life. Unfortunately, it is the second leading cause of cancer death. The screening guidelines for the diagnosis of breast cancer are continually changing. Because of increased awareness of the signs and symptoms of breast cancer and the use of screening mammograms, breast cancers are increasingly being diagnosed at earlier stages. The American Cancer Society recommends annual mammograms and clinical breast examinations for women older than 40 years. Women older than 20 years should be encouraged to do monthly breast self-examinations, and women between 20 and 39 years of age should have a clinical breast examination every 3 years. These guidelines are modified for women with risk factors, particularly those with a strong family history of breast cancer. Risk factors for breast cancer include the following:

- First-degree relative with breast cancer (especially premenopausal)
- Prior breast cancer in the patient
- Nulliparity
- First pregnancy after the age of 35 years
- Early menarche (before age 12 years)
- Late menopause (older than 50 years)
- *BRCA* gene mutation
- Age older than 50 years
- Age older than 30 at first birth
- Obesity
- High socioeconomic status
- Atypical hyperplasia on biopsy
- Ionizing radiation exposure

Apantaku LM. Breast cancer diagnosis and screening. *Am Fam Physician.* 2000;62:596–602, 605–606.

90. Which of the following foreign bodies should not be removed with irrigation from the ear?
A) Plastic bead
B) Small pebble
C) BB
D) Alkaline button battery
E) Metal part from a matchbox car

Answer and Discussion

The answer is D. Small, inorganic objects can be removed from the external auditory canal by irrigation. The irrigation solution should be at body temperature, and the stream of water should be directed along the superior margin of the external ear canal and should deliver an adequate volume of water with brisk flow. This volume can be achieved using a 20 to 50 mL syringe attached to a flexible catheter or plastic tubing from a butterfly needle. This technique is contraindicated if the tympanic membrane is perforated or the foreign body is vegetable matter or an alkaline button battery. Organic matter swells as it absorbs water, leading to further obstruction. Irrigation of the button battery enhances leakage and potential for liquefaction necrosis.

Kavanagh KT, Litovitz T. Miniature battery foreign bodies in auditory and nasal cavities. *JAMA.* 1986;255:1470.

91. Which of the following is the best time for a woman to perform breast self-examination?
A) During mid-cycle
B) One week before menses
C) During the first week after menses
D) During menstruation

Answer and Discussion

The answer is C. Breast self-examination should begin at 20 years of age and be repeated each month during the first week following menses, which is when fibrocystic changes are less prominent. The technique involves examining all quadrants of the breast in a systematic, circular motion. The tips of the middle three fingers should be used, and patients should examine themselves sitting up and in the supine position. The recommendations for mammographic screening include screening every 1 to 2 years after age 40.

If a woman has a strong family history for breast cancer, *BRCA* gene mutation, or a previous abnormal mammogram, more frequent screening may be necessary. Medicare pays for biannual screening for women older than 65 years. The false-negative rate for mammography is approximately 10% to 15%. Elderly women whose life expectancy is 5 to 10 years should continue to undergo mammographic and clinical breast examination screening.

Apantaku LM. Breast cancer diagnosis and screening. *Am Fam Physician.* 2000;62:596–602, 605–606.

92. Which of the following is associated with a positive Tinel's sign?
A) Carpal tunnel syndrome
B) Scaphoid fracture
C) de Quervain's tenosynovitis
D) Raynaud's phenomenon
E) Gamekeeper's thumb

Answer and Discussion

The answer is A. Carpal tunnel syndrome occurs when there is an entrapment of the median nerve at the level of the wrist. Symptoms include pain, numbness, and paresthesia in the distribution of the median nerve, including the palmar surface of the first three fingers. Symptoms characteristically occur at night and may awaken the patient. Symptoms may also involve the forearm or shoulder. Women are more frequently affected than men, and the condition can involve one or both hands. Percussion of the median nerve at the area of the carpal tunnel (Tinel's sign), sustained flexion of the wrist (Phalen's sign), or extension of the wrist (reverse Phalen's sign) reproduce symptoms. Other clinical findings include weakness of the thumb and thenar atrophy. Carpal tunnel syndrome is associated with continuous repetitive flexion of the wrist, pregnancy (most cases resolve after delivery), acromegaly, rheumatoid arthritis, and myxedema. Nerve conduction tests are used to help make the diagnosis but are not always necessary. Treatment includes anti-inflammatory agents, wrist braces, and steroid injections; surgery is indicated in severe cases that are unresponsive to conservative therapy.

Taylor R, David AK, Johnson TA Jr, et al., eds. *Family medicine: principles and practice*, 5th ed. New York: Springer-Verlag; 1998:576–577.

93. Which of the following is indicated immediately after a minor burn?

A) Application of butter
B) Rapid cooling with ice
C) Extensive debridement of non viable skin
D) Application of room temperature water
E) Firm washing to remove particulate matter

Answer and Discussion

The answer is D. Initial treatment of minor thermal injuries consists mainly of cooling (with room temperature water, not with ice), simple gentle cleansing with mild soap and water, and appropriate dressing. Pain management and tetanus prophylaxis are important. Extensive debridement is generally not immediately necessary and may be deferred until the initial follow-up visit.

Morgan ED, Miser WF. Treatment of minor thermal burns. Up to Date, version 14.1. Accessed 3/20/2006.

94. A 17-year-old high school football player is knocked unconscious for a brief period during a game for which you provide medical coverage. He now is doing well, and the results of his examination are normal. The most appropriate action is

A) transfer the athlete to a local emergency room
B) keep the athlete out of the game for a full quarter; if he remains normal, he may return to play
C) prohibit the athlete from returning to play for 5 to 7 days
D) allow the athlete to return to competition after 10 additional minutes of normal observation
E) prohibit the athlete from returning to play for the rest of the season

Answer and Discussion

The answer is C. If the cervical spine is not injured and the level of consciousness is not significantly altered, the athlete can be allowed to sit up and, if stable, walk off the field with support. A review of symptoms and a complete neurologic and head and neck evaluation are performed on the bench. If the examination is negative, the athlete should be observed for 15 minutes (typically one quarter of play) unless there is a history of loss of consciousness. If no loss of consciousness and no return of symptoms occur during the 15 minutes, the next step is a provocative test such as a 40-yard dash. If no symptoms return, the athlete may be returned to the game, but repeated observations must be performed. If any symptoms return, the athlete must be removed from the game. If the athlete has documented loss of consciousness or signs and symptoms that did not clear in 15 minutes or that returned with the provocative test, the athlete should not be allowed to return to competition. Any new or unusual headaches within the first 48 to 72 hours after the injury should be treated as a medical emergency. In addition, any deterioration in mental status or deterioration in physical condition is a medical emergency. When to return the athlete to play after the first concussion that resulted in loss of consciousness is controversial. Most recommend that the athlete not compete for 5 to 7 days. Before any return to competition, the athlete must be evaluated by the same clinician who performed the initial evaluation.

Wojtys EM, Hovda D, Landry G, et al. Concussion in sports. *Am J Sports Med.* 1999;27:676–687.

95. A 21 year old is brought to the emergency room by ambulance after developing sudden shortness of breath. A chest radiograph shows a 10% pneumothorax. The patient remains stable. Appropriate management includes

A) immediate chest tube placement
B) intubation and mechanical ventilation
C) pulmonary function testing
D) large-bore needle placed in the second intercostal space
E) observation

Answer and Discussion

The answer is E. Pneumothorax is the accumulation of air within the pleural space. The usual cause of pneumothorax is a penetrating wound such as a stabbing, gunshot wound, or deceleration-type injury (e.g., as seen in motor vehicle accidents). Spontaneous pneumothorax can also occur and typically affects tall, thin men or smokers (as a result of a ruptured bleb). Clinical findings include decreased breath sounds on the side affected, shortness of breath, chest pain (most common symptom), cough, distended neck veins, and hypotension. A chest radiograph is usually diagnostic. Treatment may require immediate intervention but in many cases depends on the extent of pneumothorax. If pneumothorax involves up to 15% to 20% of lung volume, observation is the only treatment necessary. Supplemental oxygen is usually administered, and most cases resolve in 10 days. For larger pneumothoraces, chest tube placement is necessary. Tension pneumothoraces require emergent decompression with a large-bore needle placed in the second intercostal space followed by chest tube placement.

Townsend CM, ed. *Sabiston textbook of surgery*, 16th ed. Philadelphia: WB Saunders; 2001:1180–1182.

96. If an unprotected individual develops minimal erythema after 20 minutes of sun exposure, after use of an SPF-8 sunscreen, minimal erythema would be expected after how many minutes exposure?

A) 60 minutes
B) 100 minutes
C) 160 minutes
D) 200 minutes
E) 300 minutes

Answer and Discussion

The answer is C. Sun protection factor (SPF) is a measure of the ability of a blocking agent (typically clothing or sunscreen) to prevent erythema in response to sun exposure. The SPF can be multiplied by the time of exposure necessary to produce minimal erythema in an unprotected individual to get the expected time until minimal erythema using that protection. As an example, if an unprotected individual develops minimal erythema after 20 minutes of sun exposure, after use of an SPF-8 sunscreen, minimal erythema would be expected after 160 minutes of exposure. However, the duration of protection with sunscreen may be shorter in many circumstances than the SPF would indicate.

Johnson KR. Sunburn. Up to Date, version 14.1. Accessed 3/20/2006.

97. The most appropriate test for the detection of a subdural hematoma is
A) skull radiographs
B) CT of the head with and without contrast
C) CT of the head without contrast
D) MRI of the head
E) lumbar puncture

Answer and Discussion

The answer is C. CT scans can be used to look for numerous intracranial processes. Intravenous contrast should be given when looking for intracranial tumors; however, the use of contrast is not necessary when looking for subdural, epidural, or intracranial hemorrhages. Blood is denser than brain tissue; thus, the color differential makes the diagnosis of intracranial blood accumulation relatively simple without contrast. Cerebral vascular accidents may not be immediately visible on CT scanning until several days after the event. Serial scans may show progressive involvement over several days if the stroke is severe. Contrast is not necessary for the detection of strokes.

Graber MA, Toth PP, Herting RL Jr. *University of Iowa: The Family Practice Handbook*, 3rd ed. St. Louis: Mosby; 1997:583.

> When performing computed tomography (CT), intravenous contrast should be given when looking for intracranial tumors; however, the use of contrast is not necessary when looking for subdural, epidural, or intracranial hemorrhages.

98. For individuals with average risk factors, screening flexible sigmoidoscopy should begin at age
A) 40 years
B) 50 years
C) 65 years
D) 70 years

Answer and Discussion

The answer is B. The U.S. Agency for Health Care Policy and Research has recommended screening for average-risk persons older than 50 years using one of the following techniques:

- fecal occult blood testing each year
- flexible sigmoidoscopy every 5 years
- fecal occult blood testing every year combined with flexible sigmoidoscopy every 5 years
- double-contrast barium enema every 5 to 10 years
- colonoscopy every 10 years

Screening of persons with risk factors should begin at an earlier age, depending on the situation. Digital rectal examinations should begin at 40 years of age. The major complication associated with flexible sigmoidoscopy is intestinal perforation, which occurs in <0.05% of cases. Polyps are usually described as sessile, broad based, or pedunculated. Polyps are usually classified histologically into hyperplastic and adenomatous types. If adenomatous polyps are noted, the patient should undergo colonoscopy to rule out synchronous polyps located more proximally in the colon. Tubular adenomas are the most common type of adenomatous polyp and have a 5% chance of malignant growth. Less commonly seen are villous-type polyps, which possess malignant cells in up to 40%. Size is also used to predict malignant potential. If the polyp is <1 cm, only 1% of polyps contain malignant growth. If the polyp is 1 to 2 cm, 10% contain malignant growth. If the polyp is >2 cm, 35% to 45% have malignant growth. Hyperplastic polyps have no malignancy potential.

Townsend CM, ed. *Sabiston textbook of surgery*, 16th ed. Philadelphia: WB Saunders; 2001:957.

99. Which of the following statements is *false* regarding the treatment of high-voltage lightning injuries?
A) Cervical spine immobilization and clearance should be performed.
B) Airway burns should be administered.
C) Tetanus immunization should be administered.
D) Serum CK-MB measurements should be measured to assess myocardial injury.
E) Cardiac monitoring should be maintained after the injury.

Answer and Discussion

The answer is D. A patient exposed to a serious electrical burn or lightning strike should be treated as a trauma patient. Resuscitation should begin with a rapid assessment of airway and cardiopulmonary status. Cervical spine immobilization and clearance should be maintained, and tetanus vaccination should be administered. Coexisting smoke inhalation or airway burns should be excluded. Patients can have spontaneous cardiac activity but paralysis of the respiratory muscles. Prompt restoration of a secure airway may prevent secondary cardiac and neurologic dysfunction or death. Coma or neurologic deficit should include brain and/or spine imaging. An extensive head-to-toe and neurologic examination should be performed. The survivor of high-energy injury should have cardiac and hemodynamic monitoring due to the high incidence of arrhythmia and autonomic dysfunction, especially if there have been arrhythmias in the field or emergency department, loss of consciousness, or if the initial ECG is abnormal. Serum CK-MB measurements and ECG changes are poor measures of myocardial injury. The diagnostic and prognostic value of cardiac troponin levels has not been evaluated in this setting.

Xenopoulos N, Movahed A, Hudson P, et al. Myocardial injury in electrocution. *Am Heart J.* 1991;122:1481.

McBride JW, Labrosse KR, McCoy HG, et al. Is serum creatine kinase-MB in electrically injured patients predictive of myocardial injury? *JAMA.* 1986;255:764.

100. An 18 year old with a history of von Willebrand's deficiency is involved in a motor vehicle accident and presents to the emergency room. There is concern about bleeding; however, the patient is stable. You want to minimize the amount of fluid the patient receives. Which of the following would be indicated to help correct the coagulation disorder?
A) Platelets
B) Cryoprecipitate

C) Whole blood
D) Fresh frozen plasma (FFP)
E) Packed RBCs

Answer and Discussion

The answer is B. The following are blood products available to treat various bleeding disorders and hemorrhagic conditions:

- *Whole blood*: Typically, whole blood is used to treat patients in an emergent setting who have lost more than 15% of their blood volume. Whole blood is less expensive than packed RBCs and plasma and has a lower infectious risk. The oxygen-carrying capacity and replacement of volume can be replaced as effectively with packed RBCs and crystalloid. However, the storage of whole blood is very inefficient, and most blood banks do not routinely store this product.
- *Packed RBCs*: Packed RBCs can be stored in cooled storage for up to 35 days; however, refrigerated temperatures cause platelets to degenerate, so banked, packed RBCs contain essentially no functioning platelets. Also, factors V and VII decrease with refrigeration; however, other factors remain unchanged. Packed RBC transfusion should be used only when time or the clinical situation precludes other therapy. Each unit of packed RBCs usually raises the hematocrit 2% to 3% in a 70-kg adult, although this varies depending on the donor, the recipient's fluid status, the method of storage, and its duration. Leukocyte-poor RBCs may be given to help reduce transfusion reactions in those who have experienced reactions with previous transfusions.
- *Platelets*: Platelet transfusions are indicated if patients have thrombocytopenia or platelet dysfunction, or both. Patients are usually administered 6 or 10 units at one time (*6-pack* or *10-pack*). Multiple-unit, single-donor platelets are harvested from one donor using apheresis. After platelet transfusion in the adult, the platelet count obtained at 1 hour should rise at least 5,000 platelets/mm^3 for each unit of platelets transfused. Patients may experience a smaller response after multiple transfusions. Platelets should not be routinely given for bleeding prophylaxis unless there is evidence of microvascular bleeding or planned surgery and the platelet count is <50,000/mm^3 or the platelet count is <10,000/mm^3 (for prophylaxis against bleeding). Previous guidelines of 20,000/mm^3 are no longer used. Patients receiving massive transfusion should not automatically receive platelets in the absence of microvascular bleeding. Additionally, body temperature can affect platelets' ability to function, and, ideally, body temperature should be restored before consideration of platelet transfusion.
- *FFP*: FFP is used to replace labile clotting factors. A unit of FFP contains near normal levels of all clotting factors, including approximately 400 mg of fibrinogen. A unit of FFP increases clotting factors by approximately 3%. Adequate clotting is usually obtained with factor levels >30% (however, higher levels are recommended before surgery). FFP is used to correct prothrombin time and activated partial thromboplastin time. FFP should not be used routinely after RBC transfusion without evidence of coagulopathy, as a volume expander, nutritional supplement, or for hypoalbuminemia. A new FFP called *solvent detergent plasma* is treated to inactivate enveloped viruses (human immunodeficiency virus; hepatitis B, C) and has virtually no risk in transmitting these viruses.
- *Cryoprecipitate*: Cryoprecipitate is useful in treating factor deficiencies such as hemophilia A, von Willebrand's disease, and hypofibrinogenemia. Because proteins are in high concentrations, a smaller volume can be used than with FFP. Cryoprecipitate is usually administered as a transfusion of 10 single units.

Townsend CM, ed. *Sabiston textbook of surgery*, 16th ed. Philadelphia: WB Saunders; 2001:70–73.

101. Which of the following medications could make the pain of acute cholecystitis worse?
A) Acetaminophen
B) Propoxyphene
C) Meperidine
D) Morphine
E) Naproxen

Answer and Discussion

The answer is D. The administration of morphine during attacks of pancreatitis can lead to spasm of the sphincter of Oddi and exacerbate pain symptoms; therefore, meperidine is typically used for the treatment of pain associated with cholecystitis. It is important to remember that meperidine (Demerol) has several disadvantages when compared with other narcotic preparations. In particular, there is potential for a neurotoxic metabolite, normeperidine, to accumulate and cause seizures, myoclonus, and tremors. This may be of specific concern for alcoholic patients who are already at risk for developing neurologic complications of ethanol withdrawal. Furthermore, meperidine has a shorter duration of action than morphine or hydromorphone and is, therefore, less effective for sustained analgesia and more likely to result in a potentially avoidable "rebound" effect. Finally, meperidine is more likely to cause muscle fibrosis than competing narcotics when administered intramuscularly.

Munoz A, Katerndahl DA. Diagnosis and management of acute pancreatitis. *Am Fam Physician.* 2000;62:164–174.

102. Which of the following is a risk factor for a near-drowning or drowning event?
A) Resident of Northeast coastal states
B) Age between 6 to 10 years
C) Low socioeconomic status
D) White/Caucasian race
E) Female sex

Answer and Discussion

The answer is C. The highest incidence of near-drowning occurs among males, African Americans, children between the ages of 1 and 5 years, persons with low socioeconomic status, and among residents of southern states. Drowning is much more common during the summer months.

Quan L, Cummings P. Characteristics of drowning by different age groups. *Inj Prev.* 2003;9:163.

Ellis AA, Trent RB. Hospitalizations for near drowning in California: incidence and costs. *Am J Public Health.* 1995; 85:1115.

103. Which of the following statements regarding acute pancreatitis is true?
A) All patients should receive nasogastric suction to maintain strict bowel rest.
B) Anticholinergics are useful in the treatment of acute pancreatitis.

C) Amylase is the most sensitive and specific test for the detection of acute pancreatitis.
D) Enteral feedings (distal to the ligament of Treitz) can be beneficial after 48 hours for severe cases.
E) Nausea and vomiting are rarely present.

Answer and Discussion

The answer is D. Acute pancreatitis usually results from alcohol abuse or bile duct obstruction. Patients with acute pancreatitis present with mild to severe epigastric pain with radiation to the flank, back, or both. Classically, the pain is characterized as constant, dull, and boring, and is worse when the patient is supine. The discomfort may lessen when the patient assumes a sitting or fetal position. A heavy meal or drinking binge often triggers the pain. Nausea and nonfeculent vomiting are present in the vast majority of patients. Serum amylase and lipase (more sensitive and specific) levels are still used to confirm the diagnosis of acute pancreatitis. Although not routinely available, the serum trypsin level is the most accurate laboratory indicator for pancreatitis. Ultrasonography, CT, and endoscopic retrograde cholangiopancreatography are used in some cases for confirming the diagnosis. Prompt identification of patients who need intensive care referral or subspecialty consultation is crucial. Intravenous rehydration should usually be aggressive, with close attention to blood pressure and cardiac and pulmonary status. Therapies such as nasogastric suctioning, anticholinergics, and histamine H_2-receptor blockers have not been shown to decrease symptoms or hospital stays in patients with acute pancreatitis. In the past, patients were routinely treated by withholding food and placing a nasogastric tube with suction for 2 to 10 days. This was done in an attempt to reduce pancreatic stimulation by food, hydrochloric acid, cholecystokinin, and secretin. Withholding food by mouth does reduce pain, but the use of a nasogastric tube with suction is no longer advocated as a routine therapeutic measure in acute pancreatitis, because it has not been shown to decrease symptoms, mortality, or hospital stay. However, a nasogastric tube may be used when the patient has protracted vomiting or if obstruction is seen on the abdominal radiograph. Anticholinergics have been used in an attempt to decrease gastric secretions and increase pH. As with the use of nasogastric tubes, anticholinergics do not decrease hospital stay or pain. In mild pancreatitis, oral intake should be withheld until the nausea and vomiting subside. Total enteral feeding beyond the ligament of Treitz administered within 48 hours of onset of severe acute pancreatitis may reduce the incidence of total and infectious complications. Systemic antibiotics (although controversial) have been found to improve outcome in patients with severe disease. With supportive care, most patients have a good clinical outcome.

Munoz A, Katerndahl DA. Diagnosis and management of acute pancreatitis. *Am Fam Physician.* 2000;62:164–174.

104. A 75 year old presents to your office complaining of anorexia, nausea, abdominal pain, and muscle weakness. Laboratory tests show an elevated calcium level. The most likely diagnosis is
A) osteoporosis
B) Paget's disease
C) hyperparathyroidism
D) myasthenia gravis
E) chronic fatigue syndrome

Answer and Discussion

The answer is C. Hyperparathyroidism is a common cause of hypercalcemia. The incidence of hyperparathyroidism increases with age. Women are more commonly affected. The hypercalcemia usually is discovered during a routine serum chemistry profile. Often, there has been no previous suspicion of this disorder. In most patients initially believed to be asymptomatic, previously unrecognized symptoms resolve with surgical correction of the disorder. In the majority of the persons affected, primary hyperparathyroidism is the result of an adenoma in a single parathyroid gland. Hypertrophy of all four parathyroid glands causes hyperparathyroidism in a smaller percentage of patients. A very small number of cases of hyperparathyroidism result from parathyroid malignancies. In addition, the incidence of hyperparathyroidism is higher in patients with type I and type II multiple endocrine neoplasia syndromes, in patients with familial hyperparathyroidism, and in patients who received radiation therapy to the head and neck area for benign diseases during childhood. Chronic renal failure, rickets, and malabsorption syndromes are the most frequent conditions leading to secondary hyperparathyroidism. The symptoms of hyperparathyroidism are vague and often similar to symptoms of depression, irritable bowel syndrome, fibromyalgia, or stress reaction. Some combination of headaches, fatigue, anorexia, nausea, paresthesias, muscular weakness, pain in the extremities, pain in the abdomen, and other such nonspecific symptoms appears to be the most common presentation of primary hyperparathyroidism. Complications of primary hyperparathyroidism include peptic ulcers, nephrolithiasis, pancreatitis, and dehydration. Intravenous hydration is the most critical treatment for a patient with an acute presentation of hyperparathyroidism and hypercalcemia. The addition of furosemide (Lasix) increases urinary calcium loss. Administration of pamidronate (Aredia) inhibits bone resorption and lowers serum calcium levels. Other drugs that have been used in the management of acute hyperparathyroidism include calcitonin (Calcimar, Miacalcin), glucocorticoids, and mithramycin (Mithracin), although use of the latter agent is limited by its toxicity. When medical management is used, routine monitoring for clinical deterioration is recommended. Surgical management is usually indicated in most cases. Preoperative localization of adenomas with technetium Tc 99m sestamibi scan is possible but may be unnecessary. An experienced surgeon should perform the parathyroidectomy.

Allerheiligen DA, Schoeber J, Houston RE, et al. Hyperparathyroidism. *Am Fam Physician.* 1998:1795.

105. Patients who have been scuba diving should wait at least _____ before flying because of the risk of decompression illness.
A) 4 hours
B) 12 hours
C) 24 hours
D) 72 hours
E) 1 week

Answer and Discussion

The answer is B. Patients who travel by air soon after scuba diving are at increased risk for developing decompression sickness (DCS) inflight. Such a passenger should be advised to wait 12 hours before flying, if he or she has been making only 1 dive/day. Individuals who have participated in multiple dives or those requiring decompression stops should consider waiting up to 48 hours before flying.

Sheffield PJ. Flying after diving guidelines: a review. *Aviat Space Environ Med.* 1990;61:1130.

Freiberger JJ, Denoble PJ, Pieper CF, et al. The relative risk of decompression sickness during and after air travel following diving. *Aviat Space Environ Med.* 2002;73:980.

106. Which of the following statements is true regarding breast implants?

A) There is a higher incidence of connective tissue disease in patients who received silicone breast implants.
B) There is a higher incidence of breast cancer in women who have had breast augmentation.
C) Mammography (with Eklund views) can be helpful in assessing breast lumps after augmentation.
D) MRI is not helpful in detecting rupture of breast implants.
E) According to the U.S. Food and Drug Administration, all women with silicone breast implants should have them removed.

Answer and Discussion

The answer is C. Women who have undergone augmentation mammoplasty with silicone gel implants may present for routine breast cancer screening or with palpable breast lumps. Conventional mammography supplemented by additional displaced or Eklund view is usually sufficient to detect most abnormalities. Ultrasonographic evaluation may be performed as an ancillary technique to characterize palpable lumps or nonpalpable lesions detected on mammography. In patients suspected of having implant rupture, conventional mammography and displaced views are performed. If clinical findings warrant, an MRI may be performed to detect intracapsular and extracapsular rupture and migration of silicone globules to the axilla, branchial plexus, and adjacent structures. A relationship between connective-tissue diseases and silicone breast implants has been the focus of controversy since the early 1990s. All studies investigated support that there is no evidence of an increased risk of any specific connective-tissue disease, all definite connective-tissue diseases combined, or other autoimmune conditions associated with the use of breast implants, including nonsilicone and silicone implants.

Janowsky EC, Kupper LL, Hulka BS, et al. Meta-analyses of the relation between silicone breast implants and the risk of connective-tissue diseases. *N Engl J Med.* 2000;342:781–790.

107. Weight-loss surgery (vertical-banded gastroplasty and gastric bypass) can be considered in individuals who have a body mass index that exceeds

A) 10 kg/mm^2
B) 20 kg/mm^2
C) 30 kg/mm^2
D) 40 kg/mm^2
E) 50 kg/mm^2

Answer and Discussion

The answer is D. For persons with very severe obesity (body mass index >40 kg/mm^2) and those with less severe obesity and serious or life-threatening complications, surgical procedures may represent an option for treatment. The procedures can result in large weight losses that are usually well maintained for more than 5 years. The most common operations—vertical banded gastroplasty and gastric bypass—radically reduce stomach volume by creating a gastric pouch of no more than 25 mL in volume. Weight loss after surgery is rapid at first, slowing gradually over a period of 2 years. It is directly proportional to the extent of obesity and usually varies between 40 and 60 kg. The weight loss is accompanied by marked improvement in medical complications as well as in mood, self-esteem, body image, activity levels, and interpersonal and vocational effectiveness. In experienced hands, preoperative and operative mortality is usually less than 1%, and operative complications are <10%. Medication can be used when the body mass index reaches 30 kg/mm^2 without comorbidities or 27 kg/mm^2 when other risk factors are present.

Beers MH, Berkow R, eds. *The Merck manual of diagnosis and therapy*, Merck Research Laboratories, 17th ed. Whitehouse Station, NJ: Merck & Co.; 1999:62.

108. How long should air travel be postponed after a patient experiences an uncomplicated myocardial infarction?

A) 1 week
B) 2 weeks
C) 1 month
D) 6 months
E) 1 year

Answer and Discussion

The answer is B. Based on consensus opinion of the ASMA, the American College of Cardiology (ACC), and the American Heart Association (AHA), patients with uncomplicated myocardial infarctions (MI) or those who have undergone uncomplicated percutaneous coronary interventions should not fly until at least 2 to 3 weeks have passed and they are tolerating their usual daily activities. The week immediately after coronary stent placement carries the highest risk for stent thrombosis, and patients should not travel by air during this period. Following an MI, a stress test is recommended in all low-risk patients. Results gained from testing help determine the patient's ability to tolerate flight. Patients with an MI complicated by severely depressed cardiac function or an untoward event during treatment should not fly until 2 weeks after they are deemed medically stable. Unstable angina is a contraindication to air travel; stable angina is generally well tolerated during flight. Severe decompensated congestive heart failure (CHF) is a contraindication to flight. Patients with class III or IV New York Heart Association CHF should be carefully assessed to determine whether they require inflight oxygen. Symptomatic valvular heart disease is a relative contraindication to airline travel.

Possick SE, Barry M. Evaluation and management of the cardiovascular patient embarking on air travel. *Ann Intern Med.* 2004;141:148.

Prout M, Pine JR. Preflight patient assessment. Up to Date, version 14.1. Accessed 3/20/2006.

> Based on consensus opinion of the ASMA, the American College of Cardiology (ACC), and the American Heart Association (AHA), patients with uncomplicated myocardial infarctions (MI) or those who have undergone uncomplicated percutaneous coronary interventions should not fly until at least 2 to 3 weeks have passed and they are tolerating their usual daily activities.

109. Which of the following is true regarding patient-controlled anesthesia (PCA)?

A) The administration is labor intensive.
B) Oversedation can usually be avoided.
C) The delivery system can usually increase the time interval between patient demand and delivery of the medication.
D) Basal infusion rates should be routinely delivered.
E) Patient response is not a good indicator of PCA effectiveness.

Answer and Discussion

The answer is B. Opioid analgesics are used in managing severe acute postoperative pain. Injectable nonsteroidal anti-inflammatory drugs (e.g., ketorolac) are also useful, and regional anesthetic techniques (e.g., local spinal anesthetic) are used in some cases. An opioid may be administered epidurally, typically administered during surgery and continued 2 to 3 days postoperatively. In the recovery room, morphine sulfate or meperidine are medication options. The dose of narcotics may have to be repeated at short intervals (e.g., every 15 to 30 minutes) until pain relief is established. On the hospital floor, parenteral morphine sulfate usually provides pain relief. Higher doses provide greater analgesia and a longer duration of effect. PCA allows self-administration of small opioid doses as needed. It has become the standard of care for the administration of postoperative narcotic analgesics for pain control. Dosage (frequency and amount) should be modified according to the patient's response. By limiting the number of doses of medication per hour, the physician can avoid oversedation of the patient. PCA pumps avoid the lag period between when the patient senses pain and initiates the call for medication and actual delivery by the nurse. It can also reduce the amount of work of drawing up and delivering multiple doses of medication by the nursing staff. PCA pumps can also deliver a constant rate of medication per hour whether or not the patient hits the demand button. Studies have shown that most patients don't benefit from the additional basal infusion rate, and oversedation may occur with it. Only patients with a high narcotic tolerance may be good candidates for basal infusion rates.

Townsend CM, ed. *Sabiston textbook of surgery*, 16th ed. Philadelphia: WB Saunders; 2001:287.

Beers MH, Berkow R, eds. *The Merck manual of diagnosis and therapy*, Merck Research Laboratories, 17th ed. Whitehouse Station, NJ: Merck & Co.; 1999:1370–1371.

110. A 31 year old is seen in the emergency room for lateral foot pain that occurred when he fell playing basketball. X-rays of the foot confirm a displaced fracture of the proximal fifth metatarsal. Appropriate management consists of

A) nonsteroidal anti-inflammatory drugs and limited weight bearing with a gradual return to usual activities in 2 to 4 weeks
B) crutches with no weight bearing for 4 to 6 weeks
C) short leg walking cast for 6 to 8 weeks
D) external reduction followed by casting for 6 to 8 weeks with limited weight bearing
E) orthopedic referral

Answer and Discussion

The answer is E. Fractures of the proximal portion of the fifth metatarsal may be classified as avulsions of the tuberosity or fractures of the shaft within 1.5 cm of the tuberosity. Tuberosity avulsion fractures cause pain and tenderness at the base of the fifth metatarsal. Bruising, swelling, and other injuries may be present. Nondisplaced tuberosity fractures are usually treated conservatively, but orthopedic referral is indicated for (a) fractures that are comminuted or displaced, (b) fractures that involve more than 30% of the cubometatarsal articulation surface, and (c) fractures with delayed union. Management and prognosis of acute (Jones fracture) and stress fracture of the fifth metatarsal within 1.5 cm of the tuberosity depend on the type of fracture, based on classification. Simple fractures are generally treated conservatively with a non-weight-bearing short leg cast for 6 to 8 weeks. Fractures with delayed union may also be treated conservatively or may be managed surgically, depending on patient preference and other factors. All displaced fractures and nonunion fractures should be managed surgically. Although most fractures of the proximal portion of the fifth metatarsal respond well to appropriate management, delayed union, muscle atrophy, and chronic pain may be long-term complications.

Strayer SM, Reece SG, Petrizzi MJ. Fractures of the proximal fifth metatarsal. *Am Fam Physician.* 1999:2516.

Chapter 6

Geriatrics

Questions

Each of the following questions or incomplete statements is followed by suggested answers or completions. Select the ONE BEST ANSWER in each case.

1. Which of the following symptoms is more likely to represent myocardial ischemia in older patients?

A) Chest pain
B) Dyspnea
C) Diaphoresis
D) Back pain
E) Jaw pain

Answer and Discussion

The answer is B. Exertional angina (chest pain) is the most common manifestation of myocardial ischemia in young and middle-age persons. Because of their more sedentary lifestyle or possibly a difference in pathophysiology, this may not be true in elderly patients. Instead of exertional chest pain, ischemia may be more commonly manifested as dyspnea in elderly patients. Other elderly patients with CAD may be completely asymptomatic, although silent ischemia may be demonstrated by stress testing or Holter monitoring.

Tresch DD. Diagnostic and prognostic value of ambulatory electrocardiographic monitoring in older patients. *J Am Geriatr Soc.* 1995;43:66–70.

Tresch DD, Saeian K, Hoffman R. Elderly patients with late onset of coronary artery disease: Clinical and angiographic findings. *Am J Geriatr Cardiol.* 1992;1:14–25.

Instead of exertional chest pain, ischemia may be more commonly manifested as dyspnea in elderly patients.

2. Which of the following statements is true regarding thrombolytic therapy when treating elderly patients with myocardial infarction (MI)?

A) Elderly patients are frequently overtreated with thrombolytics.
B) Elderly patients with non-Q-wave MIs should receive thrombolytics.
C) Streptokinase is more expensive to use than tPA.
D) tPA is associated with a higher risk of hemorrhagic stroke when compared to streptokinase in elderly patients.
E) Up to 75% of elderly patients have absolute contraindications to thrombolytics.

Answer and Discussion

The answer is D. Despite a wealth of evidence in favor of thrombolytic treatment for elderly MI patients, the therapy is commonly not used in this age group. The reasons for this are numerous and include delay in seeking medical assistance, misdiagnoses due to atypical presentation, increased contraindications, and higher prevalence of non-Q-wave MIs. Additionally, physicians are reluctant to use thrombolytics in the elderly population for fear of hemorrhage, although most studies show that intracerebral hemorrhage is not significantly increased in elderly MI patients who receive thrombolytics. Only approximately one-third of elderly patients presenting with acute MI have any contraindications to thrombolytic therapy, and less than 5% have absolute contraindications. In regard to patients with non- Q-wave infarction or unstable angina, repeated studies have demonstrated that thrombolytic therapy has no benefits in these patients regardless of age. In regard to choice of specific thrombolytic agent, initial studies comparing streptokinase (approximate cost: $200 per patient) and tissue-type plasminogen activator (approximate cost: $2,200 per patient) found that both drugs increased the survival rate equally. The Global Utilization of Streptokinase and Tissue Plasminogen Activator (tPA) for Occluded Coronary Arteries (GUSTO) trial, which was designed specifically to compare thrombolytic agents, reported a significant advantage with tPA for the overall study population. Patients over age 75, however, had a significantly higher risk of hemorrhagic stroke when treated with tPA than with streptokinase, and the incidence of death or nonfatal disabling stroke was not significantly different between the two therapies in this age group. Therefore, streptokinase may be appropriate in patients over the age of 75 years.

The GUSTO Investigators. An international randomized trial comparing four thrombolytic strategies for acute myocardial infarction. *N Engl J Med.* 1993;329:673–682.

3. A 75-year-old man presents with exertional dyspnea and generalized weakness. On examination, you discover a high-pitched, blowing diastolic murmur and a wide pulse pressure with bounding pulses. The most likely diagnosis is?
A) aortic stenosis
B) aortic insufficiency
C) mitral stenosis
D) mitral insufficiency
E) coarctation of the aorta

Answer and Discussion

The answer is B. The prevalence of aortic regurgitation increases with age. Unlike aortic valve stenosis, aortic valvular insufficiency is rarely caused by degenerative aortic valve disease. Acute aortic valvular insufficiency may be due to infective endocarditis, aortic dissection, trauma, or rupture of the sinus of Valsalva. Chronic aortic insufficiency can be caused by valve leaflet disease, including rheumatic heart disease, congenital heart disease, rheumatoid arthritis, ankylosing spondylitis, or myxomatous degeneration. Chronic aortic insufficiency may also be caused by aortic root disease secondary to systemic hypertension, syphilitic aortitis, cystic medial necrosis, ankylosing spondylitis, rheumatoid arthritis, Reiter's disease, systemic lupus erythematosus, Ehlers–Danlos syndrome, and pseudoxanthoma elasticum. Symptoms of aortic valvular insufficiency are the same in older persons as they are in younger ones. Usually, the main symptoms are related to heart failure, with exertional dyspnea and weakness being common symptoms. In some elderly patients, symptoms of dyspnea and palpitations may be more common at rest than with exertion. Nocturnal angina pectoris, often accompanied by flushing, diaphoresis, and palpitations, may occur; this is thought to be related to the slowing of the heart rate and the drop of arterial diastolic pressure. The classic findings of a high-pitched, blowing diastolic murmur and a wide pulse pressure with an abruptly rising and collapsing pulse should make the diagnosis of aortic valvular insufficiency easily recognized in elderly patients.

Tresch DD, Jamali I. Chapter 34: Cardiac Disorders. In: Duthie EH Jr, ed. *Practice of geriatrics,* 3rd ed. 1998. WB Saunders. Accessed online 4/7/06.

4. Once symptoms develop in elderly patients with aortic stenosis (without intervention), the survival is approximately
A) 6 months or less
B) 1–3 years
C) 3–5 years
D) 5–7 years
E) survival is unaffected with symptomatic aortic stenosis

Answer and Discussion

The answer is B. Once symptoms develop in patients with critical aortic valve stenosis, the clinical course is rapidly downhill. Symptoms and left ventricular dysfunction are progressive, and the average survival is approximately 1–3 years.

Tresch DD, Jamali I. Chapter 34: Cardiac Disorders. In: Duthie EH Jr, ed. *Practice of geriatrics,* 3rd ed. 1998. WB Saunders. Accessed online 4/7/06.

5. A 69-year-old female presents with peripheral edema, orthopnea, and dypsnea on exertion. She has gained 10 pounds in the last 3 days. She is otherwise healthy. You suspect congestive heart failure. Appropriate first-line medication includes which of the following?
A) Diltiazem
B) Lisinopril
C) Nitroglyercin
D) Metoprolol
E) Hydralazine

Answer and Discussion

The answer is B. Due to the results of numerous studies showing that ACE inhibitors are beneficial in relieving symptoms and preventing progressive ventricular deterioration, it is recommended that they should be the initial therapy utilized in patients with heart failure. In patients with moderate to severe heart failure due to systolic left ventricular dysfunction, the use of ACE inhibitors alone has not been found to be successful in relieving the signs and symptoms of volume overload. There is no question, however, that ACE inhibitors, such as digitalis and diuretics, are beneficial in improving the symptoms and prolonging survival in symptomatic patients with left ventricular systolic dysfunction. In the CONSENSUS trial, which demonstrated significant benefits in the use of ACE inhibitors in symptomatic patients, the mean age of the patients was over 70 years, and, at this age, ACE inhibitors were well tolerated. In asymptomatic elderly patients with depressed left ventricular systolic dysfunction, the use of ACE inhibitors is more controversial. The SOLVD trial demonstrated that asymptomatic patients with a depressed left ventricular ejection fraction of less than 35% demonstrated no benefit in survival, although a significant reduction in progression to clinical heart failure with a decrease in hospitalizations was noted. In the SAVE trial, ACE inhibitors were found to be beneficial in improving long-term survival and reducing the development of heart failure and recurrent myocardial infarction in patients with reduced left ventricular systolic function following acute MI, regardless of the patient's age.

The CONSENSUS Trial Study Group: Effects of enalapril on mortality in severe congestive heart failure. Results of the Cooperative North Scandinavian Enalapril Survival Study (CONSENSUS). *N Engl J Med.* 1987;316:1429–1435.

The SOLVD Investigators: Effect of enalapril on mortality and the development of heart failure in asymptomatic patients with reduced left ventricular ejection fractions. *N Engl J Med.* 1992;327:685–691.

Pfeffer MA, Braunwald E, Moye LA, et al. Effect of captopril on mortality and morbidity in patients with left ventricular dysfunction after myocardial infarction: Results of the Survival and Ventricular Enlargement Trial. *N Engl J Med.* 1992;327:669–677.

6. A 75-year-old man is brought in to your office by his wife. She complains that he is not the same over the last 6 months. His memory is failing him, he has difficulty walking (especially when he initiates walking), and he is incontinent of urine. Which of the following is the most likely diagnosis based on his history?
A) Alzheimer's disease
B) Parkinson's disease
C) Normal-pressure hydrocephalus
D) Pick's disease
E) Progressive supranuclear palsy

Answer and Discussion

The answer is C. Normal-pressure hydrocephalus (NPH) is a cause of dementia in the elderly. It may be caused by previous insult to the brain, usually as a result of a subarachnoid hemorrhage or diffuse meningitis that presumably results in scarring of the arachnoid villi over the brain convexities where cerebrospinal fluid (CSF) absorption usually occurs. However, elderly NPH patients seldom have a history of predisposing disease. NPH classically consists of dementia, apraxia of gait, and incontinence, but many patients with these symptoms do not have NPH. Typically, motor weakness and staggering are absent, but initiation of gait is hesitant—described as a "slipping clutch" or "feet stuck to the floor" gait—and walking eventually occurs. NPH has also been associated with various psychiatric manifestations that are not categorical. NPH should be considered in the differential diagnosis of any new mental status changes in the elderly. CT or MRI and a lumbar puncture are necessary for diagnosis. On CT or MRI, the ventricles are dilated. CSF pressure measured by a lumbar puncture is normal. A limited improvement after removing about 50 mL of CSF indicates a better prognosis with shunting. Radiographic or pressure measurements alone do not seem to predict response to shunting. Shunting CSF from the dilated ventricles sometimes results in clinical improvement, but the longer the disease has been present, the less likely shunting will be curative.

Beers MH, Porter RS, eds. *The Merck manual of diagnosis and therapy,* Merck Research Laboratories, 18th ed. Whitehouse Station, NJ: Merck & Co.; 2006:1811, 1814.

7. Which of the following is more commonly seen in patients with Lewy body dementia when compared to Alzheimer's dementia?

A) Hallucinations
B) Lip smacking
C) Tremor
D) Emotional lability
E) Repetitive behavior

Answer and Discussion

The answer is A. Although difficult to know for sure, Lewy body dementia may be the second most common dementia after Alzheimer's disease. Lewy bodies are hallmark lesions of degenerating neurons in Parkinson's disease and occur in dementia with or without features of Parkinson's disease. In Lewy body dementia, Lewy bodies may predominate markedly or be intermixed with classic pathologic changes of Alzheimer's disease. Symptoms, signs, and course of Lewy body dementia resemble those of Alzheimer's disease, except hallucinations (mainly visual) are more common and patients appear to have an exquisite sensitivity to antipsychotic-induced extrapyramidal adverse effects.

Beers MH, Porter RS, eds. *The Merck manual of diagnosis and therapy,* Merck Research Laboratories, 18th ed. Whitehouse Station, NJ: Merck & Co.; 2006:1811, 1814.

8. A patient with Pick's disease is brought in by his caregiver. She complains that he has become increasingly more apathetic and, at times, sexually inappropriate, and is smacking his lips more frequently. You suspect

A) elder abuse
B) medication side effects
C) development of Kluver–Bucy syndrome
D) toxin exposure
E) chronic hypoxia

Answer and Discussion

The answer is C. Pick's disease is a less common form of dementia, affecting the frontal and temporal regions of the cerebral cortex. Patients have prominent apathy and memory disturbances. They may show increased carelessness, poor personal hygiene, and decreased attention span. Although the clinical presentation and CT findings in Pick's disease can be quite distinctive, definitive diagnosis is possible only at autopsy. The Klüver–Bucy syndrome can occur early in the course of Pick's disease, with emotional blunting, hypersexual activity, hyperorality (bulimia and sucking and smacking of lips), and visual agnosias.

Beers MH, Porter RS, eds. *The Merck manual of diagnosis and therapy,* Merck Research Laboratories, 18th ed. Whitehouse Station, NJ: Merck & Co.; 2006:1820.

9. A 75-year-old female presents with rather severe shoulder and hip pain that has been progressively worse over the last 3 months. She complains of morning stiffness and low-grade fevers, malaise, and weight loss. She has no headache or visual disturbance, and EMG study of her lower extremities was normal. Her labs reveal a normocytic–normochromic anemia and her erythrocyte sedimentation rate (ESR) was found to be 60 mm/h. Appropriate management at this time includes

A) referral for a temporal artery biopsy
B) initiation of prednisone
C) initiation of an NSAID
D) referral to physical therapy
E) referral to orthopedics for consideration of joint replacement

Answer and Discussion

The answer is B. The true prevalence, etiology, and pathogenesis of polymyalgia rheumatica (PMR) are not entirely known. In some, the condition is a manifestation of underlying temporal arteritis. Although most patients are not at significant risk for the complications of temporal arteritis, they should be warned of the possibility and should immediately report such symptoms as headache, visual disturbance, and jaw muscle pain on chewing. PMR usually occurs in patients older than 60 years, and the female:male ratio is 2:1. Onset may be acute or subacute. PMR is characterized by severe pain and stiffness of the neck and shoulders and hips; morning stiffness; stiffness after inactivity; and systemic complaints, such as malaise, fever, depression, and weight loss. There is no selective muscle weakness or evidence of muscle disease on electromyography (EMG) or biopsy. Normochromic–normocytic anemia may be present. In most patients, the ESR is dramatically elevated, often >100 mm/h, usually >50 mm/h. C-reactive protein levels are usually elevated (>0.7 mg/dL) and may be a more sensitive marker of disease activity in certain patients than is ESR. PMR is distinguished from rheumatoid arthritis (RA by the usual absence of small joint synovitis (although some joint swelling may be present), erosive or destructive disease, rheumatoid factor, or rheumatoid nodules. PMR is differentiated from polymyositis by usually normal muscle enzymes, EMG, and muscle biopsy, as well as by the prominence of pain over weakness. Hypothyroidism can present as myalgia, with abnormal thyroid function tests and elevated creatine kinase (CK). PMR is differentiated from myeloma by the absence of monoclonal gammopathy, and from fibromyalgia by the systemic features and elevated ESR. PMR usually responds dramatically to prednisone initiated at doses of at least 15 mg/day. If temporal arteritis is suspected, treatment should be started immediately, with 60 mg/day to prevent blindness. As symptoms subside, corticosteroids are tapered to the lowest effective dose, regardless of ESR. Some patients are able to discontinue corticosteroids in less than 2 years, whereas others require small amounts for years. Rarely do patients respond adequately to salicylates or other NSAIDs.

Beers MH, Porter RS, eds. *The Merck manual of diagnosis and therapy*, Merck Research Laboratories, 18th ed. Whitehouse Station, NJ: Merck & Co.; 2006:278–279.

10. When dealing with a dying patient, the patient's family should
A) be contacted only when they request it
B) be thoroughly informed of the details that death may present to them
C) be kept away from the patient to prevent bad associations and memories
D) be contacted about an autopsy only after death has occurred
E) never be approached about organ donation until after death has occurred

Answer and Discussion

The answer is B. The family should be thoroughly informed of the changes that the patient's body may exhibit directly before and after death. They should not be surprised by irregular breathing, cool extremities, confusion, a purplish skin color, or somnolence in the last hours. A discussion about autopsy can occur either before or just after death. Families may have strong feelings, either in favor of or against it. The discussion of autopsy should not be left to a covering physician or house officer who has not had previous contact with the family. Discussions about organ donation, if appropriate, should take place before death or immediately after death.

Beers MH, Porter RS, eds. *The Merck manual of diagnosis and therapy*, Merck Research Laboratories, 18th ed. Whitehouse Station, NJ: Merck & Co.; 2006:2762–2768.

The family should be thoroughly informed of the changes that the patient's body may exhibit directly before and after death.

11. In the elderly, a rise in the systolic blood pressure with no change in the diastolic blood pressure most likely suggests
A) anemia
B) thyrotoxicosis
C) aortic insufficiency
D) stiffening of the arteries
E) none of the above

Answer and Discussion

The answer is D. Stiffened blood vessels also have an impact for blood pressure determination in later life. Systolic blood pressure rises throughout life in Western populations, whereas diastolic pressure peaks and plateaus in middle age and later life. "Normal" blood pressure has been defined by determining the cardiovascular risk associated with a given blood pressure. The presence of an isolated rise in the systolic pressure without a diastolic rise (isolated systolic hypertension) is fairly unique to older patients and, unlike younger patients, does not necessarily imply anemia, thyrotoxicosis, or aortic insufficiency, which can cause a bounding pulse and wide pulse pressure in the young.

Duthie EH Jr. Chapter 1: History and Physical Examination. In: Duthie EH Jr, ed. *Practice of geriatrics*, 3rd ed. 1998. WB Saunders. Accessed online 4/2/06.

12. Causes for orthostatic blood pressure in the elderly include all of the following except
A) declining baroreceptor sensitivity
B) decreased arterial compliance
C) increased venous tortuosity
D) decreased renal sodium conservation
E) increased plasma volume

Answer and Discussion

The answer is E. Determination of orthostatic blood pressure should be routinely performed in geriatric patients. Although a number of factors, such as declining baroreceptor sensitivity, diminished arterial compliance, increased venous tortuosity, decreased renal sodium conservation, and diminished plasma volume, could combine to cause a drop in orthostatic blood pressure among older patients, there is no clear evidence that the pressure drops solely as a function of age. However, a blood pressure drop when changing from the supine to the upright position is common among geriatric patients (possibly as many as 30% of unselected patients may experience a 20-mmHg or more drop in systolic pressure). Diseases and medications that cause the problem are common offenders.

Duthie EH Jr. Chapter 1: History and Physical Examination. In: Duthie EH Jr, ed. *Practice of geriatrics*, 3rd ed. 1998. WB Saunders. Accessed online 4/2/06.

13. When caring for the elderly, it is important to remember the following about measurement of body temperature:
A) Serious infections often adversely affect the patient's temperature.
B) Norms for fever are adjusted based on the patient's age.
C) The elderly have a tendency toward disturbances of temperature regulation.
D) Temperature variations do not occur in the elderly population based on comparisons with younger patients.
E) Temperatures should not be recorded in the elderly because of their notorious inaccuracy.

Answer and Discussion

The answer is C. Temperature determination in the elderly is the same as it is in other patients. Norms for fever or hypothermia have not been adjusted for age. Elderly people do have a tendency toward disturbances of temperature regulation (hypothermia or hyperthermia). It is possible that some elderly patients, like others, may present with serious infections that do not produce much temperature rise.

Duthie EH Jr. Chapter 1: History and Physical Examination. In: Duthie EH Jr, ed. *Practice of geriatrics*, 3rd ed. 1998. WB Saunders. Accessed online 4/2/06.

14. Which of the following is true regarding respiratory rate in the elderly?
A) Subtle differences in age-adjusted respiratory rate are present and should be adjusted for in the evaluation of the elderly patient.
B) Respiratory rates in the elderly are 5% higher than age-adjusted controls.
C) Respiratory rates and patterns do not change as the patient ages.
D) Elevated respiratory rates do not represent concern in elderly patients.
E) Respiratory rates do not correlate with disease in elderly patients.

Answer and Discussion

The answer is C. Respiratory rate and patterns do not change significantly with age. An elevated respiratory rate may be a subtle clue to a serious medical illness (e.g., acidosis, hypoxia, central nervous system disturbance) and should be detected and evaluated as in any other patient.

Duthie EH Jr. Chapter 1: History and Physical Examination. In: Duthie EH Jr, ed. *Practice of geriatrics*, 3rd ed. 1998. WB Saunders. Accessed online 4/2/06.

15. While examining a 65-year-old woman for her yearly well-woman exam, you note a palpable right ovary. The remainder of her examination is entirely normal. The most likely diagnosis is
A) cecal fecolyth
B) polycystic ovary syndrome
C) normal variant
D) ovarian carcinoma
E) fibroid tumor

Answer and Discussion

The answer is D. The presence of a palpable ovary in an elderly woman should raise a suspicion of some pathology, especially malignancy.

Duthie EH Jr. Chapter 1: History and Physical Examination. In: Duthie EH Jr, ed. *Practice of geriatrics*, 3rd ed. 1998. WB Saunders. Accessed online 4/2/06.

16. From admission to discharge, what percentage of elderly patients lose independence in one or more of the basic activities of daily living?
A) Approximately 1–3 %
B) 10%
C) 25–35%
D) 50%
E) More than 75%

Answer and Discussion

The answer is C. From hospital admission to discharge, 25% to 35% of elderly patients lose independence in one or more of the basic activities of daily living. The loss of independent functioning during hospitalization is associated with important complications including prolonged length of hospital stay, greater risk of institutionalization, and higher mortality rates.

Palmer RM. Acute hospital care of the elderly: Minimizing the risk of functional decline. *Cleve Clin J Med.* 1995;62:117–128.

17. Factors known to precipitate delirium in elderly hospitalized patients include
A) physical restraints
B) the addition of three or more medications
C) use of bladder catheter
D) malnutrition
E) all of the above

Answer and Discussion

The answer is E. Dementia is the single most important risk factor for the development of delirium or acute confused state. Delirium is found at admission or during hospitalization in about 25% of elderly patients admitted for acute medical illnesses. Patients with baseline dementia and severe systemic illness are predisposed to delirium. Factors known to precipitate delirium include the use of physical restraints, the addition of more than three medications to the regimen, the use of a bladder catheter, malnutrition, and any iatrogenic event.

Inouye SK, Charpentier PA. Precipitating factors for delirium in hospitalized elderly persons. Predictive model and interrelationship with baseline vulnerability. *JAMA.* 1996;275: 852–857.

18. A 65-year-old man presents to your office complaining of a right-hand tremor. The patient reports the tremor is worse with sustained positions and stressful situations. Surprisingly, a shot of scotch makes the tremor better. He also reports a positive family history for tremors. There are no signs of bradykinesia or rigidity. The most likely diagnosis is
A) Parkinson's disease
B) essential tremor
C) Huntington's disease
D) caffeine withdrawal
E) alcohol withdrawal

Answer and Discussion

The answer is B. Essential tremor is the most common movement disorder. This postural tremor may have its onset anywhere between the second and sixth decades of life, and its prevalence increases with age. It is slowly progressive over a period of years. An essential tremor is characterized by a rapid, fine tremor that is made worse with sustained positions. The frequency of essential tremor is 4 to 11 Hz, depending on which body segment is affected. Proximal segments are affected at lower frequencies, and distal segments are affected at higher frequencies. Although typically a postural tremor, essential tremor may occur at rest in severe and very advanced cases. It most commonly affects the hands but can also affect the head, voice, tongue, and legs. It usually affects patients older than 50 years. The tremor may be intensified by stress, anxiety, excessive fatigue, drugs (e.g., caffeine, alcohol withdrawal, steroids), or thyroid disorders. In many cases, the patient may report relief with alcohol use and a positive family history for tremors. Senile tremors tend to increase with age. Parkinson's disease is differentiated by the presence of a pill-rolling tremor at rest, masked face, bradykinesias, and rigidity. Parkinson's also shows a favorable response to the administration of L-dopamine and does not improve with the use of alcohol. Treatment of essential tremors involves the treatment of the underlying disorder and the use of propranolol (Inderal), primidone (Mysoline), diazepam (Valium), and methazolamide (Neptazane). Primidone may be preferred because of the exercise intolerance associated with the high-dose beta blockers. Patients who have a very-low-amplitude rapid tremor are generally more responsive to these agents than those who have a slower tremor with greater amplitude. Patients who have a tremor of the head and voice may also be more resistant to treatment than patients with an essential tremor of the hands. In severe cases, surgery may be considered.

Smaga S. Tremor. *Am Fam Physician.* 2003;68:1545–52,1553.

19. Which of the following tests is indicated in the initial workup of urinary incontinence?
A) Renal ultrasound
B) Urodynamic studies
C) Post-void residual
D) Urine cytology
E) Intravenous pyelogram

Answer and Discussion

The answer is C. Urinary incontinence is often seen in the elderly. In most cases, the evaluation of urinary incontinence requires only a history, physical examination, urinalysis, and measurement of post-void residual urine volume. The initial purposes of the evaluation are to identify conditions requiring referral or specialized workup and to detect and treat reversible causes that may be present. Causes may include infection, atrophic urethritis, pelvic floor weakness (usually related to previous childbirth), medications (e.g., diuretics), altered mental status, or overflow incontinence related to obstruction (e.g., fecal impaction, prostatic hypertrophy). If the patient does not require referral and a reversible cause is not identified, the next step is to categorize the patient's symptoms as typical of urge or stress incontinence and treat the patient accordingly. *Urge incontinence* results from bladder contractions that overwhelm the ability of the cerebral centers to inhibit them. These uncontrollable contractions can occur because of inflammation or irritation within the bladder resulting from calculi, malignancy, infection, or atrophic vaginitis–urethritis. They can also occur when the brain centers that inhibit bladder contractions are impaired by neurologic conditions such as stroke, Parkinson's disease, or dementia; drugs such as hypnotics or narcotics; or metabolic disorders such as hypoxemia and encephalopathy. *Stress incontinence* is caused by a malfunction of the urethral sphincter that causes urine to leak from the bladder when intraabdominal pressure increases, such as during coughing or sneezing. Classic or genuine stress incontinence is caused by pelvic prolapse, urethral hypermobility, or displacement of the urethra and bladder neck from their normal anatomic alignment. Stress incontinence can also occur as a result of intrinsic sphincter deficiency, in which the sphincter is weak because of a congenital condition or denervation resulting from α-adrenergic-blocking drugs, surgical trauma, or radiation damage. Treatment involves the strengthening of pelvic floor muscles with Kegel exercises, voiding schedules, and biofeedback. Tolterodine (Detrol) and extended-release oxybutynin chloride (Ditropan XL) are used as a first-line treatment option for overactive bladder, which contributes to incontinence because of favorable side effect profiles. A trial of therapy may be attempted before formal urodynamic studies are ordered. If treatment fails or a presumptive diagnosis of urge or stress incontinence cannot be reached, the final step would be to perform more sophisticated tests or refer the patient for testing to define the cause and determine the best treatment.

Culligan PJ, Heit M. Urinary Incontinence in Women: Evaluation and Management, *Am Fam Physician.* 2000;62:2433–44, 2447, 2452.

20. Increasing age is associated with many effects on the kidney. These effects include which of the following?

A) Increase in renal size
B) Increase in serum creatinine
C) Decreased glomerular filtration rate
D) Increase in renal blood flow
E) Decreased threshold for glucose

Answer and Discussion

The answer is C. Many changes occur within the kidney as a result of increasing age. There is a gradual decrease in renal size; a decrease in renal blood flow; and, most importantly, a decrease in glomerular filtration rate, which can have a significant effect on drug metabolism. In most cases, serum creatinine remains essentially unchanged. In many cases, the doses of renal-metabolized medications need to be reduced in patients with decreased creatinine clearance. Additionally, the renal threshold for glucose increases with increasing age, and there is a decrease in maximal urinary concentration.

Landefeld CS, Palmer R, Johnson MA. *Current Geriatric Diagnosis and Treatment.* New York: Lange Medical Books/McGraw Hill; 2004:422.

Many changes occur within the kidney as a result of increasing age. There is a gradual decrease in renal size; a decrease in renal blood flow; and, most importantly, a decrease in glomerular filtration rate, which can have a significant effect on drug metabolism. In most cases, serum creatinine remains essentially unchanged.

21. When comparing middle-age patients with hyperthyroidism to elderly patients with hyperthyroidism, elderly patients are more likely to have

A) restlessness
B) hyperactive appearance
C) atrial fibrillation
D) weight gain
E) goiter

Answer and Discussion

The answer is C. The most common cause of hyperthyroidism in the elderly is Graves' disease or toxic diffuse goiter. Graves' disease is an autoimmune disorder that results from the action of a thyroid-stimulating antibody on thyroid-stimulating hormone receptors. Thyroid-stimulating hormone receptor antibodies are detectable in the serum of approximately 80% to 100% of untreated patients with Graves' disease. Hyperthyroidism in the elderly is often more difficult to diagnose than in younger patients. Only 25% of those affected present with symptoms that are typical in younger patients, such as restlessness and hyperactive appearance. Elderly patients are more likely to show weight loss, new-onset atrial fibrillation, and withdrawal or depression. Other complications include cardiac failure, angina, myocardial infarction, and osteoporosis with an increased risk of bone fractures. Older patients have a lower incidence of goiter. Behavioral changes in younger patients include anxiety, emotional lability, insomnia, lack of concentration, restlessness, and tremulousness. In contrast, elderly patients show apathy, lethargy, pseudodementia, and depressed moods.

Landefeld CS, Palmer R, Johnson MA. *Current Geriatric Diagnosis and Treatment.* New York: Lange Medical Books/McGraw Hill; 2004:321–324.

22. Which of the following is a risk factor for the development of pressure ulcers in hospitalized patients?

A) Blanchable erythema
B) Lymphocytosis
C) Increased body weight
D) Moist skin
E) None of the above

Answer and Discussion

The answer is E. Pressure ulcers occur more often in patients who have nonblanchable erythema, lymphopenia, immobility, dry skin, and decreased body weight. Patients with these risk factors need aggressive mobilization to avoid developing pressure sores.

Landefeld CS, Palmer R, Johnson MA. *Current Geriatric Diagnosis and Treatment.* New York: Lange Medical Books / McGraw Hill; 2004:281–288.

23. When assessing for urinary retention, which of the following post-void residuals represents the *threshold* for an abnormal finding?
A) 25 ml
B) 50 ml
C) 100 ml
D) 200 ml
E) 500 ml

Answer and Discussion

The answer is D. In general, a PVR of less than 50 mL is considered adequate emptying, and a PVR greater than 200 mL is considered inadequate and suggestive of either detrusor weakness or obstruction.

Fantl, JA, Newman, DK, Colling, J, et al. Urinary Incontinence in Adults: Acute and Chronic Management. Clinical Practice Guideline, No. 2, 1996 Update, AHCPR Publication No. 96-0682, Public Health Service, Agency for Health Care Policy and Research, Rockville, MD.

24. An 80-year-old man is brought in by his wife. She complains that her husband has had a noticeable change in his personality. He is impulsive and at times inappropriate with his behavior. Although he has difficulty naming objects, his memory, ability to calculate, and his visuospatial skills appear to be intact. The most likely diagnosis is
A) Alzheimer's dementia
B) Pick's disease
C) Parkinson's disease
D) Wilson's disease
E) Lewy body dementia

Answer and Discussion

The answer is B. Pick's heterogeneous disease and other frontotemporal dementias (FTD) are a heterogeneous group of disorders that share several clinical features with AD such as rate of progression and duration. Many FTD patients are also aphasic and manifest preserved motor integrity. The language disturbance characteristic of Pick's disease initially includes anomia, but there is a more stereotyped and perseverative verbal output than that found in AD. Unlike AD, in the early stages of FTD, memory, calculation, and visuospatial function are relatively well preserved. The most striking feature of this disorder is an extravagant change in the patient's personality, including disinhibition, impulsivity, inappropriate jocularity, and intrusiveness.

Reichman WE, Cummings JL. Chapter 26: Dementia. In: Duthie EH Jr, ed. *Practice of geriatrics,* 3rd ed. 1998 WB Saunders. Accessed online 4/2/06.

25. Which of the following medications used in the treatment of benign prostatic hypertrophy (BPH) works by inhibiting the transformation of testosterone to dihydrotestosterone?
A) Finasteride (Proscar)
B) Doxazosin (Cardura)
C) Terazosin (Hytrin)
D) Tamsulosin (Flomax)
E) Prazosin (Minipress)

Answer and Discussion

The answer is A. Benign prostatic hypertrophy (BPH) is a condition associated with enlargement of the prostate gland that gives rise to obstructive urinary symptoms. The condition affects men older than 50 years and is characterized as adenomatous hyperplasia. Enlargement of the gland is usually asymptomatic until bladder outlet obstruction occurs. Symptoms reported by patients include decreased force and caliber of the urinary stream, incomplete voiding, hesitancy, frequency, overflow incontinence, retention, nocturia, and dribbling after urination. Acute urinary retention may be precipitated by prolonged attempts to retain urine, immobilization, exposure to cold, anesthetics, anticholinergic and sympathomimetic drugs, or ingestion of alcohol. Physical examination consistent with BPH shows an enlarged bladder and an enlarged prostate, which is usually firm and symmetrical. The median furrow may be absent. Hard nodules found within the gland are more worrisome for cancer. Laboratory findings may show an elevated prostate-specific antigen (PSA), usually <10 ng/dL, and elevated creatine when there is obstruction severe enough to lead to renal impairment. Post-void residuals are usually large and may predispose to infection. The most common cause of hematuria in older men is BPH. Medical treatment involves the use of 5 alpha reductase inhibitors finasteride (Proscar) or dutasteride (Avodart), which may help to shrink the prostate by blocking the transformation of testosterone to dihydrotestosterone. The drawbacks of the 5 alpha reductase inhibitors are that they require 6 to 12 months to work, they are expensive, and regrowth of the prostate occurs after the discontinuation of the medication. Other medications that help with voiding dysfunction are the α-adrenergic blockers prazosin (Minipress), doxazosin (Cardura), and terazosin (Hytrin), which are also used in the treatment of hypertension. Tamsulosin (Flomax) is a newer α-adrenergic blocker that does not significantly affect blood pressure. Definitive therapy is surgical. Although sexual potency and continence are usually retained, approximately 5% to 10% of patients experience some postsurgical problems. Transurethral resection of the prostate is preferred. Larger prostates (usually >75 g) may require open surgery using the suprapubic or retropubic approach, permitting enucleation of the adenomatous tissue from within the surgical capsule. The incidence of impotence and incontinence is much higher than after transurethral resection of the prostate. Alternative surgical approaches include intraurethral stents, microwave thermotherapy, high-intensity–focused ultrasound thermotherapy, laser ablation, electrovaporization, and radiofrequency vaporization.

Beers MH, Porter RS, eds. *The Merck manual of diagnosis and therapy,* Merck Research Laboratories, 18th ed. Whitehouse Station, NJ: Merck & Co.; 2006:2042–2045.

26. Which of the following statements regarding osteoporosis is true?
A) Routine screening of women older than 65 years is not recommended.
B) Dual-energy x-ray absorptiometry (DXA) scans result in more radiation exposure than qualitative computed tomography (CT).
C) T scores are used to diagnose osteoporosis.
D) Plain x-rays are a good diagnostic test for assessment of osteoporosis.
E) Medicare will not pay for bone-density examination.

Answer and Discussion

The answer is C. Osteoporosis afflicts 75 million persons in the United States, Europe, and Japan and results in more than 1.3 million fractures annually in the United States. Osteoporosis is defined as the loss of bone below the density for mechanical support. It occurs when there is a loss of bony matrix and mineral composition of the bone, which is defined as osteopenia. Those most commonly affected are white and Asian postmenopausal women. Bones typically affected include vertebrae, wrist, humerus, hip, and tibia. Risk factors include menopausal state, positive family history, small bone structure, decreased calcium intake, lack of exercise, smoking, excessive alcohol use, and chronic steroid use. All postmenopausal women who present with fractures, as well as younger women who have risk factors, should be evaluated for the disease. Physicians should recommend bone mineral density testing to younger women at risk and postmenopausal women younger than 65 years who have risk factors for osteoporosis other than being postmenopausal. Bone mineral density testing should be recommended to all women 65 years and older regardless of additional risk factors. The most widely used techniques of assessing bone mineral density are DXA and quantitative CT. Of these methods, DXA is the most precise and the diagnostic measure of choice. Quantitative CT is the most sensitive method but results in substantially greater radiation exposure than DXA. Bone densitometry reports provide a T score (the number of standard deviations above or below the mean bone mineral density for gender and race matched to young controls) or a Z score (comparing the patient with a population adjusted for age, gender, and race). Osteoporosis is the classification for a T score of more than 2.5 standard deviations below the gender-adjusted mean for normal young adults at peak bone mass. A T score of –1.0 to –2.5 represents osteopenia. Z scores are not used for the diagnosis. Medicare pays for bone density examination at age 65 for initial diagnosis and for follow up after 24 months. Other indications for screening at an earlier age include when estrogen deficiency is present in a woman at clinical risk for osteoporosis, vertebral abnormalities are present (e.g., osteopenia, vertebral fractures, osteoporosis), the patient has been exposed to long-term (more than 3 months' duration) glucocorticoid therapy, the patient has primary hyperparathyroidism, or the patient requires monitoring to assess response to osteoporosis drug therapy. Plain x-rays are not adequate for the detection of osteoporosis, because as much as 30% of bone mass can be lost before it becomes apparent on x-ray. More advanced cases may reveal decreased radiodensity of vertebrae, anterior wedging of vertebrae, and compression fractures. Prevention involves the use of calcium and vitamin D supplementation, exercise, and avoidance of smoking and heavy alcohol use. Thiazide diuretics may also help to decrease urinary excretion of calcium in patients with secondary hyperparathyroidism. In established cases, the bisphosphonates [alendronate (Fosamax) and risedronate (Actonel)] and a selective estrogen receptor modulator (SERM) [raloxifene (Evista)] are used for treatment. Additionally, calcitonin (Calcimar) may also be used to prevent vertebral fractures; it does not appear to prevent nonvertebral fractures.

South-Paul JE. Osteoporosis: Part 1. Evaluation and assessment. *Am Fam Physician.* 2001;63:897–904, 908.

27. Which of the following is *not* considered in deciding to screen for conditions in the elderly?
A) The exact age of the patient
B) The risk of dying from the condition
C) The potential benefits of screening
D) The direct and indirect harms of screening
E) The patient's values and preferences

Answer and Discussion

The answer is A. The decision to screen for medical conditions depends on multiple factors (i.e., burden of the disease, diagnostic accuracy of the test, consequences of false-positive and false-negative results, and the outcome of early detection of disease). In elderly patients, deciding when to discontinue specific interventions, such as cancer screening, requires individual discussion of potential benefits and risks. Steps to individualize decision making for screening tests include: (1) estimate the life expectancy of the patient; (2) estimate the risk of dying from the condition; (3) determine the potential benefits of screening; (4) weigh the direct and indirect harms of screening; and (5) assess the patient's values and preferences.

Landefeld CS, Palmer R, Johnson MA. *Current Geriatric Diagnosis and Treatment.* New York: Lange Medical Books/McGraw Hill; 2004:7–8.

28. Which one of the following statements about presbycusis is true?
A) Women are more commonly affected than men.
B) Low-frequency tones are affected first.
C) The condition cannot be treated with amplification.
D) The condition can lead to depression.
E) The condition does not affect the ability to interpret speech.

Answer and Discussion

The answer is D. Presbycusis, a progressive, high-frequency hearing loss, is the most common cause of hearing impairment in geriatric patients. Exposure to loud noises and genetic factors play a role in the etiology. Men are more commonly affected with sensory neural hearing loss. It usually begins after 20 years of age and affects the high-frequency tones first (18 to 20 kHz). Patients often report trouble hearing normal conversations in crowds. This type of hearing loss decreases the ability to interpret speech, which can lead to a decreased ability to communicate and a subsequent increased risk for social isolation and depression. Hearing loss in the elderly can also adversely affect physical, emotional, and cognitive well-being. Questionnaires such as the Hearing Handicap Inventory for the Elderly–Screening version have been shown to accurately identify persons with hearing impairment. The reference standard for establishing hearing impairment, however, remains pure tone audiometry, which can be performed in the physician's office. Combining the Hearing Handicap Inventory for the Elderly Screening version questionnaire with pure tone audiometry has been shown to improve screening effectiveness. Appropriate interventions include periodic screening to provide early detection of hearing impairment, cautious use or avoidance of ototoxic drugs, and support for the obtaining and continued use of hearing aids.

Miller KE, Zylstra RG, Standridge JB. The geriatric patient: a systematic approach to maintaining health. *Am Fam Physician.* 2000;61:1089–1104.

> Presbycusis, a progressive, high-frequency hearing loss, is the most common cause of hearing impairment in geriatric patients.

29. Which of the following statements is true regarding the abdominal aortic aneurysms (AAA)?
A) Screening has not been shown to be cost effective.
B) Computed tomography is the test recommended for screening of AAA.
C) All women and men who are 65 years or older should be screened once for AAA.
D) One-time screening with ultrasound for AAA in men 65 to 75 years of age who have ever smoked is recommended.
E) Ultrasound is specific but not sensitive for the screening of AAA.

Answer and Discussion

The answer is D. Ultrasound is the standard imaging tool for the detection of an AAA. In experienced hands, it has a sensitivity and specificity approaching 100% and 96%, respectively, for the detection of infrarenal AAA. The U.S. Preventive Services Task Force recommends screening for AAA in patients who have a relatively high risk of dying from an aneurysm. Major risk factors include age 65 years or older, male sex, and smoking at least 100 cigarettes in a lifetime. The guideline recommends one–time screening with ultrasound for AAA in men 65 to 75 years of age who have ever smoked. No recommendation was made for or against screening in men 65 to 75 years of age who have never smoked, and it recommended against screening women. Men with a strong family history of AAA should be counseled about the risks and benefits of screening as they approach 65 years of age.

U.S. Preventive Services Task Force. Screening for abdominal aortic aneurysm: recommendation statement. *Ann Intern Med.* 2005;142:198–202.

30. The threshold for considering elective repair of an AAA is
A) 4.0 cm
B) 4.5 cm
C) 5.0 cm
D) 5.5 cm
E) 6.0 cm

Answer and Discussion

The answer is D. Patients with aneurysms ≥5.5 cm should be considered for elective AAA repair. Because most clinically diagnosed AAAs are repaired, their long-term natural history is difficult to predict. The 1-year incidence of rupture is 9% for aneurysms 5.5 to 6.0 cm in diameter, 10% for 6.0 to 6.9 cm, and 33% for AAAs of 7.0 cm or more. Patients with an aneurysm <5.5 cm in diameter should have follow-up serial ultrasounds. Smoking is the biggest risk factor for the development of aneurysms.

Kent KC, Zwolak RM, Jaff MR, et al. Abdominal aortic aneurysm. *Am Fam Physician.* 2006;73:1198–1204, 1205–1206.

31. Which of the following classes of drugs has shown modest improvement in cognitive symptoms associated with Alzheimer's disease?
A) Cholinesterase inhibitors
B) Dopamine agonists
C) Norepinephrine antagonist
D) Serotonin reuptake inhibitors
E) None of the above

Answer and Discussion

The answer is A. Treatment with cholinesterase inhibitors can provide mild improvement of symptoms, temporary stabilization of cognition, or reduction in the rate of cognitive decline in some patients with mild to moderate Alzheimer's disease. Approximately 20% to 35% of patients treated with these agents exhibit a 7-point improvement on neuropsychologic tests (equivalent to 1 year's decline and representing a 5% to 15% benefit over placebo). Before treatment is started, it is important to inform the family of the expected (modest) benefits of cholinesterase inhibitors. Four cholinesterase inhibitors are currently available: donepezil (Aricept), rivastigmine (Exelon), galantamine (Reminyl), and tacrine (Cognex). These agents raise acetylcholine levels in the brain by inhibiting acetylcholinesterase.

Cummings JL, Frank JC, Cherry D. Guidelines for managing alzheimer's disease: Part II. Treatment. *Am Fam Physician.* 2002;65:2525–2534.

Rogers SL, Doody RS, Mohs RC, et al. Donepezil improves cognition and global function in Alzheimer disease: a 15-week, double-blind, placebo-controlled study. Donepezil Study Group. *Arch Intern Med.* 1998;158:1021–1031.

32. Which of the following is most consistent with signs and symptoms of retinal detachment?
A) Pain associated with the eye
B) Seeing flashes of light
C) Photophobia
D) Excessive tearing
E) Conjunctival injection

Answer and Discussion

The answer is B. Retinal detachment usually affects individuals older than 50 years. It does not cause pain or erythema of the eye. Bilateral spontaneous detachments are present in as much as 25% of those affected. Retinal detachment can be caused by retinal tears, retinal holes, or by other causes, including ocular melanoma and metastatic tumors. Warning symptoms include floaters, flashes of light (photopsia), or blurred vision. As detachment progresses, the patient may report a "curtain or shade coming down" phenomenon. Macular involvement leads to central visual loss and a worse prognosis. Patients suspected of retinal detachment should undergo emergent ophthalmologic evaluation. Prognosis is best if there is no macular involvement. Without treatment, total detachment usually occurs within 6 months. Treatment of retinal tears or holes is accomplished with laser photocoagulation, cryotherapy, or a scleral buckle. Uncomplicated retinal detachment can be repaired in up to 90% of cases.

Beers MH, Porter RS, eds. *The Merck manual of diagnosis and therapy,* Merck Research Laboratories, 18th ed. Whitehouse Station, NJ: Merck & Co.; 2006:919–920.

33. Which of the following statements about pharmacokinetics in the elderly is true?
A) Body fat stores decrease, and, thus, fat-soluble medications have decreased distribution and there is less risk for toxicity.
B) The glomerular filtration rate is reduced in the elderly, which can lead to a decreased clearance of medication and an increased risk for toxicity.
C) The volume of body water is increased in the elderly, which may require increased dosages of water-soluble medications.
D) Accumulation of active metabolites does not occur in the elderly secondary to rapid clearance.
E) Hepatic metabolism of drugs increases as patients age.

Answer and Discussion

The answer is B. In the United States, approximately two-thirds of persons 65 years or older take prescription and nonprescription (over-the-counter) medications. Women take more drugs than men, because they are, on average, older, and they use more psychoactive and antiarthritic drugs. At any given time, an average older person uses four to five prescription drugs, two over-the-counter drugs, and fills 12 to 17 prescriptions a year. The frail elderly use the most drugs. Drug use is greater in hospitals and nursing homes than in the community; typically, a nursing home resident receives seven or eight drugs. Changes that occur in the elderly often affect the medications that are administered to them. As patients age, they increase their body stores of fat. Because of this, fat-soluble medications have increased distribution and a longer half-life in the body. Although expression of drug-metabolizing enzymes in the cytochrome P-450 systems does not appear to decline with age, the overall hepatic metabolism of many drugs by these enzymes is reduced. The glomerular filtration rate in the elderly is also reduced, which can lead to a decreased clearance of medications and an increased risk for toxicity. The volume of body water is also reduced in the elderly and the administration of water-soluble medications can lead to toxicity with some medications. All these changes must be considered when administering medication to the elderly. Increased sensitivity with aging must be considered when drugs that can have serious adverse effects are used. These drugs include morphine, pentazocine, warfarin, angiotensin-converting enzyme inhibitors, diazepam (especially given parenterally), and levodopa. Some drugs' effects are reduced with aging (e.g., glyburide, β-blockers) and should also be used with caution, because serious dose-related toxicity can still occur, and signs of toxicity may be delayed. Many drugs produce active metabolites in clinically relevant concentrations. Examples are some benzodiazepines (e.g., diazepam, chlordiazepoxide), tertiary amine antidepressants (e.g., amitriptyline, imipramine), antipsychotics (e.g., chlorpromazine, thioridazine; not haloperidol), and opioid analgesics (e.g., morphine, meperidine, propoxyphene). The accumulation of active metabolites (e.g., *N*-acetylprocainamide, morphine-6-glucuronide) can cause toxicity in the elderly as a result of age-related decreases in renal clearance; toxicity is likely to be severe in those with renal disease.

Beers MH, Porter RS, eds. *The Merck manual of diagnosis and therapy,* Merck Research Laboratories, 18th ed. Whitehouse Station, NJ: Merck & Co.; 2006:2535.

34. Which one of the following features can usually distinguish delirium from dementia?
A) There is a lack of long-term memory loss with delirium.
B) The time span over which symptoms develop differs.
C) There is an absence of long-term memory loss with dementia.
D) There is a loss of orientation with delirium.
E) None of the above.

Answer and Discussion

The answer is B. Delirium is a condition that usually develops in an acute situation (over a period of hours to days) and is characterized by confusion, agitation, loss of orientation, lack of attention, hallucinations, paranoia, disturbed sleep–wake cycles, and loss of perception. The condition is a transient global disorder of cognition and consciousness. The delirious patient may also have psychomotor and emotional disturbances. In most patients, delirium due to a medical disease is reversible with treatment of the underlying condition. The symptoms of delirium tend to fluctuate in their course. The etiology may be related to toxin exposure, withdrawal from narcotics or alcohol, medications, vitamin deficiencies, infection, trauma, or structural abnormalities affecting the brain (e.g., tumor, abscess). The best treatment is to correct the underlying cause. Dementia, however, is a slow, progressive condition that may take months to years to develop.

Gleason OC. Delirium. *Am Fam Physician.* 2003;67:1027–1034.

35. Which of the following is the predominant component of dementia?
A) Confusion
B) Anxiety
C) Depression
D) Memory loss
E) Paranoia

Answer and Discussion

The answer is D. Dementia is a condition characterized by the loss of intellectual abilities and the impairment of usually short-term memory. Most patients are older than 65 years. Dementia usually has a slow, progressive, and remitting course. The condition is characterized by a decline in intellectual functioning to the extent that the patient is unable to perform the usual activities of daily living. Memory deficit is a predominant component of dementia, and the deterioration of intellectual functioning may occur over months to years. Dementing diseases in the elderly include Alzheimer's disease (now known as *dementia of the Alzheimer's type*), vascular dementia (previously called *multi-infarct dementia*), and other disorders. The precise mechanisms of the dementias are generally unclear, and no effective cures are available. There is usually no history of prior psychiatric illness, and patients affected typically perform poorly on cognitive tests. *Sundowning* (confusion, loss of orientation) at night in unfamiliar surroundings is common. As many as 15% of dementias are reversible, and, thus, physiologic causes must be ruled out. Treatable causes include medication side effects, depression, hypothyroidism, dehydration, infection, schizophrenia, Wernicke–Korsakoff syndrome, liver or kidney failure, electrolyte abnormalities, hypoglycemia, vitamin deficiency (e.g., vitamin B_{12}), subdural hematoma, normal pressure hydrocephalus, neoplasm, and stroke. The workup should be individualized but in many cases consists of electrolytes, complete blood count, thyroid-stimulating hormone, vitamin B_{12}, Venereal Disease Research Laboratory (VDRL), liver function tests, erythrocyte sedimentation rate, urine and plasma heavy metal screens, electrocardiogram, CT or magnetic resonance imaging of the head, chest x-ray, electroencephalogram, O_2 saturation, and lumbar puncture.

Santacruz KS, Swagerty D. Early diagnosis of dementia. *Am Fam Physician.* 2001; 63:703–713, 717–718.

36. Which of the following is true regarding the use of tacrine (Cognex)?
A) The drug has been shown to cause renal failure and thus serum creatinine must be monitored.
B) The drug is associated with hepatotoxicity and requires the monitoring of liver function tests.
C) The drug is favored over others in its class due to its once daily dosing.
D) The drug has an exceptionally long half-life.
E) Tacrine is considered a first-line agent in the treatment of Alzheimer's disease.

Answer and Discussion

The answer is B. The pharmacologic characteristics and side effects of tacrine make it a second-line agent. Unlike the newer cholinesterase inhibitors, tacrine causes elevation of liver enzyme levels in 40% of treated patients; thus, biweekly liver tests are necessary during the period of dosage escalations and every 3 months thereafter. Because tacrine has a short half-life, it must be administered four times daily.

Cummings JL, Frank JC, Cherry D. Guidelines for managing alzheimer's disease: Part II. Treatment. *Am Fam Physician.* 2002;65:2525–2534.

37. Which of the following is the most common cause of cognitive impairment in elderly patients?
A) Alcohol-induced encephalopathy
B) Multi-infarct dementia
C) Alzheimer's disease
D) Parkinson's associated dementia
E) Pick's disease

Answer and Discussion

The answer is C. Alzheimer's disease is the most common cause of cognitive impairment in elderly persons, with an incidence that doubles every 5 years after the age of 60 years. This disease afflicts approximately 4 million Americans and is estimated to cost the U.S. economy $60 billion annually.

Cummings JL, Frank JC, Cherry D. Guidelines for managing alzheimer's disease: Part I. Assessment. *Am Fam Physician.* 2002;65:2525–2534.

38. Which of the following is not commonly seen in Lewy body dementia?
A) Dementia
B) Delirium
C) Visual hallucinations
D) Bradykinesia
E) Tremor

Answer and Discussion

The answer is E. A useful acronym to remember the cardinal features of dementia with Lewy bodies is DDaVP: Dementia, Delirium (fluctuating cognition), and Visual hallucinations with Parkinsonism. Although bradykinesia, rigidity, and falls are common to those affected, tremor often is absent in dementia with Lewy bodies.

Neef D, Walling AD. Dementia with Lewy bodies: an emerging disease. *Am Fam Physician.* 2006;73:1223–1229, 1230.

A useful acronym to remember the cardinal features of dementia with Lewy bodies is DDaVP: Dementia, Delirium (fluctuating cognition), and Visual hallucinations with Parkinsonism.

39. The leading cause of injury-related visits (in patients older than 65 years) to the emergency room in the United States is which of the following?
A) Motor vehicle accidents
B) Falls
C) Elder abuse
D) Exposure to extremes of temperature
E) Self-induced injury related to depression

Answer and Discussion

The answer is B. Falls affecting the elderly are a major cause of morbidity. Falls are the leading cause of injury-related visits to emergency departments in the United States, and the primary etiology of accidental deaths in persons older than 65 years. They may result in severe injury, including hip or other bone fractures; bruises; and subdural hematomas, as well as dehydration and hypothermia if the patient is not found. Many factors play a role in the cause of falls, including muscle weakness, lack of coordination, poor vision, joint stiffness, autonomic dysfunction, increased reaction time, dementia or delirium, and medications. The physician should always search for precipitating causes such as stroke, cardiac arrhythmias, hypoglycemia, orthostasis, or environmental causes. Precautions should include proper lighting, short-pile carpet, railings, and walkers or canes for those with gait disorders. A visit to the patient's home or living environment may be helpful in determining dangerous conditions. All reversible problems should be corrected. When the cause of a fall is not determined or a patient remains at high risk for falls, referral to a falls prevention program may be warranted.

Fuller GF. Falls in the elderly. *Am Fam Physician.* 2000;61:2159–2168, 2173–2174.

40. Which one of the following laboratory findings is seen with aging?
A) Increase in creatinine clearance
B) Increased aspartate aminotransferase
C) Decreased serum creatinine
D) Decreased incidence of false-positive rapid plasma reagin tests
E) Increase in fasting glucose levels

Answer and Discussion

The answer is E. For the most part, many laboratory normal values remain the same for elderly patients. However, there are some exceptions. With increasing age, there is usually

1. Decline in renal function, as is evident by a 10% decrease in creatinine clearance per 10 years after 40 years of age.
2. Increasing fasting blood glucose (1 mg/dL for every 10 years), although most patients remain within the normal limit values.
3. Increased alkaline phosphatase.
4. Increased incidence of false-positive rapid plasma reagin tests for syphilis.

Other tests, including electrolytes, serum creatinine, and liver function tests, usually remain the same.

Beers MH, Porter RS, eds. *The Merck manual of diagnosis and therapy,* Merck Research Laboratories, 18th ed. Whitehouse Station, NJ: Merck & Co.; 2006:2535–2545.

41. Which one of the following defines a stage II pressure ulcer?
A) A break in the skin with surrounding erythema and induration.
B) An ulcer with penetration of the deep fascia, exposing bone or underlying muscle.
C) A localized area of nonblanchable, erythematous skin.
D) A full-thickness ulcer that extends to the subcutaneous layer but not through the underlying fascia.

Answer and Discussion

The answer is A. Pressure ulcers are quite common in elderly debilitated patients if they are not adequately cared for. Between 3% and 11% of nursing home and hospital patients suffer from pressure ulcers. Precipitating factors include constant pressure, moisture (incontinence), shearing forces, and friction. The ulcers may form as quickly as in 2 to 3 hours if the patient is not repositioned. If patients are placed on their sides, they should be positioned at a 30-degree angle to avoid excessive pressure over the greater trochanter and lateral malleolus. Soft pillows, padded chairs, and egg-crate mattresses can help decrease the risk of ulcer formation but are not a substitute for repositioning. Doughnut-type cushions are not helpful and can cause decreased circulation to the tissue in the center of the doughnut and worsening of any existing ulcers. Alternating air mattresses and waterbeds have been shown to help reduce the incidence of pressure ulcers.

Pressure ulcers are classified as follows:

Stage I—a localized area of nonblanchable, erythematous skin.
Stage II—a break in the skin with surrounding erythema and induration.
Stage III—a full-thickness ulcer that extends to the subcutaneous layer but not through the underlying fascia. Risk for infection is high, and the use of antibiotics may be required.
Stage IV—ulcer penetrates the deep fascia exposing bone or underlying muscle.

Mild pressure sores (stages I and II) require all the prophylactic measures mentioned previously to prevent necrosis. The area should be kept exposed, free from pressure, and dry. Stimulating the circulation by gentle massage can accelerate healing. Ulcers that have not advanced beyond stage III may heal spontaneously if the pressure is removed and the area is small. New hydrophilic gels and hydrocolloid dressings speed healing. Stage IV ulcers require débridement or more extensive surgery. When the ulcers are filled with pus or necrotic debris, dextranomer beads or newer hydrophilic polymers may hasten débridement without surgery. Conservative débridement of necrotic tissue with forceps and scissors should be instituted. Some ulcers may be débrided by cleansing with 1.5% hydrogen peroxide. Whirlpool baths may assist débridement. More advanced ulcers with fat and muscle involvement require surgical débridement and closure. For cellulitis, a penicillinase-resistant penicillin or a cephalosporin is necessary. A culture is generally not helpful in choosing an antibiotic, because surface growth is often polymicrobial.

Beers MH, Porter RS, eds. *The Merck manual of diagnosis and therapy*, Merck Research Laboratories, 18th ed. Whitehouse Station, NJ: Merck & Co.; 2006:1011–1017.

42. An 85-year-old nursing home patient was seen in a local physician's office during the day for a corneal abrasion. The patient had antibiotic drops instilled, and the eye was patched. At 10:00 p.m., the nursing staff calls reporting that the patient is very confused. The most appropriate action is to

A) remove the eye patch
B) prescribe haloperidol
C) have the patient taken to the emergency room
D) reassure the nursing staff and see the patient the next day
E) restrain the patient to protect him from injury

Answer and Discussion

The answer is A. Sensory deprivation, such as patching an elderly patient's eyes, may lead to an acute case of delirium. Even small alterations in the elderly patient's environment can lead to confusion. In cases of corneal abrasions, an elderly patient should receive topical ophthalmic antibiotics. Although eye patching traditionally has been recommended in the treatment of corneal abrasions, multiple well-designed studies show that patching does not help and may hinder healing. Topical anesthetics should not be used for corneal abrasions, because they interfere with the healing process; however, they may be useful in the initial evaluation to help relieve discomfort.

Wilson SA, Last A. Management of corneal abrasions. *Am Fam Physician*. 2004;70:123–128, 129–130.

43. Which of the following defines a *durable power of attorney*?

A) A written advance directive that assigns one person as a decision-making proxy should the user become incapacitated.
B) A written advance directive in which a competent person indicates health-care preferences while cognitively and physically intact.
C) A detailed written directive that describes in questionnaire format what type of treatment a person would or would not want in various medical situations.
D) The ability of attorneys to sue physicians for negligence.
E) None of the above.

Answer and Discussion

The answer is A. A *durable power of attorney* is defined as a written advance directive that assigns one person as a decision-making proxy should the user become incapacitated. A *living will* is a written advance directive in which a competent person indicates health-care preferences while cognitively and physically intact. A *medical directive* is a detailed written directive that describes in questionnaire format what type of treatment a person would or would not want in various medical situations.

Krane MK. Respecting end-of-life treatment preferences. *Am Fam Physician*. 2005;72:1263–1268, 1270.

44. You are called by the nursing supervisor at the local nursing home where you manage patients. She reports the outbreak of influenza A in three of the patients. What is your most appropriate response?

A) You place patients in isolation and call if any further episodes occur.
B) You order amantadine (Symmetrel) for all contacts.
C) You order rimantadine (Flumadine) for all contacts.
D) You order zanamivir (Relenza) for all contacts.
E) You order treatment with oseltamivir (Tamiflu) for any patients who develop symptoms of influenza.

Answer and Discussion

The answer is C. Chronically ill and elderly persons have a higher incidence of side effects while taking amantadine and rimantadine. Both medications can cause gastrointestinal effects such as anorexia and nausea. However, amantadine has significantly more side effects relating to the central nervous system than rimantadine, including confusion, anxiety, insomnia, hallucinations, and falls in nursing home residents. Amantadine also has significantly higher discontinuation rates (up to 17%). Because of this higher incidence of adverse effects and higher discontinuation rates, rimantadine should be the drug of choice in the prophylaxis and treatment of influenza A in nursing home residents.

Keyser LA, Karl M, Nafziger AN, et al. Comparison of central nervous system adverse effects of amantadine and rimantadine used as sequential prophylaxis of influenza A in elderly nursing home patients. *Arch Intern Med*. 2000;160:1485–1488.

Kingston BJ, Wright CV Jr. Influenza in the nursing home. *Am Fam Physician*. 2002;65:75–78.

45. Glucosamine has been shown to be helpful in the treatment of

A) low back pain
B) neck pain
C) hip and knee pain
D) diffuse myalgias
E) none of the above

Answer and Discussion

The answer is C. Sufficient evidence exists from studies of persons with hip or knee osteoarthritis to support the use of glucosamine as a safe and effective alternative treatment.

Towheed TE, Maxwell L, Anastassiades TP, et al. Glucosamine therapy for treating osteoarthritis. *Cochrane Database Syst Rev.* 2005;2:CD002946.

46. Which of the following is necessary to diagnose menopause?
A) Estrogen levels < 30mg/dl
B) FSH level > 35 mg/dl
C) An abnormal progesterone challenge test
D) None of the above

Answer and Discussion

The answer is D. *Menopause* is defined as the absence of menses for 6 months. The average age of onset is 51 years. Symptoms of menopause are common and include hot flashes, night sweats, mood swings with emotional lability and irritability, depression, insomnia, vaginal dryness, dyspareunia, dysuria, and urinary incontinence. Hormone replacement therapy (estrogen with or without progestin) was the primary treatment for the symptoms and long-term risks associated with menopause. However, recent evidence fails to confirm the protective effect of estrogen on cardiovascular disease risk. Menopause can be confirmed by measuring follicle-stimulating hormone levels; however, this is not necessary for the diagnosis. Follicle-stimulating hormone levels higher than 35 support a menopausal state. Also, a progesterone challenge test (13 days of progestin) resulting in no withdrawal bleeding indicates a lack of estrogen and the menopausal state.

Cutson TM, Meuleman E. Managing menopause. *Am Fam Physician.* 2000;61:1391–1340, 1405–1406.

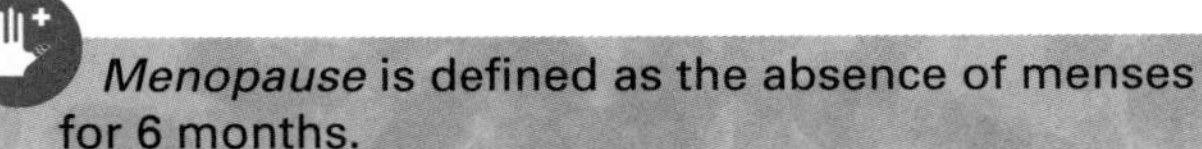

Menopause is defined as the absence of menses for 6 months.

47. Which one of the following statements concerning cataracts is true?
A) They are usually unilateral.
B) Asymptomatic lens opacities should be removed because of risk to the retina.
C) Ultraviolet light exposure may contribute to the progression of cataract formation.
D) The cataracts require a slit-lamp examination to be seen.
E) Surgery is rarely helpful for advanced cataract formation.

Answer and Discussion

The answer is C. Cataracts are lens opacities that result in a painless loss of vision in patients usually older than 60 years. The prevalence of cataract increases with age from <5% in persons younger than 65 years to approximately 50% in those 75 years of age and older. They are usually bilateral and develop gradually over many years. Exposure to ultraviolet light may contribute to the progression of cataract formation. Typical symptoms related to cataracts include decreased visual acuity, particularly at night, with excessive glare in bright light or sunlight. Most cataracts can be visualized with a handheld ophthalmoscope; however, slit-lamp examination may be more revealing. Cataract surgery is the most common surgical procedure covered by Medicare, with more than 1 million procedures performed annually. This surgery should be considered when the cataract reduces vision function to a level that interferes with everyday activities. The mere presence of lens opacities—that is, lens opacities not associated with decreased visual function—is not an indication for surgery in most instances. Cataract surgery is an outpatient procedure performed under local or topical anesthesia. More than 90% of patients undergoing cataract surgery experience visual improvement and improved quality of life if there is no ocular comorbidity. Complications of cataract surgery are unusual and occur in less than 1% of surgeries. Potentially serious complications include glaucoma, bleeding, infection, vitreous loss, retinal detachment, and loss of vision.

Landefeld CS, Palmer R, Johnson MA. *Current Geriatric Diagnosis and Treatment.* New York: Lange Medical Books/McGraw Hill; 2004:122–124.

48. A nurse calls to report that a hospitalized patient fell and is now complaining of severe left-hip pain. On arriving at the patient's room, you noticed the woman's left leg is shorter than the right and is externally rotated. The most likely diagnosis is
A) left-fibular fracture
B) stable left-hip fracture
C) left–anterior cruciate ligament injury
D) unstable left-hip fracture
E) unstable right-hip fracture

Answer and Discussion

The answer is D. Hip fractures represent significant morbidity and mortality as well as health-care costs to the elderly. Fractures of the femoral neck are classified as being stable or unstable. Stable fractures include stress or impacted fractures. Patients usually report minimal pain and may be able to walk with only mild groin pain and perhaps a limp. The physical exam is unremarkable. Both stress and impacted fractures may be treated nonoperatively; however, impacted fractures are at an increased risk to become displaced and are, therefore, usually corrected with internal fixation to stabilize a reduction and allow earlier weight bearing. Patients who are demented, nonambulatory, or poor surgical candidates should be treated by nonsurgical means. Conservative measures to protect the injured extremity, prevent decubitus ulcers, and avoid pneumonia should be instituted. Unstable fractures include displaced and comminuted fractures that can be life threatening for the elderly. Most patients report considerable pain with any movement of the hip. The physical exam usually shows the affected extremity is externally rotated and shorter in length than the unaffected side. Treatment consists of surgical reduction and internal fixation followed by traction.

Landefeld CS, Palmer R, Johnson MA. *Current Geriatric Diagnosis and Treatment.* New York: Lange Medical Books/McGraw Hill; 2004:386–388.

49. A 65-year-old woman presents to your office complaining of leakage of urine when she coughs or sneezes. The most likely diagnosis is
A) urinary tract infection
B) urge incontinence
C) neurogenic bladder
D) stress incontinence
E) interstitial cystitis

Answer and Discussion

The answer is D. *Stress urinary incontinence* is defined as bladder outlet incompetence and the loss of urine with coughing, sneezing, straining, lifting, or any activity that requires a Valsalva maneuver and associated increased abdominal pressure. In women, the usual cause is a loss in the normal posterior ureterovesical angle as a result of pelvic floor muscle laxity. Pelvic floor weakness is a common result of aging and multiparity. Treatment may involve the use of Kegel exercises (multiple contractions of the pelvic floor muscles as if the patient were shutting off the flow of urine) and α-adrenergic medications (e.g., pseudoephedrine). Estrogens may also be effective in treating women with stress incontinence. The presence of estrogen receptors in high concentrations throughout the lower urinary tract makes it possible to treat women with stress incontinence by localized estrogen replacement therapy. Estrogen replacement therapy causes engorgement of the periurethral blood supply and subsequent thickening of the urethral mucosa. Localized estrogen replacement therapy can be given in the form of estrogen cream or an estradiol-impregnated vaginal ring (Estring). Surgery (Marshall–Marchetti procedure) may be considered if the condition is severe and refractive to medication. In some cases, the use of a pessary may be beneficial. The U.S. Food and Drug Administration recently approved extracorporeal magnetic innervation, a noninvasive procedure for the treatment of incontinence caused by pelvic floor weakness. The patient sits fully clothed in a pulsating magnetic chair that stimulates the pelvic floor. A typical treatment session lasts approximately 20 minutes and includes high- and low-frequency stimulation. Preliminary results from one uncontrolled trial suggest that extracorporeal magnetic innervation may have a place in the treatment of women with stress and urge incontinence. Another minimally invasive procedure for the treatment of stress incontinence is periurethral injection. This procedure involves injection of material at the bladder neck just under the urothelium and is performed in an office setting under local anesthesia. Pharmacologic agents may be given empirically to women with symptoms of overactive bladder. Two new medications, tolterodine (Detrol) and extended-release oxybutynin chloride (Ditropan XL), have largely replaced generic oxybutynin as a first-line treatment option for overactive bladder because of favorable side effect profiles.

Culligan PJ, Heit M. Urinary incontinence in women: evaluation and management. *Am Fam Physician.* 2000;62:2433–2444, 2447, 2452.

50. An 85-year-old man complains of chronic insomnia. Based on study results, you know that

A) insomnia is relatively rare in the elderly
B) insomnia is a natural progression of aging and has little effect on the well-being of elderly patients
C) chronic insomnia is an independent risk factor for cognitive decline in elderly men
D) insomnia has no impact on the risk of falls
E) insomnia does not lead to nursing home placement

Answer and Discussion

The answer is C. Chronic insomnia is an independent risk factor for cognitive decline in patients 65 years and older, especially in men. Insomnia is often associated with dependence on sleep medications, chronic fatigue, and increased risk of falls. Chronic sleep disturbances may lead to nursing home placement.

Cricco M, Simonsick EM, Foley DJ. The impact of insomnia on cognitive functioning in older adults. *J Am Geriatr Soc.* 2001;49:1185–1189.

51. Which of the following tests may help identify elders who are at increased risk for falling?

A) Straight line test
B) One foot hop test
C) Two hand one foot test
D) Sit down and stop test
E) Get up and go test

Answer and Discussion

The answer is E. Approximately one third of noninstitutionalized elders fall each year. The annual incidence of falls approaches 50% in patients over 80 years of age. Factors contributing to falls include age-related postural changes, decreased vision, certain medications (particularly anticholinergic, sedative, and diuretic medications), and diseases affecting muscle strength and coordination. A straightforward physical examination maneuver called the "get up and go" test can help identify those at risk for falls. In this test, the patient is instructed to arise from a sitting position, walk 10 feet, turn, and return to the chair to sit. A requirement of >16 seconds to complete the process or observation of postural instability or gait impairment suggests an increased risk of falling. A number of effective interventions are available for people with a history of falls or who are at risk for falling.

Mathias, S, Nayak, US, Isaacs, B. Balance in elderly patients: the "get up and go" test. *Arch Phys Med Rehabil.* 1986;67:387.

52. A 70-year-old man is recently diagnosed with early Alzheimer's disease. His family is very concerned with his ability to drive. You explain to them

A) in the first year after the diagnosis is made, patients with Alzheimer's disease have a similar rate of accidents as registered drivers of all ages
B) the risk of accidents rarely changes as Alzheimer's patients grow older
C) the department of transportation is the only group that has a role in the determination of driving skills
D) roadside testing should not be used to determine the ability to drive
E) accident rates may be overestimated because of the number of miles elderly people drive

Answer and Discussion

The answer is A. In many situations one of the first safety issues to be confronted with elderly patients affected with dementia is their driving. In the first year after diagnosis, patients affected with Alzheimer's disease (AD) have a similar rate of accidents as registered drivers of all ages, although higher than age-matched controls. The risk of motor vehicle accidents increases dramatically in the following years. This increase is likely underrepresented in that the risk per mile driven is much greater because patients substantially reduce their driving. Discussions of driving cessation are often difficult. Patients are generally unaware of their deficits (particularly their deficits in judgment), and surrendering a license often represents a severe loss of independence. With early diagnosis, many patients will still be able to drive safely for a period of time, but all will eventually progress to the point where it is no longer safe to drive. Discussions with patients in the intermediate stages of dementia pose the greatest difficulty. Only the state of California currently has a requirement that physicians notify authorities when a patient is diagnosed with dementia. Although a number of driving safety tests have been suggested, no general guidelines have been broadly instituted. Local programs may exist to evaluate these patients with neuropsychological and roadside tests. In the absence of these programs, the department of motor vehicles often performs roadside testing, but patients must be informed that even if they pass they must be retested at regular intervals as their disease progresses. Families must be warned about potential liability for accidents. They may need to take possession of car keys, or even the cars, and restrict all driving. The American Academy of Neurology has issued guidelines for driving in patients with AD based on the clinical dementia rating scale.

Dubinsky RM, Stein AC, Lyons K. Practice parameter: risk of driving and Alzheimer's disease (an evidence-based review): report of the quality standards subcommittee of the American Academy of Neurology. *Neurology.* 2000;54:2205.

53. Which of the following statements about rehabilitation after a stroke is true?

A) Physical therapy should be instituted for stretching and strengthening once supporting muscles are strong enough to support appropriate loads.
B) Tennis ball exercises can be used to strengthen the hand muscles.
C) Most motor function improvement occurs more than 6 months after a cerebral vascular accident.
D) A walking cane used on the affected side can help with ambulation and balance.
E) Bladder or bowel incontinence has no effect on prognosis after stroke.

Answer and Discussion

The answer is A. Rehabilitation after a stroke is often a difficult and lengthy process. Most improvement in motor function occurs in the first 6 to 12 weeks after a stroke; speech may continue to improve significantly after this period. Stretching and strengthening exercises should be instituted when the supporting muscles are capable of supporting the appropriate loads. Gait training should take place as soon as the hip musculature is capable of supporting the patient's weight. In many cases, the patient can use a cane in the hand opposite to the side the stroke affected to help support the weaker side. Squeezing a tennis ball as a hand exercise should be discouraged, because it favors finger flexors over extensors and can lead to contractures. Using a team approach with a physical therapist, occupational therapist, speech therapist, and social workers is often beneficial. The outcome after a stroke is most likely to be positive when patients have bladder and bowel continence, are able to feed themselves, and have a healthy and caring spouse. Stroke rehabilitation must include the prevention or early diagnosis of medical complications, as well as patient and family education concerning the prevention of recurrent stroke.

Landefeld CS, et al. *Current Geriatric Diagnosis and Treatment.* New York: Lange Medical Books / McGraw Hill; 2004:381–382.

> Most improvement in motor function occurs in the first 6 to 12 weeks after a stroke; speech may continue to improve significantly after this period.

54. Pernicious anemia is associated with

A) vitamin B_{12} malabsorption
B) chronic blood loss
C) myelofibrosis
D) iron deficiency
E) malignancy

Answer and Discussion

The answer is A. Anemia should not be accepted as an unavoidable consequence of aging. A cause is found in approximately 80% of elderly patients. The most common causes of anemia in the elderly are chronic disease and iron deficiency. Vitamin B_{12} deficiency, folate deficiency, gastrointestinal bleeding, and myelodysplastic syndrome are among other causes of anemia in the elderly. Serum ferritin is the most useful test to differentiate iron deficiency anemia from anemia of chronic disease. The condition of pernicious anemia is the result of malabsorption or lack of ingestion of vitamin B_{12}. The lack of absorption is usually the result of atrophic gastric mucosa, which fails to produce the intrinsic factor that is required for the absorption of vitamin B_{12}. With pernicious anemia, the lack of intrinsic factor results from destruction of the gastric parietal cells by autoimmune antibodies. Previous gastrectomy, blind-loop syndrome, fish tapeworm infections, or thyroid abnormalities may also decrease intrinsic factor secretion. The anemia usually develops over time and is associated with macrocytic features, basophilic stippling of red blood cells, and an increased red blood cell distribution width index. *Achlorhydria* (lack of acid production) is usually associated with pernicious anemia. Symptoms of pernicious anemia include anorexia, constipation, diarrhea, and abdominal pain; glossitis; loss of sensation involving the distal extremities; weight loss; and generalized fatigue. Previously, the Schilling test would have been used to identify the cause of inadequate vitamin B_{12} absorption. Recent studies, however, show that high-dose oral vitamin B_{12} effectively treats the deficiency regardless of the cause. Vitamin B_{12} deficiency is effectively treated with high-dose oral or parenteral vitamin B_{12} supplementation.

Smith DL. Anemia in the elderly. *Am Fam Physician.* 2000;62: 1565–1572.

55. Which one of the following statements about Alzheimer's disease is true?

A) It is associated with microscopic senile plaques, neurofibrillary tangles, and granulovacuolar degeneration of neurons in the brain.
B) It is associated with birth trauma.
C) It is usually reversible.
D) It is associated with tremor, ataxia, and muscle rigidity.
E) It is not familial.

Answer and Discussion

The answer is A. Alzheimer's disease is a progressive, irreversible cause of dementia. It is the most common type of dementia. Symptoms include memory difficulties, disorientation, impaired judgment, aphasia, and apraxia. Histopathologic changes seen in the brain with Alzheimer's include microscopic senile plaques, neurofibrillary tangles, and granulovacuolar degeneration of neurons. A CT scan usually shows cerebral cortical atrophy and ventricular dilation. There is no identifiable cause, and other causes for dementia must be ruled out before a diagnosis of Alzheimer's disease is made. It is important to remember that 5% to 15% of dementias are reversible and may be caused by factors such as meningiomas, subdural hematomas, systemic illnesses, deficiency states and endocrinopathies, heavy metal and drug poisonings, and infections. Alzheimer's disease is familial, and no specific cause has been identified. Treatment is supportive. Efforts should be made to provide regular routines that the patient becomes accustomed to. The mainstay of treatment options is acetylcholinesterase inhibitors, which increase the duration of acetylcholine action in synapses. Tacrine (Cognex), the earliest drug in this group, has only limited benefit and a poor side effect profile, including hepatotoxicity. Donepezil (Aricept) is a highly selective acetylcholinesterase inhibitor that significantly improved cognitive scores (during phases 2 and 3 clinical trials) with a better side effect profile. A newer acetylcholinesterase inhibitor, rivastigmine (Exelon), has a good side effect profile but requires more time for dosage titration than donepezil. Estrogen therapy increases acetylcholine concentrations and has antioxidant activity, but proof of its ability to reduce the risk of Alzheimer's disease has not been shown. Anti-inflammatory drugs are under investigation. Antioxidants, including selegiline and ginkgo biloba, have demonstrated some benefits in improving cognition and delaying progression of the disease, but the outcome measures used have been variable, making treatment recommendations difficult.

O'Hara R, Mumenthaler MS, Yesavage JA. Update on Alzheimer's disease: recent findings and treatments. *West J Med.* 2000;172: 115–120.

56. Which one of the following is most likely to cause hypoglycemia in the elderly treated for diabetes mellitus?
A) Metformin (Glucophage)
B) Glyburide (Micronase, DiaBeta)
C) Glipizide (Glucotrol)
D) None of the above

Answer and Discussion

The answer is C. Diabetes in the elderly poses some additional concern. The elderly develop microvascular complications such as diabetic retinopathy and peripheral neuropathy more quickly than younger patients. Diabetes also represents a major risk factor for the development of atherosclerosis. The renal threshold for glucose is also increased in the elderly, allowing higher levels of blood glucose before glycosuria is seen. The use of glyburide has shown a twofold relative risk of hypoglycemia when compared with glipizide. Metformin does not cause hypoglycemia with monotherapy.

Landefeld CS, Palmer R, Johnson MA. *Current Geriatric Diagnosis and Treatment*. New York: Lange Medical Books/McGraw Hill; 2004:343–345.

57. An 85-year-old Alzheimer's patient is reported missing from a local nursing home. You are contacted about directions for a search. You make all of following statements *except*
A) Most people found alive are found within 24 hours.
B) Of those who die, >90% are found in natural areas.
C) Night searches should be avoided, because individuals are unlikely to wander when it is dark.
D) The first areas searched should be concentrated on open, populated areas.
E) The hottest and coldest times of the year are associated with the highest risk of death.

Answer and Discussion

The answer is C. The issue of wandering and becoming lost, with the possibility for physical harm or death, is one of the concerns that often leads families and caregivers to place demented patients in nursing homes. A review of this issue that analyzed data from several available studies produced the following observations. All persons with dementia are at risk of becoming lost. The risk may be higher for demented men than for women. Individuals residing in professional care settings are at risk as well as those at home. Wandering is only a risk factor; individuals who had never wandered have become lost. The risk of becoming lost is increased when demented persons are unattended, even in their own residences. However, about 65% of people with dementia are in the presence of a caregiver at the time they become lost. Becoming lost appears to be a highly unpredictable event and can occur even when individuals with dementia are in their own homes or are participating in activities they had routinely performed many times in the past without incident. Most individuals who are found alive remain out in the open in populated areas of the community. The risk of death is increased if the demented person ends up secluded in natural or sparsely populated areas. About 91% of persons with dementia who died were found in natural areas such as woods, fields, ditches, bodies of water (approximately 20% drowned), or abandoned vehicles. The risk of death also appears to be associated with the hottest and coldest times of the year. The time it took to search for and locate a missing person with dementia also correlated with the risk of death, as most individuals found alive were located within 24 hours, and all were found within 4 days. Locating a person with dementia who becomes lost can be difficult, and this problem is complicated by several factors related to the increased likelihood of abnormal behavior. People with dementia are often unpredictable when lost. The accuracy of the search is usually not enhanced by predictions from families and caregivers. The lost persons rarely call for help or respond to searcher's calls. Search strategies should not be based on the individual characteristics of the missing person, because the unpredictable and abnormal behavior is likely to negate any prior individual patterns. Caregivers should report the person missing immediately to local authorities. An exhaustive search should begin immediately, so that the individual has less time to find a secluded hiding place and has reduced exposure to the environment. Searches should continue through the night, as individuals often continue to wander. The initial 6 to 12 hours of the search should cover a 5-mile radius around the location where the lost person was last seen, concentrating on open, populated areas, including the inside of easily accessible buildings. If initial search efforts fail, the subsequent efforts should be devoted to an intensive foot search of natural and sparsely populated areas beginning within a 1-mile radius of the last known location and extending from there. If the person with dementia traveled by car, initial search efforts should focus on locating the vehicle. Caregivers, both formal and informal, must be informed that all persons with dementia are at risk of becoming lost, even if the individual has never wandered or exhibited "risky" behavior in the past. Because the risk is highest when persons with dementia are left unattended, every effort should be made to ensure continuous supervision. Community resources, adult day care and respite care facilities, and caregiver support groups may be utilized, if available, to reduce the burden on families and caregivers.

Rowe MA, Feinglass NG, Wiss ME. Persons with dementia who become lost in the community: a case study, current research, and recommendations. *Mayo Clin Proc.* 2004; 79:1417.

58. Which of the following supplements has been shown to decrease the risk of falls?
A) Glucosamine/chrondroitin
B) Vitamin C
C) Ginkgo biloba
D) Vitamin D
E) Vitamin B_{12}

Answer and Discussion

The answer is D. Vitamin D supplementation, with or without calcium, has been shown to decrease the risk of falls in elderly patients. A subsequent meta-analysis focused specifically on vitamin D supplementation and concluded that such supplementation reduces the risk of falls (odds ratio 0.78, 95% CI 0.64–0.92); the proposed mechanism is through improvements in muscle strength with supplementation.

Bischoff-Ferrari HA, Dawson-Hughes B, Willett WC, et al. Effect of vitamin D on falls: a meta-analysis. *JAMA*. 2004;291:1999.

59. When performing an evaluation of urinary incontinence in elderly patients which of the following tests is *not* initially indicated?
A) Urinalysis
B) Urine culture
C) Serum glucose
D) Serum calcium
E) Urodynamic testing

Answer and Discussion

The answer is E. Physicians must initiate a discussion of voiding symptoms because at least one half of incontinent individuals do not report the problem to their providers. A physical examination for incontinence should be comprehensive and extend "above the waistline." In persons with symptoms of stress incontinence a clinical stress test may be performed by having the patient (who should not have recently voided) give a single vigorous cough while standing and maintaining a relaxed perineum. Instantaneous leakage suggests stress incontinence, whereas a delay of several seconds before leakage suggests stress-induced detrusor overactivity. If urinary retention is suspected, it is important to consider post-void residual testing, either by catheterization or ultrasound. A post-void residual >200 mL suggests detrusor weakness or obstruction, and in men should prompt a renal ultrasound examination to exclude hydronephrosis. If not recorded recently, it is necessary to measure renal function, glucose, calcium, and, in older people, vitamin B_{12} levels. A urinalysis should be obtained in all patients and a urine culture if infection is suspected. Routine urodynamic testing is not recommended, and is mainly of value to provide an accurate diagnosis when surgery is being considered.

Dubeau CE. Clinical presentation and diagnosis of urinary incontinence. Up to Date Online 14.1. http://uptodateonline.com. Accessed 4/10/06.

60. A 79-year-old woman with a history of atherosclerosis and hypertension is seen in the emergency room. The patient reports she suddenly lost her vision in her left eye on awakening this morning. She reports no pain associated with the eye and has no other symptoms. Funduscopic examination shows disk swelling, extensive retinal hemorrhages, and cotton-wool spots. The most likely diagnosis is
A) cerebrovascular accident
B) central retinal vein occlusion
C) closed-angle glaucoma
D) macular degeneration
E) transient ischemic attack

Answer and Discussion

The answer is B. Central vein occlusion usually affects elderly patients with atherosclerosis. The severity is variable; older individuals are usually affected more severely. Predisposing factors include hypertension, diabetes mellitus, glaucoma, increased blood viscosity, and elevated hematocrit. Symptoms include a sudden, dramatic, painless loss of vision usually first noticed on awakening in the morning. Physical findings include disk swelling, venous dilation, retinal hemorrhages, and cotton-wool spots. Those with poor visual acuity at the onset have the worst prognosis. These patients usually have extensive hemorrhages and cotton-wool spots, indicating retinal ischemia, and they may develop neovascular (rubeotic) glaucoma within 3 months after the initial occlusion. Should this occur, laser photocoagulation should be performed; otherwise, there is no medical therapy available. Underlying predisposing factors should be ruled out and treated appropriately if present. Branch vein occlusions may show varying degrees of visual loss and have a better prognosis than central vein occlusion.

Beers MH, Porter RS, eds. *The Merck manual of diagnosis and therapy,* Merck Research Laboratories, 18th ed. Whitehouse Station, NJ: Merck & Co.; 2006:917–918.

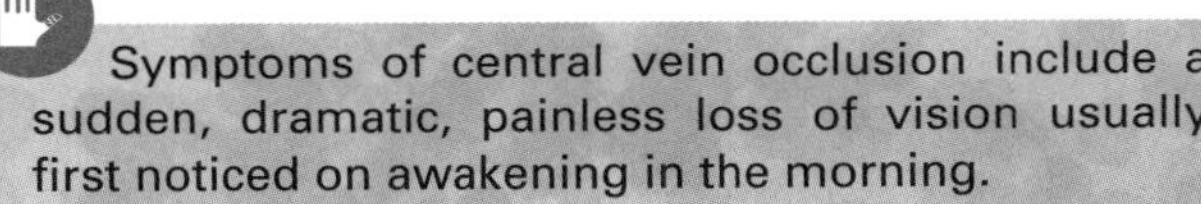
Symptoms of central vein occlusion include a sudden, dramatic, painless loss of vision usually first noticed on awakening in the morning.

61. Which of the following statements about hip fractures associated with osteoporosis is true?
A) African Americans have a higher incidence of osteoporosis and associated fractures.
B) The affected leg is usually shortened, abducted, and externally rotated.
C) Most fractures result from compression-type injuries rather than from falls laterally.
D) Bisphosphonates have not been found to be beneficial in preventing hip fractures.
E) The risk is highest for elderly men who have vision problems.

Answer and Discussion

The answer is B. Hip fractures as a result of osteoporosis represent a major morbidity for the elderly. The cost for treatment is excessive. Elderly persons are rightfully concerned about the loss of independence associated with fractures. Six months after a hip fracture, many older persons still require assistance with the activities of daily living. Furthermore, >10% of persons with hip fractures die. In the United States alone, hip fractures are responsible for 31,000 deaths each year. The risk is greatest for postmenopausal women who suffer from osteoporosis. Whites have a higher incidence of osteoporosis and associated fractures than African Americans. Most hip fractures occur as a result of falling sideways and not from compression. This mechanism of injury has a direct impact on the greater trochanter at the proximal femur. Most hip fractures present with the affected leg shortened, abducted, and externally rotated. Other fracture sites, including the spine (compression type), wrist, humerus, and tibia, are also affected. The use of estrogen replacement therapy and calcium supplementation with vitamin D in postmenopausal women has a protective effect; however, because of controversy over estrogen risk, many avoid this treatment. The use of bisphosphonates, such as alendronate (Fosamax), risidronate (Actonel), etidronate (Didronel), or once monthly ibandronate (Boniva); calcitonin (Miacalcin); or raloxifene (Evista), a selective estrogen receptor modulator, can be beneficial in preventing further bone loss. Hip protectors may also help prevent hip fractures, although recent evidence is controversial.

Kannus P, Parkkari J, Niemi S, et al. Prevention of hip fracture in elderly people with use of a hip protector. *N Engl J Med.* 2000;343:1506–1513.

62. The solid tumor malignancy most frequently diagnosed in elderly men is
A) lung cancer
B) colon cancer
C) prostate cancer
D) lymphoma
E) esophageal cancer

Answer and Discussion

The answer is C. In the United States, prostate cancer is the most common solid tumor malignancy in men and, second to lung cancer, is the leading cause of cancer deaths in this group. African Americans are at higher risk than Whites. The risk increases with age, and 70% of men older than 80 years are affected. Diagnosis is usually made by the detection of a palpable prostate nodule on physical examination followed by a PSA determination, which is elevated. The combination of a digital rectal examination and PSA test is more accurate in diagnosing early prostate cancer than either alone. The main problem with prostate cancer screening is that, although this malignancy is extremely common, it is the actual cause of death in only a small proportion of patients who have histologic evidence of prostate cancer. Prostate cancer screening programs may result in the detection and treatment of many asymptomatic cancers that have no impact on length of life. The decision to offer prostate cancer screening must be made on an individual basis, depending on the patient's age, health status, family history, risk of prostate cancer, and personal beliefs. The patient must be informed about the risks and potential benefits of screening. The patient also must be helped to realize that, although prostate cancer can grow quickly, it generally grows quite slowly.

Ultrasound examination with possible biopsy should be performed if the physical exam or PSA determination is abnormal. Metastasis is usually local extension or to bone and may manifest itself in low-back pain as the presenting complaint in an elderly man. Treatment consists of surgery, radiation, and hormonal manipulation, depending on the stage and type of tumor identified. In radical prostatectomy, the entire prostate is excised from the urethra and bladder, which are then reconnected. Severe complications from radical prostatectomy are relatively uncommon. However, damage to the urinary sphincter and penile nerves during surgery can result in postoperative urinary incontinence and impotence. External-beam radiotherapy appears to be as effective as surgery in curing prostate cancer, at least for the first 10 years after treatment. Radiotherapy is well tolerated, and it is associated with no hemorrhagic or anesthetic risks. Furthermore, this treatment option does not require hospitalization or a significant recovery period. Normal activity can usually be maintained during radiotherapy. However, treatment is administered daily for 4 to 6 weeks, and many patients report feeling fatigued at the end of this period. It is associated with severe bladder irritation (urgency, pain, and frequency) in as much as 5% of patients. Rectal irritations (diarrhea, urgency, tenesmus, and bleeding) occur in 3% to 10% of patients who receive radiotherapy for prostate cancer, and impotence is a problem in 40% to 50% of patients receiving this treatment. The two types of radiotherapy are external-beam irradiation and implantation of radioactive pellets (seeds). Although neither approach has been shown to be superior in terms of long-term outcome, seed implant therapy has been gaining in popularity since its introduction. Because of controversy surrounding outcomes and the potential for complications, the patient should be informed of the risks and benefits and participate in the decision making process.

Bhatnagar V, Kaplan RM. Treatment options for prostate cancer: evaluating the evidence. *Am Fam Physician.* 2005;71: 1915–1922, 1929–1930.

63. Which one of the following statements about herpes zoster is true?
A) The virus remains dormant in the muscle fibers and can be reactivated by stress.
B) The rash is usually maculopapular, bilateral, and typically affects the lower abdomen.
C) The virus can lead to chronic, debilitating pain for an extended period after resolution of the rash.
D) Steroids should not be used for treatment in patients older than 50 years because of their immunosuppressant properties.
E) Exposure to patients with varicella (chickenpox) can cause herpes zoster.

Answer and Discussion

The answer is C. Herpes zoster, also known as *shingles*, is caused by a reactivation of the virus that causes varicella (chickenpox). The virus remains dormant in the nerve endings and reactivates itself, in some cases, as a result of stress or infection. In most cases, a vesicular, painful rash develops in a single, unilateral, dermatomal pattern. Herpes zoster typically presents with a prodrome consisting of hyperesthesia, paresthesias, burning dysesthesias, or pruritus along the affected dermatome(s). The prodrome generally lasts 1 to 2 days but may precede the appearance of skin lesions by up to 3 weeks.

The elderly are most frequently affected. Areas of involvement usually include the trunk; however, it may occur on the face (in the distribution of the trigeminal nerve). Other symptoms include fatigue, fever, and headache. After the resolution of the rash, many patients develop postherpetic neuralgia, which can be chronic and debilitating. For acute herpes zoster, the antivirals acyclovir (Zovirax), valacyclovir (Valtrex), and famciclovir (Famvir) are useful for treatment, particularly if administered early in the course of the disease. If the use of orally administered prednisone is not contraindicated, adjunctive treatment with this agent is justified on the basis of its effects in reducing pain, despite questionable evidence for its benefits in decreasing the incidence of postherpetic neuralgia. Given the theoretic risk of immunosuppression with corticosteroids, some investigators believe that these agents should be used only in patients older than 50 years, because they are at greater risk of developing postherpetic neuralgia and prednisone may be beneficial. Treatment of postherpetic neuralgia consists of topical capsaicin (Zostrix) and amitriptyline. Pregabalin (Lyrica) is a new medication recently approved for the treatment of post herpetic neuralgia. Additionally a new immunization

(Zostavax) has been approved for the prevention of herpes zoster in patients over the age of 60. Those not immune to varicella can develop varicella after exposure to herpes zoster.

Stankus SJ, Dlugopolski M, Packer D. Management of herpes zoster (shingles) and postherpetic neuralgia. *Am Fam Physician.* 2000;61:2437–2444, 2447–2448.

64. The misuse and overprescribing of psychotropics leads to adverse effects and deteriorating medical and cognitive status. To combat the problem in the United States, nursing home reform legislation, the Omnibus Budget Reconciliation Act of 1987 (OBRA–87), mandated freedom for every resident from medically unnecessary "physical or chemical restraints imposed for purposes of discipline or convenience." After institution of this legislated action, which of the following occurred?
A) The use of SSRIs increased.
B) The use of long-acting benzodiazepines (e.g., diazepam) increased.
C) The use of neuroleptics increased.
D) Antipsychotic medication use increased.
E) There was no effect noted on physician's prescribing practices.

Answer and Discussion

The answer is A. Several multi-year, multi-facility reviews have examined the impact of OBRA regulations on psychotropic prescribing in nursing homes. These confirm an encouraging trend, including increased awareness of neuroleptic indications and side effects. Post-OBRA, overall antipsychotic use declined by nearly one-third. Antidepressant prescribing increased (by almost 85% in one study), with significant increases in the use of selective serotonin reuptake inhibitors (SSRIs), nortriptyline, and trazodone, and decreases in amitriptyline and doxepin. Anxiolytic / hypnotic prescribing patterns are less consistent. A large study documented a 12% increase in anxiolytics but decreases in particular agents (e.g., diazepam, diphenhydramine). Two studies identified the implementation of OBRA regulations alone as responsible for decreased neuroleptic dosing.

Borson S, Doane K. The impact of OBRA-87 on psychotropic drug prescribing in skilled nursing facilities. *Psychiatr Serv.* 1997;48:1289.

65. When considering treatment of hyperlipidemia in elderly patients, which of the following is true?
A) Elderly patients should not receive lipid-lowering medication over age 85 because of the risk involved with the use of the medications.
B) In the presence of a terminal illness, the use of lipid lowering medication should not be withheld.
C) The decision to use lipid-lowering medications should be individualized to the patient.
D) All patients with a history of coronary artery disease should be treated with lipid lowering medications regardless of their comorbid conditions.
E) None of the above.

Answer and Discussion

The answer is C. The decision whether to treat high or high-normal serum cholesterol in an elderly individual must be individualized, being based on both chronologic and physiologic age. As an example, a patient with a limited life span from a concomitant illness is probably not a candidate for drug therapy. However, an otherwise healthy elderly individual should not be denied drug therapy simply on the basis of age alone.

Grundy SM, Cleeman JI, Rifkind BM, et al. Cholesterol lowering in the elderly population. Coordinating Committee of the National Cholesterol Education Program. *Arch Intern Med.* 1999;159:1670.

66. Which of the following *increases* as men age?
A) Sex hormone-binding globulin (SHBG)
B) Serum free testosterone
C) Bone mineral density
D) Muscle mass
E) Muscle strength

Answer and Discussion

The answer is A. Serum sex hormone-binding globulin (SHBG) concentrations increase gradually as a function of age. The clinical implication, because SHBG binds testosterone with high affinity, is that with increasing age, less of the total testosterone is free (i.e., biologically active). Because of the increase in SHBG with age, it is not surprising that the serum free testosterone concentration decreases with increasing age to a greater degree than the total testosterone. No consequences of the decline in serum testosterone with age are known with certainty, but several parallels between the effects of aging and those of hypogonadism suggest that the decline in serum testosterone might be related to decreased frequency of orgasm or intercourse. Men with hypogonadism due to known disease also have a decline in sexual function, as illustrated by an improvement after testosterone treatment. As men age, their bone mineral density also declines. In a study of healthy men who had never had any fractures, the bone mineral density of the femur and, to a lesser extent, the spine declined from age 20 to age 90. Men who are hypogonadal due to disease or whose testosterone has been lowered surgically or medically also have a decline in bone mineral density. As men age, their muscle mass declines and fat mass increases. Hypogonadal men also have less muscle mass and more fat mass than normal men; testosterone treatment in men with hypogonadism tends to reverse these changes. Men ages 60 to 79 years have less muscle strength than those ages 20 to 39 years. The decrease in serum testosterone concentrations that occurs with aging in men may be associated with a decline in neuropsychological function.

Snyder PJ. Decline in testicular function with aging. Up to Date Online 14.1. http://uptodateonline.com. Accessed 4/10/06.

67. Which one of the following is typically associated with normal-pressure hydrocephalus?
A) Tremor
B) Small ventricles
C) Short stature
D) Urinary incontinence
E) Macrocephaly

Answer and Discussion

The answer is D. Normal pressure hydrocephalus is a relatively rare disorder characterized by the following triad: dementia, gait ataxia, and urinary incontinence. Lumbar cerebrospinal fluid (CSF) pressure must be normal, and there is usually ventricular dilation noted on the computed tomography (CT) or magnetic resonance image (MRI) examination that is disproportionate to cortical atrophy. The etiology is unknown, but there appears to be inadequate absorption of CSF, which leads to hydrocephalus. It may follow head injury, subarachnoid hemorrhage, or meningoencephalitis; however, in many cases there are no preceding conditions. The patient shows no weakness, but has a stuttering gait in which the initiation of gait is hesitant but gives way to walking. In addition, the patient may show lower-extremity spasticity and upgoing toes. Treatment has included shunting of CSF fluid from the dilated ventricles, which has shown some clinical benefit but little effect with long-standing hydrocephalus. Brief improvement after removing approximately 50 mL of CSF indicates a better prognosis with shunting. Radiographic or pressure measurements alone do not seem to predict the response to shunting. Shunting CSF from the dilated ventricles sometimes results in clinical improvement, but, the longer the disease has been present, the less likely shunting will be curative.

Beers MH, Porter RS, eds. *The Merck manual of diagnosis and therapy,* Merck Research Laboratories, 18th ed. Whitehouse Station, NJ: Merck & Co.; 2006:1811, 1814.

Normal-pressure hydrocephalus is a relatively rare disorder characterized by the following triad: dementia, gait ataxia, and urinary incontinence.

68. A 65-year-old otherwise healthy woman presents to your office complaining of dyspareunia. The examination shows a pale-pink vaginal mucosa, loss of rugae, and a friable cervix. The most appropriate treatment is
A) trichloroacetic acid application
B) cryotherapy
C) estrogen vaginal cream
D) psychotherapy
E) vaginal dilation

Answer and Discussion

The answer is C. Atrophic vaginitis is the result of a lack of estrogen on the vaginal tissue. Up to 40% of postmenopausal women have symptoms of atrophic vaginitis. Related to estrogen deficiency, the condition may occur in premenopausal women who take antiestrogenic medications [medroxyprogesterone (Provera), tamoxifen (Nolvadex), danazol (Danocrine), leuprolide (Lupron), and nafarelin (Synarel)] or who have medical or surgical conditions that result in decreased levels of estrogen. The thinned endometrium and increased vaginal pH level induced by estrogen deficiency predispose the vagina and urinary tract to infection and mechanical weakness. The earliest symptoms are decreased vaginal lubrication, followed by other vaginal and urinary symptoms that may be exacerbated by superimposed infection. Patients often report vaginal pruritus, burning, discharge, and excessive dryness with dyspareunia. Urethritis with urinary incontinence, dysuria, and frequency may also occur. Physical findings include a pale-pink vaginal mucosa with friable or atrophic cervix. Once other causes of symptoms have been eliminated, treatment usually depends on estrogen administration. Estrogen replacement therapy may be provided systemically or locally (preferred), but the dosage and delivery method must be individualized. Vaginal moisturizers and lubricants and participation in coitus may also be beneficial in the treatment of women with atrophic vaginitis.

Bachman GA, Nevadunsky NS. Diagnosis and treatment of atrophic vaginitis. *Am Fam Physician.* 2000;61:3090–3096.

69. Which of the following statements is true regarding insomnia in the elderly?
A) Men are more commonly affected.
B) The condition is associated with inadequate tryptophan ingestion.
C) Exercise before bedtime can help relieve symptoms of insomnia.
D) Low-dose trazodone (Desyrel) may be helpful for treating insomnia.
E) Small doses of alcohol given at bedtime can be used to treat insomnia.

Answer and Discussion

The answer is D. Elderly patients often sleep more than younger patients; however, some elderly patients suffer great difficulty with sleep patterns. The number of those patients receiving <5 hours per night dramatically increases as patients grow older. Women are more commonly affected. Patients with insomnia may experience one or more of the following problems: difficulty falling asleep, difficulty maintaining sleep, waking up too early in the morning, and nonrefreshing sleep. In addition, daytime consequences such as fatigue, lack of energy, difficulty concentrating, and irritability are often present. Behavior and pharmacologic therapies are used in treating insomnia. Behavior approaches take a few weeks to improve sleep but continue to provide relief even after training sessions have ended. Patients should be encouraged to keep a sleep diary for several weeks. Sleep diaries usually record bedtime, total sleep time, time until sleep onset, number of awakenings, use of sleep medications, time out of bed in the morning, and a rating of quality of sleep and daytime symptoms. The sleep diary provides a nightly record of the patient's sleep schedule and perception of sleep. Moreover, it may serve as a baseline for assessment of treatment effects. Treatment involves attention to contributing factors for insomnia, including depression, caffeine use, tobacco or alcohol use, and lack of exercise or exercise before bedtime. Medications include tricyclic antidepressants or trazodone (Desyrel) given in low doses 1 hour before bed. Zolpidem (Ambien) has less tendency for rebound and habituation and may be a suitable alternative to other medications. Other medications that are used include eszpiclone (Lunesta) and zaleplon (Sonata) and the melatonin receptor agonist ramelteon (Rozerem).

Landefeld CS, Palmer R, Johnson MA. *Current Geriatric Diagnosis and Treatment.* New York: Lange Medical Books/McGraw Hill; 2004:114–118.

70. Which of the following is a risk factor for fecal incontinence?
A) Running
B) Prolonged sitting
C) Childbirth
D) High-fiber diet

Answer and Discussion

The answer is C. Fecal incontinence is a serious and embarrassing problem that affects up to 5% of the general population and up to 39% of nursing home residents. Providing effective treatment is challenging because of the difficulties in identifying the underlying etiology. Risk factors include female gender, older age, physical limitations, and poor health. Previous studies in women have shown that obstetric or iatrogenic surgical injuries damage the internal or external sphincters, and straining or childbirth can injure the pudendal nerves. Anal ultrasound detects defects in the sphincter complex in up to 87% of incontinent women. Anorectal physiologic studies can identify pudendal nerve injuries in many of the remaining patients. Fecal incontinence may be associated with other causes, including spinal cord injuries, diabetes, dementia, fecal impaction, tumors, trauma, chronic constipation, or previous rectal surgery. All of these conditions result in a low anal sphincter resting tone. Physical examination should include a rectal examination to check for adequate anal sphincter tone and sensation. Further tests include electromyogram studies of the pelvic floor and anal manometry. Treatment involves a strict bowel program to develop predictable bowel movements. Adequate diet with fiber and bulk, proper positioning when defecating, and occasional bowel stimulants can be used to help regulate bowel movements into a regular pattern. For resistant cases, loperamide (Imodium) or diphenoxylate with atropine (Lomotil) may be used to control bowel movements. Other methods to help with rectal incontinence include Kegel exercises to strengthen the pelvic floor muscles and biofeedback; surgery can be considered for resistant cases.

Landefeld CS, Palmer R, Johnson MA. *Current Geriatric Diagnosis and Treatment*. New York: Lange Medical Books/McGraw Hill; 2004:229–230.

71. A 66-year-old otherwise healthy man presents to your office for a general examination. He had a pneumococcal vaccine 7 years ago and inquires whether he needs another one. You correctly answer

A) further immunizations are not needed
B) he should receive only one booster at 10 years
C) he should receive one more booster and no further immunizations are needed
D) he should receive boosters every 7 years indefinitely
E) he should receive boosters every 10 years indefinitely

Answer and Discussion

The answer is C. The 23-valent pneumococcal vaccine provides protection from 85% to 90% of the serotypes that cause invasive disease in the United States. The vaccine is 56% to 81% effective in preventing invasive bacteremia. Current guidelines from the Advisory Committee on Immunization Practices (ACIP) recommend that persons ages 65 or older who were vaccinated before age 65 should receive one revaccination 5 years after the initial vaccination, and previously unvaccinated individuals should receive one dose at age 65.

Center for Disease Control. Pneumococcal polysaccharide vaccine: What you need to know. Online at http://www.cdc.gov/nip/publications/VIS/vis-ppv.pdf#search='pneumococcal%20vaccine'. Accessed on 4/3/06.

72. Based on the results of the Women's Health Initiative Study, which of the following is a correct statement?

A) Those taking conjugated estrogen combined with medroxyprogesterone had an increased risk of breast cancer, coronary artery disease, stroke, and pulmonary embolism than the control group.
B) Those taking conjugated estrogen combined with medroxyprogesterone had an increased risk of breast cancer alone.
C) Those taking conjugated estrogen combined with medroxyprogesterone had an increased risk of coronary artery disease alone.
D) Those taking conjugated estrogen combined with medroxyprogesterone had an increased risk only of stroke and pulmonary embolism than controls.
E) Those taking conjugated estrogen alone had an increased risk of breast cancer, coronary artery disease, stroke, and pulmonary embolism than the control group.

Answer and Discussion

The answer is A. The conjugated estrogen/medroxyprogesterone acetate arm of the Women's Health Initiative Study was terminated early because of excess risk of breast cancer and overall risks exceeded benefits (rates of coronary artery disease, stroke, and pulmonary embolism were also higher in the control group).

Writing Group for the Women's Health Initiative Investigators: Risks and benefits of estrogen plus progestin in healthy postmenopausal women: Principal results from the Women's Health Initiative randomized controlled trial. *JAMA*. 2002; 288:321.

73. Which of the following is true regarding hospice services?

A) Patients that use hospice must be eligible for Medicare Part A.
B) Patients enrolled in hospice must be terminally ill.
C) Patients enrolled are expected to die within 6 months.
D) Patients must sign a statement choosing Hospice care instead of routine Medicare benefits for the specified illness.
E) All of the above.

Answer and Discussion

The answer is E. Medicare patients may choose to use the Medicare hospice benefit in situations of terminal illness. Terminal illness is defined as a life expectancy of 6 months or less if the condition progresses as expected. Patients who decide to use the hospice benefit must be eligible for Medicare Part A, be certified by their physician and hospice medical director as terminally ill, sign a statement choosing hospice care instead of routine Medicare benefits for the specified illness, and receive care of their terminal illness through a Medicare–approved hospice program.

Landefeld CS, Palmer R, Johnson MA. *Current Geriatric Diagnosis and Treatment*. New York: Lange Medical Books/McGraw Hill; 2004:30.

74. A 60-year-old multiparous woman presents to your office complaining of the sudden need to urinate followed by the loss of urine. The most likely diagnosis is

A) urge incontinence
B) stress incontinence
C) overflow incontinence
D) interstitial cystitis
E) multiple sclerosis

Answer and Discussion

The answer is A. There are three basic types of urinary incontinence:

1. *Urge incontinence*. Also known as *detrusor hyperactivity*, the patient suddenly feels the urge to urinate, and involuntary loss of urine follows. It is the most common form of incontinence in elderly patients. Causes include multiple sclerosis, neurogenic bladder dysfunction, interstitial cystitis, urinary obstruction, urinary stones, urinary neoplasm, and urinary infections. In most cases, the cause is idiopathic with no clear etiologic reason. Urge incontinence may occur alone or together with stress incontinence. Treatment involves determining and correcting the underlying cause. If the cause is idiopathic, a trial of anticholinergic medication such as

oxybutynin (Ditropan), imipramine (Tofranil), or propantheline (Pro-Banthine) can be used. Routine voiding schedules may also be helpful. Tolterodine (Detrol) and extended-release oxybutynin chloride (Ditropan XL) have largely replaced generic oxybutynin as a first-line treatment option for overactive bladder that contributes to incontinence because of favorable side effect profiles.

2. *Stress incontinence* occurs when there is incompetence in the urinary sphincter. The symptoms include an involuntary loss of urine with sudden and forceful Valsalva-type maneuvers such as sneezing, coughing, laughing, or lifting heavy objects. In women, pelvic floor muscle relaxation (seen with the development of cystoceles as a result of increasing age or multiparity) contributes to the symptoms. In men, who are less commonly affected, the symptoms are usually the result of previous prostate surgery that may have damaged the nerves responsible for urinary continence. Diagnosis is usually made by the observation of involuntary urinary loss with coughing while performing a pelvic examination or the loss of urine when a patient is standing and performs a Valsalva maneuver with a full bladder. Treatment involves the use of Kegel exercises (repeated tightening of the pelvic floor muscles as if one were shutting off the flow of urine), estrogen replacement, and α-adrenergic agonists (pseudoephedrine), which help improve the urinary sphincter tone. In some cases, the use of a pessary or surgical correction may be needed.

3. *Overflow incontinence* results when the bladder becomes overdistended and the pressure within the bladder increases and exceeds the pressure of the urinary sphincter, leading to involuntary incontinence. Causes include outlet obstruction as a result of severe constipation with fecal impaction, urethral strictures, or prostatic hypertrophy or carcinoma; in children, causes include urethral meatal stenosis, urethral valves, or urethral strictures. Patients often report hesitancy and incomplete voiding. Post-void residuals usually exceed 100 mL. Treatment includes the use of α-blockers such as terazosin (Hytrin), doxazosin (Cardura), and tamsulosin (Flomax). Other treatments include relieving outlet obstruction with medication such as finasteride (Proscar) and dutasteride (Avodart) or surgery.

Culligan PJ, Heit M. Urinary incontinence in women: evaluation and management. *Am Fam Physician*. 2000;62:2433–2444, 2447, 2452.

75. Which one of the following statements associated with Parkinson's disease is true?

A) The condition is associated with neurofibrillary tangles found in the substantia nigra.
B) The carbidopa component of Sinemet blocks peripheral dopa decarboxylase.
C) Amantadine (Symmetrel) is an antagonist of levodopa.
D) Benztropine (Cogentin) is helpful for the bradykinesia late in the course of Parkinson's disease.
E) Surgery for Parkinson's disease has not been shown to be beneficial.

Answer and Discussion

The answer is B. Parkinson's disease is a progressive neurologic disorder that is associated with the loss of dopamine-containing neurons in the substantia nigra. It usually affects older patients, and there is usually no family history. The diagnosis is usually made clinically. Symptoms include a resting, pill-rolling tremor, bradykinesia (the most common complaint), and cogwheel or lead-pipe rigidity. Other manifestations include infrequent blinking, a distinguishing blank stare, festinating gait (shuffling gait with a rapid initiation and the inability to stop once started), and increased salivation. The patient may also show signs of depression or dementia. Dopamine replacement is still considered the most efficacious treatment for Parkinson's disease. Because dopamine itself does not cross the blood–brain barrier, it is administered as the precursor levodopa in combination with carbidopa (Sinemet). Carbidopa blocks peripheral dopa decarboxylase, the enzyme that converts levodopa to dopamine within the blood–brain barrier. With the levodopa–carbidopa combination, more levodopa reaches the brain and is converted to dopamine. Amantadine (Symmetrel), which has a longer half-life than levodopa, appears to act synergistically with levodopa and thus has been considered useful in the treatment of early Parkinson's disease. Dopamine receptor agonists were introduced as adjuncts to levodopa therapy to help control the motor fluctuations that occur in patients with Parkinson's disease. The dopamine agonists available for the treatment of Parkinson's disease in the United States are bromocriptine (Parlodel), pergolide (Permax), pramipexole (Mirapex), and ropinirole (Requip). Dopamine enhancement through the inhibition of dopamine breakdown in the central nervous system was the mechanism behind the development of selegiline (Eldepryl), a monoamine oxidase B inhibitor. This agent is used as an adjunct to levodopa therapy. Theoretically, it allows levodopa to be administered less often, but this has not been observed in practice. Although selegiline has antioxidant properties, no evidence supports the earlier notion that the drug is neuroprotective and delays the natural progression of Parkinson's disease. Dopamine and its precursor, levodopa, are metabolized by the enzyme catechol *O*-methyltransferase in the liver, gastrointestinal tract, and other organs. By preventing this breakdown, catechol *O*-methyltransferase inhibitors [e.g., entacapone; tolcapone (Tasmar) has been associated with liver failure] enhance the amount of levodopa that reaches the central nervous system, thereby allowing more of the drug to be converted to dopamine. Although this mechanism parallels that of carbidopa, catechol *O*-methyltransferase inhibitors can be taken concurrently with the levodopa–carbidopa combination because a different enzyme is involved. Trihexyphenidyl (Artane) or benztropine (Cogentin) may be prescribed as adjunctive therapy to levodopa. Either of these anticholinergic drugs may be helpful in managing significant tremor early in the course of Parkinson's disease. Anticholinergic agents have been used with mixed results in patients with essential tremor, dystonias, and certain dyskinesias. Elderly patients are often unable to tolerate the side effects of these drugs, which include cognitive impairment, dry mouth, and urinary retention. Levodopa–carbidopa (Sinemet) should be taken with a low protein meal. Surgery is considered an option even in elderly patients as long as they meet medical screening criteria, including failure to respond to available medications and absence of cardiopulmonary risk factors for surgery. Thalamotomy effectively reduces tremor and sometimes rigidity on the contralateral side. Bilateral thalamotomy may result in speech, swallowing, and visual deficits. Thalamic stimulation can reproduce the benefits of thalamotomy without the risk of irreversible tissue loss, because no physical lesion is created. Pallidotomy is a procedure in which a portion of the globus pallidus is treated permanently. The procedure has significant associated risks, including visual field deficits and hemiparesis (because of the proximity of the medial pallidum to the optic tracts and internal capsule). Bilateral procedures have a >15% complication rate and are associated with postoperative neuropsychiatric deficits in some patients. Compared with thalamic procedures, pallidotomy is less beneficial for tremors and more beneficial for dyskinesias. Pallidal and subthalamic nucleus stimulation procedures are being accepted as less invasive, more reversible alternatives to pallidotomy. Tissue transplantation procedures are also being evaluated for the treatment of Parkinson's disease. Additional adjunctive therapies include physical therapy, nutritional counseling, and techniques to help patients manage emotional and cognitive changes related to the disease.

Landefeld CS, Palmer R, Johnson MA. *Current Geriatric Diagnosis and Treatment*. New York: Lange Medical Books/McGraw Hill; 2004:88–98.

Parkinson's disease is a progressive neurologic disorder associated with the loss of dopamine-containing neurons in the substantia nigra.

76. Which of the following statements concerning macular degeneration is true?
A) Peripheral vision is spared.
B) Drusen is a sign of late disease.
C) The exudative form is the most commonly seen.
D) Vision loss is usually sudden and irreversible.
E) Vision rehabilitation is not beneficial.

Answer and Discussion

The answer is A. Age-related macular degeneration is the leading cause of severe vision loss among the elderly. In this condition, central vision is lost, but peripheral vision almost always remains intact. Affected persons rarely require canes or guide dogs. However, the loss of central visual acuity can lead to a reduction of daily activities and mobility in the elderly and increases the risks of falls, fractures, and depression in this population. Patients with age-related macular degeneration may complain of acute loss of vision, blurred vision, scotomas (areas of lost vision), or chronic distortion of vision. All patients with vision loss should be referred to an ophthalmologist; those with acute loss of vision should be referred immediately. The diagnosis of age-related macular degeneration is based on symptoms and ophthalmoscopic findings. The disease is usually classified as early or late. Late disease can be divided into atrophic (dry) and exudative (wet) forms. In early disease, the macula shows yellowish-colored subretinal deposits called *drusen* and/or increased pigment. Drusen are thought to be byproducts of retinal pigment epithelium dysfunction. In most eyes with early disease, visual acuity remains stable for many years, and loss of vision is usually gradual. Late disease (atrophic and exudative) can lead to significant loss of vision. Exudative disease occurs in only 10% of patients with age-related macular degeneration, but it is responsible for the majority of cases of severe vision loss related to the disease. In atrophic disease, the macula usually shows areas of depigmentation. In the exudative form, fluid can accumulate underneath the retina, as in pigment epithelial detachments or subretinal neovascularization, and loss of vision is usually sudden. Fluorescein angiography can be used to help determine whether a patient has the atrophic or exudative form of the disease. The two currently proven treatments are laser photocoagulation and photodynamic therapy, but these measures are effective in only a small fraction of eyes with the exudative form of macular degeneration. Diet therapy and vitamin supplementation is still being investigated. Vision rehabilitation can help patients maximize their remaining vision and adapt so that they can perform activities of daily living. Families need encouragement in providing support and helping patients adjust to being partially sighted.

Fong DS. Age-related macular degeneration: update for primary care. *Am Fam Physician*. 2000;61:3035–3042.

77. Amyotrophic lateral sclerosis is associated with
A) sensory dysfunction
B) cerebellar dysfunction
C) atrophy of the muscles and fasciculations
D) extraocular muscle dysfunction
E) improved prognosis in elderly patients (older than 70 years)

Answer and Discussion

The answer is C. Amyotrophic lateral sclerosis (ALS, or Lou Gehrig disease) affects upper and lower motor neurons. Two-thirds of patients present with symptoms associated with the limbs, and 25% have bulbar symptoms (usually in patients older than 70 years). ALS does not affect sensory, cerebellar, or extraocular muscle function. Men are more commonly affected. Most cases occur between the ages of 40 and 70 years. Rapidly fatal disease is associated with increasing age and bulbar symptoms. Electromyogram studies show muscle denervation with preserved nerve conduction velocities. Treatment is primarily symptomatic. Attention should be focused on emotional support and "end-of-life" issues.

Beers MH, Porter RS, eds. *The Merck manual of diagnosis and therapy*, Merck Research Laboratories, 18th ed. Whitehouse Station, NJ: Merck & Co.; 2006:1897.

78. The Minimum Data Set (MDS) is
A) a document that provides a comprehensive assessment of a nursing home resident and develops a plan of care
B) a list of vital signs for the nursing home resident
C) a document that describes the activities available to a nursing home resident
D) a set of minimum requirements that a nursing home has to abide by to receive state certification
E) a group of indicators that rank nursing homes based on safety and quality

Answer and Discussion

The answer is A. A Minimum Data Set (MDS) is a federally mandated document that is based on a comprehensive resident assessment. Information from the physician's history and physical and progress notes is used to complete an MDS. The MDS is then used to develop a plan of care and also is used to determine Medicare reimbursement for the patient.

Landefeld CS, Palmer R, Johnson MA. *Current Geriatric Diagnosis and Treatment*. New York: Lange Medical Books/McGraw Hill; 2004:40.

79. Physicians are required to see nursing home patients
A) daily
B) weekly
C) monthly as long as they reside there
D) monthly for 3 months and then every 2 months thereafter
E) every 3 months

Answer and Discussion

The answer is D. Medicare regulations require that a physician make monthly visits for the first 3 months of a resident's nursing home stay and then every 2 months thereafter.

Landefeld CS, Palmer R, Johnson MA. *Current Geriatric Diagnosis and Treatment*. New York: Lange Medical Books/McGraw Hill; 2004:40.

80. Which of the following is the major feature that distinguishes delirium from dementia?
A) Cognitive changes
B) Inattention
C) Disorganized thinking
D) Altered level of consciousness
E) Acute onset and fluctuating course

Answer and Discussion

The answer is E. The distinguishing historical features of delirium are acute onset and fluctuating course, in which symptoms tend to come and go or increase and decrease in severity over a 24-hour period. This is the major feature that distinguishes delirium from dementia, which typically develops gradually and progressively over months to years. To satisfy the criteria of delirium, the change must occur in the context of a medical illness, metabolic disturbance, drug toxicity, or withdrawal.

Landefeld CS, Palmer R, Johnson MA. *Current Geriatric Diagnosis and Treatment*. New York: Lange Medical Books/McGraw Hill; 2004:55.

81. Pick's disease is
A) a hematologic disorder that causes bleeding complications
B) a malignancy associated with exposure to mining dust
C) dementia associated with the frontal lobe
D) an infection related to prior tuberculosis exposure
E) a benign condition related to underlying panic disorder

Answer and Discussion

The answer is C. Pick's disease is a less common form of dementia affecting predominantly the frontal and temporal lobes of the cortex. Symptoms include apathy, memory disturbances, increased carelessness, poor personal hygiene, and decreased attention span. Pick's disease has spongiform changes and ballooned neurons, some of which contain argyrophilic deposits known as *Pick's bodies*, which are composed of cytoskeletal proteins, neurofilament, tubulin, and tau. Frontal lobe dementias, including Pick's disease, are transmitted as an autosomal-dominant–inherited disease.

Beers MH, Porter RS, eds. *The Merck manual of diagnosis and therapy*, Merck Research Laboratories, 18th ed. Whitehouse Station, NJ: Merck & Co.; 2006:1820–1821.

82. Which of the following statements concerning advanced directives is true?
A) Once recorded, they cannot be changed.
B) Living wills are often easier for patients to complete than designating a health-care power of attorney.
C) Advanced directives should be discussed only when life-threatening illnesses are present.
D) Physicians are not automatically required to comply with patients' requests for treatment when they believe such requests are ill advised, harmful, or futile.
E) There is no need to update advance directives.

Answer and Discussion

The answer is D. An advance directive consists of a person's oral and written instructions about his or her future medical care in the event that he or she becomes unable to communicate, becomes incompetent to make health-care decisions (during a terminal illness), or is in a persistent vegetative state. There are two types of advance directives: a health-care power of attorney and a living will. The health-care ("durable") power of attorney, or *health-care proxy*, is a document by which the patient appoints a trusted person to make decisions about his or her medical care if he or she cannot make those decisions. A *living will* is a written form of advance directive in which the patient's wishes regarding the administration of medical treatment are delineated in case the patient becomes unable to communicate his or her wishes.

Discussion of advanced directives should take place early on in the care of patients to discuss the patient's wishes should they become debilitated and cannot answer for themselves. The durable power of attorney allows the patient to designate a surrogate to make medical decisions if the patient loses decision-making capacity. The durable power of attorney is often less emotionally laden than outlining specific treatments to give or withhold. The five steps identified in the ideal process of advanced care planning are as follows: (1) Raise the topic and give information regarding the advance directive and health care proxy; (2) facilitate a structured discussion; (3) complete a statement, date and record it, and have the patient supply copies to the proxy and anyone else deemed appropriate (e.g., clergy); (4) periodically review and update the directive, and initial and date all changes; and (5) implement the plan by following the patient's wishes when the appropriate time comes. Finally, physicians are not automatically obliged to comply with patients' requests for treatment when they believe such requests are ill advised, harmful, or futile. Strict adherence to such requests may interfere with the physician's autonomy and ability to provide sound medical care.

Aitken PV. Incorporating advance care planning into family practice. *Am Fam Physician*. 1999;59:605.

Silveira MJ, DiPiero A, Gerrity MS, et al. Patients' knowledge of options at the end of life: ignorance in the face of death. *JAMA*. 2000;284:2483–2488.

83. A 70-year-old man with a history of atrial fibrillation now on warfarin therapy presents with a left-sided hemiparesis and a change in personality noted by his family. The nursing home reports a fall 2 weeks ago. A CT scan from the emergency room shows a small illuminated crescentic collection of fluid that is located adjacent to the convexity of the hemisphere. The most likely diagnosis is
A) subdural hematoma
B) epidural hematoma
C) subarachnoid hemorrhage
D) subdural abscess
E) brain tumor

Answer and Discussion

The answer is A. Subdural hematomas are associated with rupturing of the bridging veins beneath the dura. The elderly and those taking anticoagulants are at increased risk. Acute subdural hematomas become symptomatic within minutes to hours after the injury. Patients may report a unilateral headache, and the examination shows a slightly enlarged pupil on the side affected. Stupor, coma, hemiparesis, and unilateral papillary enlargement are typical signs of larger hematomas. Pupillary dilation is contralateral in 5% to 10%. For the patient with a rapidly declining course, burr holes or emergency craniotomy is indicated to reduce intracerebral pressure from an expanding lesion. Most subdural hematomas appear as crescentic collections over the convexity of the hemisphere and are located in the frontotemporal region. Chronic subdural hematomas may develop as a result of mild trauma and manifest as chronic headaches, slowed thinking, change in personality, seizures, or a mild hemiparesis that develops weeks to months after the injury. Many are bilateral. Symptoms may resemble a cerebrovascular accident or transient ischemic attack. Epidural hematomas develop more quickly than subdural hematomas and are more dangerous. They occur as a result of arterial bleeding between the dura mater and skull and are less common in the elderly. Most patients are comatose when first seen. The epidural hematoma forms a lenticular-shaped clot on CT. Treatment is surgical evacuation.

Kasper DL, Braunwald E, Fauci AS, et al., eds. *Harrison's principles of internal medicine,* 16th ed. New York: McGraw Hill; 2005:2449.

84. Which of the following statements regarding home visits is true?
A) They are increasing in frequency.
B) Reimbursement has increased their use.
C) Physicians who perform home visits have increased job satisfaction.
D) Home visits are not effective at managing patients because of a lack of resources.
E) Home visits rarely identify new medical problems, but are better suited to manage chronic medical problems.

Answer and Discussion

The answer is C. Years ago, the home visit was an essential part of primary care practice. More recently, the home visit has been used less frequently. The low frequency of home visits by physicians is the result of many coincident factors, including deficits in physician compensation for these visits, time constraints, perceived limitations of technologic support, concerns about the risk of litigation, lack of physician training and exposure, and corporate and individual attitudinal biases. Physicians most likely to perform home visits are older generalists in solo practices. Health-care providers who have long-established relationships with their patients are also more likely to use house calls. Rural practice setting, older patient age, and need for terminal care correlate with an increased frequency of home visits. Studies suggest that home visits can lead to improved medical care through the discovery of undetected health-care needs. Home assessment of elderly patients with relatively good health status and function can increase the detection of new medical problems and new intervention recommendations. There is also improved effectiveness of home visits in assessing unexpected problems in patient compliance with therapeutic regimens. Additionally, specific home-based interventions such as adjusting the elderly patient's home environment to prevent falls have also yielded health benefits. Beyond the potential benefit of improved patient care, family physicians who conduct home visits report a higher level of practice satisfaction than those who do not offer this service.

Unwin BK, Jerant AF. The home visit. *Am Fam Physician.* 1999;60:1481.

85. Which of the following should be adjusted for when performing a Mini-Mental State Examination (MMSE)?
A) Location and sex of individual
B) Age and education
C) Support and living arrangement
D) Height and weight
E) Eyesight and hearing

Answer and Discussion

The answer is B. The MMSE is a 30-point tool that tests orientation, immediate recall, delayed recall, concentration/calculation, and language and visuospatial domains. Adjustments should be made for age and level of education. As a general guideline scores >26 are normal, scores of 24 to 26 may indicate mild cognitive impairment, and a score of <24 is consistent with dementia.

Landefeld CS, Palmer R, Johnson MA. *Current Geriatric Diagnosis and Treatment.* New York: Lange Medical Books/McGraw Hill; 2004:64.

The Mini-Mental State Examination (MMSE) is a 30-point tool that tests orientation, immediate recall, delayed recall, concentration/calculation, and language and visuospatial domains. Adjustments should be made for age and level of education.

86. Which of the following blood test has been correlated with an increased risk of late onset Alzheimer's disease?
A) Apolipoprotein E – E4
B) Apolipoprotein E – E2
C) Homocystine
D) Sedimentation rate
E) C-reactive protein

Answer and Discussion

The answer is A. The association between apolipoprotein E (APOE) and Alzheimer's disease is well established. The presence of one E4 allele increases the risk of Alzheimer's disease (AD) about two to three times, whereas the E2 allele may be protective. The absence of an E4 allele does not rule out the diagnosis, nor does the presence of homozygous E4/E4 rule it in. The test is considered experimental.

Landefeld CS, Palmer R, Johnson MA. *Current Geriatric Diagnosis and Treatment.* New York: Lange Medical Books/McGraw Hill; 2004:66.

87. When treating nursing home patients, it is important to remember that any antipsychotic medications must be reviewed and an attempt to withdraw or taper them made every
A) 30 days
B) 3 months
C) 6 months
D) year
E) There is no need to withdraw or taper antipsychotic medications because of the risk to patient's safety.

Answer and Discussion

The answer is C. Federal regulations require an attempt to withdraw (or decrease the dose) of medications to manage agitation or psychosis in nursing homes every 6 months.

Landefeld CS, Palmer R, Johnson MA. *Current Geriatric Diagnosis and Treatment*. New York: Lange Medical Books/McGraw Hill; 2004:68.

88. Which of the following is less likely to occur in elderly patients with influenza?
A) Headache
B) Muscle aches
C) Fatigue
D) Sore throat
E) Fever

Answer and Discussion

The answer is E. Influenza is a common respiratory infection that causes significant morbidity and mortality in older adults. Influenza is responsible for more than $1 billion in annual Medicare expenditures. Of deaths resulting from influenza, the vast majority occur in adults 65 years and older. Older adults are susceptible to severe and potentially fatal complications from this common illness because of coexisting chronic disease and weakened immunity. Older adults can benefit most from vaccination, early detection, and aggressive therapy. The signs and symptoms of influenza infection in older adults are similar to those occurring in younger patients, although a febrile response may be absent. Influenza is typically associated with rapid onset of headache, fever, chills, muscle aches, malaise, cough, and sore throat. Most people recover fully within 1 week, but older adults may develop a persistent weakness that can last for many weeks, and are also at higher risk for developing complications such as pneumonia. Diagnosis is usually made clinically. Several commercially produced rapid diagnostic tests intended for use in outpatient settings can detect influenza viruses within 30 minutes. In selected patients, obtaining a viral culture may be warranted to acquire specific information on influenza subtypes and strains. Four antiviral agents—amantadine (Symmetrel), rimantadine (Flumadine), zanamivir (Relenza), and oseltamivir (Tamiflu)—are approved for prevention or treatment of influenza. Zanamivir and oseltamivir are not approved for prophylactic use. It is unknown whether therapy with amantadine or rimantadine can prevent complications of influenza A among persons at high risk, including older adults. Rimantadine costs more than amantadine, but has fewer adverse effects on the central nervous system (e.g., confusion, nervousness, anxiety) and is less dependent on renal excretion. Zanamivir and oseltamivir are equally effective neuroaminidase inhibitors, but their place in therapy is yet to be determined. It has not yet been determined whether early initiation of treatment reduces hospital admission and mortality, particularly in elderly and high-risk patients.

Mouton CP, Bazaldua OV. Common infections in older adults. *Am Fam Physician*. 2001;63:257–268.

89. Which of the following statements regarding the treatment of prostate cancer is true?
A) Radical prostatectomy appears to have a better cure rate than radiation therapy.
B) Radiation therapy has a better cure rate than surgery.
C) Surgery is better suited for younger patients.
D) Younger patients are typically observed to prevent risks associated with surgery or radiation.
E) Metastatic disease is not treatable.

Answer and Discussion

The answer is C. Young, healthy patients are most often encouraged to undergo radical prostatectomy, and older patients are steered toward observation or radiotherapy. However, the treatment choice must be based on the patient's preference, given his understanding of the benefits and side effects of each option. Overall, cure rates for radical prostatectomy generally fall between 60% and 70%. External-beam radiotherapy appears to be as effective as surgery in curing prostate cancer, at least for the first 10 years after treatment. Radiotherapy is well tolerated, and it is associated with no hemorrhagic or anesthetic risks. Furthermore, this treatment option does not require hospitalization or a significant recovery period. Normal activity can usually be maintained during radiotherapy. However, treatment is administered daily for 4 to 6 weeks, and many patients report fatigue at the end of this period. Compared with surgery, radiotherapy has several potential disadvantages. Radical prostatectomy provides more definitive information about long-term prognosis, because the size of the tumor, the presence of cancer spread, and the presence of cancer in the lymph nodes can be determined from the surgical specimen. With radiotherapy, the post-treatment status of the tumor is unknown; serial PSA levels serve as surrogate markers to determine whether the treatment was curative. Radiotherapy can also have significant side effects. It is associated with severe bladder irritation (urgency, pain, and frequency) in as many as 5% of patients. Rectal irritations (diarrhea, urgency, tenesmus, and bleeding) occur in up to 10% of patients who receive radiotherapy for prostate cancer, and impotence is a problem in almost one-half of patients receiving this treatment. Thus, surgery is generally preferred for younger patients, whereas radiation treatment may be better suited for older patients who may not be good surgical candidates. Metastatic disease can be treated with hormonal manipulation, including surgical castration or medical castration using a luteinizing hormone releasing agonist.

Bhatnagar V, Kaplan RM. Treatment options for prostate cancer: evaluating the evidence. *Am Fam Physician*. 2005;71:1915–1922, 1929–1930.

90. The Medicare Hospice Benefit covers all of the following expenses for patients in nursing homes EXCEPT
A) all visits by hospice team members
B) the rental or purchase of durable medical equipment
C) cost of supplies that are ordered by the hospice team
D) the costs of medication (except for a small copay)
E) payment of room and board

Answer and Discussion

The answer is E. When a nursing home patient is identified as having a life-threatening illness or condition, it is appropriate to plan for end-of-life care. The Medicare Hospice Benefit can help greatly with the many tasks involved in providing palliative management of the dying patient's symptoms, attending to increased hygienic needs, and supplying bereavement services. For eligible terminally ill patients, the Medicare Hospice Benefit supplies an interdisciplinary team with skills in pain management, symptom control, and bereavement assistance. The services of the hospice team supplement the usual nursing home care at a time when staff, family members, and the patient are facing the increased and urgent needs associated with the dying process. The Medicare Hospice Benefit can make it much easier for physicians and nursing home staff to provide comprehensive palliative care for terminally ill patients. When a nursing home resident is referred for care under the Medicare Hospice Benefit, the hospice assumes responsibility for the professional management of many interdisciplinary services that supplement the usual care provided by nursing home staff. All medical treatments should have the goal of symptom control, and they should be consistent with the hospice plan of treatment. The Medicare Hospice Benefit covers all visits by hospice team members, the rental or purchase of durable medical equipment, and the cost of supplies that are ordered by the hospice team. The hospice also supplies drugs for the palliation and management of the terminal illness, a benefit that normally is not available under the regular Medicare program. For each of these drugs, the beneficiary is only responsible for a small co-payment. Thus, hospice care is not an additional expense for many nursing home residents. Payment of room and board remains the responsibility of the patient and/or the family, or government assistance programs cover it for eligible residents (e.g., under Medicaid). The Medicare Hospice Benefit cannot be provided for nursing home residents who are receiving skilled Medicare coverage if their diagnoses for hospice and nursing home skilled care are the same. Before the Medicare Hospice Benefit can be initiated, these patients may choose to use all their skilled-care days, or they may elect to waive their skilled coverage.

Keay TJ, Schonwetter RS. Hospice care in the nursing home. *Am Fam Physician.* 1998;57:491.

Landefeld CS, Palmer R, Johnson MA. *Current Geriatric Diagnosis and Treatment.* New York: Lange Medical Books/McGraw Hill; 2004:44.

91. The drug of choice for the treatment of a serious methicillin-resistant *Staphylococcus aureus* (MRSA) infection is
A) penicillin
B) ceftazidime
C) metronidazole
D) imipenem
E) vancomycin

Answer and Discussion

The answer is E. Methicillin-resistant *Staphylococcus aureus* (MRSA) is a major problem for elderly patients, especially those in institutional settings. People colonized with MRSA are at increased risk of MRSA infection. They also have a higher risk of death as a result of resistance to typical antibiotics. Poor functional status is associated with being an MRSA carrier. Therefore, nursing homes and other institutional settings must be especially careful to prevent the spread of infection caused by this organism. Hand washing, isolation of infected patients, and proper handling of body secretions are essential to prevent the spread of MRSA. The most common reservoirs for MRSA colonization are the nasal mucosa and oropharynx. Skin contamination from persons already colonized in these areas may also be a source for MRSA infection. Although colonization by MRSA does not require systemic treatment, an active serious infection with MRSA is treated with vancomycin as the preferred antibiotic. Older adults may require dosage adjustment based on renal function. Other regimens include vancomycin plus gentamicin (Garamycin) or rifampin (Rifadin), sulfamethoxazole–trimethroprim (Sulfa), doxycycline, minocyclcine, and clindamycin. Attempts to identify the original infected person (source case) should be made by swabbing the nasopharynx of patients and staff near to the outbreak and treating those found to have MRSA infection. Staff and patients who are MRSA carriers should be isolated, and some authorities recommend treatment with topical mupirocin (Bactroban), which is applied twice daily for 2 weeks to the nares or other areas of skin carriage (e.g., wounds) to reduce the shedding of MRSA. Colonization recurs in approximately one-half of treated subjects.

Mouton CP, Bazaldua OV. Common infections in older adults. *Am Fam Physician.* 2001;63:257–268.

92. The most common reason for discontinuing acetylcholinesterase inhibitors is
A) headache
B) hepatotoxicity
C) rash
D) cataracts
E) gastrointestinal side effects

Answer and Discussion

The answer is E. Gastrointestinal side effects, including nausea, vomiting, and diarrhea, are a class effect and are the most common reason for discontinuation of acetylcholinesterase inhibitors (tacrine, donepezil, rivastigmine, and galantamine). These can usually be minimized by slow titration over an 8 to 12 week period. Reversible hepatotoxicity is seen with tacrine—therefore, this drug is not generally recommended as first-line therapy.

Landefeld CS, Palmer R, Johnson MA. *Current Geriatric Diagnosis and Treatment.* New York: Lange Medical Books/McGraw Hill; 2004:69.

> Gastrointestinal side effects, including nausea, vomiting, and diarrhea, are a class effect and are the most common reason for discontinuation of acetylcholinesterase inhibitors (i.e., tacrine, donepezil, rivastigmine, and galantamine).

93. Which of the following is considered a risk factor for falls?
A) Hypothyroidism
B) Anemia
C) Addison's disease
D) Vitamin D deficiency
E) All are risk factors for falls

Answer and Discussion

The answer is E. Many conditions that affect the elderly can increase the risk for falls. Hypothyroidism, anemia, Addison's disease, vitamin B_{12} deficiency, and vitamin D deficiency are some notable causes that should be ruled out when assessing an elderly patient after a fall.

Landefeld CS, Palmer R, Johnson MA. *Current Geriatric Diagnosis and Treatment.* New York: Lange Medical Books/McGraw Hill; 2004:84.

94. An 87-year-old man is seen by you for a general examination. He has no history of coronary artery disease and remains active, playing golf three times per week. His only other medical problem is mild hypertension for which he takes hydrochlorothiazide. Which of the following statements is true regarding treatment of his elevated cholesterol, which was discovered on a recent blood test?
A) Based on his advanced age, he does not qualify for treatment of his hyperlipidemia.
B) Only lifestyle measures should be used to treat his cholesterol because of the risk of medication use.
C) The decision to treat this man should be based on national guidelines regardless of his underlying medical condition.
D) Treatment of hyperlipidemia should be individualized based on the patient's chronological and physiologic age and life expectancy.
E) The decision treat hyperlipidemia in the elderly should not be influenced by a patient's terminal diagnosis.

Answer and Discussion

The answer is D. The decision whether to treat high or high–normal serum cholesterol in an elderly individual must be individualized and based on both chronological and physiologic age of the patient. As an example, a patient with a limited life span from a concomitant illness (e.g., metastatic cancer, dementia) is probably not a candidate for drug therapy. However, an otherwise healthy elderly individual should not be denied drug therapy simply on the basis of age alone.

Grundy SM, Cleeman JI, Rifkind BM, et al. Cholesterol lowering in the elderly population. Coordinating Committee of the National Cholesterol Education Program. *Arch Intern Med.* 1999;159:1670.

Chapter 7

Pictorial Atlas

Questions

Each of the following questions or incomplete statements is followed by suggested answers or completions. Select the ONE BEST ANSWER in each case.

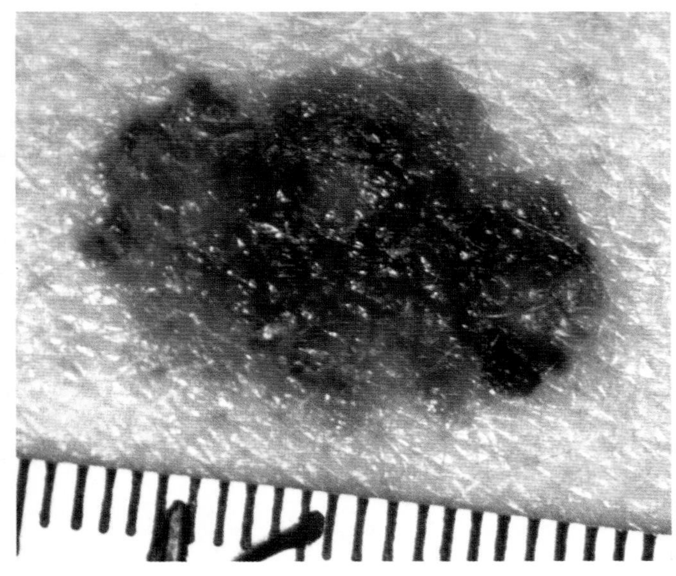

1. A 42-year-old female presents with the lesion (shown at left) on the back of her calf. She has no significant medical problems and otherwise feels well. The lesion has not bled, but seems to have grown over the last few months. Appropriate initial management of this skin lesion should be

A) observation and removal if bleeding or further change occurs
B) complete excision with normal margins
C) complete excision with wide margins
D) shave biopsy
E) electrodessication and curettage

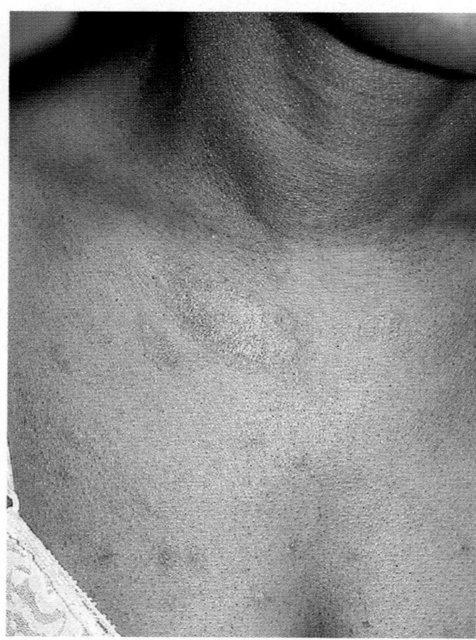

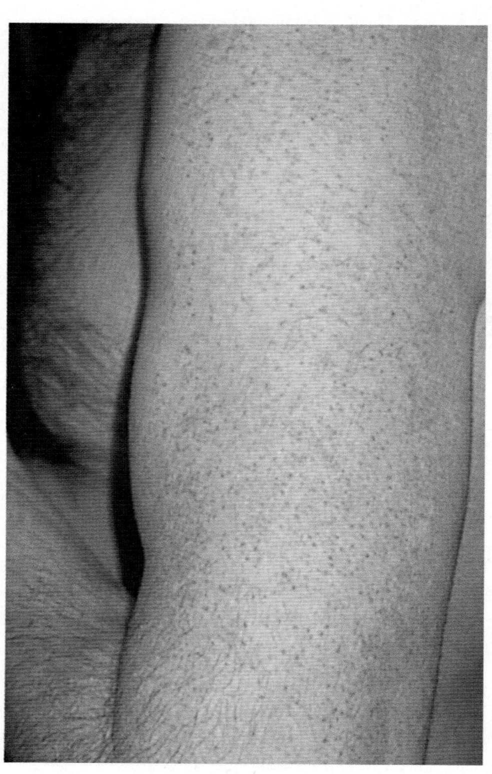

2. A 26-year-old female presents with the above rash. She states the rash is minimally pruritic and developed over the last week. She has had some virus-like symptoms and reports the rash began as a large salmon-colored patch on her chest area. The most likely diagnosis is

A) tinea versicolor
B) pityriasis rosea
C) varicella
D) psoriasis
E) cocciodiomycosis

3. An 18 year old presents to your office complaining of a sandpaper-like rash that affects his upper outer arms. He is otherwise healthy and has no other symptoms. The most likely diagnosis is

A) scarlet fever
B) infectious mononucleosis
C) keratosis pilaris
D) seborrheic dermatitis
E) psoriasis

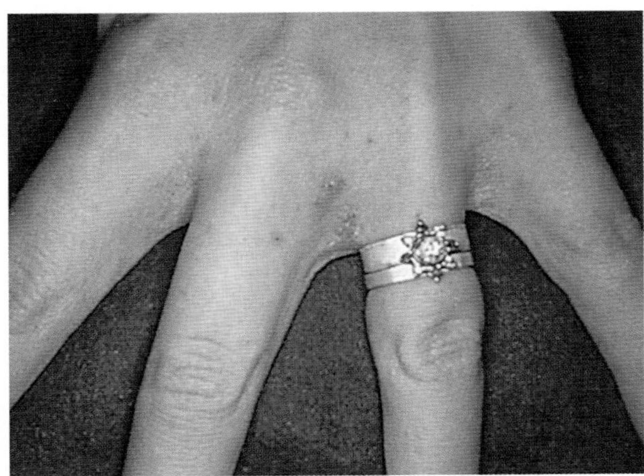

4. A 35-year-old woman presents with a pruritic rash that has been present over the last few weeks. The area affected is in the webs of the fingers, and symptoms are reported to be worse at night. Topical over-the-counter steroids have not been beneficial. The likely diagnosis is

A) poison ivy
B) dyshidrotic eczema
C) scabies
D) tinea corporis
E) psoriasis

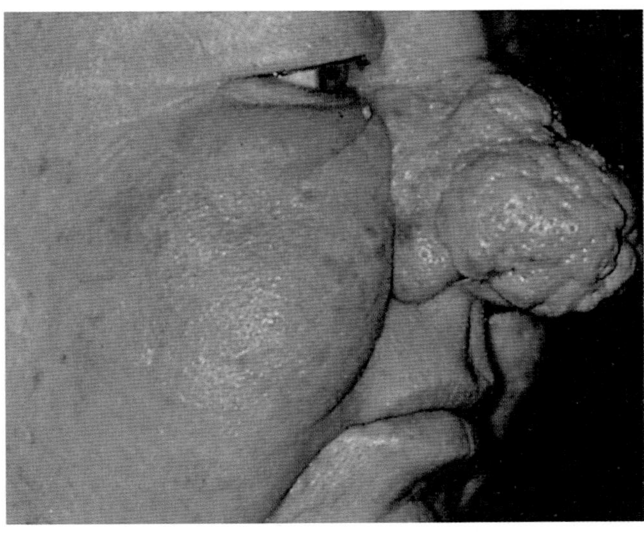

5. A 72-year-old man presents to your office complaining of an area of redness associated with the perinasal region. He states that the rash is often worse in the summer, and he has noticed that sunlight exposure makes it worse. Appropriate treatment of this condition consists of

A) hydrocortisone cream
B) tretinoin gel
C) metronidazole cream
D) mupirocin ointment
E) acyclovir ointment

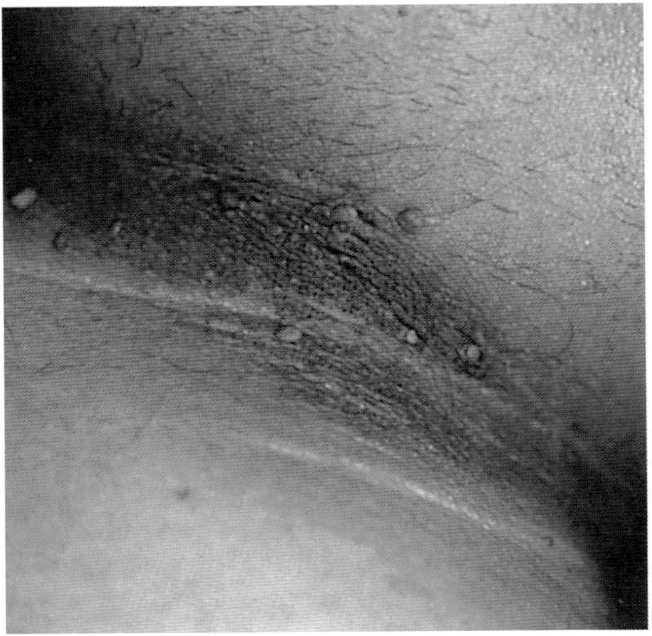

6. Which of the following malignancies is associated with the skin condition shown here?

A) Ovarian carcinoma
B) Gastric carcinoma
C) Malignant melanoma
D) Multiple myeloma
E) Hodgkin's lymphoma

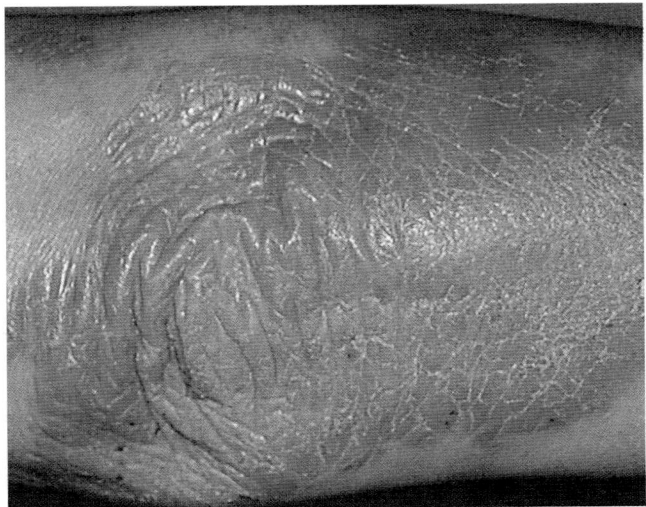

7. A 45-year-old woman presents with a localized area of erythematous scaly patches that comes and goes and typically affects the elbows. The likely diagnosis is

A) pityriasis rosacea
B) mycosis fungoides
C) tinea corpora
D) nummular eczema
E) psoriasis

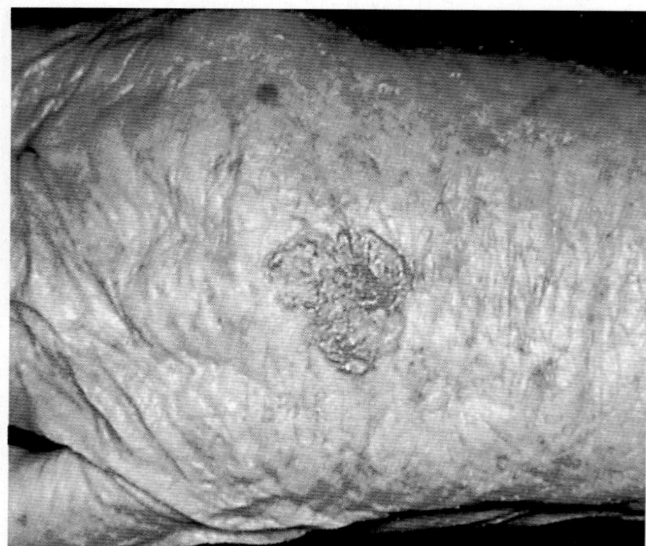

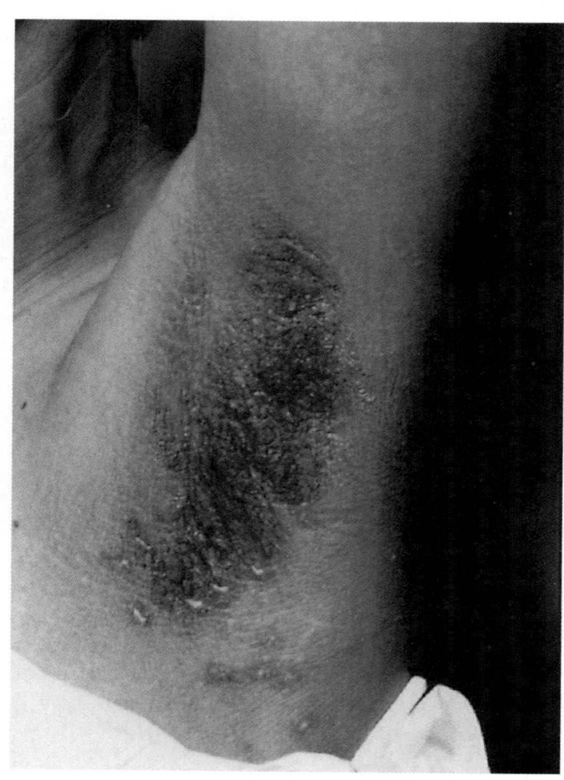

8. A 60-year-old retired construction worker presents with a non-healing skin lesion on the back of his hand that occasionally bleeds when he gets out of the shower. The most likely diagnosis is
A) basal cell carcinoma
B) squamous cell carcinoma
C) superficial spreading malignant melanoma
D) actinic keratosis
E) keratoacanthoma

9. You note the above skin disorder during a general medical evaluation. You explain to the patient they are at risk for the development of:
A) Alzheimer's disease
B) tuberculosis
C) diabetes mellitus
D) Grave's disease
E) melanoma

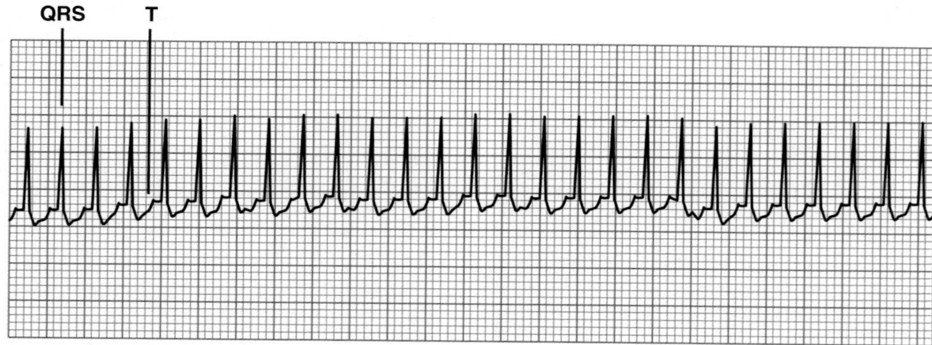

10. A 42-year-old female presents to the Emergency Room complaining of shortness of breath and palpitations. An electrocardiogram shows the above tracing. Appropriate management at this time includes:
A) Epinephrine
B) Metoprolol
C) Nitroglycerin
D) Adenosine
E) Lidocaine

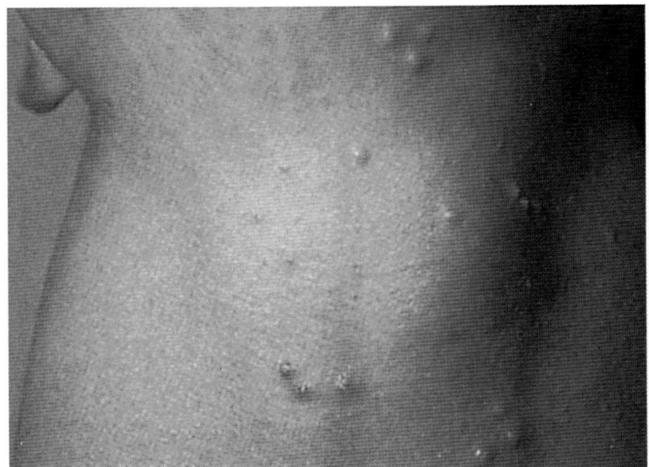

11. A 4-year-old preschooler presents with the skin lesions shown here. The area affected is just below the chin on the child's right side. The lesions have been present over the last month, and the child has reported no symptoms associated with them. The most likely diagnosis is
A) varicella
B) herpes zoster
C) *Rhus* dermatitis
D) molluscum contagiosum
E) scabies

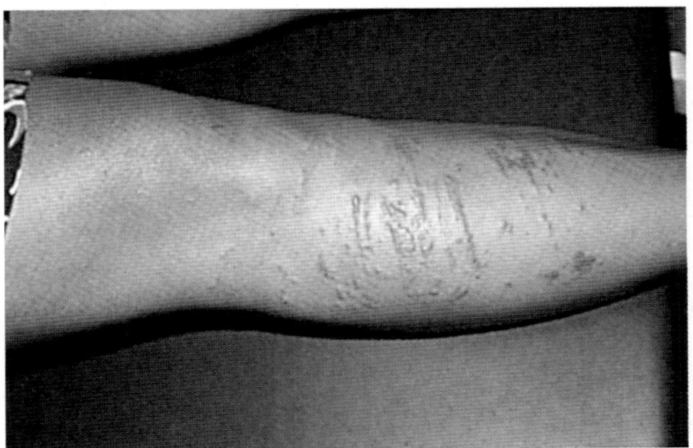

12. A 16-year-old girl who just returned from a camping trip reports an intensely pruritic vesicular rash associated with the lower extremities. The most likely diagnosis is
A) *Rhus* dermatitis
B) Lyme disease
C) chigger bite
D) brown recluse spider bite
E) black widow spider bite

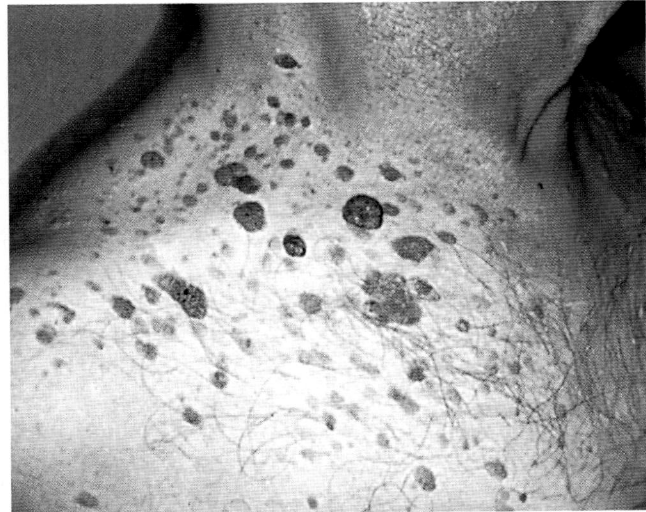

13. An 82-year-old nursing home resident is seen on monthly rounds. The floor nurse points out the skin lesions shown here. The patient is asymptomatic. Appropriate management includes
A) punch biopsy
B) topical 5-fluorouracil cream
C) cryotherapy
D) hydrocortisone cream
E) observation

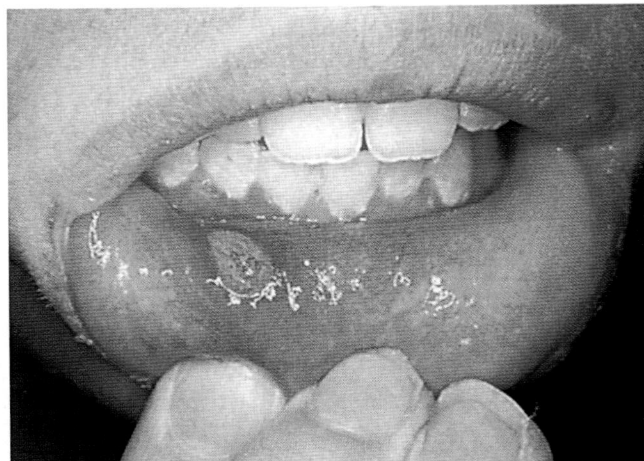

14. An 18-year-old sexually active female presents with a single ulcer that is located on the lower lip and is painful. She is a smoker and has noticed that the ulcers have been recurrent and correlate with the onset of menses. The most likely diagnosis is
A) Kawasaki disease
B) apthous stomatitis
C) squamous cell carcinoma of the lip
D) syphilis
E) Koplik's spot

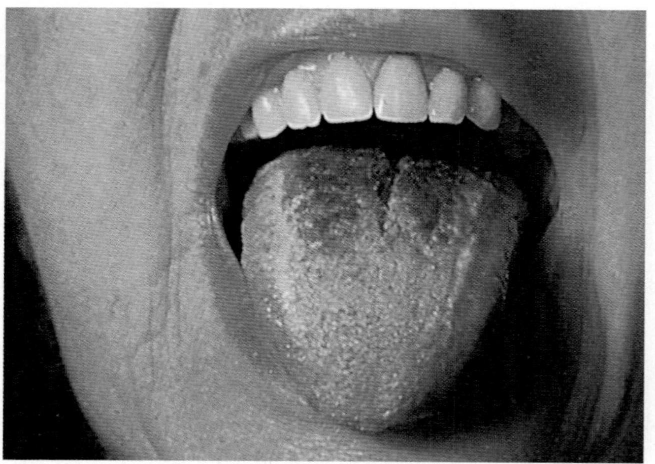

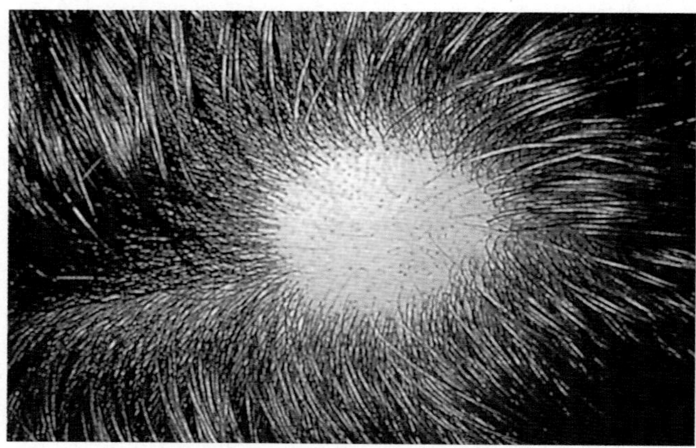

15. Which of the following conditions is the skin finding shown here associated with?

A) Prolonged antibiotic use
B) Sjögren's syndrome
C) Addison's disease
D) Chronic gastroesophageal reflux
E) Malignant melanoma

16. A 38-year-old man presents with rapid hair loss that has occurred over the last few weeks. He reports that his father had a similar condition. The most likely diagnosis is

A) alopecia areata
B) androgenic alopecia
C) tinea capitis
D) trichotillomania
E) secondary syphilis

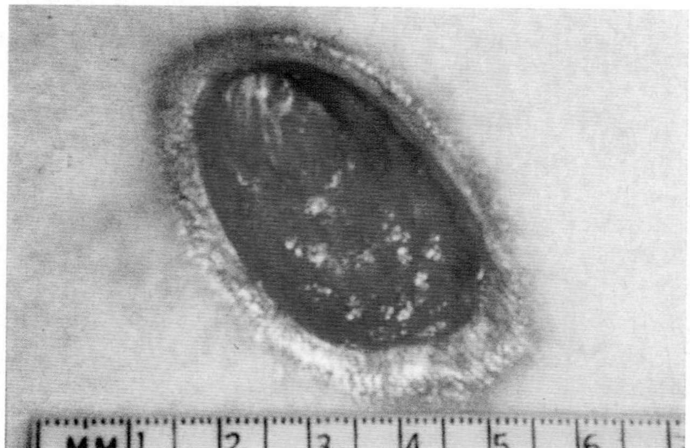

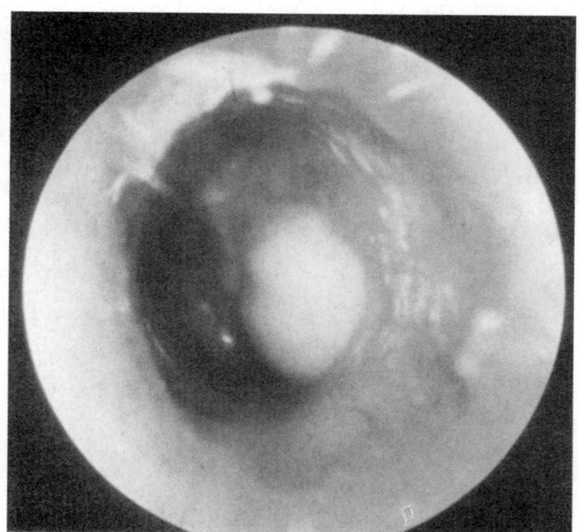

17. The condition shown here was noted associated with an 88-year-old debilitated nursing home resident. He has no evidence of bacteremia or osteomyelitis. Which of the following is an acceptable treatment?

A) application of povidone-iodine gauze two times per day
B) application of hydrogen peroxide 3 times per day
C) systemic antibiotics for 7 to 10 days
D) keeping the area clean and dry until granulation tissue forms
E) surgical debridement

18. A 35 year old presents with unilateral hearing loss that has been gradual but progressive over the last 6 months. Appropriate treatment of the above condition consists of

A) prolonged antibiotics for up to 4 weeks
B) decongestant and antihistamine administration
C) corticosteroid treatment for 2 weeks
D) hearing aid amplification
E) tympanomastoidectomy

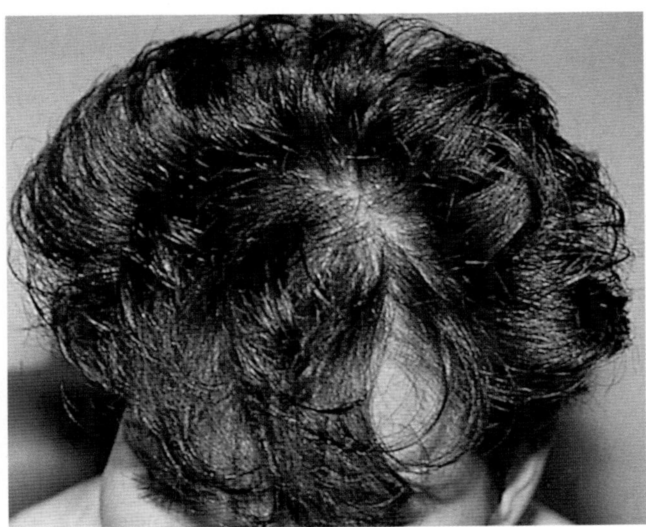

19. A 27-year-old gravida 2, para 2 woman is now 6 months postpartum and complains of excessive hair loss. The most likely diagnosis is
A) alopecia areata
B) telogen effluvium
C) trichotillomania
D) tinea capitis
E) hypothyroidism

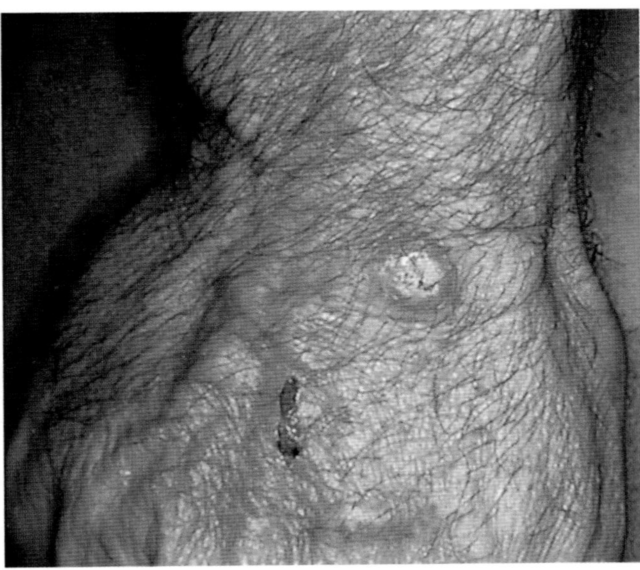

20. A 68-year-old man is seen for a general examination and reports a dome-shaped lesion on the back of the hand that has developed over the last few weeks. The lesion is rapidly becoming larger. The most likely diagnosis is
A) basal cell carcinoma
B) squamous cell carcinoma
C) seborrheic keratosis
D) actinic keratosis
E) keratoacanthoma

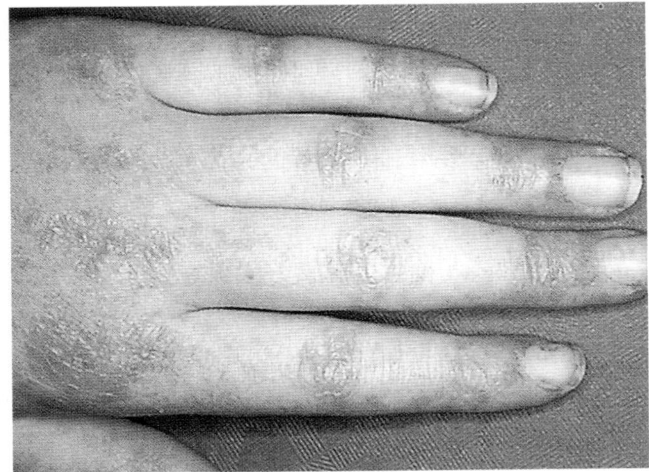

21. A 55-year-old woman complains of generalized fatigue, weakness, inability to climb stairs, arthralgias, and dysphagia. Physical examination reveals definite proximal muscle weakness, a periorbital heliotrope rash, and skin findings associated with the hands (shown here). The most likely diagnosis is
A) lupus erythematosus
B) sarcoidosis
C) Sjögren's disease
D) dermatomyositis
E) polymyalgia rheumatica

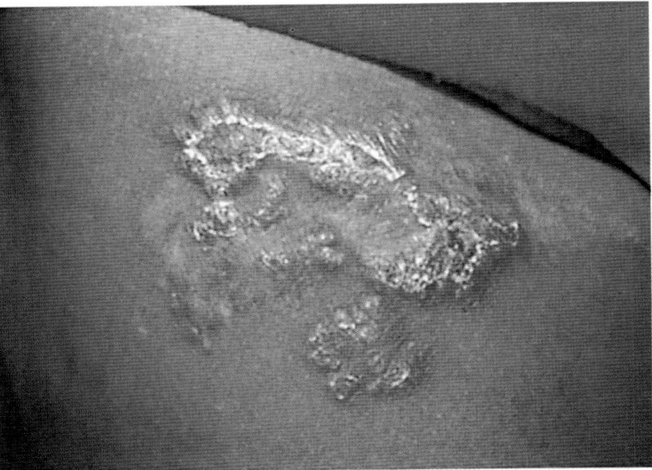

22. A 50-year-old housewife who enjoys growing roses presents to your office complaining of the lesion shown here. She reports removing a thorn from the area several weeks before. After that, a small painless lump developed that now has crusted over. The most likely diagnosis is
A) sporotrichosis
B) blastomycosis
C) Lyme disease
D) coccidioidomycosis
E) histoplasmosis

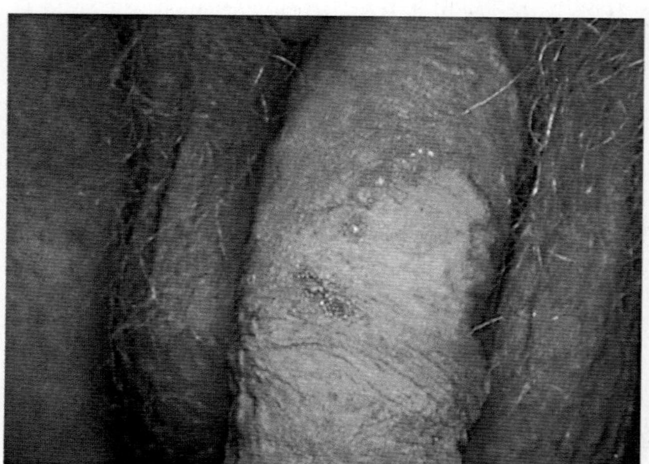

23. A 23-year-old Navy enlisted man is seen in sick bay with the recurrent lesion shown here. The patient reports pain and discomfort associated with the lesion but no dysuria. The likely diagnosis is
A) molluscum contagiosum
B) gonorrhea
C) syphilis
D) chancroid
E) herpes infection

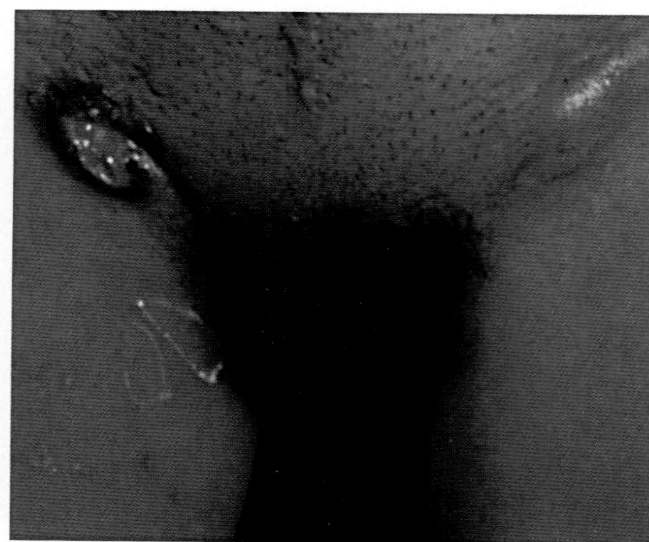

24. A 23-year-old black woman presents with a lesion affecting her groin that has developed over the last few days. Dark-field microscopic examination is negative. The etiologic agent that is responsible for the lesion is
A) *Neisseria gonorrhoeae*
B) herpes zoster
C) *Treponema pallidum*
D) molluscum contagiosum
E) *Haemophilus ducreyi*

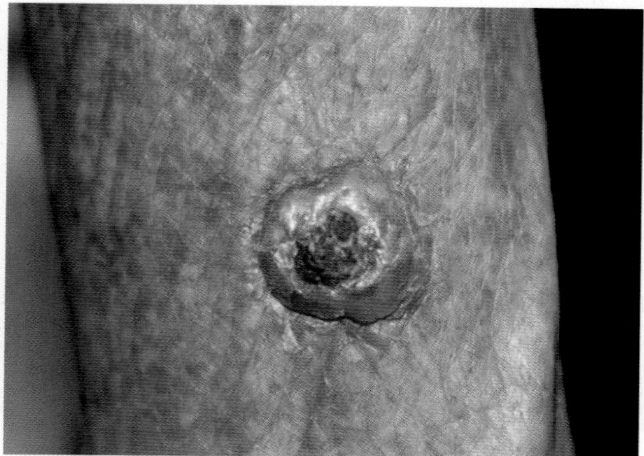

25. The pictured skin lesion developed over a 4-week time period. The most likely diagnosis is
A) melanoma
B) basal cell carcinoma
C) keratoacanthoma
D) dermatofibroma
E) molluscum contagiosum

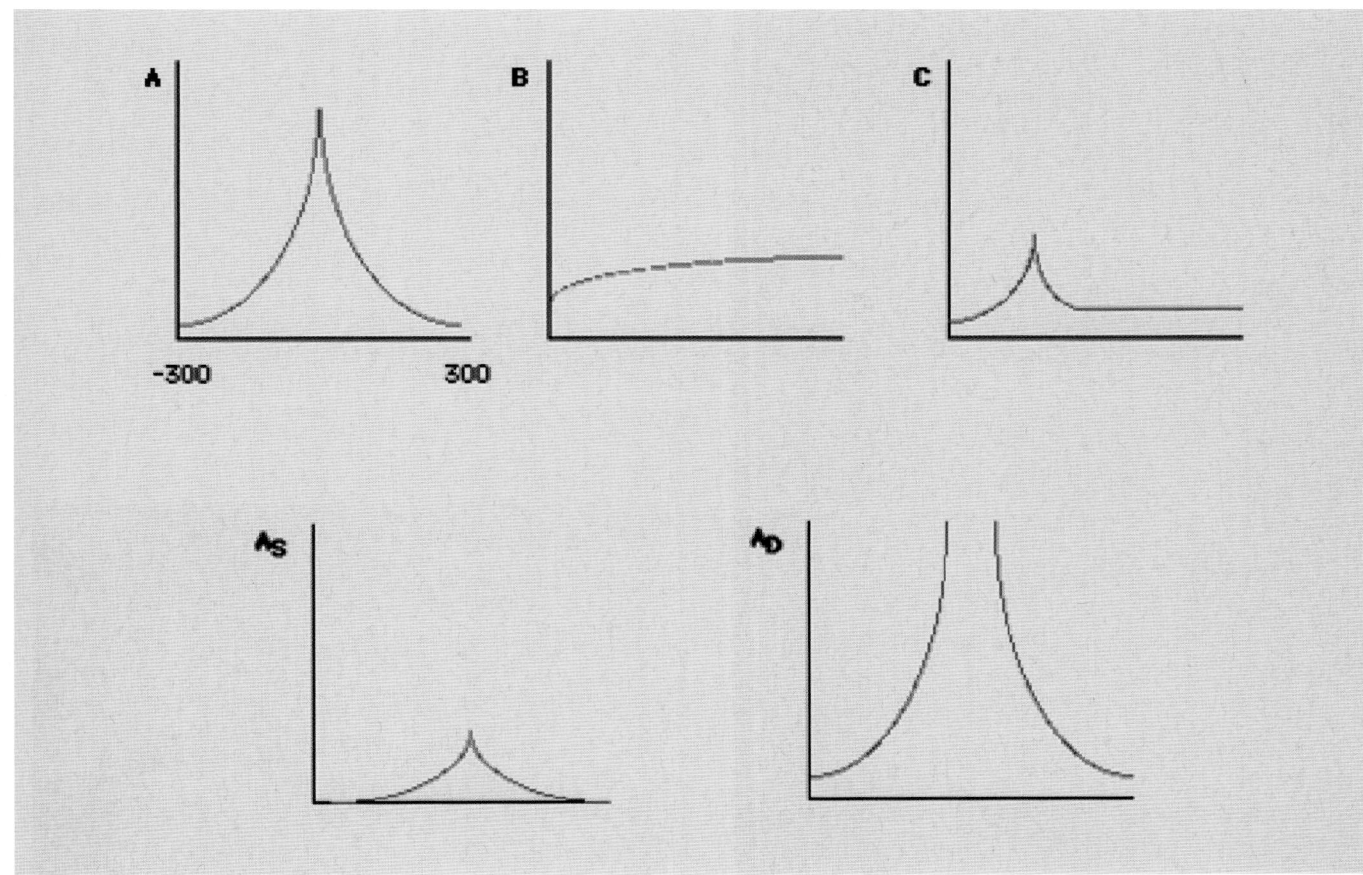

26. Which of the above audiograms represents a likely effusion behind the tympanic membrane?

A) Type A
B) Type B
C) Type C
D) Type As
E) Type Ad

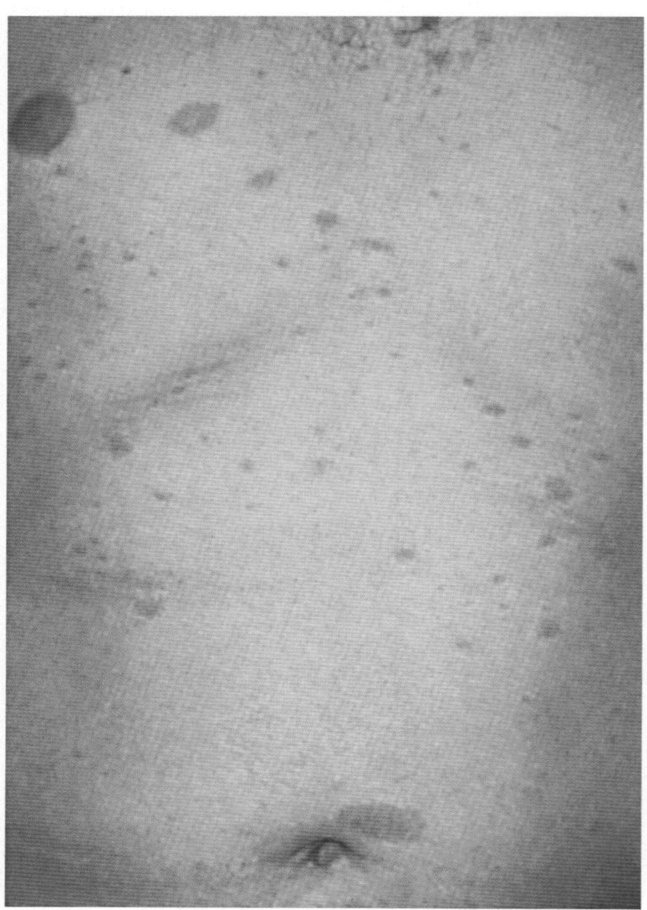

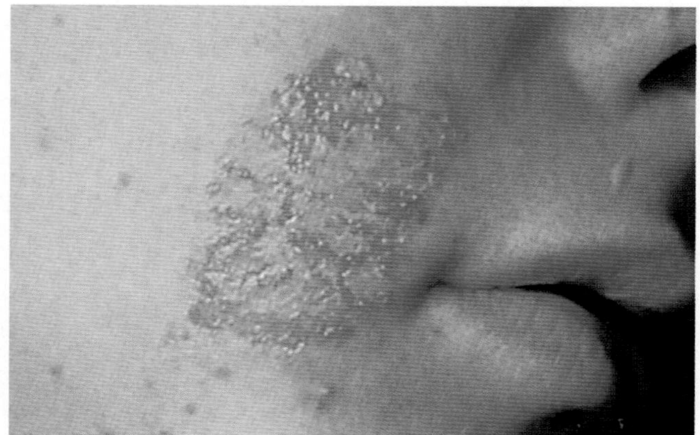

27. A 29-year-old man presents in April with the rash shown here. The rash does not itch and has been present over the last week. A large, red area developed first, followed by a more generalized rash that is now present. Physical examination shows that the rash appears in a Christmas-tree pattern on his chest and back. The most likely diagnosis is

A) pityriasis rosea
B) tinea versicolor
C) herpes zoster
D) varicella
E) Lyme disease

28. A 12-year-old boy presents with a crusted honey-brown lesion that affects his cheek. The rash began as red macules 3 days earlier. The best treatment is

A) intramuscular ceftriaxone
B) topical hydrocortisone cream
C) oral ciprofloxacin
D) topical mupirocin ointment
E) oral acyclovir

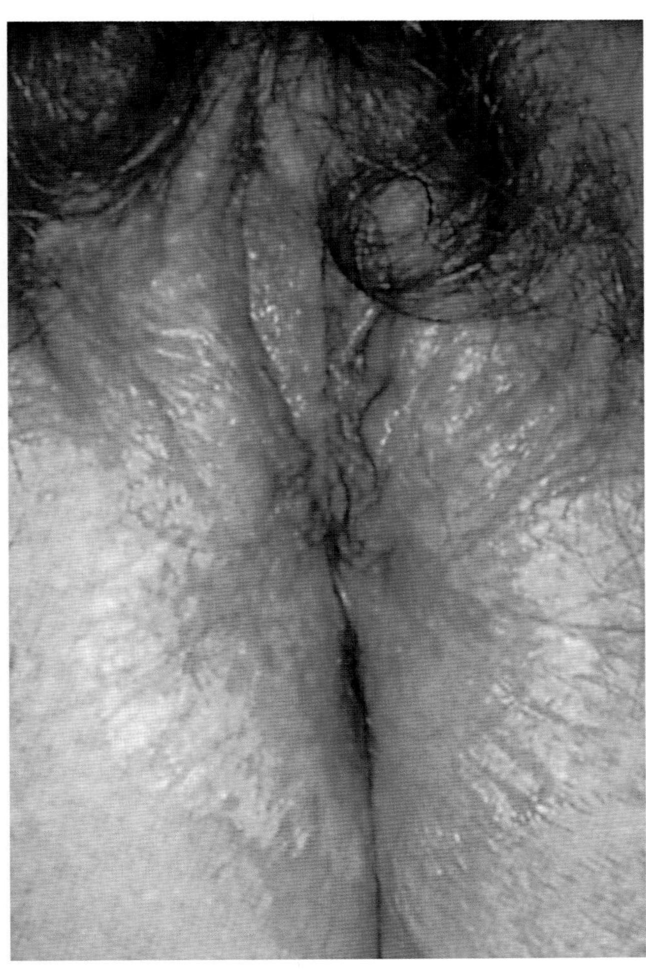

29. A 65-year-old woman presents to your office complaining of gradually increasing dyspareunia. Findings from the physical examination are pictured here. The most likely diagnosis is

A) yeast vaginitis
B) herpes genitalis
C) lichen sclerosis
D) vitiligo
E) contact dermatitis

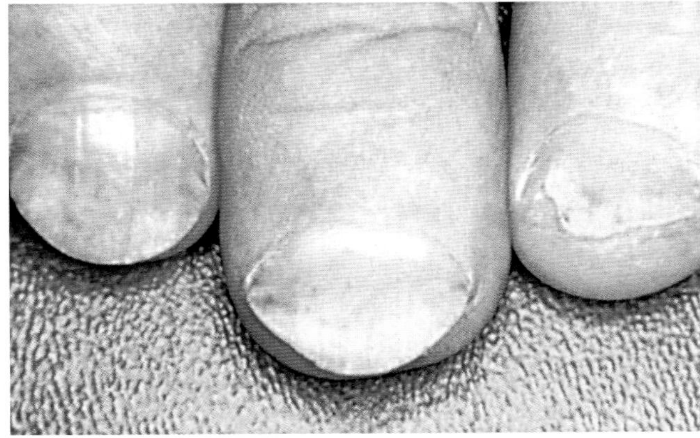

30. A 45-year-old woman presents with pitting of the nails that has developed slowly over the last few months. The most likely diagnosis is

A) psoriasis
B) onychomycosis
C) hyperthyroidism
D) chronic obstructive pulmonary disease
E) scleroderma

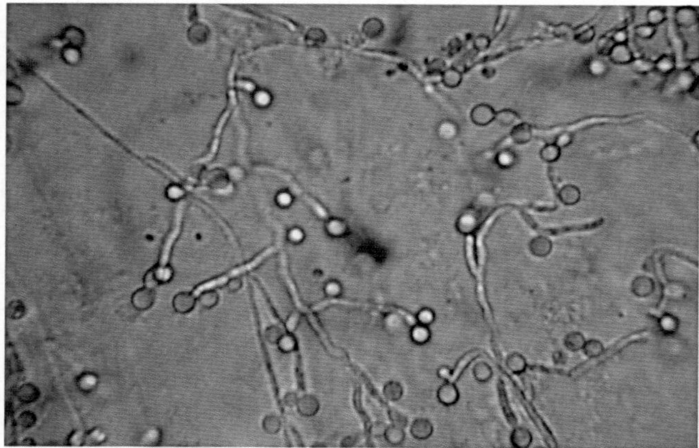

31. A sexually active 24-year-old woman presents to your office complaining of vaginal discharge. Findings from a wet prep are pictured here. The most likely diagnosis is
A) yeast vaginitis
B) *Gardnerella* infection
C) *Trichomonas* infection
D) gonorrhea
E) chlamydia

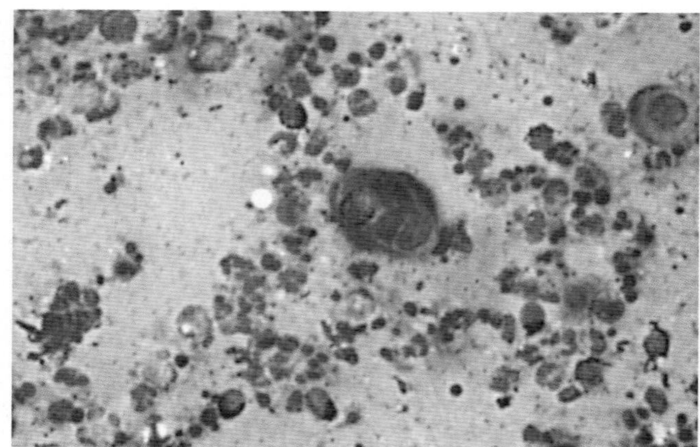

32. The sample shown here was obtained from a penile lesion of a 24-year-old sexually active male. A Tzanck smear was performed. The confirmed diagnosis is
A) gonorrhea
B) chancroid
C) herpes genitalis
D) syphilis
E) *Chlamydia*

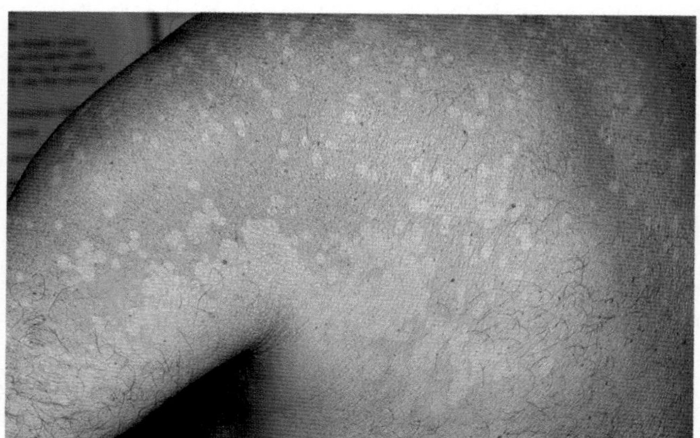

33. An 18-year-old surfer presents with the above skin condition. The most likely diagnosis is
A) pityriasis rosea
B) secondary syphilis
C) seborrheic dermatitis
D) eczema
E) tinea versicolor

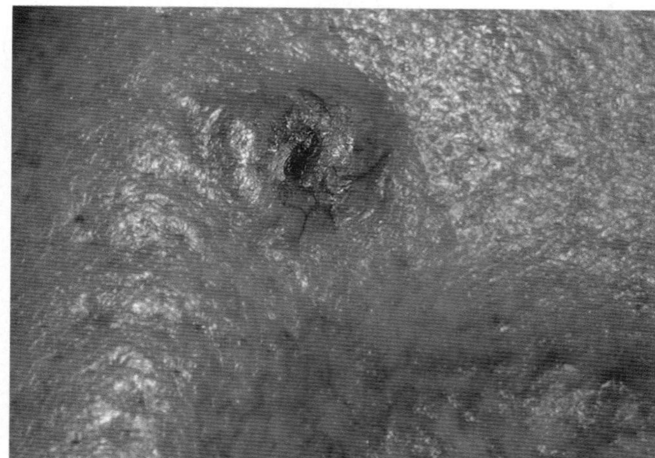

34. The most likely diagnosis is
A) pearly papule
B) basal cell carcinoma
C) molluscum contagiosum
D) squamous cell carcinoma
E) keratoacanthoma

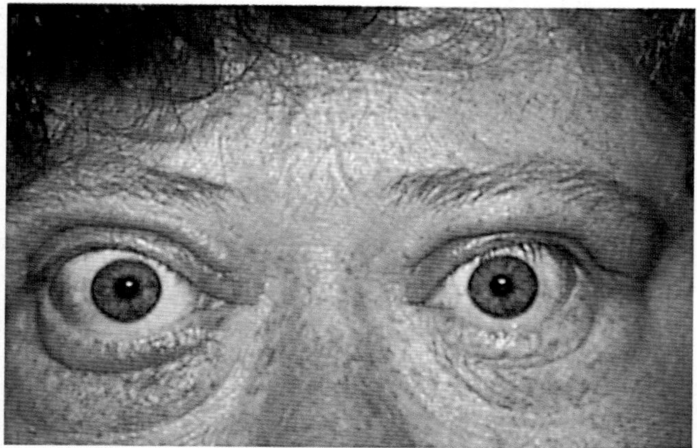

35. The eye findings pictured (at left) were seen in a 40-year-old woman who presented to the emergency room complaining of palpitations. The most likely diagnosis is
A) scleroderma
B) Graves' disease
C) amyloidosis
D) Cushing's disease
E) lupus erythematosus

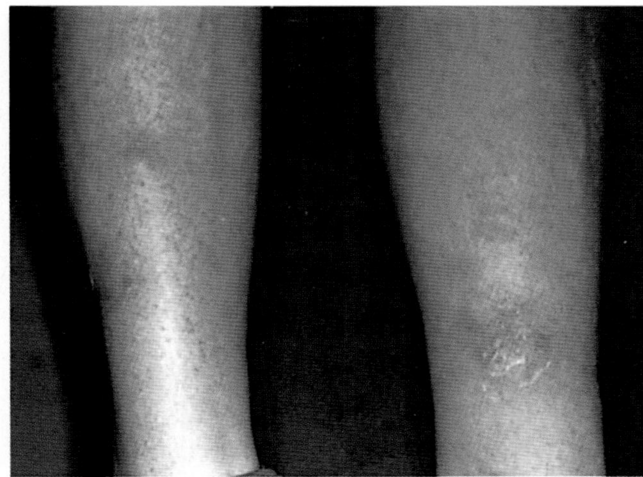

36. An 18-year-old woman presents to your office complaining of tender nodules that have developed on the lower extremities. She has no other symptoms. She continues with her oral contraceptives but has not started any new medications. She denies any fevers and has no history of recent trauma. The likely diagnosis is

A) erythema multiforme
B) erythema nodosum
C) Lyme disease
D) pyoderma gangrenosum
E) rheumatoid arthritis

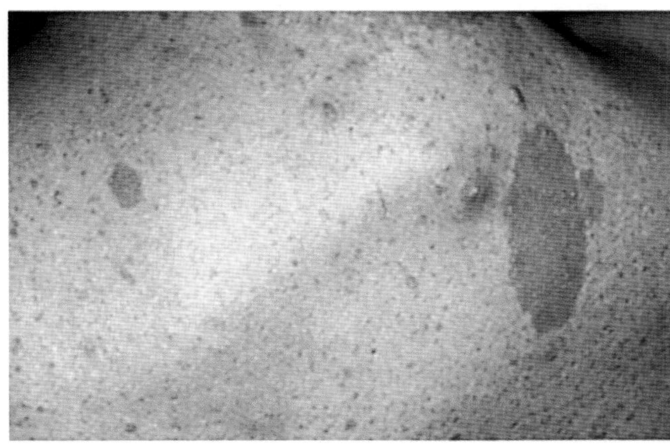

37. A 26-year-old man is seen for an upper respiratory infection. After removing his shirt, you notice the lesions shown here. He reports that his father has similar lesions. The differential diagnosis should include

A) hypothyroidism
B) Addison's disease
C) multiple sclerosis
D) neurofibromatosis
E) Gardner's syndrome

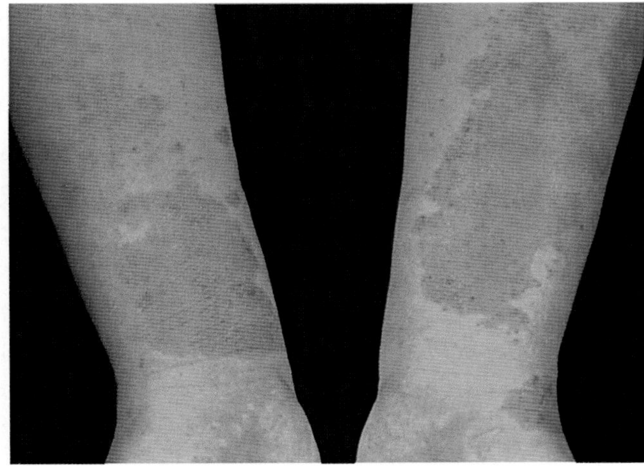

38. A 2-year-old girl is brought in by her mother. The child has an erythematous rash that is recurrent and affects the backs of the legs. The most likely diagnosis is

A) ichthyosis vulgaris
B) scabies
C) atopic dermatitis
D) dyshidrotic eczema
E) tinea corpora

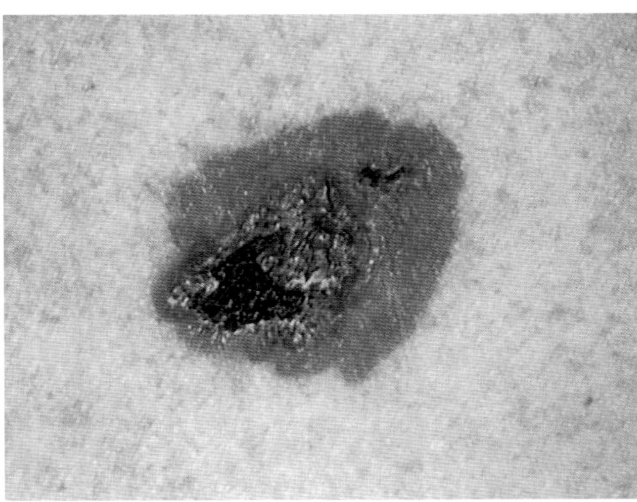

39. Appropriate management of the lesion shown here includes

A) cryotherapy
B) electrodesiccation and curettage
C) shave biopsy
D) excisional biopsy
E) laser ablation

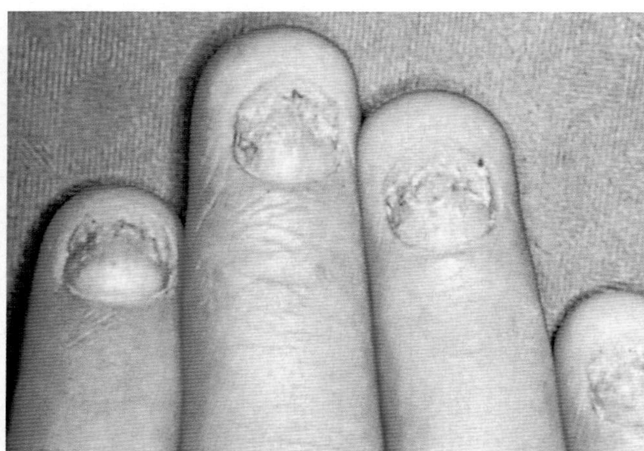

40. The most common etiologic agent that gives rise to the condition shown here is
A) *Trichophyton rubrum*
B) *Candida albicans*
C) *Epidermophytin floccosum*
D) *Aspergillus flavus*
E) *Candida glabrata*

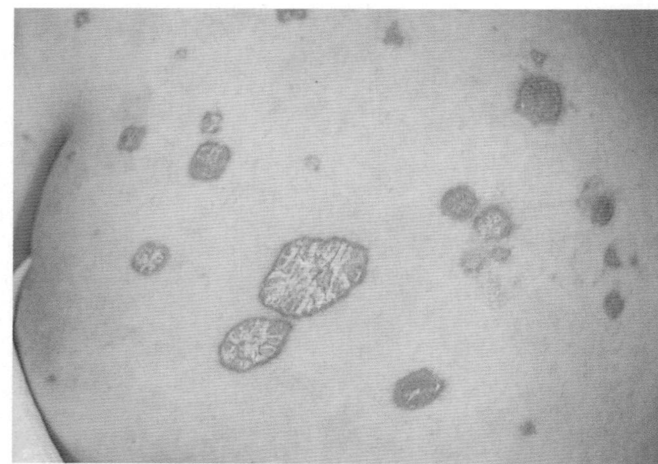

41. A 45-year-old man presents with a chronic, mildly pruritic and scaly erythematous rash. The most likely diagnosis is
A) cutaneous T-cell lymphoma
B) psoriasis
C) eczema
D) tinea versicolor
E) lichen planus

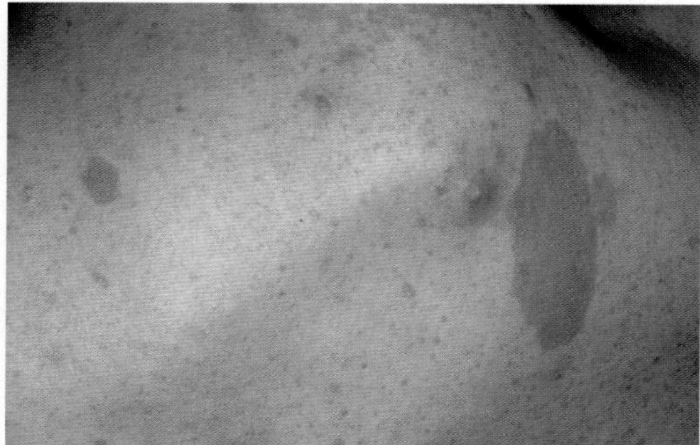

42. A 4-year-old boy is brought to your office by his parents. They are concerned about the multiple skin lesions that have been present since infancy. You explain that the lesions can be a sign for
A) dysplastic nevi syndrome
B) diabetes
C) gastrointestinal cancer
D) neurofibromatosis
E) lymphoma

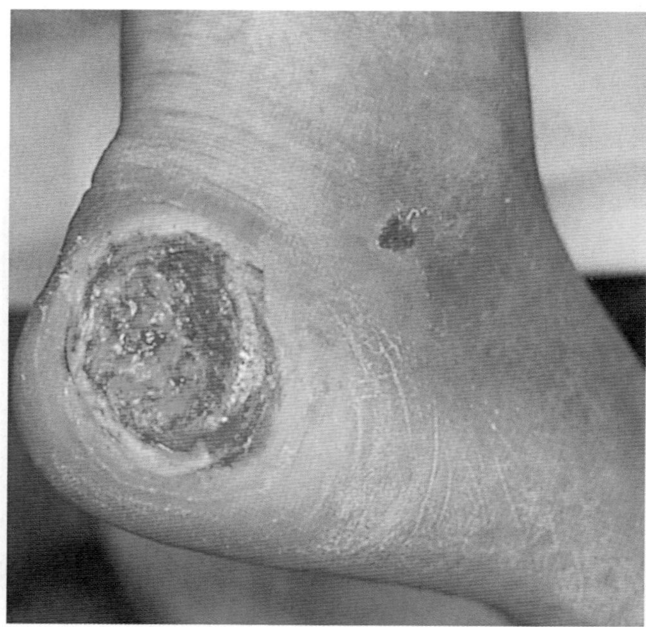

43. A 68-year-old man with a history of a previous myocardial infarction presents complaining of a painful lesion noted on his foot. He has been experiencing pain in his lower legs with ambulation over the last year. The most likely diagnosis is
A) venous stasis ulcer
B) arterial ulcer
C) basal cell carcinoma
D) livedo reticularis
E) diabetic foot ulcer

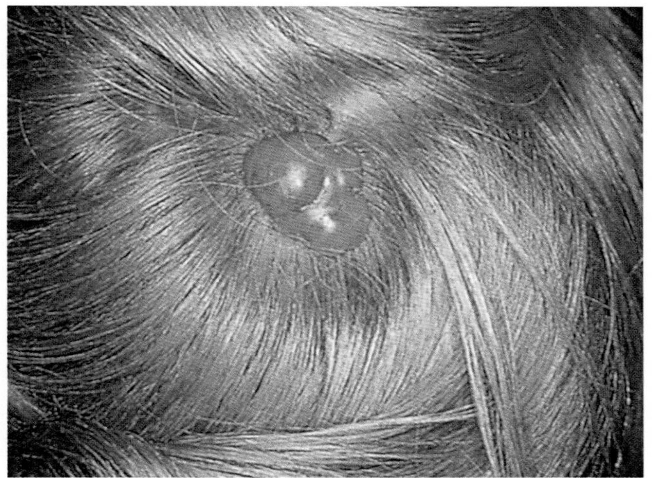

44. A 42-year-old man presents with a small lump that has formed on his scalp. The most likely diagnosis is
A) syringoma
B) cylindroma
C) trichoepithelioma
D) histiocytoma
E) dermatofibroma

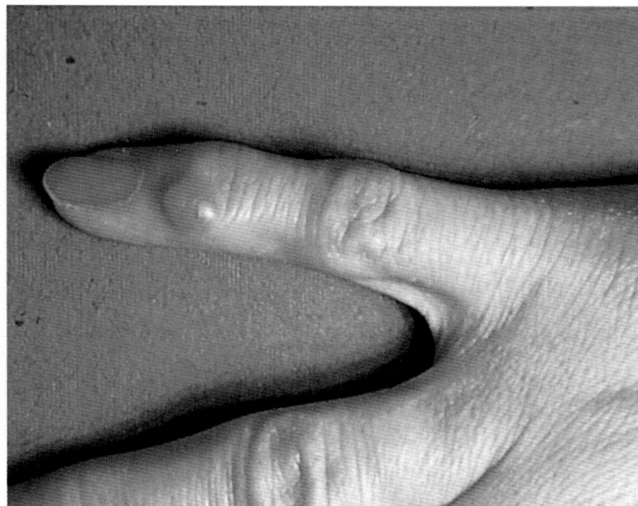

45. A 58-year-old woman presents to your office complaining of a clear fluid-filled cyst that has formed over the distal knuckle of the fifth finger of the right hand. The most likely diagnosis is
A) epidermoid cyst
B) sebaceous cyst
C) mucous cyst
D) lipoma
E) synovial cyst

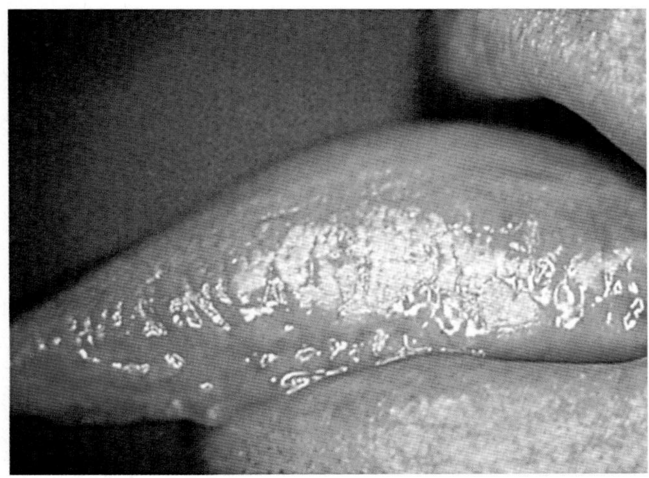

46. Which of the following conditions is associated with the skin finding shown here?
A) Vitamin B_{12} deficiency
B) Hypothyroidism
C) Human immunodeficiency syndrome
D) Periodontitis
E) Gastroesophageal reflux

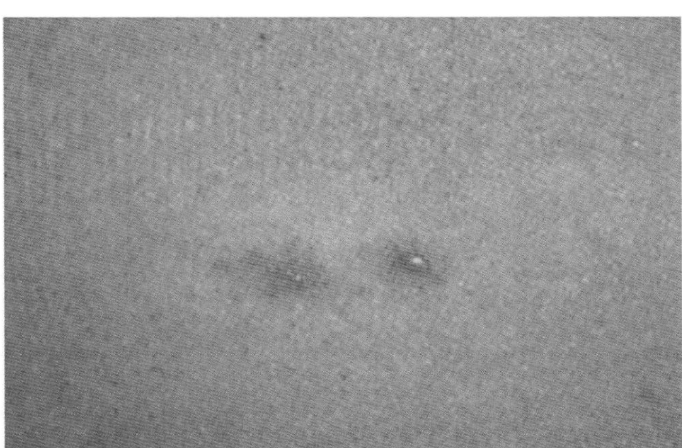

47. A 3-year-old child who attends daycare is brought in by her mother with the lesions shown here noted on the abdomen. The mother reports some low-grade fevers, and the child has not been as active as usual. The most likely diagnosis is
A) impetigo
B) coxsackievirus
C) adenovirus
D) varicella
E) scarlatina

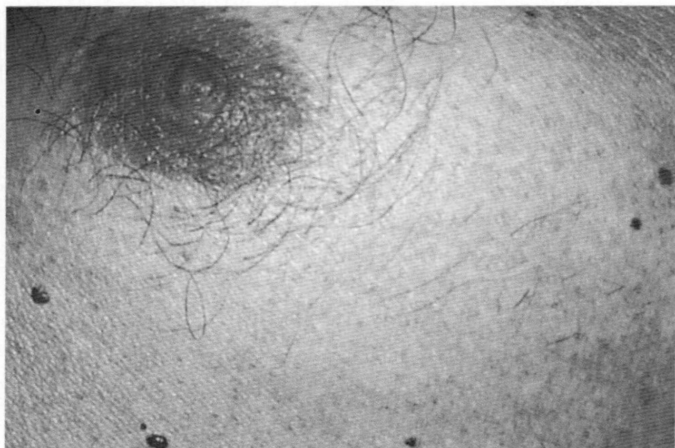

48. A 42-year-old man complains of multiple red lesions that have formed on his chest and abdomen. The most likely diagnosis is

A) scabies
B) chigger bites
C) granuloma annulare
D) cherry angiomas
E) erythroderma

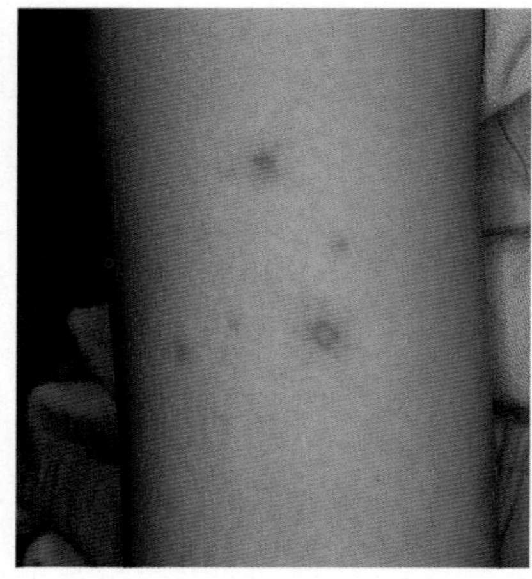

49. A 36-month-old immigrant child is brought in by his mother with a sore throat and an erythematous, pruritic rash that has developed over the last 24 hours. The most likely diagnosis is

A) varicella
B) scarlatina
C) fifth disease
D) Rocky Mountain spotted fever
E) Measles

50. A 42-year-old African American presents to your office with the above skin condition. She has a history of chronic sarcoidosis and has experienced multiple exacerbations. The most likely diagnosis is:

A) lupus pernio
B) erythema nodosum
C) erythema marginatum
D) erythema multiforme
E) psoriasis

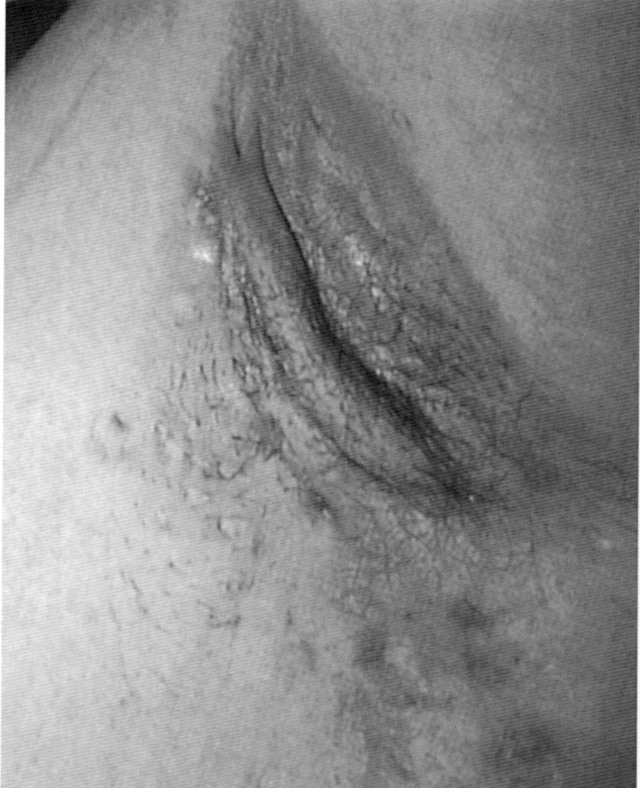

51. A 33-year-old woman presents with complaints of recurrent rashes under the arm that come and go and the development of painful cysts with scar tissue formation. The most likely diagnosis is

A) hidradenitis suppurativa
B) reaction to antiperspirant
C) impetigo
D) tinea corpora
E) scrofuloderma

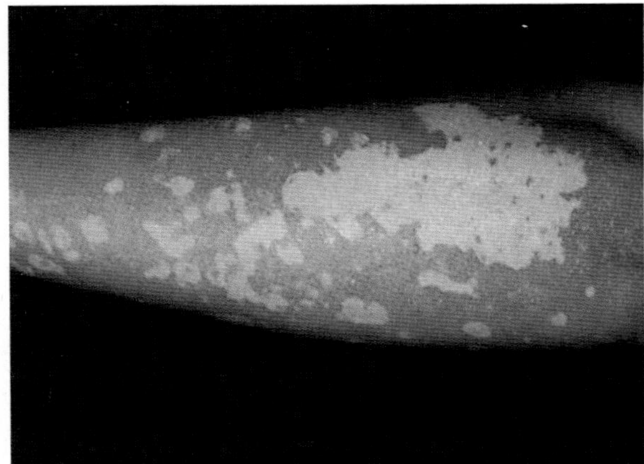

52. A 38-year-old African American presents with the lesion shown here. The lesion shows a "milk-white" fluorescence with a Wood's light examination. The most likely diagnosis is

A) tinea versicolor
B) tinea corpora
C) amelanotic melanoma
D) vitiligo
E) leprosy

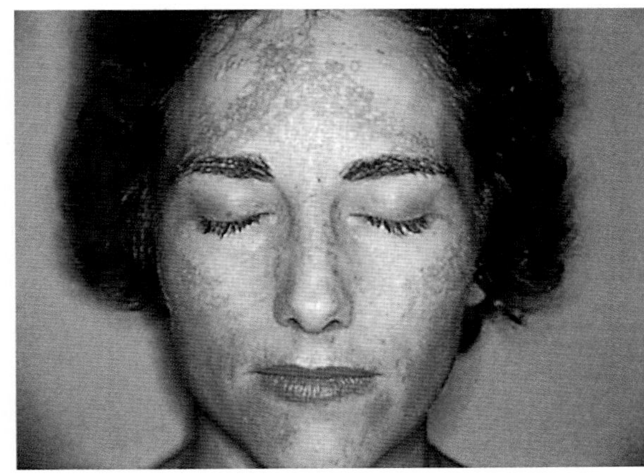

53. A 42-year-old Native American presents to your office complaining of dark spots on her face. Her medical history is unremarkable except for two previous uncomplicated pregnancies. She is now taking oral contraceptives. The most likely diagnosis is

A) solar lentigo
B) melasma
C) sunburn
D) lupus erythematosus
E) scleroderma

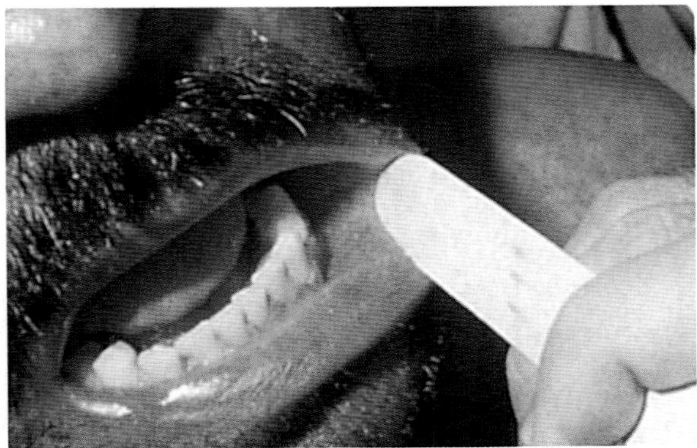

54. A 36-year-old indigent man from Mexico presents with 1-mm bluish-white macules with an erythematous oral mucosa. Two days later, an erythematous, generalized papular rash develops. The rash began on his forehead and progressed to involve his entire body. He has also had upper respiratory symptoms and a fever. The most likely diagnosis is

A) human immunodeficiency virus
B) coxsackievirus
C) rubella
D) rubeola
E) scarlet fever

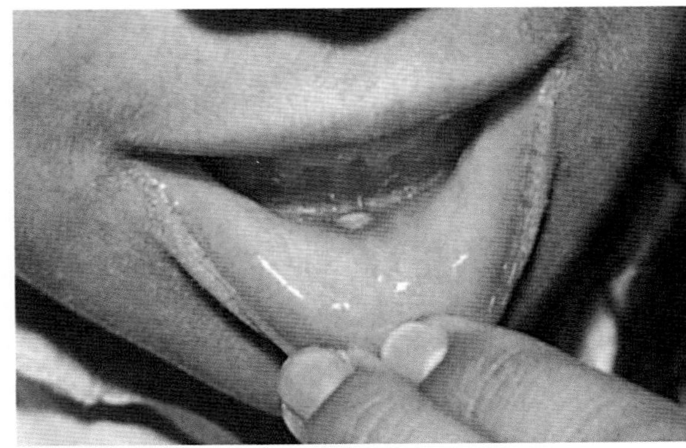

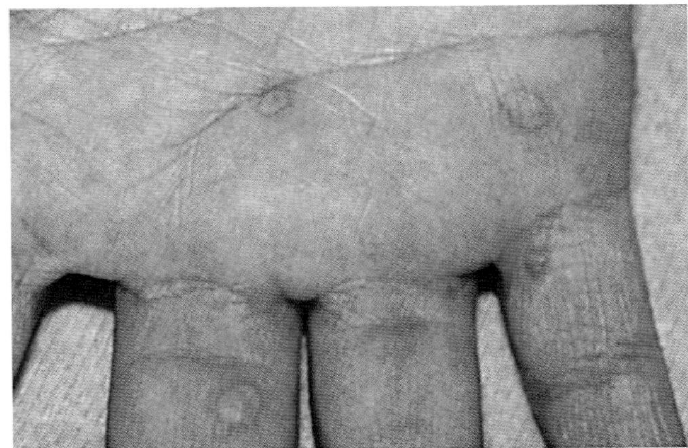

55. The most likely cause for the condition shown here is

A) herpes virus
B) coxsackievirus
C) adenovirus
D) Lyme disease
E) syphilis

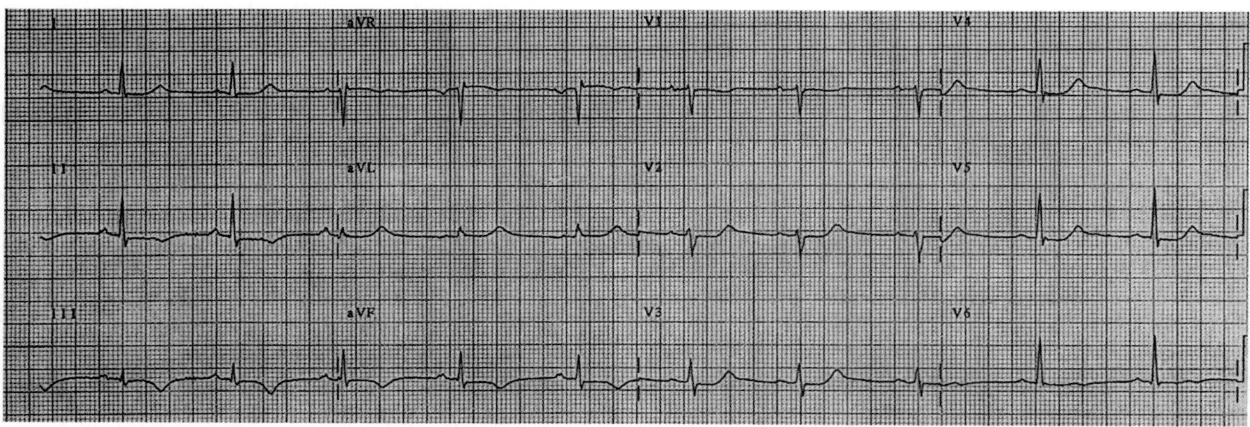

56. Based on the electrocardiographic (ECG) tracing shown here, the most likely diagnosis is
A) atrial fibrillation
B) left bundle branch block
C) third-degree heart block
D) inferior ischemia
E) left ventricular hypertrophy

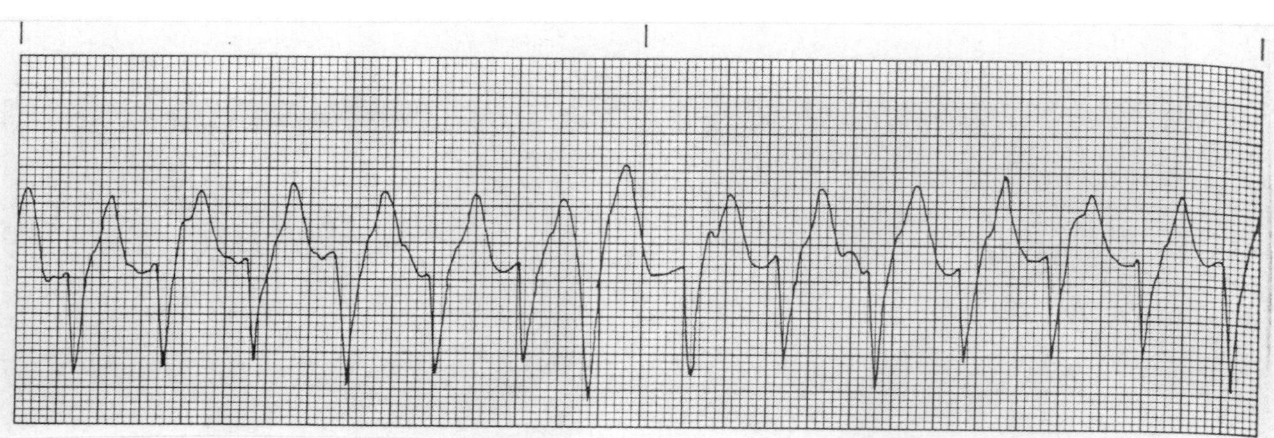

57. A 67 year old collapses in your office and the following ECG strip is obtained. The correct diagnosis is
A) atrial fibrillation
B) ventricular fibrillation
C) supraventricular tachycardia
D) ventricular tachycardia
E) atrioventricular dissociation

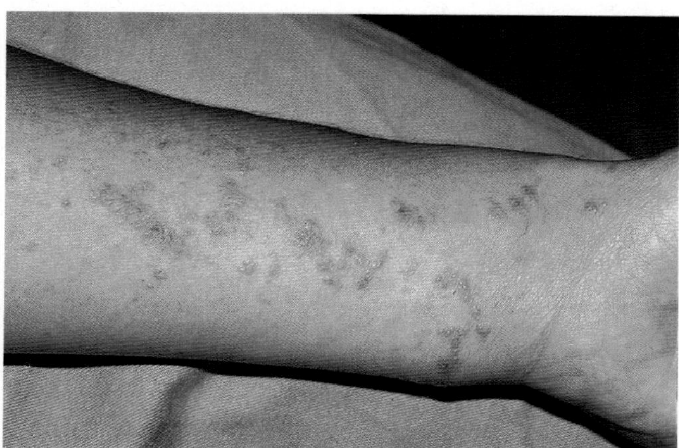

58. A 9-year-old boy is brought into your office after a weekend camping trip. He complains of a pruritic rash that has developed over the last 24 hours. The most likely diagnosis is
A) poison ivy
B) erythema multiforme
C) lichen sclerosis
D) varicella
E) herpes zoster

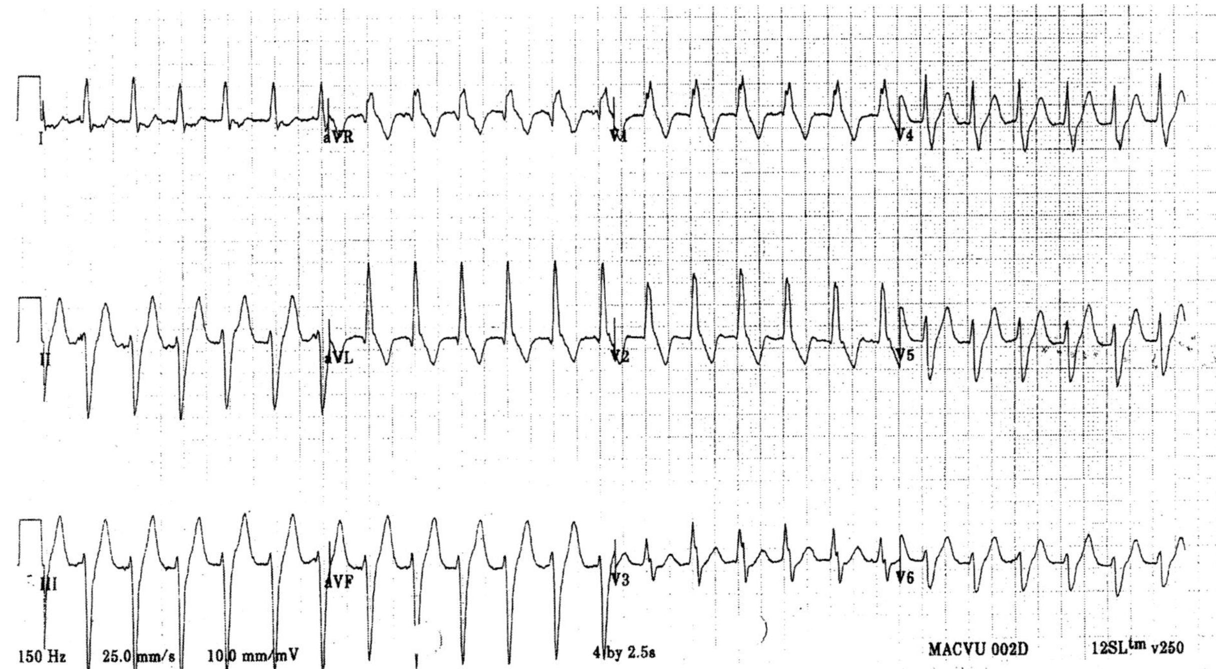

59. Please identify the rhythm shown here.
A) atrial fibrillation
B) atrial flutter
C) supraventricular tachycardia
D) ventricular fibrillation
E) ventricular tachycardia

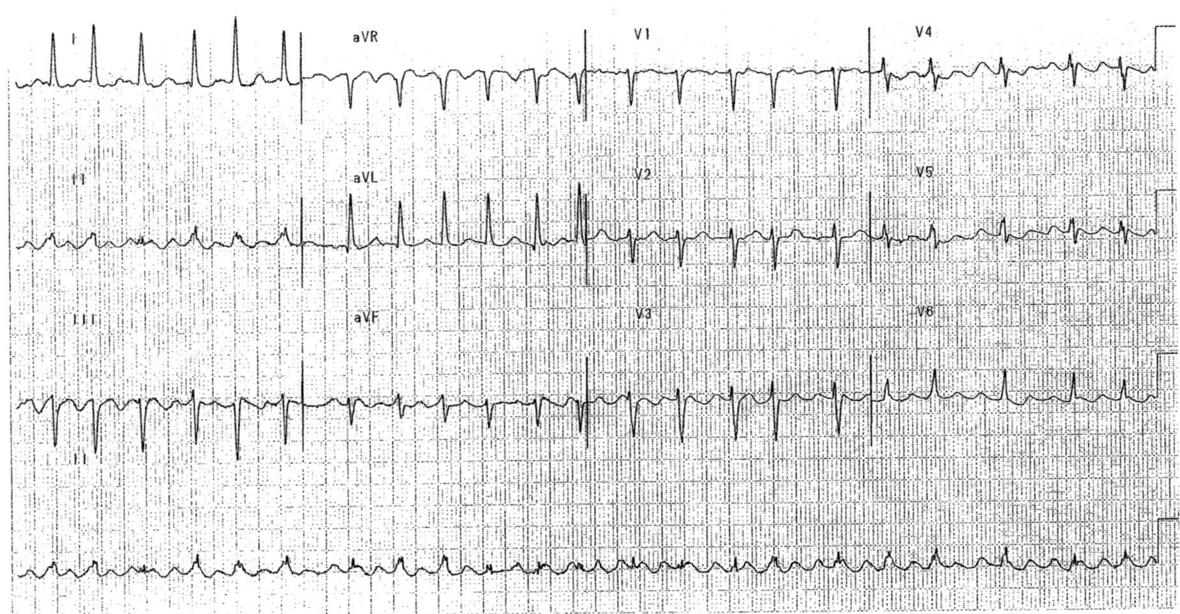

60. A 65 year old presents to the emergency room complaining of palpitations. Findings from an ECG are shown here. The most likely diagnosis is
A) acute myocardial infarction
B) atrial fibrillation
C) supraventricular tachycardia
D) ventricular fibrillation
E) ventricular tachycardia

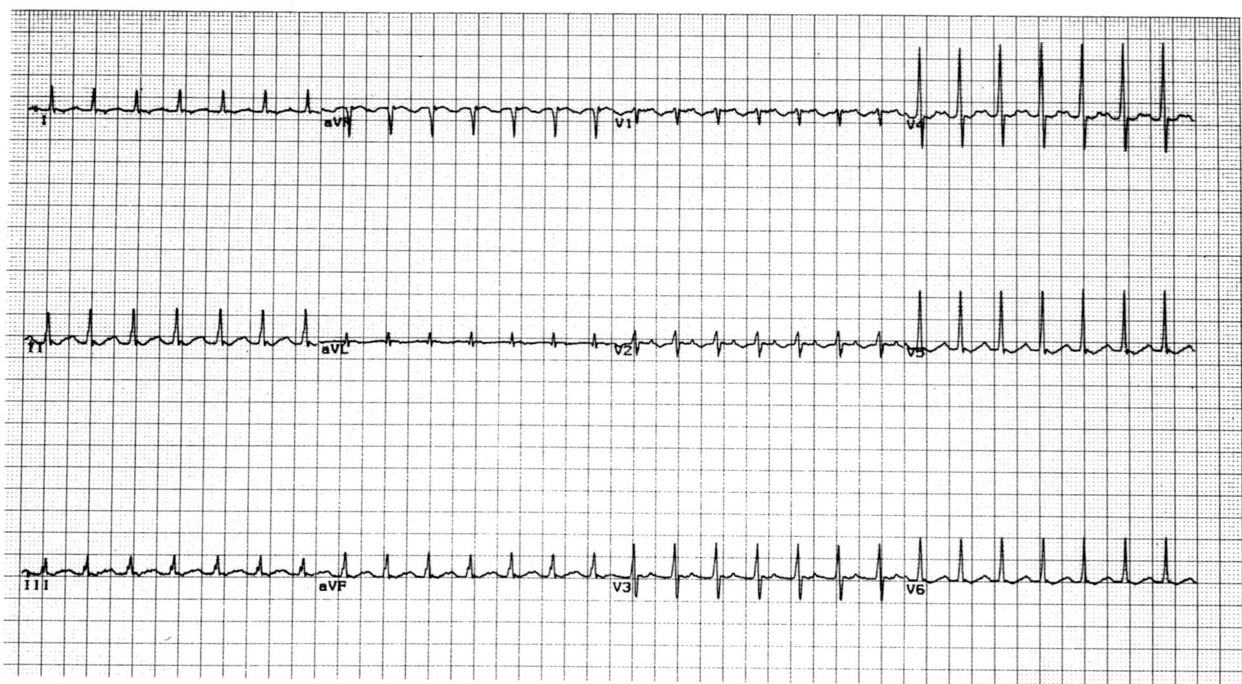

61. A 38 year old presents to the emergency room complaining of palpitations and shortness of breath. The most likely diagnosis based on the ECG findings shown here is
A) atrial fibrillation
B) supraventricular tachycardia
C) ventricular fibrillation
D) ventricular tachycardia
E) Wolff-Parkinson-White (WPW) syndrome

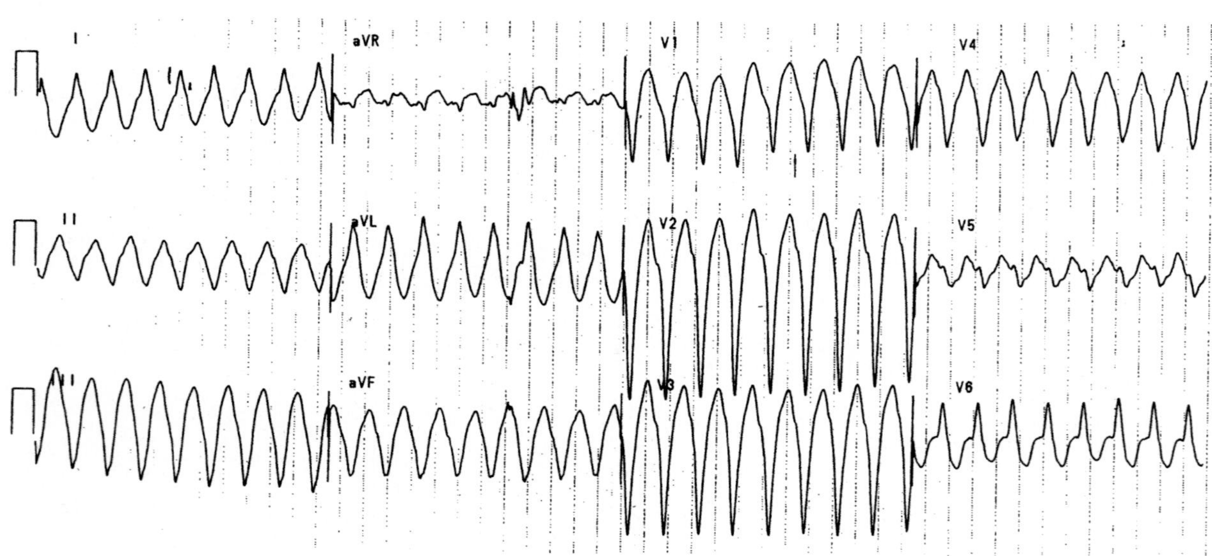

62. A 68-year-old man is found unresponsive. An initial ECG tracing is shown here. Which of the following conditions is present?
A) Atrial ventricular dissociation
B) Ventricular tachycardia
C) Ventricular fibrillation
D) Sinus tachycardia
E) Asystole

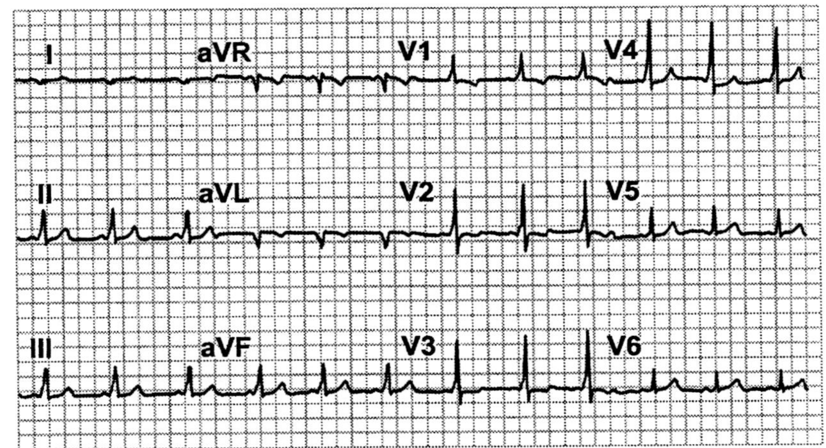

63. Please identify the condition shown here.
A) Hypothermia
B) WPW syndrome
C) Inferior myocardial infarction
D) Atrial fibrillation with 3:1 block
E) Normal sinus rhythm

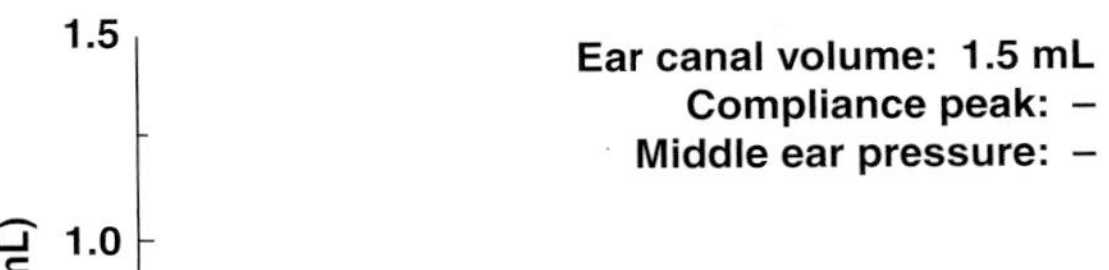

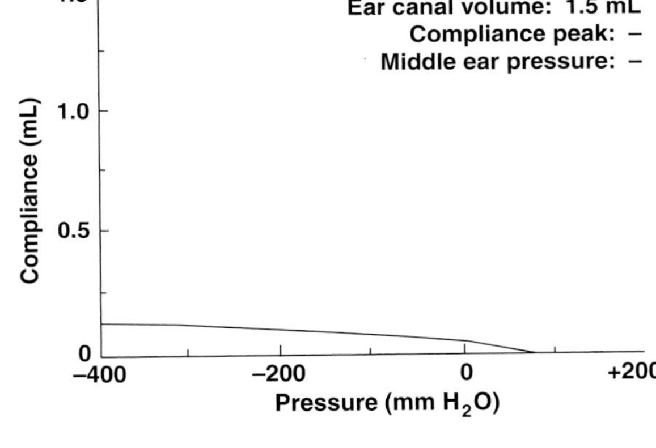

64. The tympanogram shown here would support the diagnosis of
A) normal tympanic membrane
B) fluid in the middle ear
C) negative middle ear pressure
D) hypermobile tympanic membrane
E) none of the above

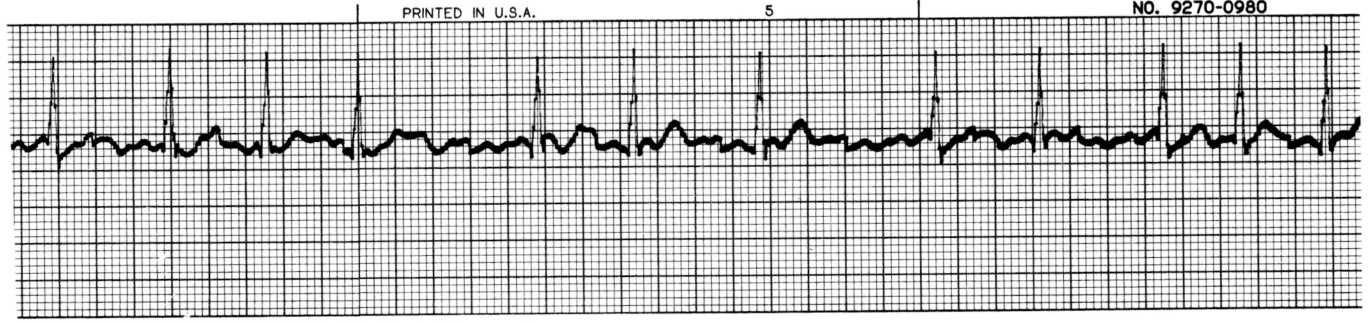

65. A 65-year-old alcoholic presents to your office with shortness of breath and generalized fatigue. An ECG is obtained. The most likely diagnosis is
A) multifocal atrial tachycardia
B) supraventricular tachycardia
C) atrial fibrillation
D) sinus tachycardia
E) pulmonary embolism

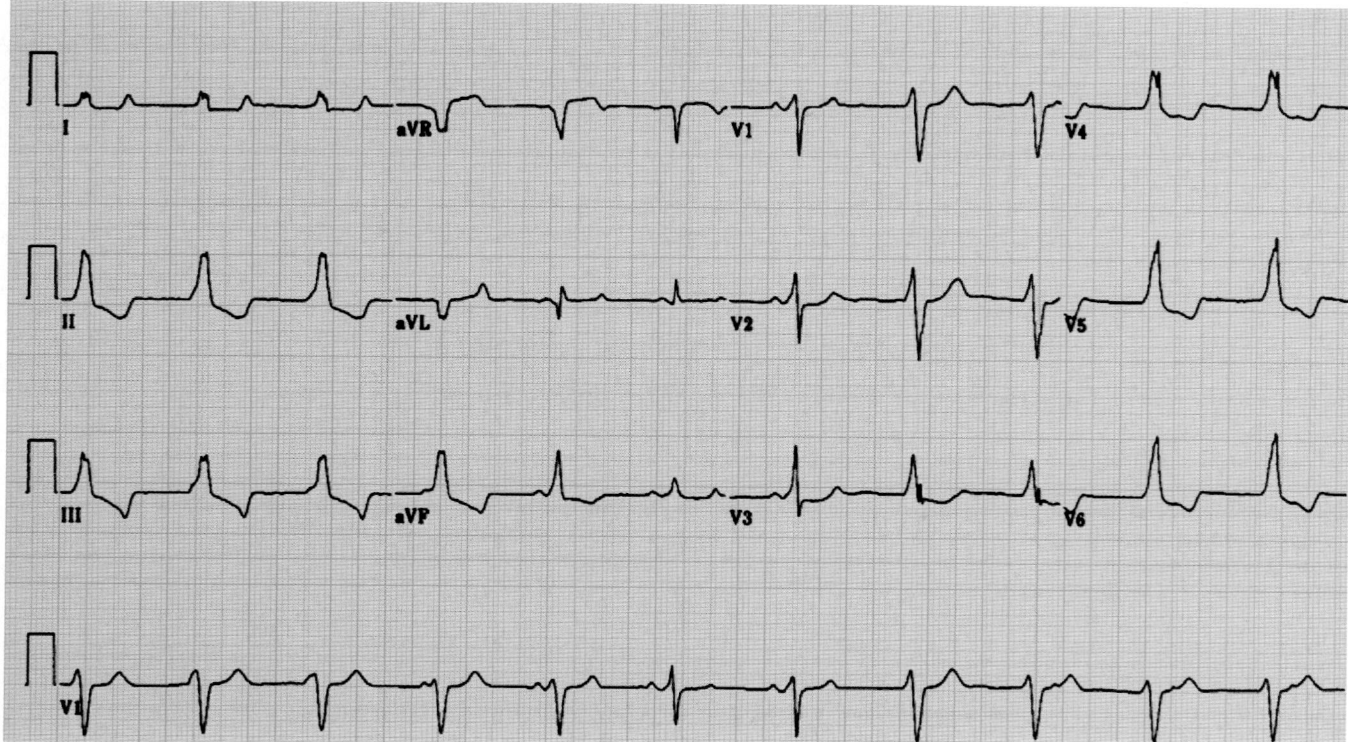

66. Based on the above ECG, the most likely diagnosis is
A) supraventricular tachycardia with 3:1 block
B) early myocardial infarction
C) incomplete right bundle branch block
D) pericarditis
E) Wolff-Parkinson-White syndrome

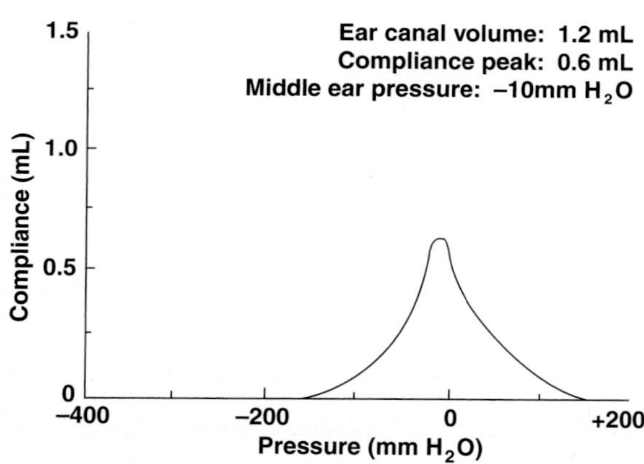

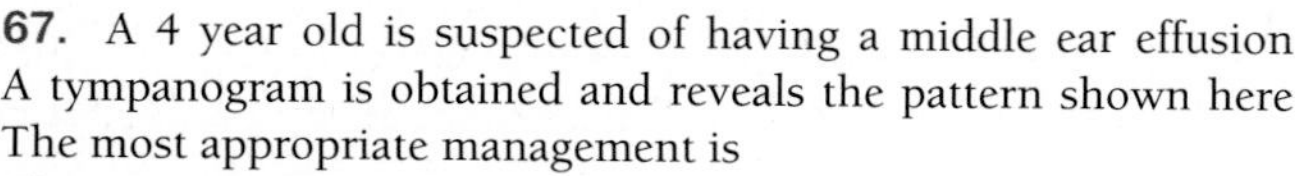

67. A 4 year old is suspected of having a middle ear effusion. A tympanogram is obtained and reveals the pattern shown here. The most appropriate management is
A) tympanocentesis
B) placement of tympanostomy tubes
C) prophylactic antibiotics for 1 year
D) decongestant use for 4 to 6 weeks
E) reassurance

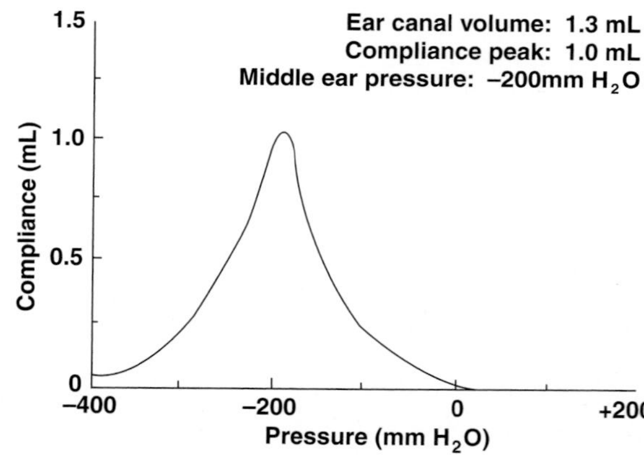

68. The tympanogram shown here was obtained on a 3-year-old girl. The likely diagnosis is
A) eustachian tube dysfunction
B) acoustic neuroma
C) middle ear effusion
D) sensorineural hearing loss
E) normal tympanogram

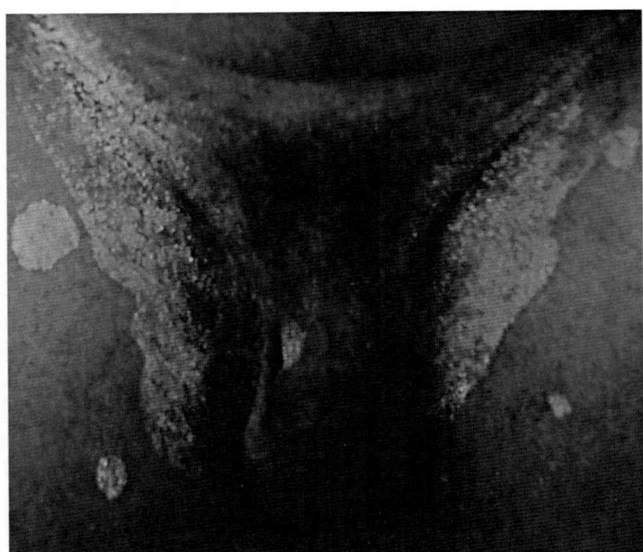

69. A 51-year-old man presents to your office complaining of a rash that affects the groin. Faint redness is noted, with fine scaling and no elevated border. Further examination under a Wood's lamp reveals a bright orange-coral fluorescence. The most likely diagnosis is

A) tinea cruris
B) mycoses fungoides
C) erythrasma
D) hidradenitis suppurativa
E) erysipelas

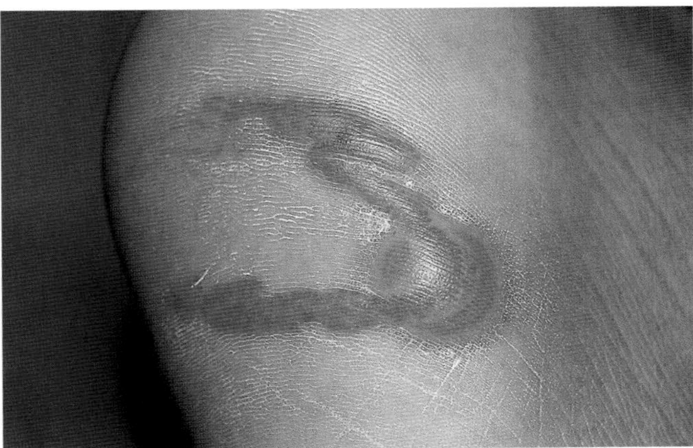

70. An 18-year-old surfer presents to your office with a rash that he noted on his foot. The vesicular rash has been present over the last week and has been enlarging. The most likely diagnosis is

A) sea lice
B) cutaneous larva migrans
C) swimming pool granuloma
D) jellyfish sting
E) bathing suit dermatitis

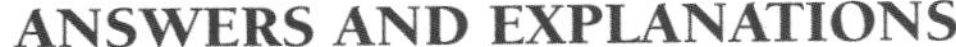

ANSWERS AND EXPLANATIONS

1. The answer is B. (*Complete excision with normal margins*) Even in the hands of experienced dermatologists, there is an approximately 15% false negative rate in determining the presence of melanoma based on examination alone; therefore, histologic confirmation is essential for both tumor diagnosis and staging. A complete excision with normal skin margins is preferable when possible as the first diagnostic step (e.g., excisional biopsy). An incisional biopsy can be performed for larger lesions when complete excision is not practical and when the suspicion of melanoma is low; incisional biopsy does not adversely affect survival. Shave biopsies should be avoided because they may not provide enough tissue for diagnosis and do not allow for accurate depth measurement. All biopsies of lesions suspected of being melanomas should provide a piece of full-thickness skin extending to the subcutaneous fat.

Sober AJ, Chuang TY, Duvic M, et al. Guidelines of care for primary cutaneous melanoma. *J Am Acad Dermatol.* 2001;45:579.

Bong JL, Herd RM, Hunter JA. Incisional biopsy and melanoma prognosis. *J Am Acad Dermatol.* 2002;46:690.

> When considering the diagnosis of melanoma, shave biopsies should be avoided because they may not provide enough tissue for diagnosis and do not allow for accurate depth measurement. All biopsies of lesions suspected of being melanomas should provide a piece of full-thickness skin extending to the subcutaneous fat.

2. The answer is B. (*Pityriasis rosea*) Pityriasis rosea is a self-limited, exanthematous skin disease that develops acutely and is characterized by the appearance of slightly inflammatory, oval, papulosquamous lesions on the trunk and proximal areas of the extremities. Pityriasis rosea is largely a disease of older children and young adults. It is more common in women than men. A prodrome of headache, malaise, and pharyngitis may occur in a small number of cases, but except for itching, the condition is usually asymptomatic. The eruption commonly begins with a "herald patch": a single round or oval, sharply demarcated pink or salmon-colored lesion on the chest, neck, or back, 2 to 5 cm in diameter. The lesion soon becomes scaly and begins to clear centrally, leaving the free edge of the scaly lesion directed inwards toward the center. A few days or a week or two later, oval lesions similar in appearance to the herald patch, but smaller, appear in crops on the trunk and proximal areas of the extremities The long axes of these oval lesions tend to be oriented along the lines of cleavage of the skin. This characteristic Christmas-tree pattern is most evident on the back, where it is emphasized by the oblique direction of the cleavage lines in that location. Most cases of pityriasis rosea need no treatment other than reassurance and proper patient education. Topical steroids with moderate potency are helpful in the control of itching. They can be applied to the pruritic areas two or three times daily. Topical antipruritic lotions such as prax, pramagel, or sarna may also be helpful.

Chuh AA. Quality of life in children with pityriasis rosea: a prospective case control study. *Pediatr Dermatol.* 2003;20:474.

3. The answer is C. (*Keratosis pilaris*) *Keratosis pilaris* is defined as hyperkeratotic follicular papules on the extensor surface of the upper arms or upper anterior thighs and occasionally on the malar area of the face. It may be associated with atopy and dry skin. A sandpaper-like feel is noted in these isolated areas. The condition is considered benign and is treated with topical lactic acid cream or lotion. Lesions that are associated with the face typically resolve at puberty.

Frankel DH. *Field Guide to Clinical Dermatology.* Philadelphia: Lippincott Williams & Wilkins; 1999:9.

4. The answer is C. (*Scabies*) The condition of scabies is associated with intense pruritus that is noted predominantly at night. The lesions are brownish in color and often form irregular burrow lines that may be marked with scaling at one end and a vesicle at the other end. The lesions are typically found in intertriginous areas and warm, protected areas such as the finger webs, inframammary areas, and axilla. The mite *Sarcoptes scabei* is responsible. Scrapings of the lesion are treated with 10% potassium hydroxide solution and studied under light microscopy. The mite is often identified. Treatment consists of permethrin cream 5% applied from head to toes and left in place for 12 hours before being washed off. Lindane can also be used as an alternative, but not in infants or in pregnant women.

Hall JC. *Sauer's Manual of Skin Diseases*, 8th ed. Philadelphia: Lippincott Williams & Wilkins; 2000:228.

5. The answer is C. (*Rosacea*) Rosacea is a common problem encountered by family physicians. The condition is associated with areas of erythema and telangiectasia on the face. It is exacerbated by sunlight, hot or spicy foods, and alcohol. Pronounced rosacea may appear as acneiform papules, pustules, or ruddiness. Northern Europeans and those of Celtic descent are most commonly affected. Treatment involves oral tetracycline or doxycycline. Topical metronidazole is also effective for milder cases.

Hall JC. *Sauer's Manual of Skin Diseases*, 8th ed. Philadelphia: Lippincott Williams & Wilkins; 2000:123.

6. The answer is B. (*Acanthosis nigricans*) Acanthosis nigricans is associated with hyperpigmented areas that typically affect flexural folds (axilla). The two basic types of acanthosis nigricans are benign and malignant. The benign form is associated with obesity, diabetes, Stein-Leventhal syndrome, Cushing's disease, Addison's disease, pituitary disorders, and hyperandrogenic syndromes. Drugs, including glucocorticoids, nicotinic acid, diethylstilbestrol, and growth hormone therapy, have also caused acanthosis nigricans. Many cases are idiopathic. Malignant acanthosis nigricans is associated with an intestinal cancer such as gastric carcinoma.

Hall JC. *Sauer's Manual of Skin Diseases*, 8th ed. Philadelphia: Lippincott Williams & Wilkins; 2000:260.

7. The answer is E. (*Psoriasis*) Psoriasis usually manifests itself as erythematous scaly patches that affect the knees or elbows. More severe cases can involve multiple areas over the entire body. Extensor surfaces are predominantly affected. Nail pitting may be present. The condition appears to be hereditary. Diagnosis is usually based on clinical findings. Skin biopsy may be helpful for definitive diagnosis. Treatment consists of topical steroids, intralesional steroids, tar preparations, anthralin, tazarotene, and calcipotriene.

Hall JC. *Sauer's Manual of Skin Diseases*, 8th ed. Philadelphia: Lippincott Williams & Wilkins; 2000:131.

Psoriasis usually manifests itself as erythematous scaly patches that affect the knees or elbows. More severe cases can involve multiple areas over the entire body. Extensor surfaces are predominantly affected. Nail pitting may be present.

8. The answer is A. (*Basal cell carcinoma*) Basal cell carcinoma is the most common form of skin cancer. The lesions are induced by ultraviolet radiation in susceptible individuals. Risk factors include age older than 40, light complexion, positive family history, and male sex. The lesion has pearly, raised borders with telangiectasia and a central ulcer that may crust. Sun-exposed areas are most commonly affected. Diagnosis is achieved with shave or excisional biopsy. Treatment is accomplished with excision, electrodessication and curettage, liquid nitrogen application, Moh's surgery, radiation treatment, and topical 5-fluorouracil cream. Almost 50% of patients with basal cell carcinoma will have another within 5 years.

Hall JC. *Sauer's Manual of Skin Diseases*, 8th ed. Philadelphia: Lippincott Williams & Wilkins; 2000:386.

9. The answer is C. (*Diabetes mellitus*) Although the majority of cases of acanthosis nigricans are benign and associated with obesity, the disease can represent the onset of malignancy as well as a variety of conditions related to insulin resistance. Acanthosis nigricans has been reported in association with a number of malignancies, particular gastrointestinal cancers (e.g., gastric, hepatocellular) and lung cancer. The suspicion for malignancy increases in patients with extensive or rapidly progressive lesions, when there is mucous membrane involvement, or when there is prominent sole and palm disease. The common finding in all non-malignancy associated cases of acanthosis nigricans is insulin resistance. This explains the relationship between this skin disorder and diseases such as diabetes mellitus, Cushing's syndrome, and hypothyroidism (most likely due to weight gain and subsequent insulin resistance), and with obesity.

Shwayder T. Disorders of keratinization: diagnosis and management. *Am J Clin Dermatol.* 2004;5:17.

10. The answer is D. (*Adenosine*) The most important step to make when a narrow QRS tachycardia is noted is whether the patient is experiencing signs and symptoms related to the rapid heart rate. These symptoms include hypotension, shortness of breath, shock, decreased level of consciousness, or chest pain suggestive of coronary ischemia. Determining whether a patient's symptoms are related to the tachycardia depends on several factors, including age and the presence of underlying cardiac disease. Paroxysmal supraventricular tachycardia (PSVT) with a heart rate of 200 bpm may be tolerated by a healthy young adult with no or few symptoms (e.g., palpitations). However, a heart rate of 120 bpm may precipitate angina in an elderly patient with significant coronary heart disease. Adenosine is approved by the Food and Drug Administration (FDA) in the United States only for the intravenous management of PSVT in which the AV node is involved. For intravenous adenosine administration, the patient should be supine and should have electrocardiographic and blood pressure monitoring. The drug is administered by rapid intravenous injection over one to two seconds at a peripheral site, followed by a normal saline flush. The usual initial dose is 6 mg, with a maximal single dose of 12 mg. The most common side effects of adenosine are facial flushing (18%), palpitations, chest pain, and hypotension. Transient asystole is a rare complication. Another important side effect of adenosine is that it may precipitate atrial fibrillation (AF). In patients with Wolf-Parkinson-White syndrome (WPW), AF can progress into ventricular fibrillation. As a result, caution should be used when giving adenosine if WPW is a possible mechanism, and emergency resuscitation equipment should be available.

Arnsdorf MF, Ganz LI. Approach to narrow QRS complex tachycardias. Up to Date, version 14.1. Accessed 5/1/06.

11. The answer is D. (*Molluscum contagiosum*) Molluscum contagiosum is a common, superficial viral infection of the skin that typically occurs in infants and preschoolers. The incidence decreases after the age of 6 to 7 years. The condition can be spread via sexual contact in young adults. The lesions are dome-shaped, waxy, or pearly-white papules with a central white core and are 1 to 3 mm in diameter. Frequently, groups of lesions are found. The lesions may resolve spontaneously. Treatment involves removal with a sharp needle or curette, application of liquid nitrogen, antiwart preparations, electrodessication and curettage, or trichloroacetic peels for extensive areas. Typically, infants or young preschool-age children should not be treated aggressively.

Hall JC. *Sauer's Manual of Skin Diseases*, 8th ed. Philadelphia: Lippincott Williams & Wilkins; 2000:188.

12. The answer is A. (*Rhus dermatitis*) Poison ivy or poison oak is also referred to as *Rhus dermatitis*. The condition is associated with intensely pruritic linear streaks of vesicles, papules, and blisters. The plants contain a resinous oil that gives rise to an allergic response approximately 2 days after exposure. Contrary to common belief, the fluid in the blisters can neither transfer the rash to others nor cause it to spread. Treatment involves topical steroid creams, Burow's solution, calamine lotion, antihistamines, cool baths with colloidal oatmeal, and oral steroids (for 2 to 3 weeks to prevent rebound dermatitis) for more widespread cases.

Goodheart HP. *A Photoguide of Common Skin Disorders: Diagnosis and Management*. Philadelphia: Lippincott Williams & Wilkins; 1999:42–43.

13. The answer is E. (*Seborrheic keratoses*) Seborrheic keratoses are common skin lesions that affect the elderly. They tend to run in families. The average diameter is 1 cm, but they can grow to 3 cm in diameter. The lesions are brown or black, oval in shape, raised, and have a "stuck on" appearance. They most commonly occur on the face, back, neck, and scalp. They may appear suddenly and become pruritic and crusted. Numerous lesions that appear rapidly may signal the development of an underlying malignancy. Treatment is cosmetic and usually reserved for those that are inflamed or causing symptoms.

Hall JC. *Sauer's Manual of Skin Diseases*, 8th ed. Philadelphia: Lippincott Williams & Wilkins; 2000:324–325.

14. The answer is B. (*Apthous stomatitis*) Apthous stomatitis, also known as *canker sores*, are painful eruptions that affect the mucosal surface of the mouth. The cause is unknown. Lesions typically develop at the same time and resolve in 5 to 10 days. A viral cause has not been proved. A streptococcal bacteria has been implicated. The lesions recur at regular intervals and may correlate with the onset of menses in some women. Treatment consists of toothpaste swish therapy, triamcinolone acetonide (Kenalog in Orabase), or tetracycline solution swish and swallow. Severe cases may respond to systemic corticosteroids.

Hall JC. *Sauer's Manual of Skin Diseases*, 8th ed. Philadelphia: Lippincott Williams & Wilkins; 2000:289–290.

15. The answer is A. (*Black tongue*) Black hairy tongue results from hyperplasia of the filiform papillae with deposition of keratin on the surface. The condition causes the tongue to have a dark, velvety, hairlike appearance. Associated conditions include smoking, consumption of coffee, prolonged use of antibiotics, and possibly acquired immunodeficiency syndrome. Treatment involves using a toothbrush to scrape off the excess keratin that forms on the tongue's surface.

Hall JC. *Sauer's Manual of Skin Diseases*, 8th ed. Philadelphia: Lippincott Williams & Wilkins; 2000:291.

16. The answer is A. (*Alopecia areata*) Alopecia areata is associated with sudden hair loss that occurs in round patches. The patches are well circumscribed and are not associated with scarring or inflammation. Patients have no other symptoms. The most common area affected is the scalp; however, the condition may also affect the eyebrows or beard. Alopecia areata usually affects children and young adults and is recurrent. A pathognomonic sign for alopecia areata is the "exclamation point" hair, which is wide distally and narrower at the base. These hairs are often found at the periphery of a patch of hair loss. Hair that regrows in the area of alopecia areata is in many cases white. Nail pitting may also be present. The treatment consists of injection of intralesional steroids and topical steroids. Most experience complete regrowth of hair.

Hall JC. *Sauer's Manual of Skin Diseases*, 8th ed. Philadelphia: Lippincott Williams & Wilkins; 2000:273.

> Alopecia areata is associated with sudden hair loss that occurs in round patches. The patches are well circumscribed and are not associated with scarring or inflammation.

17. The answer is E. (*Surgical débridement*) When treating pressure ulcers, it is important to maintain a moist environment while keeping the surrounding skin dry. This can be accomplished by loosely packing the ulcer with saline-moistened gauze. Topical antimicrobials such as silver sulfadiazine cream may be helpful in ulcers that appear infected. Topical antiseptics such as povidone-iodine or hydrogen peroxide should be not be used in the treatment of pressure ulcers. Systemic antibiotics should be reserved for serious infections (e.g., bacteremia, osteomyelitis). A 2-week trial of topical antimicrobials may be considered for ulcers that do not appear infected but are not improving. Although most patients are successfully managed without surgery, procedures may be appropriate in patients whose quality of life would be markedly improved by rapid wound closure. Stage 3 and 4 ulcers with necrotic tissue should be débrided. Ulcers with minimal exudate that are not infected can be covered with an occlusive dressing to promote autolytic débridement. Ulcers with thick exudate, slough, or loose necrotic tissue should undergo mechanical débridement. Options include wet-to-dry dressings, hydrotherapy, wound irrigation, and scrubbing the wound with gauze. Ulcers with evidence of cellulitis or deep infection should undergo sharp débridement with a scalpel or scissors. Ulcers with a thick eschar or extensive necrotic tissue should undergo sharp débridement as well. However, a thick, dry eschar covering a heel ulcer should generally be left intact. Patients without access to surgical interventions (such as in a long-term care setting) or those who may not be acceptable surgery candidates can be treated with enzymatic débriding agents. Wound débridement should stop once necrotic tissue has been removed and granulation tissue is present.

Berlowitz D. *Prevention and treatment of pressure ulcers.* Up to Date, version 14.1. Accessed 5/3/06.

18. The answer is E. (*Tympanomastoidectomy*) Cholesteatoma is a growth of desquamated, stratified, squamous epithelium within the middle ear space. The condition occurs when keratin desquamates from the epithelial lining of the sac and gradually enlarges with eventual erosion of the ossicular chain, mastoid bowl, and external auditory canal. The development of a cholesteatoma typically occurs after a retraction pocket has formed in the posterior/superior quadrant of the ear, often as a result of chronic eustachian tube dysfunction. It may also occur after tympanic membrane (TM) trauma, such as a traumatic, inflammatory, or iatrogenic perforation. Without treatment, cholesteatomas may erode the tegman (the bony covering of the middle fossa), the sigmoid sinus, or even the inner ear. As a result untreated cholesteatomas can result in lateral sinus thrombosis, sepsis, brain abscess, sensorineural hearing loss, vertigo, disequilibrium, facial paralysis, and even death. Treatment is surgical, usually involving a tympanomastoidectomy.

Weber PC. *Etiology of hearing loss in adults.* Up to Date, version 14.1. Accessed 5/3/06.

19. The answer is B. (*Telogen effluvium*) Telogen effluvium is sudden, diffuse hair loss that occurs 3 to 6 months after a stressful event. The causes include medications (heparin, coumarin, propranolol, haloperidol, and lithium), neoplasms, infection, and crash diets. The stressful event triggers the hair follicles to go into a rest phase, and once the cycle returns a larger amount of hair is lost at one time. Typically, 30% to 50% of the scalp hair is affected. No treatment is needed. Patients should be reassured that normal hair growth should resume.

Frankel DH. *Field Guide to Clinical Dermatology.* Philadelphia: Lippincott Williams & Wilkins; 1999:187–188.

20. The answer is E. (*Keratoacanthomas*) Keratoacanthomas usually develop rapidly over a 2- to 6-week time frame. The lesions are dome-shaped with a central keratin-filled plug. They occur most commonly on sun-exposed areas. Many resolve spontaneously; however, because of their similarity to squamous cell carcinomas and their ability to metastasize, they should be removed by excision. Other treatment options include intralesional methotrexate, 5-fluorouracil, interferon, systemic retinoids, or radiation therapy. Complete excision is usually curative; however, recurrences can develop at the site of treated lesions.

Hall JC. *Sauer's Manual of Skin Diseases*, 8th ed. Philadelphia: Lippincott Williams & Wilkins; 2000:338.

21. The answer is D. (*Dermatomyositis*) Dermatomyositis presents with a heliotrope rash and the presence of Gottron's papules. The rash is violaceous in color and involves the periorbital areas. Gottron's papules are erythematous or violaceous papules or plaques that form over the bony prominences, particularly the metacarpophalangeal joints, the proximal and distal interphalangeal joints. The condition is also associated with a myopathy that involves the proximal muscles. The shoulders and pelvic girdle are mainly affected in a symmetric pattern. Symptoms include fatigue, weakness, inability to climb stairs, or weakness in rising from a squatting or sitting position. Dysphagia is also seen. Approximately 20% of patients have an associated malignancy. Laboratory tests include elevated serum creatine kinase or aldolase, or both. Electromyographic studies and a muscle biopsy can also provide additional diagnostic information. The mainstays of treatment are systemic steroids. Other options include immunosuppressant agents and hydroxychloroquine. Those who are older and have severe myositis, dysphagia, associated malignancy, and a poor response to corticosteroids have a poorer prognosis.

Hall JC. *Sauer's Manual of Skin Diseases*, 8th ed. Philadelphia: Lippincott Williams & Wilkins; 2000:253.

22. The answer is A. (*Sporotrichosis*) Sporotrichosis is a granulomatous fungal infection that affects the skin. The lesion is caused by *Sporothrix schenckii*, a fungus that grows on wood and in the soil. The lesions typically affect farmers, gardeners (especially those who grow roses), laborers, and miners. A primary chancre occurs at the site of inoculation. The primary lesion is painless and forms a subcutaneous nodule that breaks down to form an ulcer. Within a few weeks multiple nodules form along the areas of draining lymphatics and break down to form streaks of ulcers, often affecting the arms or legs. The fluid from unopened ulcers can be cultured and can aid in diagnosis. Treatment consists of saturated solution of potassium iodide, ketoconazole, or itraconazole. Systemic invasion is rare.

Hall JC. *Sauer's Manual of Skin Diseases*, 8th ed. Philadelphia: Lippincott Williams & Wilkins; 2000:405.

23. The answer is E. (*Herpes infection*) Genital herpes is primarily associated with herpes simplex virus type 2. The symptoms include painful vesicles that occur in clusters, often on the shaft of the penis or vulvar areas of females. Patients often report fever, regional lymphadenopathy, and generalized fatigue in association with an outbreak. The lesions last for 2 to 3 days before the tops of the vesicles rupture. The remaining ulcers crust over and last an additional 5 to 7 days. Recurrences are common in the same area. Asymptomatic shedding of the virus can occur once the outbreak has resolved and can infect others. Diagnosis *can* be achieved with the use of Tzanck smears (which detect large bizarre mononucleate and multinucleate giant cells and nuclear changes of ballooning degeneration). Treatment is accomplished with the use of antiviral medications (acyclovir, valacyclovir, famciclovir, and topical penciclovir). Prophylactic therapy may be indicated in recurrent infections.

Hall JC. *Sauer's Manual of Skin Diseases*, 8th ed. Philadelphia: Lippincott Williams & Wilkins; 2000:176–179.

24. The answer is E. (*Haemophilus ducreyi*) Chancroid is a sexually transmitted disease that is caused by *Haemophilus ducreyi*. It has a very short (1- to 5-day) incubation period. The primary lesion occurs on the genitalia and forms a superficial or deep erosion with surrounding erythema and edema. Marked unilateral and regional lymphadenopathy are present and eventually suppurate, causing buboes in untreated cases. The organisms are arranged like "schools of fish" and are found on smears from active lesions. Treatment consists of a sulfonamide such as sulfisoxazole or third-generation cephalosporin.

Hall JC. *Sauer's Manual of Skin Diseases*, 8th ed. Philadelphia: Lippincott Williams & Wilkins; 2000:158–159.

25. The answer is C. (*Keratoacanthoma*) Keratoacanthoma (KA) is a rapidly growing hyperkeratotic nodule with a central keratin plug. A KA typically develops over 3 to 6 weeks, in contrast to the slow growth of typical SCCs over months to years. KAs occur most commonly in areas of sun-damaged skin. KAs are clinically and histologically indistinguishable from well-differentiated SCC. The etiology of KA is not certain, however; human papillomavirus DNA has been found in some cases. KAs have also occurred in skin soon after radiation therapy. Additionally, there are syndromes of multiple KAs developing over years. There is controversy regarding whether KAs are malignant or benign. Although they resemble SCCs histologically, most spontaneously regress with scar formation. There have been reported cases of invasive KAs, some with metastases, leading many experts to consider all KAs a form of SCC and treat them as such. Because of the uncertainty malignant potential of KAs, most are treated as well-differentiated SCC.

Shaw JC. *Overview of nonmelanoma skin cancers*. Up to Date, version 14.1. Accessed 5/3/06.

Keratoacanthoma (KA) is a rapidly growing hyperkeratotic nodule with a central keratin plug. A KA typically develops over 3 to 6 weeks, in contrast to the slow growth of typical squamous cell carcinomas over months to years.

26. The answer is B. (*Type B*) A flattened tympanogram is represented by choices B and is associated with fluid of perforation of the tympanic membrane.

Weber PC. *Etiology of hearing loss in adults*. Up to Date, version 14.1. Accessed 5/3/06.

27. The answer is A. (*Pityriasis rosea*) Pityriasis rosea is a common papulosquamous rash that mainly occurs on the trunks of young adults during the spring and fall. The condition begins with the onset of a "herald patch" that is oval and erythematous. Usually within 2 to 10 days, a generalized rash follows. The individual lesions have fine scaling noted around their edges. In many cases a Christmas-tree pattern is seen over the back. The lesions may continue to appear for 2 to 3 weeks. Most cases resolve by 6 to 8 weeks. Pruritus is often present. The disease is not contagious. Treatment consists of oatmeal colloidal baths, calamine lotion, antihistamines, topical steroids, and ultraviolet-B treatments. Systemic steroids may be necessary for severe cases.

Hall JC. *Sauer's Manual of Skin Diseases*, 8th ed. Philadelphia: Lippincott Williams & Wilkins; 2000:134–138.

28. The answer is D. (*Impetigo*) Impetigo is caused by group A β-hemolytic streptococci or *Staphylococcus aureus* and typically affects young children. The lesions begin as erythematous papules that expand to form crusted patches with a honey-brown appearance. More severe cases may cause bullae to form. The infection occurs more commonly around the nose and mouth and in the intertriginous areas; there are no constitutional symptoms. Examination is usually made on clinical presentation. Treatment for mild infections includes 2% topical mupirocin ointment. More severe cases respond to dicloxacillin, cephalexin, or erythromycin. Impetigo is highly contagious. Glomerulonephritis is a rare complication of impetigo that is caused by certain strains of *Streptococcus*.

Hall JC. *Sauer's Manual of Skin Diseases*, 8th ed. Philadelphia: Lippincott Williams & Wilkins; 2000:15.

29. The answer is C. (*Lichen sclerosis*) Lichen sclerosis is caused by thinning of the vulvar skin and gives rise to itching and dyspareunia. Atrophy of the skin occurs and gives rise to a shiny whitish appearance. Diagnosis is accomplished with punch biopsy. A slight increase in squamous cell carcinoma has been found in areas that are affected with lichen sclerosis. Treatment consists of potent topical corticosteroids. In addition, a topical antifungal preparation should be used to prevent secondary yeast infections.

Hall JC. *Sauer's Manual of Skin Diseases*, 8th ed. Philadelphia: Lippincott Williams & Wilkins; 2000:380.

30. The answer is A. (*Psoriasis*) Pitting of the nails is associated commonly with psoriasis. Erythematous scaly plaques are usually noted on other parts of the body. Thirty percent of patients with psoriasis have a positive family history for the condition. Males and females are affected equally. Other conditions that are related to nail pitting include alopecia areata and eczematous dermatitis. Chronic obstructive pulmonary disease is related to clubbing. Subungual hyperkeratosis is associated with onychomycosis.

Hall JC. *Sauer's Manual of Skin Diseases*, 8th ed. Philadelphia: Lippincott Williams & Wilkins; 2000:283.

31. The answer is A. (*Yeast vaginitis*) Yeast vaginitis causes approximately one-third of all vaginal infections. Risk factors include pregnancy, diabetes, use of intrauterine devices, recent antibiotic use, immune deficiency, or corticosteroid use. Diagnosis is made by examination of a vaginal smear under high-power microscopy after potassium hydroxide has been added. Budding yeast and pseudohyphae are noted. Topical antifungals are effective, as are single-dose oral antifungals.

Goodheart HP. *A Photoguide of Common Skin Disorders: Diagnosis and Management*. Philadelphia: Lippincott Williams & Wilkins; 1999:377.

32. The answer is C. (*Herpes genitalis*) Tzanck smears are used in the diagnosis of herpes infections. The preparation detects multinucleated giant cells. A sample obtained from unroofed vesicles that have appeared within 24 hours provides the best specimen for diagnosis. A #15 blade is used to scrape the base of the vesicle, and the material is spread onto a slide and allowed to dry. Giemsa's, Wright's, or methylene blue is used to stain the cells. After staining, the sample is gently flooded with tap water to remove excess stain. Oil immersion is used for viewing with the microscope.

Goodheart HP. *A Photoguide of Common Skin Disorders: Diagnosis and Management*. Philadelphia: Lippincott Williams & Wilkins; 1999:379.

33. The answer is E. (*Tinea versicolor*) Tinea versicolor is a common skin infection caused by the organism *Pityrosporum orbiculare* (also known as *Malessezia furfur, Pityrosporum ovale*, or *Malassezia ovalis*). The condition usually affects adolescents and young adults in tropical environments. The organism is a yeast that is a constituent of the normal skin flora. A number of factors may trigger conversion to the mycelial or hyphal form that is associated with clinical disease, including hot and humid weather, use of topical oils, hyperhidrosis, and immunosuppression. Tinea versicolor usually responds to medical therapy, but recurrence is common and long-term preventative treatment may be necessary. Versicolor refers to the variety and changing shades of colors present in this condition. Lesions can be hypopigmented, light brown, or salmon-colored macules. A fine scale is often noted, especially after scraping. Individual lesions are typically small, but frequently coalesce to form larger lesions. Typically the lesions are limited to the outer skin, most commonly on the upper trunk and extremities, and are less common on the face and intertriginous areas. Most patients are asymptomatic; however, some may complain of mild pruritus. The condition may occur in patients who are immunocompromised. It is most evident in the summer because the organism produces a substance which inhibits pigment transfer to keratinocytes, thus making infected skin more demarcated from uninfected, evenly pigmented skin. The diagnosis of tinea versicolor is made by microscopic examination of skin samples with 10% potassium hydroxide (KOH). Both hyphae and spores are evident in a pattern that is often described as "spaghetti and meatballs." The differential diagnosis includes seborrhea, eczema, pityriasis rosea, and secondary syphilis. Seborrheic lesions are more frequently located on the central trunk, are more erythematous, and have thicker scales. With eczema, patients usually have more scaling, pruritus, and involvement of the extremities. Patients with pityriasis usually have a herald patch, more peripheral scale around border lesions, confinement of lesions to the central trunk, and the lesions do not show hyphae on KOH prep. Secondary syphilis usually involves the hands and feet, and the lesions do not show hyphae on KOH prep. Topical antifungal therapy given for 2 weeks is the treatment of choice for patients with mild and limited disease. Virtually any topical anti-yeast preparation can be used with cure rates exceeding 70% to 80%. Patients should be informed that the healing process continues after the treatment is complete. A return to normal pigmentation may take months after the completion of successful treatment. Oral medications are more convenient for patients with extensive disease and also may be more effective in patients with recalcitrant infection. Most oral antifungal agents, with the exception of griseofulvin or terbinafine, may be used. Additionally, ketoconazole 2% shampoo in a single application or daily for 3 days may be considered as an option for treatment, especially with mild infections.

Goldstein BG, Goldstein AO. *Tinea versicolor.* Up to Date, version 14.1. Accessed 5/3/06.

34. The answer is B. (*Basal cell carcinoma*) The clinical presentation of basal cell carcinoma (BCC) can be divided into the following three groups:

1. Nodular: The most common form of BCC. It typically presents on the face as a pink or flesh-colored papule. The lesion usually has a pearly or translucent quality and a telangiectatic vessel is frequently seen within the papule. Ulceration is frequent, and the term *rodent ulcer* refers to these ulcerated nodular BCCs.
2. Superficial: The second most common subtype. Superficial BCC is most likely to occur on the trunk of the affected patient. The lesion typically presents as a slightly scaly papule or plaque that is most often pale red in color; the lesion may be atrophic in the center and usually is surrounded with fine translucent micropapules. Men are more likely to be affected.
3. Morpheaform: Also known as sclerosing BCC, this is the least common subtype. These lesions are typically smooth, flesh-colored, or very lightly erythematous papules or plaques that are frequently atrophic; they usually have a firm or indurated quality with ill-defined borders. Some experts categorize morpheaform, infiltrative, and micronodular as "aggressive-growth" BCC, because they behave similarly. Infiltrative and micronodular BCCs are less common than the morpheaform BCC.

Wrone DA, Stern RS. *Epidemiology and clinical features of basal cell carcinoma.* Up to Date, version 14.1. Accessed 5/3/06.

35. The answer is B. (*Graves' disease*) Exophthalmos can be related to hyperthyroidism (i.e., Graves' disease). Patients with hyperthyroidism may report nervousness, tremor, weight loss, hair loss, palpitations, tachycardia, and muscle weakness. Pretibial myxedema is also seen in those with Graves' disease. The eye findings are related to edema and lymphoid infiltration of the orbital tissue. Unfortunately, exophthalmos usually does not resolve after treatment.

Goodheart HP. *A Photoguide of Common Skin Disorders: Diagnosis and Management.* Philadelphia: Lippincott Williams & Wilkins; 1999:344.

36. The answer is B. (*Erythema nodosum*) Erythema nodosum is an acute inflammatory reaction of the subcutaneous fat. Women between the ages of 20 and 30 years are most likely to be affected. Causes include use of oral contraceptives or sulfonamides, pregnancy, sarcoidosis, histoplasmosis, tuberculosis, inflammatory bowel disease, lymphoma, leukemia, Behçet's disease, and streptococcal infections. Up to 40% of cases may be idiopathic. Typically, the lesions begin as bright red, tender nodules. The lesions tend to occur bilaterally on the lower extremities and occasionally on the arms. Constitutional symptoms (fever, arthralgias, and malaise) may also be present. The lesions become dark brown or violaceous during the resolution phase. Spontaneous resolution occurs in 3 to 6 weeks after onset regardless of the cause. Treatment consists of symptomatic treatment, nonsteroidal anti-inflammatory drugs, and systemic corticosteroids once an infectious cause is ruled out.

Erythema nodosum is an acute inflammatory reaction of the subcutaneous fat. Women between the ages of 20 and 30 years are most likely to be affected. Causes include use of oral contraceptives or sulfonamides, pregnancy, sarcoidosis, histoplasmosis, tuberculosis, inflammatory bowel disease, lymphoma, leukemia, Behçet's disease, and streptococcal infections. Up to 40% of cases may be idiopathic.

Hall JC. *Sauer's Manual of Skin Diseases*, 8th ed. Philadelphia: Lippincott Williams & Wilkins; 2000:109.

37. The answer is D. (*Neurofibromatosis*) Neurofibromatosis is also referred to as *von Recklinghausen's disease.* It is associated with autosomal-dominant inheritance and is characterized by multiple, macular, pigmented skin lesions called *café au lait spots* and skin tumors called *neurofibromas.* Axillary or inguinal freckling (Crowe's sign) is considered to be pathognomonic for neurofibromatosis. Ocular lesions (Lisch nodules) are asymptomatic, pigmented iris hamartomas that are seen in 80% of cases. The disease has been associated with defects on chromosomes 17 and 22. Neurofibromas may cause neurologic symptoms. Seizures, paraplegia, and mental retardation may occur secondary to the condition. Treatment consists of surgical removal of symptomatic or disfiguring lesions. Patients should be monitored for the development of neurofibrosarcomas, optic gliomas, acoustic neuromas, and pheochromocytomas. Those who are affected should also receive genetic counseling.

Goodheart HP. *A Photoguide of Common Skin Disorders: Diagnosis and Management.* Philadelphia: Lippincott Williams & Wilkins; 1999:338–339.

38. The answer is C. (*Atopic dermatitis*) Atopic dermatitis is also referred to as *atopic eczema*. The condition is associated with erythematous pruritic areas that occur in association with hay fever, asthma, allergic rhinitis, or allergic sinusitis. The flexor surfaces are commonly involved. The course is variable with flares and remissions. The condition affects children and adults. The diagnosis is made based on history and clinical presentation. Treatment consists of topical steroids, antihistamines, tar baths and ointments, and Burrow's solution. Severe cases may require systemic steroids, cyclosporine, or phototherapy.

Hall JC. *Sauer's Manual of Skin Diseases*, 8th ed. Philadelphia: Lippincott Williams & Wilkins; 2000:78.

39. The answer is D. (*Malignant melanoma*) Malignant melanoma lesions are treated with surgical excision. Biopsies must include epidermis, dermis, and subcutaneous fat. Shave biopsy should not be done. Knowledge of depth of invasion is essential for proper staging and treatment. Melanoma *in situ* (epidermal only) should be removed with margins of 0.5 cm. Melanoma that is <1.5 mm deep should be removed with a margin of 1 cm. Lesions that are 1.51 to 4 mm deep should have 1- to 2-cm margins. Lesions deeper than 4 mm should have a margin of 2 to 3 cm. Lymph node dissection is indicated if metastasis is suspected or if the lesion is of intermediate depth. Sentinel node biopsy is increasingly used in patients with proven melanoma that is >1 mm deep.

Hall JC. *Sauer's Manual of Skin Diseases*, 8th ed. Philadelphia: Lippincott Williams & Wilkins; 2000:346.

40. The answer is A. (*Trichophyton rubrum*) Onychomycosis is usually caused by *Trichophyton rubrum*. Diagnosis is generally made by clinical presentation; however, fungal elements can be confirmed with observation under a microscope using potassium hydroxide 10% preparation of nail plate scales. Nail clippings can also be used for culture.

Hall JC. *Sauer's Manual of Skin Diseases*, 8th ed. Philadelphia: Lippincott Williams & Wilkins; 2000:282.

41. The answer is B. (*Psoriasis*) Psoriasis typically involves the scalp (including the postauricular regions), the extensor surface of the extremities (particularly elbows and knees), the sacral area, buttocks, and penis. The nails, eyebrows, axillae, umbilicus, or anogenital region may also be affected. Occasionally the disease is generalized. Typical lesions are well demarcated, variously pruritic, ovoid or circular, erythematous papules or plaques covered with overlapping thick silver appearing, slightly opalescent shiny scales. Papules sometimes extend and coalesce to produce large plaques in annular patterns. The lesions heal without scarring, and hair growth is usually unaltered. Nail involvement occurs in 30% to 50% of patients and may clinically resemble a fungal infection, with stippling, pitting, fraying, discoloration or separation of the distal and lateral margins of the nail plate (onycholysis), and thickening, with hyperkeratotic material under the nail plate.

Beers MH, et al. *The Merck manual of diagnosis and therapy*, 18th ed. Whitehouse Station, NJ: Merck Research Laboratories; 2006:965–969.

42. The answer is D. (*Neurofibromatosis*) Café au lait skin lesions are seen in neurofibromatosis. The lesions are medium-brown freckle-like macules distributed most commonly over the trunk, pelvis, and flexor creases of elbows and knees; they are present at birth or develop in infancy in >90% of all patients.

Beers MH, et al. *The Merck manual of diagnosis and therapy*, 18th ed. Whitehouse Station, NJ: Merck Research Laboratories; 2006:2378.

43. The answer is B. (*Arterial ulcer*) Arterial ulcers are usually caused by atherosclerosis in the elderly. Men are more commonly affected. Pain is common, as is claudication. Distinguishing features of arterial ulcers are their sharply defined borders and round, punched-out appearance. They tend to be smaller than venous ulcers and are usually deep enough to expose muscle or tendons. Commonly affected sites include the toes, pretibial areas, and dorsum of the feet. Patients may have signs of livedo reticularis, pallor, and cyanosis. The legs may feel cold and clammy. Decreased peripheral pulses are commonly noted. Treatment consists of alleviating underlying risk factors. Pentoxifylline can be used in some cases. Surgical evaluation should be considered.

Frankel DH. *Field Guide to Clinical Dermatology.* Philadelphia: Lippincott Williams & Wilkins; 1999:173–174.

44. The answer is B. (*Cylindromas*) Cylindromas appear as numerous smooth, rounded tumors that occur in various sizes on the scalp. They have the appearance of a group of grapes. Rarely, the tumors cover the entire scalp and are referred to as *turban tumors*. Cylindromas are considered benign and can be observed.

Hall JC. *Sauer's Manual of Skin Diseases*, 8th ed. Philadelphia: Lippincott Williams & Wilkins; 2000:352.

45. The answer is E. (*Synovial cyst*) A synovial cyst appears as a translucent, pea-sized cyst that commonly forms adjacent to the joints of the fingers. The cysts form as a result of small tracts that lead from the synovial space of joints to the surface of the skin. The fluid contained is synovial fluid. Occasionally, the cysts spontaneously resolve. Aspiration can be attempted, but care must be taken not to introduce infection into the joint. Compression of the area after aspiration may help to prevent recurrence.

Hall JC. *Sauer's Manual of Skin Diseases*, 8th ed. Philadelphia: Lippincott Williams & Wilkins; 2000:329.

46. The answer is C. (*Human immunodeficiency syndrome*) Oral hairy leukoplakia is a marker for human immunodeficiency syndrome and is thought to be caused by the Epstein-Barr virus. The condition appears as white plaques that have the look of corrugated cardboard. The lesions are fixed and not friable and appear on the lateral surface of the tongue. Although the condition rarely causes symptoms, burning of the tongue can occur. Treatment consists of acyclovir, topical tretinoin, and podophyllin. Oral hairy leukoplakia can be distinguished from oral candidiasis by the fact that the latter scrapes off easily with a tongue blade. Oral candidiasis typically affects the dorsal aspect of the tongue and buccal mucosa.

Hall JC. *Sauer's Manual of Skin Diseases*, 8th ed. Philadelphia: Lippincott Williams & Wilkins; 2000:195.

47. The answer is D. (*Varicella*) Varicella (chickenpox) is described as "dew drops on rose petals" in its appearance. The lesions are red macules that progress rapidly from papules to vesicles, pustules, and then crusted lesions. The lesions are intensely pruritic. Lesions affect the entire body and oral mucosa, especially the palate. A characteristic feature is multiple lesions in varying stages of development and healing. A Tzanck smear can be helpful in confirming the diagnosis. Treatment is usually supportive but can include the use of acyclovir. Aspirin should be avoided because of the risk of developing Reye's syndrome. Varicella vaccine is recommended for all children at 12 to 18 months of age.

Goodheart HP. *A Photoguide of Common Skin Disorders: Diagnosis and Management*. Philadelphia: Lippincott Williams & Wilkins; 1999:106–109.

> Varicella (chickenpox) is described as "dew drops on rose petals" in its appearance. The lesions are red macules that progress rapidly from papules to vesicles, pustules, and then crusted lesions.

48. The answer is D. (*Cherry angiomas*) Cherry angiomas are common asymptomatic lesions that appear red in color and blanch with pressure. The diagnosis is clinical. They are more common in elderly patients. They occur more commonly on the trunk and are benign.

Frankel DH. *Field Guide to Clinical Dermatology*. Philadelphia: Lippincott Williams & Wilkins; 1999:120–121.

49. The answer is A. (*Varicella*) The manifestations of varicella in most children generally develop within 15 days after the exposure and typically include a prodrome of fever, malaise, or pharyngitis, followed by the development of a generalized vesicular rash, usually within 24 hours. The lesions are commonly pruritic and appear as groups of vesicles over a 3 to 4 day period. The patient with varicella typically has lesions in different stages of development on the face, trunk, and extremities. New lesion formation generally stops within 4 days, and most lesions have fully crusted by day 6 in normal hosts.

Straus SE, Ostrove JM, Inchauspe G, et al. NIH conference. Varicella-zoster virus infections. Biology, natural history, treatment, and prevention. *Ann Intern Med*. 1988;108:221.

50. The answer is A. (*Lupus pernio*) Lupus pernio is associated with chronic sarcoidosis and consists of indurated plaques associated with discoloration of the nose, cheeks, lips, and ears. The lesion is more common in African American women. The nasal mucosa is frequently involved. Lupus pernio is often associated with bone cysts and pulmonary fibrosis. The course of the disease with lupus pernio is prolonged; spontaneous remissions are rare.

Joint statement of the American Thoracic Society (ATS), the European Respiratory Society (ERS) and the World Association of Sarcoidosis and Other Granulomatous Disorders (WASOG): *ATS guidelines: Statement on sarcoidosis*. Up to Date, version 14.1, http://uptodateonline.com. Accessed 5/08/06.

51. The answer is A. (*Hidradenitis suppurativa*) Hidradenitis suppurativa is a painful, erythematous, and nodular condition that affects the axilla, genitalia, and perianal areas. Hallmarks for the disease include open comedones, enlarged follicular orifices, and scarring. Nodules become inflamed and pus filled, rupture, drain pus and blood, and then cause scarring. Sinus tracts can form. The disease often waxes and wanes. *Staphylococcus* bacteria is frequently the causative agent. Treatment consists of appropriate antibacterial agents based on culture and sensitivities. Intralesional corticosteroids can also be used to reduce the inflammatory response. For severe cases, excision and skin grafting may be necessary. The condition may regress as the patient approaches middle age.

Frankel DH. *Field Guide to Clinical Dermatology*. Philadelphia: Lippincott Williams & Wilkins; 1999:135–136.

52. The answer is D. (*Vitiligo*) Vitiligo is a disorder associated with depigmentation of the skin that is thought to be related to an autoimmune-mediated loss of melanocytes. Fifty percent of those who are affected have a family history of vitiligo. The lesions appear as hypopigmented chalk-white lesions and are more obvious on people who have dark complexions. The condition is bilateral and symmetric in appearance and typically forms around orifices (i.e., mouth, eyes, nose, and anus). Vitiligo is often cyclical. Some may experience partial repigmentation. Diagnosis is made clinically. A Wood's light examination reveals a "milk white" fluorescence over the lesion. Treatment is limited, but includes potent topical steroids, psoralen plus ultraviolet A photochemotherapy, minigrafting, and cosmetics to hide areas.

Hall JC. *Sauer's Manual of Skin Diseases*, 8th ed. Philadelphia: Lippincott Williams & Wilkins; 2000:242.

53. The answer is B. (*Melasma*) Melasma, also referred to as *chloasma*, is described as the "mask of pregnancy." The condition typically affects women with dark complexions and appears as hyperpigmentation of the skin, usually associated with the face. It is caused by long-term sun exposure, pregnancy, and oral contraceptives. In many cases the condition is idiopathic. Diagnosis is made clinically. Treatment involves the use of bleaching creams, hydroquinone, and chemical peels for more resistant cases. In some instances the condition disappears after pregnancy or the discontinuation of oral contraceptives.

Hall JC. *Sauer's Manual of Skin Diseases*, 8th ed. Philadelphia: Lippincott Williams & Wilkins; 2000:242.

54. The answer is D. (*Rubeola*) Rubeola, or measles, is caused by a ribonucleic acid virus that invades the respiratory epithelium of the oropharynx. Transmission occurs via a respiratory aerosol route. The condition begins with a respiratory illness prodrome (cough, coryza, and conjunctivitis—the "3 Cs") followed by discrete erythematous macules and papules that coalesce. Pruritus is usually absent. The rash lasts for up to a week and resolves with desquamation. Koplik's spots are described as 1-mm bluish-white macules that form on the oral mucosa (especially the buccal mucosa opposite the molars) 2 days before the onset of the generalized rash. The rash typically begins on the forehead or behind the ears and then spreads centrally to involve the face, trunk, arms, and legs. Pneumonia is the most common complication. No specific therapy is indicated for measles. Most cases resolve within 2 weeks. Vitamin A may decrease morbidity and mortality in severe cases. Immunization is recommended for all children who are 15 months or older.

Goodheart HP. *A Photoguide of Common Skin Disorders: Diagnosis and Management*. Philadelphia: Lippincott Williams & Wilkins; 1999:120–122.

55. The answer is B. (*Coxsackievirus*) Hand-foot-and-mouth disease is caused by coxsackievirus A16. Outbreaks commonly affect children 1 to 5 years of age during the summer or early fall. Transmission occurs via a fecal-oral route. The rash appears as shallow erosions that affect the oral mucosa. The lesions are painful and can interfere with eating. The oral lesions are followed by an exanthem that consists of oval or angulated fluid-filled vesicles that form on the palms and soles. In contrast to most viral illnesses, lymphadenopathy is minimal or absent. The diagnosis is made clinically. Cultures to confirm the infection can be obtained from the throat or stool. Treatment is supportive.

Goodheart HP. *A Photoguide of Common Skin Disorders: Diagnosis and Management*. Philadelphia: Lippincott Williams & Wilkins; 1999:110–111.

56. The answer is D. (*Inferior ischemia*) The inferior surface of the heart is usually supplied by the right coronary artery (right dominant coronary circulation). Occasionally, the inferior aspect is supplied by the circumflex artery, which branches to form the posterior descending artery (left dominant coronary circulation). Arterial occlusion related to the right coronary artery gives rise to inferior ischemic changes noted on ECG. These findings include ST-segment depression in leads II, III, and aVF.

Topol EJ, ed. *Textbook of cardiovascular medicine*. Philadelphia: Lippincott Williams & Wilkins; 1998:1569.

Arterial occlusion related to the right coronary artery gives rise to inferior ischemic changes noted on ECG. These findings include ST-segment depression in leads II, III, and aVF.

57. The answer is D. (*Ventricular tachycardia*) Ventricular tachycardia (VT) is defined as three or more successive ventricular complexes. Non-sustained VT is a series of repetitive ventricular beats which have a duration of <30 seconds, whereas sustained VT lasts >30 seconds. Typically, the rate of VT is >100 beats per minute, but may vary significantly. The rhythm is usually regular, although there may be slight irregularity of the RR intervals. The morphology of the QRS complex during VT is usually different when compared to the sinus beat. The QRS axis is typically shifted, often to the left but occasionally to the right. The width of the QRS complex is generally >0.16 sec. The VT is monomorphic when all of the QRS complexes of an episode are identical. When the QRS complexes show markedly different morphologies, the VT is said to be polymorphic and the RR intervals may be grossly irregular.

Podrid PJ. *ECG tutorial: Ventricular arrhythmias*. Up to Date, version 14.1. Accessed 5/11/06.

58. The answer is A. (*Poison ivy*) Intense pruritus and erythema are the most common presenting signs of poison ivy dermatitis. Patients develop papules, vesicles, and/or bullae, often arranged in characteristic linear or streak-like patterns where the plant has made contact with the skin. Symptoms of poison ivy in sensitized individuals generally develop within 4 to 96 hours after exposure and peak between 1 and 14 days after exposure. New lesions can present up to 21 days after exposure in previously unexposed individuals. Lesions may occur at different points in time depending on the degree of exposure to different points on the skin and the thickness of the exposed skin. This may give the impression that the poison ivy is spreading from one region to another. Blister fluid is not antigenic and is not responsible for spreading the rash. Patients may, occasionally, carry the dried antigenic resin on clothing or under fingernails, thus spreading their own dermatitis or exposing household or other contacts. Without treatment, poison ivy dermatitis usually resolves in 1 to 3 weeks. The most common complication of poison ivy dermatitis is secondary bacterial infection of the skin with *Staphylococcus aureus* or β-hemolytic group A *Streptococcus*. Bacterial infections can be polymicrobial.

McGovern TW. Dermatoses due to plants. In: Bolognia JL, Jorizzo JL, Rapini RP, et al., eds. *Dermatology*. New York: Mosby; 2003:274.

59. The answer is E. (*Ventricular tachycardia*) Ventricular tachycardia is a potentially life-threatening event. ECG changes show wide QRS complexes with no discernible P waves. The rate is >120 bpm. The patient may report palpitations, dizziness, or syncope, or circulatory collapse may occur. Asymptomatic (isolated) ventricular tachycardia is usually not treated. Sustained ventricular tachycardia can degenerate to ventricular fibrillation. Hypotensive ventricular tachycardia requires immediate treatment with synchronized direct current (DC) shock. Lidocaine is used for drug treatment. Antiarrhythmics may be needed to prevent recurrent ventricular tachycardia.

Topol EJ, ed. *Textbook of cardiovascular medicine*. Philadelphia: Lippincott Williams & Wilkins; 1998:1767.

60. The answer is B. (*Atrial fibrillation*) Atrial fibrillation is frequently seen in the offices of family physicians. ECG findings include the absence of obvious P waves and the irregularly irregular response of QRS complexes. Intra-atrial contractions may show rates of >350 bpm. The ventricular rate may vary depending on the atrioventricular nodal conduction but typically is elevated. Treatment involves the management of underlying causative disorders, control of ventricular rate, restoration of sinus rhythm if possible, and prevention of systemic emboli.

Topol EJ, ed. *Textbook of cardiovascular medicine*. Philadelphia: Lippincott Williams & Wilkins; 1998:1678.

61. The answer is B. (*Supraventricular tachycardia*) Supraventricular tachycardia is often referred to as *narrow complex tachycardia*. The condition is characterized by sustained tachyarrhythmia with a QRS complex that appears normal and has a duration >120 msec. Patients whose condition is unstable should receive immediate synchronized cardioversion. Those who are hemodynamically stable can be treated with vagal maneuvers (Valsalva, cough, carotid massage), adenosine, verapamil, or diltiazem. One should make sure that the patient does not have ventricular tachycardia, because calcium channel blockers are contraindicated.

Topol EJ, ed. *Textbook of cardiovascular medicine*. Philadelphia: Lippincott Williams & Wilkins; 1998:1735.

62. The answer is B. (*Ventricular tachycardia*) Ventricular tachycardia is a potentially life-threatening event. ECG changes show wide QRS complexes with no discernible P waves. Hypotensive ventricular tachycardia requires immediate treatment with synchronized DC shock. Lidocaine is used for drug treatment. Antiarrhythmics may be needed to prevent recurrent ventricular tachycardia.

Topol EJ, ed. *Textbook of cardiovascular medicine*. Philadelphia: Lippincott Williams & Wilkins; 1998:1773.

63. The answer is B. (*WPW syndrome*) WPW syndrome is caused by an accessory pathway that links the atria and ventricles, bypassing the atrioventricular node. The ECG shows a short PR interval and slurred upstroke at the beginning of the QRS complex known as a *delta wave* (best seen in V_2, V_3, and V_4). Antegrade and retrograde conduction both occur, causing a reciprocating tachycardia. Atrial fibrillation in the setting of WPW can be a medical emergency. Ventricular rates can be excessive and lead to ventricular fibrillation. DC cardioversion should be considered when atrial fibrillation is present in the setting of WPW.

Topol EJ, ed. *Textbook of cardiovascular medicine*. Philadelphia: Lippincott Williams & Wilkins; 1998:1738.

64. The answer is B. (*Fluid in the middle ear*) Tympanograms can help assist in the diagnosis of middle ear–related problems. A flat tympanometric pattern is typical of fluid within the middle ear. The ear volume is normal, but the mobility is greatly reduced.

Spencer JP. *The Academy Collection: Quick Reference Guide for Family Physicians, Children's Health*. Philadelphia: Lippincott Williams & Wilkins; 2000:88–89.

65. The answer is C. (*Atrial fibrillation*) Atrial fibrillation (AF) is characterized by rapid and irregular atrial fibrillatory waves at a rate of 350 to 600 impulses/minute. This is accompanied by the presence of normal atrioventricular (AV) nodal conduction, with an irregularly irregular ventricular response of 90 up to 140 to 170 bpm; however, the rate may be higher in some patients. AF in patients with intact AV nodal conduction is associated with the following characteristics on ECG tracings: P waves are absent; fibrillatory or f waves are present at a rate that is generally between 350 and 600 bpm; the f waves typically vary in amplitude, morphology, and intervals; the R-R intervals are irregularly irregular; the ventricular rate usually ranges from 90 to 170 bpm. Ventricular rates <60 bpm are seen with atrioventricular (AV) nodal disease, drugs that affect conduction, and high vagal tone as can occur in a well-conditioned athlete. Ventricular rates >200 bpm suggest catecholamine excess, parasympathetic withdrawal, or the existence of an accessory bypass tract as occurs in the preexcitation syndrome. The QRS complexes are narrow unless AV conduction is abnormal due to functional (rate-related) aberration, preexisting bundle branch or fascicular block, or preexcitation with ventricular activation via an accessory pathway.

Arnsdorf MF. *Electrocardiographic and electrophysiologic features of atrial fibrillation*. Up to Date, version 14.1. Accessed 5/11/06.

Atrial fibrillation in patients with intact AV nodal conduction is associated with the following characteristics on ECG tracings: P waves are absent; fibrillatory or f waves are present at a rate that is generally between 350 and 600 bpm; the f waves typically vary in amplitude, morphology, and intervals; the R-R intervals are irregularly irregular; the ventricular rate usually ranges from 90 to 170 bpm.

66. The answer is E. (*Wolff-Parkinson-White syndrome*) The two major features of Wolff-Parkinson-White Syndrome (WPW) include a short PR interval (<0.12 second) and a delta wave. The QRS is wide (>0.12 second) and is considered a fusion beat. The initial part of the delta wave results from rapid depolarization of the accessory pathway. Termination of ventricular depolarization is through the normal activation pathway and gives rise to a normal appearing terminal portion of the QRS complex.

Arnsdorf MF, Podrid PJ, Burke MC. *Electrocardiographic features of the Wolff-Parkinson-White Syndrome*. Up to Date, version 14.1 http://uptodateonline.com accessed 5/11/06.

67. The answer is E. (*Reasurrance*) A normal tympanogram curve is peaked, indicating normal mobility of the tympanic membrane. The peak compliance occurs at a pressure of −10 mm H_2O (normal = +100 mm H_2O to −150 mm H_2O).

Spencer JP. *The Academy Collection: Quick Reference Guide for Family Physicians, Children's Health*. Philadelphia: Lippincott Williams & Wilkins; 2000:88–89.

68. The answer is A. (*Eustachian tube dysfunction*) Eustachian tube dysfunction gives rise to a tympanogram that has a normal compliance curve, but the curve is shifted to the left, indicating a negative pressure in the middle ear. The peak occurs at –200 mm H_2O.

Spencer JP. *The Academy Collection: Quick Reference Guide for Family Physicians, Children's Health*. Philadelphia: Lippincott Williams & Wilkins; 2000:88–89.

69. The answer is C. (*Erythrasma*) Erythrasma looks very much like tinea cruris. It can affect the groin, axilla, and webs of the toes. The condition is caused by *Corynebacterium minutissimum*. The area affected fluoresces a bright reddish orange under a Wood's light. The treatment is oral or topical erythromycin.

Hall JC. *Sauer's Manual of Skin Diseases*, 8th ed. Philadelphia: Lippincott Williams & Wilkins; 2000:153–154.

70. The answer is B. (*Cutaneous larva migrans*) Cutaneous larva migrans is also called the *creeping eruption*. The causative agent is a hookworm (*Ancylostoma duodenale* and *Necator americanus*). The organisms are found in the feces of dogs, cats, cattle, and monkeys. The larvae penetrate human skin (usually the feet after walking barefoot). The condition is more common in gardeners, sea bathers, plumbers, and farmers. The lesion presents as a thin erythematous, serpiginous, raised tunnel-like lesion. The larva die in 4 to 6 weeks; thus, the eruption is typically benign and self-limited. Treatment consists of topical steroids, topical or oral thiabendazole, albendazole, or liquid nitrogen.

Beers MH, Porter RS, eds. *The Merck manual of diagnosis and therapy*, Merck Research Laboratories, 18th ed. Whitehouse Station, NJ: Merck & Co.; 2006:993–994.

Chapter 8

Clinical Problem Set 1

Note: Just prior to the publication of this study guide, the ABFM eliminated Clinical Problem Set Questions from the examinations. Despite their removal, these additional questions can be used to further your knowledge.

QUESTIONS

The following questions are designed to assess clinical problem-solving skills. For each option, select either "T" for true or "F" for false. All options are related to the specific clinical case provided. There is no penalty for guessing; however, if "T" and "F" are both marked, the response will be scored as incorrect.

PATIENT A

Options 1–15

A 65-year-old man presents with complaints of erectile dysfunction. His symptoms began approximately 4 months ago. He reports no new medications and has had no change in his medical condition. His past medical history is significant for coronary artery disease and stable angina and some benign prostatic hypertrophy. He also has a prolonged QT interval on ECG. His medications include metoprolol, nitroglycerin, atorvastatin, aspirin, lisinopril, and saw palmetto.

Appropriate laboratories at this time include

1. complete blood count (CBC)
2. electrolyte panel
3. urinalysis
4. testosterone level
5. prolactin
6. thyroid function tests
7. prostate specific antigen

After you obtain the laboratory results, you note no abnormalities. Which of the following would be appropriate treatment in this gentleman?

8. testosterone patch
9. sildenafil (Viagra)
10. tadalafil (Cialis)
11. vardenafil (Levitra)
12. vacuum erection device
13. prostaglandin injections
14. yohimbine
15. trazadone

PATIENT B

Options 16–25

A 44-year-old African American male physician is noted to be hypertensive, with blood pressure readings in the range of 160/94 mm Hg on three separate occasions. The patient drinks two cups of coffee a day, has an occasional alcoholic drink, and is 30 lb overweight. He does not have a regular exercise program, his family history is negative, and the physical examination is unremarkable.

The minimum baseline testing in the initial evaluation of this patient includes

16. urinalysis
17. 24-hour urine metanephrines
18. serum creatinine
19. electrocardiogram
20. fasting serum glucose
21. intravenous pyelogram

Appropriate management of this patient's condition includes

22. abstinence from alcohol consumption
23. initiation of an exercise program
24. high-dose zinc therapy
25. avoidance of all caffeine-containing products

PATIENT C

Options 26–33

A 52-year-old professional golfer has noted an irregular-shaped lesion on his left shoulder. He presents to your office for evaluation.

Indications for biopsy include

26. recent increase in size
27. purulent drainage from the lesion
28. variegation in color
29. irregular borders

Pathology results confirm a superficial melanoma (0.6 mm in depth). Initial treatment involves

30. excision with 1-cm borders around the lesion
31. high-dose intravenous chemotherapy

32. 5,000 rads external beam radiation
33. regional lymph node dissection

PATIENT D

Options 34–48

A 4-year-old girl is brought in by her mother because of enuresis, abdominal pain, burning with urination, and foul-smelling, cloudy urine. The child has been treated several times previously for documented and culture-proven urinary tract infections. On examination, she appears nontoxic. Mild abdominal tenderness is present with neither rebound tenderness nor costovertebral tenderness. The child does not have a fever, and she has not experienced vomiting. Dipstick urinalysis is positive for 1+ protein, positive leukocyte esterase, and positive bacteria.

Immediate diagnostic tests include

34. urine culture and sensitivity
35. further questioning about the possibility of sexual abuse
36. 24-hour urine protein collection
37. urine cytology
38. cystoscopy

Appropriate treatment for this child may include

39. amoxicillin
40. ciprofloxacin
41. tetracycline
42. nitrofurantoin
43. trimethoprim-sulfamethoxazole

Follow-up after treatment should include

44. repeat urinalysis
45. urethral dilation
46. radionuclide cystogram
47. intravenous pyelogram
48. computed tomographic (CT) scanning of the pelvis

PATIENT E

Options 49–65

A 23-year-old sexually active college student presents with a vaginal itching and discharge that has been present over the last week. She has recently had intercourse with a new partner.

Which of the following tests would be indicated?

49. chlamydia testing
50. saline wet prep test
51. culture for herpes simplex
52. HIV viral load
53. HPV typing
54. gonorrhea testing

Further evaluation shows the presence of trichomonads on microscopic evaluation. Appropriate treatment at this time includes

55. azithromycin
56. metronidazole
57. fluconazole
58. ceftriaxone

Further recommendations concerning treatment include

59. the partner should be treated
60. the patient should abstain from alcohol while taking the medication
61. the medication is considered safe during pregnancy

In women who are pregnant, trichomoniasis is associated with

62. premature rupture of membranes
63. preterm delivery
64. low birth weight
65. twin pregnancy

PATIENT F

Options 66–75

A 42-year-old woman is the lone survivor of a single-engine plane crash. She is brought to the emergency room by ambulance. Initial examination shows her to be comatose with superficial and deep partial-thickness burns (second-degree) and full-thickness (third-degree) burns over 50% of her body. Vital signs are as follows: blood pressure, 130/70 mm Hg; pulse, 110/minute; respirations, 40/minute; and temperature, 37.5°C. Immunization status is unknown.

Initial management consists of

66. endotracheal intubation
67. 1 mg lorazepam (Ativan) given orally on arrival in the emergency room
68. administration of intravenous antibiotics
69. 2 mg morphine sulfate given every 1 to 2 hours as needed
70. intravenous fluid resuscitation
71. human tetanus immune globulin
72. tetanus toxoid given intramuscularly

After relative stabilization in the first 24 hours, the patient's blood pressure remains low and her urine output is minimal. Further management consists of

73. sufficient fluid to replace evaporated and insensible fluid losses
74. low-dose dopamine
75. transfer to a local burn unit

PATIENT G

Options 76–87

Before Thanksgiving, a 67-year-old retired female secretary is seen in your office for a general examination. The patient is married, has two daughters, and has enjoyed relatively good health. Her last general examination was 6 years ago, and she has not seen a physician since then. The patient has no overall health complaints, but is interested in updating preventive health issues. Health history includes the following:

- *Surgeries*: Total abdominal hysterectomy and oophorectomy at age 42 for excessive vaginal bleeding; cholecystectomy at age 45; benign breast biopsy at age 53
- *Hospitalizations*: Vaginal childbirth at ages 21 and 25; acute pyelonephritis at age 31
- *Chronic medical problems*: Asthma as a child
- *Allergies*: Penicillin
- *Alcohol*: Social only

- *Tobacco*: None
- *Medications*: Multivitamin daily
- *Immunizations*: None over last 20 years

Based on her history, which of the following would be indicated?

76. influenza vaccination
77. pneumococcal (Pneumovax) vaccination
78. tetanus-diphtheria vaccination
79. hepatitis A vaccination
80. hepatitis B vaccination
81. purified protein derivative tuberculosis testing

A physical examination reveals the following:

- *General*: Thin female in no distress
- *Blood pressure*: 140/88 mm Hg
- *Pulse*: 82 bpm and regular
- *Respirations*: 16/minute
- *Temperature*: 37.0°C (98.6°F)
- *Height*: 5 ft, 6 in.
- *Weight*: 120 lb
- *Head, ears, eyes, nose, and throat*: Ears clear; pupils equal, round, and reactive; funduscopic examination unremarkable; nose clear; oropharynx clear
- *Neck*: Supple, no lymphadenopathy, thyroid unremarkable
- *Heart*: Regular rate and rhythm, no murmurs
- *Lungs*: Clear to auscultation
- *Breast*: No distinct masses, fibrocystic changes bilaterally
- *Abdomen*: Soft and nontender, no masses, no hepatosplenomegaly
- *Pelvis*: Unremarkable, cervix surgically absent
- *Rectum*: No stool in the rectal vault
- *Extremities*: Free range of motion
- *Neurologic*: Grossly intact
- *Skin*: No suspicious lesions

Further management of this patient should include

82. mammogram screening
83. chest x-ray
84. pulmonary function tests
85. flexible sigmoidoscopy
86. DEXA screening
87. thyroid function tests

PATIENT H

Options 88–97

A 49-year-old, overweight, sedentary male mortgage banker hired a trainer at a local gym. The patient presents to your office 2 weeks after initiating a vigorous exercise program that consists of weight lifting and aerobic exercise. Recently, the patient added a new exercise machine to his workout routine that allows the user to perform flexion and extension leg exercises against resistance. Twenty-four hours after performing this exercise, he presents to you complaining of anterior knee pain.

Likely causes of the pain include

88. injury of the muscle fibers and surrounding connective tissue
89. stress fracture of the tibial plateau
90. accumulation of lactic acid in the muscle
91. Osgood-Schlatter disease

Appropriate initial treatment for this patient may include

92. ice therapy
93. stretching exercises
94. steroid injection
95. relative rest with limited weight bearing
96. heat wraps
97. ibuprofen administration

PATIENT I

Options 98–123

You have been asked to participate in a question/answer session about current immunization practices with a local parent group at their November meeting.

The first question a parent asked is, which of the following immunizations is required at the 2-month-old well-child visit?

98. hepatitis B (Hep B)
99. diptheria and tetanus toxoid and acellular pertussis vaccine (DTaP)
100. *Haemophilus influenzae* type B conjugate vaccine (Hib)
101. inactivated polio (IPV)
102. varicella
103. meningococcal conjugate vaccine (MCV4)
104. influenza
105. hepatitis A (Hep A)
106. heptavalent pneumococcal conjugate vaccine (PCV)
107. measles, mumps, and rubella (MMR)

Another parent states that her daughter has been allergic to eggs and asks what vaccines she will likely react to?

108. hepatitis B (Hep B)
109. diptheria and tetanus toxoid and acellular pertussis vaccine (DTaP)
110. *Haemophilus influenzae* type B conjugate vaccine (Hib)
111. inactivated polio (IPV)
112. varicella
113. meningococcal conjugate vaccine (MCV4)
114. influenza
115. hepatitis A (Hep A)
116. yellow fever vaccine

The final question has to do with which of the following is a live attenuated virus type vaccine?

117. hepatitis B (Hep B)
118. diptheria and tetanus toxoid and acellular pertussis vaccine (DTaP)
119. *Haemophilus influenzae* type B conjugate vaccine (Hib)
120. measles, mumps, and rubella (MMR)
121. varicella
122. meningococcal conjugate vaccine (MCV4)
123. influenza

PATIENT J

Options 124–134

A 64-year-old wealthy socialite presents to your office for a general examination; the patient has no complaints. Past medical history includes a total abdominal hysterectomy and associated blood transfusion at age 49, mild obesity, hyperlipidemia, and borderline hypertension. The patient has traveled extensively throughout the world without significant medical problems. Medications include atorvastatin taken for cholesterol. The patient is a former smoker and admits to consuming three glasses of wine per night. Family history is noncontributory. Review of systems is unremarkable. Physical examination is normal except for her being overweight and having mild fibrocystic changes in the breasts.

The following laboratory test results were obtained:

Electrolyte Panel

Sodium (135–145 mEq/L)	140 mEq/L
Potassium (3.3–5.1 mEq/L)	4.1 mEq/L
Chloride (100–108 mEq/L)	102 mEq/L
Creatinine (0.6–0.9 mEq/L)	0.8 mEq/L
Blood urea nitrogen (6–19 mEq/L)	10 mEq/L

Liver Function Tests

AST (12–31 U/L)	82 U/L
ALT (10–45 U/L)	60 U/L
GGT (9–31 U/L)	102 U/L
Alkaline phosphatase (98–251 U/L)	232 U/L
Total bilirubin (0.1–1.1 U/L)	0.8 U/L
Direct bilirubin (0.1–0.3 U/L)	0.1 U/L
Amylase (35–115 U/L)	46 U/L

Hepatitis Screen

Hepatitis A antibody	Negative
Hepatitis B surface antigen	Negative
Hepatitis B surface antibody	Negative
Hepatitis C antibody	Negative

Possible causes of her elevated liver function tests include

124. steatohepatitis
125. cholecystitis
126. acute hepatitis A
127. chronic alcohol use
128. chronic hepatitis B
129. atorvastatin use

Further management at this point may include

130. limitation of alcohol use
131. discontinuation of atorvastatin
132. magnetic resonance imaging (MRI) of the abdomen
133. liver biopsy
134. ultrasound of the liver, pancreas, and gallbladder

PATIENT K

Options 135–152

A 21-year-old primagravida is admitted to the labor and delivery ward at 34 weeks' gestation with regular contractions that are 4 minutes apart. Until this presentation, the patient's prenatal history has been unremarkable, with appropriate weight gain and uterus size for dates. The baby has remained active; there have been no problems with blood pressure or proteinuria. Because of nausea, the patient has not been compliant in taking prenatal vitamins on a regular basis. Prenatal laboratory test results were unremarkable.

Risk factors for the development of preterm labor include

135. urinary tract infection
136. septate uterus
137. premature rupture of membranes
138. congenital anomalies
139. polyhydramnios

Physical examination of the patient reveals a blood pressure of 108/72 mm Hg and a pulse of 72 bpm. Heart and lung examinations are unremarkable. The uterus measures 34 cm above the pubic symphysis. Vaginal examination reveals 2-cm dilation and 90% effacement. The station is –2. The cervix is measured at 32 mm in length. Microscopic examination of vaginal secretions shows no evidence of ferning.

Initial testing includes

140. urinalysis with culture and sensitivity
141. vaginal cultures
142. complete blood cell count (CBC) with differential
143. fibronectin assay

Fetal monitoring shows mild to moderate contractions that occur regularly every 4 minutes. Which of the following medications is useful in stopping preterm labor?

144. terbutaline
145. magnesium sulfate
146. nifedipine
147. oxytocin
148. ritodrine

After administration of appropriate medication, preterm labor is successfully arrested. Laboratory findings include a hemoglobin of 8.7 g/dL and a urinalysis that is positive for leukocyte esterase and bacteria.

Appropriate treatment for this patient includes

149. nitrofurantoin
150. ciprofloxacin
151. trimethoprim-sulfamethoxazole
152. iron supplementation

PATIENT L

Options 153–162

In mid-January, a 24-year-old man who is a painter is brought to the emergency room by ambulance after suffering what coworkers described as seizure-like activity. The patient has been working in an enclosed house, using space heaters to keep him warm. He is drowsy on admission without further seizure-like activity. Further questioning of the family reveals no prior history of seizures in the patient and no family history of seizures.

Initial evaluation should include

153. CT of the head
154. drug screen
155. electroencephalography
156. carboxyhemoglobin level
157. serum electrolytes
158. serum glucose determination

After approximately 15 minutes, the patient becomes more alert, and further evaluation reveals that he has been suffering with nausea and headaches that occur during and immediately after work, but he denies headaches at night or on the weekend when he is not working.

Which of the following can be considered a likely diagnosis?

159. brain tumor
160. new-onset diabetes mellitus
161. migraine headaches
162. carbon monoxide poisoning

PATIENT M

Options 163–179

A 23-year-old female presents to your office with complaints of vaginal bleeding and left sided lower abdominal pain. She is sexually active. She thinks her last period was approximately 6 weeks ago. She is otherwise healthy but has been experiencing some generalized fatigue. She denies any fevers or any other symptoms.

Which of the following is indicated at this time?

163. dilation and curettage
164. vaginal cultures
165. pregnancy test
166. complete blood count
167. urinalysis

You suspect ectopic pregnancy and order further tests to confirm this. Which of the following would be appropriate at this time?

168. transvaginal ultrasound
169. CT of the abdomen
170. hysterosalpingogram
171. MRI of the fallopian tubes
172. laparoscopic exploration

She is found to have an intrauterine pregnancy and fetal heartbeat is noted. Her bleeding has stopped and she is otherwise stable.

Which of the following is indicated at this time?

173. admission for observation
174. discharge with close follow-up
175. serial quantitative β-hCG levels
176. serial transvaginal ultrasounds
177. serum estrogen levels
178. serum progesterone levels
179. dilation and curettage

PATIENT N

Options 180–194

A 17-year-old sexually active female presents to the emergency room complaining of lower abdominal pain. She is using oral contraceptive pills and denies missing any of her pills. Her last menstrual period was 1 week ago. She denies dysuria, hematuria, or flank pain, but she has had fevers. Although she has had some nausea, she denies any vomiting, diarrhea, or breast tenderness. Her last sexual encounter was 4 days ago, and she complains of dyspareunia. Physical findings include the following:

- *Temperature*: 38.9°C orally (102°F)
- *Pulse*: 110 bpm
- *Blood pressure*: 110/68 mm Hg
- *Head, ears, eyes, nose, and throat*: Unremarkable
- *Heart*: Tachycardic, no murmurs
- *Lungs*: Clear
- *Abdomen*: Positive bowel sounds, moderate diffuse tenderness in lower quadrants bilaterally, positive guarding with no rebound tenderness
- *Extremities*: Unremarkable
- *Pelvis*: Normal external genitalia, positive cervical motion tenderness, positive bilateral adnexal tenderness; fullness of the right adnexa is noted
- *Rectum*: Normal, stool guaiac negative

Which of the following tests would be indicated in the initial workup?

180. urinalysis with culture and sensitivity
181. CBC with differential
182. electrolyte panel
183. pregnancy test
184. erythrocyte sedimentation rate
185. cervical and vaginal cultures

After initial testing, pelvic inflammatory disease (PID) is diagnosed. Likely infecting organisms include

186. *Chlamydia*
187. *Ureaplasma*
188. *Neisseria gonorrhoeae*
189. *Escherichia coli*

Which of the following would be considered appropriate outpatient treatment?

190. ceftriaxone given intramuscularly once, followed by oral doxycycline given twice a day for 14 days
191. amoxicillin given orally three times a day for 21 days
192. Cefoxitin given intravenously every 6 hours, plus probenecid followed by doxycycline orally
193. ampicillin intramuscularly once, followed by metronidazole for 14 days
194. ofloxacin orally twice a day for 14 days, plus metronidazole orally daily for 14 days

PATIENT O

Options 195–209

An 8-year-old boy presents to your office with his mother. The patient complains of a recurrent cough, shortness of breath, and wheezing that has been present over the last 3 years. He denies any mucus production, fevers, or any other symptoms that are consistent with infection. The patient also has noted that with physical exertion, he has wheezing and shortness of breath.

After a complete history and physical examination, which of the following would be indicated as part of the initial evaluation of this patient?

195. spirometry
196. arterial blood gases
197. CT of the chest
198. chest radiograph
199. echocardiogram

Which of the following would be important information in the diagnosis?

200. severity of symptoms
201. frequency of exacerbations
202. triggering factors
203. family history of reactive airway disease

Once the diagnosis of asthma is made, appropriate initial management of this patient may include

204. use of a β_2-agonist inhaler
205. monitoring of peak-flow rate
206. administration of oral theophylline
207. administration of oral steroids
208. environmental control to avoid irritants and allergens
209. immunization for influenza and *Pneumococcus*

PATIENT P

Options 210–229

A 33-year-old used-car salesman presents to your office complaining of tightness in his chest, a choking sensation, shortness of breath, paresthesias of his hands, heart palpitations, and lightheadedness. The patient denies syncope. Symptoms occur suddenly, often lasting 10 to 15 minutes, and they usually occur at rest. The patient has had six episodes during the last week and describes feeling anxious after the episode of chest discomfort. He was seen by another physician 2 days ago, and a CBC, erythrocyte sedimentation rate, thyroid function tests, electrolyte panel, electrocardiogram, and chest radiograph were all normal. The physician told him that he thought his symptoms were stress-related. The patient is quite concerned, and presents to you for a second opinion. A thorough examination, including cardiac, pulmonary, and neurologic examination, is unremarkable.

A cost-effective workup of this patient may include

210. exercise echocardiogram
211. referral to a cardiologist
212. CT scan of the chest
213. further questioning about the use of diet pills, illicit drugs, or alcohol
214. serum antinuclear antibody test
215. upper extremity electromyography studies
216. lumbar puncture
217. Holter monitoring

Results from further evaluation are normal. Management at this point might include prescribing

218. paroxetine (Paxil)
219. amitriptyline (Elavil)
220. desipramine (Norpramin)
221. verapamil (Calan, Isoptin)
222. sublingual nitroglycerin
223. imipramine (Tofranil)
224. alprazolam (Xanax)

After initiation of treatment, the patient returns for follow-up as symptoms continue. Further treatment may include

225. education concerning manifestations of the illness and ways to control them
226. identification of support systems
227. use of monoamine oxidase inhibitors
228. electroconvulsive therapy
229. psychiatric referral

PATIENT Q

Options 230–244

A 75-year-old woman presents with a 3-week history of bilateral temporal headaches, diplopia, jaw pain, low-grade fevers, and generalized fatigue with weight loss. The patient's husband recently had a bout with the flu, and she believes she is developing similar symptoms. Physical examination shows the following:

- *Weight*: 60 kg (132 lb)
- *Blood pressure*: 120/80 mm Hg
- *Temperature*: 38°C (100.4°F)
- *Scalp*: Temporal tenderness
- *Eyes*: Small retinal hemorrhages
- *Nose*: Clear
- *Oropharynx*: Unremarkable
- *Neck*: Supple
- *Heart*: Regular rate and rhythm
- *Lungs*: Clear to auscultation
- *Abdomen*: Soft, nontender
- *Extremities*: Unremarkable
- *Neurologic*: Nonfocal

Appropriate initial testing would include

230. lumbar puncture
231. MRI of the head
232. erythrocyte sedimentation rate
233. CBC
234. urinalysis
235. carotid ultrasound

The diagnosis of temporal arteritis is suspected. Appropriate management at this point would be

236. broad-spectrum oral antibiotics for 10 days
237. high-dose steroid therapy
238. immediate surgical consultation for temporal artery biopsy
239. physical therapy consultation
240. initiation of anticoagulation therapy

Complications of temporal arteritis may include

241. diffuse joint pain
242. amaurosis fugax
243. blindness
244. acute myelocytic anemia

PATIENT R

Options 245–259

A newlywed couple presents to your office stating that they will be traveling to Central America for their honeymoon. They will be touring urban and rural locations. Both are concerned about the risk of traveler's diarrhea.

Which of the following recommendations should be given?

245. Avoid food from street vendors.
246. Obtain a portable filter for use with drinking water.
247. Peel all fruits before eating.
248. Carbonated beverages are generally considered safe.
249. Fluids should be iced to prevent bacterial growth.
250. Making sure to spit out the water used in brushing your teeth will prevent traveler's diarrhea.

Which of the following statements is true concerning the use of prophylactic antibiotics to prevent traveler's diarrhea?

251. Prophylactic antibiotics should be recommended for most travelers that visit developed countries, including central Europe, England, and Canada.
252. Prophylactic antibiotics are recommended for most travelers who visit third-world countries.
253. Prophylactic antibiotics may be warranted for business executives who are scheduled for important meetings or professional entertainers who are traveling abroad.
254. Prophylactic antibiotics are generally not necessary for travel abroad if hygiene and safety precautions are enforced.

Which of the following medications can be used for the prevention of traveler's diarrhea?

255. penicillin
256. erythromycin
257. bismuth subsalicylate
258. gentamicin
259. ciprofloxacin

ANSWERS AND EXPLANATIONS

Options 1–15

Answers: 1. F 2. F 3. T 4. T 5. T 6. F 7. T 8. F 9. F 10. F 11. F 12. T 13. T 14. F 15. F

A standard evaluation for erectile dysfunction (ED) should include a thorough sexual, medical, and psychosocial history, focusing on conditions such as cardiovascular disease (e.g., hypertension, atherosclerosis, hyperlipidemia), diabetes, depression, alcoholism, premature ejaculation, increased latency associated with age, psychosexual relationships, and other conditions that might be contraindications for certain drug therapies. Other risk factors for ED that may be discovered include smoking; pelvic, perianal, or penile trauma; neurologic disease; endocrinopathy; obesity; pelvic radiation therapy; Peyronie's disease; and prescription or illicit drug use. It is important to distinguish ED from problems with ejaculation or orgasm, as well as to establish the history and severity of symptoms. The physical examination should focus on the abdomen, penis, testicles, secondary sexual characteristics, and lower extremity pulses. A rectal examination, vascular and neurologic assessment, determination of prostate-specific antigen (PSA) and testosterone levels, and monitoring of nocturnal erections would be indicated in this patient. The AUA recommends that PDE5 inhibitors be offered as the first-line therapy for ED unless contraindicated. The three PDE5 inhibitors studied [i.e., sildenafil (Viagra), tadalafil (Cialis), and vardenafil (Levitra)] are metabolized by the liver, and dosage should be adjusted for patients with altered hepatic function. The side effects of all three medications include facial flushing, nasal congestion, headache, and dyspepsia. Sildenafil and vardenafil may cause visual side effects. A limited number a patients taking tadalafil report back pain. Vardenafil may cause mild prolongation of QT interval; caution should be used when prescribing this agent for patients with a history of QT prolongation or those taking medications that prolong the QT interval. Many men being treated for ED also are taking medication for treatment of hypertension or lower urinary tract symptoms. PDE5 inhibitors interact with β-blockers, a class of drugs commonly used to treat hypertension and lower urinary tract symptoms. Vardenafil should not be used by any patient taking any other medication with α-blocker activity. Any dose of tadalafil and 50- and 100-mg doses of sildenafil should be administered with caution to patients taking α-blockers. Patients taking PDE5 inhibitors should not take organic nitrates concomitantly. No safe interval between the use of nitrates and PDE5 has been determined, but it is suggested that a 24-hour interval be used for sildenafil and a 48-hour interval be used for tadalafil. It is important that physicians monitor the effectiveness, side effects, and health changes in patients using PDE5 inhibitors. This can be done at the time of prescription renewal. Patients who do not respond to PDE5 inhibitors may have modifiable risk factors such as hormonal abnormalities, food or drug interactions, incorrect dosing, lack of adequate sexual stimulation, heavy alcohol use, or relationship problems with their partner. Patients who do not respond to PDE5 inhibitors should be informed of the risks and benefits of other therapies. The panel recommends that the first dose of alprostadil intraurethral suppositories be administered under a physician's supervision because hypotension has been reported in approximately 3% of patients. Studies show that alprostadil combined with PDE5 inhibitors or a penile constriction device is more effective than the use of alprostadil alone. Intracavernous injection therapy is invasive, but it is the most effective nonsurgical treatment for ED. The most widely used drugs for this therapy are alprostadil, papaverine (Pavabid), and phentolamine. The initial dose of all intracavernous injection medications should be administered in the presence of a physician to instruct the patient on proper technique, determine the most effective dose, and monitor the patient for side effects. It is important to watch for priapism in patients taking intracavernous injection therapy. Priapism can cause corporal tissue damage but, if caught early, usually can be reversed with nonsurgical measures. Vacuum constriction devices are a low-cost treatment appropriate for some patients with ED. To avoid injury to the penis, only devices that contain a vacuum limiter should be used. Vacuum constriction devices are available with or without a prescription. Trazodone (Desyrel), testosterone (in patients with normal serum testosterone levels), and yohimbine and other herbal therapies are not recommended for treatment of ED.

Montague DK et al. *The Management of Erectile Dysfunction: An Update.* American Urological Association; 2005.

Vardenafil may cause mild prolongation of QT interval; caution should be used when prescribing this agent for patients with a history of QT prolongation or those taking medications that prolong the QT interval.

Options 16–25

Answers: 16. T 17. F 18. T 19. T 20. T 21. F 22. F 23. T 24. F 25. F

The initial management of a hypertensive patient includes the following minimal baseline tests: CBC, urinalysis, serum sodium, serum potassium, serum creatinine, fasting glucose determination, total high-density and low-density lipoprotein cholesterol, and an electrocardiogram. Other tests, including chest x-ray, ambulatory blood pressure monitoring, urine studies to rule out pheochromocytoma, and radiographic procedures to study the kidneys, are unnecessary in this patient. The patient should be counseled on weight loss with dietary modification and the institution of a regular exercise program. Sodium restriction to <2 g/day and limitation of alcohol to <1 oz/day in men and <0.5 oz/day in women should be encouraged. Home monitoring of blood pressure may be helpful in management, and the patient should have close outpatient follow-up. If these measures do not improve the patient's condition, medication can be considered. If target organ damage is present or other risk factors (e.g., diabetes) are present, or when the systolic blood pressure is ≥160 mm Hg or diastolic blood pressure is >100 mm Hg, drug therapy should not be deferred while awaiting the results of diet and exercise modification. Minimal amounts of alcohol and caffeine do not significantly alter the treatment of this individual's hypertension. High-dose vitamins and trace mineral supplementation are not recommended in the treatment. The goal is to keep blood pressure at <140/90 mm Hg or as near this level as possible in patients who are younger than 65 years of age. For those with diabetes or kidney disease, the goal should be <130/80 mm Hg. In most cases, drug therapy should be initiated with a β-blocker or diuretic unless they are contraindicated. Diuretics (e.g., hydrochlorothiazide) appear to be more effective in patients older than 60 and in African Americans. Coexisting conditions may help with the initial selection of a hypertensive agent.

Beers MH, Porter RS, eds. *The Merck manual of diagnosis and therapy*, Merck Research Laboratories, 18th ed. Whitehouse Station, NJ: Merck & Co.; 2006:604–620.

For those with diabetes or kidney disease, the blood pressure goal should be less than 130/80.

Options 26–33

Answers: 26. T 27. F 28. T 29. T 30. F 31. F 32. F 33. T

The incidence of melanoma is rising at an alarming rate. Sun exposure, familial dysplastic nevi syndrome, and a positive family history of melanoma are significant risk factors. The four histologic types are lentigo maligna melanoma, superficial spreading melanoma, nodular melanoma, and acral-lentiginous melanoma. Warning signs include the ABCDE rule: *A*symmetric lesions, lesions with irregular *B*orders, lesions with variegated *C*olor, lesions with *D*iameter greater than 6 mm, and lesions with an *E*levated surface contour. Any suspicious lesion should be biopsied. Initial treatment entails wide excision and regional node dissection. Survival rates are based on the depth of invasion.

Rakel RE, Bope ET. *Conn's Current Therapy 2005*. Philadelphia: Elsevier/Saunders; 2005:936–941.

Sun exposure, familial dysplastic nevi syndrome, and a positive family history are significant risk factors for melanoma.

Options 34–48

Answers: 34. T 35. T 36. F 37. F 38. F 39. T 40. F 41. F 42. T 43. T 44. T 45. F 46. T 47. T 48. F

Recurrent urinary tract infections in young girls should always be investigated initially with a urine culture and sensitivity. Because sexual abuse in children can present with symptoms of dysuria, enuresis, and abdominal pain, the physician should always remain alert to the possibility of sexual abuse. The most common infecting organisms include *Escherichia coli, Klebsiella, Staphylococcus*, and the enteric streptococci. Amoxicillin, nitrofurantoin, and trimethoprim-sulfamethoxazole can be used for urinary tract infections in children. Tetracycline and ciprofloxacin are contraindicated for use in children. After treatment, the child should have a repeat urinalysis. Girls have traditionally been worked up with intravenous pyelography after the second infection; however, recommendations are for further evaluation for all children after the first infection, if the first infection occurs between 2 months and 2 years of age. Renal ultrasound is often used to rule out obstruction and to determine kidney size. After age 2, some advocate further imaging only after the second infection in females. All boys should be evaluated with their first infection. Ultrasound can be done immediately; however, a voiding cystogram (used to detect posterior urethral valves) is usually done after an infection has cleared because an infection can predispose to reflux. Radionuclide cystograms can also be utilized; however, most experts prefer the voiding cystogram and use the radionuclide scan in follow-up to determine if the vesicourethral reflux has resolved. Urethral dilation and CT of the pelvis are not indicated.

Beers MH, Porter RS, eds. *The Merck manual of diagnosis and therapy*, Merck Research Laboratories, 18th ed. Whitehouse Station, NJ: Merck & Co.; 2006:2356–2358.

Because sexual abuse in children can present with symptoms of dysuria, enuresis, and abdominal pain, the physician should always remain alert to the possibility of sexual abuse.

Options 49–65

Answers: 49. T 50. T 51. F 52. F 53. F 54. T 55. F 56. T 57. F 58. F 59. T 60. T 61. T 62. T 63. T 64. T 65. T

Women presenting with vaginal symptoms following intercourse should be evaluated for chlamydia, gonorrhea, bacterial vaginosis, trichomoniasis, and *Candida* vaginitis. A culture for herpes simplex is not indicated in the absence of suspected lesions. Human papilloma virus (HPV) testing is not clinically useful in this setting, and human immunodeficiency virus (HIV) viral load assessment is not indicated in this situation. If HIV testing is performed, an HIV ELISA antibody test would be the appropriate screening test. Most men who are infected with *Trichomonas vaginalis* do not have symptoms, but others may have urethritis-type symptoms. Many infected women have a diffuse, malodorous, yellow-green discharge with vulvar irritation; however, some have minimal or no symptoms. Treatment of patients and sex partners results in relief of symptoms, cure of the condition, and reduction of transmission. Patients should be treated with oral metronidazole. The recommended regimens have resulted in cure rates of about 90% to 95%, which might increase if the treatment of sex partners is ensured. Patients should be instructed to avoid sex until they and their sex partners are cured. Follow-up is unnecessary for men and women who are initially asymptomatic or become asymptomatic after treatment. In pregnant women, vaginal trichomoniasis has been associated with premature rupture of the membranes, preterm delivery, and low birth weight. Women who are symptomatic should be treated to relieve symptoms and may be treated with oral metronidazole. Patients who have trichomoniasis and are infected with HIV should receive the same therapy as those who are not infected with HIV.

Ressel GW. CDC releases 2002 guidelines for treating STDs: Part I. Diseases characterized by vaginal discharge and PID. *Am Fam Physician.* 2002;66(9):1777–1778.

In pregnant women, vaginal trichomoniasis has been associated with premature rupture of the membranes, preterm delivery, and low birth weight.

Options 66–75

Answers: 66. T 67. F 68. T 69. T 70. F 71. T 72. T 73. T 74. T 75. T

Burns represent a special challenge to family physicians who work in emergency room settings. They are classified as follows; however, the newer terms (in parentheses) are replacing the old classification:

- *First degree (Superficial burns)*: Superficial burns that affect only the epidermis; usually resulting in mild redness and discomfort, they blanch with pressure; the protective function of the skin is maintained. There is no blister formation. An example is a mild sunburn.
- *Second degree (Superficial and Deep Partial-Thickness Burns)*: Partial-thickness burns that cause pain and blistering of the epidermis and dermis layers, they spare the hair follicles and sebaceous and sweat glands.
- *Third degree (Full-Thickness Burns)*: Involve the epidermis, dermis, and deeper structures; classically anesthetic; they appear white, dry, charred, or inelastic; regeneration of skin tissue is minimal, and skin grafting is required. They are painless and avascular; significant scarring and contractures occur.
- *Fourth degree (now included in Full-Thickness Burns)*: Involve deeper muscles, fascia, or bone. Appearance and healing are similar to that of third-degree burns. Some combine third- and fourth-degree burns together.

Physicians should stabilize all burn victims, secure the airway with endotracheal intubation when airway compromise is a possibility, and perform aggressive fluid resuscitation (including half of fluid deficits administered over the first 8 hours). The victim's clothing and any remaining hot substances should be removed and the victim covered with a sterile sheet. Copious irrigation is indicated for chemical burns. Cool compresses are used for small burns but can cause hypothermia in large burns. Transfer to a major burn center for further care is recommended for extensive burns once the patient's condition is stabilized. Severely burned patients have a generalized increase in capillary permeability throughout the body, which may lead to excessive fluid loss and development of shock. Aggressive fluid resuscitation is imperative.

Narcotic pain medication should be used to manage pain; the use of benzodiazepines for sedation is usually unnecessary. Topical antibiotic (silver sulfadiazine) is generally applied in all but first-degree burns to help prevent infection. Bacitracin ointment is a suitable alternative. If there is an extensive burned area, intravenous antibiotics are necessary to help prevent septicemia. If the patient's immunization status is unknown, tetanus immunization with tetanus toxoid and immune globulin is recommended. Further management includes aggressive management of fluids; administration of dopamine, which can increase urinary output and sustain blood pressure, can be considered. Débridement of necrotic tissue and whirlpool treatments are usually necessary.

Taylor RB, David AK, Fields SA, et al., eds. *Family medicine: principles and practice*, 6th ed. New York: Springer; 2003:431–434.

Superficial burns affect only the epidermis; usually resulting in mild redness and discomfort, they blanch with pressure; the protective function of the skin is maintained. There is no blister formation.

Options 76–87

Answers: 76. T 77. T 78. T 79. F 80. F 81. F 82. T 83. F 84. F 85. T 86. T 87. F

General health maintenance is often provided by family physicians. In this case the patient is relatively healthy, but she needs an update on some preventive health issues. Immunizations for a 67 year old should include a yearly influenza vaccination (beginning at age 50) and Pneumovax if no prior Pneumovax has been given, if the patient had a Pneumovax before age 65 and it has been more than 5 years, and if no contraindications exist (e.g., previous reaction, allergy to eggs with the influenza immunization). Hepatitis A vaccination should be considered for frequent travelers who visit Third-World and underdeveloped countries. Hepatitis B vaccination is now recommended for all schoolchildren, but is not indicated at this age unless the patient is at risk for development of hepatitis B (e.g., those with multiple sexual partners or exposure to blood and body secretions). Purified protein derivative testing for tuberculosis is not generally recommended unless the patient is at risk for tuberculosis exposure, is an immigrant, or is about to enter a nursing home. In these cases, tuberculosis screening should be considered. Further testing for this woman should include a yearly mammogram [which should begin at 50 years of age; some (ACOG/ACS) advocate starting at age 40], monthly breast self-examination, and yearly breast examination by a physician. Chest x-ray screening is not indicated in asymptomatic patients. Although this patient has a history of childhood asthma, pulmonary function testing is not indicated. Colon screening should consist of periodic bowel examination with colonoscopy or flexible sigmoidoscopy combined with yearly hemoccult testing and digital rectal examinations in patients older than 50 years of age. Barium enemas may be an option in certain patients. Unless the patient exhibits symptoms that are consistent with a thyroid disorder, the routine ordering of thyroid function tests is not indicated. DEXA screening is recommended for women over age 65.

Rakel RE. *Textbook of Family Practice.* Philadelphia: WB Saunders; 2002:170–179.

Hepatitis A vaccination should be considered for frequent travelers who visit Third-World and underdeveloped countries.

Options 88–97

Answers: 88. T 89. F 90. T 91. F 92. T 93. T 94. F 95. T 96. F 97. T

Muscle-related injuries are common in poorly conditioned individuals who start a new exercise routine. Typically, muscle fibers and surrounding connective tissue are injured. Accumulation of lactic acid in muscle tissue can also result in pain. Stress fractures occur over a period of time and are associated with chronic use and repeated trauma. Osgood-Schlatter disease is a common cause of anterior knee pain in children but not adults.

Treatment may include relative rest with limited weight bearing, ice therapy, compressive wraps, and elevation (particularly if swelling is present). Nonsteroidal anti-inflammatory agents, such as ibuprofen, should be initiated for their analgesic and anti-inflammatory properties. Stretching exercises can also be instituted. Heat therapy is usually used at least 48 hours after application of ice, and steroid injections are given if necessary for specific conditions, such as severe degenerative joint disease that is unresponsive to anti-inflammatory drugs.

Beers MH, Porter RS, eds. *The Merck manual of diagnosis and therapy*, Merck Research Laboratories, 18th ed. Whitehouse Station, NJ: Merck & Co.; 2006:2635–2636.

> Osgood-Schlatter disease is a common cause of anterior knee pain in children, but not adults.

Options 98–123

Answers: 98. T 99. T 100. T 101. T 102. F 103. F 104. F 105. F 106. T 107. F 108. F 109. F 110. F 111. F 112. F 113. F 114. T 115. F 116. T 117. F 118. F 119. F 120. T 121. T 122. F 123. F

At the 2-month-old well-child visit, the following vaccines are indicated in otherwise healthy children: hepatitis B; diphtheria, tetanus, and acellular pertussis (DTaP); *Haemophilus influenzae* type B (Hib); inactivated poliovirus (IPV); and pneumococcal vaccinations. Various combinations exist for coadministration. Varicella and hepatitis A vaccinations are normally given after 12 months of age. Influenza vaccine is given to children older than 6 months. The measles, mumps, and rubella (MMR) vaccination is given at 12 to 15 months. Egg protein is present in yellow fever and influenza vaccines and may cause reactions in egg-allergic recipients; thus, a history of allergy to the ingestion of egg should be sought prior to the administration of any egg-containing vaccine. Persons with a positive history should be evaluated by an allergist prior to vaccine administration. However, a negative history may not exclude an allergic reaction to egg protein injected with the vaccine, because vaccine recipients can be allergic to heat-labile egg proteins in raw egg, and may not think of themselves as "egg-allergic." Of the live-attenuated vaccines listed above, only varicella and the MMR vaccine are live-attenuated vaccines.

Advisory Committee on Immunization Practices, Department of Health and Human Services, Centers for Disease Control and Prevention, 2006 Recommended Childhood and Adolescent Immunization Schedule. Accessed at www.aafp.org on 5/18/06.

Kelso, JM. Raw egg allergy—a potential issue in vaccine allergy. *J Allergy Clin Immunol.* 2000;106:990.

> Egg protein is present in yellow fever and influenza vaccines and may cause reactions in egg-allergic recipients.

Options 124–134

Answers: 124. T 125. F 126. F 127. T 128. F 129. T 130. T 131. T 132. F 133. F 134. T

Elevated liver function tests can result from different causes: inflammation, medications, toxin exposures, infections, tumors, storage diseases, autoimmune diseases, congestive heart failure, muscle disease, and fatty infiltration of the liver as a result of obesity. In this case, causes that could be considered include elevations as a result of alcohol consumption, steatohepatitis, and the patient's atorvastatin use. Cholecystitis is an unlikely cause, because the alkaline phosphatase as well as the total and direct bilirubin tests are normal. If hepatitis screening tests are negative, then acute hepatitis A and chronic hepatitis B are not causes.

Further management of this patient includes weight loss counseling and a recommendation to limit or abstain from alcohol use, discontinue atorvastatin use, and repeat liver function tests. Ultrasound of the liver, pancreas, and gallbladder may be indicated. However, other tests, such as MRI or biopsy of the liver, are not indicated.

Johnston DE. Special considerations in interpreting liver function tests. *Am Fam Physician.* 1999;59:2223–2230.

> Elevated liver function tests can result from different causes: inflammation, medications, toxin exposures, infections, tumors, storage diseases, autoimmune diseases, congestive heart failure, muscle disease, and fatty infiltration of the liver as a result of obesity.

Options 135–152

Answers: 135. T 136. T 137. T 138. T 139. T 140. T 141. T 142. T 143. T 144. T 145. T 146. T 147. F 148. T 149. T 150. F 151. F 152. T

Preterm labor is defined as labor pains that occur at least every 10 minutes and last for 30 seconds accompanied by cervical dilation between 20 and 37 weeks' gestation. Causes include infections, uterine abnormalities, cervical incompetency, premature rupture of membranes, multiple gestations, and other abnormalities (e.g., polyhydramnios, fetal abnormalities). Initial management of the patient in preterm labor should consist of a sterile speculum examination to determine if there is ferning, which would indicate premature rupture of membranes; vaginal cultures to rule out vaginal infection; urinalysis with culture and sensitivity; CBC with differential; and ultrasound examination of the uterus and fetus. A long cervix (>35 mm by transvaginal ultrasound) and a negative fibronectin assay have an excellent negative predictive value for preterm labor.

Treatment of preterm labor includes appropriate care of any precipitating infections and the use of tocolytics, such as magnesium sulfate, or ritodrine and, in some cases, terbutaline. Calcium-channel blockers, (e.g., nifedipine) and indomethacin can also be used. Oxytocin is used to initiate or augment labor.

Appropriate medication for the treatment of urinary tract infections during pregnancy includes ampicillin, cephalosporins, or nitrofurantoin. Organism susceptibility should be confirmed. Quinolones, sulfonamides, and trimethoprim should be avoided. In addition, this patient should be placed on iron supplementation for anemia.

Cunningham FG, Gant NF, Leveno KJ. *Williams Obstetrics*, 21st ed. New York: McGraw-Hill; 690–718.

Preterm labor is defined as labor pains that occur at least every 10 minutes and last for 30 seconds accompanied by cervical dilation between 20 and 37 weeks' gestation.

Options 153–162

Answers: 153. T 154. T 155. F 156. T 157. T 158. T 159. F 160. F 161. F 162. T

The initial evaluation of seizure-like activity should include baseline laboratory tests: serum electrolytes, calcium, magnesium, phosphorous, CBC, BUN, serum drug screen, glucose determination, and a carboxyhemoglobin level. CT of the brain is indicated to rule out structural abnormalities. A lumbar puncture may be needed after a CT is obtained if infection is suspected. An electroencephalogram may be necessary, but is not indicated in the initial testing.

Carbon monoxide poisoning is manifested by confusion, coma, seizures, headaches, fatigue, and nausea. Diagnosis is usually made by obtaining a careful history of carbon monoxide poisoning (exposure to space heaters, furnaces, or car exhaust) and carboxyhemoglobin determination. Venous carboxyhemoglobin levels are just as good as arterial. Oxygen saturation levels are often normal. Therapy includes the administration of 100% oxygen and the consideration of hyperbaric oxygen therapy.

Brain tumors may present with progressive severe headaches. These headaches often wake the patient from sleep and are accompanied by visual disturbances, neurologic deficits, nausea, and vomiting. Diabetes may present with diabetic ketoacidosis or other symptoms, such as polyphagia, polydipsia, and polyuria. Migraine headaches are usually associated with a previous history or positive family history. Migraines may be associated with nausea, vomiting, and visual disturbances, but they are not generally associated with seizure activity.

Beers MH, Porter RS, eds. *The Merck manual of diagnosis and therapy*, Merck Research Laboratories, 18th ed. Whitehouse Station, NJ: Merck & Co.; 2006:1826.

Carbon monoxide poisoning is manifested by confusion, coma, seizures, headaches, fatigue, and nausea. Diagnosis is usually made by obtaining a careful history of carbon monoxide poisoning (exposure to space heaters, furnaces, or car exhaust) and carboxyhemoglobin determination.

Options 163–179

Answers: 163. F 164. T 165. T 166. T 167. T 168. T 169. F 170. F 171. F 172. F 173. F 174. T 175. T 176. F 177. F 178. F 179. F

Vaginal bleeding is a common concern in the first trimester of pregnancy, occurring in 20% to 40% of pregnant women. It may be light, heavy, intermittent, or constant, and there may or may not be pain. The four major causes of bleeding in early pregnancy are

1. Ectopic pregnancy
2. Threatened or impending miscarriage
3. Physiologic (i.e., related to implantation of the pregnancy)
4. Cervical, vaginal, or uterine pathology

Because the exact cause of uterine bleeding in the first trimester often cannot be determined, the goal of the evaluation is to make a definitive diagnosis when possible and exclude serious pathology in other cases. Ectopic pregnancy is especially important to exclude because it can be life-threatening.

The initial step in the evaluation is to assess the extent of bleeding. If the woman is passing blood clots or the blood is soaking through her clothes, if she feels light-headed, if she has significant pelvic pain or cramping, or if she has passed any tissue, ectopic pregnancy and miscarriage are more likely, and implantation bleeding and cervicovaginal disease (e.g., polyps, infection, cancer) are less likely. However, the presence of only light, intermittent, painless bleeding does not exclude the possibility of a life-threatening underlying disease. A past history of ectopic pregnancy or risk factors for ectopic pregnancy (e.g., pelvic inflammatory disease) increases the probability of this condition. A history of two or more consecutive pregnancy losses or a disorder associated with pregnancy loss (e.g., chromosomal translocation, antiphospholipid antibody syndrome, uterine anomaly) raise the possibility that bleeding may be related to miscarriage. Orthostatic blood pressure changes occur if bleeding has been severe. If the patient has passed tissue, it should be examined for fetal products.

The patient's abdomen should be examined prior to a vaginal examination. Midline pain is more consistent with miscarriage, whereas lateral pain is more consistent with ectopic pregnancy. An attempt should be made to determine uterine size. Typically, the uterus can be palpated abdominally after 12 weeks' gestation. If the pregnancy is at or beyond 10 to 12 weeks' gestation, a Doppler device can be used to check for the fetal heart beat. The fetal heart rate can be easily distinguished from the maternal heart rate, as it is typically in the range of 140 to 160 bpm. The absence of a previously detected fetal heartbeat should raise concern that a missed abortion has occurred. However, vaginal bleeding often occurs well before the fetal heartbeat has been detected with a Doppler device. Doppler confirmation of fetal cardiac activity is reassuring and indicates bleeding is not related to missed abortion (also called *delayed miscarriage*) or ectopic pregnancy.

After the abdominal examination, the external genitalia are examined to assess the amount and source of bleeding, and then a speculum is inserted into the vagina. If blood clots are present, these can be removed with gauze sponges on a sponge forceps. If products of conception are suspected, the specimen should always be sent for pathologic examination to look for chorionic villi and confirm the diagnosis. Physical examination may reveal a non-pregnancy-related source of bleeding associated with a wound, cervical ectropion, abnormal growth, or purulent discharge. In these cases, further evaluation depends on the nature of the findings. Appropriate testing may include also vaginal cultures and urinalysis with culture to rule out infections.

A speculum-assisted vaginal examination can provide direct visualization of a dilated cervix or the gestational sac may be sufficient to diagnose a miscarriage clinically; however, ultrasound can provide additional information such as the presence of a multiple gestation or retained products of conception.

If uterine bleeding is confirmed but the cervix appears closed and there are no obvious bleeding lesions, a bimanual pelvic examination should be performed. Ectopic pregnancy findings include adnexal, cervical motion, and/or abdominal tenderness; an adnexal mass; and mild uterine enlargement. However, in many cases the physical examination is unremarkable, especially if there is a small, unruptured ectopic pregnancy. Bleeding when the uterine size is larger than expected for dates suggests a multiple gestation with miscarriage of one of the multiples, gestational trophoblastic disease (molar pregnancy), or other uterine pathology (leiomyomas are associated with an irregularly enlarged uterus). Transvaginal ultrasonography is the cornerstone of the evaluation of bleeding in early pregnancy. Ultrasound examination is performed to determine whether the pregnancy is intrauterine or extrauterine (ectopic) and, if intrauterine, whether the pregnancy is viable (fetal cardiac activity present) or nonviable. The ultrasound finding most concerning for a diagnosis of ectopic pregnancy in the setting of first trimester vaginal bleeding is the absence of an intrauterine gestational sac, rather than the presence of an adnexal mass. Rarely, ultrasound examination reveals unusual causes of uterine bleeding, such as gestational trophoblastic disease or partial loss of a multiple gestation. In bleeding patients in whom sonography has previous confirmed a singleton intrauterine pregnancy, another examination is not necessary to confirm fetal viability if fetal heart activity can be detected by a hand-held Doppler device.

Serial measurement of human chorionic gonadotropin (hCG) levels are helpful early in pregnancy if ultrasonography is nondiagnostic (i.e., the site and viability of the pregnancy are not revealed). There is no role for monitoring hCG levels once the presence of an intrauterine pregnancy has been established sonographically. Falling β-hCG concentrations are consistent with a nonviable intrauterine pregnancy or spontaneously resolving ectopic pregnancy, but do not indicate whether the pregnancy is intrauterine or ectopic. Appropriately rising hCG levels (>66% in 48 hours) are most consistent with a viable intrauterine pregnancy. hCG levels that have plateaued or are rising slowly suggest an ectopic pregnancy. Other hormone assays (e.g., progesterone, estrogen, inhibin A, PAPP-A) are less useful.

Norwitz ER, Park JS. Overview of the etiology and evaluation of vaginal bleeding in pregnant women. Up to Date, version 14.1. Accessed 5/19/06.

The four major causes of bleeding in early pregnancy are:

1. Ectopic pregnancy
2. Threatened or impending miscarriage
3. Physiologic (i.e., related to implantation of the pregnancy)
4. Cervical, vaginal, or uterine pathology

Options 180–194

Answers: 180. T 181. T 182. F 183. T 184. T 185. T 186. T 187. T 188. T 189. T 190. T 191. F 192. T 193. F 194. T

Pelvic inflammatory disease (PID) should be considered in sexually active females who present with lower abdominal pain. Disease can manifest as any combination of endometritis, salpingitis, tuboovarian abscess, and pelvic peritonitis. Women at increased risk include those who have recently experienced childbirth or abortion, have an intrauterine device, have multiple sexual partners, have had recent menstrual periods, and have recently had pelvic surgery. Symptoms include lower abdominal pain, nausea, vomiting, fevers, vaginal discharge, and dyspareunia. Signs include lower abdominal pain with or without rebound tenderness, cervical motion tenderness, adnexal tenderness, and, in some, adnexal masses or fullness. Fever is usually present, and the white blood cell count is elevated. The differential diagnosis includes appendicitis, ectopic pregnancy, septic abortion, pyelonephritis, inflammatory bowel disease, endometriosis, hemorrhagic corpus luteum, ovarian cysts, and torsion of the ovary. Treatment is usually empiric, and antimicrobial therapy should cover *Neisseria gonorrhoeae*, *Chlamydia trachomatis*, anaerobes, gram-negative facultative bacteria, and streptococci. Parenteral therapy is required in several types of patients, including those who are pregnant; those who do not respond to or are unable to tolerate oral antimicrobial therapy; those with severe illness such as nausea, vomiting, or high fever; those with tuboovarian abscess; and patients who are immunodeficient. Sexual partners of patients with PID should be evaluated and treated. The initial workup in a case of suspected PID includes urinalysis with culture and sensitivity, CBC, pregnancy test, erythrocyte sedimentation rate, and cultures of the cervical and vaginal discharge. Likely infecting organisms include *N. gonorrhoeae*, *Chlamydia*, *Mycoplasma*, *Ureaplasma*, and gram-negative enterics and anaerobes. Outpatient treatment includes ofloxacin or levofloxacin with or without metronidazole. Ceftriaxone, or cefoxitin plus probenecid or another third-generation parenteral cephalosporin (ceftizoxime or cefotaxime), followed by doxycycline with or without metronidazole can also be used. Amoxicillin, ampicillin, and erythromycin are not considered alternatives to outpatient treatment. Complications of PID include peritonitis, increased risk of ectopic pregnancy, infertility, rupture of tuboovarian abscess, adnexal torsion, and bowel obstruction secondary to adhesions and septicemia.

Woodward C, Fisher MA. Drug treatment of common STDs (Part II). Vaginal infections, pelvic inflammatory disease and genital warts. *Am Fam Physician*. 1999;60:1716–1722.

Beers MH, Porter RS, eds. *The Merck manual of diagnosis and therapy*, Merck Research Laboratories, 18th ed. Whitehouse Station, NJ: Merck & Co.; 2006:2088.

Pelvic inflammatory disease (PID) should be considered in sexually active females who present with lower abdominal pain.

Options 195–209

Answers: 195. T 196. F 197. F 198. T 199. F 200. T 201. T 202. T 203. T 204. T 205. T 206. F 207. F 208. T 209. T

Asthma is a common problem managed by family physicians. Symptoms include cough, dyspnea, and wheezing. Wheezing may be heard with the stethoscope; some may hear it unaided. Patients with severe asthma experience such intense bronchoconstriction that wheezing is inaudible at presentation and noted only after initial treatment. Factors that trigger an asthma attack include environmental allergens (e.g., pollen, molds, pollution), hot and humid or cold conditions, exercise, and barometric changes. Important aspects of the patient's history are triggering factors, severity of symptoms, frequency of attacks, and family history of asthma. Physical findings consist of rhonchi, wheezing, and a reversal of the normal 2:1 inspiratory–expiratory ratio. Other physical findings include nasal flaring (especially in young children), use of accessory muscles for breathing, cyanosis, and altered mental status in severe cases. The initial workup should include CBC determination to rule out infection, chest x-ray, and pulmonary function tests. Initial treatment for mild asthma entails avoidance of triggering factors, proper immunization for influenza and *Pneumococcus*, monitoring of peak-flow rates, and the use of inhaled β_2 agonists. Patients with persistent asthma require medications that provide long-term control of their disease in addition to drugs that give quick relief of symptoms. Medications for long-term control of asthma include inhaled corticosteroids, cromolyn, nedocromil, leukotriene modifiers, and long-acting bronchodilators. Inhaled corticosteroids remain the most effective anti-inflammatory medications in the treatment of asthma. Quick-relief medications include the short-acting β_2 agonists. The frequent use of quick-relief medications indicates poor asthma control and the need for larger doses of drugs that provide long-term control of asthma. Guidelines from the National Asthma Education and Prevention Program Expert Panel recommend an aggressive "step-care" approach. In this approach, therapy is instituted at a step higher than the patient's current level of asthma severity, with a gradual "step down" in therapy once control is achieved. Theophylline, oral steroids, and anticholinergics are generally not considered first-line therapy.

Kasper DL, Braunwald E, Fauci AS, et al., eds. *Harrison's principles of internal medicine,* 16th ed. New York: McGraw-Hill; 2005:1515–1516.

> Inhaled corticosteroids remain the most effective anti-inflammatory medications in the treatment of asthma.

Options 210–229

Answers: 210. F 211. F 212. F 213. T 214. F 215. F 216. F 217. T 218. T 219. T 220. T 221. F 222. F 223. T 224. T 225. T 226. T 227. T 228. F 229. T

Panic disorder is a distressing and debilitating condition with a familial tendency; it may be associated with situational (agoraphobic) avoidance. The diagnosis of panic disorder requires recurrent, unexpected panic attacks and at least one of the following characteristics:

- persistent concern about having an additional attack (anticipatory anxiety)
- worry about the implications of an attack or its consequences (e.g., a catastrophic medical or mental consequence)
- making a significant change in behavior as a consequence of the attacks

No organic factor is found to account for the symptoms, which may include dyspnea, dizziness, light-headedness, palpitations, trembling, sweating, choking, nausea or abdominal discomfort, paresthesias, chest discomfort, and fear of uncontrolled behavior. Workup should be focused and must be adequate enough to rule out underlying organic disorders. In this case, a Holter monitor may help to reassure the patient and physician that there are no cardiac arrhythmias contributing to the patient's symptoms. Other testing listed would be considered excessive. Questioning the patient about drug use, alcohol abuse, and the use of diet pills is necessary; many of the symptoms may be similar to those of panic disorder and panic attacks. Extensive and exhaustive workups are unnecessary and should be avoided. Treatment involves the use of tricyclic antidepressants, serotonin reuptake inhibitors, high-potency benzodiazepines, and, for resistant cases, monoamine oxidase inhibitors. The serotonin reuptake inhibitors are an appropriate first consideration. A high-potency benzodiazepine given at the minimum therapeutic dose may be a useful adjunct to antidepressant therapy if prompt relief is indicated. However, the treatment plan should include discontinuing the benzodiazepine when the antidepressant's maximal effects are expected (i.e., approximately 4–6 weeks) to minimize the risks of discontinuation difficulties that are associated with the benzodiazepines. Further treatment should focus on educating the patient about the disorder and the types of symptoms to expect. The physician should also help identify support systems in the patient's life. If further counseling and medication are unsuccessful, psychiatric referral may be necessary.

Kasper DL, Braunwald E, Fauci AS, et al., eds. *Harrison's principles of internal medicine,* 16th ed. New York: McGraw-Hill; 2005:2547.

> The diagnosis of panic disorder requires recurrent, unexpected panic attacks and at least one of the following characteristics: persistent concern about having an additional attack (anticipatory anxiety), worry about the implications of an attack or its consequences (e.g., a catastrophic medical or mental consequence), and making a significant change in behavior as a consequence of the attacks. No organic factor is found to account for the symptoms.

Options 230–244

Answers: 230. F 231. F 232. T 233. T 234. F 235. F 236. F 237. T 238. T 239. F 240. F 241. T 242. T 243. T 244. F

Temporal arteritis (also known as *giant cell arteritis*) is seen predominantly in elderly patients. Women are more commonly affected than men. The condition results from inflammation of the cranial arteries; veins are usually spared. Symptoms include severe headache, temporal tenderness, claudication of the jaw muscles, and visual disturbances, including amaurosis fugax, diplopia, scotomas, ptosis, and visual blurring. Untreated, the condition may lead to blindness. Other symptoms may include generalized arthralgias, low-grade fevers, weight loss, and generalized fatigue. Physical examination usually shows temporal artery tenderness, and the temporal artery may be palpable. Eye examination may show loss of disk margins and hemorrhages. Laboratory testing reveals a normocytic, normochromic anemia and a markedly elevated erythrocyte sedimentation rate (often >100 mm/hour). Definitive diagnosis is made by temporal artery biopsy. Treatment to prevent blindness should begin once the diagnosis is suspected. Treatment consists of high-dose steroid therapy (prednisone, 60 mg/day). This high-dose therapy is usually maintained for 2 to 4 weeks and is then tapered gradually. In many cases, the steroid taper takes months; in some, it may take years. If symptoms flare with reduction of steroid dose, the dose should be increased until symptoms are controlled, followed by continuation of a slow taper.

Beers MH, Porter RS, eds. *The Merck manual of diagnosis and therapy*, Merck Research Laboratories, 18th ed. Whitehouse Station, NJ: Merck & Co.; 2006:2547.

> Laboratory testing for temporal arteritis reveals a normocytic, normochromic anemia and a markedly elevated erythrocyte sedimentation rate (often >100 mm/hour).

Options 245–259

Answers: 245. T 246. F 247. T 248. T 249. F 250. F 251. F 252. F 253. T 254. T 255. F 256. F 257. T 258. F 259. T

Traveler's diarrhea affects as many as 30% to 50% of travelers who visit Third-World countries. Common pathogens in traveler's diarrhea include enterotoxigenic *Escherichia coli, Campylobacter, Shigella, Salmonella, Yersinia*, and many other species. Viruses and protozoa are the cause in many cases. Those who travel abroad should avoid drinking water in developing countries. If used, the water must be boiled for at least 10 minutes. Filters are not recommended because small viruses can often pass through the filter pores. In addition, travelers should be advised to avoid street vendors, peel all fruit before eating, and avoid using the water for brushing teeth. Ice cubes can also be contaminated and should be avoided. Carbonated beverages are generally considered safe. The use of prophylactic antibiotics is not recommended for travel abroad except in some circumstances, which may include business executives scheduled for important business meetings that cannot be missed or for professional entertainers performing abroad who also cannot afford to suffer from traveler's diarrhea. Although drug prophylaxis is discouraged, treatment with loperamide (in the absence of dysentery) and a fluoroquinolone, such as ciprofloxacin, is usually safe and effective in adults with traveler's diarrhea. Trimethoprim-sulfamethoxazole and doxycycline are alternatives, but resistance increasingly limits their usefulness. Antibiotic treatment is best reserved for cases that fail to respond to loperamide quickly. Bismuth subsalicylate (Pepto-Bismol), four times a day (taken with meals and in the evening), can prevent traveler's diarrhea.

Kasper DL, Braunwald E, Fauci AS, et al., eds. *Harrison's principles of internal medicine,* 16th ed. New York: McGraw-Hill; 2005:758–759.

> Filters are not recommended for the prevention of traveler's diarrhea because small viruses can often pass through the filter pores.

Chapter 9

Clinical Problem Set 2

QUESTIONS

The following questions are designed to assess clinical problem-solving skills. For each option, select either "T" for true or "F" for false. All options are related to the specific clinical case provided. There is no penalty for guessing; however, if "T" and "F" are both marked, the response will be scored as incorrect.

PATIENT A

Options 1–9

An 85-year-old nursing home patient resides at a nursing home. You are the medical director for the facility. The facility is about to undergo a state inspection and you have been reviewing guidelines for the care of nursing home patients.

Which of the following is true?

1. Patients who are admitted to a nursing home must undergo a comprehensive evaluation at the time of admission.
2. Patients should be restrained if they are confused or wander to protect their safety.
3. An attempt to taper or discontinue psychiatric medications should not be attempted because of the risk of psychosis.
4. A Minimal Data Set (MDS) typically is filled out by nursing home staff within 14 days of admission and subsequently on a quarterly basis.

Just before Thanksgiving, you are called by the Director of Nursing about an outbreak of influenza A in the facility.

Which of the following is appropriate?

5. Infection can be rapidly detected with a blood test that looks for antibodies to influenza A.
6. Amantadine can be used for prophylaxis in exposed contacts.
7. Rimantadine can be used for prophylaxis and is associated with fewer side effects than amantadine.
8. All nursing home residents should receive prophylaxis with medication regardless if they have been exposed to the virus.
9. A decline in functional status can signal an influenza infection.

PATIENT B

Options 10–24

A 28-year-old married woman with four children presents to the emergency room with abdominal pain and cramping, which has been present for 3 months. The patient describes episodes of diarrhea alternating with constipation and a 10-lb weight loss over the last 8 weeks. Mild dysuria over the last few days without back pain or fever has been noted. The patient has no new sexual partners or previous surgeries. Her last menstrual period was 6 weeks ago; periods have otherwise been normal. Physical examination, including pelvic examination, is unremarkable except for some mild right upper abdominal pain (without peritoneal signs).

Appropriate diagnostic tests at this point include

10. urinalysis with culture and sensitivity
11. pregnancy test
12. computed tomography (CT) scan of the abdomen
13. ultrasound of the right upper quadrant
14. stool hemoccult testing
15. intravenous pyelography

The initial workup is unremarkable. Further review of her history reveals a fractured wrist 6 months ago from a fall when she tripped on the stairs. The medical assistant also reports that there is mild ecchymosis affecting her left cheek, which she has covered with makeup. When questioned about this finding, the patient reports that her child hit her with a baseball, and she appears uncomfortable when asked the question.

Further questioning of this patient should include

16. a family history of bleeding disorders
17. discussion of possible spousal abuse
18. drug and alcohol history
19. history of child abuse affecting the family
20. discussion of the patient's support system at home

Further management of this patient may involve

21. hospitalization
22. social service consult

23. referral to a gynecologist
24. frequent follow-up visits in your office

PATIENT C

Options 25–34

A 5-year-old girl is brought to your office by her mother. The mother reports that the child has had vulvar itching and irritation for the last 5 days. The patient's mother denies any prior symptoms or vaginal discharge and reports no pain with urination. Bowel movements have been normal. The patient's mother denies any history of child or sexual abuse, and the child's history is otherwise unremarkable. The patient has no history of recent trauma to the pelvic area.

The initial workup of this patient should include

25. Papanicolaou smear
26. vaginal cultures for chlamydia
27. intravenous pyelography
28. digital vaginal examination
29. biopsy of the irritated area

Treatment of this child should include

30. topical estrogen cream application
31. administration of oral sulfa-containing medication
32. a discussion of perineal hygiene
33. a report to child abuse authority
34. referral to a pediatric gynecologist

PATIENT D

Options 35–49

A 63-year-old banker presents to the emergency room with midsternal chest pain that radiates to the neck and left arm, as well as mild shortness of breath. The pain began at 6 a.m. and has been constant for the last 20 minutes. Physical findings include the following:

- *Vitals*: Temperature, 38°C; blood pressure, 160/92 mm Hg; pulse, 92 bpm; respirations, 20; weight, 245 lb
- *General appearance*: Nervous, diaphoretic
- *Head, ears, eyes, nose, and throat*: Negative
- *Neck*: Supple, faint left carotid bruit, positive jugular venous distention
- *Heart*: Regular rhythm, positive S_3 sound
- *Lungs*: Crackles in bases bilaterally
- *Abdomen*: Soft, mild, right upper quadrant tenderness
- *Pulses*: Intact and equal bilaterally
- *Rectum*: Hemoccult negative, positive hemorrhoids
- *Extremities*: 1+ pitting ankle edema
- *Neurologic*: Nonfocal

Initial assessment for this man should include the following:

35. oxygen saturation
36. chest x-ray
37. partial prothrombin time
38. cardiac enzymes
39. exercise echocardiogram
40. electrocardiogram

Which of the following medications can be used in the initial treatment of this patient?

41. Verapamil
42. Nitroglycerin
43. Aspirin
44. Heparin
45. Captopril

Coronary angiography reveals that the patient has multiple occluded coronary arteries. He subsequently undergoes coronary artery bypass surgery. Six weeks later he returns to your office for follow-up. He is doing well and has no complaints.

Important aspects of this follow-up visit may include

46. consideration of an ultrasound of the gallbladder, pancreas, and liver to rule out cholelithiasis
47. determination of cardiac risk factors and lifestyle modification
48. regular exercise program and diet modification
49. repeat cardiac enzyme tests

PATIENT E

Options 50–59

A 19-year-old college student presents to your office complaining of profuse vaginal bleeding for the past 7 days. She denies being sexually active. Her periods began at 12 years of age and they have been irregular with intervals ranging from 14 to 28 days. She does have a lot of cramping with her periods and she reports the flow is heavy. She denies any abdominal pain or urinary symptoms. On examination, she appears pale and afebrile, pulse is 118 beats/minute, and her respirations are normal. A pelvic examination reveals clots of dark blood in the vaginal vault and a normal-size uterus with a closed cervical os. There is no adnexal tenderness or masses and the ovaries are not palpated.

Which of the following tests would be appropriate at this time?

50. β-hCG level
51. CBC
52. Blood typing and screening
53. endometrial biopsy
54. coagulation studies
55. pelvic CT scan

Following your workup, you diagnose the patient with dysfunctional uterine bleeding.

Initial treatment may consist of

56. intramuscular medroxyprogesterone acetate (Depo-Provera)
57. dilation and curettage
58. high dose intravenous estrogen
59. bromocriptine

PATIENT F

Options 60–74

An 82-year-old female nursing home patient complains of dysuria and urinary frequency. She has no fevers and no nausea or vomiting. Physical examination shows mild suprapubic tenderness but no costovertebral tenderness. A dipstick urinalysis is positive for leukocyte esterase, nitrite, and white and red blood cells.

Diagnostic tests that are appropriate for this patient include

60. intravenous pyelography
61. renal ultrasound

62. urine culture and sensitivity
63. urine cytology
64. complete blood cell count (CBC) with differential

Appropriate treatment medication for this patient includes

65. amoxicillin (Amoxil)
66. trimethoprim-sulfamethoxazole (Bactrim, Septra)
67. nitrofurantoin (Macrodantin)
68. erythromycin (EES)
69. ciprofloxacin (Cipro)

Six months after treatment, the nursing staff calls once again to report that the patient has cloudy urine. The patient complains of no further symptoms.

Appropriate management at this point includes

70. urologic referral
71. cystoscopy
72. urine culture and sensitivity
73. renal ultrasound
74. observation

PATIENT G

Options 75–86

A 60-year-old farmer who has smoked 2 packs of cigarettes/day for 45 years presents to your office complaining of exertional dyspnea that has been gradually worsening over the past year. The patient reports that he can only walk halfway across his cornfield before he gets short of breath. He has also noted a gradually increasing productive cough that is pronounced in the morning and has been present for at least a year.

Physical examination and diagnostic tests reveal the following:

- *Temperature*: 37.0°C (98.6°F)
- *Pulse*: 78 bpm, regular
- *Blood pressure*: 120/86 mm Hg
- *Respirations*: 20/minute
- *Heart*: Regular rate and rhythm (heard sounds distant)
- *Chest*: Barrel shaped, decreased breath sounds
- *Extremities*: No edema
- *Chest x-ray*: Normal heart size, flattened diaphragm, prominent pulmonary arteries
- *Arterial blood gases on room air*: Partial pressure of oxygen (PaO_2), 62 mm Hg; partial pressure of carbon dioxide ($PaCO_2$), 44 mm Hg; pH, 7.41; hemoglobin, 14.8 g/dL
- *Pulmonary function tests*: Vital capacity, 3.16 L (predicted 3.50 L); forced expiratory volume in 1 second (FEV_1), 1.78 L (predicted 2.45); FEV_1/FVC, 56% (predicted >70%)

Initial treatment would consist of

75. oral furosemide (Lasix)
76. yearly influenza vaccine
77. intravenous antibiotics
78. counseling for smoking cessation
79. prednisone taper
80. pneumovax vaccination
81. ipratropium bromide (Atrovent) inhaler

Six months after his initial visit, the patient returns, complaining of chills, fever, productive cough with green sputum, dyspnea, and generalized weakness. You decide to admit the patient.

Appropriate medications may include

82. metronidazole
83. nebulized albuterol
84. cefuroxime
85. methylprednisolone
86. erythromycin

PATIENT H

Options 87–96

A 2-year-old boy is brought into your office. The mother reports that the child has a fever to 104.5°F. The child also has been vomiting and has increasing lethargy. Physical examination shows an inactive child with dry mucous membranes and a positive Brudzinski's sign.

Which of the following would be considered a likely diagnosis?

87. streptococcal pharyngitis
88. viral gastroenteritis
89. dehydration
90. bacterial meningitis
91. giardiasis

Appropriate treatment for this child includes

92. oral amoxicillin
93. oral rehydration
94. intravenous rehydration
95. intravenous administration of ceftriaxone (Rocephin)
96. intravenous administration of erythromycin

PATIENT I

Options 97–105

A 42-year-old school teacher who presents with a 3-month history of difficulty with sleeping and predominantly early morning awakenings with a loss of appetite and 10-lb weight loss and lack of interest in her usual activities. She is recently divorced. She has had at least two documented episodes of depression in the past requiring medication that she stopped on her own after several months of therapy. She states she does not smoke and consumes one glass of wine nightly. She takes atorvastatin for her cholesterol. Her physical examination is unremarkable. Laboratory tests including thyroid testing are normal.

Prior to starting the patient on an antidepressant, which of the following would be considered appropriate?

97. An MRI of the brain
98. Neuropsychometric testing
99. Discussing with the patient that alcohol may interrupt sleep patterns
100. Discontinuing atovastatin
101. Inquiry about suicidal thoughts or plans

She returns to your office 6 weeks later reporting significant improvement, and she is tolerating the medication without difficulty. Continued management for this patient includes

102. long-term psychoanalytic therapy
103. life-long antidepressant therapy
104. tapering and discontinuing the antidepressant medication
105. consideration of electroconvulsant therapy (ECT)

PATIENT J

Options 106–115

A 59-year-old secretary with a history of hyperlipidemia presents to your office complaining of severe upper abdominal pain, which has been present for the last 6 months. The patient describes the pain as periodic in nature, worse after meals, and associated with nausea and vomiting. Over the course of the last 4 months she has lost 15 lb. The patient has many responsibilities with work, but denies any excessive stress. The patient's medical history is unremarkable except for two uncomplicated vaginal deliveries and tobacco abuse. The abdomen is soft, with mild, diffuse, upper abdominal discomfort with palpation but no peritoneal signs. No masses are present, and the rest of the examination is unremarkable.

Which of the following initial tests would be appropriate for this patient?

106. Magnetic resonance imaging of the abdomen
107. CT scan of the abdomen
108. Ultrasound of the liver, pancreas, and gallbladder
109. Upper gastrointestinal series
110. Renal ultrasound

After further evaluation, the patient's tests are found to be normal except for mild bowel wall inflammation. Hemoccult stool samples are negative.

Appropriate management at this point would include

111. ultrasound of the abdominal vessels
112. exploratory laparotomy
113. elective cholecystectomy
114. endoscopic retrograde cholangiopancreatography
115. observation

PATIENT K

Options 116–125

A 34-year-old man presents with facial pain, sinus congestion, a productive cough of greenish-yellow sputum, fever to 101°F, and generalized fatigue. Physical findings include the following:

- *Appearance*: Mildly to moderately ill
- *Weight*: 185 lb
- *Eyes*: Pupils equal, round, and reactive; extraocular muscles intact
- *Ears*: Minimal erythema associated with tympanic membranes
- *Nose*: Bilateral mucosal thickening with positive maxillary sinus tenderness with palpation
- *Throat*: Normal tonsils and pharynx; postnasal discharge noted
- *Neck*: Shoddy anterior cervical nodes palpable
- *Heart*: Regular rate and rhythm
- *Lungs*: Clear to auscultation
- *Abdomen*: Soft, nontender, no hepatosplenomegaly

Further evaluation that is required for this patient would include

116. sinus x-ray
117. CT scan of the sinuses
118. otorhinolaryngology referral
119. sinus lavage
120. chest x-ray

Appropriate first-line treatment regimens for this patient would include

121. 875 mg amoxicillin orally, two times a day for 21 days
122. double-strength trimethoprim-sulfamethoxazole orally, two times a day for 21 days
123. 500 mg levofloxacin orally, once a day for 3 weeks
124. 500 mg cefuroxime axetil orally, two times a day for 3 weeks
125. 400 mg cefixime orally, once a day for 3 weeks

PATIENT L

Options 126–135

A 52-year-old man is brought to the emergency room after being found staggering and confused in a city park by the police. Vital signs include the following: temperature, 37.0°C (98.6°F); pulse, 96 bpm; respirations, 16/minute; blood pressure, 120/80 mm Hg. The patient has a strong smell of alcohol on his breath. He is disoriented, confused, and drowsy, but is able to be aroused. He is unable to ambulate because of his unsteady gait, and he has vomited three times in the emergency room. Ophthalmology examination shows six-beat nystagmus with lateral gaze bilaterally and bilateral sixth-nerve ophthalmoplegia. The remainder of his examination is unremarkable except for a sensory bilateral lower extremity peripheral neuropathy.

Appropriate initial management of this patient would include

126. drug screen
127. serum alcohol level
128. administration of intravenous glucose
129. arterial blood gas determination
130. administration of intravenous thiamine

After hospitalization, the patient's wife reports that he has recently lost his job, has become despondent, and has been drinking heavily. Two months ago, he attempted suicide with an overdose of over-the-counter medication.

Appropriate treatment of the patient would include

131. alcohol rehabilitation program
132. psychotherapy
133. antidepressant medication
134. major tranquilizers
135. electroconvulsive therapy

PATIENT M

Options 136–149

A 56-year-old state employee with a history of type 2 diabetes mellitus is seen in a follow up to a recent fasting blood test. She is overweight but has no history of cardiovascular disease. Her blood pressure is 138/86. She is on no medications at the present time. She has not seen a doctor recently.

Laboratory Findings

Hemoglobin A1C	8.2%
Total cholesterol	226 mg/dL
HDL cholesterol	46 mg/dL
LDL cholesterol	110 mg/dL
Triglycerides	265 mg/dL
Serum creatinine	0.6 mg/dL (normal 0.6–1.5)

Which of the following statements is true regarding this patient's condition?

136. Her diabetic management is under acceptable control.
137. Her blood pressure is acceptable.
138. Her LDL cholesterol is acceptable.

Which of the following medications should be recommended at this time?

139. A statin
140. An ACE inhibitor
141. Glucophage (metformin)
142. Insulin
143. β-Blocker

Other tests that are appropriate in this individual include

144. ultrasound of the kidney
145. urine for microalbumin
146. filament testing for peripheral neuropathy
147. treadmill exercise testing
148. ophthalmology evaluation
149. 24-hour urine for creatinine clearance

PATIENT N

Options 150–159

A grandmother presents to your office with her 2-year-old grandson. The child has been extremely restless, especially at night, and has been unable to sleep for the last 4 nights. The grandmother also reports that he has been scratching his genitalia and rectal area. Physical examination reveals a well-nourished, well-developed child with no abnormal findings other than excoriations around the genitalia and perianal area.

Workup at this time should include

150. skin biopsy of excoriated areas
151. Scotch-tape test
152. flashlight examination of the child's rectal area at night
153. CBC, including eosinophil count
154. stool cultures for ova and parasites

Appropriate treatment for this child includes

155. topical hydrocortisone cream
156. antifungal topical cream
157. mebendazole (Vermox)
158. pyrantel pamoate (Antiminth)
159. thiabendazole (Mintezol)

PATIENT O

Options 160–168

A 27-year-old woman (gravida 2, para 2) presents to your office with complaints of a 1-week history of vaginal itching and discharge. The discharge is present daily and is minimally foul-smelling. She is married and is using a diaphragm and contraceptive foam for birth control. She denies any extramarital affairs and does not suspect her husband of any. In addition, her husband has not reported any symptoms. Physical findings include the following:

- *Labia*: Mildly erythematous, no lesions noted
- *Vagina*: White vaginal discharge present in the posterior vault
- *Cervix*: Multiparous, nontender, no lesions
- *Adnexa*: No masses or tenderness
- *Rectal and vaginal examination*: Unremarkable

A urinalysis was performed showing 0 to 3 white blood cells (WBC) per high-power field, trace ketones, and no bacteria.

The differential diagnosis includes

160. vaginal candidiasis
161. vaginitis secondary to chemical irritation
162. herpes genitalis
163. human papillomavirus
164. bacterial vaginosis

A vaginal smear is obtained and shows the presence of clue cells under the microscope.

Appropriate treatment at this time would include

165. clotrimazole (Gyne-Lotrimin) vaginal suppositories
166. oral metronidazole (Flagyl)
167. intramuscular ceftriaxone (Rocephin)
168. oral trimethoprim-sulfamethoxazole (Bactrim)

PATIENT P

Options 169–178

A 26-year-old woman (gravida 1, para 0) presents to your office at 34 weeks' gestation after slipping on wet pavement and falling to the ground. On arrival, she reports some vaginal spotting and some lower abdominal cramping, which has been present over the last hour. She has noted fetal movement since her fall but is worried that she has had a miscarriage. Physical findings include the following:

- *Blood pressure*: 120/80 mm Hg
- *Temperature*: 37.0°C (98.6°F)
- *Pulse*: 96 bpm
- *Respirations*: 16/minute
- *Fetal monitor*: 150/minute with adequate variability and normal reactivity; two minor contractions in 1 hour
- *Heart*: Regular rate and rhythm
- *Lungs*: Clear to auscultation
- *Abdomen*: Soft, mild diffuse tenderness, no peritoneal signs

Appropriate management at this point would include

169. sterile speculum examination
170. continued external monitoring of uterine contractions and fetal heart rate
171. administration of magnesium sulfate
172. close observation with the patient in a left lateral decubitus position
173. emergent cesarean section

Appropriate laboratory testing may include

174. CBC with differential
175. Rh typing
176. Kleihauer-Betke test
177. amniocentesis for fetal maturity tests
178. obstetric ultrasound

PATIENT Q

Options 179–188

A 78-year-old woman presents to your office complaining of low back pain. She reports that she was planting flowers in her garden last week when the pain began. The pain is aggravated by twisting motions of the back and alleviated by lying still on a flat, firm surface. Physical examination reveals a thin woman who appears her stated age. Back examination reveals point tenderness over L1 vertebrae. Neurologic examination is unremarkable, and she has a negative straight leg–raising test. An x-ray of the spine confirms an L1 compression fracture.

Complications of this condition include

179. nerve root irritation
180. disc herniation
181. back pain for 6 to 8 weeks
182. urinary incontinence
183. peripheral neuropathy

Appropriate treatment for this patient includes

184. strict bed rest for 6 to 8 weeks
185. pain medications
186. gradual increase of activity as tolerated by the patient
187. vertebroplasty
188. laminectomy

PATIENT R

Options 189–198

An 18-year-old college freshman presents to your office complaining of a swollen, erythematous, and painful ankle. He has no history of trauma and states that the condition developed rapidly over the last 48 hours. He has no prior history of joint swelling.

The differential diagnosis may include

189. gonorrhea
190. Lyme disease
191. streptococcal infection
192. Reiter's syndrome
193. rheumatoid arthritis

Appropriate workup for this patient includes

194. CBC with differential
195. monospot
196. erythrocyte sedimentation rate
197. rheumatoid factor
198. joint aspiration with Gram's stain and culture of fluid

PATIENT S

Options 199–212

A 54-year-old obese woman presents with urinary frequency, polyphagia, and blurred vision. Her symptoms have gradually worsened over the last 6 months. Physical examination is unremarkable except for the patient's obesity and decreased pinprick sensation associated with the lower extremities.

Appropriate laboratory testing includes

199. fasting glucose
200. glycosylated hemoglobin
201. thyroid-stimulating hormone
202. urinalysis
203. antinuclear antibody
204. lipid profile

Test results confirm the diagnosis of new-onset type II diabetes mellitus.

Appropriate management of this patient should include

205. regular exercise
206. diet modification to promote weight loss
207. ophthalmologic evaluation
208. audiologic evaluation

After a 3-month trial of diet and exercise, the patient is started on oral medication.

Appropriate management would include

209. weekly monitoring of fasting glucose until the patient's glucose levels are well controlled
210. repeat glycosylated hemoglobin in 8 to 12 weeks
211. continued exercise and diet therapy
212. endocrinology referral

ANSWERS AND EXPLANATIONS

Options 1–9

Answers: 1. T 2. F 3. T 4. T 5. F 6. T 7. T 8. T 9. T

In the United States, as a result of the need to provide a systematic assessment for the basis of care planning in nursing homes, the Omnibus Reconciliation Act of 1987 (OBRA 87) mandated that nursing homes complete a comprehensive evaluation of residents at the time of admission.

Physical and chemical restraints are not the solution to wandering. They infringe on patient autonomy and, in the United States, violate OBRA legislation governing skilled nursing facilities. OBRA 87 defines a *physical restraint* as a device that restricts a resident's freedom of movement or access to his/her body and is intended to restrict movement of the resident. The federal regulations state that restraints (e.g., belts, vests, cuffs, bedrails) cannot be used without a physician's order and that physicians cannot order restraints without clear medical justification. Additionally, psychotropic medications should be reviewed on a regular basis, and an attempt should be made to reduce the dosage or eliminate the medication.

The minimal data set (MDS) typically is filled out by nursing home staff within 14 days of admission and subsequently on a quarterly basis. It can be a useful tool for the physician by providing valuable background information. In addition, if a problem is identified or triggered by the MDS, the companion Resident Assessment Protocols (RAPs) specify how the nursing staff should proceed. In the majority of nursing homes where the physician rounds only once every 30 or 60 days (as required by state law) and is often not available to evaluate an acute problem at its inception, these protocols help ensure good patient care.

Influenza virus is often brought into the nursing home by staff or visitors and spreads quickly among the residents who share rooms and eat in a common dining area. Hospitalization rates rise significantly during epidemics. Many who are frail develop cardiac complications, including myocardial infarction and congestive heart failure, and pulmonary complications, particularly bronchospasm and pneumonia (either due to influenza or from bacterial superinfection with organisms such as *Staphylococcus aureus*). Additionally, many nursing home residents affected with influenza infection experience a decline in functional status, including a decrease in independent functioning such as bathing, dressing, and ambulation. With this in mind, it is important to vaccinate both residents and staff against influenza in the early fall. If an outbreak of respiratory illness characterized by fever, nonproductive cough, and myalgias occurs, influenza should be suspected. Infection can be confirmed by culture of throat and nose swabs or more rapidly using an enzyme linked immunosorbent assay (ELISA). If influenza A is documented, all exposed residents should be treated with amantadine or rimantadine until the outbreak subsides. Rimantadine, although more expensive, is preferred over amantadine because it is less likely to cause delirium in frail nursing home residents. Neuraminidase inhibitors zanamivir (inhaled) and oseltamivir (oral) have been developed for the treatment and prevention of both influenza A and B with fewer side effects than amantadine and rimantadine. The neuraminidase inhibitors are a useful alternative to amantadine or rimantadine, particularly when influenza B is the source of infection or when there is resistance to these drugs. Additional infection control measures should be instituted in the event of an influenza outbreak and include avoiding new admissions to the affected units and limiting the movement of both residents and staff from affected to unaffected parts of the nursing home.

Gillick MR. *Medical care of the nursing home patient.* Up to Date, version 14.1. Accessed 5/19/06.

The minimal data set (MDS) typically is filled out by nursing home staff within 14 days of admission and subsequently on a quarterly basis.

Options 10–24

Answers: 10. T 11. T 12. F 13. T 14. T 15. F 16. F 17. T 18. T 19. T 20. T 21. T 22. T 23. F 24. T

Abdominal pain in young, sexually active females has an extensive differential diagnosis. Causes may include bowel-related conditions: infections, including appendicitis and gastroenteritis; irritable bowel syndrome or inflammatory bowel disease; cholecystitis; or peptic ulcer disease. Pelvic pathology may include ectopic pregnancy, torsion of an ovary, ovulation, pelvic inflammatory disease, endometriosis, and menstrual-related problems. Also, urinary causes, such as infection, renal stones, or interstitial cystitis, can be included in the differential. Appropriate initial testing in this patient includes electrolytes because of the diarrhea, a urinalysis with culture and sensitivity, stool for hemoccult blood, CBC with differential, liver function tests, alkaline phosphatase, lipase, amylase, pregnancy test, and abdominal x-ray. Because of the location of the patient's abdominal pain (right upper quadrant), an abdominal ultrasound would be appropriate to rule out cholecystitis. A CT scan of the abdomen and intravenous pyelography are not recommended at this point in the evaluation. The patient's history is also suspicious for spousal abuse. Further questioning of the patient should include a discussion about the possibility of abuse (spousal, sexual, or child), a drug and alcohol history, and a discussion about the patient's living arrangements and support network. The first step in the treatment of a patient who has been abused is to remove her from her dangerous environment and provide safety. Hospitalization is often used to ensure the patient's safety. The physician should make a social service consult to assist in follow-up, and the abuse should always be reported to the proper authorities. Once the patient is released from the hospital, it is important to arrange frequent and close follow-up.

Beers MH, Porter RS, eds. *The Merck manual of diagnosis and therapy*, Merck Research Laboratories, 18th ed. Whitehouse Station, NJ: Merck & Co.; 2006:94–98.

The first step in the treatment of a patient who has been abused is to remove her from her dangerous environment and provide safety.

Options 25–34

Answers: 25. F 26. F 27. F 28. F 29. F 30. F 31. F 32. T 33. F 34. F

Nonspecific perineal irritation (vulvovaginitis) in young girls is common and is usually caused by inadequate perineal hygiene. Excessive irritation by urine on the vulvar area or constricting clothing that does not allow proper ventilation usually causes vulvar irritation. The discharge is characteristically brown or green, has a fetid odor, and is associated with a vaginal pH of 4.7 to 6.5. Parents should be instructed to teach young girls to wipe the perineum from front to back after each urination. Children should wear cotton underwear, and underwear should be changed daily (and more often if exposed to moisture). Parents should be instructed to avoid bubble baths and strong soaps or creams that contain irritating perfumes. The child's perineum should be inspected by the physician; however, further evaluation is unnecessary unless initial attempts at treatment fail. Estrogen cream is used as the drug of choice for recurrent vulvovaginitis secondary to labial adhesions.

Behrman RE, Kliegman RM, Jenson HB. *Nelson Textbook of Pediatrics*, 17th ed. Philadelphia: Saunders; 2004:1828–1832.

Nonspecific perineal irritation (vulvovaginitis) in young girls is common and is usually caused by inadequate perineal hygiene.

Options 35–49

Answers: 35. T 36. T 37. T 38. T 39. F 40. T 41. F 42. T 43. T 44. T 45. F 46. F 47. T 48. T 49. F

Chest pain and associated myocardial infarction is a relatively common problem seen by family physicians. Patients usually present with shortness of breath and substernal pressure or pain that radiates to the neck or upper extremities. In many cases, the patient is anxious and diaphoretic. The physical findings (i.e., jugular venous distention, mild right upper abdominal distention secondary to hepatic congestion, S_3 heart sound, crackles in the lungs, and 1+ pitting edema in the lower extremities) in this patient reveal mild congestive heart failure in addition to a likely myocardial infarction. Initial assessment for this patient should include electrolyte panel, CBC, partial thromboplastin time, cardiac enzymes, oxygen saturation, electrocardiogram, and chest x-ray. Data from clinical trials suggest that troponin I and troponin T provide more prognostic information than the patient's demographic characteristics or the electrocardiographic findings at presentation. Myoglobin may be helpful for the early diagnosis of reperfusion. Troponin I and troponin T have been found to be highly cardiac specific and particularly efficient for the diagnosis of myocardial infarction. CK-MB subforms are also efficient for early diagnosis (within 6 hours) of myocardial infarction. An exercise echocardiogram is not indicated.

Medications that are used in the initial treatment of this patient include intravenous nitroglycerin, a vasodilator; aspirin, an antiplatelet agent; and intravenous heparin. A thrombolytic, such as streptokinase or tissue plasminogen activator, may be indicated in select cases. Percutaneous transluminal coronary angioplasty (PTCA) can be considered an alternative to thrombolytic therapy in patients with ST-segment elevation or new (or presumed new) left bundle branch block, provided that angioplasty of the infarct-related artery can be performed within 12 hours of the onset of symptoms or beyond 12 hours if ischemic symptoms persist. In addition, PTCA can be an alternative in patients who are within 36 hours of an acute ST-elevation/Q-wave or new left bundle branch block infarction who develop cardiogenic shock, are younger than 75 years, and in whom revascularization can be performed within 18 hours of shock. PTCA may be appropriate in other situations as well. Glycoprotein IIb/IIIa inhibitors (abciximab [Reopro], eptifibatide [Integrilin], and tirofiban [Aggrastat]) are used in combination with heparin in patients with a myocardial infarction who have some high-risk features or refractory ischemia, or both, provided that they do not have a major contraindication due to a bleeding risk. The drugs are given prior to revascularization. Captopril, an angiotensin-converting enzyme inhibitor that assists in the remodeling process of the myocardium, should be started once the patient's condition has stabilized. β-blockers should also be started if no contraindications (e.g., asthma, congestive heart failure) exist. Verapamil, a calcium-channel blocker, has negative inotropic and chronotropic properties that may exacerbate congestive heart failure, and thus is not indicated for this patient.

Appropriate follow-up management after coronary bypass surgery should include risk factor assessment and lifestyle modification, including establishment of a regular exercise program and diet modification. An ultrasound and cardiac enzyme testing in this patient are not indicated at the time of follow-up.

Morey SS. Practice guidelines: ACC/AHA guidelines on the management of acute myocardial infarction. *Am Fam Physician.* 2000;61:1901–1902.

Topol EJ, et al. Multi-year follow-up of abciximab therapy in three randomized, placebo-controlled trials of percutaneous coronary revascularization. *Am J Med.* 2002;113:1–6.

Troponin I and troponin T have been found to be highly cardiac specific and particularly efficient for the diagnosis of myocardial infarction.

Options 50–59

Answers: 50. T 51. T 52. T 53. F 54. T 55. F 56. F 57. T 58. T 59. F

After the diagnosis of pregnancy has been ruled out, the most common cause of vaginal bleeding in young women is dysfunctional uterine bleeding. Initial evaluation should focus on weather the patient is clinically stable. Some will need to be monitored in a hospital setting. Appropriate laboratory tests include a β-hCG level to rule out pregnancy, CBC, coagulation studies to look for a coagulopathy, and blood typing and screening in case transfusion is necessary. Dysfunctional uterine bleeding results from inadequate estrogen in the setting of a proliferating endometrium. Appropriate treatment in this patient consists of a combination oral hospitalization with administration of high dose intravenous estrogen. If bleeding does not stop, dilation and curettage can be performed. Following the cessation of bleeding, shedding of the endometrium can be triggered by the administration and withdrawal of medroxyprogesterone.

Goldman L, Ausiello D, eds. *Cecil textbook of medicine*, 22nd ed. Philadelphia: Saunders; 2004:1501.

Dysfunctional uterine bleeding results from inadequate estrogen in the setting of a proliferating endometrium.

Options 60–74

Answers: 60. F 61. F 62. T 63. F 64. F 65. T 66. T 67. F 68. F 69. T 70. F 71. F 72. F 73. F 74. T

Urinary tract infections in elderly women are usually manifested by mild suprapubic discomfort, dysuria, urinary frequency or hesitancy, and incontinence. Initial diagnostic tests should include a urinalysis with culture and sensitivity. Further testing based on these findings is unnecessary. Appropriate treatment may include amoxicillin, trimethoprim-sulfamethoxazole, and fluoroquinolones (e.g., ciprofloxacin). Erythromycin does not provide adequate coverage; nitrofurantoin has a high rate of adverse reactions in elderly patients and should be avoided. *Asymptomatic bacteriuria* is defined as the presence of more than 100,000 colony-forming units/mL of voided urine in persons with no symptoms of urinary tract infection. The largest patient population at risk for asymptomatic bacteriuria is the elderly. Up to 40% of elderly men and women may have bacteriuria without symptoms. Aggressively screening elderly persons for asymptomatic bacteriuria and subsequent treatment of the infection have not been found to reduce either infectious complications or mortality.

Screening for asymptomatic bacteriuria: a brief evidence update for the U.S. Preventive Services Task Force. Agency for Healthcare Research and Quality, 2004. Accessed online 8/2/2006, at: http://www.preventiveservices.ahrq.gov.

Aggressively screening elderly persons for asymptomatic bacteriuria and subsequent treatment of the infection have not been found to reduce either infectious complications or mortality.

Options 75–86

Answers: 75. F 76. T 77. F 78. T 79. F 80. T 81. T 82. F 83. T 84. T 85. T 86. T

Chronic obstructive pulmonary disease (COPD) is a common finding in long-term smokers. Symptoms include dyspnea, increasing cough, and generalized fatigue. The physical examination may reveal an increased anteroposterior chest diameter, decreased breath sounds, and distant heart sounds. Pulmonary function tests often show a normal or decreased FVC, decreased FEV_1, and decreased FEV_1/FVC ratio. Initial treatment of COPD would include the use of ipratropium bromide, pneumococcal and yearly influenza vaccination, and counseling concerning smoking cessation for those patients who continue to smoke. In this case, antibiotics, prednisone, and the use of furosemide are not warranted. On return, the patient has classic symptoms for a COPD exacerbation.

Initial therapy should focus on maintaining oxygen saturation at 90% or higher. Oxygen status can be monitored clinically as well as by pulse oximetry. Oxygen supplementation by nasal cannula or facemask is frequently required. With more severe exacerbations, intubation or a positive-pressure mask ventilation method (e.g., continuous positive airway pressure) is often necessary to provide adequate oxygenation. Inhaled β_2 agonists should be administered as soon as possible during an acute exacerbation of COPD. Use of a nebulizer to provide albuterol (Ventolin) or a similar agent with saline and oxygen enhances delivery of the medication to the airway. Orally administered β_2 agonists have more side effects than inhaled forms; therefore, oral agents generally are not used to treat exacerbations of COPD. Compared with β_2 agonists, inhaled anticholinergics such as ipratropium provide the same or greater bronchodilation. These agents have been shown to be beneficial in patients with COPD. Anticholinergics can be delivered by nebulizer or metered-dose inhaler. In inhaled forms, anticholinergics have few adverse effects because of minimal systemic absorption. Use of a combination product such as ipratropium-albuterol (Combivent) may simplify the medication regimen, thereby improving compliance. All patients without serious contraindications should receive systemic corticosteroids for severe exacerbations of COPD. The use of methylxanthines such as aminophylline and theophylline is controversial in patients with exacerbations of COPD. Although methylxanthines can be of some help in improving diaphragmatic function, they are potentially toxic and are associated with serious drug effects. With close monitoring and attention to potential adverse effects, methylxanthines may have a place in the treatment of patients who do not respond to other bronchodilators. Antibiotic therapy is directed at the most common pathogens, including *Streptococcus pneumoniae*, *Haemophilus influenzae*, and *Moraxella catarrhalis*. Mild to moderate exacerbations of COPD are usually treated with broad-spectrum antibiotics such as doxycycline, trimethoprim-sulfamethoxazole, and amoxicillin-clavulanate potassium. Treatment with augmented penicillins, respiratory fluoroquinolones, third-generation cephalosporins, or aminoglycosides can be considered in patients with more severe exacerbations. Newer macrolides offer coverage for atypical organisms. Metronidazole is not indicated in the initial treatment of COPD exacerbation.

Hunter MH, King DE. COPD: management of acute exacerbations and chronic stable disease. *Am Fam Physician*. 2001;64: 603–612, 621–622.

Pulmonary function tests associated with chronic obstructive pulmonary disease often show a normal or decreased FVC, decreased FEV_1, and decreased FEV_1/FVC ratio.

Options 87–96

Answers: 87. F 88. F 89. T 90. T 91. F 92. F 93. F 94. T 95. T 96. F

Bacterial meningitis is a serious and life-threatening problem that affects young children. The most common infecting organisms include *H. influenzae, Neisseria meningitidis*, and *S. pneumoniae*. In many cases, children present with signs of dehydration (e.g., dry mucous membranes, sunken fontanels, lethargy, and decreased urine output) secondary to vomiting and fever. Signs of meningitis include nuchal rigidity, headache, lethargy, and decreased feeding. Other signs of meningitis include a positive Brudzinski's sign (neck flexion in a supine patient results in involuntary flexion of the hips and knees) and a positive Kernig's sign (attempts to extend the knees from a flexed-thigh position are met with passive resistance). Because neonates usually do not have meningismus, a change in the child's affect or state of alertness is one of the most important signs. The most sensitive and commonly used test that is currently available is the latex agglutination test, which detects the antigens of the common meningeal pathogens such as *H. influenzae* type b (Hib), *S. pneumoniae*, *N. meningitidis*, *Escherichia coli* K1, and *Streptococcus agalactiae*. The emergence of antibiotic-resistant bacterial strains in recent years has necessitated the development of new strategies for empiric antimicrobial therapy for bacterial meningitis. Specifically, the emergence of strains of *S. pneumoniae* that are resistant to penicillin and the cephalosporins have led to empiric therapy for patients with pneumococcal meningitis consisting of vancomycin with or without rifampin plus a third-generation cephalosporin pending susceptibility testing. Third-generation cephalosporins are also effective as empiric therapy against other pathogens that cause community-acquired bacterial meningitis, with the exception of *Listeria monocytogenes*, for which ampicillin or penicillin G is the antimicrobial agent of choice. Adjunctive dexamethasone should be administered to infants and children with suspected or proven *H. influenzae* type b meningitis to reduce audiologic and neurologic sequelae; administration concomitant with or just before the first dose of the antimicrobial agent is optimal for best results. Treatment must be initiated immediately with first suspicion. Oral administration of antibiotics is insufficient for treatment of this child. Erythromycin is not acceptable for the treatment of bacterial meningitis. Institution of recommended immunization has decreased the incidence of meningitis caused by *H. influenzae* type b, *S. pneumoniae*, and *N. meningitides*.

Tunkel AR, Scheld WM. Issues in the management of bacterial meningitis. *Am Fam Physician*. 1997;56(5):1355–1362.

Signs of meningitis include a positive Brudzinski's sign (neck flexion in a supine patient results in involuntary flexion of the hips and knees) and a positive Kernig's sign (attempts to extend the knees from a flexed-thigh position are met with passive resistance).

Options 97–105

Answers: 97. F 98. F 99. T 100. F 101. T 102. F 103. T 104. F 105. F

This patient has symptoms consistent with a diagnosis of major depression. When evaluating depressed patients it is imperative to ask about and document any suicidal thoughts or plans. Beyond normal screening tests including chemistry panel, complete blood count, and thyroid function tests, further workup is not necessary unless the history physical or baseline laboratory tests show abnormalities that suggest underlying disease. Alcohol may interrupt sleep patterns but atorvastatin should not have deleterious effects on this patient and does not require discontinuation of the medication. Neuropsychiatric testing would not be indicated in this situation. In the situation where the patient has had more than two episodes of major depression, the risk of recurrence is sufficiently high to warrant lifetime medication. Tapering and discontinuation of the medication is not indicated in this scenario. Although short-term psychiatric intervention may be helpful, long-term psychoanalytic therapy and electroconvulsant therapy (ECT) is not indicated.

Rakel RE, Bope ET, eds. *Conn's current therapy 2004*. 2004: 1161–1166.

When evaluating depressed patients, it is imperative to ask about and document any suicidal thoughts or plans.

Options 106–115

Answers: 106. F 107. T 108. T 109. T 110. F 111. T 112. F 113. F 114. F 115. F

Acute occlusion of the superior mesenteric artery is usually the result of embolism, acute thrombosis in a narrowed artery, or aortic dissection. Chronic occlusion most often stems from arteriosclerosis and less often from fibromuscular hyperplasia or external compression by mass lesions. Stenosis of the superior mesenteric artery causes postprandial abdominal pain (intestinal angina) that can result in significant weight loss. The pain is usually severe and begins 30 to 60 minutes after eating. Patients become fearful of eating, and weight loss, often severe, is the rule. Intestinal malabsorption may contribute to weight loss. Doppler ultrasonography of the superior mesenteric artery and celiac axis may accurately detect reduced flow through these vessels. Mesenteric arteriography is crucial in demonstrating the presence and severity of the occlusion and the suitability for surgery. Nitroglycerin may provide relief. In severely symptomatic patients, surgical revascularization of the superior mesenteric artery and celiac axis can usually be achieved. The differential diagnosis for this patient may include cholecystitis, pancreatic cancer, peptic ulcer disease, and lymphoma. Appropriate initial diagnostic tests would include CT scan of the abdomen; ultrasound of the liver, pancreas, and gallbladder; and an upper gastrointestinal series. Magnetic resonance imaging is more costly than CT imaging and is not recommended as an initial test. In addition, there is no evidence that this patient has renal dysfunction; therefore, a renal ultrasound would not be appropriate. Based on the patient's presenting symptoms and lack of findings with initial tests, appropriate further workup would include a mesenteric angiogram. Other options listed would not be considered appropriate at this point in the patient's diagnostic evaluation.

Beers MH, Porter RS, eds. *The Merck manual of diagnosis and therapy*, Merck Research Laboratories, 18th ed. Whitehouse Station, NJ: Merck & Co.; 2006:98–100.

Stenosis of the superior mesenteric artery causes postprandial abdominal pain (intestinal angina) that can result in significant weight loss. The pain is usually severe and begins 30 to 60 minutes after eating. Patients become fearful of eating, and weight loss, often severe, is the rule.

Options 116–125

Answers: 116. F 117. F 118. F 119. F 120. F 121. T 122. T 123. F 124. F 125. F

Acute sinusitis is a common problem seen in a family physician's office. Symptoms include facial fullness, purulent nasal discharge, fever, facial headache aggravated by bending forward, and usually a history of a recent upper respiratory illness. The sinuses are normally sterile. This sterility is maintained by factors such as the mucociliary clearance system, endogenous concentrations of nitric oxide, and immunologic defense mechanisms. Inflammatory swelling of the nasal mucosa can constrict the ostia and hamper sinus drainage. Predisposing conditions, such as a viral upper respiratory tract infection and allergic and nonallergic rhinitis, may cause edema that obstructs the ostia. Ostial obstruction often is exacerbated by anatomic defects, such as septal deviation, traumatic fractures, polyps, and concha bullosa (an aerated turbinate) that limit the dimensions of outflow channels. The environment within the enclosed sinus cavities then becomes hypoxic and acidic, providing a stable medium for the growth of bacteria such as *S. pneumoniae* and *H. influenzae*. The maxillary and ethmoid sinuses are the most developed in childhood and are the only sinuses that are large enough at birth to be clinically significant in rhinosinusitis. The sphenoidal and frontal sinuses are very small or nonexistent at birth and enlarge with age, becoming well developed by the ages of 7 and 12 years, respectively. Physical findings may include nasal mucosal thickening, sinus tenderness with percussion or palpation, purulent nasal discharge, and postnasal discharge. A reliable history and supporting clinical findings are all that are needed to make the diagnosis of acute sinusitis. First-line treatment is amoxicillin or a double-strength oral dose of trimethoprim-sulfamethoxazole for 14 to 21 days. Second-line treatment may include amoxicillin-clavulanate, cefuroxime axetil, or cefixime. Newer-generation fluoroquinolone antibiotics gatifloxacin (Tequin), levofloxacin (Levaquin), and moxifloxacin (Avelox) are effective against the usual pathogens that are responsible for acute rhinosinusitis but are often more expensive. Expectorants and decongestants have not been proved effective in amelioration of symptoms or in hastening cure of acute bacterial rhinosinusitis.

Semchenko A, Baroody F, Culpepper L. Management of acute sinusitis and acute otitis media. *Am Fam Physician*. Monograph No. 1, 2001.

The maxillary and ethmoid sinuses are the most developed in childhood and are the only sinuses that are large enough at birth to be clinically significant in rhinosinusitis.

Options 126–135

Answers: 126. T 127. T 128. F 129. T 130. T 131. T 132. T 133. T 134. F 135. F

Wernicke's syndrome is associated with alcoholism and consists of vomiting, horizontal nystagmus, unilateral or bilateral sixth-nerve ophthalmoplegia, fever, ataxia, and progressive global confusion. Initial evaluation of this patient should include a laboratory workup that includes electrolytes, glucose, arterial blood gases, hemoglobin, and WBC count. In addition, the patient should have a drug screen, serum alcohol level, and CT scan of the head to rule out other precipitating causes of confusion. The cause of Wernicke's encephalopathy is the lack of thiamine, which leads to progressive neurologic deficits. Therefore, before administration of glucose-containing fluids, thiamine should be administered immediately through an intravenous route. The patient should be monitored carefully for the development of delirium tremens and, on discharge, should be enrolled in an alcohol rehabilitation program. The patient also shows signs and symptoms that are consistent with major depression. Treatment should consist of antidepressant medication and psychotherapy. The use of electroconvulsive therapy is reserved for patients who fail medical management. The use of major tranquilizers is not indicated. Korsakoff's syndrome occurs in approximately 80% of patients with Wernicke's encephalopathy. Symptoms and signs include highly characteristic memory defects. Immediate memory is severely affected, but long-term memory is less affected.

Beers MH, Porter RS, eds. *The Merck manual of diagnosis and therapy*, Merck Research Laboratories, 18th ed. Whitehouse Station, NJ: Merck & Co.; 2006:1688–1689.

Wernicke's syndrome is associated with alcoholism and consists of vomiting, horizontal nystagmus, unilateral or bilateral sixth-nerve ophthalmoplegia, fever, ataxia, and progressive global confusion.

Options 136–149

Answers: 136. F 137. F 138. F 139. T 140. T 141. T 142. F 143. F 144. F 145. T 146. T 147. F 148. T 149. F

The guidelines for diabetes management recommend a hemoglobin A1C below 7%. Values in the 7% to 8% range are acceptable; however, values >8% require a change in management. Goals for blood pressure in diabetics have also been lowered based on new guidelines. Currently the goal is to maintain levels <130/80 mm Hg. Cholesterol goals include an LDL <100 mg/dL and the target may eventually be even lower. Clearly, this patient's LDL is above goal. Management for this patient would include a statin to lower cholesterol and ACE inhibitor for its reno-protective effect and also blood pressure reduction and the initiation of metformin (Glucophage), which may help the patient to lose weight and will help treat her diabetes. A β-blocker would not be first-line treatment for this individual. Further testing should include a "spot" urine for microalbumin, filament testing for peripheral neuropathy, and ophthalmologic evaluation. Although this patient is at risk for the development of kidney disease and cardiovascular disease the other tests listed would not be indicated.

American Diabetes Association: standards of medical care for patients with diabetes. *Diabetes Care*. 2005;28 (supplement 1): S4–S36.

The guidelines for diabetes management recommend a hemoglobin A1C below 7%. Values in the 7% to 8% range are acceptable; however, values >8% require a change in management.

Options 150–159

Answers: 150. F 151. T 152. T 153. F 154. F 155. F 156. F 157. T 158. T 159. F

Pinworm (*Enterobius vermicularis*) infections occur worldwide and are especially common in children. Humans are infected by ingesting the eggs, which are carried on the fingernails, clothing, bedding, or house dust. Eggs hatch in the stomach, and larva migrate to the cecum, where they mature into adult worms. Females migrate at night to the anal region, where they deposit eggs. Clinical manifestations include nocturnal anal pruritus and sleeplessness. Diagnosis is made by applying adhesive cellophane tape (Scotch-tape test) to the perianal area early in the morning and microscopic or visual examination for the worm or its eggs. Flashlight examination of the child's perianal area at night may also reveal the presence of a pinworm infection. Because tissue invasion does not occur in most cases of enterobiasis, eosinophilia is not observed. In addition, stool cultures may be difficult to obtain, are expensive, and are generally unnecessary for diagnosis. Treatment consists of mebendazole, albendazole, or pyrantel pamoate. Doses are repeated 2 weeks after initial treatment. In some cases, other family members may require treatment.

Behrman RE, Kliegman RM, Jenson HB. *Nelson Textbook of Pediatrics*, 17th ed. Philadelphia: Saunders; 2004:1159.

Because tissue invasion does not occur in most cases of enterobiasis, eosinophilia is not observed.

Options 160–168

Answers: 160. T 161. T 162. F 163. F 164. T 165. F 166. T 167. F 168. F

Bacterial vaginosis is a common diagnosis for vaginal irritation in women. The cause is usually a *Gardnerella* or *Trichomonas* infection. Symptoms include vaginal itching, irritation, and discharge that produces a characteristic fishy odor when mixed with potassium hydroxide. Microscopic examination of vaginal smears confirms the diagnosis if clue cells are present. The vaginal discharge pH is >4.5. The lack of lesions noted in this patient would exclude the diagnosis of herpes genitalis and human papillomavirus, although vaginal candidiasis and chemical irritation from the diaphragm or contraceptive foam should be considered. Appropriate treatment includes the use of oral or topical metronidazole or clindamycin.

Kasper DL, Braunwald E, Fauci AS, et al., eds. *Harrison's principles of internal medicine*, 16th ed. New York: McGraw-Hill; 2005:7767–7768.

When diagnosing bacterial vaginosis, the vaginal discharge pH is >4.5.

Options 169–178

Answers: 169. T 170. T 171. F 172. T 173. F 174. T 175. T 176. F 177. F 178. T

Minor trauma may occur in pregnancy and is usually benign. Complications include maternal anxiety, premature onset of labor, and placental abruption. The workup should consist of external fetal monitoring, sterile speculum examination, and laboratory tests that include CBC with differential, Rh typing, and ultrasound examination (to determine fetal well-being and assess for placental abruption). The Kleihauer-Betke test (to determine fetal-to-maternal hemorrhage) has been shown to have little use in the setting of acute trauma. The mother should be reassured to help relieve anxiety, and she should be monitored in a left lateral position for at least 4 hours. Delivery should not be attempted unless there is a life-threatening situation. Amniocentesis could be performed to confirm hemorrhagic amniotic fluid, but not to assess fetal lung maturity.

Cunningham FG, Gant NF, et al. *Williams Obstetrics*, 21st ed. New York: McGraw-Hill; 2001:1175.

The Kleihauer-Betke test (to determine fetal-to-maternal hemorrhage) has been shown to have little use in the setting of acute trauma.

Options 179–188

Answers: 179. F 180. F 181. T 182. F 183. F 184. F 185. T 186. T 187. T 188. F

Compression fractures of the spine are relatively common in elderly women who have osteoporosis. Vertebral crush fractures may develop with minimal or no trauma, usually in weight-bearing vertebrae (T8 and below); isolated fractures of T4 or above suggest malignancy. When symptomatic, the pain is of acute onset, usually does not radiate, is aggravated by weight bearing, may be associated with local tenderness, and generally begins to subside in 1 week. However, residual pain may last for more than 3 months. Multiple compression fractures eventually may lead to dorsal kyphosis with exaggerated cervical lordosis ("dowager's hump"). Abnormal stress on the spinal muscles and ligaments may cause chronic, dull, aching pain, particularly prominent in the lower thoracic and lumbar area. Fractures at other sites, commonly the hip or distal radius, usually result from a fall. Nerve root irritation and associated disc herniation with possible urinary incontinence are not usually associated with compression fractures. Pain may at times be severe and may require adequate pain medications. Patients should be encouraged to return to normal activities as tolerated once their pain subsides. Strict bed rest is contraindicated and may lead to progressive weakness. Surgery is not indicated, although treatment for osteoporosis should be considered. Vertebroplasty is beneficial in select cases.

Beers MH, Porter RS, eds. *The Merck manual of diagnosis and therapy*, Merck Research Laboratories, 18th ed. Whitehouse Station, NJ: Merck & Co.; 2006:306, 308, 325.

Nerve root irritation and associated disc herniation with possible urinary incontinence are not usually associated with compression fractures.

Options 189–198

Answers: 189. T 190. T 191. T 192. T 193. T 194. T 195. F 196. T 197. T 198. T

Septic arthritis can result from hematogenous dissemination of bacteria, contiguous spread of an osteomyelitis, or direct inoculation of microorganisms into the joint space as a result of penetrating trauma. Infectious arthritis, if untreated, can lead to irreversible joint damage. Symptoms of septic joint include acute onset of symptoms, history of previously abnormal joint, immunocompromised status, or intravenous drug use. Physical findings such as fever, warmth, and erythema over the involved joint, coupled with the absence of ligamentous or meniscal findings, suggest an infectious etiology. Radiographs are usually normal. The most important test is joint fluid evaluation. Findings that indicate infection include effusion, WBC count >50,000/mm^3 (50×10^9/L), organisms present on Gram's stain, and positive cultures. An elevated peripheral WBC and erythrocyte sedimentation rate also support an infectious process. Causative agents may include *H. influenzae* type b, *Staphylococcus aureus*, *S. pneumoniae*, and *Neisseria gonorrhoeae* (especially in sexually active adolescents). *Borrelia burgdorferi*, the causative agent of Lyme disease, may also cause septic arthritis. If the joint effusion recurs despite appropriate therapy, evaluation for fungal infection, tuberculosis, and Lyme disease should be undertaken. The differential in this patient should also include other conditions, such as Reiter's syndrome (urethritis, arthritis, and ocular inflammation) and early onset of rheumatoid arthritis. The workup should consist of a CBC with differential, erythrocyte sedimentation rate, rheumatoid factor, and joint aspiration with Gram's stain and culture of fluid.

Johnson MW. Acute knee effusions: a systemic approach to diagnosis. *Am Fam Physician*. 2000;61:2391–2400.

Septic arthritis can result from hematogenous dissemination of bacteria, contiguous spread of an osteomyelitis, or direct inoculation of microorganisms into the joint space as a result of penetrating trauma.

Options 199–212

Answers: 199. T 200. F 201. T 202. T 203. F 204. T 205. T 206. T 207. T 208. F 209. T 210. T 211. T 212. F

Type II diabetes mellitus (formerly called *non-insulin-dependent diabetes*) causes abnormal carbohydrate, lipid, and protein metabolism associated with insulin resistance and impaired insulin secretion. Insulin resistance is a major contributor to progression of the disease and to complications of diabetes. Obesity increases the risk for development of type II diabetes. Symptoms include polyphagia, urinary frequency, and often blurred vision. The diagnosis of diabetes is confirmed by two fasting glucose levels of >126 mg/dL. Initial evaluation usually consists of fasting glucose determination, lipid profile, thyroid function tests, and urinalysis. An antinuclear antibody test is not indicated. Most patients are given a trial of diet and exercise before initiation of medication if the fasting glucose is <200 mg/dL. In addition, the patient should be evaluated for end-organ damage with serum creatinine and ophthalmologic evaluation. Hearing loss is not routinely associated with the development of adult-onset diabetes mellitus; thus, audiology evaluation is unnecessary. Once medication is started, the patient should continue with diet and exercise modification. The patient should also be monitored regularly with fasting glucoses performed at least weekly until glucose levels are controlled and every 8 to 12 weeks with glycosylated hemoglobin determination. Glycosylated hemoglobin levels are not used to diagnose diabetes mellitus. In most cases, the family physician can successfully treat adult-onset diabetes mellitus without an endocrinology referral.

Beers MH, Porter RS, eds. *The Merck manual of diagnosis and therapy*, Merck Research Laboratories, 18th ed. Whitehouse Station, NJ: Merck & Co.; 2006:1275, 1279.

Glycosylated hemoglobin levels are not used to diagnose diabetes mellitus.

Chapter 10

Clinical Problem Set 3

QUESTIONS

The following questions are designed to assess clinical problem-solving skills. For each option, select either "T" for true or "F" for false. All options are related to the specific clinical case provided. There is no penalty for guessing; however, if "T" and "F" are both marked, the response will be scored as incorrect.

PATIENT A

Options 1–11

A 55-year-old female has recently been divorced and has moved to the West Coast to assume a sales position after losing her job with another company. Her children are in college and the rest of her family is located on the East Coast. She is under considerable financial strain after her divorce and her supervisor has been inquiring about her multiple days of unexplained absenteeism. She is having difficulty sleeping and trouble concentrating and often feels anxious. Other than some chronic constipation she is otherwise healthy.

Which of the following disorders may be present?

1. Depression
2. Panic disorder
3. Schizophrenia
4. Substance abuse
5. Generalized anxiety

Which of the following would be indicated for treating this patient?

6. SSRI antidepressant
7. Exercise
8. Tricyclic antidepressant
9. Short-term hypnotic [e.g., zolpidem (Ambien)]
10. Counseling
11. A long-acting benzodiazepine

PATIENT B

Options 12–26

A 6-month-old male infant is brought to your office by the parents for his 6-month well-child visit. The birth was a vacuum-assisted vaginal delivery. The child weighed 8 lb, 5 oz; Apgar scores were 8 and 9. The child has done well since delivery, and the parents have no concerns.

Which of the following developmental milestones are considered appropriate for this child's age?

12. Reaches and grasps objects
13. Sits alone without support
14. Crawls
15. Poor neck tone when pulled to a sitting position
16. Says "mama" and "dada"

Important anticipatory guidance recommendations at this age should include

17. advising the use of shoes
18. advising the use of an infant car seat
19. advising parents to keep a supply of ipecac syrup at home
20. advising parents to supplement feedings with whole milk
21. discussing the use of fluoride supplementation if indicated

Appropriate immunizations for the child would include

22. diphtheria-tetanus-acellular pertussis
23. polio immunization
24. measles-mumps-rubella
25. varicella
26. Pneumovax

PATIENT C

Options 27–41

A 3-year-old girl is brought to your office by her parents. They report that the patient has been complaining of left-sided ear pain over the last 24 hours. She has had a nonproductive cough and runny nose over the last week but has had no diarrhea or vomiting. Physical examination includes the following:

- *General*: Child is clinging to mother but appears alert.
- *Ears*: Erythematous, bulging tympanic membrane is noted on left with decreased mobility; right tympanic membrane appears unremarkable.
- *Nose*: Dry, crusted yellow mucus is present.

- *Mouth*: Membranes are moist; tonsils and pharynx are mildly erythematous; there are no exudates.
- *Neck*: Supple bilateral lymphadenopathy is present.
- *Heart*: Regular rate and rhythm.
- *Lungs*: Scattered rhonchi, no wheezing.
- *Abdomen*: Soft, nontender; no organomegaly.

Appropriate management of this child consists of

27. reassuring parents and continuing observation without further medical therapy
28. oral antibiotics for 10 days
29. analgesic ear drops
30. lumbar puncture with examination of cerebrospinal fluid
31. immediate hospitalization

After treatment, the child returns to the physician on three occasions in the next 6 months with similar symptoms.

Appropriate management at this time includes

32. antibiotic prophylaxis continued through the respiratory illness season
33. tympanocentesis
34. referral to an allergy specialist
35. hospitalization for intravenous antibiotic treatment
36. referral to ear-nose-throat specialist for tympanostomy tube placement

Complications of otitis media include

37. perforation of the tympanic membrane
38. hearing loss
39. mastoiditis
40. cholesteatoma formation
41. facial nerve paralysis

PATIENT D

Options 42–51

A 72-year-old previously healthy man presents to the emergency room with sudden onset of left-sided paralysis. The patient's wife reports that he was watching television when his symptoms began. The patient is confused, with a facial droop and increased reflexes on the left. Blood pressure is 190/108 mm Hg.

Appropriate initial management of this patient includes

42. laboratory tests, including complete blood cell count (CBC) with differential, electrolytes, and coagulation studies (prothrombin time: international normalized ratio and partial thromboplastin time)
43. immediate treatment with sublingual nifedipine to lower blood pressure to $<$140/90 mm Hg
44. initiation of intravenous heparin
45. emergent computed tomography (CT) scan of the head
46. electrocardiogram

Further studies confirm the presence of an evolving nonhemorrhagic cerebrovascular accident.

Appropriate treatment at this point consists of

47. hospitalization with telemetry monitoring
48. initiation of intravenous heparin
49. transesophageal echocardiogram
50. carotid ultrasound
51. neurologic consultation

PATIENT E

Options 52–62

A 42-year-old police officer presents to the emergency room complaining of left calf pain that has been present over the last 3 days.

Which of the following would be appropriate questions to be asked at the time of his evaluation?

52. Recent long flights?
53. Prolonged sitting?
54. Chest pain?
55. Shortness of breath?
56. Trauma associated with the leg?
57. Visual changes?

He is treated with anti-inflammatories and sent home. Ten days later he presents to your office complaining of shortness of breath. His vital signs include a respiratory rate of 26/min and a pulse of 115 bpm. Although he is having some respiratory distress, on examination you find his lungs are clear.

Appropriate tests at this time include

58. spiral CT of the lungs
59. sedimentation test
60. Factor 8 level
61. pulmonary function tests
62. pulmonary angiogram

PATIENT F

Options 63–79

A 17-year-old girl (gravida 1, para 0) presents to your office for an initial obstetric visit. The patient is at 8 weeks' gestation and unmarried. She admits to multiple sexual partners over the last 6 months and does not know who is the father of the child; she has decided to give the baby up for adoption.

Appropriate laboratory tests include

63. CBC
64. urinalysis
65. ABO blood type
66. serum α-fetoprotein
67. hepatitis B surface antigen
68. human immunodeficiency virus (HIV) antibody testing
69. cytomegalovirus titers

Tests show that the mother is Rh negative. Appropriate management includes

70. repeat antibody screen at 26 weeks' gestation
71. administration of 300 mg Rh_o (D) immune globulin (RhoGAM) intramuscularly if *no* antibody is present
72. administration of 600 mg Rh_o (D) immune globulin intramuscularly if antibody is present
73. after delivery, check the fetal ABO/Rh type, and if the infant is Rh positive, the mother receives 300 mg Rh_o (D) immune globulin intramuscularly within 72 hours
74. a Kleihauer-Betke test if fetal-maternal hemorrhage occurs during pregnancy

You remain concerned that gestational diabetes may develop.

Which of the following are risk factors for the development of gestational diabetes?

75. Maternal age younger than 20 years
76. Obesity
77. Family history of diabetes mellitus
78. First pregnancy
79. Smoking

PATIENT G

Options 80–89

A 62-year-old housewife with a history of depression and known diverticulosis presents to the emergency room complaining of vomiting, fevers, and left lower abdominal pain. Her last bowel movement was 4 days ago. Physical examination includes the following:

- *Head, ears, eyes, nose, and throat*: Oral mucosa dry, otherwise unremarkable
- *Heart*: Tachycardic
- *Lungs*: Clear to auscultation
- *Abdomen*: Soft, mildly distended; decreased, high-pitched bowel sounds; diffuse tenderness localized to the left lower abdomen with slight fullness noted
- *Pelvis*: Normal-appearing external genitalia, no cervical motion tenderness, no adnexal masses or tenderness
- *Rectum*: Positive hemorrhoids, stool guaiac positive
- *Extremities*: Unremarkable
- *Neurologic*: Nonfocal

Initial treatment of this patient should consist of

80. clear liquid diet only
81. morphine sulfate for pain control
82. contrast barium enema
83. administration of broad-spectrum intravenous antibiotics
84. colonoscopy

Three days after admission, the patient's condition has not improved, and she continues to have high fevers, left lower abdominal pain, and no bowel movements.

Appropriate management at this time includes

85. ultrasound of the liver, gallbladder, and pancreas
86. colonoscopy
87. CT scan of the abdomen
88. upper gastrointestinal series with small bowel follow-through
89. surgical consultation

PATIENT H

Options 90–104

A 17-year-old woman is brought to the emergency room after taking an overdose of acetaminophen. The patient's family reports that she has been distraught over the recent breakup with her boyfriend. On arrival, her vital signs are stable, and she is alert and oriented. Physical examination is unremarkable. Laboratory tests, including liver function tests and serum creatinine, are normal.

Initial management of this patient in the emergency room should consist of

90. gastric lavage
91. administration of sodium bicarbonate
92. administration of charcoal
93. administration of ipecac syrup
94. reassurance to the patient and family, with discharge home and close follow-up
95. hospitalization in a monitored bed

Four hours after ingestion a plasma acetaminophen assay is drawn. A significantly high value of 250 μg/mL is obtained.

Appropriate treatment should consist of

96. administration of intravenous deferoxamine
97. oral administration of acetylcysteine
98. intravenous steroids
99. hemodialysis
100. forced diuresis

The most common complications that are associated with acetaminophen toxicity include

101. renal failure
102. hepatic failure
103. tinnitus
104. peripheral neuropathy

PATIENT I

Options 105–121

An otherwise healthy 59-year-old factory worker presents with complaints of erectile dysfunction. His past medical history is significant for a prior appendectomy, mild hypertension, and benign prostatic hypertrophy. He denies any cardiac disease. He smokes 1 pack of cigarettes per day and drinks an occasional beer. His medications consist of terazosin (Hytrin) once daily. Occasionally, he has noted some low blood pressures but reports no syncopal or near-syncopal episodes.

An appropriate problem-focused exam should include

105. opthalmology evaluation
106. abdominal evaluation
107. evaluation of peripheral pulses
108. evaluation of pinprick sensation in the peripheral extremities
109. evaluation of deep tendon reflexes

Your findings are normal. Appropriate laboratory tests include:

110. fasting glucose level
111. lipid profile
112. erythrocyte sedimentation rate (ESR)
113. serum cortisol level
114. serum testosterone level
115. urinalysis

The laboratory tests come back normal. Which of the following may be indicated?

116. Sildenafil (Viagra)
117. Tadalafil (Cialis)
118. Vardenafil (Levitra)
119. Alprostadil (Muse)
120. Vacuum erection device (VED)
121. Monthly testosterone injections

PATIENT J

Options 122–135

A 47-year-old woman presents to your office complaining of generalized fatigue, insomnia, the inability to concentrate, and a 10-lb weight gain over the last 6 months. Her husband, a local politician, recently told her that he has been having sexual relations with a young intern at his office. The wife reports that she is not suicidal but is under a great deal of stress. She has had frequent crying episodes and mood swings.

Appropriate initial evaluation for this patient includes

122. CT scan of the head
123. CBC
124. thyroid-stimulating hormone (TSH)
125. sleep study
126. neuropsychometric testing

Further testing is unremarkable. Appropriate treatment at this point includes

127. inpatient observation
128. psychiatric counseling
129. electroconvulsive shock treatment
130. initiation of diet and exercise program
131. initiation of antidepressant medication

Four weeks after a selective serotonin reuptake inhibitor (SSRI) is initiated, the patient presents to the emergency room with agitation, anxiety, confusion, tremors, tachycardia, hypertension, excessive salivation, and hyperthermia.

Appropriate treatment consists of

132. increasing the dose of antidepressant
133. applying cooling blankets
134. administering diazepam (Valium)
135. stabilizing the patient, lowering the dose of the SSRI, and adding a nonselective monoamine oxidase inhibitor

PATIENT K

Options 136–145

You have been asked to perform sports physicals for the local high school football team. During these examinations, you discover a systolic murmur in a 16-year-old boy. The murmur becomes louder with Valsalva maneuver. The boy has neither cardiac symptoms nor a history of cardiac problems. He denies any family history of cardiac problems before the age of 50.

Appropriate management of this patient includes

136. reassurance to patient and parents with approval to play
137. recommendation of subacute bacterial endocarditis prophylaxis and limitation of the patient's playing time to one quarter per game
138. ordering a cardiolyte (sestamibi radionuclide) stress test
139. ordering an echocardiogram
140. allowing the patient to participate in noncontact sports only

Additional laboratory tests that should be checked include

141. electrolyte panel
142. fasting serum glucose
143. CBC
144. urinalysis
145. thyroid-stimulating hormone

PATIENT L

Options 146–155

A 65-year-old woman presents with a 20-lb weight gain over the last year, generalized fatigue, cold intolerance, dry skin, constipation, and problems with concentration. She denies being depressed but is concerned about her health.

Physical examination includes the following:

- *Head, ears, eyes, nose, and throat*: Unremarkable except for periorbital swelling
- *Neck*: Supple; thyroid unremarkable; no carotid bruits
- *Heart*: Regular rate and rhythm
- *Lungs*: Clear to auscultation
- *Abdomen*: Soft, nontender; no organomegaly
- *Pelvis*: Atrophic external genitalia; no adnexal masses or tenderness
- *Rectum*: Stool guaiac positive
- *Extremities*: Unremarkable
- *Neurologic*: Prolonged relaxation of deep tendon reflexes, otherwise nonfocal
- *Skin*: Hair is sparse; skin is coarse, dry, scaly, and thick

Appropriate laboratory tests include the following:

146. CBC
147. thyroid function tests
148. serum follicle-stimulating hormone level
149. serum estrogen level
150. antinuclear antibody

Laboratory tests confirm your suspicions. Further treatment of this patient may include

151. colonoscopy
152. initiation of levothyroxine
153. administration of propylthiouracil
154. administration of potassium iodide
155. administration of propranolol

PATIENT M

Options 156–165

A 93-year-old debilitated and bedridden nursing home patient is noted to have a sacral decubitus ulcer.

Contributing factors for the development of decubitus ulcers include

156. fecal incontinence
157. skin colonization by *Staphylococcus aureus*
158. inability to reposition oneself
159. poor nutrition
160. recent antibiotic use

Further care of this patient should include

161. use of a doughnut cushion
162. frequent repositioning
163. nutrition evaluation
164. débridement of necrotic tissue
165. application of topical antibiotic

PATIENT N

Options 166–180

A 31-year-old homosexual man presents to your office complaining of generalized weakness, malaise, anorexia, myalgias, nonproductive cough, and a 15-lb weight loss over the last 2 months. You suspect

HIV infection. A chest radiograph obtained by another physician shows bilateral interstitial infiltrates.

Appropriate laboratory tests at this time include

166. CBC
167. $CD4^+$ T-cell count
168. enzyme-linked immunosorbent assay (ELISA) for HIV antibodies
169. TSH
170. Western blot assay

Your suspicion is confirmed with further testing. The patient is HIV positive.

You explain that the following are considered modes of transmission from contamination:

171. blood
172. semen
173. vaginal secretions
174. breast milk
175. sweat

Which of the following can be considered in the treatment of HIV complicated with Pneumocystis infection?

176. Nucleoside derivatives (retroviral agents)
177. Protease inhibitors
178. Combination therapy (retroviral agents and protease inhibitors)
179. Trimethoprim-sulfamethoxazole (Bactrim, Septra)
180. Aerosolized pentamidine (Pentam 300)

PATIENT O

Options 181–194

A 46-year-old rancher presents to the emergency room. The rancher reports that he suffered a laceration to the right leg 1 hour ago while working on the farm. The laceration was caused by rusted barbed-wire fence. He does not recall having had a tetanus immunization within the last 20 years. Physical examination shows a 3-cm laceration that extends into the subcutaneous fat layer. Examination of the distal extremity reveals that tendons are intact and there are no neurovascular deficits.

Appropriate treatment involves

181. copious irrigation of wound site
182. exploration of wound site for foreign bodies
183. débridement of nonviable tissue
184. suturing of laceration
185. plastic surgery referral

Before treating the laceration, you instill lidocaine 1% with epinephrine to provide anesthesia to the wound site. In which of the following sites would you avoid the use of lidocaine with epinephrine?

186. Fingers
187. Nose
188. Penis
189. Toes
190. Neck

Appropriate immunization for this patient would include

191. tetanus and diphtheria toxoid only
192. tetanus immune globulin only
193. tetanus and diphtheria toxoid plus tetanus immune globulin
194. no further immunization

PATIENT P

Options 195–204

A 27-year-old nursing student presents to your employee health clinic after suffering a needle-stick injury. The student reports that she was assisting a laceration repair and was stuck with a solid-bore needle. The patient is reported to be otherwise healthy and has no known history of HIV or hepatitis B. The student is likewise healthy, but has not had hepatitis B immunization.

Which of the following statements is true?

195. The student is at more risk to have contracted HIV than hepatitis B virus.
196. The student is at more risk to have contracted hepatitis B virus than HIV.
197. The student is at equal risk to have contracted HIV as well as hepatitis B.
198. A solid-bore needle-stick is more likely to transmit HIV than a hollow-bore needle-stick.
199. A hollow-bore needle-stick is more likely to transmit HIV than a solid-bore needle-stick.

Appropriate laboratory tests for the student would include

200. ELISA test for HIV
201. Western blot test for HIV
202. antibody to hepatitis B surface antigen
203. hepatitis B surface antigen
204. immunoglobulin M antibodies to hepatitis B core antigen

ANSWERS AND EXPLANATIONS

Options 1–11

Answers: 1. T 2. T 3. F 4. T 5. T 6. T 7. T 8. F 9. T 10. T 11. F

This patient has undergone life events associated with major psychological stress including divorce, loss of job, relocation, and loss of support from friends and family. Based on her reported symptoms it is likely this patient may have depression, generalized anxiety with possible panic disorder, or substance abuse. Psychotic illness such as schizophrenia is unlikely. Appropriate treatment for this individual would include SSRI antidepressants. Because of her constipation a tricyclic antidepressant should be avoided. Other treatments may include regular exercise, a short term hypnotic to help establish a sleeping pattern, and counseling. Long acting benzodiazepines would not be appropriate at this time for this patient.

Moore DP, Jefferson JW. *Handbook of Medical Psychiatry,* 2nd ed. St. Loius: Mosby; 2004:176–177.

Tricyclic antidepressants can cause significant constipation.

Options 12–26

Answers: 12. T 13. T 14. F 15. F 16. F 17. F 18. T 19. T 20. F 21. T 22. T 23. T 24. F 25. F 26. F

A 6-month well-child visit should consist of evaluation of developmental milestones. Appropriate development in the child would include reaching to grasp objects, rolling over, showing no head lag when pulled to a sitting position, sitting without support, bearing some weight on the lower extremities, playing with feet, and laughing, squealing, or babbling. Crawling is usually not accomplished until 9 months of age. Saying "mama" and "dada" discriminately occurs at approximately 10 months of age. Appropriate anticipatory guidance counseling should consist of the use of infant car seats, the availability of ipecac syrup at home, and the use of fluoride supplement if indicated. The use of shoes is not necessary, and whole milk should be added to the infant's diet after 1 year of age. Appropriate immunizations for this child should include diphtheria-tetanus-acellular pertussis, inactivated polio immunization, *Haemophilus influenzae*, hepatitis B vaccination, and pneumococcal 7–valent conjugate vaccine (Prevnar). Measles-mumps-rubella (MMR) immunization is given at 12 to 15 months, and varicella is given after 1 year of age. Pneumococcal (Pneumovax 23) polysaccharide isolate vaccination is not given to children who are younger than 2 years old.

Behrman RE, Kliegman RM, Jenson HB. *Nelson Textbook of Pediatrics*, 17th ed. Philadelphia: Saunders; 2004:1174–1184.

> Saying "mama" and "dada" discriminately occurs at approximately 10 months of age.

Options 27–41

Answers: 27. F 28. T 29. T 30. F 31. F 32. T 33. F 34. F 35. F 36. F 37. T 38. T 39. T 40. T 41. T

Acute otitis media is a problem that is commonly encountered in a family physician's office. Symptoms include ear pain, fever, hearing loss, vomiting, and diarrhea and are commonly preceded by upper respiratory symptoms. The classic findings of acute otitis media, such as fever and earache, are sometimes absent even in cases confirmed by tympanocentesis. A bulging, red, immobile tympanic membrane is highly associated with acute otitis media. However, many physicians rely on redness of the eardrum as the main diagnostic clue. Crying (most young children cry when their ears are examined), removal of cerumen with associated irritation of the auditory canal, and fever can all cause redness of the eardrum in the absence of middle ear infection. Common bacterial organisms that are responsible for otitis media in this age group are *Streptococcus pneumoniae* (40% to 50%), *H. influenzae* (20% to 25%), *Moraxella catarrhalis* (10% to 15%), group A *Streptococcus* (2%), and enteric gram-negative bacteria (1%). *Mycoplasma pneumoniae* and various viruses are other causative agents. Acute otitis media is defined by the presence of symptoms of acute illness and signs (full or bulging) of a tympanic membrane under positive pressure. Otitis media with effusion is defined by the absence of symptoms and signs of acute infection (other than reduced hearing) and the presence of signs (retracted or neutral position) of a tympanic membrane under negative pressure or no pressure and fluid in the middle ear space. Antibiotics are traditionally indicated for acute otitis media but can often be appropriately deferred if otitis media with effusion is present. Treatment consists of antibiotic coverage (amoxicillin, trimethoprim-sulfamethoxazole, erythromycin-sulfisoxazole) given orally for 5 to 10 days (10 days being standard). Amoxicillin remains the antibiotic of first choice, although a higher dosage (80 mg/kg/day) may be indicated to ensure eradication of resistant *S. pneumoniae*. Oral cefuroxime or amoxicillin-clavulanate and intramuscular ceftriaxone are suggested second-line choices for treatment failure. Risk factors for resistant pathogens include recent antibiotic treatment of acute otitis media, children in daycare facilities, wintertime infections, and acute otitis media in children who are younger than 2 years of age. Compliance with antibiotic regimens is enhanced by selecting agents that require less frequent dosing (such as 1 or 2 times a day) and by prescribing shorter (5 days) treatment courses. Selective use of tympanocentesis if the patient does not respond to empiric therapy can help to confirm the diagnosis and guide effective therapy. Analgesic eardrops or oral analgesics may help to alleviate the patient's discomfort. Recurrent otitis media (three or more episodes in 6 months or four episodes in 1 year) can be treated with prophylactic antibiotics (amoxicillin, sulfisoxazole) and continued through the respiratory illness season. Recurrent otitis media despite prophylactic therapy requires evaluation by an ear-nose-throat specialist; tympanostomy tube placement may be needed. Complications of otitis media include perforation of the tympanic membrane, hearing loss, mastoiditis, meningitis, epidural abscess formation, cholesteatoma formation, facial nerve paralysis, language delay, labyrinthitis, lateral sinus thrombosis, and otic hydrocephalus.

Pichichero ME. Acute otitis media (Pt I). Improving diagnostic accuracy. *Am Fam Physician*. 2000;61:2051–2056.

Pichichero ME. Acute otitis media (Pt II). Treatment in an era of increasing antibiotic resistance. *Am Fam Physician*. 2000; 61:2410–2416.

> Risk factors for resistant pathogens in otitis media include recent antibiotic treatment, children in daycare facilities, wintertime infections, and acute otitis media in children who are younger than 2 years of age.

Options 42–51

Answers: 42. T 43. F 44. F 45. T 46. T 47. T 48. T 49. T 50. T 51. T

The initial management of a cerebrovascular accident consists of ordering laboratory studies: CBC with differential, electrolytes, pulse oximetry or arterial blood gas, glucose, prothrombin time/international normalized ratio, partial thromboplastin time, chest radiograph, and electrocardiogram. Before consideration of anticoagulation, an emergent CT of the head (magnetic resonance imaging is more sensitive for detecting infarction or masses, but CT is preferred because of the difficulty of obtaining a magnetic resonance image emergently) is necessary to rule out hemorrhage. It is important to correct hypertension slowly and gently after a cerebrovascular accident to avoid extending the infarcted area as a result of decreased perfusion pressure. Sublingual nifedipine should not be used. Once the stroke is determined to be nonhemorrhagic, intravenous heparin can be initiated if the patient is a candidate for anticoagulation and has a low risk for development of a hemorrhage. In some cases, patients may be candidates for thrombolytic therapy. The patient should be hospitalized and monitored for arrhythmias on a telemetry bed. Also, a transesophageal echocardiogram can determine if cardiac thrombi have developed; a carotid ultrasound can determine if carotid occlusive disease is present. Angiography may be necessary to confirm a carotid lesion. A neurology consultation is appropriate, and a physical therapist can be involved to help with the patient's rehabilitation.

Papadakis MA, McPhee SJ. *2006 Current Consult Medicine*. New York: Lange/McGraw-Hill; 2006:212–213.

It is important to correct hypertension slowly and gently after a cerebrovascular accident to avoid extending the infarcted area as a result of decreased perfusion pressure.

Options 52–62

Answers: 52. T 53. T 54. T 55. T 56. T 57. F 58. T 59. F 60. F 61. F 62. F

Risk factors for deep venous thrombosis (DVT) include prolonged sitting such as during long car rides or flights, surgery (especially orthopedic), family or personal history of coagulopathy, and malignancy. Symptoms often present with unilateral swelling usually of the lower extremity with or without discomfort. The major life threatening complication of DVT is pulmonary embolism. If a pulmonary embolus occurs patients may present with shortness of breath, tachypnea, chest pain, and tachycardia. The appropriate testing to order in this individual is a spiral CT of the lungs. Nondiagnostic pulmonary angiography can assist in confirming or alleviating the diagnosis but should be reserved until after a spiral CT is obtained.

Papadakis MA, McPhee SJ. *2006 Current Consult Medicine*. New York: Lange/McGraw-Hill; 2006:280–281.

Risk factors for deep venous thrombosis (DVT) include prolonged sitting, such as during long car rides or flights; surgery (especially orthopedic); and family or personal history of coagulopathy and malignancy.

Options 63–79

Answers: 63. T 64. T 65. T 66. F 67. T 68. T 69. F 70. T 71. T 72. F 73. T 74. T 75. F 76. T 77. T 78. F 79. F

Laboratory tests to be ordered with the first prenatal visit include a Papanicolaou smear, CBC, urinalysis and screen for bacteriuria, ABO blood type, antibody screen (indirect Coombs' test), Venereal Disease Research Laboratory (VDRL), rubella antibody titer, HIV testing, and hepatitis B surface antigen. When indicated, cervical cultures for gonorrhea and chlamydia should be ordered; in this case, because of the patient's multiple sexual partners, they should be included. The patient does not have risk factors for cytomegalovirus; thus, testing is unnecessary. A serum triple screen (α-fetoprotein, β–human chorionic gonadotropin, and estradiol) is measured at 15 to 20 weeks' gestation. Because of the patient's Rh-negative status, she needs repeat antibody screening at 26 weeks' gestation. If the test is negative, she should receive 300 mg Rh_o (D) immune globulin intramuscularly. If the test is positive for antibodies, she should be referred to a specialist. After delivery, it is important to check the fetal ABO/Rh type. If the infant is Rh positive, the mother should receive 300 mg Rh_o (D) immune globulin intramuscularly within 72 hours of delivery. If an Rh-negative mother has evidence of fetal maternal hemorrhage, a Kleihauer-Betke test should be obtained; this test measures the amount of fetal blood that has entered the maternal circulation. The dose of Rh_o (D) immune globulin that is required can then be calculated from this value. Risk factors for the development of gestational diabetes include maternal age older than 25 years, obesity, positive family history of diabetes, previous history of gestational diabetes, macrosomic infant or stillborn, and signs or symptoms of diabetes with glycosuria.

Cunningham FG, Gant NF, et al. *Williams Obstetrics*, 21st ed. New York: McGraw-Hill; 2001:1056, 984.

A serum triple screen (α-fetoprotein, β-human chorionic gonadotropin, and estradiol) is measured at 15 to 20 weeks' gestation.

Options 80–89

Answers: 80. F 81. F 82. F 83. T 84. F 85. F 86. F 87. T 88. F 89. T

The diagnosis of diverticulitis is suggested by abdominal pain that is initially hypogastric but then localizes to the left lower quadrant. Urinary symptoms may occur if the affected colonic segment is close to the bladder. A lower quadrant abdominal or rectal mass may be palpated, but associated rectal bleeding is uncommon and suggests an alternative diagnosis. Other symptoms include fever, constipation, or frequent defecation. Approximately 85% of cases of acute diverticulitis involve the descending or sigmoid colon; however, right-sided disease may also occur and is reported more frequently in persons of Asian descent. Abscess formation can occur and lead to bowel obstruction, which is characterized by vomiting, decreased or high-pitched bowel sounds, inadequate response to broad-spectrum antibiotic administration, and lack of bowel movements or flatulence. Previously, diverticular disease was diagnosed using a contrast barium enema. However, because of the possibility of an obstructing fecolith being dislodged by insufflation and causing bowel perforation, CT scanning is now the diagnostic procedure of choice. Besides being safe and cost effective, CT can also be used to assist percutaneous drainage of an abscess. Treatment of diverticulitis can take place on an outpatient basis for a patient with a mild first attack who is able to tolerate oral hydration and an antibiotic. Treatment consists of a liquid diet and 7 to 10 days of therapy with broad-spectrum antimicrobials such as metronidazole and ciprofloxacin. Patients with more severe illness (as seen in the example), those who cannot tolerate oral hydration, or those who have pain that is severe enough to require narcotic analgesia should be hospitalized. Patients should receive nothing by mouth and should be treated with intravenous triple therapy consisting of ampicillin, gentamicin, and metronidazole. Alternative monotherapy includes piperacillin or tazobactam. If narcotics are required for pain control, meperidine is recommended because morphine sulfate can lead to colonic spasm. If pain, fever, and leukocytosis do not resolve within 3 days, further imaging studies are indicated. If an abscess is present and is >5 cm in size, CT-guided drainage and adequate antibiotic coverage should be considered. Colonoscopy is generally not indicated in the initial treatment of diverticulitis. Complications of diverticular disease include bowel perforation and fistula formation. Bowel resection is usually recommended for recurrent episodes of diverticulitis or if fistulas are present. Resection with primary anastomosis is now the procedure of choice unless generalized peritonitis has occurred, in which case a two-stage procedure is usually necessary. Rarely is the older three-stage Hartmann's procedure required.

Kasper DL, Braunwald E, Fauci AS, et al., eds. *Harrison's principles of internal medicine*, 16th ed. New York: McGraw-Hill; 2005:1795–1796.

The diagnosis of diverticulitis is suggested by abdominal pain that is initially hypogastric, but then localizes to the left lower quadrant.

Options 90–104

Answers: 90. T 91. F 92. T 93. F 94. F 95. T 96. F 97. T 98. F 99. F 100. F 101. F 102. T 103. F 104. F

Acetaminophen toxicity is a potentially life-threatening condition. An oral dose of acetaminophen of ≥150 mg/kg in a child is considered toxic. In adults, ≥150 mg/kg acetaminophen or a total dose of 7.5 g, regardless of the mg/kg amount, is considered toxic. Symptoms are usually mild until 48 hours or more after ingestion and include abdominal symptoms as well as nausea and vomiting. Treatment at home can be initiated with ipecac syrup to induce vomiting. Once patients reach the emergency room, they should undergo gastric lavage with administration of activated charcoal. They should be hospitalized in a monitored setting and observed closely. Acetaminophen levels should be measured 3 to 4 hours after ingestion and plotted on the Rumack-Matthew nomogram. If the plasma level is within the high-risk zone (≥150 μg/mL), the patient should receive acetylcysteine (Mucomyst) orally or by gastric tube. Intravenous administration has also been used, but the U.S. Food and Drug Administration has not approved this route, and it is not commercially available. Repeated doses should be given every 4 hours. Forced diuresis may be harmful and is not helpful. Hemodialysis is ineffective. The use of steroids, deferoxamine, and sodium bicarbonate is not included in the treatment of acetaminophen toxicity. The most common complication of acetaminophen toxicity is hepatic failure. Patients with fulminant hepatic failure are often candidates for liver transplantation.

Beers MH, Porter RS, eds. *The Merck manual of diagnosis and therapy*, Merck Research Laboratories, 18th ed. Whitehouse Station, NJ: Merck & Co.; 2006:2658–2660.

When treating an overdose acetaminophen levels should be measured 3 to 4 hours after ingestion and plotted on the Rumack-Matthew nomogram. If the plasma level is within the high-risk zone (≥150 μg/mL), the patient should receive acetylcysteine (Mucomyst).

Options 105–121

Answers: 105. F 106. T 107. T 108. F 109. T 110. T 111. T 112. F 113. F 114. T 115. T 116. F 117. F 118. F 119. F 120. T 121. F

The evaluation of erectile dysfunction can be conducted with a problem-focused examination that includes examination of the breast, penis, testes, hair distribution, palpation of the peripheral pulses, and testing of the genital and perineal sensation. Laboratory tests that should be conducted in a fasting state include a urinalysis, CBC, serum glucose, creatinine, lipid profile, and testosterone level. In this scenario the patient is taking an α-blocker for his hypertension and prostate related symptoms and because of his borderline low blood pressure would not be a good candidate for treatment with phosphodiesterase type 5 inhibitors (sildenafil, tadalafil, vardenafil) because of the potential to cause hypotension. Additionally, alprostadil can also cause hypotension and would not be a good selection. Monthly testosterone injections would not be indicated in this patient because there is no evidence of testosterone deficiency. Of the following choices listed, a vacuum erection device is the only suitable option.

Lue TF. Erectile dysfunction. *N Engl J Med*. 2000;342(24):1802–1813.

Kasper DL, Braunwald E, Fauci AS, et. al., eds. *Harrison's principles of internal medicine*, 16th ed. New York: McGraw-Hill; 2005:273, 2188.

The evaluation of erectile dysfunction can be conducted with a problem-focused examination that includes examination of the breast, penis, testes, hair distribution, palpation of the peripheral pulses, and testing of the genital and perineal sensation.

Options 122–135

Answers: 122. F 123. T 124. T 125. F 126. F 127. F 128. T 129. F 130. T 131. T 132. F 133. T 134. T 135. F

Depression is often manifested by symptoms such as depressed mood, loss of interest or pleasure in all or almost all activities, significant weight loss or gain, decreased appetite, insomnia or hypersomnia, fatigue, diminished ability to concentrate, or feelings of worthlessness. Appropriate initial evaluation of the patient would include a CBC to rule out anemia (which can cause fatigue) and a measure of TSH to rule out thyroid dysfunction (which could cause similar symptoms). A CT of the head, a sleep study, and neuropsychometric testing are not indicated. Appropriate treatment for this patient would include psychiatric counseling, regular exercise, diet modification, and initiation of an antidepressant medication. Serotonin syndrome is a condition that is associated with the use of selective SSRIs. Symptoms include altered mental status, anxiety, agitation, confusion, hyperreflexia, myoclonus, diaphoresis, hyperthermia, abnormal neuromuscular activity, salivation, diarrhea, tachycardia, and hypertension. Seizures and death may occur. Treatment consists of managing adequate airway, breathing, and circulation. The patient should be rapidly cooled in the setting of hyperthermia, and serotonin antagonists (e.g., benzodiazepines, cyproheptadine, propranolol, methysergide) should be administered. The concomitant use of fluoxetine and nonselective monoamine oxidase inhibitors has resulted in the serotonin syndrome. Because of the long half-life of fluoxetine (2 to 3 days) and its active metabolite norfluoxetine (half-life of 7 to 9 days), fluoxetine interactions theoretically can occur weeks after the drug is discontinued. It is generally accepted that all combinations of nonselective monoamine oxidase inhibitors and SSRIs are contraindicated.

Ament PW, Bertolino JG, Liszewski JL. Clinically significant drug interactions. *Am Fam Physician*. 2000;61:1745–1754.

Symptoms of serotonin syndrome include altered mental status, anxiety, agitation, confusion, hyperreflexia, myoclonus, diaphoresis, hyperthermia, abnormal neuromuscular activity, salivation, diarrhea, tachycardia, and hypertension. Seizures and death may occur.

Options 136–145

Answers: 136. F 137. F 138. F 139. T 140. F 141. F 142. F 143. F 144. F 145. F

Each autumn, family physicians perform sports examinations for athletic teams. In evaluating athletes, it is important to obtain an accurate history and to perform an adequate physical examination to determine if the patient is at risk during sports participation. The presence of a systolic murmur that becomes louder with Valsalva maneuver is a hallmark warning sign for hypertrophic obstructive cardiomyopathy, a potentially fatal condition that may affect young, seemingly healthy athletes. Evaluation of this finding should consist of an echocardiogram; if the condition is present, refer the patient to a cardiologist before allowing the athlete to participate in sports. Further laboratory testing is not recommended for sports examinations unless the history and physical examination suggest abnormalities; it is cost prohibitive, and there is a high rate of false-positive results.

Beers MH, Porter RS, eds. *The Merck manual of diagnosis and therapy*, Merck Research Laboratories, 18th ed. Whitehouse Station, NJ: Merck & Co.; 2006:2631, 2669.

The presence of a systolic murmur that becomes louder with Valsalva maneuver is a hallmark warning sign for hypertrophic obstructive cardiomyopathy, a potentially fatal condition that may affect young, seemingly healthy athletes.

Options 146–155

Answers: 146. T 147. T 148. F 149. F 150. F 151. T 152. T 153. F 154. F 155. F

Hypothyroidism is manifested by lethargy, constipation, cold intolerance, stiffness and cramping of muscles, carpal tunnel syndrome, menorrhagia, weight gain, dry skin, and decreased concentration. Prolonged relaxation of deep tendon reflexes may also be seen. Although unrelated to the patient's hypothyroidism, the patient also has an occult source for gastrointestinal blood loss indicated by the guaiac-positive stool. Appropriate laboratory tests include a CBC and thyroid function tests. Although the patient is postmenopausal and has evidence of lack of estrogen (i.e., vaginal atrophy), measurement of hormone levels is unnecessary. In addition, an antinuclear antibody test is unnecessary. Treatment consists of colonoscopy to evaluate further for a gastrointestinal bleeding source and the administration of levothyroxine to treat hypothyroidism. Propylthiouracil, potassium iodide, and propranolol are used to treat thyroid storm.

Kasper DL, Braunwald E, Fauci AS, et al., eds. *Harrison's principles of internal medicine*, 16th ed. New York: McGraw-Hill; 2005:2109.

Hypothyroidism is manifested by lethargy, constipation, cold intolerance, stiffness and cramping of muscles, carpal tunnel syndrome, menorrhagia, weight gain, dry skin, and decreased concentration. Prolonged relaxation of deep tendon reflexes may also be seen.

Options 156–165

Answers: 156. T 157. F 158. T 159. T 160. F 161. F 162. T 163. T 164. T 165. F

Decubitus ulcers may affect elderly, bedridden nursing home patients who are in a poor nutritional state. Risk factors include fecal incontinence, lack of ability to reposition oneself, and malnutrition. The classification of decubitus ulcers consists of four stages:

- *Stage 1*: Nonblanchable erythema
- *Stage 2*: Partial-thickness skin loss
- *Stage 3*: Full-thickness skin loss
- *Stage 4*: Full-thickness skin loss with extensive destruction

Treatment consists of frequent repositioning of the patient, nutrition assessment, use of pressure-relieving devices (e.g., foam- or air-fluidized mattresses), débridement of necrotic tissue, and close follow-up. Doughnut cushions are not recommended because they decrease blood flow to the ulcer and prevent the healing process. The application of a topical antibiotic may interfere with granulation tissue formation and has no significant benefit to healing. Mild pressure sores (stages 1 and 2) require all the prophylactic measures above to prevent necrosis. The area should be kept exposed, free from pressure, and dry. Stimulating the circulation by gentle massage can accelerate healing. Ulcers that have not advanced beyond stage 3 may heal spontaneously if the pressure is removed and the area is small. New hydrophilic gels and hydrocolloid dressings speed healing. Stage 4 ulcers require débridement or more extensive surgery. When the ulcers are filled with pus or necrotic debris, dextranomer beads or newer hydrophilic polymers may hasten débridement without surgery. Conservative débridement of necrotic tissue with forceps and scissors should be instituted. Some ulcers can be débrided by cleansing with hydrogen peroxide 1.5%. Whirlpool baths may assist débridement. More advanced ulcers with fat and muscle involvement require surgical débridement and closure. For cellulitis, an oral or parenteral penicillinase-resistant penicillin or a cephalosporin is necessary.

Beers MH, Porter RS, eds. *The Merck manual of diagnosis and therapy*, Merck Research Laboratories, 18th ed. Whitehouse Station, NJ: Merck & Co.; 2006:1011–1017.

Doughnut cushions are not recommended for the prevention of decubitus ulcers because they decrease blood flow to the ulcer and prevent the healing process.

Options 166–180

Answers: 166. T 167. F 168. T 169. T 170. F 171. T 172. T 173. T 174. T 175. F 176. T 177. T 178. T 179. T 180. T

HIV and associated acquired immunodeficiency syndrome are the leading cause of death for men ages 25 to 44 years and the eighth leading cause of death for all ages in the United States. The appropriate screening test for HIV antibodies is ELISA. If this test is positive, the results are then confirmed by a Western blot assay. In the initial testing, $CD4^+$ T-cell counts and viral load titers are unnecessary until the presence of HIV is determined. In this patient, because of his symptoms, a CBC and TSH would be acceptable screening tests in addition to the ELISA test for HIV. Infected body fluids that play a role in the transmission of the virus include blood, semen, vaginal secretions, and breast milk. Sweat has not been implicated in the transmission of HIV. Appropriate treatment for this patient who has documented HIV and suspected *Pneumocystis jiroveci* (formerly known as *Pneumocystis carinii*) pneumonia based on his symptoms of a dry cough and x-ray findings would include the use of nucleoside derivatives (retroviral agents: zidovudine, abacavir, didanosine, emtricitabine, stavudine, zalcitabine, and lamivudine) and protease inhibitors: saquinavir (Invirase), ritonavir (Novir), indinavir (Crixivan), and others. Other treatment modalities may include combination therapy with antiretroviral therapy and protease inhibitors. Other antiretroviral medications are used as well. Treatment of *Pneumocystis jiroveci* consists of the use of trimethoprim-sulfamethoxazole (Bactrim, Septra). Trimethoprim-sulfamethoxazole (Bactrim, Septra) is the drug of choice, because it is efficacious and treats systemically, but dapsone, with or without other drugs, and aerosolized pentamidine (NebuPent) are still acceptable treatments in patients who are unable to tolerate trimethoprim-sulfamethoxazole. Non-life-threatening adverse reactions to trimethoprim-sulfamethoxazole, such as maculopapular skin rash, are not contraindications to the medication unless the patient finds the side effect unacceptable even with use of an appropriate antihistamine. Desensitization to trimethoprim-sulfamethoxazole should be considered in patients who have mild or moderate adverse reactions to trimethoprim-sulfamethoxazole.

Beers MH, Porter RS, eds. *The Merck manual of diagnosis and therapy*, Merck Research Laboratories, 18th ed. Whitehouse Station, NJ: Merck & Co.; 2006:1625–1642.

The appropriate screening test for HIV antibodies is ELISA. If this test is positive, the results are then confirmed by a Western blot assay.

Options 181–194

Answers: 181. T 182. T 183. T 184. T 185. F 186. T 187. T 188. T 189. T 190. F 191. F 192. F 193. T 194. F

Simple lacerations are often repaired by family physicians in the emergency room or in their office. Repair of lacerations initially involves copious irrigation of the wound site with sterile saline. The wound site should be gently explored after anesthesia is administered to rule out the presence of foreign bodies. Any nonviable tissue should be removed by sharp débridement. Most simple lacerations can be sutured with interrupted nylon sutures, with special care to avoid excess tension when approximating the edges of the wound site. Anesthesia before wound repair can be accomplished with one of the two classes of local anesthetics: esters (e.g., procaine) and amides (e.g., lidocaine). Anesthesia is usually accomplished by local infiltration. Buffering the solution with sodium bicarbonate may help decrease the pain. Warming the anesthetic solution also decreases pain with infiltration. Prior administration of topical anesthetics such as tetracaine 1% can ameliorate injection pain. Alternative methods for local anesthesia include topical and regional applications. A topical combination of tetracaine, adrenaline, and cocaine has been shown to be an effective anesthetic in children and patients with face or scalp lacerations; however, serious adverse events have been reported. Local anesthetic (EMLA) cream has been useful, but the onset of anesthesia is delayed. Local anesthetics can also be administered regionally by infiltrating around a regional sensory nerve. This technique is most useful when dealing with multiple lacerations or when large areas of skin must be débrided or scrubbed. Postoperative care need not include routine use of prophylactic antibiotics unless evidence of bacterial contamination or a risk host factor is evident. Sutured or stapled lacerations should be covered with a protective nonadherent dressing for at least 24 to 48 hours to avoid gross contamination. Patients should be instructed to observe the wound for the presence of warmth, redness, swelling, or drainage. Sutures or staples should be removed after approximately 7 days. Facial sutures should be removed within 3 to 5 days. Sutures in areas that are subject to high tension should be left in place for 10 to 14 days. Lidocaine with epinephrine should be avoided in areas such as the fingers, nose, penis, or toes, or any other distal appendage that may be at risk for ischemia if vasoconstriction occurs. The neck would not be considered at risk for ischemia. A dirty wound caused by an object such as rusted barbed wire should be treated with tetanus and diphtheria toxoid as well as tetanus immune globulin if the patient is unsure of his or her immunization status. Close follow-up to ensure appropriate wound healing and observation for infection are necessary for any laceration repair.

Rakel RE. *Textbook of Family Practice*, 6th ed. Philadelphia: WB Saunders; 2002:660–661.

Facial sutures should be removed within 3 to 5 days. Sutures in areas that are subject to high tension should be left in place for 10 to 14 days.

Options 195–204

Answers: 195. F 196. T 197. F 198. F 199. T 200. T 201. F 202. T 203. T 204. T

Needle-stick injuries are a relatively common occurrence in hospitals and doctors' offices. All health-care providers should receive training on proper disposal of needles and on universal contamination precautions. In addition, all health-care workers should receive hepatitis B immunization. The risk of transmission of HIV by accidental needle-stick is estimated at approximately 1 in 300 accidents. However, the risk for transmission of hepatitis B is higher, presumably because of the relatively low number of HIV virions in blood. In addition, the risk of transmission may be increased by deep injections or injections of blood. With this in mind, the use of hollow-bore needles has an associated higher risk for transmission of disease than solid-bore needles. In this individual, it would be important to document her current HIV status by obtaining an ELISA test for HIV antibodies. The Western blot test is used as a confirmatory test if the initial ELISA test is positive. In addition, documenting her hepatitis status by obtaining tests for hepatitis B surface antigen, antibodies to hepatitis B surface antigen, and immunoglobulin M antibody to hepatitis core antigen is helpful in documenting previous infection. Combinations of a protease inhibitor with two nucleoside reverse transcriptase inhibitors for one month are currently recommended for postexposure prophylaxis of relatively high-risk exposures. Because some women in early pregnancy are offered postexposure prophylaxis before their pregnancy is suspected or confirmed, special caution must be exercised in treating potentially pregnant women. Additional problems arise when the source or HIV status of blood is unknown, but identification of the source and testing of that person for HIV infection should be vigorously pursued.

Beers MH, Porter RS, eds. *The Merck manual of diagnosis and therapy*, Merck Research Laboratories, 18th ed. Whitehouse Station, NJ: Merck & Co.; 2006:1639–1640.

In needle-stick injuries, the use of hollow-bore needles has an associated higher risk for transmission of disease than solid-bore needles.

Index

Note: Page numbers followed by *f* indicate figures.

Continuing Medical Education (CME) Overview

Lippincott CME Institute, Inc. (LCMEI) is accredited by the Accreditation Council for Continuing Medical Education to provide continuing medical education for physicians.

LCMEI designates this educational activity for a maximum of 20 *AMA PRA Category 1 Credits*™. Physicians should only claim credit commensurate with the extent of their participation in the activity.

Faculty Credentials and Disclosure Information: Robert L. Bratton, M.D., is Chair and Associate Professor, Department of Family Medicine, Mayo Clinic Arizona, Scottsdale/Phoenix.

Dr. Bratton has disclosed that he has no financial interests in or relationships with any commercial companies pertaining to this educational activity.

Target Audience: This Continuing Medical Education (CME) activity is intended for family physicians with an interest in studying for the annual American Board of Family Medicine (ABFM) certification and recertification examinations.

Statement of Need: Each year, approximately 5,000 physicians take the American Board of Family Medicine Certification Examination and Recertification Examination to obtain and keep Diplomate status (board certification). Recertification is required every 7 to 10 years with the option to take the examination at 6 years. Although the test is not exceedingly difficult, there is a core body of knowledge that must be mastered and maintained in order to pass the examination. Approximately 3% to 5% of those taking the exam for the first time fail to pass (Reference: https://www.theabfm.org/about/stats_exams.aspx). Failure to pass the examination can result in loss of Diplomate status at the ABFM. Increasingly, HMOs, hospitals, and other health care institutions are requiring board certification for employment and participation in health care plans. The purpose of this text is to prepare those who are about to sit for the certification examination, recertification, and in-training examination. The Family Medicine Board Review covers major areas including internal medicine, pediatrics, obstetrics and gynecology, psychiatry, surgery, and geriatrics. This text gives the test taker a feel for the actual examination through the use of a similar format and similar topics covered. The CME credit earned from completion of this review will allow the test taker the opportunity to report 20 hours of dedicated medical review time while preparing for the examination. Participants in previous CME-accredited editions of *Bratton's Family Practice Board Review* textbook have indicated, through evaluation assessment questionnaire responses, that the use of this CME activity is valuable in preparing for the Family Medicine Board Review.

General Learning Objectives: After completing *Bratton's Family Medicine Review*, the physician will be able to:

1. Identify common presenting signs and symptoms of various disease process that involve internal medicine, pediatrics, obstetrics and gynecology, psychiatry, surgery, and geriatrics
2. Recognize common skin lesions and their presentation and treatment
3. Identify up-to-date immunization schedules
4. Discuss optimal testing for age-adjusted health care maintenance and screening
5. Recognize signs and symptoms of physical and sexual abuse
6. Interpret common electrocardiogram rhythms
7. Name risk factors for cardiovascular and cerebrovascular disease
8. Select appropriate tests for the evaluation and treatment of common outpatient problems
9. Discriminate between normal and abnormal physical findings
10. Recognize presenting signs and symptoms of human immunodeficiency virus (HIV)
11. Identify the appropriate treatment for hypertension, hyperlipidemia, and diabetes based on national guidelines

12. Recognize appropriate child development
13. Identify signs and symptoms of mental illness (i.e., depression, anxiety)
14. Identify substance abuse and treat it effectively
15. Recognize common diseases that affect the elderly and appropriate testing for this group

Method of Physician Participation: To earn CME credit, participants must first read the text and complete the CME examination and evaluation assessment questionnaire. Participants can mail a photocopy of the Answer Sheet and Evaluation Assessment Form, along with a check or money order for the $ 20.00 processing fee, to Lippincott CME Institute, Inc., 770 Township Line Road, Suite 300, Yardley, PA 19067. Entries must be received by LCMEI by the expiration date of **March 31, 2010.** Acknowledgment will be sent to participants within 6 to 8 weeks of participation. For more information, call (267) 757-3531.

Continuing Medical Education Activity Evaluation

Please take the time to help us continue to publish the most effective CME materials available. Your responses to this survey will provide us with information necessary to evaluate the content and effectiveness of this CME activity.

Name: ______________________________

Address: ______________________________

____

Phone: ______________________________

E-mail: ______________________________

Specialty: ______________________________

Activity: **Bratton's Family Medicine Board Review**

Date: ______________________________

Your evaluation of this CME activity will help guide future planning. Please respond to the following questions:

1. Did the content of this activity meet the stated learning objectives?

   [ ] Yes [ ] No

2. On a scale of 1 to 5, with 5 being the highest, how do you rank the overall quality of this educational activity?

   [ ] 5 [ ] 4 [ ] 3 [ ] 2 [ ] 1

3. As a result of meeting the learning objectives of this educational activity, will you be changing your practice behavior in a manner that improves your patient care?

   [ ] Yes [ ] No

Please explain your answer:

____

____

____

4. Did you perceive any evidence of bias for or against any commercial products? If yes, please explain.

   [ ] Yes   [ ] No

____

____

____

5. How long did it take you to complete this CME activity?

   _____ hour(s)   _____ minutes

6. Please state one or two topics that you would like to see addressed in future editions.

____

____

____

Thank you.

Bratton's Family Medicine Board Review

Continuing Medical Education Answer Sheet

Please circle the correct answer.

Part 1
Multiple-Choice Questions

Internal Medicine

1. A B C D E
2. A B C D E
3. A B C D E
4. A B C D E
5. A B C D E
6. A B C D E
7. A B C D E
8. A B C D E
9. A B C D E
10. A B C D E
11. A B C D E
12. A B C D E
13. A B C D E
14. A B C D E
15. A B C D E
16. A B C D E
17. A B C D E
18. A B C D E
19. A B C D E
20. A B C D E
21. A B C D E
22. A B C D E
23. A B C D E
24. A B C D E
25. A B C D E
26. A B C D E
27. A B C D E
28. A B C D E
29. A B C D E
30. A B C D E
31. A B C D E
32. A B C D E
33. A B C D E
34. A B C D E
35. A B C D E
36. A B C D E
37. A B C D E
38. A B C D E
39. A B C D E
40. A B C D E
41. A B C D E
42. A B C D E
43. A B C D E
44. A B C D E
45. A B C D E
46. A B C D E
47. A B C D E
48. A B C D E
49. A B C D E
50. A B C D E
51. A B C D E
52. A B C D E
53. A B C D E
54. A B C D E
55. A B C D E
56. A B C D E
57. A B C D E
58. A B C D E
59. A B C D E
60. A B C D E
61. A B C D E
62. A B C D E
63. A B C D E
64. A B C D E
65. A B C D E
66. A B C D E
67. A B C D E
68. A B C D E
69. A B C D E
70. A B C D E
71. A B C D E
72. A B C D E
73. A B C D E
74. A B C D E
75. A B C D E
76. A B C D E
77. A B C D E
78. A B C D E
79. A B C D E
80. A B C D E
81. A B C D E
82. A B C D E
83. A B C D E
84. A B C D E
85. A B C D E
86. A B C D E
87. A B C D E
88. A B C D E
89. A B C D E
90. A B C D E
91. A B C D E
92. A B C D E
93. A B C D E
94. A B C D E
95. A B C D E
96. A B C D E
97. A B C D E
98. A B C D E
99. A B C D E
100. A B C D E
101. A B C D E
102. A B C D E
103. A B C D E
104. A B C D E
105. A B C D E
106. A B C D E
107. A B C D E
108. A B C D E
109. A B C D E
110. A B C D E
111. A B C D E
112. A B C D E
113. A B C D E
114. A B C D E
115. A B C D E
116. A B C D E
117. A B C D E
118. A B C D E
119. A B C D E
120. A B C D E
121. A B C D E
122. A B C D E
123. A B C D E
124. A B C D E
125. A B C D E
126. A B C D E
127. A B C D E
128. A B C D E
129. A B C D E
130. A B C D E
131. A B C D E
132. A B C D E
133. A B C D E
134. A B C D E
135. A B C D E
136. A B C D E
137. A B C D E
138. A B C D E
139. A B C D E
140. A B C D E
141. A B C D E
142. A B C D E
143. A B C D E
144. A B C D E
145. A B C D E
146. A B C D E
147. A B C D E
148. A B C D E
149. A B C D E
150. A B C D E
151. A B C D E
152. A B C D E
153. A B C D E
154. A B C D E
155. A B C D E
156. A B C D E
157. A B C D E
158. A B C D E
159. A B C D E
160. A B C D E
161. A B C D E
162. A B C D E
163. A B C D E
164. A B C D E
165. A B C D E
166. A B C D E
167. A B C D E
168. A B C D E
169. A B C D E
170. A B C D E
171. A B C D E
172. A B C D E
173. A B C D E
174. A B C D E
175. A B C D E
176. A B C D E
177. A B C D E
178. A B C D E
179. A B C D E
180. A B C D E
181. A B C D E
182. A B C D E
183. A B C D E
184. A B C D E
185. A B C D E
186. A B C D E
187. A B C D E
188. A B C D E
189. A B C D E
190. A B C D E
191. A B C D E
192. A B C D E
193. A B C D E
194. A B C D E
195. A B C D E
196. A B C D E
197. A B C D E
198. A B C D E
199. A B C D E
200. A B C D E
201. A B C D E
202. A B C D E
203. A B C D E
204. A B C D E
205. A B C D E
206. A B C D E
207. A B C D E
208. A B C D E
209. A B C D E
210. A B C D E
211. A B C D E
212. A B C D E
213. A B C D E
214. A B C D E
215. A B C D E
216. A B C D E
217. A B C D E
218. A B C D E
219. A B C D E
220. A B C D E
221. A B C D E
222. A B C D E
223. A B C D E
224. A B C D E
225. A B C D E
226. A B C D E
227. A B C D E
228. A B C D E
229. A B C D E
230. A B C D E
231. A B C D E
232. A B C D E
233. A B C D E
234. A B C D E
235. A B C D E
236. A B C D E
237. A B C D E
238. A B C D E
239. A B C D E
240. A B C D E
241. A B C D E
242. A B C D E
243. A B C D E
244. A B C D E
245. A B C D E
246. A B C D E

247. A B C D E
248. A B C D E
249. A B C D E
250. A B C D E
251. A B C D E
252. A B C D E
253. A B C D E
254. A B C D E
255. A B C D E
256. A B C D E
257. A B C D E
258. A B C D E
259. A B C D E
260. A B C D E
261. A B C D E
262. A B C D E
263. A B C D E
264. A B C D E
265. A B C D E
266. A B C D E
267. A B C D E
268. A B C D E
269. A B C D E
270. A B C D E
271. A B C D E
272. A B C D E
273. A B C D E
274. A B C D E
275. A B C D E
276. A B C D E
277. A B C D E
278. A B C D E
279. A B C D E
280. A B C D E
281. A B C D E
282. A B C D E
283. A B C D E
284. A B C D E
285. A B C D E
286. A B C D E
287. A B C D E
288. A B C D E
289. A B C D E
290. A B C D E
291. A B C D E
292. A B C D E
293. A B C D E
294. A B C D E
295. A B C D E
296. A B C D E
297. A B C D E
298. A B C D E
299. A B C D E
300. A B C D E
301. A B C D E
302. A B C D E
303. A B C D E
304. A B C D E
305. A B C D E
306. A B C D E
307. A B C D E
308. A B C D E
309. A B C D E
310. A B C D E
311. A B C D E
312. A B C D E
313. A B C D E
314. A B C D E
315. A B C D E
316. A B C D E
317. A B C D E
318. A B C D E
319. A B C D E
320. A B C D E
321. A B C D E
322. A B C D E
323. A B C D E
324. A B C D E
325. A B C D E
326. A B C D E
327. A B C D E
328. A B C D E
329. A B C D E
330. A B C D E
331. A B C D E
332. A B C D E
333. A B C D E
334. A B C D E
335. A B C D E
336. A B C D E
337. A B C D E
338. A B C D E
339. A B C D E
340. A B C D E
341. A B C D E
342. A B C D E
343. A B C D E
344. A B C D E
345. A B C D E
346. A B C D E
347. A B C D E
348. A B C D E
349. A B C D E
350. A B C D E
351. A B C D E
352. A B C D E
353. A B C D E
354. A B C D E
355. A B C D E
356. A B C D E
357. A B C D E
358. A B C D E
359. A B C D E
360. A B C D E
361. A B C D E
362. A B C D E
363. A B C D E
364. A B C D E
365. A B C D E
366. A B C D E
367. A B C D E
368. A B C D E
369. A B C D E
370. A B C D E
371. A B C D E
372. A B C D E
373. A B C D E
374. A B C D E
375. A B C D E
376. A B C D E
377. A B C D E
378. A B C D E
379. A B C D E
380. A B C D E
381. A B C D E
382. A B C D E
383. A B C D E
384. A B C D E
385. A B C D E
386. A B C D E
387. A B C D E
388. A B C D E
389. A B C D E
390. A B C D E

Pediatrics

1. A B C D E
2. A B C D E
3. A B C D E
4. A B C D E
5. A B C D E
6. A B C D E
7. A B C D E
8. A B C D E
9. A B C D E
10. A B C D E
11. A B C D E
12. A B C D E
13. A B C D E
14. A B C D E
15. A B C D E
16. A B C D E
17. A B C D E
18. A B C D E
19. A B C D E
20. A B C D E
21. A B C D E
22. A B C D E
23. A B C D E
24. A B C D E
25. A B C D E
26. A B C D E
27. A B C D E
28. A B C D E
29. A B C D E
30. A B C D E
31. A B C D E
32. A B C D E
33. A B C D E
34. A B C D E
35. A B C D E
36. A B C D E
37. A B C D E
38. A B C D E
39. A B C D E
40. A B C D E
41. A B C D E
42. A B C D E
43. A B C D E
44. A B C D E
45. A B C D E
46. A B C D E
47. A B C D E
48. A B C D E
49. A B C D E
50. A B C D E
51. A B C D E
52. A B C D E
53. A B C D E
54. A B C D E
55. A B C D E
56. A B C D E
57. A B C D E
58. A B C D E
59. A B C D E
60. A B C D E
61. A B C D E
62. A B C D E
63. A B C D E
64. A B C D E
65. A B C D E
66. A B C D E
67. A B C D E
68. A B C D E
69. A B C D E
70. A B C D E
71. A B C D E
72. A B C D E
73. A B C D E
74. A B C D E
75. A B C D E
76. A B C D E
77. A B C D E
78. A B C D E
79. A B C D E
80. A B C D E
81. A B C D E
82. A B C D E
83. A B C D E
84. A B C D E
85. A B C D E
86. A B C D E
87. A B C D E
88. A B C D E
89. A B C D E
90. A B C D E
91. A B C D E
92. A B C D E
93. A B C D E
94. A B C D E
95. A B C D E
96. A B C D E
97. A B C D E
98. A B C D E
99. A B C D E
100. A B C D E
101. A B C D E
102. A B C D E
103. A B C D E
104. A B C D E
105. A B C D E
106. A B C D E
107. A B C D E
108. A B C D E
109. A B C D E
110. A B C D E
111. A B C D E
112. A B C D E
113. A B C D E
114. A B C D E
115. A B C D E
116. A B C D E
117. A B C D E
118. A B C D E
119. A B C D E
120. A B C D E
121. A B C D E
122. A B C D E
123. A B C D E
124. A B C D E
125. A B C D E
126. A B C D E
127. A B C D E
128. A B C D E
129. A B C D E
130. A B C D E

131. A B C D E
132. A B C D E
133. A B C D E
134. A B C D E
135. A B C D E
136. A B C D E
137. A B C D E
138. A B C D E
139. A B C D E
140. A B C D E
141. A B C D E
142. A B C D E
143. A B C D E
144. A B C D E
145. A B C D E
146. A B C D E
147. A B C D E
148. A B C D E
149. A B C D E
150. A B C D E
151. A B C D E
152. A B C D E
153. A B C D E
154. A B C D E
155. A B C D E
156. A B C D E
157. A B C D E
158. A B C D E
159. A B C D E
160. A B C D E
161. A B C D E
162. A B C D E
163. A B C D E
164. A B C D E
165. A B C D E
166. A B C D E
167. A B C D E
168. A B C D E
169. A B C D E
170. A B C D E
171. A B C D E
172. A B C D E
173. A B C D E
174. A B C D E
175. A B C D E
176. A B C D E
177. A B C D E
178. A B C D E
179. A B C D E
180. A B C D E
181. A B C D E
182. A B C D E
183. A B C D E
184. A B C D E
185. A B C D E
186. A B C D E
187. A B C D E
188. A B C D E
189. A B C D E
190. A B C D E
191. A B C D E
192. A B C D E
193. A B C D E
194. A B C D E
195. A B C D E
196. A B C D E
197. A B C D E
198. A B C D E
199. A B C D E
200. A B C D E
201. A B C D E
202. A B C D E
203. A B C D E
204. A B C D E
205. A B C D E
206. A B C D E
207. A B C D E
208. A B C D E

Obstetrics and Gynecology

1. A B C D E
2. A B C D E
3. A B C D E
4. A B C D E
5. A B C D E
6. A B C D E
7. A B C D E
8. A B C D E
9. A B C D E
10. A B C D E
11. A B C D E
12. A B C D E
13. A B C D E
14. A B C D E
15. A B C D E
16. A B C D E
17. A B C D E
18. A B C D E
19. A B C D E
20. A B C D E
21. A B C D E
22. A B C D E
23. A B C D E
24. A B C D E
25. A B C D E
26. A B C D E
27. A B C D E
28. A B C D E
29. A B C D E
30. A B C D E
31. A B C D E
32. A B C D E
33. A B C D E
34. A B C D E
35. A B C D E
36. A B C D E
37. A B C D E
38. A B C D E
39. A B C D E
40. A B C D E
41. A B C D E
42. A B C D E
43. A B C D E
44. A B C D E
45. A B C D E
46. A B C D E
47. A B C D E
48. A B C D E
49. A B C D E
50. A B C D E
51. A B C D E
52. A B C D E
53. A B C D E
54. A B C D E
55. A B C D E
56. A B C D E
57. A B C D E
58. A B C D E
59. A B C D E
60. A B C D E
61. A B C D E
62. A B C D E
63. A B C D E
64. A B C D E
65. A B C D E
66. A B C D E
67. A B C D E
68. A B C D E
69. A B C D E
70. A B C D E
71. A B C D E
72. A B C D E
73. A B C D E
74. A B C D E
75. A B C D E
76. A B C D E
77. A B C D E
78. A B C D E
79. A B C D E
80. A B C D E
81. A B C D E
82. A B C D E
83. A B C D E
84. A B C D E
85. A B C D E
86. A B C D E
87. A B C D E
88. A B C D E
89. A B C D E
90. A B C D E
91. A B C D E
92. A B C D E
93. A B C D E
94. A B C D E
95. A B C D E
96. A B C D E
97. A B C D E
98. A B C D E
99. A B C D E
100. A B C D E
101. A B C D E
102. A B C D E
103. A B C D E
104. A B C D E
105. A B C D E
106. A B C D E
107. A B C D E
108. A B C D E
109. A B C D E
110. A B C D E
111. A B C D E
112. A B C D E
113. A B C D E
114. A B C D E
115. A B C D E
116. A B C D E
117. A B C D E
118. A B C D E
119. A B C D E
120. A B C D E
121. A B C D E
122. A B C D E
123. A B C D E
124. A B C D E
125. A B C D E
126. A B C D E
127. A B C D E
128. A B C D E
129. A B C D E
130. A B C D E
131. A B C D E
132. A B C D E
133. A B C D E
134. A B C D E
135. A B C D E
136. A B C D E
137. A B C D E
138. A B C D E
139. A B C D E
140. A B C D E
141. A B C D E
142. A B C D E
143. A B C D E
144. A B C D E
145. A B C D E
146. A B C D E
147. A B C D E
148. A B C D E
149. A B C D E
150. A B C D E
151. A B C D E
152. A B C D E
153. A B C D E
154. A B C D E
155. A B C D E
156. A B C D E
157. A B C D E
158. A B C D E
159. A B C D E
160. A B C D E
161. A B C D E
162. A B C D E
163. A B C D E
164. A B C D E
165. A B C D E
166. A B C D E
167. A B C D E
168. A B C D E
169. A B C D E
170. A B C D E
171. A B C D E
172. A B C D E
173. A B C D E
174. A B C D E
175. A B C D E
176. A B C D E
177. A B C D E
178. A B C D E
179. A B C D E
180. A B C D E
181. A B C D E
182. A B C D E
183. A B C D E
184. A B C D E
185. A B C D E
186. A B C D E
187. A B C D E
188. A B C D E
189. A B C D E
190. A B C D E

Psychiatry

1. A B C D E
2. A B C D E
3. A B C D E
4. A B C D E
5. A B C D E
6. A B C D E
7. A B C D E
8. A B C D E
9. A B C D E

10. A B C D E
11. A B C D E
12. A B C D E
13. A B C D E
14. A B C D E
15. A B C D E
16. A B C D E
17. A B C D E
18. A B C D E
19. A B C D E
20. A B C D E
21. A B C D E
22. A B C D E
23. A B C D E
24. A B C D E
25. A B C D E
26. A B C D E
27. A B C D E
28. A B C D E
29. A B C D E
30. A B C D E
31. A B C D E
32. A B C D E
33. A B C D E
34. A B C D E
35. A B C D E
36. A B C D E
37. A B C D E
38. A B C D E
39. A B C D E
40. A B C D E
41. A B C D E
42. A B C D E
43. A B C D E
44. A B C D E
45. A B C D E
46. A B C D E
47. A B C D E
48. A B C D E
49. A B C D E
50. A B C D E
51. A B C D E
52. A B C D E
53. A B C D E
54. A B C D E
55. A B C D E
56. A B C D E
57. A B C D E
58. A B C D E
59. A B C D E
60. A B C D E
61. A B C D E
62. A B C D E
63. A B C D E
64. A B C D E
65. A B C D E
66. A B C D E
67. A B C D E
68. A B C D E
69. A B C D E
70. A B C D E
71. A B C D E
72. A B C D E
73. A B C D E
74. A B C D E
75. A B C D E
76. A B C D E
77. A B C D E
78. A B C D E
79. A B C D E
80. A B C D E
81. A B C D E
82. A B C D E
83. A B C D E
84. A B C D E
85. A B C D E
86. A B C D E
87. A B C D E
88. A B C D E
89. A B C D E
90. A B C D E
91. A B C D E
92. A B C D E
93. A B C D E
94. A B C D E
95. A B C D E
96. A B C D E
97. A B C D E
98. A B C D E
99. A B C D E
100. A B C D E
101. A B C D E
102. A B C D E
103. A B C D E
104. A B C D E
105. A B C D E
106. A B C D E
107. A B C D E
108. A B C D E
109. A B C D E

Surgery

1. A B C D E
2. A B C D E
3. A B C D E
4. A B C D E
5. A B C D E
6. A B C D E
7. A B C D E
8. A B C D E
9. A B C D E
10. A B C D E
11. A B C D E
12. A B C D E
13. A B C D E
14. A B C D E
15. A B C D E
16. A B C D E
17. A B C D E
18. A B C D E
19. A B C D E
20. A B C D E
21. A B C D E
22. A B C D E
23. A B C D E
24. A B C D E
25. A B C D E
26. A B C D E
27. A B C D E
28. A B C D E
29. A B C D E
30. A B C D E
31. A B C D E
32. A B C D E
33. A B C D E
34. A B C D E
35. A B C D E
36. A B C D E
37. A B C D E
38. A B C D E
39. A B C D E
40. A B C D E
41. A B C D E
42. A B C D E
43. A B C D E
44. A B C D E
45. A B C D E
46. A B C D E
47. A B C D E
48. A B C D E
49. A B C D E
50. A B C D E
51. A B C D E
52. A B C D E
53. A B C D E
54. A B C D E
55. A B C D E
56. A B C D E
57. A B C D E
58. A B C D E
59. A B C D E
60. A B C D E
61. A B C D E
62. A B C D E
63. A B C D E
64. A B C D E
65. A B C D E
66. A B C D E
67. A B C D E
68. A B C D E
69. A B C D E
70. A B C D E
71. A B C D E
72. A B C D E
73. A B C D E
74. A B C D E
75. A B C D E
76. A B C D E
77. A B C D E
78. A B C D E
79. A B C D E
80. A B C D E
81. A B C D E
82. A B C D E
83. A B C D E
84. A B C D E
85. A B C D E
86. A B C D E
87. A B C D E
88. A B C D E
89. A B C D E
90. A B C D E
91. A B C D E
92. A B C D E
93. A B C D E
94. A B C D E
95. A B C D E
96. A B C D E
97. A B C D E
98. A B C D E
99. A B C D E
100. A B C D E
101. A B C D E
102. A B C D E
103. A B C D E
104. A B C D E
105. A B C D E
106. A B C D E
107. A B C D E
108. A B C D E
109. A B C D E
110. A B C D E

Geriatrics

1. A B C D E
2. A B C D E
3. A B C D E
4. A B C D E
5. A B C D E
6. A B C D E
7. A B C D E
8. A B C D E
9. A B C D E
10. A B C D E
11. A B C D E
12. A B C D E
13. A B C D E
14. A B C D E
15. A B C D E
16. A B C D E
17. A B C D E
18. A B C D E
19. A B C D E
20. A B C D E
21. A B C D E
22. A B C D E
23. A B C D E
24. A B C D E
25. A B C D E
26. A B C D E
27. A B C D E
28. A B C D E
29. A B C D E
30. A B C D E
31. A B C D E
32. A B C D E
33. A B C D E
34. A B C D E
35. A B C D E
36. A B C D E
37. A B C D E
38. A B C D E
39. A B C D E
40. A B C D E
41. A B C D E
42. A B C D E
43. A B C D E
44. A B C D E
45. A B C D E
46. A B C D E
47. A B C D E
48. A B C D E
49. A B C D E
50. A B C D E
51. A B C D E
52. A B C D E
53. A B C D E
54. A B C D E
55. A B C D E
56. A B C D E

57. A B C D E
58. A B C D E
59. A B C D E
60. A B C D E
61. A B C D E
62. A B C D E
63. A B C D E
64. A B C D E
65. A B C D E
66. A B C D E
67. A B C D E
68. A B C D E
69. A B C D E
70. A B C D E
71. A B C D E
72. A B C D E
73. A B C D E
74. A B C D E
75. A B C D E
76. A B C D E
77. A B C D E
78. A B C D E
79. A B C D E
80. A B C D E
81. A B C D E
82. A B C D E
83. A B C D E
84. A B C D E
85. A B C D E
86. A B C D E
87. A B C D E
88. A B C D E
89. A B C D E
90. A B C D E
91. A B C D E
92. A B C D E
93. A B C D E
94. A B C D E

Pictorial Atlas

1. A B C D E
2. A B C D E
3. A B C D E
4. A B C D E
5. A B C D E
6. A B C D E
7. A B C D E
8. A B C D E
9. A B C D E
10. A B C D E
11. A B C D E
12. A B C D E
13. A B C D E
14. A B C D E
15. A B C D E
16. A B C D E
17. A B C D E
18. A B C D E
19. A B C D E
20. A B C D E
21. A B C D E
22. A B C D E
23. A B C D E
24. A B C D E
25. A B C D E
26. A B C D E
27. A B C D E
28. A B C D E
29. A B C D E
30. A B C D E
31. A B C D E
32. A B C D E
33. A B C D E
34. A B C D E
35. A B C D E
36. A B C D E
37. A B C D E
38. A B C D E
39. A B C D E
40. A B C D E
41. A B C D E
42. A B C D E
43. A B C D E
44. A B C D E
45. A B C D E
46. A B C D E
47. A B C D E
48. A B C D E
49. A B C D E
50. A B C D E
51. A B C D E
52. A B C D E
53. A B C D E
54. A B C D E
55. A B C D E
56. A B C D E
57. A B C D E
58. A B C D E
59. A B C D E
60. A B C D E
61. A B C D E
62. A B C D E
63. A B C D E
64. A B C D E
65. A B C D E
66. A B C D E
67. A B C D E
68. A B C D E
69. A B C D E
70. A B C D E

Part II Clinical Problem Sets

Please circle TRUE or FALSE

Set #1

1. TRUE FALSE
2. TRUE FALSE
3. TRUE FALSE
4. TRUE FALSE
5. TRUE FALSE
6. TRUE FALSE
7. TRUE FALSE
8. TRUE FALSE
9. TRUE FALSE
10. TRUE FALSE
11. TRUE FALSE
12. TRUE FALSE
13. TRUE FALSE
14. TRUE FALSE
15. TRUE FALSE
16. TRUE FALSE
17. TRUE FALSE
18. TRUE FALSE
19. TRUE FALSE
20. TRUE FALSE
21. TRUE FALSE
22. TRUE FALSE
23. TRUE FALSE
24. TRUE FALSE
25. TRUE FALSE
26. TRUE FALSE
27. TRUE FALSE
28. TRUE FALSE
29. TRUE FALSE
30. TRUE FALSE
31. TRUE FALSE
32. TRUE FALSE
33. TRUE FALSE
34. TRUE FALSE
35. TRUE FALSE
36. TRUE FALSE
37. TRUE FALSE
38. TRUE FALSE
39. TRUE FALSE
40. TRUE FALSE
41. TRUE FALSE
42. TRUE FALSE
43. TRUE FALSE
44. TRUE FALSE
45. TRUE FALSE
46. TRUE FALSE
47. TRUE FALSE
48. TRUE FALSE
49. TRUE FALSE
50. TRUE FALSE
51. TRUE FALSE
52. TRUE FALSE
53. TRUE FALSE
54. TRUE FALSE
55. TRUE FALSE
56. TRUE FALSE
57. TRUE FALSE
58. TRUE FALSE
59. TRUE FALSE
60. TRUE FALSE
61. TRUE FALSE
62. TRUE FALSE
63. TRUE FALSE
64. TRUE FALSE
65. TRUE FALSE
66. TRUE FALSE
67. TRUE FALSE
68. TRUE FALSE
69. TRUE FALSE
70. TRUE FALSE
71. TRUE FALSE
72. TRUE FALSE
73. TRUE FALSE
74. TRUE FALSE
75. TRUE FALSE
76. TRUE FALSE
77. TRUE FALSE
78. TRUE FALSE
79. TRUE FALSE
80. TRUE FALSE
81. TRUE FALSE
82. TRUE FALSE
83. TRUE FALSE
84. TRUE FALSE
85. TRUE FALSE
86. TRUE FALSE
87. TRUE FALSE
88. TRUE FALSE
89. TRUE FALSE
90. TRUE FALSE
91. TRUE FALSE
92. TRUE FALSE
93. TRUE FALSE
94. TRUE FALSE
95. TRUE FALSE
96. TRUE FALSE
97. TRUE FALSE
98. TRUE FALSE
99. TRUE FALSE
100. TRUE FALSE
101. TRUE FALSE
102. TRUE FALSE
103. TRUE FALSE
104. TRUE FALSE
105. TRUE FALSE
106. TRUE FALSE
107. TRUE FALSE
108. TRUE FALSE
109. TRUE FALSE
110. TRUE FALSE
111. TRUE FALSE
112. TRUE FALSE
113. TRUE FALSE
114. TRUE FALSE
115. TRUE FALSE
116. TRUE FALSE
117. TRUE FALSE
118. TRUE FALSE
119. TRUE FALSE
120. TRUE FALSE
121. TRUE FALSE
122. TRUE FALSE
123. TRUE FALSE
124. TRUE FALSE
125. TRUE FALSE
126. TRUE FALSE
127. TRUE FALSE
128. TRUE FALSE
129. TRUE FALSE
130. TRUE FALSE
131. TRUE FALSE
132. TRUE FALSE
133. TRUE FALSE
134. TRUE FALSE
135. TRUE FALSE
136. TRUE FALSE
137. TRUE FALSE
138. TRUE FALSE
139. TRUE FALSE
140. TRUE FALSE
141. TRUE FALSE
142. TRUE FALSE
143. TRUE FALSE
144. TRUE FALSE
145. TRUE FALSE
146. TRUE FALSE
147. TRUE FALSE
148. TRUE FALSE
149. TRUE FALSE
150. TRUE FALSE
151. TRUE FALSE

152. TRUE FALSE
153. TRUE FALSE
154. TRUE FALSE
155. TRUE FALSE
156. TRUE FALSE
157. TRUE FALSE
158. TRUE FALSE
159. TRUE FALSE
160. TRUE FALSE
161. TRUE FALSE
162. TRUE FALSE
163. TRUE FALSE
164. TRUE FALSE
165. TRUE FALSE
166. TRUE FALSE
167. TRUE FALSE
168. TRUE FALSE
169. TRUE FALSE
170. TRUE FALSE
171. TRUE FALSE
172. TRUE FALSE
173. TRUE FALSE
174. TRUE FALSE
175. TRUE FALSE
176. TRUE FALSE
177. TRUE FALSE
178. TRUE FALSE
179. TRUE FALSE
180. TRUE FALSE
181. TRUE FALSE
182. TRUE FALSE
183. TRUE FALSE
184. TRUE FALSE
185. TRUE FALSE
186. TRUE FALSE
187. TRUE FALSE
188. TRUE FALSE
189. TRUE FALSE
190. TRUE FALSE
191. TRUE FALSE
192. TRUE FALSE
193. TRUE FALSE
194. TRUE FALSE
195. TRUE FALSE
196. TRUE FALSE
197. TRUE FALSE
198. TRUE FALSE
199. TRUE FALSE
200. TRUE FALSE
201. TRUE FALSE
202. TRUE FALSE
203. TRUE FALSE
204. TRUE FALSE
205. TRUE FALSE
206. TRUE FALSE
207. TRUE FALSE
208. TRUE FALSE
209. TRUE FALSE
210. TRUE FALSE
211. TRUE FALSE
212. TRUE FALSE
213. TRUE FALSE
214. TRUE FALSE
215. TRUE FALSE
216. TRUE FALSE
217. TRUE FALSE
218. TRUE FALSE
219. TRUE FALSE
220. TRUE FALSE
221. TRUE FALSE
222. TRUE FALSE
223. TRUE FALSE
224. TRUE FALSE
225. TRUE FALSE
226. TRUE FALSE
227. TRUE FALSE
228. TRUE FALSE
229. TRUE FALSE
230. TRUE FALSE
231. TRUE FALSE
232. TRUE FALSE
233. TRUE FALSE
234. TRUE FALSE
235. TRUE FALSE
236. TRUE FALSE
237. TRUE FALSE
238. TRUE FALSE
239. TRUE FALSE
240. TRUE FALSE
241. TRUE FALSE
242. TRUE FALSE
243. TRUE FALSE
244. TRUE FALSE
245. TRUE FALSE
246. TRUE FALSE
247. TRUE FALSE
248. TRUE FALSE
249. TRUE FALSE
250. TRUE FALSE
251. TRUE FALSE
252. TRUE FALSE
253. TRUE FALSE
254. TRUE FALSE
255. TRUE FALSE
256. TRUE FALSE
257. TRUE FALSE
258. TRUE FALSE
259. TRUE FALSE

Set #2

1. TRUE FALSE
2. TRUE FALSE
3. TRUE FALSE
4. TRUE FALSE
5. TRUE FALSE
6. TRUE FALSE
7. TRUE FALSE
8. TRUE FALSE
9. TRUE FALSE
10. TRUE FALSE
11. TRUE FALSE
12. TRUE FALSE
13. TRUE FALSE
14. TRUE FALSE
15. TRUE FALSE
16. TRUE FALSE
17. TRUE FALSE
18. TRUE FALSE
19. TRUE FALSE
20. TRUE FALSE
21. TRUE FALSE
22. TRUE FALSE
23. TRUE FALSE
24. TRUE FALSE
25. TRUE FALSE
26. TRUE FALSE
27. TRUE FALSE
28. TRUE FALSE
29. TRUE FALSE
30. TRUE FALSE
31. TRUE FALSE
32. TRUE FALSE
33. TRUE FALSE
34. TRUE FALSE
35. TRUE FALSE
36. TRUE FALSE
37. TRUE FALSE
38. TRUE FALSE
39. TRUE FALSE
40. TRUE FALSE
41. TRUE FALSE
42. TRUE FALSE
43. TRUE FALSE
44. TRUE FALSE
45. TRUE FALSE
46. TRUE FALSE
47. TRUE FALSE
48. TRUE FALSE
49. TRUE FALSE
50. TRUE FALSE
51. TRUE FALSE
52. TRUE FALSE
53. TRUE FALSE
54. TRUE FALSE
55. TRUE FALSE
56. TRUE FALSE
57. TRUE FALSE
58. TRUE FALSE
59. TRUE FALSE
60. TRUE FALSE
61. TRUE FALSE
62. TRUE FALSE
63. TRUE FALSE
64. TRUE FALSE
65. TRUE FALSE
66. TRUE FALSE
67. TRUE FALSE
68. TRUE FALSE
69. TRUE FALSE
70. TRUE FALSE
71. TRUE FALSE
72. TRUE FALSE
73. TRUE FALSE
74. TRUE FALSE
75. TRUE FALSE
76. TRUE FALSE
77. TRUE FALSE
78. TRUE FALSE
79. TRUE FALSE
80. TRUE FALSE
81. TRUE FALSE
82. TRUE FALSE
83. TRUE FALSE
84. TRUE FALSE
85. TRUE FALSE
86. TRUE FALSE
87. TRUE FALSE
88. TRUE FALSE
89. TRUE FALSE
90. TRUE FALSE
91. TRUE FALSE
92. TRUE FALSE
93. TRUE FALSE
94. TRUE FALSE
95. TRUE FALSE
96. TRUE FALSE
97. TRUE FALSE
98. TRUE FALSE
99. TRUE FALSE
100. TRUE FALSE
101. TRUE FALSE
102. TRUE FALSE
103. TRUE FALSE
104. TRUE FALSE
105. TRUE FALSE
106. TRUE FALSE
107. TRUE FALSE
108. TRUE FALSE
109. TRUE FALSE
110. TRUE FALSE
111. TRUE FALSE
112. TRUE FALSE
113. TRUE FALSE
114. TRUE FALSE
115. TRUE FALSE
116. TRUE FALSE
117. TRUE FALSE
118. TRUE FALSE
119. TRUE FALSE
120. TRUE FALSE
121. TRUE FALSE
122. TRUE FALSE
123. TRUE FALSE
124. TRUE FALSE
125. TRUE FALSE
126. TRUE FALSE
127. TRUE FALSE
128. TRUE FALSE
129. TRUE FALSE
130. TRUE FALSE
131. TRUE FALSE
132. TRUE FALSE
133. TRUE FALSE
134. TRUE FALSE
135. TRUE FALSE
136. TRUE FALSE
137. TRUE FALSE
138. TRUE FALSE
139. TRUE FALSE
140. TRUE FALSE
141. TRUE FALSE
142. TRUE FALSE
143. TRUE FALSE
144. TRUE FALSE
145. TRUE FALSE
146. TRUE FALSE
147. TRUE FALSE
148. TRUE FALSE
149. TRUE FALSE
150. TRUE FALSE
151. TRUE FALSE
152. TRUE FALSE
153. TRUE FALSE
154. TRUE FALSE
155. TRUE FALSE

156. TRUE FALSE
157. TRUE FALSE
158. TRUE FALSE
159. TRUE FALSE
160. TRUE FALSE
161. TRUE FALSE
162. TRUE FALSE
163. TRUE FALSE
164. TRUE FALSE
165. TRUE FALSE
166. TRUE FALSE
167. TRUE FALSE
168. TRUE FALSE
169. TRUE FALSE
170. TRUE FALSE
171. TRUE FALSE
172. TRUE FALSE
173. TRUE FALSE
174. TRUE FALSE
175. TRUE FALSE
176. TRUE FALSE
177. TRUE FALSE
178. TRUE FALSE
179. TRUE FALSE
180. TRUE FALSE
181. TRUE FALSE
182. TRUE FALSE
183. TRUE FALSE
184. TRUE FALSE
185. TRUE FALSE
186. TRUE FALSE
187. TRUE FALSE
188. TRUE FALSE
189. TRUE FALSE
190. TRUE FALSE
191. TRUE FALSE
192. TRUE FALSE
193. TRUE FALSE
194. TRUE FALSE
195. TRUE FALSE
196. TRUE FALSE
197. TRUE FALSE
198. TRUE FALSE
199. TRUE FALSE
200. TRUE FALSE
201. TRUE FALSE
202. TRUE FALSE
203. TRUE FALSE
204. TRUE FALSE
205. TRUE FALSE
206. TRUE FALSE
207. TRUE FALSE
208. TRUE FALSE
209. TRUE FALSE
210. TRUE FALSE
211. TRUE FALSE
212. TRUE FALSE

Set #3

1. TRUE FALSE
2. TRUE FALSE
3. TRUE FALSE
4. TRUE FALSE
5. TRUE FALSE
6. TRUE FALSE
7. TRUE FALSE
8. TRUE FALSE
9. TRUE FALSE
10. TRUE FALSE
11. TRUE FALSE
12. TRUE FALSE
13. TRUE FALSE
14. TRUE FALSE
15. TRUE FALSE
16. TRUE FALSE
17. TRUE FALSE
18. TRUE FALSE
19. TRUE FALSE
20. TRUE FALSE
21. TRUE FALSE
22. TRUE FALSE
23. TRUE FALSE
24. TRUE FALSE
25. TRUE FALSE
26. TRUE FALSE
27. TRUE FALSE
28. TRUE FALSE
29. TRUE FALSE
30. TRUE FALSE
31. TRUE FALSE
32. TRUE FALSE
33. TRUE FALSE
34. TRUE FALSE
35. TRUE FALSE
36. TRUE FALSE
37. TRUE FALSE
38. TRUE FALSE
39. TRUE FALSE
40. TRUE FALSE
41. TRUE FALSE
42. TRUE FALSE
43. TRUE FALSE
44. TRUE FALSE
45. TRUE FALSE
46. TRUE FALSE
47. TRUE FALSE
48. TRUE FALSE
49. TRUE FALSE
50. TRUE FALSE
51. TRUE FALSE
52. TRUE FALSE
53. TRUE FALSE
54. TRUE FALSE
55. TRUE FALSE
56. TRUE FALSE
57. TRUE FALSE
58. TRUE FALSE
59. TRUE FALSE
60. TRUE FALSE
61. TRUE FALSE
62. TRUE FALSE
63. TRUE FALSE
64. TRUE FALSE
65. TRUE FALSE
66. TRUE FALSE
67. TRUE FALSE
68. TRUE FALSE
69. TRUE FALSE
70. TRUE FALSE
71. TRUE FALSE
72. TRUE FALSE
73. TRUE FALSE
74. TRUE FALSE
75. TRUE FALSE
76. TRUE FALSE
77. TRUE FALSE
78. TRUE FALSE
79. TRUE FALSE
80. TRUE FALSE
81. TRUE FALSE
82. TRUE FALSE
83. TRUE FALSE
84. TRUE FALSE
85. TRUE FALSE
86. TRUE FALSE
87. TRUE FALSE
88. TRUE FALSE
89. TRUE FALSE
90. TRUE FALSE
91. TRUE FALSE
92. TRUE FALSE
93. TRUE FALSE
94. TRUE FALSE
95. TRUE FALSE
96. TRUE FALSE
97. TRUE FALSE
98. TRUE FALSE
99. TRUE FALSE
100. TRUE FALSE
101. TRUE FALSE
102. TRUE FALSE
103. TRUE FALSE
104. TRUE FALSE
105. TRUE FALSE
106. TRUE FALSE
107. TRUE FALSE
108. TRUE FALSE
109. TRUE FALSE
110. TRUE FALSE
111. TRUE FALSE
112. TRUE FALSE
113. TRUE FALSE
114. TRUE FALSE
115. TRUE FALSE
116. TRUE FALSE
117. TRUE FALSE
118. TRUE FALSE
119. TRUE FALSE
120. TRUE FALSE
121. TRUE FALSE
122. TRUE FALSE
123. TRUE FALSE
124. TRUE FALSE
125. TRUE FALSE
126. TRUE FALSE
127. TRUE FALSE
128. TRUE FALSE
129. TRUE FALSE
130. TRUE FALSE
131. TRUE FALSE
132. TRUE FALSE
133. TRUE FALSE
134. TRUE FALSE
135. TRUE FALSE
136. TRUE FALSE
137. TRUE FALSE
138. TRUE FALSE
139. TRUE FALSE
140. TRUE FALSE
141. TRUE FALSE
142. TRUE FALSE
143. TRUE FALSE
144. TRUE FALSE
145. TRUE FALSE
146. TRUE FALSE
147. TRUE FALSE
148. TRUE FALSE
149. TRUE FALSE
150. TRUE FALSE
151. TRUE FALSE
152. TRUE FALSE
153. TRUE FALSE
154. TRUE FALSE
155. TRUE FALSE
156. TRUE FALSE
157. TRUE FALSE
158. TRUE FALSE
159. TRUE FALSE
160. TRUE FALSE
161. TRUE FALSE
162. TRUE FALSE
163. TRUE FALSE
164. TRUE FALSE
165. TRUE FALSE
166. TRUE FALSE
167. TRUE FALSE
168. TRUE FALSE
169. TRUE FALSE
170. TRUE FALSE
171. TRUE FALSE
172. TRUE FALSE
173. TRUE FALSE
174. TRUE FALSE
175. TRUE FALSE
176. TRUE FALSE
177. TRUE FALSE
178. TRUE FALSE
179. TRUE FALSE
180. TRUE FALSE
181. TRUE FALSE
182. TRUE FALSE
183. TRUE FALSE
184. TRUE FALSE
185. TRUE FALSE
186. TRUE FALSE
187. TRUE FALSE
188. TRUE FALSE
189. TRUE FALSE
190. TRUE FALSE
191. TRUE FALSE
192. TRUE FALSE
193. TRUE FALSE
194. TRUE FALSE
195. TRUE FALSE
196. TRUE FALSE
197. TRUE FALSE
198. TRUE FALSE
199. TRUE FALSE
200. TRUE FALSE
201. TRUE FALSE
202. TRUE FALSE
203. TRUE FALSE
204. TRUE FALSE

RRS0908